ORTHOPEDIC
PHYSICAL
ASSESSMENT

ORTHOPEDIC PHYSICAL ASSESSMENT

FIFTH EDITION

David J. Magee, PhD, BPT

Professor
Department of Physical Therapy
Faculty of Rehabilitation Medicine
University of Alberta
Edmonton, Alberta, Canada

SAUNDERS

ELSEVIER

SAUNDERS
ELSEVIER

11830 Westline Industrial Drive
St. Louis, Missouri 63146

ORTHOPEDIC PHYSICAL ASSESSMENT, ED 5

ISBN-13: 978-0-7216-0571-5
ISBN-10: 0-7216-0571-0

Notice

Neither the Publisher nor the Authors assume any responsibility for any loss or injury and/or damage to persons or property arising out of or related to any use of the material contained in this book. It is the responsibility of the treating practitioner, relying on independent expertise and knowledge of the patient, to determine the best treatment and method of application for the patient.

The Publisher

ISBN-13: 978-0-7216-0571-5
ISBN-10: 0-7216-0571-0

Previous editions copyrighted 1987, 1992, 1997, 2006

Vice President and Publisher: Linda Duncan
Acquisitions Editor: Kathy Falk
Publishing Services Manager: Julie Eddy
Project Manager: Rich Barber
Designer: Julia Dummitt

Working together to grow
libraries in developing countries

www.elsevier.com | www.bookaid.org | www.sabre.org

ELSEVIER   BOOK AID International   Sabre Foundation

Printed in Canada

Last digit is the print number: 9 8 7 6 5 4 3 2 1

To my parents,
Who taught me to pick a goal in life
and to take it seriously

To my family, Bernice, Wendy, Shawn,
Dolly and Theo
My reason for being

Spanning the Generations
(92 years – 2 weeks)

Preface

This fifth edition is a culmination of a dream I have had for many years. When the first edition was published in 1987, I hoped, at that time, that I would be able to develop a series of books that would meet the needs of rehabilitation clinicians in the area of musculoskeletal conditions. With the assistance of the other two editors, James Zachazewski and Sandy Quillen, along with a number of experts in their respective fields, my dream has become a reality with the **Musculoskeletal Rehabilitation Series**.

In this edition of *Orthopedic Physical Assessment*, information has been updated in all of the chapters. In addition, and in response to a number of requests, I have included tables on the reliability and validity of many of the special tests. In addition, I changed one of the chapters that was previously entitled "Preparticipation Evaluation" to a chapter on primary care assessment, because many clinicians, in additional to physicians, are moving into the area of primary care.

Thanks to Elsevier, this edition is in full color, which has necessitated taking many new photographs and adding colored line drawings. Although some black and white photographs still remain, I believe these colored additions greatly enhance the book.

I am grateful to the people who have provided input and constructive criticism to make the book better. The support of these people, my students, and family are greatly appreciated. The book is what it is because of you.

David J. Magee

Acknowledgments

The writing of a book like this, although undertaken by one person, is in reality the bringing together of ideas, concepts, and teachings developed and put forward by colleagues, friends, clinicians, and experts in the field of musculoskeletal assessment. When the book was first published in 1987, I had no idea of how successful it would be. It has succeeded in becoming more than I could have ever imagined in seven languages.

In particular, for this edition, I would like to thank the following people:

• My family, for putting up with my moods and idiosyncrasies, especially at 4 AM!

• Bev Evjen, my irreplaceable developmental editor and friend. Without her help, encouragement, persistence, and eye for detail, this edition, and in fact, the whole musculoskeletal rehabilitation series, would not be what it is.

• My undergraduate, graduate, and postgraduate students from Canada, the United States, Brazil, Chile, and Japan, who provided me with many ideas for revisions, who collected many of the articles used as references, and helped me with many of the tables.

• The many authors and publishers who were kind enough to allow me to use their photographs, drawings, and tables in the text so that explanations could be more easily understood. Without these additions, the book would not be what I hoped for.

• My photographer, James Tennant, whose photographic talents along with those of Ted Huff, my artist, add immeasurably to the book.

• My models, Tanya Beasley, Chelsey Brown, Lisa Burrows, Judy Chepeha, Paul Caines, Lee-Anne Clayholt, Devon Fraser, Nathaniel Hay, Sarah Kazmir, Tysen LeBlanc, Dolly Magee, Shawn Magee, Theo Magee, Judy Sara, Paula Shoemaker, Ryley Tennant, Brandon Thome, and Joan Matthews White. Your patience, agreement to participate and help is very much appreciated.

• My colleagues who contributed ideas, suggestions, radiographs, and photographs, and who typed and reviewed the manuscripts.

• The people at WB Saunders (Elsevier) – especially Kathy Falk and Marion Waldman, for their ideas, suggestions, assistance, and patience.

• My teachers, colleagues, and mentors, who encouraged me to pursue my chosen career.

To these people and many others – thank you for your help, ideas, and encouragement. Your support played a large part in the success and completion of this book.

David J. Magee

Contents

Principles and Concepts

A musculoskeletal assessment requires a proper and thorough systematic examination of the patient. A correct diagnosis depends on a knowledge of functional anatomy, an accurate patient history, diligent observation, and a thorough examination. The differential diagnosis process involves the use of clinical signs and symptoms, physical examination, a knowledge of pathology and mechanisms of injury, provocative and palpation (motion) tests, and laboratory and diagnostic imaging techniques. It is only through a complete and systematic assessment that an accurate diagnosis can be made. The purpose of the assessment should be to fully and clearly understand the patient's problems, from the patient's perspective as well as the clinician's, and the physical basis for the symptoms that have caused the patient to complain. As James Cyriax stated, "Diagnosis is only a matter of applying one's anatomy."[1]

One of the more common assessment recording techniques is the problem-oriented medical records method, which uses "SOAP" notes.[2] SOAP stands for the four parts of the assessment: Subjective, Objective, Assessment, and Plan. This method is especially useful in helping the examiner to solve a problem. In this book, the subjective portion of the assessment is covered under the heading Patient History, objective under Observation, and assessment under Examination.

Although the text deals primarily with musculoskeletal physical assessment on an outpatient basis, it can easily be adapted to evaluate inpatients. The primary difference is in adapting the assessment to the needs of a bedridden patient. Often, an inpatient's diagnosis has been made previously, and any continuing assessment is modified to determine how the patient's condition is responding to treatment. Likewise, an outpatient is assessed continu-

ally during treatment, and the assessment is modified to reflect the patient's response to treatment.

Regardless of which system is selected for assessment, the examiner should establish a **sequential method** to ensure that nothing is overlooked. The assessment must be organized, comprehensive, and reproducible. In general, the examiner compares one side of the body, which is assumed to be normal, with the other side of the body, which is abnormal or injured. For this reason, the examiner must come to understand and know the wide variability in what is considered normal. In addition, the examiner should focus attention on only one aspect of the assessment at a time, for example, ensuring a thorough history is taken before completing the examination component. When assessing an individual joint, the examiner must look at the joint and injury in the context of how the injury may affect other joints in the kinetic chain. These other joints may demonstrate changes as they try to compensate for the injured joint.

Total Musculoskeletal Assessment

- Patient history
- Observation
- Examination of movement
- Special tests
- Reflexes and cutaneous distribution
- Joint play movements
- Palpation
- Diagnostic imaging

Each chapter ends with a summary, or précis, of the assessment procedures identified in that chapter. This section enables the examiner to quickly review the pertinent steps of assessment for the joint or structure being assessed. For further information, the examiner can refer to the more detailed sections of the chapter.

Patient History

A complete medical and injury history should be taken and written to ensure reliability. This requires effective and efficient communication on the part of the examiner and the ability to develop a good rapport with the patient and, in some cases, family members and other members of the health care team. This includes speaking at a level and using terms the patient will understand; taking the time to listen; and being empathic, interested, caring, and professional.[3] Naturally, emphasis in taking the history should be placed on the portion of the assessment that has the greatest clinical relevance. Often the examiner can make the diagnosis by simply *listening to the patient*. No subject areas should be skipped. Repetition helps the examiner to become familiar with the characteristic history of the patient's complaints so that unusual deviation, which often indicates problems, is noticed immediately. Even if the diagnosis is obvious, the history provides valuable information about the disorder, its present state, its prognosis, and the appropriate treatment. The history also enables the examiner to determine the type of person the patient is, his or her language and cognitive ability, the patient's ability to articulate, any treatment the patient has received, and the behavior of the injury. In addition to the history of the present illness or injury, the examiner should note relevant past history, treatment, and results. Past medical history should include any major illnesses, surgery, accidents, or allergies. In some cases, it may be necessary to delve into the social and family histories of the patient if they appear relevant. Lifestyle habit patterns, including sleep patterns, stress, workload, and recreational pursuits, should also be noted.

It is important that the examiner politely but firmly keeps the patient focused and discourages irrelevant information. Questions and answers should provide practical information about the problem. At the same time, to obtain optimum results in the assessment, it is important for the examiner to establish a good rapport with the patient. In addition, the examiner should listen for any potential **"red flag"** signs and symptoms (Table 1-1) that would indicate the problem is not a musculoskeletal one or a more serious problem that should be referred to the appropriate health care professional.[4] **"Yellow flag"** signs and symptoms (Table 1-2) are also important for the examiner to note as they denote problems that may be more severe or may involve more than one area requiring a more extensive examination, or they may relate to cautions and contraindications to treatment that the examiner might have to consider.

Table 1-1
"Red Flag" Findings in Patient History That Indicate Need for Referral to Physician

Cancer	Persistent pain at night
	Constant pain anywhere in the body
	Unexplained weight loss (e.g., 4.5 to 6.8 kg [10 to 15 lb] in 2 weeks or less)
	Loss of appetite
	Unusual lumps or growths
	Unwarranted fatigue
Cardiovascular	Shortness of breath
	Dizziness
	Pain or a feeling of heaviness in the chest
	Pulsating pain anywhere in the body
	Constant and severe pain in lower leg (calf) or arm
	Discolored or painful feet
	Swelling (no history of injury)
Gastrointestinal/ Genitourinary	Frequent or severe abdominal pain
	Frequent heartburn or indigestion
	Frequent nausea or vomiting
	Change in or problems with bowel and/or bladder function (e.g., urinary tract infection)
	Unusual menstrual irregularities
Miscellaneous	Fever or night sweats
	Recent severe emotional disturbances
	Swelling or redness in any joint with no history of injury
	Pregnancy
Neurological	Changes in hearing
	Frequent or severe headaches with no history of injury
	Problems with swallowing or changes in speech
	Changes in vision (e.g., blurriness or loss of sight)
	Problems with balance, coordination, or falling
	Faint spells (drop attacks)
	Sudden weakness

Data from Stith JS, Sahrmann SA, et al: Curriculum to prepare diagnosticians in physical therapy, *J Phys Ther Educ* 9:50, 1995.

The patient's history is usually taken in an orderly sequence. It offers the patient an opportunity to describe the problem and the limitations caused by the problem as he or she perceives them. To achieve a good functional outcome, it is essential that the clinician heed to the patient's concerns and expectations for treatment. After all, the history is the patient's report of his or her own condition. The clinician should ask questions that

Table 1-2
"Yellow Flag" Findings in Patient History That Indicate a More Extensive Examination May Be Required
Abnormal signs and symptoms (unusual patterns of complaint)
Bilateral symptoms
Symptoms peripheralizing
Neurological symptoms (nerve root or peripheral nerve)
Multiple nerve root involvement
Abnormal sensation patterns (do not follow dermatome or peripheral nerve patterns)
Saddle anesthesia
Upper motor neuron symptoms (spinal cord) signs
Fainting
Drop attacks
Vertigo
Autonomic nervous system symptoms
Progressive weakness
Progressive gait disturbances
Multiple inflamed joints
Psychosocial stresses
Circulatory or skin changes

are easy to understand and should not lead the patient. For example, the examiner should not say, "Does this increase your pain?" It would be better to say, "Does this alter your pain in any way?" The examiner should ask one question at a time and receive an answer to each question before proceeding with another question. Open-ended questions ask for narrative information; closed or direct questions ask for specific information. Direct questions are often used to fill in details of information given in open-ended questions, and they frequently require only a one-word answer, such as yes or no. In any musculoskeletal assessment, the examiner should seek answers to the following pertinent questions.

1. *What is the patient's age and sex?* Many conditions occur within certain age ranges. For example, various growth disorders, such as Legg-Perthes disease or Scheuermann's disease, are seen in adolescents or teenagers. Degenerative conditions, such as osteoarthritis and osteoporosis, are more likely to be seen in an older population. Shoulder impingement in young people (15 to 35 years) is more likely to result from muscle weakness, primarily in the muscles controlling the scapula, whereas the condition in older people (40+ years) is more likely to be the result of degenerative changes in the shoulder complex. Some conditions show sex and even race differences. For example, some cancers are more prevalent in men (e.g., prostrate, bladder), whereas others occur more frequently in women (e.g., cervical, breast), yet still others are more common in whites.

2. *What is the patient's occupation?* What does the patient do at work? What is the working environment like? What are the demands and postures assumed?[5] For example, a laborer probably has stronger muscles than a sedentary worker and may be less likely to suffer a muscle strain. However, laborers are more susceptible to injury because of the types of jobs they have. Because sedentary workers usually have no need for high levels of muscle strength, they may overstress their muscles or joints on weekends because of overactivity or participation in activity they are not used to. Habitual postures and repetitive strain caused by some occupations may indicate the location or source of the problem.

3. *Why has the patient come for help?* This is often referred to as the **history of the present illness** or **chief complaint.** This part of the history provides an opportunity for patients to describe in their own words what is bothering them and the extent to which it bothers them. It is important for the clinician to determine what the patient wants to be able to do functionally and what the patient is unable to do functionally. This information can help the examiner determine whether the patient's expectations for the following treatment are realistic and what direction functional treatment should take to ensure the patient can, if at all possible, return to his or her previous level of activity.

4. *Was there any inciting trauma (macrotrauma) or repetitive activity (microtrauma)?* In other words, what was the **mechanism of injury**, and were there any predisposing factors? If the patient was in a motor vehicle accident, for example, was the patient the driver or the passenger? Was he or she the cause of the accident? What part of the car was hit? How fast were the cars going? Was the patient wearing a seat belt? When asking questions about the mechanism(s) of injury, the examiner must try to determine the direction and magnitude of the injuring force and how the force was applied. By carefully listening to the patient, the examiner can often determine which structures were injured and how severely by knowing the force and mechanism of injury. For example, anterior dislocations of the shoulder usually occur when the arm is abducted and laterally rotated beyond the normal range of motion, and the "terrible triad" injury to the knee (i.e., medial collateral ligament, anterior cruciate ligament, and medial meniscus injury) usually results from a blow to the lateral side of the knee while the knee is flexed, the full weight of the patient is on the knee, and the foot is fixed. Likewise, the examiner should determine whether there were any predisposing, unusual, or new factors, such as sustained postures or repetitive activities, general health, or familial or genetic problems that may have led to the problem.[6]

5. *Was the onset of the problem slow or sudden?* Did the condition start as an insidious, mild ache and then progress to continuous pain, or was there a specific episode in which the body part was injured? If inciting trauma has occurred, it is often relatively easy to determine the location of the problem. Does the pain get worse as the day progresses? Was the sudden onset caused by trauma, or was it sudden with locking because of muscle spasm (spasm lock) or pain? Is there anything that relieves the symptoms? Knowledge of these facts helps the examiner make a differential diagnosis.

6. *Where are the symptoms that bother the patient?* If possible, have the patient point to the area. Does the patient point to a specific structure or a more general area? The latter may indicate a more severe condition or referral of symptoms (**yellow flag**). The way in which the patient describes the symptoms often helps to delineate problems. Has the dominant or nondominant side been injured? Injury to the dominant side may lead to greater functional limitations.

7. *Where was the pain or other symptoms when the patient first had the complaint?* Pain is subjective, and its manifestations are unique to each individual. It is a complex experience involving several dimensions (Figure 1-1). If the intensity of the pain or symptoms is such that the patient is unable to move in a certain direction or to hold a particular posture because of the symptoms,

the symptoms are said to be severe. If the symptoms or pain become progressively worse with movement or the longer a position is held, the symptoms are said to be irritable.[7,8] Acute pain is new pain which is often severe, continuous, and perhaps disabling, and is of sufficient quality or duration that the patient seeks help. Acute injuries tend to be more irritable resulting in pain earlier in the movement, or minimal activity will bring on symptoms and often the pain will remain after movement has stopped.[3] Chronic pain is more aggravating, is not as intense, has been experienced before, and in many cases, the patient knows how to deal with it. Acute pain is more often accompanied by anxiety, whereas chronic pain is associated with depression.[9] Has the pain moved or spread? The location and spread of pain may be marked on a body chart, which is part of the assessment sheet (Appendix 1-1). The examiner should ask the patient to point to exactly where the pain was and where it is now. Are trigger points present? Trigger points are localized areas of hyperirritability within the tissues; they are tender to compression, are often accompanied by tight bands of tissue, and, if sufficiently hypersensitive, may give rise to referred pain that is steady, deep, and aching. These trigger points can lead to a diagnosis, because pressure on them reproduces the patient's symptoms. Trigger points are not found in normal muscles.[10]

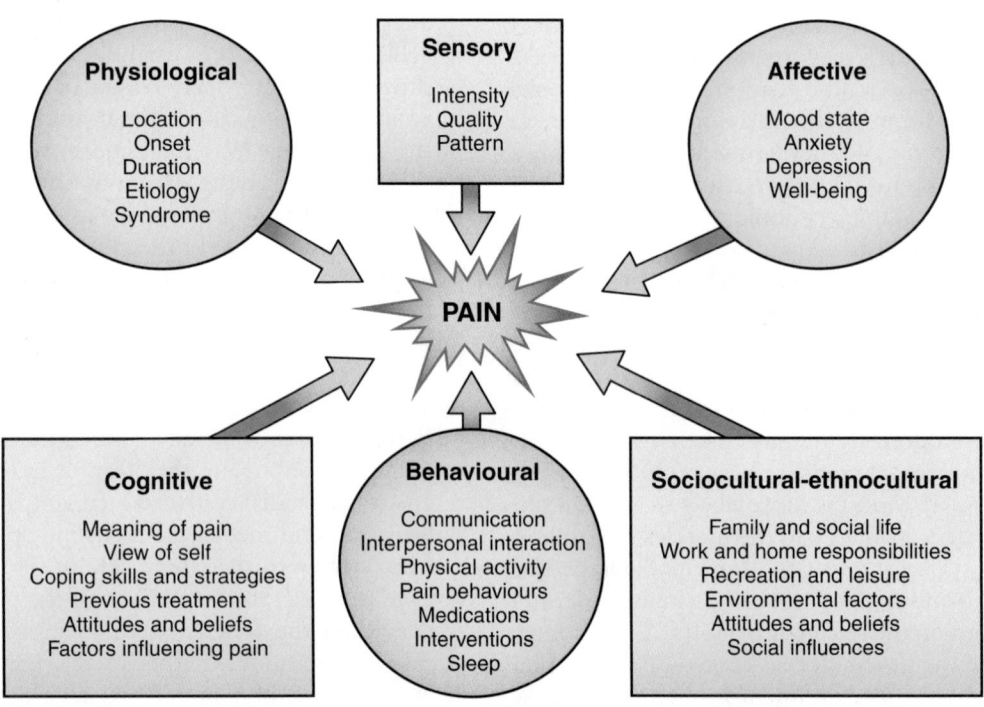

Figure 1-1

The dimensions of pain. (Redrawn from Petty NJ and Moore AP: *Neuromusculoskeletal examination and assessment: a handbook for therapists*, p. 8, London, 1998, Churchill-Livingstone.)

In general, the area of pain enlarges or becomes more distal as the lesion worsens and becomes smaller or more localized as it improves. Some examiners call the former **peripheralization** of the symptoms and the latter, **centralization** of symptoms.[11,12] The more distal and superficial the problem, the more accurately the patient can determine the location of the pain. In the case of referred pain, the patient usually points out a general area; with a localized lesion, the patient points to a specific location. Referred pain tends to be felt deeply; its boundaries are indistinct, and it radiates segmentally without crossing the midline. The term **referred pain** means that the pain is felt at a site other than the injured tissue because the same or adjacent neural segments supply the referred site. Pain also may shift as the lesion shifts. For example, with an internal derangement of the knee, pain may occur in flexion one time and in extension another time if it is caused by a loose body within the joint. The examiner must clearly understand where the patient feels the pain. For example, does the pain occur only at the end of the range of motion (ROM), in part of the range, or throughout the ROM?[6]

8. *What are the exact movements or activities that cause pain?* At this stage, the examiner should not ask the patient to do the movements or activities; this will take place during the examination. However, the examiner should remember which movements the patient says are painful so that when the examination is carried out, the patient can do these movements last to avoid an overflow of painful symptoms. With cessation of the activity, does the pain stay the same, or how long does it take for the pain to return to its previous level? Are there any other factors that aggravate or help to relieve the pain? Do these activities alter the intensity of the pain? The answers to these questions give the examiner some idea of the irritability of the joint. They also help the examiner to differentiate between musculoskeletal or mechanical pain and systemic pain, which is pain arising from one of the body's systems other than the musculoskeletal system (Table 1-3).[12] Functionally, pain can be divided into different levels, especially for repetitive stress conditions.

9. *How long has the problem existed?* What are the duration and frequency of the symptoms? Answers to these questions help the examiner to determine whether the condition is acute, subacute, chronic, or acute on chronic and to develop some understanding of the patient's tolerance to pain. Generally, **acute conditions** are those that have been present for 7 to 10 days, **subacute conditions** have been present for 10 days to 7 weeks, and **chronic conditions** or symptoms have been present for longer than 7 weeks. In acute or chronic cases, the injured tissues

---

Pain and Its Relation to Severity of Repetitive Stress Activity

- Level 1: Pain after specific activity
- Level 2: Pain at start of activity resolving with warmup
- Level 3: Pain during and after specific activity that does not affect performance
- Level 4: Pain during and after specific activity that does affect performance
- Level 5: Pain with activities of daily living (ADL)
- Level 6: Constant dull aching pain at rest that does not disturb sleep
- Level 7: Dull aching pain that does disturb sleep

NOTE: Level 7 indicates highest level of severity.

---

usually have been reinjured. This knowledge is also beneficial in terms of how vigorously the patient can be examined. For example, the more acute the condition, the less stress the examiner is able to apply to the joints and tissues during the assessment. A full examination may not be possible in very acute conditions. In that case, the examiner must select those procedures of assessment that will give the greatest amount of information with the least stress to the patient. Does the patient protect or support the injured part? If so, this behavior signifies discomfort

Table 1-3
Differentiation of Systemic and Musculoskeletal Pain

Systemic	Musculoskeletal
Disturbs sleep	Generally lessens at night
Deep aching or throbbing	Sharp or superficial ache
Reduced by pressure	Usually decreases with cessation of activity
Constant or waves of pain and spasm	Usually continuous or intermittent
Is not aggravated by mechanical stress	Is aggravated by mechanical stress
Associated with the following:	
Jaundice	
Migratory arthralgias	
Skin rash	
Fatigue	
Weight loss	
Low-grade fever	
Generalized weakness	
Cyclic and progressive symptoms	
Tumors	
History of infection	

From Meadows JT: *Orthopedic differential diagnosis in physical therapy: a case study approach*, p. 100, New York, 1999, McGraw Hill. Reproduced with permission of the McGraw-Hill Companies.

and fear of pain if the part moves, usually indicating a more acute condition.

10. *Has the condition occurred before?* If so, what was the onset like the first time? Where was the site of the original condition, and has there been any radiation (spread) of the symptoms? If the patient is feeling better, how long did the recovery take? Did any treatment relieve symptoms? Does the current problem appear to be the same as the previous problem, or is it different? If it is different, how is it different? Answers to these questions help the examiner to determine the location and severity of the injury.

11. *Are the intensity, duration, or frequency of pain or other symptoms increasing?* These changes usually mean the condition is getting worse. A decrease in pain or other symptoms usually means the condition is improving. Is the pain static? If so, how long has it been that way? This question may help the examiner to determine the present state of the problem. These factors may become important in treatment and may help to determine whether a treatment is helping. Are pain or other symptoms associated with other physiological functions? For example, is the pain worse with menstruation? If so, when did the patient last have a pelvic examination? Questions such as these may give the examiner an indication of what is causing the problem or what factors may affect the problem. It is often worthwhile to give the patient a pain questionnaire, visual-analog scale (VAS), numerical rating scale, box scale, or verbal rating scale that can be completed while the patient is waiting to be assessed.[13,14] The McGill-Melzack pain questionnaire and its short form (Figures 1-2 and 1-3)[15-17] provide the patient with three major classes of word descriptors—sensory, affective, and evaluative—to describe their pain experience. These designations are used to differentiate patients who have a true sensory pain experience from those who think they have experienced pain (affective pain state). Other pain-rating scales allow the patient to visually gauge the amount of pain along a solid 10-cm line (visual analog scale) (Figure 1-4) or on a thermometer-type scale (Figure 1-5).[18] It has been shown that an examiner should consistently use the same pain scales when assessing or reassessing patients to increase consistent results.[19-22] The examiner can use the completed questionnaire or scale as an indication of the pain as described or perceived by the patient. Alternatively, a self-report pain drawing (see Appendix 1-1), which, with the training and guidelines of the raters, has been shown to have reliability, can be used for the same purpose.[23]

12. *Is the pain constant, periodic, episodic (occurring with certain activities), or occasional?* Does the condition bother the patient at that exact moment? If the patient is not bothered at that exact moment, the pain is not constant. **Constant pain** suggests chemical irritation, tumors, or possibly visceral lesions.[12] It is always there, although its intensity may vary. If **periodic or occasional pain** is present, the examiner should try to determine the activity, position, or posture that irritates or brings on the symptoms as this may help determine what tissues are at fault. This type of pain is more likely to be mechanical and related to movement and stress.[12] **Episodic pain** is related to specific activities. At the same time, the examiner should be observing the patient. Does the patient appear to be in constant pain? Does the patient appear to be lacking sleep because of pain? Does the patient move around a great deal in an attempt to find a comfortable position?

13. *Is the pain associated with rest? Activity? Certain postures? Visceral function? Time of day?* Pain on activity that decreases with rest usually indicates a mechanical problem interfering with movement, such as adhesions. Morning pain with stiffness that improves with activity usually indicates chronic inflammation and edema, which decrease with motion. Pain or aching as the day progresses usually indicates increased congestion in a joint. Pain at rest and pain that is worse at the beginning of activity than at the end implies acute inflammation. Pain that is not affected by rest or activity usually indicates bone pain or could be related to organic or systemic disorders such as cancer or diseases of the viscera. Chronic pain is often associated with multiple factors such as fatigue or certain postures or activities. If the pain occurs at night, how does the patient lie in bed: supine, on the side, or prone? Does sleeping alter the pain, or does the patient wake when he or she changes position? Intractable pain at night may indicate serious pathology (e.g., a tumor). Movement seldom affects visceral pain unless the movement compresses or stretches the structure.[7] Symptoms of peripheral nerve entrapment (e.g., carpal tunnel syndrome) and thoracic outlet syndromes tend to be worse at night. Pain and cramping with prolonged walking may indicate lumbar spinal stenosis (neurogenic intermittent claudication) or vascular problems (circulatory or vascular intermittent claudication). Intervertebral disc pain is aggravated by sitting and bending forward. Facet joint pain is often relieved by sitting and bending forward and is aggravated by extension and rotation. What type of mattress and pillow does the patient use? Foam pillows often cause more problems for persons with cervical disorders because these pillows have more "bounce" to them than do feather or buckwheat pillows. Too many pillows, pillows improperly positioned, or too soft a mattress may also cause problems.

14. *What type or quality of pain is exhibited?* **Nerve pain** tends to be sharp (lancinating), bright, and burning and also tends to run in the distribution of

McGill-Melzack
PAIN QUESTIONNAIRE

Patient's name _____ Age _____

File No. _____ Date _____

Clinical category (e.g., cardiac, neurological, etc.):

Diagnosis : _____ _____

Analgesic (if already administered):

1. Type _____
2. Dosage _____
3. Time given in relation to this test _____

Patient's intelligence: circle number that represents best estimate

1 (low)   2   3   4   5 (high)

****

This questionnaire has been designed to tell us more about your pain. Four major questions we ask are:

1. Where is your pain?
2. What does it feel like?
3. How does it change with time?
4. How strong is it?

It is important that you tell us how your pain feels now. Please follow the instructions at the beginning of each part.

© R. Melzack, Oct. 1970

Part 1.   Where Is Your Pain?

Please mark, on the drawings below, the areas where you feel pain. Put E if external, or I if internal, near the areas which you mark. Put EI if both external and internal.

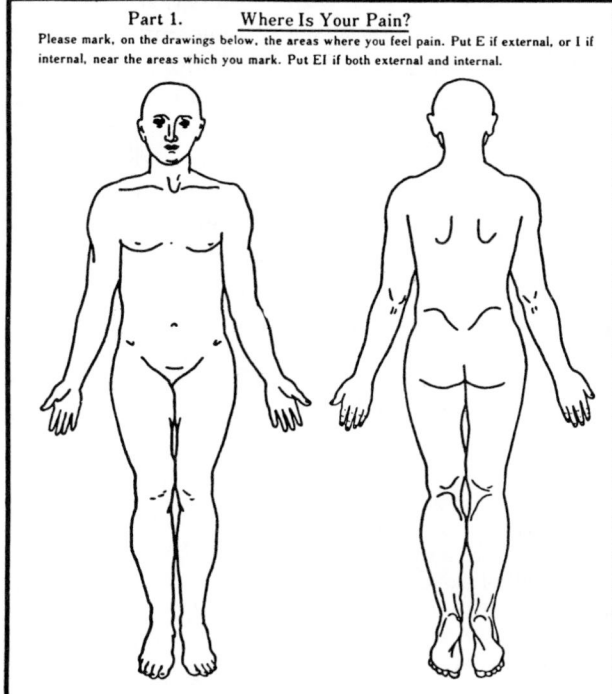

Part 2.   What Does Your Pain Feel Like?

Some of the words below describe your present pain. Circle ONLY those words that best describe it. Leave out any category that is not suitable. Use only a single word in each appropriate category—the one that applies best.

1	2	3	4
Flickering	Jumping	Pricking	Sharp
Quivering	Flashing	Boring	Cutting
Pulsing	Shooting	Drilling	Lacerating
Throbbing		Stabbing	
Beating		Lancinating	
Pounding			

5	6	7	8
Pinching	Tugging	Hot	Tingling
Pressing	Pulling	Burning	Itchy
Gnawing	Wrenching	Scalding	Smarting
Cramping		Searing	Stinging
Crushing			

9	10	11	12
Dull	Tender	Tiring	Sickening
Sore	Taut	Exhausting	Suffocating
Hurting	Rasping		
Aching	Splitting		
Heavy			

13	14	15	16
Fearful	Punishing	Wretched	Annoying
Frightful	Gruelling	Blinding	Troublesome
Terrifying	Cruel		Miserable
	Vicious		Intense
	Killing		Unbearable

17	18	19	20
Spreading	Tight	Cool	Nagging
Radiating	Numb	Cold	Nauseating
Penetrating	Drawing	Freezing	Agonizing
Piercing	Squeezing		Dreadful
	Tearing		Torturing

Part 3.   How Does Your Pain Change With Time?

1. Which word or words would you use to describe the pattern of your pain?

1	2	3
Continuous	Rhythmic	Brief
Steady	Periodic	Momentary
Constant	Intermittent	Transient

2. What kind of things relieve your pain?

3. What kind of things increase your pain?

Part 4.   How Strong Is Your Pain?

People agree that the following 5 words represent pain of increasing intensity. They are:

1	2	3	4	5
Mild	Discomforting	Distressing	Horrible	Excruciating

To answer each question below, write the number of the most appropriate word in the space beside the question.

1. Which word describes your pain right now?   _____
2. Which word describes it at its worst?   _____
3. Which word describes it when it is least?   _____
4. Which word describes the worst toothache you ever had?   _____
5. Which word describes the worst headache you ever had?   _____
6. Which word describes the worst stomach-ache you ever had?   _____

Figure 1-2

McGill-Melzack Pain Questionnaire. (From Melzack R: The McGill pain questionnaire: Major properties and scoring methods, *Pain* 1:280–281, 1975.)

---

specific nerves. Thus, the examiner must have detailed knowledge of the sensory distribution of nerve roots (dermatomes) and peripheral nerves as the different distributions may tell where the pathology or problem is if the nerve is involved. **Bone pain** tends to be deep, boring, and localized. **Vascular pain** tends to be diffuse, aching, and poorly localized and may be referred to other areas of the body. **Muscle pain** is usually hard to localize, is dull and aching, is often aggra-vated by injury, and may be referred to other areas (Table 1-4). If a muscle is injured, when the muscle contracts or is stretched, the pain will increase. Inert tissue such as ligaments, joint capsules, and bursa tend to exhibit pain similar to muscle pain and may be indistinguishable from muscle pain in the resting state (e.g., when the examiner is taking the history); however, pain in inert tissue is increased when the structures are stretched or pinched. Each of these specific tissue

SHORT-FORM McGILL PAIN QUESTIONNAIRE
RONALD MELZACK

PATIENT'S NAME: _____   DATE: _____

	NONE	MILD	MODERATE	SEVERE
THROBBING	0) ____	1) ____	2) ____	3) ____
SHOOTING	0) ____	1) ____	2) ____	3) ____
STABBING	0) ____	1) ____	2) ____	3) ____
SHARP	0) ____	1) ____	2) ____	3) ____
CRAMPING	0) ____	1) ____	2) ____	3) ____
GNAWING	0) ____	1) ____	2) ____	3) ____
HOT-BURNING	0) ____	1) ____	2) ____	3) ____
ACHING	0) ____	1) ____	2) ____	3) ____
HEAVY	0) ____	1) ____	2) ____	3) ____
TENDER	0) ____	1) ____	2) ____	3) ____
SPLITTING	0) ____	1) ____	2) ____	3) ____
TIRING-EXHAUSTING	0) ____	1) ____	2) ____	3) ____
SICKENING	0) ____	1) ____	2) ____	3) ____
FEARFUL	0) ____	1) ____	2) ____	3) ____
PUNISHING-CRUEL	0) ____	1) ____	2) ____	3) ____

NO PAIN ├───────────────────────────┤ WORST POSSIBLE PAIN

P P I

0 NO PAIN	____
1 MILD	____
2 DISCOMFORTING	____
3 DISTRESSING	____
4 HORRIBLE	____
5 EXCRUCIATING	____

Figure 1-3
The short-form McGill Pain Questionnaire (SF-MPQ). Descriptors 1 to 11 represent the sensory dimension of pain experience and 12 to 15 represent the affective dimension. Each descriptor is ranked on an intensity scale of 0 = none, 1 = mild, 2 = moderate, 3 = severe. The Present Pain Intensity (PPI) of the standard long-form McGill Pain Questionnaire (LF-MPQ) and the visual analogue (VA) are also included to provide overall intensity scores. (From Melzack R: The short-form McGill pain questionnaire, *Pain* 30:193, 1987.)

pains is sometimes grouped as **neuropathic pain** and follows specific anatomical pathways and affect specific anatomical structures.[12] **Somatic pain,** on the other hand, is a severe chronic or aching pain that is inconsistent with injury or pathology to specific anatomical structures and cannot be explained by any physical cause because the sensory input can come from so many different structures supplied by the same nerve root.[12] Superficial somatic pain may be localized, but deep somatic pain is more diffuse and may be referred.[24] On examination, somatic pain may be reproduced, but visceral pain is not reproduced by movement.[24]

15. *What types of sensations does the patient feel, and where are these abnormal sensations?* If the problem is in bone, there usually is very little radiation of pain. If pressure is applied to a nerve root, radicular pain (radiating pain) results from pressure on the dura mater, which is the outermost covering of the spinal cord. If there is pressure on the nerve trunk, no pain occurs, but there is paresthesia or an abnormal sensation such as a "pins and needles" feeling or tingling. Paresthesia is an unpleasant sensation that occurs without an apparent stimulus or cause (to the patient). Autonomic pain is more likely to be a burning type of pain. If the nerve

On the line provided, please mark where your "pain status" is today.

No pain   Most severe pain
0   10

On the line provided, please mark where your "pain status" was when it was at its most severe on any occasion.

No pain   Most severe pain
0   10

Figure 1-4
Visual-analog scales for pain. Example only. For an actual examination, lines would be 10 cm long.

Pain Rating Scale

Instructions:
Below is a thermometer with various grades of pain on it from "No pain at all" to "The pain is almost unbearable." Put an X by the words that describe your pain best. Mark how bad your pain is **at this moment in time.**

— The pain is almost unbearable

— Very bad pain

— Quite bad pain

— Moderate pain

— Little pain

— No pain at all

Figure 1-5
"Thermometer" pain rating scale. (Redrawn from Brodie DJ et al: Evaluation of low back pain by patient questionnaires and therapist assessment, *J Orthop Sports Phys Ther* 11:528, 1990.)

itself is affected, regardless of where the irritation occurs along the nerve, the brain perceives the pain as coming from the periphery. This is an example of **referred pain.**

Table 1-4
Pain Descriptions and Related Structures

Type of Pain	Structure
Cramping, dull, aching	Muscle
Dull, aching	Ligament, joint capsule
Sharp, shooting	Nerve root
Sharp, bright, lightning-like	Nerve
Burning, pressure-like, stinging, aching	Sympathetic nerve
Deep, nagging, dull	Bone
Sharp, severe, intolerable	Fracture
Throbbing, diffuse	Vasculature

16. *Does a joint exhibit locking, unlocking, twinges, instability, or giving way?* Seldom does locking mean that the joint will not move at all. **Locking** may mean that the joint cannot be fully extended, as is the case with a meniscal tear in the knee, or it may mean that it does not extend one time and does not flex the next time **(pseudolocking),** as in the case of a loose body moving within the joint. Locking may mean that the joint cannot be put through a full ROM because of muscle spasm or because the movement was too fast; this is sometimes referred to as **spasm locking. Giving way** is often caused by reflex inhibition or weakness of the muscles, so that the patient feels that the limb will buckle if weight is placed on it or because pain will be too great. Inhibition may be caused by anticipated pain or instability.

In nonpathological states, excessive ROM in a joint is called **laxity** or **hypermobility.** Laxity implies the patient has excessive range of motion but can control movement in that range and no pathology is present. It is a function of the ligaments and joint capsule resistance.[25] This differs from flexibility, which is the range of motion available in one or more joints and is a function of contractile tissue resistance primarily as well as ligament and joint capsule resistance.[25] Gleim and McHugh[25] describe flexibility in two parts: static and dynamic. Static flexibility is related to the ROM available in one or more joints; dynamic flexibility is related to stiffness and ease of movement. Laxity may be caused by familial factors or may be job or activity (e.g., sports) related. In any case, laxity, when found, should be considered normal (Figure 1-6). If symptoms occur, then laxity is considered to be hypermobility and has a pathological component, which commonly indicates the patient's inability to control the joint during movement, especially at end range, which, in turn, implies instability of the joint. Instability can cover a wide range of pathological hypermobility from a loss of control of

Figure 1-6
Congenital laxity at the elbow leading to hyperextension. This may also be called nonpathological hypermobility.

arthrokinematic joint movements to anatomical instability where subluxation or dislocation is imminent or has occurred. For assessment purposes, instability can be divided into translational (loss of arthrokinematic control) and anatomical (dislocation or subluxation) instability.[26] **Translational instability** (also called pathological or mechanical instability) refers to loss of control of the small, arthrokinematic joint movements (e.g., spin, slide, roll, translation) that occur when the patient attempts to stabilize (statically or dynamically) the joint during movement. **Anatomical instability** (also called clinical or gross instability, or pathological hypermobility) refers to excessive or gross physiological movement in a joint where the patient becomes apprehensive at the end of the ROM because a subluxation or dislocation is imminent. It should be noted that there is confusion in the application of the terms used to describe the two types of instability. For example, mechanical instability is sometimes used to mean anatomical instability because of anatomical or pathological dysfunction. **Functional instability** may mean either or both types of instability and implies an inability to control either arthrokinematic or osteokinematic movement in the available ROM either consciously or unconsciously during functional movement. These

instabilities are more likely to be evident during high-speed or loaded movements. Both types of instability can cause symptoms, and treatment centers on teaching the patient to develop muscular control of the joint and to improve reaction time and proprioceptive control. Both types of instability may be voluntary or involuntary. **Voluntary instability** is initiated by muscle contraction, and **involuntary instability** is the result of positioning. Another concept worth remembering during assessment for instability is the **circle concept of instability** originally developed from shoulder studies[27,28] but equally applicable to other joints. This concept states that injury to structures on one side of a joint leading to instability can, at the same time, cause injury to structures on the other side or other parts of the joint. Thus, an anterior shoulder dislocation can lead to injury of the posterior capsule. Similarly, anterolateral rotary instability of the knee leads to injury to posterior structures (e.g., arcuate-popliteus complex, posterior capsule) as well as anterior (e.g., anterior cruciate ligament) and lateral (e.g., lateral collateral ligament) structures. Thus, the examiner must be aware of potential injuries on the opposite side of the joint even if symptoms are predominantly on one side, especially when the mechanism of injury is trauma.

17. *Has the patient experienced any bilateral spinal cord symptoms, fainting, or drop attacks?* Is bladder function normal? Is there any "saddle" involvement (abnormal sensation in the perianal region, buttocks, and superior aspect of the posterior thighs) or vertigo? "Vertigo" and "dizziness" are terms often used synonymously, although vertigo usually indicates more severe symptoms. The terms describe a swaying, spinning sensation accompanied by feelings of unsteadiness and loss of balance. These symptoms indicate severe neurological problems, such as cervical myelopathy, which must be dealt with carefully and can (e.g., in cases of altered bladder function) be emergency conditions potentially requiring surgery. Drop attacks occur when the patient suddenly falls without warning or provocation but remains conscious.[12] It is caused by neurological dysfunction especially in the brain.

18. *Are there any changes in the color of the limb?* Ischemic changes resulting from circulatory problems may include white, brittle skin; loss of hair; and abnormal nails on the foot or hand. Conditions such as reflex sympathetic dystrophy, which is an autonomic nerve response to trauma, however minor, can cause these symptoms, as can circulatory problems such as Raynaud's disease.

19. *Has the patient been experiencing any life or economic stresses?* These psychological stressors are sometimes considered to be **yellow flags** that alter both the assessment and subsequent treatment.[29,30] Divorce, marital

problems, financial problems, or job stress or insecurity can contribute to increasing the pain or symptoms because of psychological stress. What support systems and resources are available? Are there any cultural issues one should be aware of? Does the patient have an easily accessible living environment? Each of these issues may increase stress to the patient. Pain is often accentuated in patients with anxiety, depression, or hysteria, or patients may exaggerate their symptoms (symptom magnification) in the absence of objective signs, which may be called **psychogenic pain**.[3,31,32] Waddell and Main[29] consider illness behavior normal with patients who are exhibiting both a physical problem and varying degrees of illness behavior (Table 1-5). In these cases, it may be beneficial to determine the level of psychological stress or to refer the patient to another appropriate health care professional.[30] When symptoms such as pain appear to be exaggerated, the examiner must also consider the possibility that the patient

is malingering. Malingering implies trying to obtain a particular gain by a conscious effort to deceive.[33]

Reactions to Stress

- Aches and pains
- Anxiety
- Changed appetite
- Chronic fatigue
- Difficulty concentrating
- Difficulty sleeping
- Irritability and impatience
- Loss of interest and enjoyment in life
- Muscle tension (headaches)
- Sweaty hands
- Trembling
- Withdrawal

Table 1-5

Spectrum of Clinical Symptoms and Signs

	Physical Disease	Illness Behavior
Pain		
Pain drawing	Localized Anatomic	Nonanatomic Regional Magnified
Pain adjectives	Sensory	Emotional
Symptoms		
Pain	Musculoskeletal or neurological distribution	Whole leg pain Pain at the tip of the tailbone
Numbness	Dermatomal	Whole leg numbness
Weakness	Myotomal	Whole leg giving way
Time pattern	Varies with time and activity	Never free of pain
Response to treatment	Variable benefit	Intolerance of treatments Emergency hospitalization
Signs		
Tenderness	Musculoskeletal distribution	Superficial Nonanatomic
Axial loading	Neck pain	Low back pain
Simulated rotation	Nerve root pain	Low back pain
Straight leg raising	Limited on formal examination No improvement on distraction	Marked improvement with distraction
Motor	Myotomal	Regional, jerky, giving way
Sensory	Dermatomal	Regional

From Waddell G and Main CJ: Illness behavior. In Waddell G, editor: *The back pain revolution.* Edinburgh, 1998, Churchill Livingstone, p. 162.

20. *Does the patient have any chronic or serious systemic illnesses or adverse social habits (e.g., smoking, drinking) that may influence the course of the pathology or the treatment?* In some cases, the examiner may use a medical history screening form (Figure 1-7) to determine the presence of conditions that may affect treatment or require referral to another health care professional.

21. *Is there anything in the family or developmental history that may be related, such as tumors, arthritis, heart disease, diabetes, allergies, and congenital anomalies?* Some disease processes and pathologies have a familial incidence.

22. *Has the patient undergone an x-ray examination or other imaging techniques?* If so, x-ray overexposure must be considered; if not, an x-ray examination may help yield a diagnosis.

23. *Has the patient been receiving analgesic, steroid, or any other medication? If so, for how long?* High dosages of steroids taken for long periods may lead to problems such as osteoporosis. Has the patient been taking any other medication that is pertinent? Anticoagulants such as aspirin or anticoagulant therapy increase the chance of bruising or hemarthrosis because the clotting mechanism is altered. Patients may not regard over-the-counter formulations, birth control pills, and so on as medications. If such medications have been taken for a long period, their use may not seem pertinent to the patient. How long has the patient been taking the medication? When did he or she last take the medication? Did the medication help?[34] It is also important to determine whether medication is being taken for the condition under review. If analgesics or anti-inflammatories were taken just before the patient's visit for the assessment, some symptoms may be masked.

24. *Does the patient have a history of surgery or past/ present illness?* If so, when was the surgery performed,

Date:			
Patient's Name:	DOB:	Age:	
Diagnosis:	Date of Onset:		
Physician:	Therapist:	Precautions:	

Medical History		*Do Not Complete, For Clinician*		
Have you or any immediate family member ever been told you have:	Circle one:	*Relation to Patient*	*Date of Onset*	*Current Status*
Cancer	Yes No			
Diabetes	Yes No			
Hypoglycemia	Yes No			
Hypertension or high blood pressure	Yes No			
Heart disease	Yes No			
Angina or chest pain	Yes No			
Shortness of breath	Yes No			
Stroke	Yes No			
Kidney disease/stones	Yes No			
Urinary tract infection	Yes No			
Allergies	Yes No			
Asthma, hay fever	Yes No			
Rheumatic/scarlet fever	Yes No			
Hepatitis/jaundice	Yes No			
Cirrhosis/liver disease	Yes No			
Polio	Yes No			
Chronic bronchitis	Yes No			
Pneumonia	Yes No			
Emphysema	Yes No			
Migraine headaches	Yes No			
Anemia	Yes No			
Ulcers/stomach problems	Yes No			
Arthritis/gout	Yes No			
Other	Yes No			

Medical Testing

1. Are you taking any prescription or over-the-counter medications? Yes No
   If yes, please list:
2. Have you had any x-rays, sonograms, computed tomography (CT) Yes No
   scans, or magnetic resonance imaging (MRI) done recently?
   If yes, when? Where? Results?
3. Have you had any laboratory work done recently (urinalysis or blood tests)? Yes No
   If yes, when? Where? Results?
4. Please list any operations that you have ever had and the date(s) of surgery.
   Surgery/Date:

General Health

1. Have you had any recent illnesses within the last 3 weeks (e.g., colds, Yes No
   influenza, bladder or kidney infection)?

Figure 1-7

Medical history screening card. (From Goodman CC and Snyder TK: *Differential diagnosis in physical therapy,* Philadelphia, 1990, WB Saunders.)

Continued

2.	Have you noticed any lumps or thickening of skin or muscle anywhere on your body?	Yes	No
3.	Do you have any sores that have not healed or any changes in size, shape, or color of a wart or mole?	Yes	No
4.	Have you had any unexplained weight loss in the last month?	Yes	No
5.	Do you smoke or chew tobacco?	Yes	No
	If yes, how many packs/day?		
	For how many months or years?		
6.	How much alcohol do you drink in the course of a week?		
7.	How much caffeine to you consume daily (including soft drinks, coffee, tea, or chocolate)?		
8.	Are you on any special diet prescribed by a physician?	Yes	No

Special Questions for Women

1.	Last Pap smear:		
2.	Last breast examination:		
3.	Do you perform a monthly self-breast examination?	Yes	No
4.	Do you take birth control pills or do you use an intrauterine device (IUD)?	Yes	No

Special Questions for Men

1.	Do you ever have difficulty with urination (e.g., difficulty in starting or continuing flow or a very slow flow or urine)?	Yes	No
2.	Do you ever have blood in your urine?	Yes	No
3.	Do you ever have pain on urination?	Yes	No

Work Environment

1.	Occupation:		
2.	Does your job involve:		
	prolonged sitting (e.g., desk, computer, driving)	Yes	No
	prolonged standing (e.g., equipment operator, sales clerk)	Yes	No
	prolonged walking (e.g., mill worker, delivery service)	Yes	No
	use of large or small equipment (e.g., telephone, fork lift, typewriter, drill press, cash register)	Yes	No
	lifting, bending, twisting, climbing, turning	Yes	No
	exposure to chemicals or gases	Yes	No
	other: please describe		
3.	Do you use any special supports:		
	back cushion, neck cushion	Yes	No
	back brace, corset	Yes	No
	other kind of brace or support for any body part	Yes	No

For Clinician

Vital signs:

Resting pulse rate:

Oral temperature:

Blood pressure: 1st reading: 2nd reading:

Position: Extremity:

Figure 1-7 cont'd

what was the site of operation, and what condition was being treated? Sometimes, the condition the examiner is asked to treat is the result of the surgery. Has the patient ever been hospitalized? If so, why? Health conditions such as high blood pressure, heart and circulatory problems, and systemic diseases (e.g., diabetes) should be noted because of their effect on healing, exercise prescription, and functional activities.[3]

It is evident that the taking of an accurate, detailed history is very important. ***Listen to the patient—he or she is telling you what is wrong!*** With experience, the examiner should be able to make a **preliminary "working" diagnosis** from the history alone. The observation and examination phases of the assessment are then used to confirm, alter, or refute the possible diagnoses. What an examiner looks for in observation and tests for in examination is often related to what she or he has found when taking a history.

Observation

In an assessment, observation is the "looking" or inspection phase. Its purpose is to gain information on visible defects, functional deficits, and abnormalities of alignment. Much of the observation phase involves assessment of **normal standing posture** (see Chapter 15). Normal posture covers a wide range, and asymmetric findings are common. The key is to determine whether these findings are related to the pathology being presented. The examiner should note the patient's way of moving as well as the general posture, manner, attitude, willingness to cooperate, and any signs of overt pain behavior.[35] Observation may begin in the waiting room or as the patient is being taken to the assessment area. Often the patient is unaware that observation is occurring at this stage and may present a different picture. The patient must be adequately undressed in a private assessment area to be observed properly. Male patients should wear only shorts, and female patients should wear a bra or halter top and shorts. Because the patient is in a state of undress, it is essential for the examiner to explain that observation and detailed looking at the patient are integral parts of the assessment. This explanation may prevent a potentially embarrassing situation that can have legal ramifications.

As the patient enters the assessment area, the examiner should observe his or her gait (see Chapter 14). This initial gait assessment is only a cursory one; however, problems such as Trendelenburg sign or drop foot are easily noticed. If there appears to be an abnormality, the gait may be checked in greater detail after the patient has undressed.

The examiner should be positioned so that the dominant eye is used, and both sides of the patient should be compared simultaneously. During the observation stage,

Overt Pain Behavior[35]

- Guarding. Abnormally stiff, interrupted or rigid movement while moving the joint or body from one position to an other
- Bracing. A stationary position in which a fully extended limb supports and maintains an abnormal distribution of weight
- Rubbing. Any contact between hand and injured area (i.e., touching, rubbing, or holding the painful area)
- Grimacing. Obvious facial expression of pain that may include furrowed brow, narrowed eyes, tightened lips, corners of mouth pulled back and clenched teeth
- Sighing. Obvious exaggerated exhalation of air usually accompanied by the shoulders first rising and then falling; patients may expand their cheeks first

the examiner is only looking at the patient and does not ask the patient to move; the examiner usually does not palpate, except possibly to learn whether an area is warm or hot or to find specific landmarks.

After the patient has undressed, the examiner should observe the posture and attempt to answer the following questions.

1. What is the normal body alignment? Anteriorly, the nose, xiphisternum, and umbilicus should be in a straight line. From the side, the tip of the ear, the tip of the acromion, the high point of the iliac crest, and the lateral malleolus (anterior aspect) should be in a straight line.

2. Is there any obvious deformity? Deformities may take the form of restricted ROM (e.g., flexion deformity), malalignment (e.g., genu varum), alteration in the shape of a bone (e.g., fracture), or alteration in the relationship of two articulating structures (e.g., subluxation, dislocation). **Structural deformities** are present even at rest; examples include torticollis, fractures, scoliosis, and kyphosis. **Functional deformities** are the result of assumed postures and disappear when posture is changed. For example, a scoliosis due to a short leg seen in an upright posture disappears on forward flexion. A pes planus (flatfoot) on weight bearing may disappear on non-weight-bearing. **Dynamic deformities** are caused by muscle action and are present when muscles contract or joints move. Therefore, they are not usually evident when the muscles are relaxed. Dynamic deformities are more likely to be seen during the examination phase.

3. Are the bony contours of the body normal and symmetric, or is there an obvious deviation? The body is not perfectly symmetric, and deviation may have no clinical implications. For example, many people have a lower shoulder on the dominant side or demonstrate a slight scoliosis of the spine adjacent to the heart. However, any deviation should be noted, because it may contribute to a more accurate diagnosis.

4. Are the soft-tissue contours (e.g., muscle, skin, fat) normal and symmetric? Is there any obvious muscle wasting?

5. Are the limb positions equal and symmetric? The examiner should compare limb size, shape, position, any atrophy, color, and temperature.

6. Are the color and texture of the skin normal? Does the appearance of the skin differ in the area of pain or symptoms, compared with other areas of the body? Ecchymosis or bruising indicates bleeding under the skin from injury to tissues (Figure 1-8). In some cases, this ecchymosis may track away from the injury site because of gravity. Trophic changes in the skin resulting from peripheral nerve lesions include loss of skin elasticity, shiny skin, hair loss on the skin, and skin that breaks down easily and heals slowly. The nails may become brittle and ridged. Skin disorders such as psoriasis may affect joints (psoriatic arthritis). Cyanosis, or a bluish color to the skin, is usually an indication of poor blood perfusion. Redness indicates increased blood flow or inflammation.

7. Are there any scars that indicate recent injury or surgery? Recent scars are red because they are still healing and contain capillaries; older scars are white and primarily avascular. Fibers of the dermis (skin) tend to run in one direction, along so-called cleavage or tension lines. Lacerations or surgical cuts along these lines produce less scarring. Cuts across joint flexion lines frequently produce excessive (hypertrophic) scarring. Some individuals are also prone to keloid (excessive) or hypertrophic scarring. Hypertrophic scars are scars that have excessive scar tissue but stay within the margins of the wound. Keloid scars expand beyond the margins of the wound. Are there any callosities, blisters, or inflamed bursae, indicative of excessive pressure or friction to the skin? Are there any sinuses that may indicate infection? If so, are the sinuses draining or dry?

8. Is there any crepitus, snapping, or abnormal sound in the joints when the patient moves them? Sounds, by themselves, do not necessarily indicate pathology. Sounds on movement only become significant when they are related to the patient's symptoms. Crepitus may vary from a loud grinding noise to a squeaking noise. Snapping, especially if not painful, may be caused by a tendon moving over a bony protuberance. Clicking is sometimes heard in the temporomandibular joint and may be an indication of early nonsymptomatic pathology.

9. Is there any heat, swelling, or redness in the area being observed? All of these signs along with pain and loss of function are indications of inflammation or an active inflammatory condition.

10. What attitude does the patient appear to have toward the condition or toward the examiner? Is the patient apprehensive, restless, resentful, or depressed? These questions give the examiner some indication of the patient's psychological state and how he or she will respond to the examination and treatment.

11. What is the patient's facial expression? Does the patient appear to be apprehensive, in discomfort, or lacking sleep?

12. Is the patient willing to move? Are patterns of movement normal? If not, how are they abnormal? Any alteration should be noted and included in the observation portion of the assessment.

On completion of the observation phase of the assessment, the examiner should return to the original preliminary working diagnosis made at the end of the history to see if any alteration in the diagnosis should be made with the additional information found in this phase.

Examination

Principles

Because the examination portion of the assessment involves touching the patient and may, in some cases, cause the patient discomfort, the examiner must obtain a valid consent to perform the examination before it begins. A valid consent must be voluntary, must cover the procedures to be done (informed consent), and the patient must be legally competent to give the consent (Appendix 1-2).[36,37]

Figure 1-8
Ecchymosis around the knee following rupture of the quadriceps and dislocation of the patella. Note how the ecchymosis is tracking distally toward the foot because of gravity from the leg hanging dependent.

The examination is used to confirm or refute the suspected diagnosis, which is based on the history and observation. The examination must be performed systematically, with the examiner looking for a consistent pattern of signs and symptoms that leads to a differential diagnosis. Special care must be taken if the condition of the joint is irritable or acute. This is especially true if the area is in severe spasm or if the patient complains of severe unremitting pain that is not affected by position or medication, severe night pain, severe pain with no history of injury, or nonmechanical behavior of the joint.

"Red Flags" in Examination Indicating the Need for Medical Consultation

- Severe unremitting pain
- Pain unaffected by medication or position
- Severe night pain
- Severe pain with no history of injury
- Severe spasm
- Inability to urinate or hold urine
- Elevated temperature (especially if prolonged)
- Psychological overlay

In the examination portion of the assessment, a number of principles must be followed.

1. Unless bilateral movement is required, the normal side is tested first. Testing the normal side first allows the examiner to establish a baseline for normal movement for the joint being tested and shows the patient what to expect, resulting in increased patient confidence and less patient apprehension when the injured side is tested.

2. The patient does active movements before the examiner does passive movements. Passive movements are followed by resisted isometric movements (see later discussion). In this way, the examiner has a better idea of what the patient thinks he or she can do before the structures are fully tested.

3. Any movements that are painful are done last, if possible, to prevent an overflow of painful symptoms to the next movement which, in reality, may be symptom free.

4. If active ROM is not full, overpressure is applied only with extreme care to prevent the exacerbation of symptoms.

5. During active movements, if the ROM is full, overpressure may be carefully applied to determine the end feel of the joint. This often negates the need to do passive movements.

6. Each active, passive, or resisted isometric movement may be repeated several times or held (sustained) for a certain amount of time to see whether symptoms increase or decrease, whether a different pattern of movement results, whether there is increased weakness, or whether

there is possible vascular insufficiency. This repetitive or sustained activity is especially important if the patient has complained that repetitive movement or sustained postures alter symptoms.

7. Resisted isometric movements are done with the joint in a neutral or resting position so that stress on the inert tissues is minimal. Any symptoms produced by the movement are then more likely to be caused by problems with contractile tissue.

8. For passive ROM or ligamentous tests, it is not only Mhe degree (i.e., the amount) of the opening but also the quality (i.e., the end feel) of the opening that is important.

9. When the examiner is testing the ligaments, the appropriate stress is applied gently and repeated several times. The stress is increased up to but not beyond the point of pain, thereby demonstrating maximum instability without causing muscle spasm.

10. When testing **myotomes** (groups of muscles supplied by a single nerve root), each contraction is held for a minimum of **5 seconds** to see whether weakness becomes evident. Myotomal weakness takes time to develop.

11. At the completion of an assessment, because a good examination commonly involves stressing different tissues, the examiner must warn the patient that symptoms may exacerbate as a result of the assessment. This will prevent the patient from thinking any initial treatment may have made the patient worse and thus be hesitant to return for further treatments.

12. If, at the conclusion of the examination, the examiner has found that the patient has presented with unusual signs and symptoms or if the condition appears to be beyond his or her scope of practice, the examiner should not hesitate to refer the patient to another appropriate health care professional.

Principles of Examination

- Tell the patient what you are doing.
- Test the normal (uninvolved) side first.
- Do active movements first, then passive movements, then resisted isometric movements.
- Do painful movements last.
- Apply overpressure with care to test end feel.
- Repeat movements or sustain certain postures or positions if history indicates.
- Do resisted isometric movements in a resting position.
- Remember that with passive movements and ligamentous testing, both the degree and quality (end feel) of opening are important.
- With ligamentous testing, repeat with increasing stress.
- With myotome testing, make sure that contractions are held for 5 seconds.
- Warn the patient of possible exacerbations.
- Maintain the patient's dignity.
- Refer if necessary.

Vital Signs

In some cases, the examiner may want to begin the examination by taking the patient's vital signs to establish the patient's baseline physiological parameters and vital signs (Table 1-6) and review the medical history screening card (see Figure 1-7). These include the pulse (most commonly the radial pulse at the wrist is used), blood pressure, respiratory rate, temperature (98.4°F or 37°C is normal but may range from 96.5°F [35.8°C] to 99.4°F [37.4°C]), and weight. Table 1-7 outlines guidelines for blood pressure measurement. High blood pressure values should be checked several times at 15- to 30-minute intervals, with the patient resting in between to determine whether a high reading is accurate or is being caused by anxiety ("white coat syndrome") or some similar reason. If three consecutive readings are high, the patient is said to have high blood pressure (hypertension) (Table 1-8). If the readings remain high, further investigation may be warranted.[38-40]

Scanning Examination

The examination described in this book emphasizes the joints of the body, their movement and stability. It is necessary to examine all appropriate tissues to delineate the affected area, which can then be examined in detail. Application of tension, stretch, or isometric contraction to specific tissues produces either a normal or an appropriate abnormal response. This action enables the examiner to determine the nature and site of the present symptoms and the patient's response to these symptoms. The examination shows whether certain activities provoke or change the patient's pain; in this way, the examiner can focus on the subjective response (i.e., the patient's feelings or opinions) as well as the test findings. The patient must be clear about his or her side of the examination. For instance, the patient must not confuse questions about movement-associated pain ("Does the movement make any difference to the pain?" "Does the movement bring on or change the pain?") with questions about already existing pain. In addition, the examiner attempts to see whether patient responses are measurably abnormal. Do the movements cause any abnormalities in function? A loss of movement or weakness in muscles can be measured and therefore is an objective response. Throughout the assessment, the examiner looks for two sets of data: (1) what the patient feels (subjective) and (2) responses that can be measured or are found by the examiner (objective).

When to Use the Scanning Examination

- There is no history of trauma.
- There are radicular signs.
- There is trauma with radicular signs.
- There is altered sensation in the limb.
- There are spinal cord ("long track") signs.
- The patient presents with abnormal patterns.
- There is suspected psychogenic pain.

Table 1-6

Vital Sign Normal Ranges

Age Group	Respiratory Rate	Heart Rate	Diastolic Blood Pressure	Systolic Blood Pressure	Temperature	Weight (kg)	Weight (lbs)
Newborn	30–50	120–160	Varies	50–70	97.7°F (36.5°C)	2–3	4.5–7
Infant (1–12 months)	20–30	80–140	Varies	70–100	98.6°F (37.0°C)*	4–10	9–22
Toddler (1–3 years)	20–30	80–130	48–80	80–110	98.6°F (37.0°C)*	10–14	22–31
Preschooler (3–5 years)	20–30	80–120	48–80	80–110	98.6°F (37.0°C)*	14–18	31–40
School Age (6–12 years)	20–30	70–110	50–90	80–120	98.6°F (37.0°C)*	20–42	41–92
Adolescent (13–17 years)	12–20	55–105	60–92	110–120	98.6°F (37.0°C)*	>50	>110
Adults (18+ years)	18–20	60–100	<85	<130	98.6°F (37.0°C)*	Varies	Depends on body size

*Ranges from 97.8°F to 99.1°F (36.5°C to 37.3°C).

Remember these points:

The patient's normal range should always be taken into consideration.

Heart rate, blood pressure and respiratory rate are expected to increase during times of fever or stress.

Respiratory rate for infants should be counted for a full 60 seconds.

Table 1-7

Guidelines for Measurement of Blood Pressure

Posture	Blood pressure obtained in the sitting position is recommended. The subject should sit quietly for 5 minutes, with the back supported and the arm supported at the level of the heart, before blood pressure is recorded.
Circumstances	No caffeine during the hour preceding the reading. No smoking during the 30 minutes preceding the reading. A quiet, warm setting.
Equipment	Cuff size: the bladder should encircle and cover two thirds of the length of the arm; if it does not, place the bladder over the brachial artery. If bladder is too short, misleading high readings may result. Manometer: aneroid gauges should be calibrated every 6 months against a mercury manometer.

Technique	Number of readings:
	  On each occasion, take at least two readings, separated by as much time as is practical. If readings vary by more than 5 mm Hg, take additional readings until two consecutive readings are close.
	  If the initial values are elevated, obtain two other sets of readings at least 1 week apart.
	  Initially, take pressure in both arms; if the pressures differ, use the arm with the higher pressure.
	  If the arm pressure is elevated, take the pressure in one leg (particularly in patients younger than 30 years of age).
	Performance:
	  Inflate the bladder quickly to a pressure 20 mm Hg above the systolic pressure, as recognized by disappearance of the radial pulse.
	  Deflate the bladder by 3 mm Hg every second.
	  Record the Korotkoff phase V (disappearance), except in children, in whom use of phase IV (muffling) may be preferable if disappearance of the sounds is not perceived.
	  If the Korotkoff sounds are weak, have the patient raise the arm and open and close the hand 5 to 10 times, and then reinflate the bladder quickly.

Recordings	Blood pressure, patient position, arm and cuff size.

From Kaplan NM et al: Systemic hyperextension, *Med Sci Sports Exerc* 26:S269, 1994.

Table 1-8

Classification of Hypertension by Age

		Magnitude of Hypertension			
	Normal	Mild, Stage 1	Moderate, Stage 2	Severe, Stage 3	Very Severe, Stage 4
Child (6–9 years)					
Systolic	80–120	120–124	125–129	130–139	≥140
Diastolic	50–75	75–79	80–84	85–89	≥90
Child (10–12 years)					
Systolic	80–120	125–129	130–134	135–144	≥145
Diastolic	50–80	80–84	85–89	90–94	≥95
Adolescent (13–15 years)					
Systolic	110–120	135–139	140–149	150–159	≥160
Diastolic	60–85	85–89	90–94	95–99	≥100
Adolescent (16–18 years)					
Systolic	110–120	140–149	150–159	160–179	≥180
Diastolic	60–90	90–94	95–99	100–109	≥110
Adult (>18 years)					
Systolic	110–130	140–159	160–179	180–209	≥210
Diastolic	80–90	90–99	100–109	110–119	≥120

Reprinted, by permission, from McGrew CA: Clinical implications of the AHA preparticipation cardiovascular screening guidelines, *Athletic Ther Today* 5(4):55, 2000.

To ensure that all possible sources of pathology are assessed, the examination must be extensive. This is especially true if there are symptoms when no history of trauma is present. In this case, a scanning or screening examination is performed to rule out the possibility of referral of symptoms, especially from the spine. Similarly, if there is any doubt about where the pathology is located, the scanning examination is essential to ensure a correct diagnosis. The scanning examination is a "quick look" or scan of a part of the body involving the spine and extremities. It is used to rule out symptoms, which may be referred from one part of the body to another. It is divided into two scans: the upper limb scan and the lower limb scan. It is part of the examination that is used, where necessary, along with a detailed and focused examination of one or more of the joints.

As with all assessments, the use of a scanning examination depends on what the examiner found in the history and observation. For assessment of the spine, the scanning examination is integrated into the examination as a regular part of the cervical or lumbar assessment (Figure 1-9, *A*) and includes a peripheral joint scan, myotome testing, and a sensory scan. If, when assessing the peripheral joints, the examiner suspects a problem is being referred from the spine, the scanning examination is "inserted" into the examination of that joint (Figure 1-9, *B*). For the scanning examination, the peripheral joints are "scanned," with the patient doing only a few key movements at each joint. The movements should include those that may be expected to exacerbate symptoms that are derived from the history. The examiner then tests the upper or lower limb myotomes (key muscles representing a specific nerve root). After these tests, a sensory scanning examination (sensory scan) can be performed that may include the appropriate reflexes, the sensory distributions of the dermatomes and peripheral nerve

Figure 1-9

The scanning examination used to rule out referral of symptoms from the spine. **A,** Spinal assessment (i.e., based on the history, the clinician feels the problem is in the spine). **B,** Peripheral joint assessment (i.e., based on the history, the clinician feels the problem is in a peripheral joint). (* These are done if scanning examination is not done.)

distribution, and selected neurodynamic tests (e.g., upper limb tension test, slump test) if the examiner suspects some neurological involvement. At this point, the examiner makes a decision or an "educated guess" as to whether the problem is in the cervical spine, lumbar spine, or the peripheral joint, based on the information gained. Once the decision is made, the examiner either completes the spinal assessment (in the case of a suspected spinal problem) or turns instead to completing the assessment of the appropriate peripheral joint (see Figure 1-9). The scanning examination should add no more than 5 or 10 minutes to the assessment.

The idea of the scanning examination was developed by James Cyriax,[1] who also, more than any other author, originated the concepts of "contractile" and "inert" tissue, "end feel," and "capsular patterns" and contributed greatly to development of a comprehensive and systematic physical examination of the moving parts of the body. Although several of his constructs and paradigms have been questioned,[41-43] the basic principles of ensuring that all tissues are tested remains sound.

Spinal Cord and Nerve Roots

To further comprehend and ensure the value of the scanning examination, the examiner must have a clear understanding of signs and symptoms arising from the spinal cord and nerve roots of the body and those arising from peripheral nerves. The scanning examination helps to determine whether the pathology is caused by tissues innervated by a nerve root or peripheral nerve that is referring symptoms distally.

The nerve root is that portion of a peripheral nerve that "connects" the nerve to the spinal cord. Nerve roots arise from each level of the spinal cord (e.g., C3, C4), and many, but not all, intermingle in a plexus (brachial, lumbar, or lumbosacral) to form different peripheral nerves (Figure 1-10). This arrangement can result in a single nerve root supplying more than one peripheral nerve. For example, the median nerve is derived from the C6, C7, C8, and T1 nerve roots, whereas the ulnar nerve is derived from C7, C8 and T1 (Table 1-9). For this reason, if pressure is applied to the nerve root, the distribution of the sensation or motor function is often felt or exhibited in more than one peripheral nerve distribution (Table 1-10). Therefore, although the symptoms seen in a nerve root lesion (e.g., paresthesia, pain, muscle weakness) may be similar to those seen in peripheral nerves, the signs (e.g., area of paresthesia, where pain occurs, which muscles are weak) are commonly different. The examiner must be able to differentiate a dermatome (nerve root) from the sensory distribution of a peripheral nerve, and a myotome (nerve

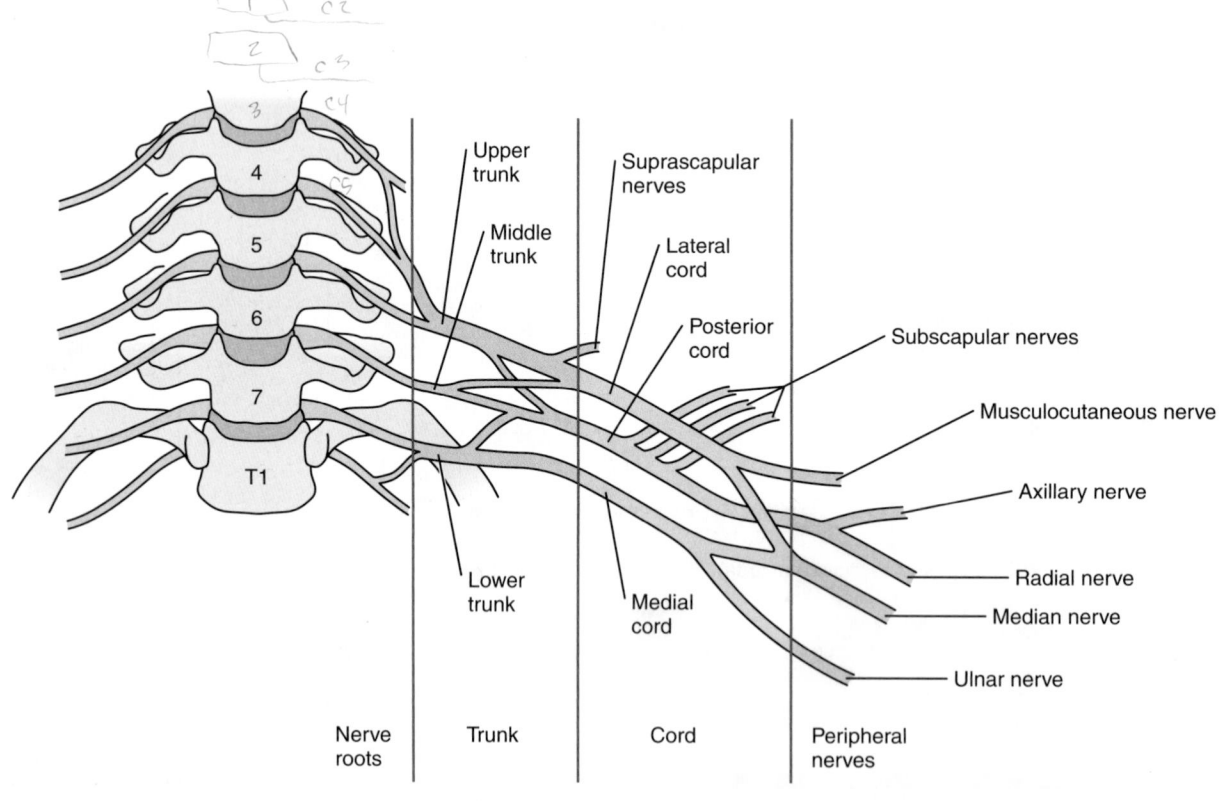

Figure 1-10

The interrelationship of the spinal nerve roots, plexus, and peripheral nerves, using cervical spine and brachial plexus as an example.

Table 1-9

Common Peripheral Nerves and Their Nerve Root Derivation

Peripheral Nerve	Nerve Root Derivation
Axillary	C5,6
Supraclavicular	C3,4
Suprascapular	C5,6
Subscapular	C5,6
Long thoracic	C5,6,7
Musculocutaneous	C5,6,7
Medial cutaneous nerve of forearm	C8,T1
Lateral cutaneous nerve of forearm	C5,6
Posterior cutaneous nerve of forearm	C5,6,7,8
Radial	C5,6,7,8,T1
Median	C6,7,8,T1
Ulnar	C(7)8,T1
Pudendal	S2,3,4
Lateral cutaneous nerve of thigh	L2,3
Medial cutaneous nerve of thigh	L2,3
Intermediate cutaneous nerve of thigh	L2,3
Posterior cutaneous nerve of thigh	S1,2,3
Femoral	L2,3,4
Obturator	L2,3,4
Sciatic	L4,5,S1,2,3
Tibial	L4,5,S1,2,3
Common peroneal	L4,5,S1,2
Superficial peroneal	L4,5,S1
Deep peroneal	L4,5,S1,2
Lateral cutaneous nerve of leg (calf)	L4,5,S1,2
Saphenous	L3,4
Sural	S1,2
Medial plantar	L4,5
Lateral plantar	S1,2

root) from muscles supplied by a specific peripheral nerve. In addition, neurological signs and symptoms such as paresthesia and pain may result from inflammation or irritation of tissues such as facet joints and interspinous ligaments or other tissues supplied by the nerve roots, and they may be demonstrated in the dermatome, myotome, or sclerotome supplied by that nerve root. This irritation can contribute to the referred pain (see later discussion).

Nerve roots are made up of anterior (ventral) and posterior (dorsal) portions that unite near or in the intervertebral foramen to form a single **nerve root** or **spinal nerve** (Figure 1-11). They are the most proximal parts of the peripheral nervous system.

The human body has 31 nerve root pairs: 8 cervical, 12 thoracic, 5 lumbar, 5 sacral, and 1 coccygeal. Each nerve root has two components: a **somatic** portion, which innervates the skeletal muscles and provides sensory input from the skin, fascia, muscles, and joints, and a **visceral** component, which is part of the autonomic nervous system.[44] The autonomic system supplies the blood vessels, dura mater, periosteum, ligaments, and intervertebral discs, among many other structures.

The sensory distribution of each nerve root is called the **dermatome.** A dermatome is defined as the area of skin supplied by a single nerve root. The area innervated by a nerve root is larger than that innervated by a peripheral nerve.[45] The descriptions of dermatomes in the following chapters should be considered as examples only, because slight differences occur with each patient, and dermatomes also exhibit a great deal of overlap.[46] The variability in dermatomes was aptly demonstrated by Keegan and Garrett in 1948 (Figure 1-12).[47] The overlap may be demonstrated by the fact that, in the thoracic spine, the loss of one dermatome often goes unnoticed because of the overlap of the adjacent dermatomes.

Spinal nerve roots have a poorly developed epineurium and lack a perineurium. This development makes the nerve root more susceptible to compressive forces, tensile deformation, chemical irritants (e.g., alcohol, lead, arsenic), and metabolic abnormalities. For example, compression of the nerve root could occur with a posterolateral intervertebral disc herniation, a "burner" or stretching of the nerve roots or the brachial plexus in a football player or alcoholic neuritis in an alcoholic. Pressure on nerve roots leads to loss of muscle tone and mass, but the loss is often not as obvious as when pressure is applied to a peripheral nerve. Because the peripheral nerve that innervates the muscle is usually supplied by more than one nerve root, more muscle fibers are likely to be affected and wasting or atrophy is more evident if the peripheral nerve itself is damaged. In addition, the pattern of weakness (i.e., which muscles are affected) is different for an injury to a nerve root and to a peripheral nerve, because a nerve root supplies more than one peripheral nerve. Pressure on a peripheral nerve resulting in a neuropraxia leads to temporary nonfunction of the nerve. With this type of injury, there is primarily motor involvement, with little sensory or autonomic involvement, and although weakness may be demonstrated, muscle atrophy may not be evident. With more severe peripheral nerve lesions (e.g., axonotmesis and neurotmesis), atrophy is evident.

Myotomes are defined as groups of muscles supplied by a single nerve root. A lesion of a single nerve root is usually associated with paresis (incomplete paralysis) of the myotome (muscles) supplied by that nerve root. It therefore takes time for any weakness to become evident on resisted isometric or myotome testing, and for this

Table 1-10

Nerve Root Dermatomes, Myotomes, Reflexes, and Paresthetic Areas

Nerve Root	Dermatome*	Muscle Weakness (Myotome)	Reflexes Affected	Paresthesias
C1	Vertex of skull	None	None	None
C2	Temple, forehead, occiput	Longus colli, sternocleidomastoid, rectus capitis	None	None
C3	Entire neck, posterior cheek, temporal area, prolongation forward under mandible	Trapezius, splenius capitis	None	Cheek, side of neck
C4	Shoulder area, clavicular area, upper scapular area	Trapezius, levator scapulae	None	Horizontal band along clavicle and upper scapula
C5	Deltoid area, anterior aspect of entire arm to base of thumb	Supraspinatus, infraspinatus, deltoid, biceps	Biceps, brachioradialis	None
C6	Anterior arm, radial side of hand to thumb and index finger	Biceps, supinator, wrist extensors	Biceps, brachioradialis	Thumb and index finger
C7	Lateral arm and forearm to index, long, and ring fingers	Triceps, wrist flexors (rarely, wrist extensors)	Triceps	Index, long, and ring fingers
C8	Medial arm and forearm to long, ring, and little fingers	Ulnar deviators, thumb extensors, thumb adductors (rarely, triceps)	Triceps	Little finger alone or with two adjacent fingers; *not* ring or long fingers, alone or together (C7)
T1	Medial side of forearm to base of little finger	Disc lesions at upper two thoracic levels do not appear to give rise to root weakness. Weakness of intrinsic muscles of the hand is caused by other pathology (e.g., thoracic outlet pressure, neoplasm of lung, and ulnar nerve lesion). Dural and nerve root stress has T1 elbow flexion with arm horizontal. T1 and T2 scapulae forward and backward on chest wall. Neck flexion at any thoracic level.		
T2	Medial side of upper arm to medial elbow, pectoral and midscapular areas			
T3-T12	T3-T6, upper thorax; T5-T7, costal margin; T8-T12, abdomen and lumbar region	Articular and dural signs and root pain are common. Root signs (cutaneous analgesia) are rare and have such indefinite area that they have little localizing value. Weakness is not detectable.		
L1	Back, over trochanter and groin	None	None	Groin; after holding posture, which causes pain
L2	Back, front of thigh to knee	Psoas, hip adductors	None	Occasionally anterior thigh
L3	Back, upper buttock, anterior thigh and knee, medial lower leg	Psoas, quadriceps, thigh atrophy	Knee jerk sluggish, PKB positive, pain on full SLR	Medial knee, anterior lower leg
L4	Medial buttock, lateral thigh, medial leg, dorsum of foot, big toe	Tibialis anterior, extensor hallucis	SLR limited, neck flexion pain, weak or absent knee jerk, side flexion limited	Medial aspect of calf and ankle
L5	Buttock, posterior and lateral thigh, lateral aspect of leg, dorsum of foot, medial half of sole, first, second, and third toes	Extensor hallucis, peroneals, gluteus medius, dorsiflexors, hamstring and calf atrophy	SLR limited one side, neck flexion painful, ankle decreased, cross-leg raising—pain	Lateral aspect of leg, medial three toes

Continued

Table 1-10—cont'd

Nerve Root	Dermatome*	Muscle Weakness (Myotome)	Reflexes Affected	Paresthesias
S1	Buttock, thigh, and leg posterior	Calf and hamstring, wasting of gluteals, peroneals, plantar flexors	SLR limited, Achilles reflex weak or absent	Lateral two toes, lateral foot, lateral leg to knee, plantar aspect of foot
S2	Same as S1	Same as S1 except peroneals	Same as S1	Lateral leg, knee, and heel
S3	Groin, medial thigh to knee	None	None	None
S4	Perineum, genitals, lower sacrum	Bladder, rectum	None	Saddle area, genitals, anus, impotence, massive posterior herniation

*In any part of which pain may be felt.
PKB = prone knee bending; SLR = straight leg raising.

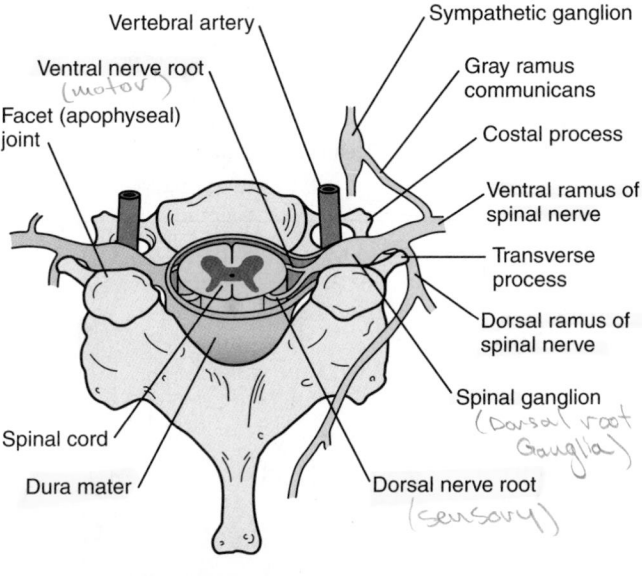

Figure 1-11
Spinal cord, nerve root portions, and spinal nerve in the cervical spine and their relation to the vertebra and vertebral artery.

Examples of Autonomic Nervous System Involvement ("Yellow Flags")

- Ringing in the ears
- Dizziness
- Blurred vision
- Photophobia (sensitivity to light)
- Rhinorrhea (runny nose)
- Sweating
- Lacrimation (tearing)
- Generalized loss of muscle strength
- Increase in heart rate
- Flushing (vasodilatation)

reason, the isometric testing of myotomes is held for *at least 5 seconds*. On the other hand, a lesion of a peripheral nerve leads to complete paralysis of the muscles supplied by that nerve, especially if the injury results in an axonotmesis or neurotmesis, and the weakness therefore is evident right away. Differences in the amount of resulting paralysis arise from the fact that more than one myotome contributes to the formation of a muscle embryologically.

A **sclerotome** is an area of bone or fascia supplied by a single nerve root (Figure 1-13). As with dermatomes, sclerotomes can show a great deal of variability among individuals.

It is the complex nature of the dermatomes, myotomes, and sclerotomes supplied by the nerve root that can lead to **referred pain,** which is pain felt in a part of the body that is usually a considerable distance from the tissues that have caused it. Referred pain is explained as an error in perception on the part of the brain. Usually, pain can be referred into the appropriate myotome, dermatome, or sclerotome from any somatic or visceral tissue innervated by a nerve root, but, confusingly, it sometimes is not referred according to a specific pattern.[48] It is not understood why this occurs, but clinically it has been found to be so.

Many theories of the mechanism of referred pain have been developed, but none has been proven conclusively. Generally, referred pain may involve one or more of the following mechanisms:

1. Misinterpretation by the brain as to the source of the painful impulses
2. Inability of the brain to interpret a summation of noxious stimuli from various sources
3. Disturbance of the internuncial pool by afferent nerve impulses.

Figure 1-12

The variability of dermatomes at C8 and S1 as found by four researchers. Similar variability is demonstrated in most cervical, lumbar, and sacral vertebrae. (Redrawn from Keegan JJ and Garrett FD: The segmental distribution of the cutaneous nerves in the limbs of man, *Anat Rec* 101:430, 433, 1948. Copyright © 1948. This material is used by permission of Wiley-Liss, a subsidiary of John Wiley & Sons.)

POSTERIOR   ANTERIOR

Figure 1-13 ▓

Sclerotomes of the body. Lines show areas of bone and fascia supplied by individual nerve roots.

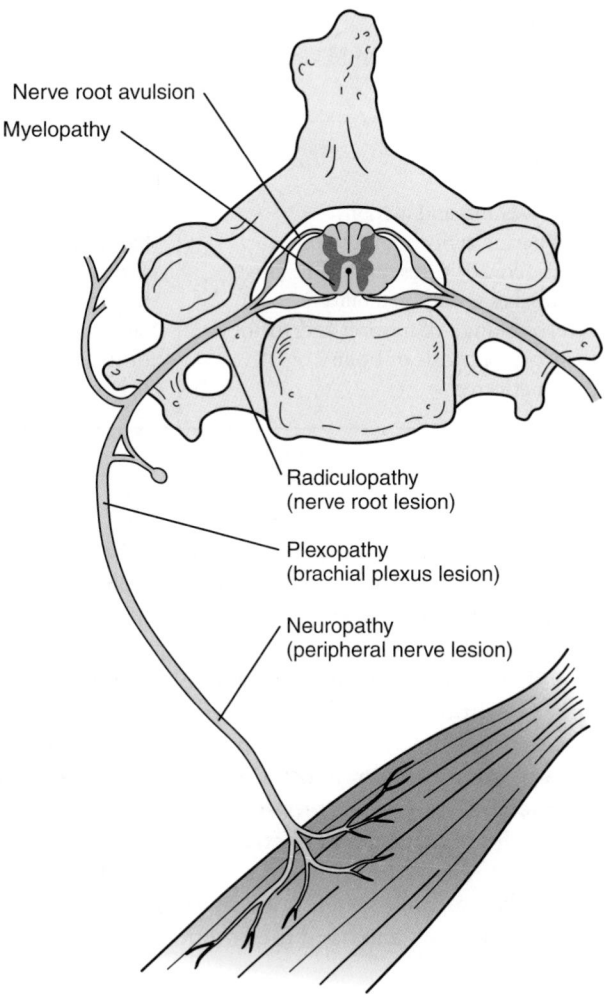

Figure 1-14 ▓

Path of neurological tissue from spinal cord to muscles, showing sites of neurological lesions.

Referral of pain is a common occurrence in problems associated with the musculoskeletal system. Pain is often felt at points remote from the site of the lesion. The site to which pain is referred is an indicator of the segment that is at fault: it indicates that one of the structures innervated by a specific nerve root is causing signs and symptoms in other tissues supplied by that same nerve root. For example, pain in the L5 dermatome could arise from irritation around the L5 nerve root, from an L5 disc causing pressure on the L5 nerve root, from facet joint involvement at L4-L5 causing irritation of the L5 nerve root, from any muscle supplied by the L5 nerve root, or from any visceral structures having L5 innervation. Referred pain tends to be felt deeply; its boundaries are indistinct, and it radiates segmentally without crossing the midline. **Radicular** or **radiating pain,** a form of referred pain, is a sharp, shooting pain felt in a dermatome, myotome, or sclerotome because of direct involvement of a spinal nerve or nerve root.[34] A **radiculopathy** refers to radiating paresthesia, numbness or weakness but not pain.[49] A **myelopathy** is a neurogenic disorder involving the spinal cord or brain and resulting in an upper motor neuron lesion; the patterns of pain or symptoms are different from that of radicular pain, and often both upper and lower limbs are affected (Figure 1-14).

Peripheral Nerves

Peripheral nerves are a unique type of "inert" tissue (see the later discussion) in that they are not contractile tissue but they are necessary for the normal functioning of voluntary muscle. The examiner must be aware of potential injury to nervous tissue when examining both contractile and inert tissue. Table 1-11 shows some of the tissue changes that result when a peripheral nerve lesion occurs.

Table 1-11

Signs and Symptoms of Mixed Peripheral Nerve (Lower Motor Neuron) Lesions[*]

Motor	Sensory	Sympathetic
Flaccid paralysis	Loss of or abnormal sensation	Loss of sweat glands (dryness)
Loss of reflexes	Loss of vasomotor tone: warm flushed	Loss of pilomotor response
Muscle wasting and atrophy	(early); cold, white (later)	
Lost synergic action of muscles	Skin may be scaly (early); thin, smooth	
Fibrosis, contractures, and adhesions	and shiny (later)	
Joint weakness and instability	Shallower skin creases	
Decreased range of motion and stiffness	Nail changes (striations, ridges, dry,	
Disuse osteoporosis of bone	brittle, abnormal curving, luster lost)	
Growth affected	Ulceration	

*Primarily axonotmesis and neurotmesis.

In peripheral nerves, the epineurium consists of a loose areolar connective tissue matrix surrounding the nerve fiber. It allows changes in growth length of the bundled nerve fibers (funiculi) without allowing the bundles to be strained. The perineurium protects the nerve bundles by acting as a diffusion barrier to irritants and provides tensile strength and elasticity to the nerve. Peripheral nerves therefore are most commonly affected by pressure, traction, friction, anoxia, or cutting. Examples include pressure on the median nerve in the carpal tunnel, traction to the common peroneal nerve at the head of the fibula during a lateral ankle sprain, friction to the ulnar nerve in the cubital tunnel, anoxia of the anterior tibial nerve in a compartment syndrome, and cutting of the radial nerve with a fracture of the humeral shaft. Cooling, freezing, and thermal or electrical injury may also affect peripheral nerves.

Nerve injuries are usually classified by the systems of Seddon[50] or Sunderland.[51] Seddon, whose system is most commonly used, classified nerve injuries into neuropraxia (most common), axonotmesis, and neurotmesis (Table 1-12). Sunderland followed a similar system but divided axonotmesis and neurotmesis into two levels each. Any examination of a joint must include a thorough peripheral nerve examination, especially if there are neurological signs and symptoms. The examiner must be able not

Table 1-12

Classification of Nerve Injuries According to Seddon

Grade of Injury	Definition	Signs and Symptoms
Neuropraxia (Sunderland 1°)	A transient physiological block caused by ischemia from pressure or stretch of the nerve with no wallerian degeneration	Pain No or minimal muscle wasting Muscle weakness Numbness Proprioception affected Recovery time: minutes to days
Axonotmesis (Sunderland 2° and 3°)	Internal architecture of nerve preserved, but axons are so badly damaged that wallerian degeneration occurs	Pain Muscle wasting evident Complete motor, sensory, and sympathetic functions lost (see Table 1-11) Recovery time: months (axon regenerates at rate of 1 inch/month, or 1 mm/day) Sensation is restored before motor function
Neurotmesis (Sunderland 4° and 5°)	Structure of nerve is destroyed by cutting, severe scarring, or prolonged severe compression	No pain (anesthesia) Muscle wasting Complete motor, sensory, and sympathetic functions lost (see Table 1-11) Recovery time: months and only with surgery

Data from Seddon HJ: Three types of nerve injury, *Brain* 66:17-28, 1943.

only to differentiate inert tissue lesions from contractile tissue lesions but also to determine whether a contractile tissue malfunction is the result of the contractile tissue itself or a peripheral nerve lesion or a nerve root lesion.

Sensory loss combined with motor loss should alert the examiner to lesions of nervous tissue.[52-54] Injury to a single peripheral nerve (e.g., the median nerve) is referred to as a **mononeuropathy.** Systemic diseases (e.g., diabetes) may affect more than one peripheral nerve. In this case, the pathology is referred to as a **polyneuropathy.** Careful mapping of the area of sensory loss and testing of the muscles affected by the motor loss allow the examiner to differentiate between a peripheral nerve lesion and a nerve root lesion. (An example is shown in Table 1-13.) If electromyographic studies are to be used to determine the grade of nerve injury, denervation cannot be evaluated for at least 3 weeks after injury to allow wallerian degeneration to occur and to allow regeneration (if any) to begin.[55-57] Muscle wasting usually becomes obvious after 4 to 6 weeks and progresses to reach its maximum by about 12 weeks following injury. Circulatory changes after nerve injury vary with time. In the initial or early stages, the skin is warm, but after about 3 weeks, the skin becomes cooler as a result of decreased circulation. Because of the decreased circulation and altered cell metabolism, trophic changes occur to the skin and nails.

When assessing a patient, the examiner must also be aware of what has been called the double-crush syndrome or double-entrapment neuropathy.[58-61] The theory of this lesion (which has not yet been proved but has clinical supporting evidence) is that, whereas compression at one point along a peripheral nerve or nerve root may not be sufficient to cause signs and symptoms, compression at two or more points may lead to a cumulative effect that results in apparent signs and symptoms. Because of this cumulative effect, signs and symptoms may indicate one area of involvement (e.g., the carpal tunnel), whereas other areas (e.g., cervical spine, brachial plexus, thoracic outlet) may be contributing to the problem. Similarly, cervical lesions may be involved in tennis elbow (lateral epicondylitis) syndromes. Upton and McComas[58] believed that compression proximally on the nerve trunk could increase the vulnerability of the peripheral nerves or nerve roots at distal points along their paths because axonal transport would be disrupted. In addition, diseased nerves are more susceptible to injury; thus, the presence of systemic disease (e.g., diabetes, thyroid dysfunction) may make the nerve more susceptible to compression somewhere along its path.[53] Finally, the signs and symptoms could potentially be arising from both a nerve root lesion and a peripheral nerve lesion. Only with meticulous assessment can the clinician delineate where the true problems lie.

Similarly, the loss of extensibility of the nervous tissue at one site may produce increasing tensile loads when the peripheral nerve or nerve root is stretched, leading to mechanical dysfunction.[62] This is the principle behind the **neural tension** or **neurodynamic tests,** such as the straight leg raise, slump test, and upper limb tension test,[62-64] and may provide a partial explanation for lesions such as cervical spine lesions mimicking tennis elbow and carpal tunnel syndrome. These tests put neural tissue (e.g., neuraxis [CNS], meninges, nerve roots, peripheral nerves) under tension when they are performed and may duplicate symptoms

Table 1-13

Comparison of Signs and Symptoms for C7 Nerve Root Lesion and Median Nerve Lesion at Elbow

	C7 Nerve Root	**Median Nerve**
Sensory alteration	Lateral arm and forearm to index, long, and ring fingers on palmar and dorsal aspect	Palmar aspect of thumb, index, middle, and half of ring finger Dorsal aspect of index, middle, and possibly half of ring finger
Motor alteration	Triceps Wrist flexors Wrist extensors (rarely)	Pronator teres Wrist flexors (lateral half of flexor digitorum profundus) Palmaris longus Pronator quadratus Flexor pollicis longus and brevis Abductor pollicis brevis Opponens pollicis Lateral two lumbricals
Reflex alteration	Triceps may be affected	None*
Paresthesia	Index, long, and ring fingers on palmar and dorsal aspect	Same as sensory alternation

*No "common" reflexes are affected; if the examiner tested the tendon reflexes of the muscles listed, they would be affected.

that result during functional activity.[62,64,65] For example, sitting in a car is closely mimicked by the action of the slump test and straight leg raising.

Neural tissue moves toward the joint at which elongation is initiated. Thus, if cervical flexion is initiated, the nerve roots, even those in the lumbar spine, move toward the cervical spine. Likewise, flexion of the whole spine causes movement toward the lumbar spine, and extension of the knee or dorsiflexion of the foot causes neural movement toward the knee or ankle.[62,64,65] These "tension points" can potentially help determine where the restriction to movement is occurring. Normally, tension tests are not painful, although the patient is often aware of increased tension or discomfort in the spine or the limb. As tension tests indicate neural mobility and sensitivity to mechanical stresses, they are considered positive only if they reproduce the patient's symptoms, or if the patient's response is altered by movement of a body part distal to where the symptoms are felt (e.g., foot dorsiflexion causing symptoms in the lumbar spine), or if there is asymmetry in the response.[62] When doing tension tests, the examiner should note the angle or position at which the restriction occurs and what the resistance feels like. With irritable conditions, only those parts of the test that are needed to cause positive results should be performed. For example, in the slump test, if neck flexion and slumping cause positive signs, there is no need to cause further discomfort to the patient by doing knee extension and foot dorsiflexion.

In the examination, testing of neurological tissue occurs during active, passive, and resisted isometric movement, as well as during functional testing, specific tests, reflexes, and cutaneous distribution and palpation.

Examination of Specific Joints

The examiner should use an unchanging, systematic approach to the examination that varies only slightly to elaborate certain clues given by the history or by asymmetric responses. For example, if the history is characteristic of a disc lesion, the examination should be a detailed one of all the tissues that may be affected by the disc and a brief one of all the other joints to exclude contradictory signs. If the history suggests arthritis of the hip, the examination should be a detailed one of the hip and a brief one of the other joints—again, to exclude contradictory signs. As the movements are tested, the examiner is looking sometimes for the patient's subjective responses and sometimes for clinical objective findings. For example, if examination of the cervical spine shows clear signs of a disc problem, as the examination is continued down the arm, the examiner looks more for muscle weakness (objective) rather than for elicitation of pain (subjective). In contrast, if the history suggests a muscle lesion, pain will probably be provoked when the arm is examined.

In either case, the structures expected to be normal are not omitted from the examination. There are only a few situations in which deviation from this systematic routine should occur: when there is uncertainty about where the pathology lies (in which case, a scanning examination must be performed, with combined assessment of the spine and one or more peripheral joints); when there is no history of trauma or indication of pathology in a specific joint yet the patient complains of pain in that joint (again, a scanning examination is performed); or when the joint to be assessed is too acutely injured or irritable to do the total systematic examination.

If there is an organic lesion, some active, passive, or resisted isometric movements will be abnormal or painful and others will not. Negative findings must balance positive ones, and the examination must be extensive enough to allow characteristic patterns to emerge. Determination of the problem is not made on the strength of the first positive finding; it is made only after it is clear that there are no other contradictory signs. Movements may be repeated several times quickly to rule out any problem such as vascular insufficiency or if the patient has indicated in the history that repetitive movements increase the symptoms. Likewise, sustained postures may be held for several seconds or combined movements may be performed if the history indicates increased symptoms with those postures or movements.

Contractile tissues may have tension placed on them by stretching or contraction.[1] These structures include the muscles, their tendons, and their attachments into the bone. **Nervous tissues** and their associated sheaths also have tension put on them by stretching and pinching, as do **inert tissues.** Inert tissues include all structures that would not be considered contractile or neurological, such as joint capsules, ligaments, bursae, blood vessels, cartilage, and dura mater. Table 1-14 demonstrates differential diagnosis of injuries to contractile tissue (strains and paratenonitis) and inert tissue (sprains). Some examiners separate vascular tissues from the other inert tissues; however, for the most part, when doing a musculoskeletal examination, they can be grouped with the other inert tissues with the understanding that they do present their own unique signs and symptoms.

When doing movement testing, the examiner should note whether pain or restriction predominate. If pain predominates, the condition is more acute and gentler assessment and treatment are required. If restriction predominates, the condition is subacute or chronic and more vigorous assessment and treatment can be performed.

Active Movements

Active movements are "actively" performed by the patient's voluntary muscles and have their own special value in that they combine tests of joint range, control,

Table 1-14

Differential Diagnosis of Muscle Strains, Tendon Injury, and Ligament Sprains

	1° Strain	2° Strain	3° Strain (Rupture)	Paratenonitis[a] Tendinosis[b]	1° Sprain	2° Sprain	3° Sprain
Definition	Few fibers of muscle torn	About half of muscle fibers torn	All muscle fibers torn (rupture)	[a]Inflammation of tendon [b]Intratendinous degeneration	Few fibers of ligament torn	About half of ligament torn	All fibers of ligament torn
Mechanism of Injury	Overstretch Overload	Overstretch Overload Crushing	Overstretch Overload	Overuse Overstretch Overload [b]Aging	Overload Overstretch	Overload Overstretch	Overload Overstretch
Onset	Acute	Acute	Acute	Chronic Acute	Acute	Acute	Acute
Weakness	Minor	Moderate to major (reflex inhibition)	Moderate to major	Minor to moderate	Minor	Minor to moderate	Minor to moderate
Disability	Minor	Moderate	Major	Minor to major	Minor	Moderate	Moderate to major
Muscle Spasm	Minor	Moderate to major	Moderate	Minor	Minor	Minor	Minor
Swelling	Minor	Moderate to major	Moderate to major	[a]Minor to major (thickening) [b]No	Minor	Moderate	Moderate to major
Loss of Function	Minor	Moderate to major	Major (reflex inhibition)	Minor to major	Minor	Moderate to major	Moderate to major (instability)
Pain on Isometric Contraction	Minor	Moderate to major	No to minor	Minor to major	No	No	No
Pain on Stretch	Yes	Yes	No*	Yes	Yes	Yes	No*
Joint Play	Normal	Normal	Normal	Normal	Normal	Normal	Normal to excessive
Palpable Defect	No	No	Yes (if early)	[b]May have palpable module	No	No	Yes (if early)
Crepitus	No	No	No	Possible	No	No	No
ROM	Decreased	Decreased	May increase or decrease depending on swelling	Decreased	Decreased	Decreased	May increase or decrease depending on swelling Dislocation or subluxation possible

*Not if it is the only tissue injured; however, often with 3° injuries, other structures will suffer 1° or 2° injuries and be painful.

muscle power, and the patient's willingness to perform the movement. These movements are sometimes referred to as **physiological movements.** The end of active movement is sometimes referred to as the **physiological barrier.** Contractile, nervous, and inert tissues are involved or moved during active movements. When active movements occur, one or more rigid structures (bones) move, and such movement results in movement of all structures that attach to or are in close proximity to that bone. Although active movements are usually the first movements done, they either are not performed at all or are performed with caution during fracture healing or if the movement could put stress on newly repaired soft tissues. The examiner should note which movements, if any, cause pain or other symptoms and the amount and quality of pain that results. For example, small, unguarded movements causing intense pain indicate an acute, irritable joint. If the condition is very irritable or acute, it may not be possible to elicit all the movements desired. In this case, only those movements that provide the most useful information should be performed. The examiner should note the rhythm of movement along with any pain, limitation, or unusual (e.g., instability jog) or trick movements that occur. Trick movements are modified movements that the patient consciously or unconsciously uses to accomplish what the examiner has asked the patient to do. For example, in the presence of deltoid paralysis, if the examiner asks the patient to abduct the arm, the patient can accomplish this movement by laterally rotating the shoulder and using the biceps muscle to abduct the arm.

Active movement may be abnormal for several reasons, and the examiner must try to differentiate the cause. Pain is a common cause for abnormal movement as is muscle weakness, paralysis, or spasm. Other causes include tight or shortened tissues, altered length-tension relationships, modified neuromuscular factors, and joint-muscle interaction.

The active movement component of the examination is a functional test of the anatomical and dynamical aspects of the body and joints while demonstrating correct or incorrect motor function, which is the ability to demonstrate skillful and efficient movement patterns while maintaining control of voluntary postures.[5,66] The examiner should ensure the movement is performed at a smooth constant speed in the desired direction using the most efficient pathway through full ROM.[67,68] This will involve the integration and synchronization of prime movers and synergists through the whole or part of the kinetic chain involved in the movement.

When testing active movements, the examiner should note where in the arc of movement the symptoms occur. For example, pain occurs during abduction of the shoulder between 60° and 120° if there is impingement under the acromion process or coracoacromial ligament. Any increase in intensity and quality of pain should also be noted. This information helps the examiner determine the particular tissue at fault. For example, bone pain, except in the case of a fracture or tumor, often is not altered with movement. By observing the patient's reaction to pain, the examiner can get some idea of how much the condition is affecting the patient and the patient's pain threshold. By noting the pattern of movement, the quality and rhythm of the movement, the movements in other joints, and the observable restriction, the examiner can tell if the patient is "cheating" (using accessory muscles or muscle substitution) to do the movement and what tissues are affected. For example, "shoulder hiking" may indicate a capsular pattern of the shoulder or incorrect sequential firing of different muscles.

Generally, active movements are performed once or twice in each desired direction while the examiner notes

---

Examiner Observations during Active Movement

- When and where during each of the movements the onset of pain occurs
- Whether the movement increases the intensity and quality of the pain
- The reaction of the patient to pain
- The amount of observable restriction and its nature
- The pattern of movement
- The rhythm and quality of movement
- The movement of associated joints
- The willingness of the patient to move the part

---

the pattern of movement and any discrepancies or cheating/substitution movements. If the patient has noted pain or difficulty with any particular movements, these movements should be done last to ensure no overflow of symptoms to other movements. If the patient has complained that certain repetitive movements or sustained postures are the problem, the examiner should ensure that the movements are repeated (5 to 10 times) or sustained (usually 5 to 20 seconds but may depend on history) until the symptoms are demonstrated.

There are standard movements for each joint, and these movements tend to follow cardinal planes (i.e., they are single plane movements). However, if the patient complains of problems outside these standard movements or if symptoms are more likely to be elicited by combined movements (i.e., movements in multiple planes or around combined axes), repeated movements, movements with speed, or movements under compression, then these should be performed.[69–71] McKenzie has reported that repeated movements increase symptoms in irritable acute tissues or in internal derangements,[11] whereas postural dysfunctions change little with repeated movements.

In some cases, especially if the joints are not too reactive or irritable, overpressure may carefully be applied at the end of the active ROM. If the overpressure does not produce symptoms and the end feel is normal, the movement is considered normal and the examiner may decide that passive movements are unnecessary.

Passive Movements

With passive movement, the examiner puts the joint through its ROM while the patient is relaxed. These movements may also be referred to as **anatomical movements.** The end of passive movement is sometimes referred to as the **anatomical barrier.** Normally, the physiological barrier (active movement) occurs before the anatomical barrier (passive movement) so that passive movement is always slightly greater than active movement. The movement must proceed through as full a range as possible and should, if possible, involve the same motions as were performed actively. Positioning the patient (e.g., sitting, lying supine) may have an effect on active and passive ROM, so the examiner must consider positioning. Differences in ROM between active and passive movements may be caused by muscle contraction or spasm, muscle deficiency, neurological deficit, contractures, or pain. Active and passive ROM may be measured by goniometer, inclinometer, examiner estimation ("eyeballing"), or a similar measure.[72,73] With most of these methods, it is difficult to show consistent differences of less than 5°.[74,75] Goniometry is especially useful for measuring and recording joint or fracture deformities and has been shown to have a satisfactory level of intratester reliability,[75-77] although this may depend on the motion measured.[77] Measurements at different times show progression or regression of the deformity. Although there are sources that describe ROMs for various joints, the values given are averages and do not necessarily constitute the ROM needed to do specific activities or the ROM that is present in a specific patient. Normal mobility is relative. For example, gymnasts tend to be classed as lax (nonpathological hypermobility) in most joints, whereas elderly persons tend to be classed as hypomobile. For these individual populations, however, the available ROM may be considered normal. In reality, the important question is, does the patient have the range of motion available to do what he or she wants to do functionally? Certain pathological states may also affect ROM. For example, Ehlers-Danlos syndrome, a connective tissue disorder, results in hypermobility not only of joints but of the skin as well.

Examiner Observations during Passive Movement

- When and where during each of the movements the pain begins
- Whether the movement increases the intensity and quality of pain
- The pattern of limitation of movement
- The end feel of movement
- The movement of associated joints
- The range of motion available

Each movement must be compared with the same movement in the opposite joint or, secondarily, with accepted norms. Although passive movement must be gentle, the examiner must determine whether there is any limitation of range (**hypomobility**) or excess of range (**hypermobility** or **laxity**) and, if so, whether it is painful. Hypermobile joints tend to be more susceptible to ligament sprains, joint effusion, chronic pain, recurrent injury, paratenonitis resulting from lack of control (instability), and early osteoarthritis. Hypomobile joints are more susceptible to muscle strains, pinched nerve syndromes, and paratenonitis resulting from overstress.[78,79]

Myofascial hypomobility results from adaptive shortening or hypertonicity of the muscles or from posttraumatic adhesions or scarring. **Pericapsular hypomobility** has a capsular or ligamentous origin and may result from adhesions, scarring, arthritis, arthrosis, fibrosis, or tissue adaptation. Restriction may be in all directions but not the same amount in each direction (e.g., capsular pattern). **Pathomechanical hypomobility** occurs as a result of joint trauma (micro or macro) leading to restriction in one or more directions.[12] Hypermobility is not the same as instability. Instability covers a wide range of pathological hypermobility. Although there are tests[80,81] to demonstrate general hypermobility, these tests should be interpreted with caution because patients demonstrate a wide range of variability between joints and within joints. With careful assessment, one often finds that a joint may be hypermobile in one direction and hypomobile in another direction. It must also be remembered that evidence of hypomobility or hypermobility does not necessarily indicate a pathological state in the person being assessed. The examiner should attempt to determine the cause of the limitation (e.g., pain, spasm, adhesions, compression) or hypermobility (e.g., injury, occupational, genetic, disease) and the quality of the movement (e.g., lead pipe, cogwheel).

End Feel[1]. When assessing passive movement, the examiner should apply overpressure at the end of the ROM to determine the quality of end feel (the sensation the examiner "feels" in the joint as it reaches the end of the ROM) of each passive movement (Table 1-15). Care must be taken when testing end feel, however, to be sure that

Table 1-15

Normal and Abnormal End Feels

End Feel	Example
Normal	
Bone to bone	Elbow extension
Soft tissue approximation	Knee flexion
Tissue stretch	Ankle dorsiflexion, shoulder lateral rotation, finger extension
Abnormal	
Early muscle spasm	Protective spasm following injury
Late muscle spasm	Spasm resulting from instability or pain
"Mushy" tissue stretch	Tight muscle
Spasticity	Upper motor neuron lesion
Hard capsular	Frozen shoulder
Soft capsular	Synovitis, soft tissue edema
Bone to bone	Osteophyte formation
Empty	Acute subacromial bursitis
Springy block	Meniscus tear

severe symptoms are not provoked. If the patient is able to hold a position at the end of the physiological ROM (end range of active movement) without provoking symptoms or if the symptoms ease quickly after returning to the resting position, then the end feel can be tested. Pain with pathological end feels is common.[42] If, however, the patient has severe pain at end range, end feel should only be tested with extreme care. A proper evaluation of end feel can help the examiner to assess the type of pathology present, determine a prognosis for the condition, and learn the severity or stage of the problem. By determining if pain or restriction is the main problem, the examiner can determine if a more gentle treatment should be given (pain predominating) or a more vigorous treatment (restriction predominantly). The end feel sensations that the examiner experiences are subjective, so intrarater reliability tends to be good, whereas interrater reliability is poor.[41] Many clinicians develop their own classification with the most common ones used[42] developed by Cyriax,[1] Kaltenborn,[69] and Paris.[82]

Cyriax described three classic normal end feels:[1]

Bone to Bone. This is a "hard," unyielding sensation that is painless. An example of normal bone-to-bone end feel is elbow extension.

Soft-Tissue Approximation. With this type of end feel, there is a yielding compression (mushy feel) that stops further movement. Examples are elbow and knee flexion, in which movement is stopped by compression of the soft tissues, primarily the muscles. In a particularly slim person with little muscle bulk, the end feel of elbow flexion may be bone to bone.

Tissue Stretch. There is a hard or firm (springy) type of movement with a slight give. Toward the end of ROM, there is a feeling of springy or elastic resistance. The normal tissue stretch end feel has a feeling of "rising tension or stiffness". This changing tension has led to this end feel sometimes being divided into two types: **elastic (soft)** and **capsular (hard)**. This feeling depends on the thickness and type of tissue being stretched, and it may be very elastic, as in the Achilles tendon stretch, or slightly elastic, as in wrist flexion (tissue stretch), or hard as in knee extension. A hard end feel is firm with a definite stopping point, whereas soft end feel implies a softer end feel without a definite stopping place.[83] Tissue stretch is the most common type of normal end feel; it is found when the capsule and ligaments are the primary restraints to movement. Examples are lateral rotation of the shoulder, and knee and metacarpophalangeal joint extension.

In addition to the three normal types of end feel, Cyriax described five classic abnormal end feels,[1] several of which have subdivisions and each of which is commonly associated with some degree of pain or restricted movement.[1,84]

Muscle Spasm. This end feel is invoked by movement, with a sudden dramatic arrest of movement often accompanied by pain. The end feel is sudden and hard.

Cyriax called this a "vibrant twang."[1] Some examiners divide muscle spasm into different parts. **Early muscle spasm** occurs early in the ROM, almost as soon as movement starts; this type of muscle spasm is associated with inflammation and is seen in more acute conditions. **Late muscle spasm** occurs at or near the end of the ROM. It is usually caused by instability and the resulting irritability caused by movement. An example is muscle spasm occurring during the apprehension test for anterior dislocation of the shoulder. Both types of muscle spasm are the result of the subconscious efforts of the body to protect the injured joint or structure, and their occurrence may be related to how quickly the examiner does the movement. **Spasticity** is slightly different and is seen with upper motor neuron lesions. It is a form of muscle hypertonicity that offers increased resistance to stretch involving primarily the flexors in the upper limb and extensors in the lower limb and may be associated with muscle weakness. The Ashworth scale is sometimes used to measure spasticity and resistance to passive movement, but its reliability has been questioned.[85,86] A **tight muscle** may give its own unique end feel. This is similar to normal tissue stretch, but it does not have as great an elastic feel.

Capsular. Although this end feel is similar to tissue stretch, it does not occur where one would expect (i.e., it occurs earlier in the ROM) and it tends to have a thicker feel to it. ROM is obviously reduced, and the capsule can be postulated to be at fault. Muscle spasm usually does not occur in conjunction with the capsular type of end feel except if the movement is fast and the joint acute. Some examiners divide this end feel into **hard capsular,** in which the end feel has a thicker stretching quality to it, and **soft capsular** (boggy), which is similar to normal tissue stretch end feel but with a restricted ROM. The hard capsular end feel is seen in more chronic conditions or in full-blown capsular patterns. The limitation comes on rather abruptly after a smooth, friction-free movement. The soft capsular end feel is more often seen in acute conditions, with stiffness occurring early in the range and increasing until the end of range is reached. Maitland calls this "resistance through range."[87] Some authors interpret this soft, boggy end feel as being the result of synovitis, soft-tissue edema or hemarthrosis.[88] Major injury to ligaments and the capsule often causes a **soft end feel** until the tension is taken up by other structures.[89]

Bone-to-Bone. This abnormal end feel is similar to the normal bone-to-bone type, but the restriction occurs before the end of ROM would normally occur or where a bone-to-bone end feel would not be expected. An example is a bone-to-bone end feel in the cervical spine resulting from osteophyte formation.

Empty. The empty end feel is detected when movement produces considerable pain. The movement cannot be performed or stops because of the pain, although no real mechanical resistance is being detected. Examples include an acute subacromial bursitis or a tumor. Patients often have difficulty describing the empty end feel, and there is no muscle spasm involved.

Springy Block. Similar to a tissue stretch, this occurs where one would not expect it to occur; it tends to be found in joints with menisci. There is a rebound effect with a thick stretching feel although it is not as stretchy as a hard capsular end feel, and it usually indicates an internal derangement within the joint. A springy block end feel may be found with a torn meniscus of a knee when it is locked or unable to go into full extension.

Capsular Patterns[1]. With passive movement, a full ROM must be carried out in several directions. A short, too-soft movement in the midrange does not achieve the proper results or elicit potential findings. In addition to evaluating the end feel, the examiner must look at the **pattern of limitation or restriction.** If the capsule of the joint is affected, the pattern of limitation is the feature that indicates the presence of a **capsular pattern** in the joint. This pattern is the result of a total joint reaction, with muscle spasm, capsular contraction (the most common cause), and generalized osteophyte formation being possible mechanisms at fault. Each joint has a characteristic pattern of limitation. The presence of this capsular pattern does not indicate the type of joint involvement; only an analysis of the end feel can do that. Only joints that are controlled by muscles have a capsular pattern; joints such as the sacroiliac and distal tibiofibular joints do not exhibit a capsular pattern. Dutton pointed out that capsular patterns are based on empirical findings rather than research, and this may be the reason capsular patterns may be different or inconsistent.[3] In fact, Hayes et al.[41] felt the pattern of limitation was useful but the proportional limitation concept should not be used. Table 1-16 illustrates some of the common capsular patterns seen in joints.

Noncapsular Patterns[1]. The examiner must also be aware of **noncapsular patterns,** for example, a limitation that exists but does not correspond to the classic capsular

Table 1-16
Common Capsular Patterns of Joints

Joint	Restriction*
Temporomandibular	Limitation of mouth opening
Atlanto-occipital	Extension, side flexion equally limited
Cervical spine	Side flexion and rotation equally limited, extension
Glenohumeral	Lateral rotation, abduction, medial rotation
Sternoclavicular	Pain at extreme of range of movement
Acromioclavicular	Pain at extreme of range of movement
Ulnohumeral	Flexion, extension
Radiohumeral	Flexion, extension, supination, pronation
Proximal radioulnar	Supination, pronation
Distal radioulnar	Full range of movement, pain at extremes of rotation
Wrist	Flexion and extension equally limited
Trapeziometacarpal	Abduction, extension
Metacarpophalangeal and interphalangeal	Flexion, extension
Thoracic spine	Side flexion and rotation equally limited, extension
Lumbar spine	Side flexion and rotation equally limited, extension
Sacroiliac, symphysis pubis, and sacrococcygeal	Pain when joints are stressed
Hip†	Flexion, abduction, medial rotation (but in some cases, medial rotation is most limited)
Knee	Flexion, extension
Tibiofibular	Pain when joint stressed
Talocrural	Plantar flexion, dorsiflexion
Talocalcaneal (subtalar)	Limitation of varus range of movement
Midtarsal	Dorsiflexion, plantar flexion, adduction, medial rotation
First metatarsophalangeal	Extension, flexion
Second to fifth metatarsophalangeal	Variable
Interphalangeal	Flexion, extension

*Movements are listed in order of restriction.
†For the hip, flexion, abduction, and medial rotation are always the movements most limited in a capsular pattern. However, the order of restriction may vary.

pattern for that joint. In the shoulder, abduction may be restricted but with very little rotational restriction (e.g., subacromial bursitis). Although a total capsular reaction is absent, there are other possibilities, such as ligamentous adhesions, in which only part of a capsule or the accessory ligaments are involved. There may be a local restriction in one direction, often accompanied by pain, and full, pain-free ROM in all other directions. A second possibility is **internal derangement,** which commonly affects only certain joints, such as the knee, ankle, and elbow. Intracapsular fragments may interfere with the normal sequence of motion. Movements causing impingement of the fragments will be limited, whereas other motions will be free. In the knee, for example, a torn meniscus may cause a blocking of extension, but flexion is usually free. Loose bodies cause limitation when they are caught between articular surfaces. A third possibility is **extra-articular lesions.** These lesions are revealed by disproportionate limitation, extra-articular adhesions, or an acutely inflamed structure limiting movement in a particular direction. For example, limited straight leg raising in the lumbar disc syndrome is referred to as a **constant length phenomenon.** This phenomenon results when the limitation of movement in one joint depends on the position in which another joint is held. The restricted tissue (in this case, the sciatic nerve) must lie outside the joint or joints (in this case, hip and knee) being tested. The constant length phenomenon may also result from muscle adhesions that cause restriction of motion.

Inert Tissue[1]. After the active and passive movements are completed, the examiner should be able to determine whether there are problems with any of the **inert tissues.** The examiner makes such a determination by judging the degree of pain and the limitation of movement within the joint. For lesions of inert tissue, the examiner may find that active and passive movements are painful in the same direction. Usually pain occurs as the limitation of motion approaches. Resisted isometric movements (discussed later) are not usually painful unless some compression is occurring. During the examination, inert tissues are tested or stressed during active and passive movements, functional testing, selected special tests, joint play testing, and palpation.

Inert tissue refers to all tissue that is not considered contractile or neurological. Four classic patterns may be seen in lesions of inert issue, according to the ROM available (or restriction present) and the amount of pain produced.[1]

1. If the **range of movement is full and there is no pain,** there is no lesion of the inert tissues being tested by that passive movement; however, there may be lesions of inert tissue in other directions or around other joints.

2. The next possible pattern is one of **pain and limitation of movement in every direction.** In this pattern, the entire joint is affected, indicating arthritis or capsulitis. Each joint has its own capsular pattern (see Table 1-16), and the amount of limitation is not usually the same in each direction; however, although there is a set pattern for each joint, other directions may also be affected. All movements of the joint may be affected, but the motions described for the capsular pattern usually occur in the particular order listed. For example, the capsular pattern of the shoulder is lateral rotation most limited, followed by abduction and medial rotation. In early capsular patterns, only one movement may be restricted; this movement is usually the one that has the potential for the greatest restriction. For example, in an early capsular pattern of the shoulder, only lateral rotation may be limited, and the limitation may be slight.

3. A patient with a lesion of inert tissue may experience **pain and limitation or excessive movement in some directions but not in others,** as in a ligament sprain or local capsular adhesion. In other words, a noncapsular pattern is presented. Movements that stretch, pinch, or move the affected structure cause the pain. Internal derangement that results in the blocking of a joint is another example of a lesion of inert tissue that produces a variable pattern. Extra-articular limitation occurs when a lesion outside the joint affects the movement of that joint. Because these movements pinch or stretch the involved structure (e.g., bursitis in the buttock, acute subacromial bursitis), pain and limitation of movement occur on stretch or compression of these structures. If a structure such as a ligament has been torn, the ROM may increase if swelling is minimal, especially right after injury, indicating instability (pathological hypermobility) of the joint and can be seen in spinal or peripheral joints. Swelling often masks instability because it puts the tissues under tension. Pathological hypermobility, if present, results in greater than normal movement at the joint, causes pain, puts neurogenic structures at risk, and can result in progressive deformity and degeneration.[90]

4. The final inert tissue pattern is **limited movement that is pain free.** The end feel for this type of condition is often of the abnormal bone-to-bone type, and it usually indicates a symptomless osteoarthritis—that is, osteophytes are present and restrict movement, but they are not pinching or compressing any sensitive structures. If this situation is encountered, it should be left alone because it is not causing the patient any problem other than restricted ROM and attempts at treatment could lead to further problems.

Patterns of Inert Tissue Lesions

- Pain-free, full range of motion
- Pain and limited range of motion in every direction
- Pain and excessive or limited range of motion in some directions
- Pain-free, limited range of motion

Resisted Isometric Movements

Resisted isometric movements are the movements tested last in the examination of the joints. This type of movement consists of a strong, static (isometric), voluntary muscle contraction, and it is used primarily to determine whether the contractile tissue is the tissue at fault, although the nerve supplying the muscle is also tested. If the muscle, its tendon, or the bone into which they insert is at fault, pain and weakness result; the amount of pain and weakness is related to the degree of injury and the patient's pain threshold. If movement is allowed to occur at the joint, inert tissue around the joint will also move, and it will not be clear whether any resulting pain arises from contractile or inert tissues. The joint, therefore, is put in a neutral or resting position (see Table 1-32) so that minimal tension is placed on the inert tissue. The patient is asked to contract the muscle as strongly as possible while the examiner resists to prevent any movement from occurring and to ensure that the patient is using maximum effort. To keep movement to a minimum, it is best for the examiner to position the joint properly in the resting position and then to say to the patient, "Don't let me move you." In this way, the examiner can ensure that the contraction is isometric and can control the amount of force exerted. Movement cannot be completely eliminated, but this method minimizes it. Some compression of the inert tissues (e.g., cartilage) occurs with the contraction, and there may be some joint shear as well, but it will be minimal if done as described.

Table 1-17

Muscle Test Grading

Grade	Value	Movement Grade
5+	Normal (100%)	Complete range of motion against gravity with maximal resistance
4	Good (75%)	Complete range of motion against gravity with some (moderate) resistance
3+	Fair +	Complete range of motion against gravity with minimal resistance
3	Fair (50%)	Complete range of motion against gravity
3–	Fair –	Some but not complete range of motion against gravity
2+	Poor +	Initiates motion against gravity
2	Poor (25%)	Complete range of motion with gravity eliminated
2–	Poor –	Initiates motion if gravity is eliminated
1	Trace	Evidence of slight contractility but no joint motion
0	Zero	No contraction palpated

If, as advocated, this isometric hold method is used, then movement against this resistance would require muscle strength of grade 3 to 5 on the muscle test grading scale (Table 1-17).[91] If the muscle strength is less than grade 3, then the methods advocated in muscle testing manuals[88,92] must be used. If the examiner is having difficulty differentiating between grade 4 and grade 5, an eccentric break method of muscle testing may be used. This method starts as an isometric contraction, but then the examiner applies sufficient force to cause an eccentric contraction or a "break" in the patient's isometric contraction. This method provides a more recognizable threshold for maximum isometric contraction.[91] It must be recognized, however, that all three methods are subjective for normal and good values. When a muscle is tested in the resting position, it is usually being tested in its position of optimum length so that maximum force, if necessary, can be elicited. In some cases, however, a muscle, because of pathology, may become lengthened or shortened leading to weakness when tested in the normal resting position. Testing a muscle in the fully lengthened position tightens the inert components of muscle and puts more stress on the contractile tissues, whereas testing it in a shortened position puts it in its weakest position. Kendall et al.,[93] for example, called muscle weakness that results from muscle lengthening **stretch weakness** or **positional weakness.** Thus, if the examiner has found range of motion to be limited or excessive during passive movement testing, consideration should be given to performing the isometric tests in different positions of the ROM to see if the problem is not one of strength but of muscle length. This action will also help differentiate between weakness throughout the ROM (**pathological weakness**) from weakness only in certain positions (**positional weakness**). If, in the history, the patient has complained of symptoms in a different position than those commonly tested, the examiner may modify the isometric test position to try to elicit the symptoms. If the patient has complained that a concentric, eccentric, or econcentric contraction has caused the problem, the examiner may include these movements, with or without load, in the examination, but only after the isometric tests have been completed. Econcentric or pseudo-isometric contraction involves two-joint muscles in which the muscle is acting concentrically at one joint and eccentrically at the other joint, the result being minimal or no change in muscle length. Two-joint muscles are among the most frequently injured muscles (e.g., hamstrings, biceps, gastrocnemius) often because of the different actions occurring over the two joints at the same time.

In some cases, machines may be used to measure muscle strength, but care should be taken, because these tests are often not isometric, and they are often not performed in functional positions nor at functional speeds. They do, however, provide a comparison or ratio between right and left and between different movements.

Muscle weakness, if elicited, may be caused by an upper motor neuron lesion, injury to a peripheral nerve, pathology at the neuromuscular junction, a nerve root lesion, or a lesion or disease (myopathy) of the muscle, its tendons, or the bony insertions themselves. For the first four of these causes, the system of muscle test grading may be used. For nerve root lesions, myotome testing is the method of choice. When testing for muscle lesions, it is more appropriate to test the resisted movements isometrically first, to determine which movements are painful, then perform individual muscle tests, as advocated in texts such as that of Daniels and Worthingham,[92] to determine exactly which muscle is at fault.

If the contraction appears weak, the examiner must make sure that the weakness is not caused by pain or by the patient's fear, unwillingness, or malingering. The examiner can often resolve such a finding by having the patient make a contraction on the good side first, which normally will not cause pain. Weakness that is not associated with pain or disuse is a positive neurological sign indicating that a nerve root, peripheral nerve, or upper motor neuron lesion is at least part of the problem.

Contractile Tissue.[1] With resisted isometric testing, the examiner is looking for problems of **contractile tissue,** which consists of muscles, their tendons, and attachments (e.g., bone), and the nervous tissue supplying the contractile tissue. Both active movements and resisted isometric testing demonstrate symptoms if contractile tissue is affected. Other parts of the examination, which will test contractile tissue, include passive movement, functional testing, specific

special tests, and palpation. Usually, passive movements are normal—that is, passive movements are full and pain free, although pain may be exhibited at the end of the ROM when the contractile or nervous tissue is stretched. If contractile tissue has been injured, active movement is painful in one direction (contraction) and passive movement, if painful, is painful in the opposite direction (stretch). Resisted isometric testing is painful in the same direction as active movement. If the muscles are tested as previously described, not all movements will be found to be affected, except in patients with psychogenic pain and sometimes in patients with an acute joint lesion, in which even a small amount of tension on the muscles around the joint provokes pain. However, if the joint lesion is acutely severe, passive movements, when tested, will be markedly affected, and there will be no confusion as to where the lesion lies. As with inert tissue, four classic patterns have been identified with lesions of contractile and nervous tissue.[1] (In this case, however, one is dealing with pain and strength rather than pain and altered ROM.)

1. Movement that is **strong and pain free** indicates that there is no lesion of the contractile unit being tested or the nervous tissue supplying that contractile unit, regardless of how tender the muscles may be when touched. The muscles and nerves function painlessly and are not the source of the patient's discomfort.

2. Movement that is **strong and painful** indicates a local lesion of the muscle or tendon. Such a lesion could be a first- or second-degree muscle strain. The amount of strength is usually determined by the amount of pain the patient feels on contraction, which results from reflex inhibition that leads to weakness or cogwheel contractions. A second-degree strain produces greater weakness and more pain than a first-degree strain. Similarly, tendinosis, tendinitis, paratenonitis, or paratenonitis with tendinosis (Table 1-18) all may lead to contractions that are strong (relative) and painful, but one that is not usually as strong as on the good side, and the pain is in or around the tendon, not the muscle.[94,95] If there is a partial avulsion fracture, again, the movement will be strong and painful. However, if the avulsion is complete, the movement will be weak and painful (see later discussion). Typically, there is no primary limitation of passive

Table 1-18

Bonar's Modification of Clancy's Classification of Tendinopathies

Pathological Diagnosis	Concept (Macroscopic Pathology)	Histological Appearance
Tendinosis	Intratendinous degeneration (commonly caused by aging, microtrauma, and vascular compromise)	Collagen disorientation, disorganization, and fiber separation with an increase in mucoid ground substance, increased prominence of cells and vascular spaces with or without neovascularization, and focal necrosis or calcification
Tendinitis/partial rupture	Symptomatic degeneration of the tendon with vascular disruption and inflammatory repair response	Degenerative changes as noted above with superimposed evidence of tear, including fibroblastic and myofibroblastic proliferation, hemorrhage, and organizing granulation tissue
Paratenonitis	Inflammation of the outer layer of the tendon (paratenon) alone, regardless of whether the paratenon is lined by synovium	Mucoid degeneration in the areolar tissue is seen; a scattered mild mononuclear infiltrate with or without focal fibrin deposition and fibrinous exudate is also seen
Paratenonitis with tendinosis	Paratenonitis associated with intratendinous degeneration	Degenerative changes as noted for tendinosis with mucoid degeneration with or without fibrosis and scattered inflammatory cells in the paratenon alveolar tissue

From Khan KM et al: Histopathology of common tendinopathies: update and implications for clinical management, *Sports Med* 27:399, 1999.

movement when contractile tissue is injured although end range may be painful (stretch), except, for example, in the case of a gross muscle tear with hematoma where the muscle, which is often in spasm, is being stretched. In this case, the patient may develop joint stiffness secondary to disuse. This is often caused by protective muscle spasm of adjacent muscles that allow, for example, some joint contracture to be superimposed on the muscle lesion. This stiffness then takes precedence in the treatment. One should always remember that it is easier to maintain physiological function than it is to restore it.

3. Movement that is **weak and painful** indicates a severe lesion around that joint, such as a fracture. The weakness that results is usually caused by reflex inhibition of the muscles around the joint, secondary to pain.

4. Movement that is **weak and pain free** indicates a rupture of a muscle (third-degree strain) or its tendon or involvement of the peripheral nerve or nerve root supplying that muscle. If the movement is weak and pain free, neurological involvement or a tendon rupture should be suspected first. With neurological involvement, the examiner must be able to differentiate between the muscle innervation of a nerve root (myotome) and the muscle innervation of a peripheral nerve (see Table 1-13 as an example). Also, the examiner should be able to differentiate between upper and lower motor neuron lesions (see Table 1-11). Third-degree strains are sometimes masked, because if the force is great enough to cause a complete tear of a muscle, the surrounding muscles, which assisted the movement, may also be injured (first- or second-degree strain). The pain from these secondary muscles can mask the third-degree strain to the primary mover.

The tested weakness, however, would be greater with the third-degree strain (and its lack of pain). Although significant pain can occur at the time of the third-degree injury, this pain usually quickly subsides to a dull ache, even when the muscle is contracting, because there is no tension on the muscle, which no longer has two attachment (origin and insertion) points. For this reason, a gap or hole in the muscle may be palpated. When the third-degree injured muscle does contract, the muscle may bunch up or bulge, giving an obvious deformity (Figure 1-15).

Patterns of Contractile Tissue and Nervous Tissue Lesions

- No pain, and movement is strong
- Pain, and movement is relatively strong (but not as strong as it should be)
- Pain, and movement is weak
- No pain, and movement is weak

Signs and Symptoms of Upper Motor Neuron Lesions

- Spasticity
- Hypertonicity
- Hyperreflexia (deep tendon reflexes)
- Positive pathological reflexes (e.g., Babinski, Hoffman)
- Absent or reduced superficial reflexes
- Extensor plantar response (bilateral)

Figure 1-15
Rupture (3° strain) of right adductor muscle. Note the bulge in the muscle caused when the patient is asked to contract the muscle.

Table 1-19
Functional Division of Muscle Groups*

Muscles Prone to Tightness (Postural Muscles)	Muscles Prone to Weakness (Phasic Muscles)
Gastrocnemius and soleus	Peronei
Tibialis posterior	Tibialis anterior
Short hip adductors	Vastus medialis and lateralis
Hamstrings	Gluteus maximus, medius, and minimus
Rectus femoris	
Iliopsoas	Rectus abdominis
Tensor fasciae latae	External oblique
Piriformis	Serratus anterior
Erector spinae (especially lumbar, thoracolumbar, and cervical portions)	Rhomboids
	Lower portion of trapezius
	Short cervical flexors
Quadratus lumborum	Extensors of upper limb
Pectoralis major	
Upper portion of trapezius	
Levator scapulae	
Sternocleidomastoid	
Scalenes	
Flexors of the upper limb	

Modified from Jull G and Janda V: Muscles and motor control in low back pain. In Twomey LT and Taylor JR, editors: *Physical therapy for the low back: clinics in physical therapy*, p. 258, New York, 1987, Churchill Livingstone.
*Janda considered all other muscles neutral.

If all movements around a joint appear painful, the pain is often a result of fatigue, emotional hypersensitivity, or emotional problems. Patients may equate effort with discomfort, and they must be told that they are not necessarily the same.

Janda put forth an interesting concept by dividing muscles into two groups: postural and phasic.[96] He believed that **postural** or **tonic muscles,** which are the muscles responsible for maintaining upright posture, have a tendency to become tight and hypertonic with pathology and to develop contractures but are less likely to atrophy, whereas **phasic muscles,** which include almost all other muscles, tend to become weak and inhibited with pathology. The examiner must be careful to note the type of muscle affected and the ROM available (active movements) as well as the strength and production of pain (resisted isometric movements) when testing contractile tissue. Table 1-19 shows the muscles that are postural and prone to tightness and those that are phasic and prone to weakness. Table 1-20 shows the characteristics of postural and phasic muscles. If a muscle imbalance is present, the tight muscles must first be stretched to their normal length and tone before strength can be equalized.[97,98]

Janda and his associates further expanded this concept with the "upper crossed syndrome" and "pelvic crossed syndrome," which show muscles (primarily postural) on one diagonal at a joint to be tight and hypertonic, whereas muscles on the other diagonal are weak and lengthened (Figure 1-16).[98,99] This concept of tight and hypertonic muscles in one aspect of a joint with weak lengthened muscles in the opposite aspect is one that examiners should remember for all joints, especially when looking at chronic joint injuries as both types of muscles tend to be present and require different treatment approaches.

Table 1-20
Characteristics of Postural and Phasic Muscle Groups

Muscles Prone to Tightness (Postural Muscles)	Muscles Prone to Weakness (Phasic Muscles)
Predominantly postural function	Primarily phasic function
Associated with flexor reflexes	Associated with extensor reflexes
Primarily two-joint muscles	Primarily one-joint muscles
Readily activated with movement (shorter chronaxie)	Not readily activated with movement (longer chronaxie)
Tendency to tightness, hypertonia, shortening, or contractures	Tendency to hypotonia, inhibition, or weakness
Resistance to atrophy	Atrophy occurs easily

Modified from Jull G and Janda V: Muscles and motor control in low back pain. In Twomey LT and Taylor JR, editors: *Physical therapy for the low back: clinics in physical therapy*, New York, 1987, Churchill Livingstone.

Figure 1-16
Postural and phasic muscle response to pathology producing "crossed syndromes."

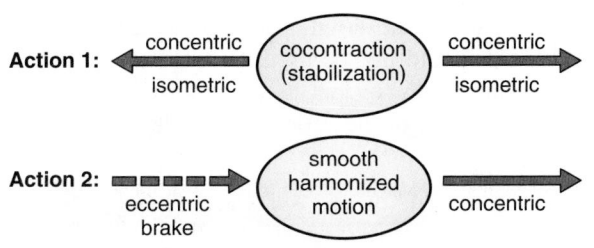

Figure 1-17
Force couple action.

In addition, the examiner should always consider the action of **force couples** surrounding a joint. Force couples are counteracting groups of muscles functioning either by co-contraction to stabilize a joint or by one group acting concentrically and the opposing group acting eccentrically to cause a controlled joint motion that is smooth and harmonized (Figure 1-17).[100] Pathology to one of the force couple muscles or to one of the force couples acting about a joint can lead to muscle imbalance, instability, and loss of smooth coordinated movement.

Other Findings during Movement Testing

When carrying out the examination of the joints, the examiner must be aware of other findings that may become evident and may help to determine the nature and location of the problem. For example, it should be noted whether there is excessive ROM (hypermobility or laxity) within the joints. Comparison of the normal side with the involved side of the body gives some indication as to whether the findings on the affected side would be considered normal. For example, an apparently excessive range (laxity) may just be the normal ROM for that patient. It must also be remembered that joints on the nondominant side tend to be more flexible than those on the dominant side.

It is also important to note whether a **painful arc** is present; this finding indicates that an internal structure is being squeezed or pinched in part of the ROM. **Sounds** such as crepitus, clicking, or snapping should be noted. To be pathologically significant however, these sounds must be related to the patient's symptoms. They may be caused by structures slipping over one another (e.g., tendons slipping over bone), loose bodies or arthritic changes in the joint, abnormal movement of structures (e.g., meniscus click on opening or closing of the temporomandibular joint), or a tear in a structure (e.g., a tear in the triangular cartilaginous disc of the wrist). **Pain at the extreme of range of motion** may be caused by squeezing or stretching of structures around the joint or even in the joint, especially if the movement takes the joint into its close packed position.

Functional Assessment

Functional assessment plays an important role in the evaluation of the patient. It is different from the analysis of specific movement patterns of active, passive, and resisted isometric movements used to differentiate between inert, neurological, and contractile tissue. Functional assessment may involve task analysis, observation of certain patient activities, or a detailed evaluation of the effect of the injury or disability on the patient's ability to function in everyday life. Determining what the patient hopes is an appropriate functional outcome, and what the patient can and cannot do functionally can be extremely important in the choice of treatments that will be successful. Primarily, functional assessment helps the examiner establish what is important to the patient and the patient's expectations. It represents a measurement of a **whole-body task performance ability,** as opposed to isolated examination of a joint. Because it is part of each individual joint assessed, the functional testing should demonstrate whether an isolated impairment affects the patient's ability to perform everyday activities.

The examiner should attempt to establish what functional factors are important to the patient. For example, functional testing may include movements under different loads to determine the patient's ability to work or play. Likewise, repeated movements and sustained postures may be necessary for work, recreational, or social activities. In some cases, movements at different speeds or under different loads may be necessary to determine pathology.[71] Atraumatic shoulder instability, for example, may not be evident in a swimmer except when he or she is actually doing the activity at the speed and load at which the activity is done in the water.

Because functional testing relates to the effect of the injury on the patient's life, those activities that cause symptoms, those that are restricted by symptoms, and the factors (e.g., strength, power, flexibility) that are needed to perform the activities must be considered. For example, if the patient is seated normally while a history is taken, the

Table 1-21

Examples of Functional and Clinical Outcomes

Clinical Outcomes	Functional Outcomes
Strength	Power
Range of motion	Agility
Proprioception	Kinesthetic awareness
Endurance (muscular)	Endurance (muscular and cardiovascular)
Swelling	Speed
Pain	Activity specificity
Psychological overlay	Pain
	Skill level required for activity
	Psychological preparedness
	Daily living skills

examiner knows the patient has the functional ROM (agility) for sitting with 90° of hip and knee flexion. Table 1-21 lists some functional outcome measures that should be considered. The activities should be simple, patient-oriented, and based on coordinated functional movement of the joints, and they should be activities the patient wants to do. Although most functional outcomes or tests are subjective, this does not make them any less effective.[101]

The functional assessment is important to determine the effect of the condition or injury on the patient's daily life, including his or her sex life. Functional impairment may be slightly annoying or completely disabling for the patient. Functional activities that should be tested, if appropriate, include self-care activities such as walking, dressing, daily hygiene (e.g., washing, bathing, shaving, combing hair), eating, and going to the bathroom; recreational activities such as reading, sewing, watching television, gardening, and playing a musical instrument; and activities such as driving, dialing a telephone, getting groceries, preparing meals, and hanging clothes. Goldstein nicely divided activities of human function into four broad areas, which are then broken down into more discrete levels (Table 1-22).[102] The examiner should consider which of these are important to the patient and ensure that they are considered in the assessment. Figure 1-18 shows some of the daily living skills and mobility questions that may be of concern to both the examiner and the patient. The short musculoskeletal function assessment (SMFA) helps to determine how much the patient is bothered by functional problems (Figure 1-19).[103] Other functional assessment tool examples that are available include the functional capacity evaluation (FCE),[102] the functional independence measure (FIM),[104] the physical performance test,[105] the functional status test,[106] the arthritis impact measurement scale (AIMS 2),[107] the functional assessment tool (FAT),[108] the SF-36 Health Status Survey,[109,110] the Sickness Impact Profile,[111] the Short Musculoskeletal

Functional Assessment Questionnaire,[112] and the Sock Test.[113] The particular tool used depends on the needs of the patient and the presenting pathological problem.

Part of this functional assessment occurs during the history, when the examiner asks the patient which activities can be done easily, which with some difficulty, and which not at all. During the observation, the examiner notes what the patient can and cannot do within the confines of the assessment area. Finally, during the examination, functional testing or a work analysis may be performed. For example, when examining the hand, the examiner notes the power and dexterity exhibited during performance of fundamental maneuvers such as gripping and pinching. Below is an example of a work activity analysis, which may be evaluated if the patient is hoping to return to that activity and to do it successfully.[114] Regardless of which functional test is used, the examiner must understand the purpose of the test. A functional test should not be done just because it is available. It should not be used in isolation but rather in conjunction with the overall assessment, so that a complete assessment picture of the patient can be developed.

Example of an Analysis of Work Activity

Job title: *Packer*
Essential function: *Packing individual cobbler cups for shipping*
Steps

1. Select a box.
2. Place the box on the conveyor side rack.
3. Pick up one cobbler cup in each hand.
4. Place the cups into the packing box.
5. Repeat steps 3 and 4 until 36 cups are in a box.
6. Place the filled box on the "sealing table."
7. Fold the short flaps of the box lid.
8. Fold the longer flaps of the box lid.
9. Tape down the long flaps of the box using the manual taping machine.
10. Place the sealed box on the pallet.

From Ellexson MT: Analyzing an industry: job analysis for treatment, prevention, and placement, *Orthop Phys Ther Clin* 1:17, 1992.

Numerical scoring systems are often used as part of the functional assessment. These scoring systems are often more related to function as it applies to a specific joint and often a specific activity rather than to the whole body (Figure 1-20),[115] and for many, functional assessment plays only a small part. With these numerical systems, the clinician must ensure that the scoring systems really measure what they say they measure. To be effective, a numerical scoring system must demonstrate universality, practicality, reliability, reproducibility, effectiveness, and inclusiveness, and it must have been validated.[116] The terminology and methods must be described precisely; the criteria should be related to functional outcome (what the patient desires) rather than clinical outcome (what the clinician desires), and

Table 1-22
Goldstein's Divisions of Human Function

Function: Basic or Personal Activities of Daily Living (ADLs)			
Activity	**Examples**	**Activity**	**Examples**
Bed activities	Moving in bed Managing pillows and blankets Reaching for objects Sitting up	Dressing activities	Putting on clothes Tying laces Putting on socks and shoes
Hygiene activities	Brushing teeth Bathing and showering Washing Toileting Combing hair Shaving Putting on makeup	Transfer activities Walking activities	Bed to chair Sit to stand Getting into car Level and uneven surfaces Curbs and stairs Opening doors Walking and carrying items Distance and velocity
Eating activities	Using utensils Cutting meat Managing glass and cup		Assistive devices Gait deviations

Function: Instrumental (Advanced) Activities of Daily Living (IADLs)			
Activity	**Examples**	**Activity**	**Examples**
Meal preparation	Cutting vegetables Turning on oven Measuring ingredients	Having sex Driving car	Manipulating clothing Changing positions Getting in and out Turning wheel Adjusting pedals, mirrors
Light housework	Dusting Washing dishes Mopping floors	Gardening	Kneeling Raking Digging Watering
Check writing	Manipulating pen Adding and subtracting		
Shopping	Pushing cart Carrying groceries Reaching Getting money out of pocket	Communicating	Using writing tools Using telephone

Function: Work Activities			
Activity	**Examples**	**Activity**	**Examples**
Lifting	From table and from floor	Kneeling	On all fours and just knees
Carrying	Small and large objects	Manipulating objects	Pen, salt shaker
Stooping	Wiping floor	Climbing	Stairs and ladder
Pushing	Broom	Standing	
Pulling	Drawer and door	Walking	Slow and fast
Reaching	Into cupboard		

Function: Sport and Recreational Activities			
Activity	**Examples**	**Activity**	**Examples**
Walking	Forward and backward Sideways Level and uneven surfaces	Hitting	Baseball bat Tennis racquet Golf club
Jogging and sprinting	Different surfaces In water	Swimming	Different strokes Different kicks

Continued

Table 1-22—cont'd

Goldstein's Divisions of Human Function

Activity	Examples	Activity	Examples
Cutting	Circles Figure-eights Crossover and sidestep	Agility Open and closed kinetic chain Speed and power	Specific drills Throwing and pushing Moving different sized objects at different speeds
Jumping and hopping	Vertical and distance Forward and backward Level and uneven surfaces	Endurance	Aerobic and anaerobic Cardiovascular and muscle
Throwing	Underhand and overhand Two-handed Different objects	Reaction time and proprioception	Blinking lights
Catching	One- and two-handed Different sizes and weights		

Data from Goldstein TS: *Functional rehabilitation in orthopedics*, pp. 19–23, Gaithersburg, MD, 1995, Aspen.

the measures must be sensitive enough to show a difference.[117] Figure 1-21 shows a functional assessment involving the entire upper limb.[118] Table 1-23 demonstrates tests that could be used in an examination of simulated activities of daily living.[119] Similar charts can and have been developed for almost all joints of the body. However,

many of these numerical scoring systems have been developed from the clinician's perspective rather than from what the patient thinks is important.

Functional tests may also be used as provocative tests to bring on the symptoms the patient has complained of or to determine how the patient is progressing or whether he

Daily Living Skill and Mobility Questions for Functional Assessment

Daily Living Skills	Mobility
Feeding (7) Are you able to feed yourself from a tray or table using ordinary utensils? Can you cut meat? Can you pour liquids from open containers? (4) If you use a spork or rocker knife or other helpful aid, are you able to feed yourself in a reasonable length of time? (2) Are you able to feed yourself with some help from another person, for example, to help you raise a cup to your mouth or to cut meat? (0) Do you depend on another person to feed you?	***Supine to Sit*** (7) When you are lying on your back, can you sit up without using your arms or without rolling to the side? Can you do this smoothly and easily? (4) Do you use your arms to help you sit up, or do you roll to the side before sitting up? Do you have to try several times before sitting up? (2) Does someone help you to sit up? (0) Are you unable to sit up?
Dress Upper Body (7) Are you able to get clothes out of your closets and drawers and put them on and remove them from your upper body by yourself, including bra, slip, pullovers, and front opening shirts and blouses, as well as managing zippers, buttons, and snaps? (4) If someone lays your clothes out for you or hands them to you, are you able to dress your upper body by yourself even if it takes a little more time, or do you need some help with closures, such as buttons, zippers, snaps, or hooks? Do you use aids such as reachers, dressing hooks, button hooks, or zipper pulls? (2) Does someone help you put on your blouse or shirt or sweater because you are limited by pain, lack of strength, or limited range of motion? (0) Do you depend on another person to dress your upper body?	***Sitting to Standing*** (7) Are you able to stand up from a regular chair without using your arms? (4) Do you need to use your arms to help you stand up, or do you need to try several times? (2) Does someone need to help you stand up out of a chair? (0) Do you depend on someone else entirely to get you out of a chair? ***Transfer—Toilet*** (7) Are you able to get on and off the toilet easily and without using your hands? (4) Do you need to use your arms to help you get on and off the toilet, or do you require assistive devices such as elevated toilet seats or grab bars? (2) Does someone need to help you get on and off the toilet? (0) Are you unable to use the toilet?

Figure 1-18 ▬▬▬▬

Daily living skill and mobility questions for function assessment. (Modified from Convery FR et al: Polyarticular disability: a functional assessment, *Arch Phys Med Rehab* 58:498, 1977.)

Continued

Daily Living Skills	Mobility

Dress Lower Body

(7) Are you able to put on undergarments, slacks, socks, nylons, and shoes by yourself? Can you tie shoelaces?

(4) Are you able to put on undergarments, slacks, socks, nylons, and shoes by yourself if they are laid out for you or handed to you? Do you use dressing aids such as long handled reachers? Do you avoid shoes that have laces or buckles, or do you use elastic laces or Velcro shoe closures by yourself?

(2) Does someone help you to put on undergarments, slacks, nylons, or shoes?

(0) Do you depend on another person to dress your lower body?

Grooming

(7) Are you able to comb and brush and shampoo your hair, shave, apply makeup, clean your teeth or dentures, and manage nail care by yourself without adaptations or modifications?

(4) Do you use assistive devices or adapted methods for grooming: If someone places what you need within reach, are you then able to complete grooming activities unaided? Do you use long-handled combs or brushes, suction brushes for cleaning nails or dentures, adapted shaving equipment or adapted key for rolling toothpaste tubes?

(2) Does someone actually help you shampoo or brush your hair, shave, apply makeup, clean your teeth or dentures, or manicure your nails?

(0) Do you depend on someone else entirely for your grooming needs?

Care of Perineum/Clothing at Toilet

(7) Are you able to go to the bathroom by yourself including managing your clothes, wiping yourself (and placing sanitary napkins or tampons)?

(4) Are you able to manage your clothing at the toilet and wipe yourself independently although it may be difficult, or do you use aids such as an extended reacher for wiping yourself or clothing aids?

(2) Does someone help you with your clothing at the toilet or assist you with wiping yourself (or in placement of sanitary napkins or tampons)?

(0) Do you depend on someone else to manage your clothes at the toilet for you or to wipe you (or to place sanitary napkins or tampons)?

Wash or Bathe

(7) Are you able to wash and dry your entire body by yourself, including your back and feet? Are you able to turn water faucets?

(4) Do you use bathing aids such as long handled bath brushes or sponges? Are you unable to reach some parts of your body for bathing or drying thoroughly but can still manage without help?

(2) Are you able to bathe and dry most parts of your body and have someone help you with the rest?

(0) Does someone else bathe you?

Vocational

(2) Are you employed full-time in your usual occupation? Are you a full-time homemaker and require no assistance? Are you retired for other than medical reasons?

(0) Not able to do the above

Transfer—Tub or Shower

(7) Are you able to get in and out of a tub or shower safely?

(4) Can you get in and out of a tub or shower using aids such as grab bars or special seat or lift?

(2) Does someone need to help you to get in and out of the tub or shower?

(0) Are you unable to get in and out of the tub or shower?

Transfer—Automobile

(7) Can you get in and out of a car easily, including opening and closing the door?

(4) Can you get in and out of a car by yourself if you use aids such as grab bars or if someone opens the door for you?

(2) Does someone help you get in and out of a car?

(0) Are you unable to get in and out of a car even with assistance?

Walk on Level

(7) Are you able to walk two blocks at an even pace without using a cane, crutches, walker, or adapted shoes?

(4) Do you need a cane, crutches, or walker to walk two blocks?

(2) Can you walk one block with assistance?

(0) Are you unable to walk one block even with assistance?

Walk Outdoors

(7) Are you able to walk outdoors at least two blocks without avoiding rough terrain such as grass, sand, gravel, curbs, ramps, or hills?

(4) Do you try to avoid uneven terrain? Do you use a crutch or cane for safety or balance purposes only when outside?

(2) Must you use a cane or crutches to walk at least two blocks on uneven terrain?

(0) Are you unable to walk on uneven terrain?

Up and Down Stairs

(7) Can you go up and down at least five steps safely, step over step without using the hand rail or other support?

(4) Are you able to go up and down at least five steps if you use a hand rail, cane, or crutches or if you go one step at a time?

(2) Do you need someone to help you go up and down at least five steps?

(0) Are you unable to go up and down at least five steps even with help?

Wheelchair/10 Yards

(7) Are you able to push your wheelchair without help for 10 yards? Can you turn corners and get close to bed, table, and toilet?

(4) Do you use a motorized wheelchair?

(2) Do you need someone to help you maneuver your wheelchair around corners or to help you position it?

(0) Are you unable to push your wheelchair 10 yards?

Figure 1-18 cont'd ▮

Short Musculoskeletal Function Assessment (SMFA)

Instructions

We are interested in finding out how you are managing with your injury or arthritis this week. We would like to know about any problems you may be having with your daily activities because of your injury or arthritis.

Please answer each question by putting a check in the box corresponding to the choice that best describes you.

These questions are about how much difficulty you may be having <u>this week</u> with your daily activities because of your injury or arthritis.

	Not at All Difficult	A Little Difficult	Moderately Difficult	Very Difficult	Unable To Do
1. How difficult is it for you to get in or out of a low chair?	☐	☐	☐	☐	☐
2. How difficult is it for you to open medicine bottles or jars?	☐	☐	☐	☐	☐
3. How difficult is it for you to shop for groceries or other things?	☐	☐	☐	☐	☐
4. How difficult is it for you to climb stairs?	☐	☐	☐	☐	☐
5. How difficult is it for you to make a tight fist?	☐	☐	☐	☐	☐
6. How difficult is it for you to get in or out of the bathtub or shower?	☐	☐	☐	☐	☐
7. How difficult is it for you to get comfortable to sleep?	☐	☐	☐	☐	☐
8. How difficult is it for you to bend or kneel down?	☐	☐	☐	☐	☐
9. How difficult is it for you to use buttons, snaps, hooks, or zippers?	☐	☐	☐	☐	☐
10. How difficult is it for you to cut your own fingernails?	☐	☐	☐	☐	☐
11. How difficult is it for you to dress yourself?	☐	☐	☐	☐	☐
12. How difficult is it for you to walk?	☐	☐	☐	☐	☐
13. How difficult is it for you to get moving after you have been sitting or lying down?	☐	☐	☐	☐	☐
14. How difficult is it for you to go out by yourself?	☐	☐	☐	☐	☐
15. How difficult is it for you to drive?	☐	☐	☐	☐	☐
16. How difficult is it for you to clean yourself after going to the bathroom?	☐	☐	☐	☐	☐
17. How difficult is it for you to turn knobs or levers (for example, to open doors or to roll down car windows)?	☐	☐	☐	☐	☐
18. How difficult is it for you to write or type?	☐	☐	☐	☐	☐
19. How difficult is it for you to pivot?	☐	☐	☐	☐	☐
20. How difficult is it for you to do your usual physical recreational activities, such as bicycling, jogging, or walking?	☐	☐	☐	☐	☐
21. How difficult is it for you to do your usual leisure activities, such as hobbies, crafts, gardening, card-playing, or going out with friends?	☐	☐	☐	☐	☐
22. How much difficulty are you having with sexual activity?	☐	☐	☐	☐	☐
23. How difficult is it for you to do <u>light</u> housework <u>or</u> yard work, such as dusting, washing dishes, or watering plants?	☐	☐	☐	☐	☐
24. How difficult is it for you to do <u>heavy</u> housework <u>or</u> yard work, such as washing floors, vacuuming, or mowing lawns?	☐	☐	☐	☐	☐
25. How difficult is it for you to do your usual work, such as a paid job, housework, or volunteer activities?	☐	☐	☐	☐	☐

Figure 1-19 ▬

Short Musculoskeletal Function Assessment (SMFA). (From Swiontkowski MF et al: Short musculoskeletal function assessment questionnaire: the validity, reliability, and responsiveness, *J Bone Joint Surg Am* 81: 1256–1258, 1999.)

Continued

These next questions ask how often you are experiencing problems <u>this week</u> because of your injury or arthritis.

	None of the Time	A Little of the Time	Some of the Time	Most of the Time	All of the Time
26. How often do you walk with a limp?	☐	☐	☐	☐	☐
27. How often do you avoid using your painful limb(s) or back?	☐	☐	☐	☐	☐
28. How often does your leg lock or give-way?	☐	☐	☐	☐	☐
29. How often do you have problems with concentration?	☐	☐	☐	☐	☐
30. How often does doing too much in one day affect what you do the next day?	☐	☐	☐	☐	☐
31. How often do you act irritable toward those around you (for example, snap at people, give sharp answers, or criticize easily)?	☐	☐	☐	☐	☐
32. How often are you tired?	☐	☐	☐	☐	☐
33. How often do you feel disabled?	☐	☐	☐	☐	☐
34. How often do you feel angry or frustrated that you have this injury or arthritis?	☐	☐	☐	☐	☐

These questions are about how much you are bothered by problems you are having <u>this week</u> because of your injury or arthritis.

	Not at All Bothered	A Little Bothered	Moderately Bothered	Very Bothered	Extremely Bothered
35. How much are you bothered by problems using your hands, arms, or legs?	☐	☐	☐	☐	☐
36. How much are you bothered by problems using your back?	☐	☐	☐	☐	☐
37. How much are you bothered by problems doing work around your home?	☐	☐	☐	☐	☐
38. How much are you bothered by problems with bathing, dressing, toileting, or other personal care?	☐	☐	☐	☐	☐
39. How much are you bothered by problems with sleep and rest?	☐	☐	☐	☐	☐
40. How much are you bothered by problems with leisure or recreational activities?	☐	☐	☐	☐	☐
41. How much are you bothered by problems with your friends, family or other important people in your life?	☐	☐	☐	☐	☐
42. How much are you bothered by problems with thinking, concentrating, or remembering?	☐	☐	☐	☐	☐
43. How much are you bothered by problems adjusting or coping with your injury or arthritis?	☐	☐	☐	☐	☐
44. How much are you bothered by problems doing your usual work?	☐	☐	☐	☐	☐
45. How much are you bothered by problems with feeling dependent on others?	☐	☐	☐	☐	☐
46. How much are you bothered by problems with stiffness and pain?	☐	☐	☐	☐	☐

Figure 1-19 cont'd

Shoulder Evaluation Form

Diagnosis:	Patient's Name:
Aim of Procedure:	Hospital Unit #:
Operation:	Date of Operation:
Shoulder: right: left:	Date of Follow-up:
Arm Dominance: right: left:	Surgeon:
	Preoperative rating:
The rating in each category can be adjusted according to the AIM of the procedure	Postoperative rating:
	Patient's Evaluation (circle):
	Exc. Good Fair Poor

Unit Rating
(circle one in
each category)

Unit Rating
(circle one in
each category)

I. PAIN (15)

1.	None	15
2.	Slight during activity	12
3.	Increased pain during activities	6
4.	Moderate/severe pain in activity	3
5.	Severe pain, dependent on medication	0 ___

II. STABILITY (25)

1.	Normal. Shoulder stable and strong in all positions	25
2.	Mild apprehension in normal use of arm. No subluxation or dislocation	20
3.	Avoids elevation and external rotation. Rare subluxation	10
4.	Recurrent subluxations ("Dead arm syndrome"). Positive apprehension test or recurrent dislocation	5
5.	Recurrent dislocation	0 ___

III. FUNCTION (25)

1.	Normal function. All activities of daily living. Performs all work, sport/recreation prior to injury. Lifting 30+ lb. Swimming, tennis, throwing. Combat	25
2.	Mild limitation in sports and work. Can throw, but limited in baseball. Strong in tennis, football, swimming, lifting (15–20 lb) and combat. Performs all personal care	20
3.	Moderate limitation in overhead work and lifting (10 lb) and athletics. Unable to throw or serve in tennis. Swims sidestroke. Difficulty with body care (perineal care, back pocket, combing hair, reaching back). Aid necessary at times	10
4.	Severe limitations. Unable to perform usual work or lifting. No athletics. Sedentary occupation. Unable to perform body care without aid. Can feed self and comb hair.	5
5.	Complete disability of extremity	0 ___

IV. MOTION (25)

Abduction and forward flexion

151 to 170°	15
121 to 150°	12
91 to 120°	10
61 to 90°	7
31 to 60°	5
Less than 30°	0 ___

IR	Thumb to scapula	5
	Thumb to sacrum	3
	Thumb to trochanter	2
	Less than trochanter	0 ___

ER	(with arm at side)	
	80°	5
	60°	3
	30°	2
	Less than 30°	0 ___

V. STRENGTH (10) (compared to opposite shoulder)

(specify method = manual, spring gauge, Cybex)

Normal	10
Good	6
Fair	4
Poor	0 ___

TOTAL UNITS

Excellent	(100–85 units)	—
Good	(84–70 units)	
Fair	(69–50 units)	
Poor	(49 units or less)	

Figure 1-20 ▬▬▬▬▬

Shoulder evaluation form. (Modified from Rowe CR: *The shoulder*, p. 632, Edinburgh, 1988, Churchill Livingstone.)

or she is ready to return to activity. Examples of these tests include the hop test and disco test for the knee. These tests, in reality, could be used for all the weight-bearing (lower limb) joints. However, it must be remembered that many of these provocative or stress tests are designed for very active persons and are not suitable for all populations.

Special (Diagnostic) Tests

After the examiner has completed the history, observation, and evaluation of movement, special tests may be performed for the involved joint. Many special tests are available for each joint to determine whether a particular type of disease, condition, or injury is present. They are

Upper Extremity Function Test

Basic Function	*Date* _____	
	Right	Left
Grasp		
1. Block 4 in. (Item 1)		
2. Block 3 in. (Item 2)		
3. Block 2 in. (Item 3)		
4. Block 1 in. (Item 4)		
Grip		
5. Pipe 1¾ in. (Item 5)		
6. Pipe ¾ in. (Item 6)		
Lateral Prehension		
7. Slate 1 × ⅝ × 4 in. (Item 7)		
Pinch		
8. Ball 3 in. (Item 8)		
Marble ⅝ in. (Item 9)		
9. Index finger and thumb		
10. Middle finger and thumb		
11. Ring finger and thumb		
12. Small finger and thumb		
Ball-bearing ⁷⁄₁₆ in. (Item 10)		
13. Index finger and thumb		
14. Middle finger and thumb		
15. Ring finger and thumb		
16. Small finger and thumb		
Ball-bearing ¼ in. (Item 11)		
17. Index finger and thumb		
18. Middle finger and thumb		
19. Ring finger and thumb		
20. Small finger and thumb		
Ball-bearing ⁵⁄₃₂ in. (Item 12)		
21. Index finger and thumb		
22. Middle finger and thumb		
23. Ring finger and thumb		
24. Small finger and thumb		
Placing		
25. Washer over nail (Item 13)		
26. Iron to shelf (Item 14)		
Supination and Pronation		
27. Pour water from pitcher to glass		
28. Pour water from glass to glass (pronation)		
29. Pour water back to first glass (supination)		
30. Place hand behind head		
31. Place hand on top of head		
32. Hand to mouth		
33. Write name _____		
	TOTAL _____	

Smedly Dynamometer Reading:
Does pain interfere with function?

Scoring: 3—Performs test normally
2—Completes test, but takes abnormally long time or has great difficulty
1—Performs test partially
0—Can perform no part of test

Score: 0–25: Trace
26–50: Very poor
51–75: Poor
76–89: Partial
90–98: Functional
99–100: Maximal (dominant hand) (96-nondominant hand)

Figure 1-21 ▮▮▮▮▮▮▮▮

Upper extremity function test. (Modified by permission of the publisher from Carroll D: A quantitative test of upper extremity function, *J Chron Dis* 18:482, Copyright 1965 by Elsevier Science.)

Table 1-23

Summary Description of Tests in Simulated Activities of Daily Living Examination (SADLE)

Test	Measure	Units	Instrumentation
Two leg standing, eyes open	Maximum time of three 30-second trials	Seconds	Stopwatch
One leg standing, eyes open	Maximum time of three 30-second trials	Seconds	Stopwatch
Two leg standing, eyes closed	Maximum time of three 30-second trials	Seconds	Stopwatch
One leg standing, eyes closed	Maximum time of three 30-second trials	Seconds	Stopwatch
Tandem walking with supports	Time to take 10 heel-to-toe steps	Steps/sec	Stopwatch and parallel bars
Tandem walking without supports	Time to take 10 heel-to-toe steps	Steps/sec	Stopwatch and parallel bars
Putting on a shirt	Average time of two trials	Seconds	Stopwatch and shirt
Managing three visible buttons	Average time of two trials	Seconds	Stopwatch and cloth with three buttons mounted on a board
Zipping a garment	Average time of two trials	Seconds	Stopwatch and cloth with zipper mounted on a board
Putting on gloves	Average time of two trials	Seconds	Stopwatch and two garden gloves
Dialing a telephone	Average time of two trials	Seconds	Stopwatch and telephone
Tying a bow	Average time of two trials	Seconds	Stopwatch and large shoelaces mounted on a board
Manipulating safety pins	Average time of two trials	Seconds	Stopwatch and two safety pins
Picking up coins	Average time of two trials	Seconds	Stopwatch and four coins placed on a plastic sheet
Threading a needle	Average time of two trials	Seconds	Stopwatch, thread, and large-eyed needle
Unwrapping a Band-Aid	Time for one trial	Seconds	Stopwatch and one Band-Aid
Squeezing toothpaste	Average time of two trials	Seconds	Stopwatch, tube of toothpaste, and a board
Cutting with a knife	Average time of two trials	Seconds	Stopwatch, plate, fork, knife, and Permoplast
Using a fork	Average time of two trials	Seconds	Stopwatch, plate, fork, and Permoplast

Modified from Potvin AR et al: Simulated activities of daily living examination, *Arch Phys Med Rehab* 53:478, 1972.

sometimes called clinical accessory, provocative, motion, palpation, or structural tests. These tests, although strongly suggestive of a particular disease or condition when they yield positive results, do not necessarily rule out the disease or condition when they yield negative results. This will depend on the test. When deciding to use these diagnostic tests, the examiner must determine if the test will give reliable and useful information that will help in the diagnosis and subsequent treatment.[120,121] To be useful, diagnostic tests must give reliable data (i.e., consistent results regardless of who does the test), must be valid (i.e., test what it says it tests), and must be accurate to maximize patient outcomes.[120,122] Reliability is determined by the cooperation of the patient, which may be influenced by the patient's ability to relax, pain, apprehension, and sincerity; the skill of the clinician, which may be influenced by experience, his or her ability to relax, and confidently do the test; and calibration of the equipment.[120] Several methods are used to determine reliability, but the intraclass correlation coefficient (ICC) is the preferred index because it reflects both agreement and correlation among ratings.[123] It is calculated through analysis of variance (ANOVA) using variance estimates.[123] Table 1-24 shows ICC agreement values that are illustrative for diagnostic tests. With nominal data, the kappa statistic (K) is applied after the percentage agreement between testers has been determined.[123]

When performing a test, it is also useful, in terms of reliability, to know the standard error of measurement (SEM).[123] The SEM reflects the reliability of the response when the test is performed many times. It is an indication of how much change there might be when a test is repeated. If the SEM is small, then the test is stable with minimal variability between tests.[123]

Table 1-24

Benchmark Intraclass Correlation Coefficient Values

Value	Description
<0.75	Poor to moderate agreement
>0.75	Good agreement
>90	Sufficient agreement to ensure reasonable validity of clinical measurements

Data from Portney LG and Walkins MP: *Foundations of clinical research: applications to practice*, Upper Saddle River, N.J., 2000, Prentice Hall, p. 201.

Diagnostic tests should be evaluated on their diagnostic accuracy or ability to determine which people have the condition or disease and those who do not as this will have an impact on subsequent treatment and patient outcomes.[124] The most useful methods of determining whether a test is a good test for the pathology under consideration are sensitivity, specificity, and likelihood ratios.[120–132] Sensitivity implies the ability of a test to identify the person who has a particular condition, dysfunction, or disease when they do (i.e., a true positive).[120,122,123,128,132] Specificity, on the other hand, is used to determine which people do not have a particular condition, dysfunction, or disease (i.e., a true negative).[120,122,123,128,132] Sensitivity and specificity values for tests are usually based on a gold standard, or reference test[132] (e.g., diagnostic imaging, what was found at surgery). If the clinician is unsure that the patient has a particular condition, dysfunction or disease, then the examiner would want to use a test of exclusion or discovery that has a high sensitivity as it will rule out those people who do not have the problem, provided the test's specificity is equal to or higher than another test testing for the same thing.[127] On the other hand, if the examiner has a high level of suspicion (based on the preceding history, observation, and examination) that the problem is present and wants to confirm that decision (confirmation test), then the examiner would want a test with higher specificity to "rule in" those people who do have the problem, provided the test's sensitivity is equal to or higher than another test testing for the same thing.[122,127] This is especially true if further evaluation or treatment is expensive or dangerous. To prevent healthy people from receiving unnecessary expensive or dangerous treatment, high specificity is desired.[128] In an ideal world, one would want a test that has both high sensitivity and high specificity. To try to solve these differences in levels of sensitivity and specificity, likelihood ratios are often recommended as determinants of the usefulness of a test.[120,122,124,127,129,133] Likelihood ratios are based on determining the odds that a condition, dysfunction, or disease is present by combining sensitivity and specificity to indicate whether the test will raise or lower the probability of the patient having the condition, dysfunction, or disease.[120,129] The higher the likelihood ratio, the greater is the likelihood that the patient has the problem.

There are two other issues that the clinician should be aware of when considering special or diagnostic tests. Although beyond the scope of this book, clinicians should also consider responsiveness, which is the ability of a test to detect a clinically important change, and the minimal clinical important difference (MCID), which is the smallest difference in the result of a test that the clinician perceives as beneficial or significant in the context that it may result in a particular treatment or change in treatment.[125,126]

Tests can be more accurately performed right after injury (during the period of tissue shock—5 to 10 minutes after injury), under anesthesia, or in chronic conditions. Each examiner tends to use those tests he or she has found to be clinically effective. Under no circumstances should special tests be used in isolation, nor is it necessary to learn all of the special tests. They should be viewed as an integral part of a total examination.[134] They should be considered as tests to confirm a tentative diagnosis, to make a differential diagnosis, to differentiate between structures, to understand unusual signs, or to unravel difficult signs and symptoms.[70]

For each joint examination described in this book, specific tests are mentioned for specific conditions. Tests that the author has found to be particularly effective and provide useful and reliable information have been highlighted, but this does not rule out the use of other tests. Many of the tests are similar and show similar results; which ones to

Special Test Uses[70]

- To confirm a tentative diagnosis
- To make a differential diagnosis
- To differentiate between structures
- To understand unusual signs
- To unravel difficult signs and symptoms

use depends on which give the best results for the individual examiner and which tests provide the most useful and reliable information. For example, both the Lachman test and anterior drawer test may be used to test the anterior cruciate ligament, although the literature indicates the Lachman test is more sensitive.

If desired, the examiner can design his or her own special tests or modify the described tests. Sometimes, the examiner can reproduce the same movement the patient described as the mechanism of injury, which may provoke the symptoms. However, the addition of too many special tests only makes the picture more confusing and the diagnosis more difficult. Also, care should be taken when performing these tests, because they are usually provocative tests and will provoke signs and symptoms, including pain and apprehension. Thus, special tests should be done with caution and may be contraindicated in the presence of severe pain, acute and irritable conditions of the joints, instability, osteoporosis, pathological bone diseases, active disease processes, unusual signs and symptoms, major neurological signs, and patient apprehension.

In addition to the special tests, the examiner may also make use of **laboratory tests** ordered by a physician for specific conditions. With osteomyelitis, for example, a positive blood culture is likely to be obtained, the white blood cell count will be elevated, and the erythrocyte sedimentation rate will be increased. The examiner, if a physician, may decide to draw fluid out of a joint (aspirate) with a hypodermic needle to view the synovial fluid. Tables 1-25, 1-26, and 1-27 present normal laboratory values, laboratory findings in some bone diseases, and a classification of synovial fluid as examples of laboratory tests and values.

Reflexes and Cutaneous Distribution

After the special tests, the examiner can test the superficial, deep tendon, or pathological reflexes to obtain an indication of the state of the nerve or nerve roots supplying the reflex. If the neurological system is thought to be normal, there is no need to test the reflexes or cutaneous distribution. If, however, the examiner is unsure whether there is neurological involvement, both reflexes and sensation should be tested to clarify the problem and where the problem actually is.

Most often, the deep tendon reflexes (sometimes referred to as muscle stretch reflexes)[24] are tested with

a reflex hammer. A deep tendon reflex can be elicited from almost any tendon with practice. The more common deep tendon reflexes tested are shown in Table 1-28. Tables 1-29 and 1-30 demonstrate superficial and pathological reflexes. Superficial reflexes are provoked by superficial stroking, usually with a sharp object. A pathological reflex is not normally present, except in the very young (<5-7 months) in whom the cerebrum is not developed enough to suppress this reflex.[24] If it is present in adults and children, it often signals a pathological condition.

With a loss or abnormality of nerve conduction, there is a diminution (hyporeflexia) or loss (areflexia) of the stretch reflex. Aging also causes a decreased response. Upper motor neuron lesions produce findings of spasticity, hyperreflexia, hypertonicity, extensor plantar responses, reduced or absent superficial reflexes, and weakness of muscles distal to the lesion. Lower motor neuron lesions involving nerve roots or peripheral nerves produce findings of flaccidity, hyporeflexia or areflexia, hypotonicity, fasciculation, fibrillations, and weakness and atrophy of the involved muscles (see Table 1-11).[135]

Deep tendon reflexes are performed to test the integrity of the spinal reflex, which has a sensory (afferent) and motor (efferent) component.[7] Abnormal deep tendon reflexes are not clinically relevant unless they are found with sensory or motor abnormalities. To properly test the deep tendon reflexes, the patient must be relaxed and the examiner must ensure that the muscle of the tendon to be tested is relaxed. The tendon to be tested is put on slight stretch, and an adequate stimulus is applied by dropping the reflex hammer onto the tendon. The examiner should tap the tendon five or six times to uncover any fading reflex response, indicative of developing nerve root signs. If the deep tendon reflexes are difficult to elicit, the reflexes often can be enhanced by having the patient clench the teeth or squeeze the hands together (**Jendrassik maneuver**) when testing the lower limb or squeeze the legs together when testing the upper limb. These activities increase the facilitative activity of the spinal cord and thereby accentuate minimally active reflexes.[136]

Superficial reflexes are tested by stroking the skin with a moderately sharp object that does not break the skin. The expected responses are shown in Table 1-29. A great deal of practice is needed to become proficient in testing the superficial reflexes.

Pathological reflexes, which are not usually evident because they are suppressed by the cerebrum at the brain stem or spinal cord level (see Table 1-30), may indicate upper motor neuron lesions if present on both sides or lower motor neuron lesions if present on only one side.[24] Improper stimulation (e.g., too much pressure) may lead to voluntary withdrawal in normal subjects, and the examiner must take care not to confuse this reaction with the pathological response. The two most commonly

Table 1-25

Normal Laboratory Values Used in Orthopedic Medicine*

Laboratory Test	Normal Range
White blood cell (WBC) count	$4–9 \times 10^9$/L
Red blood cell (RBC) count	$4.3–5.4 \times 10^{12}$/L (male)
	$3.8–5.2 \times 10^{12}$/L (female)
Hematocrit (HCT)	38–50% (male)
	34–46% (female)
Hemoglobin (Hgb)	130–170 g/L (male)
	115–160 g/L (female)
Erythrocyte sedimentation rate (ESR)	0–10 mm/hr (male)
	0–15 mm/hr (female
	0–10 mm/hr (children)
Myoglobin (Mb)	30–90 ng/ml
Ferritin	25–465 μg/ml (male)
	15–200 μg/ml (female)
Platelet count	140,000–350,000/mm³
Calcium	8.5–10.5 mg/dl
Ionized calcium	4.2–5.4 mg/dl
Alkaline phosphatase	25–92 U/L
Antinuclear antibodies screen	Negative
Uric acid	3.5–7.2 mg/dl (male)
	2.6–6.0 mg/dl (female)
Rheumatoid arthritis factor	<1.20

*Values may vary slightly depending on equipment used.

Table 1-26

Laboratory Findings in Bone Disease

Condition	Calcium	Inorganic Phosphorus	Alkaline Phosphatase	Calcium	Phosphorus
Hyperparathyroidism, primary	↑	↓	↑	↑	↑
Hyperparathyroidism, secondary	N- ↓	↑	R ↑	↑	↑
Hyperthyroidism, marked	N	N	↑	↑	↑
Hypothyroidism	N	N	N	N	N
Senile osteoporosis	N	N-O ↓	N	N	N
Rickets (child)	↓	↓	↑	N	N
Osteomalacia (adult)	N- ↓	↓	↑	N	N
Paget's disease	R ↑	R ↓	↑	N	N
Multiple myeloma	↑	N- ↑	R ↑	↑	↑

Adapted from Quinn J: Introduction to the musculoskeletal system. In Meschan I: *Synopsis of analysis of roentgen signs in general radiology*, p.27, Philadelphia, 1976, WB Saunders.
N = normal; O = occasionally; R = rarely; ↑ = increased; ↓ = decreased.

Table 1-27

Classification of Synovial Fluid

Type	Appearance	Significance
Group 1	Clear yellow	Noninflammatory states, trauma
Group 2*	Cloudy	Inflammatory arthritis; excludes most patients with osteoarthritis
Group 3	Thick exudate, brownish	Septic arthritis; occasionally seen in gout
Group 4	Hemorrhagic	Trauma, bleeding disorders, tumors, fractures

From Curran JF et al: Rheumatologic aspects of painful conditions affecting the shoulder, *Clin Orthop Relat Res* 173:28, 1983.
*Inflammatory fluids will clot and should be collected in heparin-containing tubes. All group 2 or 3 fluids should be cultured if the diagnosis is uncertain.

tested pathological reflexes are the Babinski reflex (lower limb) and the Hoffman reflex (upper limb).

To be of clinical significance, findings must show asymmetry between bilateral reflexes unless there is a central lesion. The eliciting of reflexes often depends on the skill of the examiner. The examiner should not be overly concerned if the reflexes are absent, diminished, or excessive on both sides, especially in young people, unless a central lesion is suspected. Exercise just before testing or patient anxiety or tenseness may lead to accentuated tendon reflexes.[64] Hyporeflexia or areflexia indicates a lesion of a peripheral nerve or spinal nerve root as a result of impingement, entrapment, or injury. Examples would be nerve root compression, cauda equina syndrome, or peripheral neuropathy. Hyporeflexia or areflexia may be seen in the absence of muscle weakness or atrophy because of the involvement of the efferent loop of the reflex arc in the reflex. Hyperactive or exaggerated reflexes (hyperreflexia) indicate upper motor neuron lesions as seen in neurological disease and cerebral or brain stem impairment. In the cervical spine, if a disc herniation and compression occur above the cervical enlargement, the reflexes of the upper extremity are exaggerated. If the cervical enlargement is involved (which is more commonly the case), then some reflexes are exaggerated and some are decreased.[137]

Deep Tendon Reflex Grading

- 0—Absent (areflexia)
- 1—Diminished (hyporeflexia)
- 2—Average (normal)
- 3—Exaggerated (brisk)
- 4—Clonus, very brisk (hyperreflexia)

At the same time, the examiner can perform a **sensory scanning examination** by checking the cutaneous distribution of the various peripheral nerves and the dermatomes around the joint being examined. The sensory examination is performed for several reasons. First, it is used to determine the extent

Table 1-28

Common Deep Tendon Reflexes

Reflex	Site of Stimulus	Normal Response	Pertinent Central Nervous System Segment
Jaw	Mandible	Mouth closes	Cranial nerve V
Biceps	Biceps tendon	Biceps contraction	C5-C6
Brachioradialis	Brachioradialis tendon or just distal to the musculotendinous junction	Flexion of elbow and/or pronation of forearm	C5-C6
Triceps	Distal triceps tendon above the olecranon process	Elbow extension/muscle contraction	C7-C8
Patella	Patellar tendon	Leg extension	L3-L4
Medial hamstrings	Semimembranosus tendon	Knee flexion/muscle contraction	L5, S1
Lateral hamstrings	Biceps femoris tendon	Knee flexion/muscle contraction	S1-S2
Tibialis posterior	Tibialis posterior tendon behind medial malleolus	Plantar flexion of foot with inversion	L4-L5
Achilles	Achilles tendon	Plantar flexion of foot	S1-S2

Table 1-29

Superficial Reflexes

Reflex	Normal Response	Pertinent Central Nervous System Segment
Upper abdominal	Umbilicus moves up and toward area being stroked	T7-T9
Lower abdominal	Umbilicus moves down and toward area being stroked	T11-T12
Cremasteric	Scrotum elevates	T12, L1
Plantar	Flexion of toes	S1-S2
Gluteal	Skin tenses in gluteal area	L4-L5, S1-S3
Anal	Contraction of anal sphincter muscles	S2-S4

of sensory loss, whether that loss is caused by nerve root lesions, peripheral nerve lesions, or compressive tunnel syndromes. Second, because function is often tied to sensation, it is used to determine the degree of functional impairment. Third, because sensory function returns before motor function, it can be used to determine nerve recovery after injury or repair as well as when reeducation can commence. Also, if sensory function remains after injury to the spinal cord, it is a good indication that some motor function, at least, will be restored.[138] Finally, it is part of the total assessment and is often necessary for medicolegal reasons. Although the sensory distribution of peripheral nerves may vary from person to person, they tend to be more consistent than dermatomes.[47,139] The examiner must be able to differentiate between sensory loss involving a nerve root (dermatome) and that involving a peripheral nerve (see Table 1-13 for an example).

The sensory examination begins with a quick scan of sensation. To do this, the examiner runs his or her relaxed hands relatively firmly over the skin to be tested bilaterally and asks the patient whether there are any differences in sensation. The patient's eyes may be open for the scan. If the patient notes any differences in sensation between the affected and unaffected sides, then a more detailed sensory assessment is performed. The examiner should note the patient's ability to perceive the sensation being tested and the difference, if any, between the two sides of the body. In addition, distal and proximal sensitivities should be compared for each form of sensation tested. During the detailed sensory testing, the patient should keep his or her eyes closed so that the results will indicate the patient's perception and interpretation of the stimuli, not what the patient sees happening. With the detailed sensory testing, the examiner marks out, or delineates, the specific area of altered sensation and then correlates the area with the known dermatome and peripheral nerve distribution. The examiner must be aware, however, that the abnormal sensation does not necessarily come from the indicated nerve root or peripheral nerve; because of referred pain, it may come from any structure supplied by that nerve root. In some cases, the paresthesia may involve no specific pattern, or it may involve the entire circumference of a limb. This "opera glove" or "stocking" paresthesia or anesthesia may result from vascular insufficiency or systemic disease.

Table 1-30

Pathological Reflexes[*]

Reflex	Elicitation	Positive Response	Pathology
Babinski[†]	Stroking of lateral aspect of sole of foot	Extension of big toe and fanning of four small toes Normal reaction in newborns	Pyramidal tract lesion Organic hemiplegia
Chaddock's	Stroking of lateral side of foot beneath lateral malleolus	Same response as above	Pyramidal tract lesion
Oppenheim's	Stroking of anteromedial tibial surface	Same response as above	Pyramidal tract lesion
Gordon's	Squeezing of calf muscles firmly	Same response as above	Pyramidal tract lesion
Piotrowski's	Percussion of tibialis anterior muscle	Dorsiflexion and supination of foot	Organic disease of central nervous system
Brudzinski's	Passive flexion of one lower limb	Similar movement occurs in opposite limb	Meningitis
Hoffman's (Digital)[‡]	"Flicking" of terminal phalanx of index, middle, or ring finger	Reflex flexion of distal phalanx of thumb and of distal phalanx of index or middle finger (whichever one was not "flicked")	Increased irritability of sensory nerves in tetany Pyramidal tract lesion
Rossolimo's	Tapping of the plantar surface of toes	Plantar flexion of toes	Pyramidal tract lesion
Schaeffer's	Pinching of Achilles tendon in middle third	Flexion of foot and toes	Organic hemiplegia

[*]Bilateral positive response indicates an upper motor neuron lesion. Unilateral positive response may indicate a lower motor neuron lesion.
[†]Tests most commonly performed in the lower limb.
[‡]Tests most commonly performed in the upper limb.

Superficial tactile (light touch) sensation, which is commonly the first sensation affected, can be tested with a wisp of cotton, soft hairbrush, or small paint or makeup brush. Superficial pain can be tested with a flagged pin (holding a piece of tape attached to a pin), pinwheel, or other sharp object. Only light tapping should be used. About 2 seconds should elapse between each stimulus to avoid summation. It is the group II afferent fibers (Table 1-31) that are being tested. Perception to pin prick may range from absence of awareness, through pressure sensation, hyperanalgesia with or without radiation, localization, and sensation of sharpness, to normal perception.

If desired, the examiner may also test other sensations. Two test tubes (one with hot water, one with cold) are used to assess sensitivity to temperature (lateral spinothalamic tract and group III fibers), one containing hot water and one containing cold water. A normal response to this test does not necessarily mean that the patient has normal temperature sensation. Rather, the patient can distinguish between hot and cold, each at one level in the range, but not necessarily between different degrees of hot and cold. Sensitivity to vibration (i.e., how long until vibration stops) may be tested by holding a tuning fork (usually 30- or 256-cps tuning forks are used) against bony prominences; this tests the integrity of group II fibers and the dorsal

column and medial lemniscal systems. Deep pressure pain (group II Aβ fibers) can be tested by squeezing the Achilles tendon, the trapezius muscle, or the web space between the thumb and index finger or by applying a knuckle to the sternum. To test proprioception

Table 1-31

Nerve Fiber Classification

Sensory Axons	Axon Diameter (μm)	Conduction Velocity (m/sec)	Innervation
Ia (Aα)	12–22	65–130	Muscle spindles (annulospiral endings)
Ib (Aα)	12–22	65–130	Golgi tendon organs
II (Aβ)	5–15	20–90	Pressure, touch, vibration (flower spray endings)
III (Aδ)	2–10	6–45	Temperature, fast pain
IV (C)	0.2–1.5	0.2–2.0	Slow pain, visceral, temperature, crude touch

and motion (i.e., the skin and joint receptors, muscle spindles, dorsal column and medial lemniscal systems, and group I and II fibers), the patient's fingers or toes are passively moved, and the patient is asked to indicate the direction of movement and final position while keeping the eyes closed. To ensure that pressure on the patient's skin cannot be used as a clue to direction of movement, the test digit should be grasped between the examiner's thumb and index finger.

Cortical and discriminatory sensations may be tested by two-point discrimination, point localization, texture discrimination, stereognostic function (i.e., identification of familiar objects held in the hand), and graphesthesia (i.e., recognition of letters or numbers written with a blunt object on the patient's palms or other body parts). These techniques also test the integrity of the dorsal column and lemniscal systems.

Joint Play Movements

All synovial and secondary cartilaginous joints, to some extent, are capable of an active ROM, termed "voluntary movement" (also called active physiological movement) through the action of muscles crossing over the joint. In addition, there is a small ROM that can be obtained only passively by the examiner; this movement is called **joint play** or **accessory movement.** These accessory movements are not under voluntary control; they are necessary, however, for full painless function of the joint and full ROM of the joint. **Joint dysfunction** signifies a loss of joint play movement.

The existence of joint play movement is necessary for full, pain-free voluntary movement to occur. An essential part of the detailed assessment of any joint includes an examination of its joint play movements. If any joint play movement is found to be absent or decreased, this movement must be restored before the patient can regain functional voluntary movement. In most joints, this movement is normally less than 4 mm in any one direction.

In some cases, joint play movements may be similar to or the same as movements tested during passive movements or ligamentous testing. This is most obvious in joints that have minimal movement and in joints that do not have muscles acting directly on them, such as the sacroiliac joints and superior tibiofibular joints.

Loose Packed (Resting) Position

To test joint play movement, the examiner places the joint in its resting position, which is the position in its ROM at which the joint is under the least amount of stress; it is also the position in which the joint capsule has its greatest capacity.[141] The resting position (sometimes called the loose packed or maximum loose packed position) is one of minimal congruency between the articular surfaces and the joint capsule, with the ligaments being in the posi-

Mennell's Rules for Joint Play Testing[140]
• The patient should be relaxed and fully supported.
• The examiner should be relaxed and should use a firm but comfortable grasp.
• One joint should be examined at a time.
• One movement should be examined at a time.
• The unaffected side should be tested first.
• One articular surface is stabilized while the other surface is moved.
• Movements must be normal and not forced.
• Movements should not cause undue discomfort.

tion of greatest laxity and passive separation of the joint surfaces being the greatest. This position may be the anatomical resting position, which is usually considered in the midrange, or it may be just outside the range of pain and spasm. The advantage of the loose packed position is that the joint surface contact areas are reduced and are always changing to decrease friction and erosion in the joints. The position also provides proper joint lubrication and allows the arthrokinematic movements of spin, slide, and roll. It is therefore the most common position used for treatment using joint play mobilizations. Examples of resting positions are shown in Table 1-32.

Close Packed (Synarthrodial) Position

The close packed position should be avoided as much as possible during an assessment except to stabilize an adjacent joint, because in this position, the majority of joint structures are under maximum tension. In this position, the two joint surfaces fit together precisely—that is, they are fully congruent. The joint surfaces are tightly compressed; the ligaments and capsule of the joint are maximally tight; and the joint surfaces cannot be separated by distractive forces. It is the position of maximum joint stability. Thus, this position is commonly used during treatment to stabilize the joint, if an adjacent joint is being treated. Ligaments, bone, or other joint structures, if injured, become more painful as the close packed position is approached. If a joint is swollen, the close packed position cannot be achieved.[89] In the close packed position, no accessory movement is possible. Examples of the close packed positions of most joints are shown in Table 1-33.

Palpation

Initially, palpation for tenderness plays no part in the assessment, because referred tenderness is real and can be misleading. Only after the tissue at fault has been identified is palpation for tenderness used to determine the exact extent of the lesion within that tissue, and then palpation is done only if the tissue lies superficially and

Table 1-32

Resting (Loose Packed) Position of Joints

Joint	Position
Facet (spine)	Midway between flexion and extension
Temporomandibular	Mouth slightly open (freeway space)
Glenohumeral	55° abduction, 30° horizontal adduction
Acromioclavicular	Arm resting by side in normal physiological position
Sternoclavicular	Arm resting by side in normal physiological position
Ulnohumeral (elbow)	70° flexion, 10° supination
Radiohumeral	Full extension, full supination
Proximal radioulnar	70° flexion, 35° supination
Distal radioulnar	10° supination
Radiocarpal (wrist)	Neutral with slight ulnar deviation
Carpometacarpal	Midway between abduction-adduction and flexion-extension
Metacarpophalangeal	Slight flexion
Interphalangeal	Slight flexion
Hip	30° flexion, 30° abduction, slight lateral rotation
Knee	25° flexion
Talocrural (ankle)	10° plantar flexion, midway between maximum inversion and eversion
Subtalar	Midway between extremes of range of movement
Midtarsal	Midway between extremes of range of movement
Tarsometatarsal	Midway between extremes of range of movement
Metatarsophalangeal	Neutral
Interphalangeal	Slight flexion

Table 1-33

Close Packed Position of Joints

Joint	Position
Facet (spine)	Extension
Temporomandibular	Clenched teeth
Glenohumeral	Abduction and lateral rotation
Acromioclavicular	Arm abducted to 90°
Sternoclavicular	Maximum shoulder elevation
Ulnohumeral (elbow)	Extension
Radiohumeral	Elbow flexed 90°, forearm supinated 5°
Proximal radioulnar	5° supination
Distal radioulnar	5° supination
Radiocarpal (wrist)	Extension with radial deviation
Metacarpophalangeal (fingers)	Full flexion
Metacarpophalangeal (thumb)	Full opposition
Interphalangeal	Full extension
Hip	Full extension, medial rotation*
Knee	Full extension, lateral rotation of tibia
Talocrural (ankle)	Maximum dorsiflexion
Subtalar	Supination
Midtarsal	Supination
Tarsometatarsal	Supination
Metatarsophalangeal	Full extension
Interphalangeal	Full extension

*Some authors include abduction (e.g., Kaltenborn[141]).

2. Distinguish differences in tissue texture. For example, the examiner can, in some cases, palpate the direction of fibers or presence of fibrous bands.

3. Identify shapes, structures, and tissue type and thereby detect abnormalities. For example, bone deformities such as myositis ossificans may be palpated.

Examiner Observations When Palpating a Patient

- Differences in tissue tension and texture
- Differences in tissue thickness
- Abnormalities
- Tenderness
- Temperature variation
- Pulses, tremors, and fasciculations
- Pathological state of tissues
- Dryness or excessive moisture
- Abnormal sensation

within easy reach of the fingers. Palpation is an important assessment technique that must be practiced if it is to be used effectively.[142-144] Tenderness often does enable the examiner to name the affected ligament or the specific section or exact point of the tearing or bruising.

To palpate properly, the examiner must ensure that the area to be palpated is as relaxed as possible. For this to be done, the body part must be supported as much as possible. As the ability to perform palpation develops, the examiner should be able to accomplish the following:

1. Discriminate differences in tissue tension (e.g., effusion, spasm) and muscle tone (i.e., spasticity, rigidity, flaccidity). Spasticity refers to muscle tonus in which there may be a collapse of muscle tone during testing. Rigidity refers to involuntary resistance being maintained during passive movement and without collapse of the muscle. Flaccidity means there is no muscle tone.

4. Determine tissue thickness and texture and determine whether it is pliable, soft, and resilient. Is there any obvious swelling? Edema is an abnormal accumulation of fluid in the intercellular spaces; swelling, on the other hand, is

the abnormal enlargement of a body part. It may be the result of bone thickening, synovial membrane thickening, or fluid accumulation in and around the joint. It may be intracellular or extracellular (edema), intracapsular or extracapsular. Swelling may be localized (encapsulated), which may indicate intra-articular swelling, a cyst, or a swollen bursa. Visualization of swelling depends on the depth of the tissue (a swollen olecranon bursa is more obvious than a swollen psoas bursa) and the looseness of the tissues (swelling is more evident on the dorsum of the hand than on the palmar aspect because the dorsal tissues are not "held down" to adjacent tissue). Swelling that develops immediately or within 2 to 4 hours of injury is probably caused by blood extravasation into the tissues (ecchymosis) or joint. Swelling that becomes evident after 8 to 24 hours is caused by inflammation and, in a joint, by synovial swelling. Bony or hard swelling may be caused by osteophytes or new bone formation (e.g., in myositis ossificans). Soft-tissue swelling such as edematous synovium produces a boggy, spongy feeling (like soft sponge rubber), whereas fluid swelling is a softer and more mobile, fluctuating feeling. Blood swelling is usually a harder, thick, gel-like feeling, and the overlying skin is usually warmer. Pus is thick and less fluctuant; the overlying skin is warm, and the temperature is usually elevated. Older, longstanding soft-tissue swelling, such as a skin callus, feels like tough, dry leather. Synovial hypertrophy has a hard, thick feeling to it with little give. The more leathery the thickening feels, the more likely it is to be chronic and caused by local symptoms. Softer thickenings tend to be more acute and associated with recent symptoms.[87] Pitting edema is thick and slow moving, leaving an indentation after pressure is applied and removed. It is commonly caused by circulatory stasis and is most commonly seen in the distal extremities. Long-lasting swelling may cause reflex inhibition of the muscles around the joint, leading to atrophy and weakness. Blood swelling within a joint is usually aspirated because of the irritating and damaging effect it has on the joint cartilage.

Swelling

- Comes on soon after injury → blood
- Comes on after 8 to 24 hours → synovial
- Boggy, spongy feeling → synovial
- Harder, tense feeling with warmth → blood
- Tough, dry → callus
- Leathery thickening → chronic
- Soft, fluctuating → acute
- Hard → bone
- Thick, slow-moving → pitting edema

5. Determine joint tenderness by applying firm pressure to the joint. The pressure should always be applied with care, especially in the acute phase.

Grading Tenderness When Palpating

- *Grade I.* Patient complains of pain.
- *Grade II.* Patient complains of pain and winces.
- *Grade III.* Patient winces and withdraws the joint.
- *Grade IV.* Patient will not allow palpation of the joint.

6. Feel variations in temperature. This determination is usually best done by using the back of the examiner's hand or fingers and comparing both sides. Joints tend to be warm in the acute phase, in the presence of infection, with blood swelling, after exercise, or if they have been covered (for example, with an elastic bandage).

7. Feel pulses, tremors, and fasciculations. Fasciculations result from contraction of a number of muscle cells innervated by a single motor axon. The contractions are localized, are usually subconscious, and do not involve the whole muscle. Tremors are involuntary movements in which agonist and antagonist muscle groups contract to cause rhythmic movements of a joint. Pulses indicate circulatory sufficiency and should be tested for rhythm and strength if circulatory problems are suspected. Table 1-34 indicates the more commonly palpated pulses that may be used to determine circulatory sufficiency and location.

8. Determine the pathological state of the tissues in and around the joint. The examiner should note any tenderness, tissue thickening, or other signs or symptoms that would indicate pathology. Painful scars or neuromas may be diagnosed using the **thumbnail test**. This test involves running the dorsum of the thumbnail over the scar. If this action elicits a sharp pain, it is a possible indication of a neuroma within the scar. Diffuse sensitivity may suggest complex regional pain syndrome (reflex sympathetic dystrophy).

Table 1-34

Common Circulatory Pulse Locations

Artery	Location
Carotid	Anterior to sternocleidomastoid muscle
Brachial	Medial aspect of arm midway between shoulder and elbow
Radial	At wrist, lateral to flexor carpi radialis tendon
Ulnar	At wrist, between flexor digitorum superficialis and flexor carpi ulnaris tendons
Femoral	In femoral triangle (sartorius, adductor longus, and inguinal ligament)
Popliteal	Posterior aspect of knee (deep and hard to palpate)
Posterior tibial	Posterior aspect of medial malleolus
Dorsalis pedis	Between first and second metatarsal bones on superior aspect

9. Feel dryness or excessive moisture of the skin. For example, acute gouty joints tend to be dry, whereas septic joints tend to be moist. Nervous patients usually demonstrate increased moisture (sweating) in the hands.

10. Note any abnormal sensation such as dysesthesia (diminished sensation), hyperesthesia (increased sensation), anesthesia (absence of sensation), or crepitus. Soft, fine crepitus may indicate roughening of the articular cartilage, whereas coarse grating may indicate badly damaged articular cartilage or bone. A creaking, leathery crepitus (snowball crepitation) is sometimes felt in tendons and indicates pathology. Tendons may "snap" over one another or over a bony prominence. Loud, snapping, pain-free noises in joints are usually caused by cavitation, in which gas bubbles form suddenly and transiently owing to negative pressure in the joint.

Palpation of a joint and surrounding area must be carried out in a systematic fashion to ensure that all structures are examined. This procedure involves having a starting point and working from that point to adjacent tissues to assess their normality or the possibility of pathological involvement. The examiner must work slowly and carefully, applying light pressure initially and working into a deeper pressure of palpation, then "feeling" for pathological conditions or changes in tissue tension.[142] The uninvolved side should be palpated first so that the patient has some idea of what to expect and to enable the examiner to know what "normal" feels like. Any differences or abnormalities should be noted and contribute to the diagnosis.

Diagnostic Imaging

Although it is important, the diagnostic imaging portion of the examination is usually used only to confirm a clinical opinion and must be interpreted within the context of the whole examination.[145] As with special tests, diagnostic imaging should be viewed as one part of the assessment, to be used when it will help confirm or establish a diagnosis.[146] In some cases, clinical decision rules have been developed (e.g., Ottawa ankle and foot rules). These rules increase the accuracy of diagnostic assessments, but the examiner should be aware that the rules apply primarily to acute, first-time injuries.[145] Although this book has examples of diagnostic imaging in each chapter, the reader is advised to consult more detailed texts on the subject for more in-depth knowledge.[147–149]

Plain Film Radiography

Conventional plain film radiography (also called x-rays) is the primary means of diagnostic imaging for musculoskeletal problems. It offers the advantages of being readily available, being relatively cheap, and providing good anatomical resolution. On the negative side, it does expose the patient to radiation, and it offers poor differentiation of soft-tissue structures and is not sensitive to subtle pathology.[145] Radiographs are not taken indiscriminately. Because x-rays have the potential for causing cell damage, there should be a clear indication of need before a radiograph is taken, and the process should not be considered routine.[150]

Normally, the clinician orders two projections at 90° orientation to each other—most commonly, anteroposterior (AP) and lateral projections. Two views are necessary because x-rays take planar images, so that all structures in the path of the x-ray beam are superimposed on each other and abnormalities may be difficult to evaluate with only one view. Two views give information concerning the dimensions of a structure, whether foreign bodies or lesions are present and their location, and to determine the alignment of fractures.[149] Other views may be obtained, depending on clinical circumstances and specific needs.[150–153] In the lumbar spine, AP, lateral, and oblique views are commonly taken.

X-rays are part of the electromagnetic spectrum and have the ability to penetrate tissue to varying degrees. X-ray imaging is based on the principle that different tissues have different densities and produce images in different shades of gray.[154] The greater the density of the tissue, the less penetration of x-rays there is, and the whiter its image appears on the film. In order of descending degree of density are the following structures: metal, bone, soft tissue, water, fat, and air. These differences give the six basic densities on the x-ray plate. When viewing the x-rays, the examiner must identify the film, noting the name, age, date, and sex of the patient, and must identify the type of projection taken (e.g., AP, lateral, tunnel, skyline, weight-bearing, stress-type).

The x-ray plates that are developed after exposure to the roentgen rays enables the examiner to see any fractures, dislocations, foreign bodies, or radiopaque substances that may be present. The main function of plain x-ray examination is to rule out or exclude fractures or serious disease such as infection (osteomyelitis), ankylosing spondylitis, or tumors and structural body abnormalities such as developmental anomalies, arthritis, and metabolic bone diseases. Commonly, an ABCs search pattern is used when looking at radiological images (Table 1-35).[149] With soft-tissue injuries, clinical findings should take precedence over x-ray findings. It is desirable to know whether an x-ray has been taken so the examiner can obtain the films if necessary. The examiner should be aware of obvious and unusual x-ray findings that distract attention from other tissue that is actually the cause of the pain; such x-ray abnormalities are significant only if clinical examination bears out their relevance. With experience, the examiner becomes able to detect many important soft-tissue changes on x-ray examination, such as effusion in joints, tendinous calcifications, ectopic bone in muscle, tissue displaced by tumor, and the presence of air or foreign body material in the tissues. Radiographs

Table 1-35

ABCs Search Pattern for Radiological Image Interpretation

Division	Evaluates	Look For Normal Findings	Look For Variations/Abnormalities
A: Alignment	General skeletal architecture	Gross normal size of bones Normal number of bones	Supernumerary (extra) bones Absent bones Congenital deformities Developmental deformities Cortical fractures
	General contour of bone	Smooth and continuous cortical outlines	Avulsion fractures Impaction fractures Spurs Breaks in cortex continuity
	Alignment of bones to adjacent bones	Normal joint articulations Normal spatial relationships	Markings of past surgical sites Fracture Joint subluxation Joint dislocation
B: Bone Density	General bone density	Sufficient contrast between soft-tissue shade of gray and bone shade of gray Sufficient contrast within each bone, between cortical shell and cancellous center	General loss of bone density resulting in poor contrast between soft tissues and bone Thinning or absence of cortical margins
	Texture abnormalities	Normal trabecular architecture	Appearance of trabeculae altered; may look thin, delicate, lacy, coarsened, smudged, fluffy
	Local bone density changes	Sclerosis at areas of increased stress, such as weight-bearing surfaces or sites of ligamentous, muscular, or tendinous attachments	Excessive sclerosis (increase in bone density) Reactive sclerosis that walls off a lesion (e.g., tumor) Osteophytes
C: Cartilage Spaces	Joint space width	Well-preserved joint spaces imply normal cartilage or disk thickness	Decreased joint spaces imply degenerative or traumatic conditions
	Subchondral bone	Smooth surface	Excessive sclerosis as seen in degenerative joint disease Erosions as seen in the inflammatory arthritides
	Epiphyseal plates	Normal size relative to epiphysis and skeletal age	Compare contralaterally for changes in thickness that may be related to abnormal conditions or trauma
D: Soft Tissues	Muscles	Normal size of soft-tissue image	Gross wasting Gross swelling
	Fat pads and fat lines	Radiolucent crescent parallel to bone Radiolucent lines parallel to length of muscle	Displacement of fat pads from bony fossae into soft tissues indicates joint effusion Elevation or blurring of fat planes indicates swelling of nearby tissues
	Joint capsules	Normally indistinct	Observe whether effusion or hemorrhage distends capsule
	Periosteum	Normally indistinct Solid periosteal reaction is normal in fracture healing	Observe periosteal reactions: solid, laminated or onionskin, spiculated or sunburst, Codman's triangle
	Miscellaneous soft-tissue findings	Soft tissues normally exhibit a water-density shade of gray	Foreign bodies evidenced by radiodensity Gas bubbles appear radiolucent Calcifications/ossification appear radiopaque

Modified from McKinnis LN: *Fundamentals of musculoskeletal imaging,* pp. 40–41, Philadelphia, 2005, FA Davis.

may also be used to indicate bone loss. For osteoporosis to be evident on x-ray, approximately 30% to 35% of the bone must be lost (Figure 1-22).

Examiner Observations When Viewing an X-ray

- Overall size and shape of bone
- Local size and shape of bone
- Number of bones
- Alignment of bones
- Thickness of the cortex
- Trabecular pattern of the bone
- General density of the entire bone
- Local density change
- Margins of local lesions
- Any break in continuity of the bone
- Any periosteal change
- Any soft-tissue change (e.g., gross swelling, periosteal elevation, visibility of fat pads)
- Relation among bones
- Thickness of the cartilage (cartilage space within joints)
- Width and symmetry of joint space
- Contour and density of subchondral bone

The examiner should keep in mind the maturity of the patient when viewing films. Skeletal changes occur with age,[155] and the appearance and fusion of the epiphyses, for example, may be important in interpreting the pathol-ogy of the condition seen. Soft-tissue structures as well as bone can be seen, provided there is something to outline them. For example, the joint capsule may be silhouetted by the pericapsular fat, or air in the lungs may silhouette a cardiac shadow. Anatomical variations and anomalies must be ruled out before pathology can be ruled in; for example, accessory navicular, bipartite patella, and os trigonum may be confused with fractures by the unsuspecting examiner. The fabella is often confused with a loose body in the knee in the AP projection x-ray film.

Radiographs may also be used to determine the maturity index of a patient. A special film of the wrist is taken to assess skeletal maturity (Figure 1-23). These films can be compared with established films in a bone atlas such as that compiled by Gruelich and Pyle.[155] This is often done before epiphysiodesis and leg-lengthening procedures to ensure that the child is of a suitable skeletal age to do the procedure.

Arthrography

Arthrography is an invasive technique in which air, a water-soluble contrast material containing iodine, or a combination of the two (double contrast) is injected into a joint space and a radiograph is taken of the joint. The air or contrast material outlines the structures within the joint or communicating with the joint (Figure 1-24). It is especially useful in detecting abnormal joint and bursal communications, synovial abnormalities, articular cartilage lesions, and the extent of or pathology to the

A　　　　　　　　　　　　**B**

Figure 1-22
Osteoporosis of immobilization and disuse. Radiographs obtained immediately before wrist ligament reconstruction (**A**) and 2 months later (**B**) are shown. Observe in (**B**) the extent of the osteopenia. (From Resnick D and Kransdorf MJ: *Bone and joint imaging*, p. 547, Philadelphia, 2005, Elsevier.)

A   **B**   **C**

Figure 1-23

X-ray films showing skeletal maturity. **A,** Male, newborn. **B,** Male, 5 years old. **C,** Female, 17 years old.

Figure 1-24

Normal arthrogram, shoulder in lateral rotation. Note the good dependent fold *(wide arrow)* and the outline of the bicipital tendon *(narrow arrow).* (From Neviaser TJ: Arthrography of the shoulder, *Orthop Clin North Am* 11:209, 1980.)

capsule.[149] It is used primarily in the hip, knee, ankle, shoulder, elbow, and wrist.[150]

Computed Arthrography (CT-Arthrography)

This technique combines arthrography and computed tomography (CT). This method provides a three-dimen-sional definition of the joint, and the dye helps to delineate articular surfaces and joint margins. It is usually reserved for those cases in which conventional CT scanning has not provided adequate anatomical detail (e.g., shoulder instability).[26,150,153]

Venogram and Arteriogram

With a venogram or an arteriogram, radiopaque dye is injected into specific vessels to outline abnormal con-ditions (Figure 1-25). This technique may be used to diagnose arteriosclerosis, investigate tumors, and dem-onstrate blockage after traumatic injury.

Myelography

Myelography is an invasive imaging technique that is used to visualize the soft tissues within the spine. A water-soluble radiopaque dye is injected into the epidu-ral space by spinal puncture and allowed to flow to dif-ferent levels of the spinal cord, outlining the contour of the thecal sac, nerve roots, and spinal cord. A plain x-ray film is then taken of the spine (Figures 1-26 and 1-27). In many cases today, CT scans and MRI have taken the place of myelograms.[150] This technique is used to detect disc disease, disc herniation, nerve root entrapment, spinal stenosis, and tumors of the spinal cord. The clini-cian should be aware that myelograms can have adverse side effects. Grainger[156] reported that 20% to 30% of patients receiving myelograms complained of headache, dizziness, nausea, vomiting, and seizures.[154]

A   B

Figure 1-25

Occlusion of brachial artery. **A,** Arteriogram of a young man with a previously reduced elbow dislocation and an ischemic hand shows an occluded brachial artery. **B,** A later film shows fresh clot *(arrow)* in the brachial artery and reconstituted radial and ulnar arteries. Primary repair and thrombectomy treated the ischemic symptoms. (From McLean G and Frieman DB: Angiography of skeletal disease, *Orthop Clin North Am* 14:267, 1983.)

Figure 1-26

Myelogram of cervical spine. Note how radiopaque dye fills root sheaths *(arrow)*.

Figure 1-27

Myelogram of lumbar spine showing extrusion of nucleus pulposus of L4-L5 *(large arrow)*. Note how radiopaque dye fills dural recesses *(small arrow)*. (From Selby DK et al: Water-soluble myelography, *Orthop Clin North Am* 8:82, 1977.)

Tomography and Computed Tomography

Tomography has become a common imaging technique for musculoskeletal disorders, especially when computer enhanced (CT scan). It produces cross-sectional images of the tissues. Conventional tomography, which is also called thin-section radiography or linear tomography, tends to show one small area or plane in focus with other areas or planes appearing fuzzy or blurred. The conventional tomogram is seldom used today except when subtle bone density alterations are sought.

The CT scan involves the same thin cross sections or "slices" taken at specific levels (Figure 1-28). CT scans produce cross-sectional images based on x-ray attenuation. Because of computer enhancement, CT produces superior tissue contrast resolution compared with conventional x-rays, thus enabling greater details of subtle bone pathology.[145] CT provides excellent bony architecture detail and has good resolution of soft-tissue structures. Its disadvantages include limited scanning plane, cost, exposure to radiation (dosage similar to or greater than that of plain x-rays), alteration of the image by artifacts, and degradation of soft-tissue resolution in obese people.[26,150] The CT scan, or computed axial tomography (CAT) scan, is a radiological technique that may be used to assess for disc protrusions, facet disease, or spinal stenosis.[157] The technique may also be used to assess complex fractures, especially those involving joints, dislocations, patellofemoral alignment and tracking, osteonecrosis, tumors, and osteomyelitis. Because only a small cross-sectional area in one plane is viewed with each scan, multiple images or scans are taken to get a complete view of the area.[26]

Figure 1-28

A, Normal computed tomographic (CT) image at the level of the mid acetabulum obtained with soft-tissue window settings shows the homogenous, intermediate signal of musculature. a = common femoral artery; gd = gluteus medius; gn = gluteus minimus; gx = gluteus maximus; ip = iliopsoas; oi = obturator internus; ra = rectus abdominis; rf = rectus femoris; s = sartorius; t = tensor fascia lata; v = common femoral vein.
B, Axial CT at bone window settings reveals improved delineation of cortical and medullary osseous detail. Note anterior and posterior semilunar acetabular articular surfaces and the central nonarticular acetabular fossa.
C, Normal midacetabular T1-weighted axial 0.4-T magnetic resonance image (MRI) (TR, 600 msec; TE, 20 msec) of a different patient shows a normal, high-signal-intensity image of fatty marrow (adult pattern) and subcutaneous tissue, low-signal-intensity image of muscle, and absence of signal in the cortical bone. The thin articular hyaline cartilage is of intermediate signal intensity *(arrow)*. **D,** T2-weighted MRI (TR, 2,000 msec; TE, 80 msec) shows decreasing high signal intensity in fatty marrow and subcutaneous tissue with increased signal intensity in the fluid-filled urinary bladder. (From Pitt MJ et al: Imaging of the pelvis and hip, *Orthop Clin North Am* 21:553, 1990.)

Radionuclide Scanning (Scintigraphy)

With bone scans (osteoscintigraphy), chemicals labeled with isotopes (radioactive tracers) such as technetium-99m–labeled methyl diphosphonate complexes are intravenously injected several hours before the scan to localize specific organs that concentrate the particular chemical. The isotope is then localized where there is a high level of activity (e.g., bone turnover) relative to the rest of the bone. The radiograph reveals a "hot spot" (Figure 1-29) indicating areas of increased mineral turnover.[149] Although plain film radiographs do not show bone disease or stress fractures until there is 30% to 50% bone loss, bone scans show bone disease or stress fractures with as little as 4% to 7% bone loss (Figure 1-30).[157] Because the isotope is excreted by the kidneys, the kidneys and bladder are often visible in bone scans. Bone scans are used for lytic (bone-loss) diseases, infection, fractures, and tumors. They are highly sensitive to bone abnormalities but do not tell what the abnormality is. The whole body may be imaged, and a gamma camera picks up the tracer.[150]

Discography

The technique of discography involves injecting a small amount of radiopaque dye into the nucleus pulposus of an intervertebral disc (Figure 1-31) under radiographic guidance. It is not a commonly used technique but may be used to determine disruptions in the nucleus pulposus or the annular fibrosus and is sometimes used as a provocative test to see whether injection into the disc brings on the patient's symptoms.[150]

Magnetic Resonance Imaging

Magnetic resonance imaging (MRI) is a noninvasive, painless imaging technique that uses exposure to magnetic fields, not ionizing radiation, to obtain an image of bone and soft tissue. MRI is based on the effect of a strong magnetic field on hydrogen atoms. T1 images show good anatomical detail of soft tissues (Figure 1-32), whereas T2 images are used to demonstrate soft-tissue pathology that alters tissue water content.[26,156] MRI

A   **B**   **C**

Figure 1-29

Whole body bone scans. **A,** Normal adult anterior scan. **B,** Normal adult posterior scan. **C,** Posterior scan showing joint involvement of rheumatoid arthritis. (From Goldstein HA: Bone scintigraphy, *Orthop Clin North Am* 14:244, 250, 1983.)

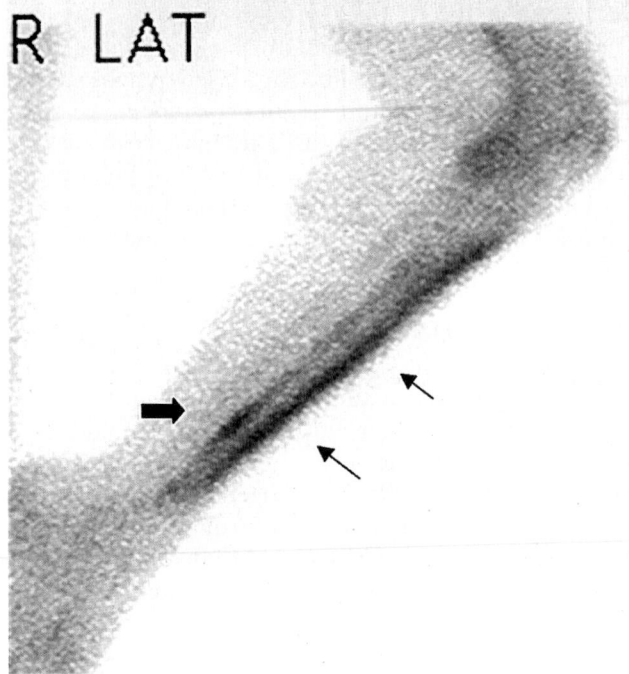

Figure 1-30

Stress fracture of the tibia and anterior shin splint. A short fusiform area of increased uptake in the posterior aspect of the distal shaft of the tibia represents a stress fracture (*large arrow*). A long longitudinal area of increased uptake in the anterior aspect of the tibial shaft is consistent with a shin splint (*small arrow*). (From Resnick D and Kransdorf MJ: *Bone and joint imaging*, p. 103, Philadelphia, 2005, Elsevier.)

Figure 1-31

Normal discogram shown with barium paste. (From Farfan HF: *Mechanical disorders of the low back*, p. 96, Philadelphia, 1973, Lea & Febiger.)

offers excellent tissue contrast, is multiplanar (i.e., can image in any plane), and has no known adverse effects. In some patients, claustrophobia is a problem, and artifacts may result if the patient does not remain still.[156]

MRI is used to assess for spinal cord tumors, intracranial disease, and some types of central nervous system diseases (e.g., multiple sclerosis); it largely replaced myelography in the evaluation of disc pathology. It also aids in the diagnosis of muscle, meniscal and ligamentous tears, synovial pathology, abnormal patellofemoral tracking, joint pathology, bone marrow pathology, osteonecrosis, stress fractures, and osteochondral lesions.[26]

On the negative side, MRI is expensive, and specificity of pathology (e.g., tendon strain versus tendinitis) may not be possible with its use. The presence of some metallic objects such as cardiac pacemakers may make its use contraindicated because of the magnetic pull, especially if the objects are not solidly fixed to bone. It has been reported that MRI is safe with prosthetic joints and internal fixation devices provided they are stable.[150]

Fluoroscopy

Fluoroscopy is a technique that is used to show motion in joints through x-ray imaging; it also may be used as a guidance technique for injections (e.g., in discography). It is only rarely used because of the amount of radiation exposure. It is sometimes used to position fracture fragments and to demonstrate abnormal motion.

Diagnostic Ultrasound

Like therapeutic ultrasound, diagnostic ultrasound involves transmission of high-frequency sound waves (5 to 10 MHz) into the tissues by a transducer through a coupling agent, with calculation of the time it takes for the echo to return to the transducer from different interfaces. The depth of the structure is determined, and an image is formed. Each tissue has a unique echo texture that relates to its internal structure (Figure 1-33).[26,158]

In the hands of an experienced operator, ultrasound can provide good image detail and cross-sectional images in different planes. No radiation is used, and no harmful biological effects have been reported. It has the advantage of providing dynamic (moving) real-time images, so that tissues can be visualized as they move. It also allows localization of any tenderness or palpable mass[26,158] and therefore is used to assess soft-tissue injury such as tendon, ligament, or muscle pathology, soft-tissue masses (e.g., tumor, ganglion, cyst, inflamed bursa), effusion, and congenital dislocation of the hip.

The disadvantages of diagnostic ultrasound include limited contrast resolution, limited depth of penetration, small viewing field, and lack of penetration of bone.[26,158] The use of diagnostic ultrasound has a difficult learning curve, and the quality and interpretation of the images depend on the operator.

Figure 1-32
Magnetic resonance T1-weighted coronal oblique images from anterior (**A**) to posterior (**C**). T = trapezius muscle; A = acromion; SS = supraspinatus muscle; D = deltoid muscle; C = coracoid; SB = subscapularis muscle; sbt = subscapularis tendon; AC = acromioclavicular joint; sst = supraspinatus tendon; sdb = subdeltoid-subacromial bursa; H = humerus; G = glenoid of scapula; ist = infraspinatus tendon; IS = infraspinatus muscle. (From Mayer SJ and Dalinka MK: Magnetic resonance imaging of the shoulder, *Orthop Clin North Am* 21:500, 1990.)

Xeroradiography

Xeroradiography is a technique in which a xeroradiographic plate replaces the normal x-ray film. On the plate, there is a thin layer of a photoconductor material, which enhances the image (Figure 1-34). This technique is used when the margins between areas of different densities need to be exaggerated.[153,159]

Précis

Each chapter ends with a précis of the assessment to serve as a quick reference. The précis does not follow the text description exactly but is laid out so that each assessment involves minimal movement of the patient, to decrease patient discomfort. For example, all aspects of the

Figure 1-33

Diagnostic ultrasound—patellar tendon. A longitudinal extended field of view of a normal patellar tendon shows a well-defined hyperechoic tendon with a fine intrasubstance fibrillar pattern (*arrows*). Note the infrapatellar fat pad (Hoffa's FP), the inferior pole of the patella (P), and the tibial tubercle (T). (From Resnick D and Kransdorf MJ: *Bone and joint imaging*, p. 81, Philadelphia, 2005, Elsevier.)

examination that are performed with the patient standing are done first, followed by those done with the patient sitting, and so on.

Case Studies

Case studies are provided as written exercises to help the examiner develop skills in assessment. Based on the presented case study, the reader should develop a list of appropriate questions to ask in the history based on the pathology of the conditions, what should especially be noted in observation, and what part of the examination is essential to make a definitive diagnosis. Where appropriate, example diagnoses are given in parentheses at the end of each question. At the end of the case study, the reader can develop a table showing the differential diagnosis for the case described. Tables 1-36 and 1-37 illustrate such differential diagnosis charts.

A   B

Figure 1-34

Xeroradiography. **A,** Normal examination. Note the ability to demonstrate both soft tissues and bony structures on a single examination. The halo effect *(arrow)* around the bony cortices is an example of edge enhancement. **B,** Hyperparathyroid bone changes shown on xeroradiography. The subperiosteal bone resorption *(arrow)* and distal tuft erosion are well shown. (**A** from Weissman BNW and Sledge CB: *Orthopedic radiology*, Philadelphia, 1986, WB Saunders, p. 11. **B** from Seltzer SE et al: Improved diagnostic imaging in joint diseases, *Semin Arthritis Rheum* 11:315, 1982.)

Table 1-36
Differential Diagnosis of Claudication and Spinal Stenosis

Vascular Claudication	Neurogenic Claudication	Spinal Stenosis
Pain* is usually bilateral	Pain is usually bilateral but may be unilateral	Usually bilateral pain
Occurs in the calf (foot, thigh, hip, or buttocks)	Occurs in back, buttocks, thighs, calves, feet	Occurs in back, buttocks, thighs, calves, and feet
Pain consistent in all spinal positions	Pain decreased in spinal flexion Pain increased in spinal extension	Pain decreased in spinal flexion Pain increased in spinal extension
Pain brought on by physical exertion (e.g., walking)	Pain increased with walking	Pain increased with walking
Pain relieved promptly by rest (1 to 5 minutes)	Pain decreased by recumbency	Pain relieved with prolonged rest (may persist hours after resting)
Pain increased by walking uphill		Pain decreased when walking uphill
No burning or dysesthesia	Burning and dysesthesia from the back to buttocks and leg or legs	Burning and numbness present in lower extremities
Decreased or absent pulses in lower extremities	Normal pulses	Normal pulses
Color and skin changes in feet—cold, numb, dry, or scaly skin, poor nail and hair growth	Good skin nutrition	Good skin nutrition
Affects ages from 40 to over 60	Affects ages from 40 to over 60	Peaks in seventh decade of life; affects men primarily

*"Pain" associated with vascular claudication may also be described as an "aching," "cramping," or "tired" feeling.
Modified from Goodman CC and Snyder TE: *Differential diagnosis in physical therapy*, ed 2, p. 539, Philadelphia, 1995, WB Saunders.

Table 1-37
Differential Diagnosis of Contractile Tissue (Muscle) and Inert Tissue (Ligament) Pathology

	Muscle	Ligament
Mechanism of Injury	Overstretching (overload) Crushing (pinching)	Overstretching (overload)
Contributing Factors	Muscle fatigue Poor reciprocal muscle strength Inflexibility Inadequate warmup	Muscle fatigue Hypermobility
Active Movement	Pain on contraction (1°, 2°) Pain on stretch (1°, 2°) No pain on contraction (3°) Weakness on contraction (1°, 2°, 3°)	Pain on stretch or compression (1°, 2°) No pain on stretch (3°) ROM decreased
Passive Movement	Pain on stretch Pain on compression	Pain on stretch (1°, 2°) No pain on stretch (3°) ROM decreased
Resisted Isometric Movement	Pain on contraction (1°, 2°) No pain on contraction (3°) Weakness on contraction (1°, 2°, 3°)	No pain (1°, 2°, 3°)
Special Tests	If test isolates muscle, weakness and pain on contraction (1°, 2°) or weakness and no pain on contraction (3°)	If test isolates ligament, ROM and pain affected

Continued

Table 1-37—cont'd

	Muscle	Ligament
Reflexes	Normal unless 3°	Normal
Cutaneous Distribution	Normal	Normal
Joint Play Movement (in Resting Position)	Normal	Increased ROM, unless restricted by swelling
Palpation	Point tenderness at site of injury Gap if palpated early Swelling (blood—ecchymosis late) Spasm	Point tenderness at site of injury Gap if palpated early Swelling (blood/synovial fluid)
Diagnostic Imaging	MRI, arthrogram, and CT scan show lesion	MRI, arthrogram, and CT scan show lesion Stress x-ray shows increased ROM

CT = computed tomography; MRI = magnetic resonance imaging; ROM = range of motion.

Conclusion

Having completed all parts of the assessment, the examiner can look at the pertinent objective and subjective facts, note the significant signs and symptoms to determine what is causing the patient's problems, and design a proper treatment regimen based on the findings. This is the normal and correct reasoning process.[160,161] If the assessment is not followed through completely, the treatment regimen may not be implemented properly, and this may lead to unwarranted extended care of the patient and increased health care costs.

Occasionally, patients present with a mixture of signs and symptoms that indicates two or more possible problem areas. Only by adding the positive findings and subtracting the negative findings can the examiner determine the probable cause of the problem. In many cases, the decision may be an "educated guess," because few problems are "textbook perfect". Only the examiner's knowledge, clinical experience, and diagnosis, followed by trial treatment, can conclusively delineate the problem.

Finally, when the assessment has been completed, the clinician should warn the patient about a possible exacerbation of symptoms and should not hesitate to refer the patient to another health care professional if the patient has presented with unusual signs and symptoms or if the condition appears to be beyond the scope of the examiner's practice.

References

To enhance this text and add value for the reader, all references have been incorporated into a CD-ROM that is provided with this text. The reader can view the reference source and access it online whenever possible. There are a total of 161 cited references and other general references for this chapter.

APPENDIX 1-1

EXAMPLE OF AN ASSESSMENT FORM

DATE:

NAME:

AGE:

OCCUPATION:

HISTORY

Mechanism of Injury:

Aggravating/Easing Factors or Movements:

24-Hour History:

Improving/Static/Worse

New/Old Injury

Past History (include social and family history):

Diagnostic Imaging:

OBSERVATION (POSTURE)

EXAMINATION

ACTIVE MOVEMENTS   PASSIVE MOVEMENTS

EXT   EXT
L   R   L   R

FLEX   FLEX

Comments:

End Feel:

Capsular Pattern:

Mark where symptoms are:

VAS: Intensity of Pain

no
pain
0

pain as bad
as it could
possibly get
10

Pain: constant, periodic, episodic, occasional

RESISTED ISOMETRIC MOVEMENTS	FUNCTIONAL TESTING
Comments:	

NEUROLOGICAL TESTS

Sensory Scan:

Reflexes:

Neurological Special Tests:

SPECIAL TESTS

JOINT PLAY MOVEMENTS

PALPATION

Tenderness, Effusion

(use reverse side for other comments)

APPENDIX 1-2

Example of Informed Consent/Patient Authorization

PATIENT AUTHORIZATION

I hereby authorize and grant permission to _____,

a _____, to carry out any assessment and examination, procedures, and
occupation

treatments as may be necessary to assess and treat my condition or injury.

The above-named _____ has agreed to provide me with understandable:
occupation

information on:

- my diagnosis, as known
- the treatment being suggested
- significant risks, benefits of treatment, and possible alternatives to this treatment
- reasonable additional procedures which may be necessary
- the potential risks of foregoing the suggested care

I hereby authorize and grant permission to the above-named _____ to
occupation

communicate with any health care professional that rehabilitation of my condition may indicate.

I hereby authorize and grant permission to the above-named _____ to
occupation

release information regarding my condition and my ability to return to normal activity or work to my

insurance company/employer/lawyer or their representative.

I, _____, understand the conditions and information as
patient's name

verbally provided and voluntarily give my consent to the above authorizations.

_____   _____   _____
date   signature   witness

HEAD AND FACE

Casualty officers and clinicians working in emergency care settings are often the ones who assess the head and face. In these settings, the assessment involves the bony aspects of the head and face as well as the soft tissues. The soft-tissue assessment involves primarily the sensory organs such as the skin, eyes, nose, and ears, whereas the muscles are tested only as they relate to injury to these structures. Joints and their integrity are not the main objects of the assessment. Because the temporomandibular joints and cervical spine are discussed in Chapters 3 and 4, this chapter deals with only the head, the face, and their associated structures.

Applied Anatomy

The head and face are made up of the cranial vault and facial bones. The **cranial vault,** or skull, is composed of several bones: one frontal, two sphenoid, two parietal, two temporal, and one occipital (Figure 2-1). Of these, the strongest is the occipital bone, and the weakest are the temporal bones. The frontal bone forms the forehead, and the temporal and sphenoid bones form the anterolateral walls of the skull, or the temples of the head. The parietal bones form the top and posterolateral portions of the skull, and the occipital bones form the posterior portion of the skull. The cranial vault reaches 90% of its ultimate size by age 5.

In addition to the cranial vault bones, there are 14 **facial bones.** These bones develop more slowly than the cranial bones, reaching only 60% of their ultimate size by age 6. The facial skeleton is composed of the mandible, which forms the lower jaw; the maxilla, which forms the upper jaw on each side; the nasal bones, which form the bridge of the nose; and the palatine, lacrimal, zygomatic,

and ethmoid bones, which form the remainder of the face. It is the zygomatic bone that gives the cheek its prominence. The sphenoid bones also form part of the orbital cavity. The facial skull has several cavities for the eyes (orbital), nose (nasal), and mouth (oral), as well as spaces for nerves and blood vessels to penetrate the bony structure. Weight is saved in the skull area by the addition of sinus cavities (Figure 2-2).

The muscles of the head and face are controlled primarily by the 12 **cranial nerves.** The cranial nerves and their chief functions are shown in Table 2-1. The cranial nerves generally contain both sensory and motor fibers. However, some cranial nerves are strictly sensory (olfactory and optic), whereas others are strictly motor (oculomotor, trochlear, and hypoglossal).

The **external eye** is composed of the eyelids (upper and lower), conjunctiva (a transparent membrane covering the cornea, iris, pupil, lens, and sclera), lacrimal gland, eye muscles, and bony skull orbit (Figure 2-3). Muscles of the eye, their actions, and their nerve supply are shown in Table 2-2. The muscles and movements of the eye are shown in Figure 2-4. To produce some of the actions, the various muscles of the eye must work in concert. The **eyelids** protect the eye from foreign bodies, distribute tears over the surface of the eye, and limit the amount of light entering the eye. The **conjunctiva** is a thin membrane covering the majority of the anterior surface of the eye. It helps to protect the eye from foreign bodies and desiccation (drying up). The lacrimal gland provides tears, which keep the eye moist (Figure 2-5). The eye itself is made up of the sclera, cornea, and iris as well as the lens and retina (Figure 2-6). The **sclera** is the dense white portion of the eye that physically supports the internal structures. The **cornea** is very sensitive to pain (e.g., the extreme

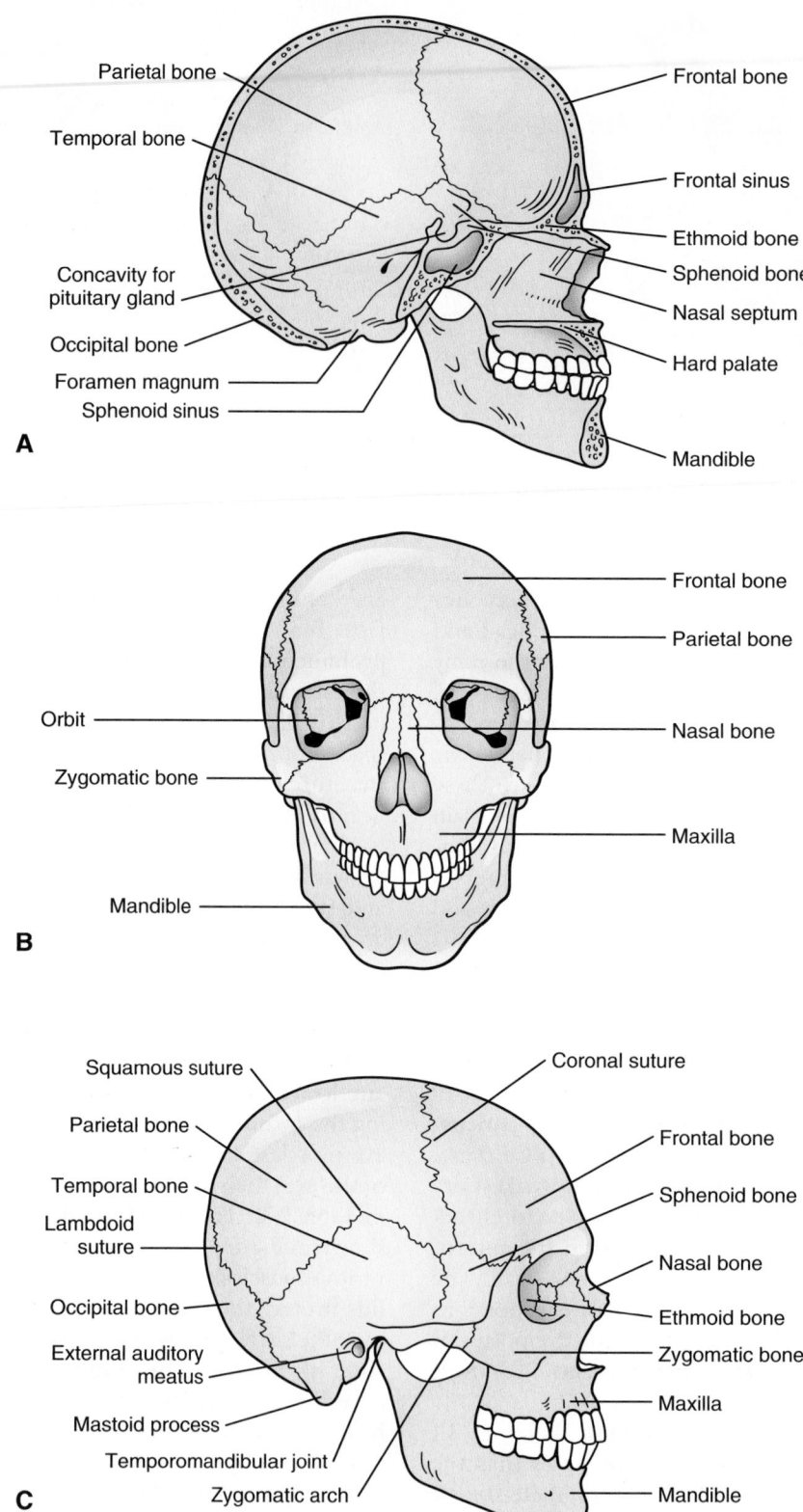

Figure 2-1

Bones of the head and face. **A,** Interior view. **B,** Anterior view. **C,** Lateral view. (Redrawn from Jenkins DB: *Hollinshead's functional anatomy of the limbs and back*, pp. 332–333, Philadelphia, 1991, WB Saunders.)

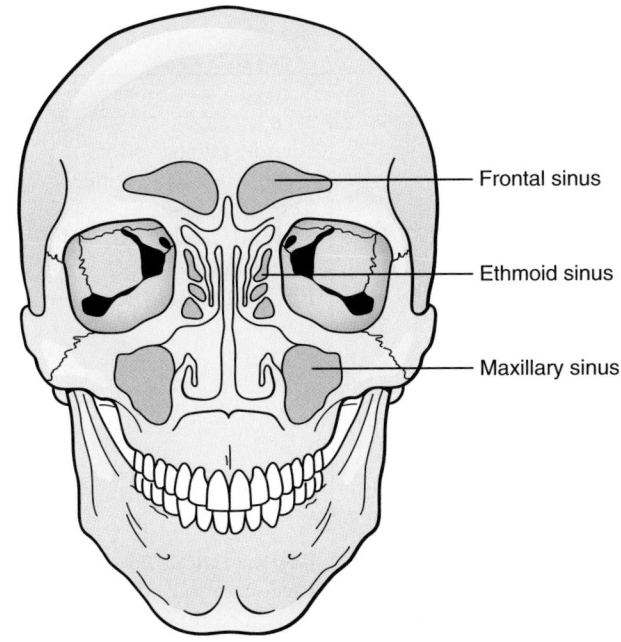

Figure 2-2
The nasal sinuses. (Modified from Swartz HM: *Textbook of physical diagnosis*, p. 166, Philadelphia, 1989, WB Saunders.)

pain that accompanies corneal abrasion) and separates the watery fluid of the anterior chamber of the eye from the external environment. It permits transmission of light through the lens to the retina. The **iris** is a circular, contractile muscular disc that controls the amount of light entering the eye and contains pigmented cells that give color to the eye. The **lens** is a crystalline structure located immediately behind the iris that permits images from varied distances to be focused on the retina. It is primarily the lens and its supporting ligaments that separate the eye into chambers: the anterior chamber (aqueous humor) and the posterior chamber (vitreous humor). Finally, the **retina** is the primary sensory structure of the eye that transforms light impulses into electrical impulses that are then transmitted by the optic nerve to the brain, which interprets the impulses as the objects seen.

The **external ear** consists of cartilage covered with skin. Its primary purpose is to direct sound and to protect the external auditory meatus, through which sound is transmitted to the eardrum. The external ear, which is sometimes called the pinna, auricle, or trumpet, consists of the helix and lobule around the outside and the triangular fossa, antihelix, concha, tragus (a cartilaginous projection anterior to external auditory meatus), and antitragus on the inside (Figure 2-7). The **middle ear** structures consist of the tympanic membrane, or eardrum, which vibrates when sound hits it and sends vibrations through the ossicles—called the malleus (hammer), incus (anvil), and stapes (stirrup)—to the cochlea. The cochlea, which

is part of the **inner ear**, transmits the sound waves to the vestibulocochlear nerve (cranial nerve VIII), which transmits electrical impulses to the brain for interpretation. The semicircular canals, the other part of the inner ear, play a significant role in maintaining balance.

The **external nose,** like the external ear, consists primarily of cartilage covered with skin. However, its proximal portion contains bone covered with skin. Figure 2-8 shows the bone and cartilage makeup of the nose. The floor of the nose consists of the hard and soft palates and forms the roof of the mouth (Figure 2-9). Cartilage and the nasal, frontal, ethmoid, and sphenoid bones form the roof of the nose. The frontal and maxillary bones form the nasal bridge. Three bony structures called turbinates (superior, middle, and inferior) form the lateral aspects of the nose, which increase the surface area of the nose and thereby warm, humidify, and filter more of the inspired air. The nose is divided into two chambers (vestibules) by a septum. These chambers are lined with a mucous membrane containing hairs that collect debris and other foreign substances from the inspired air. The cribriform plate of the ethmoid bone contains the sensory fibers of the olfactory nerve (cranial nerve I) for smell.

Patient History

In addition to the questions listed under Patient History in Chapter 1, the examiner should obtain the following information from the patient who has sustained an injury to the head or the face:

1. *What happened?* This question determines the mechanism of injury and, potentially, the area of the brain or face injured (Table 2-3). A forceful blow to a resting, movable head usually produces maximum brain injury beneath the point of impact (Figure 2-10). This type of injury, called a **coup injury,** is usually caused by linear or translational acceleration.[1] It often causes focal ischemic lesions, especially in the cerebellum, leading to alterations in smooth, coordinated movements, equilibrium, and posture. If the head is moving and strikes an unyielding object such as the ground, maximum brain injury is usually sustained in an area opposite the site of impact. This **contrecoup injury** is the result of impact deceleration. The injury occurs on the side of the head opposite to that receiving the blow because the head is accelerating before impact, which squeezes the cerebrospinal fluid away from the trailing edge (the side away from the impact). The fluid moves toward the impact side, thereby thickening the cerebrospinal fluid and offering a cushioning effect at the point of impact. Because of the lack of cushioning on the trailing edge, greater injury is likely to occur to the brain on the side opposite the impact. The brain may also experience a "shaking" caused by repeated

Table 2-1

Cranial Nerves and Methods of Testing

Nerve	Afferent (Sensory)	Efferent (Motor)	Test
I. Olfactory	Smell: Nose	—	Identify familiar odors (e.g., chocolate, coffee)
II. Optic	Sight: Eye	—	Test visual fields
III. Oculomotor	—	Voluntary motor: Levator of eyelid; superior, medial, and inferior recti; inferior oblique muscle of eyeball Autonomic: Smooth muscle of eyeball	Upward, downward, and medial gaze Reaction to light
IV. Trochlear		Voluntary motor: Superior oblique muscle of eyeball	Downward and lateral gaze
V. Trigeminal	Touch, pain: Skin of face, mucous membranes of nose, sinuses, mouth, anterior tongue	Voluntary motor: Muscles of mastication	Corneal reflex Face sensation Clench teeth; push down on chin to separate jaws
VI. Abducens		Voluntary motor: Lateral rectus muscle of eyeball	Lateral gaze
VII. Facial	Taste: Anterior tongue	Voluntary motor: Facial muscles Autonomic: Lacrimal, submandibular, and sublingual glands	Close eyes tight Smile and show teeth Whistle and puff cheeks Identify familiar tastes (e.g., sweet, sour)
VIII. Vestibulocochlear (acoustic nerve)	Hearing: Ear Balance: Ear	—	Hear watch ticking Hearing tests Balance and coordination test
IX. Glossopharyngeal	Touch, pain: Posterior tongue, pharynx Taste: Posterior tongue	Voluntary motor: Unimportant muscle of pharynx Autonomic: Parotid gland	Gag reflex Ability to swallow
X. Vagus	Touch, pain: Pharynx, larynx, bronchi Taste: Tongue, epiglottis	Voluntary motor: Muscles of palate, pharynx, and larynx Autonomic: Thoracic and abdominal viscera	Gag reflex Ability to swallow Say "Ah"
XI. Accessory	—	Voluntary motor: Sternocleidomastoid and trapezius muscle	Resisted shoulder shrug
XII. Hypoglossal	—	Voluntary motor: Muscles of tongue	Tongue protrusion (if injured, tongue deviates toward injured side)

Adapted from Hollinshead WH and Jenkins DB: *Functional anatomy of the limbs and back*, Philadelphia, 1981, WB Saunders, p. 358; and Reid DC: *Sports injury assessment and rehabilitation*, p. 860, New York, 1992, Churchill Livingstone.

reverberation within the brain after the head has been struck. This type of injury often results in the signs and symptoms of a concussion, with the degree of the concussion depending on the severity of the injury (Table 2-4). Concussion severity is only determined after signs and symptoms have disappeared and any neurological and cognitive testing is normal.[2] If the cervical spine is taken beyond its normal range of motion, especially into rotation or side flexion, there may be a twisting of the cerebral hemisphere, brain stem, carotid artery, or carotid sinus that can result in injury to these structures or ischemia to the brain.

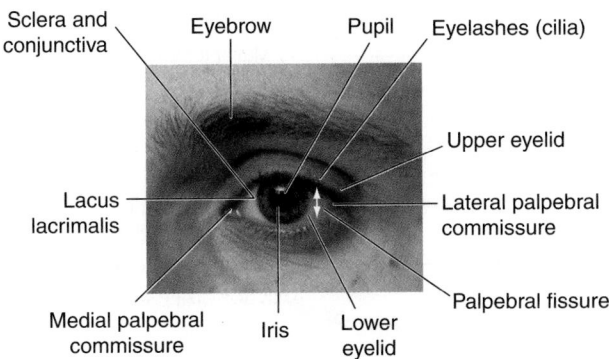

Figure 2-3
External features of the eye.

Those areas of the brain that are most susceptible to damage include the temporal lobes, anterior frontal lobe, posterior occipital lobe, and upper portion of the midbrain.[3]

2. *Did the patient lose consciousness? If so, how long was the patient unconscious? Has the patient suffered a concussion before?* These questions are often difficult for the patient to answer or the examiner to know, because the patient may have been momentarily stunned and the time may have been so short that the patient believed there was no loss of consciousness. In other words, loss of consciousness may have been only momentary or, more traditionally, it may have lasted seconds to minutes. If the examiner is working with a sports team, accurate records are essential to record the severity (see later discussion) and the number of concussions suffered by the athlete and to ensure that proper care is instituted so that the athlete is not allowed to return to competition too soon.

Table 2-2

Muscles of the Eye: Their Actions and Nerve Supply

Action	Muscles Acting	Nerve Supply
Moves pupil upward	Superior rectus	Oculomotor (CN III)
Moves pupil downward	Inferior rectus	Oculomotor (CN III)
Moves pupil medially	Medial rectus	Oculomotor (CN III)
Moves pupil laterally	Lateral rectus	Abducens (CN VI)
Moves pupil downward and laterally	Superior oblique	Trochlear (CN IV)
Moves pupil upward and laterally	Inferior oblique	Oculomotor (CN III)
Elevates upper eyelid	Levator palpebrae superioris	Oculomotor (CN III)

CN = cranial nerve.

A

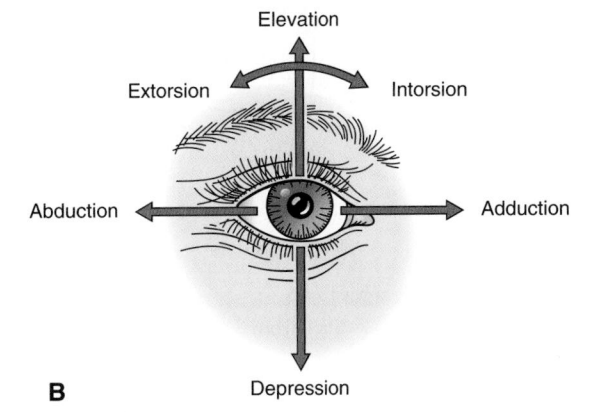

B

Figure 2-4
Muscles (**A**) and movements (**B**) of the eye. (Modified from Swartz HM: *Textbook of physical diagnosis*, pp. 125–126, Philadelphia, 1989, WB Saunders.)

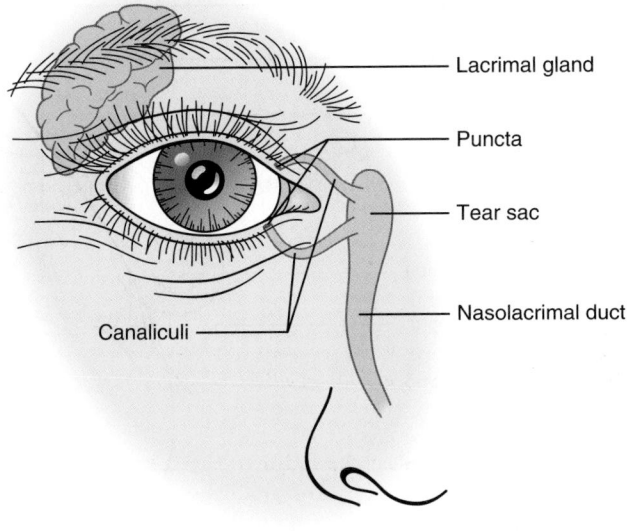

Figure 2-5
The lacrimal apparatus. (Modified from Swartz HM: *Textbook of physical diagnosis*, p. 126, Philadelphia, 1989, WB Saunders.)

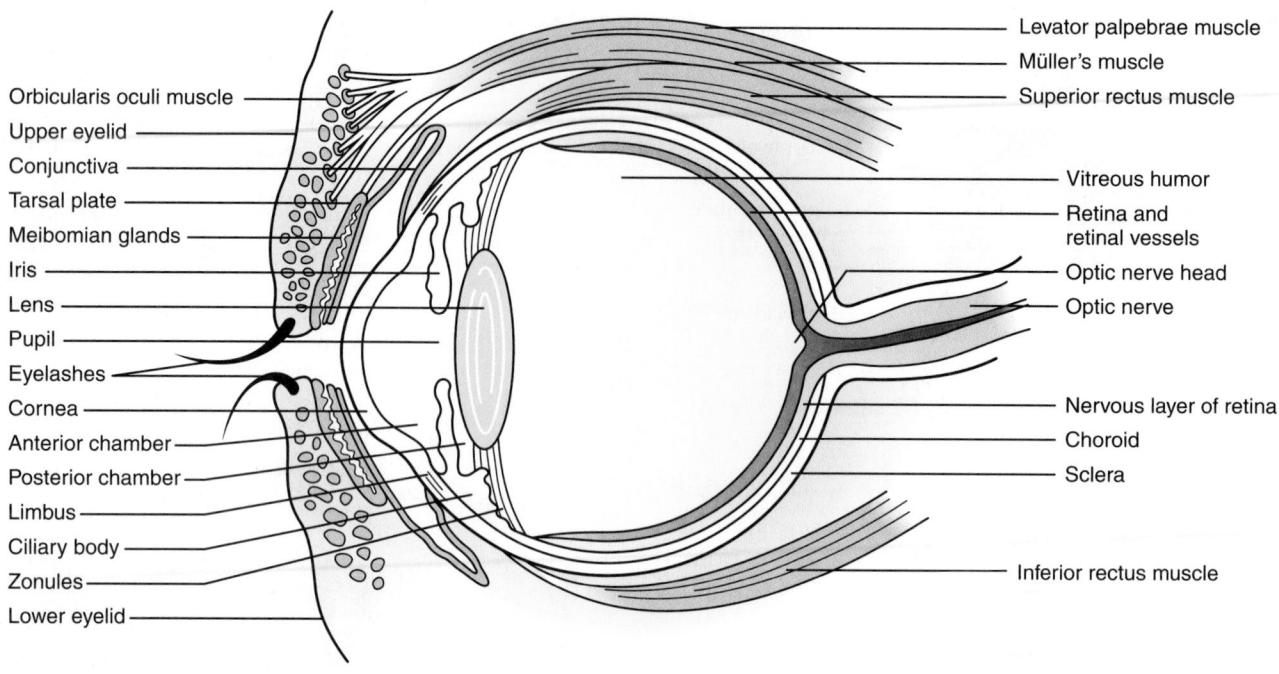

Figure 2-6

Cross section of the eye. (Modified from Swartz HM: *Textbook of physical diagnosis*, p. 132, Philadelphia, 1989, WB Saunders.)

Figure 2-7

A cross-sectional view through the ear.

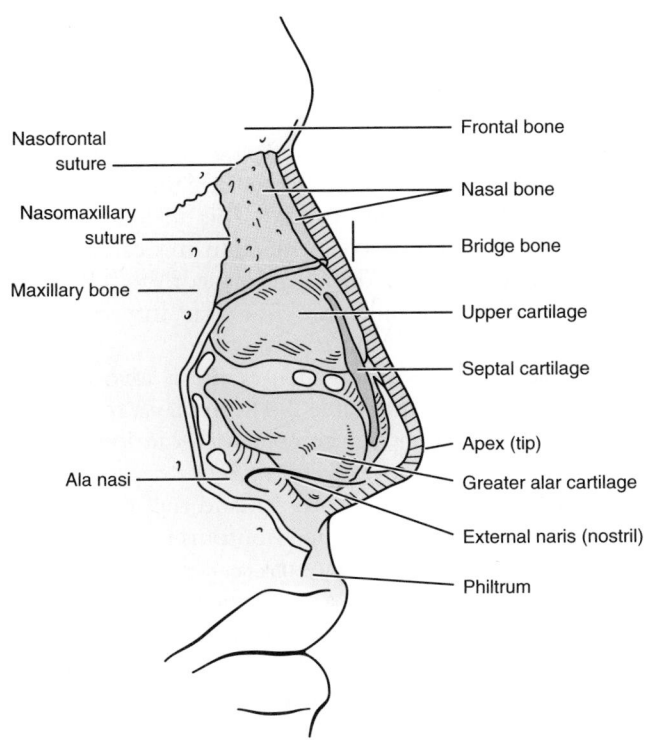

Figure 2-8
The bony and cartilaginous structures of the nose.

Concussions (which are examples of diffuse brain injuries) are the most common cause of loss of consciousness after trauma. They are defined as any alteration in cerebral function resulting from direct or indirect force to the head. Signs and symptoms of concussions are shown in Table 2-5.[4-6] **Concussions** can result from a blow to the head or jaw or a fall on the buttocks from a height and can result in an inability to process information. Their effect is cumulative, and the risk of having another concussion following an initial concussion is four to six times greater than someone who has not had a concussion.[5,7] Concussions can lead to continued and severe problems (e.g., postconcussion syndrome, second-impact syndrome).[5,7-9] To be maximally effective, athletes should have done baseline tests in their preparticipation evaluation and have an extensive concussion history taken covering somatic, neurobehavioral, and cognitive symptoms (see Table 2-6 for example).[2,5,10-13] The International Conference on Concussion in Sport in 2004 developed the sideline concussion assessment tool (SCAT) (Figure 2-11). Kelly and Rosenberg[5,6] have developed a Standardized Assessment of Concussion (SAC) (Figure 2-12),[14,15] which provides a concise evaluation method for concussion by including measures of orientation, immediate memory, concentration, delayed recall, and other

Figure 2-9
Cross section of the nose and nasopharynx.

Table 2-3

Areas of the Brain and Their Function

Cerebrum	Cognitive aspects of motor control
	Memory
	Sensory awareness (e.g., pain, touch)
	Speech
	Special senses (e.g., taste, vision)
Cerebellum	Coordinate and integrate motor behavior
	Balance
	Motor learning
	Motor control (muscle contraction and force production)
Diencephalon (thalamus)	Regulation of body temperature and water balance
	Control of emotions
	Information processing to cerebrum
Brain stem	Control of respiratory and heart rates
	Peripheral blood flow control

parameters. Lovell and Burke have developed a similar form for ice hockey.[16]

There are several different grading systems for concussions (Table 2-7). It should be pointed out, however, that the International Conference on Concussion in Sport[2] recommended that grade scales be abandoned as concussion severity can only be determined retrospectively after all signs and symptoms have cleared, the neurological examination is normal, and cognitive function has returned to normal.[17] The conference group felt concussions should be grouped as simple or complex. Simple concussion implies that the injury resolves over 7 to 10 days without complications. Neurophysiological screening does not play a role, but mental status screening is part of the assessment. Complex concussions are those in which persistent symptoms and specific sequelae (i.e., convulsions, loss of consciousness for longer than 1 minute, prolonged cognitive impairment) occur.[2] This includes people with more than one concussion. In this case, neurophysiological testing does play a role.[13,18–21] Table 2-8 shows some neurophysiological tests that could be used for postconcussion assessment.

Grades of concussion such as those advocated by Torg (see below and Table 2-4) can play a role in the acute phase but should be used with caution if making return to activity decisions.[22] With each grade, the signs and symptoms worsen and the sequelae are more evident. No signs and symptoms under exertion (i.e., simulating the activity the person will return to) should be evident, even with simple concussions.

With a **grade I concussion,** the patient is slightly confused and may have a dazed look. The patient is completely lucid within 5 to 15 minutes; has no amnesia, sequelae, or residual symptoms; and has had no loss of consciousness. Some people refer to the grade I concussion as the patient's having his or her "bell rung."

With a **grade II concussion,** there is slight confusion, and posttraumatic amnesia becomes evident. **Posttraumatic (anterograde) amnesia** is the loss of memory for events occurring immediately after wakening or from the moment of injury. Posttraumatic amnesia is considered to be the length of time from injury until conscious memory returns. In the acute state, it may take time for posttraumatic amnesia to become obvious. Sometimes, the patient will remember what happened immediately after the injury, but as time goes on (up to 1 to 2 hours after the injury),

LINEAR ACCELERATION
(Coupe injury)

IMPACT DECELERATION
(Contracoupe injury)

ROTATIONAL ACCELERATION
(Rotation and side flexion of head)

Figure 2-10

Mechanisms of injury to the brain.

Table 2-4
Signs and Symptoms* of Concussion (Torg Classification)

	Grade 1	Grade 2	Grade 3	Grade 4	Grade 5
Confusion	None or momentary	Slight	Moderate	Severe	Severe
Amnesia	No	Posttraumatic amnesia <30 min	Posttraumatic amnesia <30 min Retrograde amnesia	Posttraumatic amnesia >30 min Retrograde amnesia	Posttraumatic amnesia >24 hours Retrograde amnesia
Residual symptoms	No	Perhaps	Sometimes	Yes	Yes
Loss of consciousness	No	No	No	Yes (<5 min)	Yes (>5 min)
Tinnitus	No	Mild	Moderate	Severe	Often severe
Dizziness	No	Mild	Moderate	Severe	Usually severe
Headache	No	May be present (dull)	Often	Often	Often
Disorientation and unsteadiness	None or minimal	Some	Moderate	Severe (5–10 min)	Often severe (>10 min)
Blurred vision	No	No	No	Not usually	Possible
Postconcussion syndrome	No	Possible	Possible	Possible	Possible
Personality changes	No	No	No	Possible	Possible

Data from Vegso JJ and Torg JS: Field evaluation and management of intracranial injuries. In Torg JS, editor: *Athletic injuries to the head, neck and face*, pp. 226–227, St. Louis, 1991, Mosby.
*These signs and symptoms should only be used as a guide in acute situations.

Table 2-5
Signs and Symptoms of Concussions

Acute	Late (Delayed)
Lightheadedness	Persistent low-grade headache
Delayed motor or verbal responses	Easy fatigability
Memory or cognitive dysfunction	Sleep irregularities
Disorientation	Inability to perform daily activities
Amnesia	Depression/anxiety
Headache	Lethargy
Balance problems/ incoordination	Memory dysfunction
Vertigo/dizziness	Lightheadedness
Concentration difficulties	Personality changes
Loss of consciousness	Low frustration tolerance/ irritability
Blurred vision	Intolerance to bright lights, loud sounds
Vacant stare (befuddled facial expression)	
Photophobia	
Tinnitus	
Nausea	
Vomiting	
Increased emotionality	
Slurred or incoherent speech	

posttraumatic amnesia becomes evident. This is one of the reasons it is advisable to reassess acute head injuries every 15 to 30 minutes. Manzi and Weaver reported that a patient who had sustained a period of posttraumatic amnesia of less than 60 minutes was considered to have sustained a mild head injury.[23] If the period of posttraumatic amnesia lasted from 1 to 24 hours, moderate head injury was considered

Table 2-6
Concussion Symptoms

Somatic	Neurobehavioral	Cognitive
Headache Nausea Vomiting Balance problems Light/sound sensitivity Numbness/ tingling	Sleeping more than usual Drowsiness Fatigue Sadness Nervousness Trouble falling asleep	Feeling "slowed down" Feeling "in a fog" Concentration difficulty Remembering difficulty

Data from Piland SG et al: Structural validity of a self-report concussion-related symptoms scale, *Med Sci Sports Exerc* 38:27–32, 2006.

Sport Concussion Assessment Tool (SCAT)

This tool represents a standardized method of evaluating people after concussion in sport. This tool has been produced as part of the Summary and Agreement Statement of the Second International Symposium on Concussion in Sport, Prague 2004

  IIHF

The SCAT Card
(Sport Concussion Assessment Tool)
Athlete Information

What is a concussion? A concussion is a disturbance in the function of the brain caused by a direct or indirect force to the head. It results in a variety of symptoms (like those listed below) and may, or may not, involve memory problems or loss of consciousness.

How do you feel? You should score yourself on the following symptoms, based on how you feel now.

Post Concussion Symptom Scale

	None		Moderate			Severe	
Headache	0	1	2	3	4	5	6
"Pressure in head"	0	1	2	3	4	5	6
Neck pain	0	1	2	3	4	5	6
Balance problemsor dizzy	0	1	2	3	4	5	6
Nausea or vomiting	0	1	2	3	4	5	6
Vision problems	0	1	2	3	4	5	6
Hearing problems/ringing	0	1	2	3	4	5	6
"Don't feel right"	0	1	2	3	4	5	6
Feeling "dinged"or "dazed"	0	1	2	3	4	5	6
Confusion	0	1	2	3	4	5	6
Feeling slowed down	0	1	2	3	4	5	6
Feeling like "in a fog"	0	1	2	3	4	5	6
Drowsiness	0	1	2	3	4	5	6
Fatigue or low energy	0	1	2	3	4	5	6
More emotional than usual	0	1	2	3	4	5	6
Irritability	0	1	2	3	4	5	6
Difficulty concentrating	0	1	2	3	4	5	6
Difficulty remembering	0	1	2	3	4	5	6

(follow up symptoms only)

Sadness	0	1	2	3	4	5	6
Nervous or anxious	0	1	2	3	4	5	6
Trouble falling asleep	0	1	2	3	4	5	6
Sleeping more than usual	0	1	2	3	4	5	6
Sensitivity to light	0	1	2	3	4	5	6
Sensitivity to noise	0	1	2	3	4	5	6
Other: _____	0	1	2	3	4	5	6

Sports concussion is defined as a complex pathophysiological process affecting the brain, induced by traumatic biomechanical forces. Several common features that incorporate clinical, pathological and biomechanical injury constructs that may be utilized in defining the nature of a concussive head injury include:

1. Concussion may be caused either by a direct blow to the head, face, neck or elsewhere on the body with an "impulsive" force transmitted to the head.
2. Concussion typically results in the rapid onset of short-lived impairment of neurological function that resolves spontaneously.
3. Concussion may result in neuropathological changes but the acute clinical symptoms largely reflect a functional disturbance rather than structural injury.
4. Concussion results in a graded set of clinical syndromes that may or may not involve loss of consciousness. Resolution of the clinical and cognitive symptoms typically follows a sequential course.
5. Concussion is typically associated with grossly normal structural neuroimaging studies.

Post Concussion Symptoms

Ask the athlete to score themselves based on how they eel now. It is recognized that a low score may be normal for some athletes, but clinical judgment should be exercised to determine if a change in symptoms has occurred following the suspected concussion event.

It should be recognized that the reporting of symptoms may not be entirely reliable. This may be due to the effects of a concussion or because the athlete's passionate desire to return to competition outweighs their natural inclination to give an honest response.

If possible, ask someone who knows the athlete well about changes in affect, personality, behavior, etc.

Remember, concussion should be suspected in the presence of ANY ONE or more of the following:
- Symptoms (such as headache), or
- Signs (such as loss of consciousness), or
- Memory problems

Any athlete with a suspected concussion should be monitored for deterioration (i.e., shouldnot be left alone) and should not drive a motor vehicle.

For more information see the "Summary and Agreement Statement of the Second International Symposium on Concussion in Sport" in the April 2005 edition of the *Clinical Journal of Sport Medicine* (vol 15), *British Journal of Sports Medicine* (vol 39), *Neurosurgery* (vol 59) and the *Physician and Sportsmedicine* (vol 33). This tool may be copied for distribution to teams, groups and organizations. ©2005 Concussion in Sport Group

What should I do?
Any athlete suspected of having a concussion should be removed from play, and then seek medical evaluation.

Signs to watch for:
Problems could arise over the first 24-48 hours.You should not be left alone and must go to a hospital at once if you:
- Have a headache that gets worse
- Are very drowsy or can't be awakened (woken up)
- Can't recognize people or places
- Have repeated vomiting
- Behave unusually or seem confused; are very irritable
- Have seizures (arms and legs jerk uncontrollably)
- Have weak or numb arms or legs
- Are unsteady on your feet; have slurred speech

Remember, it is better to be safe. Consult your doctor after a suspected concussion.

What can I expect?
Concussion typically results in the rapid onset of short-lived impairment that resolves spontaneously over time.You can expect that you will be told to rest until you are fully recovered (that means resting your body and your mind).Then, your doctor will likely advise that you go through a gradual increase in exercise over several days (or longer) before returning to sport.

Figure 2-11

© Concussion in Sport Group.

Sport Concussion Assessment Tool (SAC) and instructions. (From McCrory PK et al: Summary and agreement statement of the 2nd International Conference on Concussion in Sport, Prague 2004, *Clin J Sports Med* 15:48–55, 2005.)

Sport Concussion Assessment Tool (SCAT)

  IIHF

The SCAT Card
(Sport Concussion Assessment Tool)
Medical Evaluation

Name: _____ Date _____

Sport/Team: _____ Mouth guard? Y N

1) SIGNS
Was there loss of consciousness or unresponsiveness? Y N
Was there seizure or convulsive activity? Y N
Was there a balance problem / unsteadiness? Y N

2) MEMORY
Modified Maddocks questions (check correct)

At what venue are we? __; Which half is it? __; Who scored last?__

What team did we play last? __; Did we win last game? __

3) SYMPTOM SCORE
Total number of positive symptoms (from reverse side of the card) = _____

4) COGNITIVE ASSESSMENT

5-word recall	(Examples)	Immediate	Delayed (after concentration tasks)
Word 1 _____	cat	___	___
Word 2_____	pen	___	___
Word 3 _____	shoe	___	___
Word 4 _____	book	___	___
Word 5 _____	car	___	___

Months in reverse order :
Jun-May-Apr-Mar-Feb-Jan-Dec-Nov-Oct-Sep-Aug-Jul (circle incorrect)

or

Digits backwards (check correct)
5-2-8   3-9-1   _____
6-2-9-4   4-3-7-1   _____
8-3-2-7-9   1-4-9-3-6   _____
7-3-9-1-4-2 5-1-8-4-6-8 _____

Ask delayed 5-word recall now

5) NEUROLOGIC SCREENING

	Pass	Fail
Speech	___	___
Eye Motion and Pupils	___	___
Pronator Drift	___	___
Gait Assessment	___	___

Any neurologic screening abnormality necessitates formal neurologic or hospital assessment

6) RETURN TO PLAY
Athletes should not be returned to play the same day of injury.
When returning athletes to play, they should follow a stepwise symptom-limited program, with stages of progression. For example:
1. rest until asymptomatic (physical and mental rest)
2. light aerobic exercise (e.g., stationary cycle)
3. sport-specific exercise
4. non-contact training drills (start light resistance training)
5. full contact training after medical clearance
6. return to competition (game play)

There should be approximately 24 hours (or longer) for each stage and the athlete should return to stage 1 if symptoms recur. Resistance training should only be added in the later stages. Medical clearance should be given before return to play.

Instructions:
This side of the card is for the use of medical doctors, physiotherapists or athletic therapists. In order to maximize the information gathered from the card, it is strongly suggested that all athletes participating in contact sports complete a baseline evaluation prior to the beginning of their competitive season. This card is a suggested guide only for sports concussion and is not meant to assess more severe forms of brain injury. **Please give a COPY of this card to the athlete for their information and to guide follow-up assessment.**

Signs:
Assess for each of these items and circle Y (yes) or N (no).

Memory: If needed, questions can be modified to make them specific to the sport (e.g. "period" versus "half")

Cognitive Assessment:
Select any 5 words (an example is given). Avoid choosing related words such as "dark" and "moon," which can be recalled by means of word association. Read each word at a rate of oneword per second. The athlete should not be informed of the delayed testing of memory (to be done after the reverse months and/or digits). Choose a different set of words each time you perform a follow-up exam with the same candidate.
Ask the athlete to recite the months of the year in reverse order, starting with a random month. Do not start with December or January. Circle any months not recited in the correct sequence.
For digits backwards, if correct, go to the next string length. If incorrect, read trial 2. Stop after incorrect on both trials.

Neurologic Screening:
Trained medical personnel must administer this examination. These individuals might include medical doctors, physiotherapists or athletic therapists. Speech should be assessed for fluency and lack of slurring. Eye motion should reveal no diplopia in any of the 4 planes of movement (vertical, horizontal and both diagonal planes). The pronator drift is performed by asking the patient to hold both arms in front of them, palms up, with eyes closed. A positive test is pronating the forearm, dropping the arm, or drift away from midline. For gait assessment, ask the patient to walk away from you, turn and walk back.

Return to Play:
A structured, graded exertion protocol should be developed, individualized on the basis of sport, age and the concussion history of the athlete. Exercise or training should be commenced only after the athlete is clearly asymptomatic with physical and cognitive rest. Final decision for clearance to return to competition should ideally be made by a medical doctor.

For more information see the "Summary and Agreement Statement of the Second International Symposium on Concussion in Sport" in the April 2005 *Clinical Journal of Sport Medicine* (vol 15), *British Journal of Sports Medicine* (vol 39), *Neurosurgery* (vol 59) and the *Physician and Sportsmedicine* (vol 33). ©2005 Concussion in Sport Group

Figure 2-11 cont'd

SAC: Standardized Assessment of Concussion

NAME: _____

AGE: ____ SEX: ____ EXAMINER: _____

Nature of Injury: _____

Date of Exam: _____ Time: _____ No. _____

1) ORIENTATION:

Month: _____	0	1
Date: _____	0	1
Day of Week: _____	0	1
Year: _____	0	1
Time (within 1 hour): _____	0	1

Orientation Total Score _____ /5

2) IMMEDIATE MEMORY: (all 3 trials are completed regardless of score on trials 1 & 2; score equals sum across all 3 trials)

LIST	TRIAL 1	TRIAL 2	TRIAL 3
Elbow	0 1	0 1	0 1
Apple	0 1	0 1	0 1
Carpet	0 1	0 1	0 1
Saddle	0 1	0 1	0 1
Bubble	0 1	0 1	0 1
Total			

Immediate Memory Score _____ /15

3) CONCENTRATION:

Digits Backward: (If correct, go to next string length. If incorrect, read trial 2. Stop after incorrect on both trials.)

4-9-3	6-2-9	0	1
3-8-1-4	3-2-7-9	0	1
6-2-9-7-1	1-5-2-8-6	0	1
7-1-8-4-6-2	5-3-9-1-4-8	0	1

Months in Reverse Order: (entire reverse sequence correct for 1 point)
DEC-NOV-OCT-SEP-AUG-JUL
JUN-MAY-APR-MAR-FEB-JAN   0   1

Concentration Total Score _____ /5

EXERTIONAL MANEUVERS (when appropriate):

5 jumping jacks	5 push-ups
5 sit-ups	5 knee-bends

4) DELAYED RECALL

Elbow	0	1
Apple	0	1
Carpet	0	1
Saddle	0	1
Bubble	0	1

Delayed Recall Score _____ /5

SUMMARY OF TOTAL SCORES:

Orientation	_____ / 5
Immediate Memory	_____ / 15
Concentration	_____ / 5
Delayed Recall	_____ / 5
OVERALL TOTAL SCORE	_____ / 30

Figure 2-12

Standardized Assessment of Concussion (SAC). (Redrawn from McCrea M et al: Standard assessment of concussion in football players, *Neurology* 48:586–588, 1997.)

to have occurred. If the posttraumatic amnesia lasted for more than 1 week, the patient was considered to have sustained a serious head injury. If the duration of the posttraumatic amnesia was more than 7 days, full return to neurological function was highly unlikely.[23] With a grade II concussion, the patient may experience mild tinnitus (ringing in the ears), mild dizziness, and a dull headache with some disorientation.

The patient who experienced a grade II concussion may also develop a **postconcussion syndrome** (i.e., have continual neurological problems after the concussion), which is observed in about 10% of concussion cases. The signs and symptoms of this syndrome include persistent headaches, especially with exertion; inability to concentrate; and irritability. The symptoms may last from several weeks to several years.

Head Injury Severity Based on Length of Posttraumatic Amnesia

<60 minutes:	Mild
1–24 hours:	Moderate
>1 week:	Serious (full return of neurological function unlikely)

A patient with a **grade III concussion** has the same symptoms as someone with a grade II concussion and also experiences retrograde amnesia. **Retrograde amnesia** is loss of memory of events that occurred before the injury. It may take 5 to 10 minutes for retrograde amnesia to develop after the concussion, and amnesia may involve only a few minutes before the injury. For this reason, the patient should be questioned frequently about what happened before the injury occurred and how it occurred, to see if there is any change in the patient's memory pattern. There is always some degree of permanent retrograde amnesia with these patients.

With a **grade IV concussion,** the patient loses consciousness for 5 minutes or less. The level of consciousness may vary; the patient may be comatose, stuporous, obtunded, lethargic, confused, or fully alert. The patient goes through the following stages of recovery: unconsciousness (also called paralytic coma), stupor, obtundity, lethargy, confusion (with or without delirium), near lucidity with automatism, and finally full alertness. **Stupor** implies that the patient is only partially conscious and has reduced responsiveness. **Obtundity** implies the patient has reduced sensitivity to painful or unpleasant stimuli. **Lethargy** implies a state of sluggishness, dullness, or serious drowsiness. **Confusion** implies that the patient is disoriented in terms of time, place, or person. **Delirium** means that the patient may experience illusions, hallucinations, restlessness, or incoherence. **Lucidity with automatism** implies that the patient appears to be alert and fully recovered but acts only mechanically and is not really aware of what he or she is doing. With a grade IV concussion, there may be subtle changes in the patient's personality and memory function. Both retrograde and posttraumatic amnesia are evident, and the patient demonstrates mental confusion and complains of tinnitus and dizziness to a greater degree than is seen with a grade III concussion. The patient also has residual headaches and are unsteady for 5 to 10 minutes after regaining consciousness. The literature has reported that loss of consciousness, by itself, is not a good predictor of the degree of neurophysiological loss or damage with a head injury.[24] The severity of the head injury is best determined by the administration of different neurophysiological tests (e.g., GOAT test,[25] Hopkins Verbal Learning Test,[26] Trail Making Test, Wisconsin Card Sorting Test, Digit Symbol Substitution Test [DSST],[27] measures of decision time[27]) as well as considering all signs and symptoms the patient demonstrates.[28] To ensure adequate data, however, these tests must also have been administered before the injury (e.g., in a preparticipation evaluation in sports).[4]

Table 2-7

Classification Systems for Concussions

System	Grade I (Mild)	Grade Ia	Grade II (Moderate)	Grade III (Severe)	Grade IV
Cantu	No LOC or PTA <30 min	N/A	LOC <5 min, PTA 30 min to 24 h	LOC >5 min, PTA >24 h	N/A
Torg	(Grade I to II) No LOC or amnesia (except PTA)	N/A	(Grade III-IV) LOC <few minutes, PTA or retrograde amnesia	(Grade V-VI) LOC/coma, confusion, amnesia	N/A
Colorado Consortium	Confusion without amnesia, no LOC	N/A	Confusion and amnesia, no LOC	LOC	N/A
Virginia Neurological Institute	Short LOC, PTA <1 h, GCS score = 15	Short LOC, PTA 1 to 24 h, GCS score = 15	LOC <5 min, PTA ≥ 24 h, GCS score >15 for <5 min	LOC <5 min, PTA N/A, GCS score <15 for <1 h	LOC 5 to 60 min, PTA N/A, GCS score <12 for >5 min or <15 for >1 h
American Academy of Neurology	No LOC, Sxs <15 min	N/A	No LOC, Sxs >15 min	Any LOC	N/A

From Durand P and Adamson GJ: On-the-field management of athletic head injuries, *J Am Acad Orthop* Surg 12:194, 2004. Adapted with permission from Macciocchi SN et al: Outcome after mild head injury, *Clin Sports Med* 17:27–36, 1998.

LOC = loss of consciousness; PTA = posttraumatic amnesia; GCS = Glasgow Coma Scale; Sxs = signs and symptoms.

Table 2-8

Examples of Neurophysiological Tests

Test	Ability Evaluated
Continuous Performance Test	Sustained attention, reaction time
Controlled Oral Word Association Test	Word fluency, word retrieval
Delayed Recall (from Hopkins Verbal Learning Test)	Delayed learning from previously learned word list
Digit Span (from Wechsler Memory Scale, revised)	Attention span
Grooved-Pegboard Test	Motor speed and coordination
Hopkins Verbal Learning Test	Verbal memory (memory for words)
Immediate Measurement of Performance and Cognitive Testing (IMPACT)	Attention span, sustained and selective attention, reaction time, memory
Number/Symbol Matching	Processing speed, visual motor speed
Orientation Questionnaire	Orientation, posttraumatic amnesia
Sequential Digit Tracking	Sustained attention, reaction time
Stroop Test	Mental flexibility, attention
Symbol Digit Modalities	Visual scanning, attention
Symbol Memory	Immediate visual memory
Trail-making Test	Visual scanning, mental flexibility
Verbal Working Memory	Word memory, working memory
Visual Span	Visual attention, immediate memory
Visual Symbol Search	Visual scanning, reaction time
Word/Colour Tracking	Focused attention, response inhibition

Data from Maroon JC et al: Cerebral concussion in athletes: evaluation and neurophysiological testing, *Neurosurg* 47:659–672, 2000.

Levels of Consciousness

Alertness	Is readily aroused, oriented and fully aware of surroundings
Confusion	Memory is impaired Is confused and disoriented
Lethargy	Sleeps when not stimulated Is drowsy and inattentive Responds to name Loses train of thought Shows decreased spontaneous movement Has slow and fuzzy thinking
Obtundity	Responds to loud voice or shaking Responds to painful stimulus (withdrawal) Is confused when aroused Talks in monosyllables Mumbles and is incoherent Needs constant stimulation to cooperate
Stupor (semicoma)	Responds to painful stimuli (withdrawal), shaking Groans, mumbles Exhibits reflex activity
Coma	Does not respond to painful or any other stimuli

With a **grade V concussion,** the patient has experienced a paralytic coma or unconsciousness for 5 minutes or longer. This grade of concussion involves bruising of the brain, and there is prolonged retrograde amnesia as well as posttraumatic amnesia. The patient complains of severe tinnitus, unsteadiness for longer than 10 minutes, blurred vision, poor light accommodation, and a headache that feels "different" from most headaches. Both the autonomic and the peripheral nervous systems can be affected through their control by the brain. These patients may also experience nausea, vomiting, and sometimes convulsions. The recovery after a grade V concussion may be one of two types. In type A, the patient goes from a paralytic coma through stupor, confusion, lucidity, and full alertness, which is similar to a grade IV concussion but more severe. The individual with a type B grade V concussion experiences a paralytic coma that is associated with secondary cardiorespiratory collapse and is of much greater concern to the examiner, especially during the initial assessment, when the body's essential functions must be maintained.

More severe diffuse brain injuries are associated with more severe neurological dysfunction. With these injuries, loss of consciousness lasts for more than 24 hours and recovery is never complete, leading to deficits in intelligence, reasoning, and memory and to changes in personality. Shearing brain injuries tend to be more severe than diffuse brain injuries and lead to abnormal brain stem signs such as decerebrate rigidity.[22]

3. *If the patient has had an injury to the head, are there any associated symptoms in the neck or problems with breathing, altered vision, discharge from the nose or ears, or urinary or fecal incontinence?* These symptoms indicate severe brain or spinal cord injury, and the patient must be handled with extreme care.

4. *What are the sites and boundaries of pain?* This question helps the examiner determine what structures have been injured. It is important to keep in mind that the patient may be experiencing a referral of pain.

5. *What type of pain is the patient experiencing?* The type of pain indicates the type of structure injured (see Table 1-4).

6. *Is there any paresthesia, abnormal sensation, or lack of sensation?* Are smell (cranial nerve I), vision (cranial nerve II), taste (cranial nerve VII), and hearing (cranial nerve VIII) normal? These questions give the examiner some idea of whether neurological structures (especially the cranial nerves) have been injured and, if so, which ones.

Head Signs and Symptoms Requiring Specialist Care

- Presence of amnesia
- Prolonged residual symptoms
- Loss of consciousness
- Prolonged headache
- Postconcussion syndrome
- Personality changes
- More than one first- or second-degree concussion
- Prolonged disorientation, unsteadiness, or confusion (>2–3 min)
- Blurred vision
- Dizziness (>5 min)
- Tinnitus (>5 min)

7. *What activities aggravate the particular problem?*
8. *What activities ease the particular problem?*
9. *Does the patient have a **headache** and, if so, where (Tables 2-9 and 2-10)? Is the headache tolerable?* What type of headache is it? Is it a throbbing, pounding, boring, shocklike, dull, nagging, or constant-pressure type of headache? Is the pain of the headache aggravated by movement or by rest? What is the exact location of the headache? Is the headache affected by position or time of day (Table 2-11)? Does it cover the entire head, the sinus region, or behind the eyes? Does it present a "hat band" distribution, or does it affect

Table 2-9

Type of Headache Pain and Usual Causes

Type of Pain	Usual Causes
Acute	Trauma, acute infection, impending cerebrovascular accident, subarachnoid hemorrhage
Chronic, recurrent	Migraine (definite pattern of irregular interval); eyestrain; noise; excessive eating, drinking, or smoking; inadequate ventilation
Continuous, recurrent	Trauma
Severe, intense	Meningitis, aneurysm (ruptured), migraine, brain tumor
Intense, transient, shocklike	Neuralgia
Throbbing, pulsating (vascular)	Migraine, fever, hypertension, aortic insufficiency, neuralgia
Constant, tight (bandlike), bilateral	Muscle contraction

Table 2-10

Location of Headache and Usual Causes

Location	Usual Causes
Forehead	Sinusitis, eye or nose disorder, muscle spasm of occipital or suboccipital region
Side of head	Migraine, eye or ear disorder, auriculotemporal neuralgia
Occipital	Myofascial problems, herniated disc, eyestrain, hypertension, occipital neuralgia
Parietal	Hysteria (viselike), meningitis, constipation, tumor
Face	Maxillary sinusitis, trigeminal neuralgia, dental problems, tumor

Table 2-11

Effect of Position or Time of Day on Headache

Position or Time of Day When Headache Is Worst	Usual Causes
Morning	Sinusitis, migraine, hypertension, alcoholism, sleeping position
Afternoon	Eyestrain, muscle tension
Night	Intracranial disease, osteomyelitis, nephritis
Bending	Sinusitis
Lying horizontal	Migraine

the neck or the occiput area? It is important for the examiner to record the location, character, duration, and frequency of the headache, as well as any factors that appear to either aggravate or relieve the pain, so that a diagnosis can be made and any changes can be noted (Table 2-12).

10. *Is the patient dizzy or unsteady or having problems with balance?* The examiner should also note whether the dizziness occurs when the patient suddenly stands up, turns, or bends, or whether it occurs without movement. Remember that "dizziness" is a word that patients sometimes use to indicate unsteadiness in walking. Dizziness is usually associated with problems of the middle ear, vertebrobasilar insufficiency, or problems in the upper cervical spine. Vertigo implies a rotary component; the patient's environment seems to whirl around the patient, or the patient's body seems to rotate in relation to the environment. If the patient complains of dizziness or vertigo, the time of onset and duration of these attacks should be noted. A description of the type of motion that occurs and any other associated symptoms should be included. Balance may be affected by problems within the brain or the semicircular canals in the inner ear. The examiner should also note whether the patient is talking about unsteadiness, loss of balance, or actual falling.

11. *Is the patient unduly irritated or having trouble concentrating?* The patient's state indicates the severity of the injury.

12. *Does the patient know where he or she is, who he or she is, the day, and the time of day?* Does the patient have some idea of what was happening when the injury occurred? These types of questions reveal the severity of the injury.

13. *Does the patient have any memory of past events or what occurred before or after the injury?* This type of question tests for retrograde amnesia, posttraumatic amnesia, and injury severity, which can be determined by asking the patient straightforward questions about events in the patient's own past, such as birth date or year of graduation from high school or university. The examiner may also ask questions about the injury, preceding events, and posttraumatic events. Questions such as "What day is it?" "Who is the opposition?" "Who is winning?" and "What is your telephone number and address?" test the patient's static memory ability. The examiner must ensure that he or she or someone present at the time of the examination knows the answer to these questions. The examiner can test **recent memory** by asking the patient to remember the names for two to five persons or common objects, such as the color "red," the number "five," the name "Mr. Smith," and the word "pride," and then asking the patient to name them 5 or 10 minutes later. The patient may be asked to repeat the words two or

three times when the examiner initially says them to test immediate recall or to ensure that the patient can say and recall the words. **Immediate recall,** another form of memory, is best tested by asking the patient to repeat a series of single digits. Normally, a person can repeat at least six digits, and many people can repeat eight or nine. The examiner may also ask the patient to repeat the months of the year backward in a similar type of test. Memory is generally thought to be formed and stored in certain regions of the temporal lobes. The parietal lobe of the brain is thought to enable one to appreciate the environment, to interpret visual stimuli, and to communicate.

Common Head Injury Tests

- Static memory (What day is it? Who's winning?)
- Immediate recall (repeat series of single digits)
- Recent memory (recall three common objects or names after 15 minutes)
- Short term memory (What is the game plan?)
- Processing and concentration ability (minus-7 test, multiplying)
- Abstract relationships
- Coordination (eye-hand tests)
- Balance (Romberg test)
- Myotomes
- Eye coordination
- Visual disturbance tests

---

14. *Can the patient solve simple problems?* Because concussions reduce one's ability to process information, it is important to determine the patient's **reasoning and processing ability.** For example, does the patient know his or her home telephone number? Is the patient able to do the "minus 7" or "serial 7" test (i.e., count backward from 100 by sevens)? This test gives the examiner some idea of the patient's calculating ability and concentration skills. Mathematic ability (the ability to add, subtract, multiply, and divide) can also be evaluated to test processing ability. In addition, the examiner can ask the patient to name several important people from the present in reverse chronological order (e.g., the last three presidents of the United States) or to give the names of some familiar capital cities. Finally, the patient should be tested on his or her ability to comprehend abstract relations. For example, the examiner may quote a common proverb such as "A bird in the hand is worth two in the bush" and then ask the patient to explain what the expression means. Patients with organic mental impairment and certain patients with schizophrenia may give a concrete answer, failing to recognize the abstract principle involved.[23] The ability to conceptualize, abstract, plan

Table 2-12

Headaches: A Differential Diagnosis

Disorder	Sex/Age Predominance	Nature of Pain	Frequency	Location	Duration	Prodromal Events	Precipitating Factors	Cause	Familial Predisposition	Other Possible Symptoms
Migraine	Female/20 to 40 years	Builds to throbbing and intense	Usually not more than twice a week May be nocturnal	Usually unilateral	Several hours to days	Visual disturbances can occur contralateral to pain site	Unknown, may be physical, emotional, hormonal, dietary	Vasomotor	Yes	Nausea, vomiting, pallor, photophobia, mood disturbances, fluid retention
Cluster (histamine) headache	Male/40 to 60 years	Excruciating, stabbing, burning, pulsating	One to four episodes per 24 hours Nocturnal manifestation	Unilateral, eye, temple, forehead	Minutes to hours	Sleep disturbances or personality changes can occur	Unknown, may be serotonin, histamine, hormonal blood flow	Vasomotor	Minor	Ipsilateral sweating of face, lacrimation, nasal congestion or discharge
Hypertension headache	None	Dull, throbbing, nonlocalized	Variable	Entire cranium, especially occipital region	Variable	None	Activity that increases blood pressure	High blood pressure; diastolic > 120 mm Hg	Only as related to hypertension	
Trigeminal neuralgia (tic douloureux)	Female/40 to 60 years	Excruciating, spontaneous, lancinating, lightning	Can occur many (12 or more) times per day	Unilateral along trigeminal nerve area	30 seconds to 1 minute	Disagreeable tingling	Touch (cold) to affected area	Neurological	None	Reddened conjunctiva, lacrimation
Glossopharyngeal neuralgia	Male/40 to 60 years	Excruciating, spontaneous, lancinating, lightning	Can occur many (12 or more) times per day	Unilateral retrolingual area to ear	30 seconds to 1 minute	None	Movement or contact of the pharynx	Neurological	None	

Continued

Table 2-12—cont'd

Headaches: A Differential Diagnosis

Disorder	Sex/Age Predominance	Nature of Pain	Frequency	Location	Duration	Prodromal Events	Precipitating Factors	Cause	Familial Predisposition	Other Possible Symptoms
Cervical neuralgia	None	Dull pain or pressure in head		Bilateral, occipital, frontal, or facial	Variable	None	Posture or head movement	Neurological, pressure on roots of spinal nerves	None	Dizziness, auditory disturbances
Eye disorders	None	Generalized discomfort in or around the eyes	Intensify with sustained visual effort	Entire cranium	During and after visual effort	None	Impairment of eye function	Cornea, iris, or intraocular pain	Possible	Diminished vision, sensitivity to light
Sinus, ear, and nasal disorders	None	Dull, persistent	Variable	Frontal, temporal, ear, nose, occipital	Variable	None	Infection, allergy, chemical, bending, straining	Blockage, inflammation, infection	None	

Modified from Esposito CJ et al: Headaches: a differential diagnosis, *J Craniomand Pract* 4:320–321, 1986.

ahead, and formulate rational judgments of problems or events is largely a function of the frontal lobes.

15. *Can the patient talk normally?* Patients with lesions of the parietal lobe have difficulty communicating and understanding what is occurring around them. **Dysarthria** indicates defects in articulation, enunciation, or rhythm of speech. It usually results from extraneural problems such as poor-fitting dentures, malformation of the oral structures, or impairment of the musculature of the tongue, palate, pharynx, or lips because of incoordination, weakness, or abnormal innervation. It is characterized by slurring, slowness of speech, indistinct speech, and breaks in normal speech rhythm. **Dysphonia** is a disorder of vocalization characterized by the abnormal production of sounds from the larynx. Dysphonia is usually caused by various abnormalities of the larynx itself or of its innervation. The principal complaint of dysphonia is hoarseness, ranging from mild roughness of the voice to an inability to produce sound. **Dysphasia** denotes the inability to use and understand written and spoken words as a result of disorders involving cortical centers of speech or their interconnections in the dominant cerebral hemisphere. With all of these conditions, the peripheral mechanisms for speech remain intact.

16. *Does the patient have any allergies, or is the patient receiving any medication?* Allergies may affect the eyes and nose, as may medications. Medications themselves may mask some symptoms.

17. *Is the patient having any problems with the eyes?* Monocular **diplopia** (blurred vision when looking with one eye) may result from hyphema, a detached lens, or other trauma to the globe of the eye.[29] Binocular diplopia (blurred vision when looking through both eyes) occurs in 10% to 40% of patients with a zygoma fracture. It may be caused by soft-tissue entrapment, neuromuscular injury (intraorbital or intramuscular), hemorrhage, or edema. It disappears when one eye is closed. Double vision, which occurs when the good eye is closed, indicates that some structure of the eye is injured. If it occurs with both eyes open, something is affecting the free movement of the eyes (Tables 2-13 and 2-14).

18. *Does the patient wear glasses or contact lenses?* If the patient wears glasses, are the lenses treated (hardened) or made of polycarbonate? If they are hardened, how long ago were they treated? If the patient wears contact lenses, are they hard, soft, or extended-wear lenses? Did the patient wear eye protectors? If so, what type were they? Are the patient's eyes watering? Is there any pain in the eyes? Small perforating injuries may be painless. If the patient complains of flashes of bright light, "a curtain falling in front of the eye," or floating black specks, these findings may indicate retinal detachment. These questions tell the examiner whether the eyewear or eyes need to be examined in greater detail.

Table 2-13

Common Visual Eye Symptoms and Disease States

Visual Symptom	Associated Causes
Loss of vision	Optic neuritis
	Detached retina
	Retinal hemorrhage
	Central retinal vascular occlusion
Spots	No pathological significance*
Flashes	Migraine
	Retinal detachment
	Posterior vitreous detachment
Loss of visual field or presence of shadows or curtains	Retinal detachment
	Retinal hemorrhage
Glare, photophobia	Iritis (inflammation of the iris)
	Meningitis (inflammation of the meninges)
Distortion of vision	Retinal detachment
	Macular edema
Difficulty seeing in dim light	Myopia
	Vitamin A deficiency
	Retinal degeneration
Colored haloes around lights	Acute narrow angle glaucoma
	Opacities in lens or cornea
Colored vision changes	Cataracts
	Drugs (digitalis increases yellow vision)
Double vision	Extraocular muscle paresis or paralysis

From Swartz MH: *Textbook of physical diagnosis*, p. 132, Philadelphia, 1989, WB Saunders.

*May precede a retinal detachment or be associated with fertility drugs.

19. *Is the patient having any problem with hearing?* Does the patient complain of an earache? If so, when was the onset and what is the duration of the earache? Does the patient complain of pain or a discharge from the ear? Is the earache associated with an upper respiratory tract infection, swimming, or trauma? The patient should also be questioned on his or her method of cleaning the ear. If there appears to be a hearing loss, the patient should be asked whether the hearing loss came on quickly or slowly, whether the patient hears best on the telephone (amplified sound) or in a quiet or noisy environment, and whether speech is heard soft or loud. Does the patient use a hearing aid?

20. *Is the patient having any problems with the nose?* Has the patient used nose drops or spray? If so, how much, how often, and for how long? Does the patient have any nasal discharge, and if so, is its character watery, mucoid, purulent, crusty, or bloody? Does the discharge have any odor (indicative of infection), and is it unilateral or bilateral? Does the patient exhibit any

Table 2-14
Common Nonvisual Eye Symptoms and Disease States

Nonvisual Symptom	Associated Causes
Itching	Dry eyes
	Eye fatigue
	Allergies
Tearing	Emotional states
	Hypersecretion of tears
	Blockage of drainage
Dryness	Sjögren's syndrome
	Decreased secretion as a result of aging
Sandiness, grittiness	Conjunctivitis
Fullness of eyes	Proptosis (bulging of the eyeball)
	Aging changes in the lids
Twitching	Fibrillation of orbicularis oculi
Eyelid heaviness	Fatigue
	Lid edema
Dizziness	Refractive error
	Cerebellar disease
Blinking	Local irritation
	Facial tic
Lids sticking together	Inflammatory disease of lids or conjunctivae
Foreign body sensation	Foreign body
	Corneal abrasion
Burning	Uncorrected refractive error
	Conjunctivitis
	Sjögren's syndrome
Throbbing, aching	Acute iritis (inflammation of the iris)
	Sinusitis (inflammation of the sinuses)
Tenderness	Lid inflammations
	Conjunctivitis
	Iritis
Headache	Refractive errors
	Migraine
	Sinusitis
Drawing sensation	Uncorrected refractive errors

From Swartz MH: *Textbook of physical diagnosis*, p. 133, Philadelphia, 1989, WB Saunders.

associated nasal symptoms such as sneezing, nasal congestion, itching, or mouth breathing? Does the patient complain of a nosebleed, and has the patient had many nosebleeds? If so, how frequent are the nosebleeds, what is the amount of the bleeding, and what appears to be causing the bleeding? Positive responses to any of these questions indicate that the nose must be examined in greater detail.

21. *If the examiner is concerned about the mouth and teeth or the temporomandibular joints, questions related to these areas can be found in Chapter 4.* It is important, however, to ensure that the patient's dental occlusion and biting alignment have not been altered. Are all the teeth present, and are they symmetrical? Is there any swelling or bleeding around the teeth? Are the teeth mobile or is part of a tooth missing? Is the pulp exposed? Each of these questions helps determine whether the teeth have been injured. Teeth that have been avulsed, if intact, should be reimplanted as quickly as possible. If reimplanted after cleansing (rinsed in saline solution or water) within less than 30 minutes, the tooth has a 90% chance of being retained. If it is not possible to reimplant the tooth, it should be kept moist in saline, or the patient should keep it between the gum and cheek while dental care is sought.

22. *Questions concerning the neck and cervical spine can be found in Chapter 3.*

Observation

For proper observation[30–33] of the head and face, any hat, helmet, mouth guard, or face guard should be removed. If a neck injury is suspected or if the patient presents an emergency situation, the examiner may take the time to remove only those items that are interfering with immediate emergency care. If a neck injury is suspected, extreme caution should be observed when removing the item. When assessing the head and face, the examiner must also observe and assess the posture of the cervical spine and the temporomandibular joints; see Chapters 3 and 4 for detailed descriptions of observation of these areas.

When observing the head and face, it is essential that the examiner look at the face to note the position and shape of the eyes, nose, mouth, teeth, and ears and look for deformity, asymmetry, facial imbalance, swelling, lacerations, foreign bodies, or bleeding during rest, with movement, or with different facial expressions.[34] One should also note, as much as possible, the individual's normal facial expression. A patient's facial expression often reflects the patient's general feeling and well-being. A dazed or vacant look often indicates problems. While talking to the patient, the examiner should watch for any asymmetry of facial motion or change in facial expression when the patient answers; slight facial asymmetry is common. In addition, small degrees of paralysis may not be obvious unless one attempts an exaggerated expression. If some facial paralysis is suspected, the examiner should ask the patient to make exaggerated facial expressions that will demonstrate the paralysis. If facial asymmetry is present, one should note whether all of the features on one side of the face are affected or only a portion of the face is affected. For example, with facial nerve (cranial nerve VII) paralysis, the entire side of the face is affected, although the most noticeable differences will occur around one eye and one side of the mouth. If only one side of the mouth is involved, then a problem with the trigeminal nerve (cranial nerve V) should be suspected. Any changes in the shape of the face or unusual features such as masses, edema, puffiness, coarseness, prominent eyes, amount of facial hair, excessive perspiration, or skin color should be noted. Eye puffiness is often one of the earliest signs of edema in the face. Skin color may include cyanosis, pallor, jaundice, or pigmentation, and each may be indicative of different systemic problems.

The examiner should view the patient from the front, side, behind, and above, noting the area behind the ears, at the hairline, and around the crown of the head as well as on the face (Figure 2-13). An examiner who suspects a skull (cranial vault) injury should look behind the ears, at the hairline, and around the crown of the head for any deformity, bruising, or laceration.

Viewing from the front, the examiner should observe the patient's hairline, noting any abnormalities. The soft tissues such as the eyelids, eyebrows, cheeks, lips, nose, and chin should be inspected for lacerations, bruising, or hematoma (Figures 2-14 and 2-15). The eyes should be level. For example, a zygoma fracture causes the eye on the affected side to drop (Figure 2-16). The two eyes should be compared for prominence or retraction (Figure 2-17). If there appears to be any bulging, especially unilaterally, the examiner should tilt the patient's head forward or back and, looking from above, compare each cornea with the lid below, noting whether one or both corneas bulge beyond the lid margins. If one or

both eyes appear to bulge, the examiner can use a pocket ruler to roughly measure the distance from the angle of the eye to the corneal apex.

Immediate referral for further examination by a specialist is required for an embedded corneal foreign body; haze or blood in the anterior chamber (hyphema); decreased or partial vision; irregular, asymmetric, or poor pupil action; diplopia or double vision; laceration of the eyelid or impaired lid function; perforation or laceration of the globe; broken contact lens or shattered eyeglass in the eye; unexplained eye pain that is stabbing or deep and throbbing; blurred vision that does not clear with blinking; loss of all or part of the visual field; protrusion of one eye relative to the other; an injured eye that does not move as fully as the uninjured eye; or abnormal pupil size or shape. A teardrop pupil usually indicates iris entrapment in a corneal or scleral laceration. In addition, the eyes should be observed from the lateral aspect. The normal distance from the cornea to the angle of the eye is 16 mm or less. The distances between the upper and lower lids should be the same for both eyes. When the eyes open, the superior eyelid should cover a portion of the iris but not the pupil itself. If it covers more of the iris than the other upper eyelid does, or if it extends over the iris or pupil, ptosis or drooping of that eyelid should be suspected. If the eyelid does not cover part of the iris, retraction of the eyelid should be suspected. Are the eyelids everted or inverted? Normally, they are neither. The examiner should also note whether the patient can close both eyes completely. If an eye injury is suspected,

A   **B**   **C**

Figure 2-13
Views of the head and face. **A,** Anterior. **B,** Side. **C,** Posterior.

Figure 2-14
Lacerations to the upper eyelid and eyebrow.

Figure 2-15
Contusion to the forehead caused by a racquetball ball.

Figure 2-16
Inferior displacement of the zygoma (1) results in depression of the lateral canthus and pupil (2) because of depression of the suspensory ligaments that attach to the lateral orbital (Whitnall's) tubercle. (Modified from Ellis E: Fractures of the zygomatic complex and arch. In Fonseca RJ and Walker RV, editors: *Oral and maxillofacial trauma*, p. 446, Philadelphia, 1991, WB Saunders.)

Figure 2-17
A severe glancing or direct blow to this right eye has resulted in a ruptured globe. Note the depressed eye. (From Pashby TJ and Pashby RC: Treatment of sports eye injuries. In Schneider RC et al, editors: *Sports injuries: mechanisms, prevention and treatment*, p. 589, Baltimore, 1985, Williams & Wilkins.)

Figure 2-18
Black eye (periorbital ecchymosis).

this action should be done carefully, because closing the eyes can increase intraocular pressure. The lids should be pressed together only enough to bring the eyelashes together. Any inflammation or masses, especially on the lid margin, should be noted. If present, a "black eye," or periorbital contusion, should also be noted (Figure 2-18). The lashes should be viewed to see if there is even distribution along the lid margins. "Raccoon eyes," which are purple discolorations of the eyelids and orbital regions, may indicate orbital fractures, basilar skull fractures, or a fracture of the base of the anterior cranial fossa.[30] This sign takes several hours to develop.

The conjunctiva should be inspected for hemorrhage, laceration, and foreign bodies.[34] If the patient complains of "something in the eye," eversion of the upper

Eye Signs and Symptoms Requiring Specialist Care

- Foreign body that is not easily removed
- Eye does not move properly
- Altered pupil action
- Abnormal pupil size or shape
- Double vision
- Blurred vision
- Decreased or partial vision
- Loss of part or all of visual field
- Laceration of eye or eyelid
- Blood between cornea and iris (hyphema)
- Impaired eyelid function
- Penetration of eye or eyelid
- Eye pain
- Sharp or throbbing eye pain
- Protrusion or retraction of eye

eyelid usually reveals a foreign body that can often be easily brushed away. Displaced contact lenses are often found in this upper area of the eye. The conjunctival covering of the lower lid may be examined by having the patient look upward while the examiner draws the lower lid downward. The conjunctiva should be examined as being a continuous sheet of epithelium from the globe to the lids. The color of the sclera should also be noted. Posttraumatic conjunctival hemorrhage (Figure 2-19) and possible scleral lacerations (Figure 2-20) should be noted, if present. In dark-skinned patients, pigmented areas may show up as small dark spots or patches near the limbus. The shape and color of the cornea should be inspected. The anterior chambers of the eye should be inspected and compared for clarity and depth.[35] If present, hyphema in the form of haze or actual blood pooling (Figure 2-21) in the anterior eye chamber should be noted.[29] If there is any potential for or evidence of bleeding in the anterior chamber of the eye, the patient's activity should be curtailed, because increased activity increases the chances of secondary hemorrhage during the first week after injury. Examination of the cornea with a penlight shone obliquely on the eye should be carried out to look for foreign bodies, abrasions, or lacerations. Corneal injuries can lead to lacrimation (tearing), photophobia (intolerance to light), or blepharospasm (spasm of the eyelid orbicular muscle) as well as extreme pain from exposure of sensory nerve endings. A fluorescein strip dipped into tears that are exposed as the lower lid is pulled downward will readily outline abrasions.

A

B

C

Figure 2-19

A, Posttraumatic conjunctival hemorrhage without other ocular or orbital damage. **B,** Posttraumatic conjunctival hemorrhage from blunt injury, with a small hyphema *(arrow)*. In this case, the injury was significant because of the presence of blood in the anterior chamber. **C,** Subconjunctival ecchymosis with no lateral limit should suggest osseous orbital fractures. (**A** and **B** from Paton D and Goldberg MF: *Management of ocular injuries*, Philadelphia, 1976, WB Saunders, p. 182. **C** from Lew D and Sinn DP: *Diagnosis and treatment of midface fractures.* In Fonseca RJ and Walker RV, editors: *Oral and maxillofacial trauma*, p. 250, Philadelphia, 1991, WB Saunders.)

Figure 2-20

Scleral rupture *(arrow)* at the limbus after blunt trauma. The iris and ciliary body have prolapsed into the subconjunctival space. (From Paton D and Goldberg MF: *Management of ocular injuries,* p. 310, Philadelphia, 1976, WB Saunders.)

Figure 2-21

Hyphema in the anterior chamber of the eye. (From Easterbrook M and Cameron J: Injuries in racquet sports. In Schneider RC et al, editors: *Sports injuries—mechanisms, prevention and treatment,* p. 556, Baltimore, 1985, Williams & Wilkins.)

The pupillary size (diameter range, 2 to 6 mm; mean, 3.5 mm), shape (round), and symmetry should be compared with those of the other eye. Elliptical pupils often indicate a corneal laceration. The color of the irises of the eyes should be compared. When looking at the pupils, the examiner should note whether the pupils are equal. Are the pupils smaller or larger than normal? Are they round or irregularly shaped? The pupils are normally slightly unequal in 5% of the population, but inequality of pupil size should initially be viewed with suspicion. For example, unilateral dilation may be the result of a sympathetic nerve response following a blow to the face.[3] Pupils tend to be smaller in infants, the elderly, and persons with hyperopia (farsightedness), whereas they tend to be slightly dilated in persons with myopia (nearsightedness) or light-colored irises.

The nose should be inspected for any deviations in shape, size, or color.[34] The skin should be smooth without swelling and should conform to the color of the face. The airways are usually oval and symmetrically proportioned. If a discharge is present, its character (i.e., color, smell, texture) should be noted and described. Bloody discharge occurs as a result of epistaxis or trauma such as a nasal fracture, zygoma fracture, or skull fracture. Mucoid discharge is typical of rhinitis. Bilateral purulent discharge can occur with upper respiratory tract infection. Unilateral purulent, thick, greenish, and often malodorous discharge usually indicates the presence of a foreign body.

Depression of the nasal bridge can result from a fracture of the nasal bone. Nasal flaring is associated with respiratory distress, whereas narrowing of the airways on inspiration may indicate chronic nasal obstruction and be associated with mouth breathing. The nasal mucosa should be deep pink and glistening. A film of clear discharge is often apparent on the nasal septum. The nasal septum should be close to midline and fairly straight, appearing thicker anteriorly than posteriorly. If present, a hematoma in the septal area should be noted. Asymmetric posterior nasal cavities may indicate a deviation of the nasal septum.

With the patient's mouth closed, the lips should be observed for symmetry, color, edema, and surface abnormalities. Lipstick should be removed before the assessment. The lips should be pink and have vertical and horizontal symmetry, both at rest and with movement. Dry, cracked lips may be caused by dehydration from wind or low humidity, whereas deep fissures at the corners of the mouth may indicate overclosure of the mouth or riboflavin deficiency.

Drooping of the mouth on one side, sagging of the lower eyelid, and flattening of the nasolabial fold suggest possible facial nerve (cranial nerve VII) involvement. The patient is also unable to pucker the lips to whistle.

The shape and position of the jaw and teeth should also be noted anteriorly and from the side.[34] Asymmetry may indicate a fracture of the jaw (Figure 2-22), whereas bleeding around the gums of the teeth may indicate fracture, avulsion, or loosening of the teeth (Figure 2-23). If teeth are missing, they must be accounted for. If they are not accounted for, an x-ray may be required to ensure that the teeth have not entered the abdominal or chest cavity. Pain on percussion of the teeth often indicates damage to the periodontal ligament.

Figure 2-22

Fracture of the neck of the condyle on the right *(upper arrows)* with fracture through the mandible on the same side *(lower arrow)*. When one fracture is shown in the mandible, search carefully for the second. (From O'Donoghue DH: *Treatment of injuries to athletes*, p. 115, Philadelphia, 1984, WB Saunders.)

A

B

Figure 2-23

A 9-year-old boy was hit in the mouth with a ball while he was playing baseball. The right maxillary central and lateral incisors were chipped. **A,** Avulsed teeth reimplanted with finger pressure. **B,** Radiograph of root canal with wide-open apex. Reimplanted quickly, these teeth may not require root canal treatment. (From Torg JS: *Athletic injuries to the head, neck and face*, p. 247, Philadelphia, 1982, Lea & Febiger.)

From the side, the examiner should look for any asymmetry or depression, which may indicate pathology. The examiner should inspect the auricles of the ears for size, shape, symmetry, landmarks, color, and position on the head. To determine the position of the auricle, the examiner can draw an imaginary line between the outer canthus of the eye and occipital protuberance (Figure 2-24). The top of the auricle should touch or be above this line.[28] The examiner can then draw another imaginary line perpendicular to the previous line and just anterior to the auricle. The auricle's position should be almost vertical. If the angle is more than 10° posterior or anterior, it is considered abnormal. An auricle that is set low or is at an unusual angle may indicate chromosomal aberrations or renal disorders. In addition, the lateral and medial surfaces and surrounding tissues should be examined, noting any deformities, lesions, or nodules. The auricles should be the same color as the facial skin without moles, cysts, or other lesions or deformities. Athletes, especially wrestlers, may exhibit a cauliflower ear (hematoma auris), which is a keloid scar forming in the auricle because of friction to or twisting of the ear (Figure 2-25). Blueness may indicate some degree of cyanosis. Pallor or excessive redness may be the result of vasomotor instability or increased temperature. Frostbite can cause extreme pallor or blistering (Figure 2-26).

The examiner should look posteriorly for any asymmetry or depression. The positions of the ears (height, protrusion) can be compared by observing them from behind. A low hairline may indicate conditions such as Klippel-Feil syndrome. The examiner should also look for the presence of **Battle's sign.** This sign, which takes as long as 24 hours to appear, is demonstrated by purple and blue discoloration of the skin in the mastoid area and may indicate a temporal bone or basilar skull fracture.

The examiner then views the patient from overhead (superior view) to note any asymmetry from above (Figure 2-27). This method is especially useful when looking for a possible fracture of the zygoma (Figure 2-28). The deformity is easier to detect if the examiner carefully places the index fingers below the infraorbital margins along the zygomatic bodies and then gently pushes into the edema to reduce the effect of the edema (Figure 2-29).

> ▼ **Signs and Symptoms of Maxillary and Zygomatic Fractures**
>
> - Facial asymmetry
> - Loss of cheek prominence
> - Palpable steps
>   - Infraorbital rim (zygomaticomaxillary suture)
>   - Lateral orbital rim (frontozygomatic suture)
>   - Root of zygoma intraorally
>   - Zygomatic arch between the ear and the eye (zygomatico-temporal suture)
> - Hypoesthesia/anesthesia
>   - Cheek, side of nose, upper lip, and teeth on the injured side
>   - Compression of the infraorbital nerve as it courses along the floor of the orbit to exit into the face via the foramen beneath the orbital rim

Figure 2-25
Cauliflower ear (hematoma auris).

Figure 2-24
Auricle alignment. Normal position shown.

Figure 2-26
Auricular frostbite with development of massive vesicles that are beginning to resolve spontaneously. (From Schuller DE and Bruce RA: Ear, nose, throat and eye. In Strauss RH, editor: *Sports medicine*, p. 191, ed 2, Philadelphia, 1991, WB Saunders.)

Examination

The examination of the head and face differs from the orthopedic assessment of other areas of the body because the assessment does not involve joints. The only joints that could be included in the assessment are the temporomandibular joints, and these joints are discussed in Chapter 4.

Examination of the Head

Many problems in the head and face may be problems referred from the cervical spine, temporomandibular

joint, or teeth. However, if one suspects a head injury, it is necessary to keep a close watch on the patient, noting any changes and when these changes occur. The examiner should implement a **neural watch** so that any changes that occur over time can be determined easily (Table 2-15). The testing should occur at 15- or 30-minute intervals, depending on the severity of the injury and the changes recorded.

Figure 2-27
View of the patient from above to look for bilateral symmetry of the face.

Head Examination

- Concussion
- Headache
- Memory tests
- Neural watch (Glasgow Coma Scale)
- Expanding intracranial lesion
- Proprioception
- Coordination
- Head injury card

The issue of whether a patient should be allowed to return to competition or high-level activity following a concussion, and how soon, is one that has not been completely settled, although clinicians are becoming more concerned about the consequences of concussions (Table 2-16).[4,36-42] Research has shown that the brain is vulnerable to reinjury for 3 to 5 days following concussions because of altered blood flow and metabolic dysfunction.[4] If the examiner is contemplating allowing the patient to return to activity because all symptoms have disappeared, provocative stress tests should be considered before allowing the patient to return. These tests are commonly related to the sport but may include jumping jacks, situps, pushups, deep knee bends, and lying supine for 1 minute with feet elevated or similar activities that may be

Figure 2-28
Typical fracture of zygomatic arch on the right *(arrow)*. Note normal arch on the left. (From O'Donoghue DH: *Treatment of injuries to athletes*, p. 114, Philadelphia, 1984, WB Saunders.)

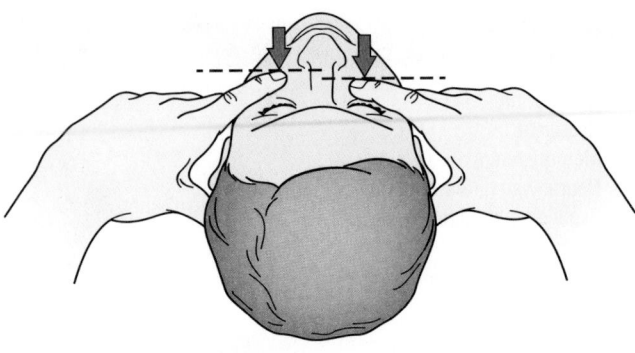

Figure 2-29
Method of assessing posterior displacement of the zygomatic complex from behind the patient. The examiner should firmly but carefully depress the fingers into the edematous soft tissues while palpating along the infraorbital areas. (Modified from Ellis E: Fractures of the zygomatic complex and arch. In Fonseca RJ and Walker RV, editors: *Oral and maxillofacial trauma*, p. 443, Philadelphia, 1991, WB Saunders.)

related to what the patient will return to functionally (e.g., rapid head movements, straining or holding breath). These activities should be viewed as actions that increase intracranial pressure and can cause a different physiological response in concussed athletes,[45] which may lead to symptoms.[3,46] Although the guidelines outlined in Table 2-17 may appear excessively precautionary, they are designed to prevent **second impact syndrome,** which is potentially catastrophic injury with a mortality rate close to 50% or permanent brain injury.[8,36,47–51]

The examiner should always be looking for the possibility of an expanding intracranial lesion resulting from a leaking or torn blood vessel. Normally, the brain has a fixed volume that is enclosed in a nonexpansile structure, namely, the skull and dura mater. These lesions may be caused by epidural hemorrhage (usually tearing of one of the meningeal arteries as a result of high-speed

Table 2-15

Neural Watch Chart

Unit		Time 1 ( )	Time 2 ( )	Time 3 ( )	Unit		Time 1 ( )	Time 2 ( )	Time 3 ( )
I Vital signs	Blood pressure Pulse Respiration Temperature				VI Pupils	Size on right Size on left Reacts on right Reacts on left			
II Conscious and	Oriented Disoriented Restless Combative				VII Ability to move	Right arm Left arm Right leg Left leg			
III Speech	Clear Rambling Garbled None				VII Sensation	Right side (normal/ abnormal) Left side (normal/ abnormal) Dermatome affected (specify) Peripheral nerve affected (specify)			
IV Will awaken to	Name Shaking Light pain Strong pain								
V Nonverbal reaction to pain	Appropriate Inappropriate "Decerebrate" None								

Modified from American Academy of Orthopedic Surgeons: *Athletic Training and Sports Medicine*, p. 399, Park Ridge, Ill., 1984, AAOS.

Table 2-16

Return to Play Protocol

When a patient shows *any* symptoms or signs of a concussion:

1. The patient should *not* be allowed to return to play in the current game, practice or any strenuous activity.

2. The patient should *not* be left alone, and regular monitoring for deterioration is essential over the initial few hours following injury.

3. The patient should be medically evaluated following the injury.

4. Return to play must follow a *medically supervised* stepwise process.

A patient should never return to play while symptomatic. "When in doubt, sit them out."

As described above, the majority of injuries will be **simple concussions** and such injuries recover spontaneously over several days. In these situations, it is expected that a patient will proceed rapidly through the stepwise return to play strategy.[43]

During this period of recovery in the first few days following an injury, it is important to emphasize to the patient that physical *and* cognitive rest is required. Activities that require concentration and attention may exacerbate the symptoms and as a result delay recovery.

The return to play following a concussion follows a stepwise process:

1. No activity, complete rest. Once asymptomatic, proceed to next level[44]

2. Light aerobic exercise such a walking or stationary cycling, no resistance training

3. Sport specific exercise (e.g., skating in hockey, running in soccer), progressive addition of resistance training at steps 3 or 4

4. Noncontact training drills

5. Full-contact training after medical clearance

6. Game play

With this stepwise progressive, the patient should continue to proceed to the next level if asymptomatic at the current level. If any postconcussion symptoms occur, the patient should drop back to the previous asymptomatic level and try to progress again after 24 hours.

NOTE 1: In cases of **complex concussion**, the rehabilitation will be more prolonged and return to play advice will be more circumspect. Complex cases should be managed by physician specialists with a specific expertise in the management of such injuries.

NOTE 2: Patient should not only be symptom free but also should not be taking any pharmacological agents/medications that may affect or modify the symptoms of concussion. Where antidepressant therapy may be commenced during the management of a **complex concussion**, the decision to return to play while still on such medication must be considered carefully by the clinical concerned.

Adapted from McCrory PK et al: Summary and agreement statement of the 2nd International Conference on Concussion in Sport, Prague 2004, *Clin J Sports Med* 15:48–55, 2005.

impact), subarachnoid hemorrhage (usually as a result of an aneurysm), or subdural hemorrhage (usually as a result of tearing of bridging veins between the brain and cavernous sinus).[36] These injuries are emergency conditions that must be looked after immediately because of their high mortality rate (as much as 50%). An **expanding intracranial lesion** is indicated by an altered lucid state (state of consciousness), development of inequality of the pupils, unusual slowing of the heart rate that primarily occurs after a lucid interval, irregular eye movements, and eyes that no longer track properly. There is also a tendency for the patient to demonstrate increased body temperature and irregular respirations. Normal intracranial pressure measures from 4 to 15 mm Hg, and an intracranial pressure of more than 20 mm Hg

is considered abnormal. Intracranial pressure of 40 mm Hg causes neurological dysfunction and impairment. Although in the emergency care setting there is no way of determining the intracranial pressure, the signs and symptoms mentioned indicate that the pressure is increasing. Most patients who experience an increase in intracranial pressure complain of severe headache, and this symptom is often followed by vomiting (sometimes projectile vomiting). Finally, an expanding intracranial lesion causes increased weakness on the side of the body opposite that on which the lesion has occurred.

Signs and symptoms that indicate a good possibility of recovery from a head injury, especially after the patient experiences unconsciousness, include response to noxious stimuli, eye opening, pupil activity, spontaneous eye

Table 2-17
Return-to-Play Guidelines

Grade of Concussion	On-the-Field Treatment	First Concussion	Second Concussion	Third Concussion
Simple: Loss of consciousness <1 minute; posttraumatic amnesia <30 minutes	Remove athlete from the competition	Athlete may return to play if asymptomatic for 1 week	Obtain CT scan; athlete may return in 2 weeks if asymptomatic for 1 week	Athlete sidelined a minimum of 1 month; may return then if asymptomatic for 1 week
Complex: Loss of consciousness >1 minute; posttraumatic amnesia >30 minutes	Remove athlete from the competition; transport athlete to a hospital for emergency evaluation of the player by a neurosurgeon and to obtain diagnostic neuroimaging	Obtain CT scan, remove from play for a minimum of 1 month; athlete may then return to play if asymptomatic for 1 week	Obtain CT scan; consider terminating for season	Terminate athlete for season; athlete may return next season if asymptomatic, but permanent retirement from contact sports should be considered

Data from Warren WL et al: Guidelines for safe return to play after athletic head and neck injuries. In Cantu RC, editor: *Neurologic athletic head and spine injuries*, Philadelphia, 2000, WB Saunders.

movement, intact oculovestibular reflexes, and appropriate motor function responses. Neurological signs that indicate a poor prognosis after a head injury include nonreactive pupils, absence of oculovestibular reflexes, severe extension patterns or no motor function response at all, and increased intracranial pressure.[23]

Signs and Symptoms of an Expanding Intracranial Lesion

- Altered state of consciousness
- Nystagmus
- Pupil inequality
- Irregular eye movements
- Abnormal slowing of heart
- Irregular respiration
- Severe headache
- Intractable vomiting
- Positive expanding intracranial lesion tests (lateralizing)
- Positive coordination tests
- Decreasing muscle strength
- Seizure

It is important when examining the unconscious or conscious patient for a possible head injury to determine the individual's level of consciousness, which may be determined using the **Glasgow Coma Scale** (Table 2-18). The first test relates to eye opening. Eye opening may occur spontaneously, in response to speech, or in response to pain, or there may be no response at all. Each of these responses is given a numerical value: spontaneous eye opening, 4; response to speech, 3; response to pain, 2; and no response, 1. Spontaneous opening of the eyes indicates functioning of the ascending reticular activating system. This finding does not necessarily mean that the patient is aware of the surroundings or of what is happening, but it does imply that the patient is in a state of arousal. A patient who opens his or her eyes in response to the examiner's voice is probably responding to the stimulus of sound, not necessarily to the command to open the eyes. If unsure, the examiner may use different sound-making objects (e.g., bell, horn) to elicit an appropriate response.

The second test involves motor response; the patient is given a grade of 6 if there is a response to a verbal command. Otherwise, the patient is graded on a 5-point scale depending on the motor response to a painful stimulus (see Table 2-18). When scoring motor responses, it is the ease with which the motor responses are elicited that constitutes the criterion for the best response. Commands given to the patient should be simple, such as, "Move your arm." The patient should not be asked to squeeze the examiner's hand, nor should the examiner place something in the patient's hand and then ask the patient to grasp it. This action may cause a reflex grasp, not a response to a command.[23]

If the patient does not give a motor response to a verbal command, then the examiner should attempt to elicit a motor response to a painful stimulus. It is the type and quality of the patient's reaction to the painful

Table 2-18

Glasgow Coma Scale*

				Time 1 ( )	Time 2 ( )
Eyes	Open	Spontaneously	4		
		To verbal command	3		
		To pain	2		
		No response	1	————	————
Best motor response	To verbal command	Obeys	6		
	To painful stimulus†	Localizes pain	5		
		Flexion—withdrawal	4		
		Flexion—abnormal (decorticate rigidity)	3		
		Extension (decerebrate rigidity)	2		
		No response	1	————	————
Best verbal response‡		Oriented and converses	5		
		Disoriented and converses	4		
		Inappropriate words	3		
		Incomprehensible sounds	2		
		No response	1	————	————
Total			3–15		

*The Glasgow Coma Scale, which is based on eye opening and verbal and motor responses, is a practical means of monitoring changes in level of consciousness. If responses on the scale are given numerical grades, the overall responsiveness of the patient can be expressed in a score that is the summation of the grades. The lowest score is 3, and the highest is 15.
†Apply knuckles to sternum; observe arms.
‡Arouse patient with painful stimulus if necessary.

stimulus that constitute the scoring criteria. The stimulus should not be applied to the face, because painful stimulus in the facial area may cause the eyes to close tightly as a protective reaction. The painful stimulus may consist of applying a knuckle to the sternum, squeezing the trapezius muscle, or squeezing the soft tissue between the thumb and index finger (Figure 2-30). If the patient moves a limb when the painful stimulus is applied to more than one point or tries to remove the examiner's hand that is applying the painful stimulus, the patient is localizing, and a value of 5 is given. If the patient withdraws from the painful stimulus rapidly, a normal reflex withdrawal is being shown, and a value of 4 is given.

However, if application of a painful stimulus creates a decorticate or decerebrate posture (Figure 2-31), an abnormal response is being demonstrated, and a value of 3 is given for the decorticate posture (injury above red nucleus) or a value of 2 is given for decerebrate posture (brain stem injury). **Decorticate posturing** results from lesions of the diencephalon area, whereas decerebrate posturing results from lesions of the midbrain. With decorticate posturing, the arms, wrists, and fingers are flexed, the upper limbs are adducted, and the legs are extended, medially rotated, and plantar flexed. **Decerebrate posturing,** which has a poorer prognosis,

involves extension, adduction, and hyperpronation of the arms, whereas the lower limbs are the same as for decorticate posturing.[52] Decerebrate rigidity is usually bilateral. If the patient exhibits no reaction to the painful stimulus, a value of 1 is given. It is important to be sure the "no" response is caused by a head injury and not a spinal cord injury leading to lack of feeling or sensation. Any difference in reaction between limbs should be carefully noted; this finding may indicate a specific focal injury.[23]

In the third test, verbal response is graded on a 5-point scale to measure the patient's speech in response to simple questions such as "Where are you?" or "Are you winning the game?" For verbal responses, the patient who converses appropriately shows proper orientation, being aware of oneself and the environment and is given a grade of 5. The patient who is confused is disoriented and unable to completely interact with the environment; this patient is able to converse using the appropriate words and is given a grade of 4. The patient exhibiting inappropriate speech is unable to sustain a conversation with the examiner; this person would be given a grade of 3. A vocalizing patient only groans or makes incomprehensible sounds; this finding leads to a grade of 2. Again, the examiner should note any possible mechanical reason for the inability to verbalize. If the patient makes no sounds and thus has no verbal response, a grade of 1 is assigned.

Figure 2-30

Examples of painful stimuli applied by the examiner. **A,** Knuckle to sternum. **B,** Squeezing trapezius muscle. **C,** Squeezing tissue between the thumb and index finger. **D,** Squeezing a fingertip. **E,** Squeezing an object between two fingers.

Figure 2-31
A, Decorticate rigidity. **B,** Decerebrate rigidity.

Table 2-19
Rancho Los Amigos Scale of Cognitive Function

Level I	No response
Level II	Generalized response
Level III	Localized response
Level IV	Confused, agitated
Level V	Confused, inappropriate
Level VI	Confused, appropriate
Level VII	Automatic, appropriate
Level VIII	Purposeful, appropriate

From Hagen C et al: Levels of cognitive functioning.
In *Rehabilitation of the brain injured adult: comprehensive management.* Professional Staff Association of Rancho Los Amigos, Downey, CA., 1980.

It is vital that the initial score on the Glasgow Coma Scale be obtained as soon as possible after the onset of the injury. The scale can then be repeated at 15- or 30-minute intervals, especially in the early stages, if changes are noted. If the score is between 3 and 8, emergency care is required. With the Glasgow Coma Scale, the initial score is used as a basis for determining the severity of the patient's head injury. Patients who maintain a score of 8 or lower on the Glasgow Coma Scale for 6 hours or longer are considered to have a serious head injury. A patient who scores between 9 and 11 is considered to have a moderate head injury, and one who scores 12 or higher is considered to have a mild head injury.[23]

Head Injury Severity Based on Score Maintained on Glasgow Coma Scale (6 Hr+)

8 or less:	Severe head injury
9–11:	Moderate head injury
12+:	Mild head injury

The Rancho Los Amigos Scale of Cognitive Function may also be used to assess the patient's cognitive abilities. This scale is an eight-level progression from level I, in which the patient is nonresponsive, to level VIII, in which the patient's behavior is purposeful and appropriate (Table 2-19). The Rancho Los Amigos scale provides an assessment of cognitive function and behavior only, not of physical functioning.[23]

If a person receives a head injury such as a mild concussion and is not referred to the hospital, the examiner should ensure that someone accompanies the person home and that someone at home knows what has happened so he or she can monitor the patient in case the patient's condition worsens. Appropriate written instructions should be sent home concerning the individual. The **Head Injury Card** is such an example (Figure 2-32).

Levin and colleagues reported the use of the Galveston Orientation and Amnesia Test (GOAT),[25] which they believe measures orientation to person, place, and time, and the memory of events preceding and following head trauma (Figure 2-33). As the patient improves, the total GOAT score should increase.

The examiner may also wish to determine whether the patient has suffered an upper motor neuron lesion. Testing the deep tendon reflexes (see Table 1-28) or the pathological reflexes (see Table 1-30) or having the patient perform various balance and coordination tests may help to determine whether this type of lesion has occurred. However, the pathological reflexes may not be elicited owing to shock. Deep tendon reflexes are accentuated on the side of the body opposite that on which the brain injury has occurred. Balance can play an important role in the assessment of a head-injured patient. Balance involves the integration of several inputs (e.g., visual, proprioceptive, and vestibular systems) that are analyzed by the brain to allow a proper action. For example, in standing, the body is inherently unstable, and only the integration of input from various sources enables the patient to stand and to make appropriate corrections to maintain proper standing posture. Balance and coordination can be tested in several ways. The examiner can ask the patient to stand and walk a straight line with the eyes open and then with the eyes closed. The examiner should note any difference. He or she can then ask the patient to bring the finger to the nose or the heel of the foot to the opposite knee with the eyes closed (Figure 2-34). These

---

Home Health Care Guidelines: Head Injury Care

The person you have been asked to watch has suffered a head injury, which at this time does *not* appear to be severe. However, to ensure proper care, please ensure that the following guidelines are followed for the next 24 hours.

1. Limited physical activity for at least 24 hours. (rest quietly, do not drive a vehicle)

2. Liquid diet only for the next 8 to 24 hours (no alcohol).

3. Apply ice to the head for approximately 15 minutes every hour to relieve discomfort and swelling.

4. Tylenol may be given as needed but NO aspirin. No other medication for 24 hours without doctor's approval.

5. Awaken the patient every 2 hours during the next _____ hours and be aware of any symptoms in #6.

6. Appearance of any of the following signs and symptoms means that you should consult a doctor or go to an emergency room at a hospital **immediately:**

   • Nausea and/or vomiting
   • Weakness or numbness in arm, leg, or any other body part
   • Any visual difficulties or dizziness
   • Ringing in the ears
   • Mental confusion or disorientation, irritability, restlessness, forgetfulness
   • Loss of coordination
   • Unusual sleepiness or difficulty in awakening
   • Progressively worsening headache
   • Persistent intense headache after 48 hours
   • Unequal pupil size; slow or no pupil reaction to light
   • Difficulty breathing
   • Irregular heartbeat
   • Convulsions or tremors

7. Call to arrange an appointment with your doctor or the team physician/therapist* for a follow-up visit. If unable to contact your doctor, go to an emergency room as soon as possible for an evaluation.

   *Consult: _____ at _____
   phone number

   or: _____ at _____
   phone number

SPECIAL INSTRUCTIONS, APPOINTMENTS:

Figure 2-32 ▬▬▬▬

Home health care guidelines for patients with head injuries. (Modified from Allman FL and Crow RW: On-field evaluation of sports injuries. In Griffin LY, editor: *Orthopedic knowledge update: sports medicine*, p. 14, Rosemont, IL., American Academy of Orthopaedic Surgeons, 1994.)

---

tests and others described under Special Tests assess balance and coordination.

Muscle tone and strength may also play a role in assessing the patient for head injury. Increased unilateral muscle tone usually implies contralateral cerebral peduncle compression. Flaccid muscle tone implies brain stem infarction, spinal cord transaction, or spinal shock. Unilateral effects such as hemiparesis may be seen with a stroke.

Examination of the Face[31–35,53]

Once a head injury has been ruled out or if no head injury is suspected, the examiner can inspect the face for injury. Major trauma and subsequent injury to the face should be assessed first. If major trauma has not occurred, only those areas of the face that have been affected by the trauma (e.g., eyes, nose, ears) need be assessed. The patient may initially be tested for fractures with the use of a tongue depressor, if the patient can open her or his mouth. The patient is asked to bite down as hard as possible on the tongue depressor (Figure 2-35, *A*). The examiner should note whether the patient is able to bite down strongly and hold the contraction and where any pain is elicited.

Facial Examination

• Bone and soft tissue contours
• Fractures
• Mandible
• Maxilla
• Zygoma
• Skull
• Cranial nerves
• Facial muscles

To test for a maxillary fracture, the examiner grasps the anterior aspect of the maxilla with the fingers of one hand and places the fingers of the other hand over the bridge of the patient's nose or forehead. The examiner then gently pulls the maxilla forward (Figure 2-36). If the fingers of the other hand at the nose feel movement or the examiner feels the test hand moving forward, a Le Fort II or III fracture may be present (Figure 2-37). If the maxilla moves without movement at the nose, either the maxilla is horizontally fractured or a Le Fort I fracture is present. With a Le Fort I fracture, the palate is separated from the superior portion of the maxilla, and the upper tooth-bearing segment of the face moves alone. The nasal bones, midportion of the face, and maxilla move if a Le Fort II fracture is

Galveston Orientation and Amnesia Test (GOAT)

Name _____ Date of test _____

Age _____ Sex M F Day of the week S M T W Th F S

Date of birth _____ Time AM PM

Diagnosis _____ Date of injury _____

Error points

1. What is your name? (2) _____ When were you born? (4) _____ _____

   Where do you live? (4) _____

2. Where are you now? (city) (5) _____ Location (e.g., hospital) (5) _____ _____
   (unnecessary to state name of hospital)

3. On what date were you admitted to this hospital? (5) _____ _____

   How did you get here? (5) _____

4. What is the first event you can remember *after* the injury? (5) _____ _____
   Can you describe in detail (e.g., date, time, companions) the first event you can recall after injury?

   (5) _____

5. Can you describe the last event you recall *before* the accident? (5) _____ _____
   Can you describe in detail (e.g., date, time, companions) the first event you can recall before injury?

   (5) _____

6. What time is it now? _____ (1 for each 1/2 hour removed from correct time, to maximum of 5) _____

7. What day of the week is it? _____ (1 for each day removed from correct one) _____

8. What day of the month is it? _____ (1 for each day removed from correct date, to maximum _____
   of 5)

9. What is the month? _____ (5 for each month removed from correct one, to maximum of 15) _____

10. What is the year? _____ (10 for each year removed from correct one, to maximum of 30) _____

Total error points _____

Total GOAT score (100 minus total error points) _____

Figure 2-33 ▬▬▬▬
Galveston Orientation and Amnesia Test. Examiner adds up only error points, not positive responses.
For example, if patient remembers the first name but not the last name, he or she would get 1 error point.
(Modified from Levin HS et al: The Galveston Orientation and Amnesia Test: a practical scale to assess
cognition after head injury, *J Nerve Ment Dis* 167:677, 1979.)

present. With a Le Fort III fracture, the middle third of the face separates from the upper third of the face; this is often called a craniofacial separation. The patient may complain of lip or cheek anesthesia and double vision (diplopia) with any of these fractures.

The examiner then asks the patient to open his or her mouth slightly. The examiner carefully applies pressure bilaterally at the angles of the mandible (Figure 2-35, *B*). Localized pain, lower lip anesthesia, and intraoral laceration may indicate a fracture of the mandible.

Figure 2-34
Performing coordination exercises. **A,** Touching knee with opposite heel. **B,** Touching nose with index finger with eyes closed.

Malocclusion of the teeth is often seen with fractures of the mandible or maxilla (Figure 2-38). Alterations in smell (cranial nerve I) are often seen with frontobasal and nasoethmoid fractures. Skull fractures are often associated with clear nasal discharge (spinal fluid rhinorrhea), clear ear discharge (otorrhea), or a salty taste. If blood accompanies the fluid, the examiner can use a gauze pad to collect the fluid. If cerebrospinal fluid is mixed with the blood, the examiner may observe a "halo" effect as the fluid collects on the gauze pad (Figure 2-39). If the eardrum has not been perforated, blood may be visible behind it. Skull fractures may also result in blurred or double vision, loss of smell (anosmia), dizziness, tinnitus, and nausea and vomiting as well as signs and symptoms of concussion. Orbital floor fractures or dislocations are often accompanied by anesthesia of the skin in the midface or anesthesia of the cheek, lip, maxillary teeth, and gingiva.[54] Zygoma fractures are detected by observation (see Figure 2-29). They may also cause unilateral epistaxis, double vision, and anesthesia and be associated with eye injuries. Mouth opening may also be affected.

After major trauma has been ruled out, the examiner may test the muscles of the face (Table 2-20), especially if injury to these structures is suspected. The muscles of the face are different from most muscles in that they move

Figure 2-35
Testing for mandibular fracture. **A,** Patient bites down on tongue depressor while examiner tries to pull it away. **B,** Pressure at the angles of the mandible.

the skin and soft tissues rather than joints, if one excludes the temporomandibular joint. For example, the frontalis muscle may be weak if the eyebrows do not raise symmetrically. The corrugator muscle draws the eyebrows medially and downward (frowning). The orbicularis oris muscle approximates and compresses the lips, whereas the zygomaticus muscles raise the lateral angle of the mouth (smiling).

Examination of the Eye[31-34]

If the eyelids are swollen shut, the examiner should initially assume that the globe has been ruptured. A penetrating wound of the eyelid should be assessed carefully,

Stabilize

Figure 2-36
Testing for maxillary fracture.

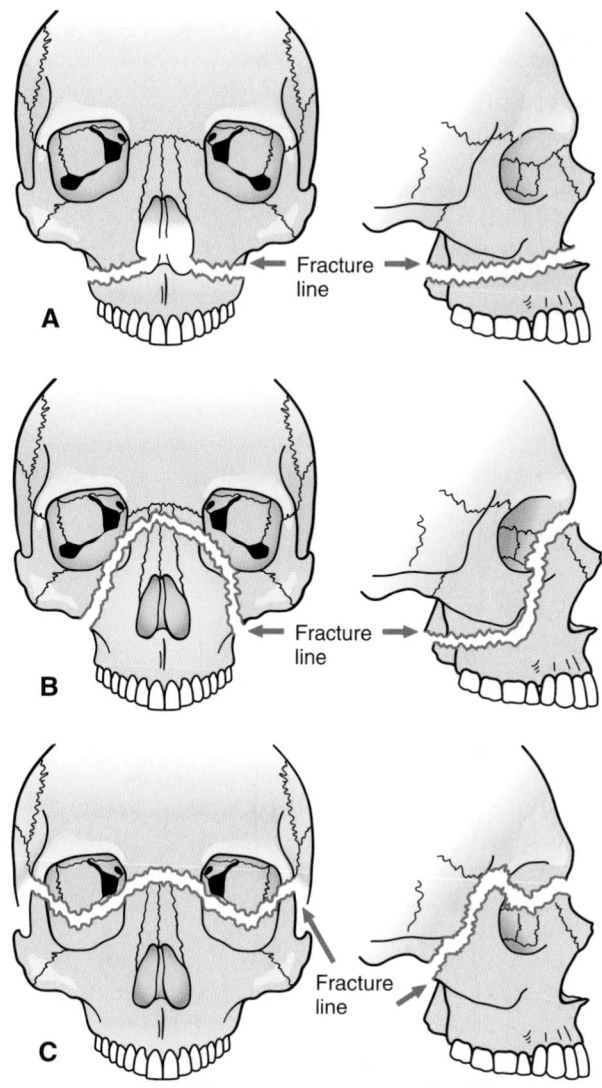

Figure 2-37
Le Fort fractures. **A**, Le Fort I. **B**, Le Fort II. **C**, Le Fort III.

because it may be associated with a globe injury. The examiner should not force the eyelid open, because intraocular pressure can force extrusion of the ocular contents if the globe has been ruptured. The patient should also be instructed not to squeeze the eyelids tight, because this action can increase the intraocular pressure from a normal value of 15 mm Hg up to approximately 70 mm Hg.

To examine the normal functioning of the eye muscles and several of the cranial nerves (II, III, IV, and VI), the examiner asks the patient to move through the six cardinal positions of gaze (Figure 2-40). The examiner holds the patient's chin steady with one hand and asks the patient to follow the examiner's other hand while the examiner traces a large "H" in the air. The examiner should hold the index finger or pencil approximately 25 cm (10 inches) from the patient's nose. From the midline, the finger or pencil is moved approximately 30 cm (12 inches) to the patient's right and held. It is then moved up approximately 20 cm (8 inches) and held, moved down 40 cm (16 inches) (20 cm relative to midline) and held, and moved slowly back to midline. The same movement is repeated on the other side. The examiner should observe movement of both eyes, noting whether the eyes follow the finger or pencil smoothly. The examiner should also observe any parallel movement of the eyes in all directions. If the eyes do not move in unison or if only one eye moves, something is affecting the action of the muscles. One of the most common causes of one eye's not moving after trauma to the eye is a blowout fracture of the orbital floor (Figure 2-41). Because the inferior muscles become "caught" in the fracture site, the affected eye demonstrates limited movement (Figure 2-42), especially upward. The patient with this type of fracture may also demonstrate depression of the eye globe, blurred vision, double vision, and conjunctival hemorrhage.

Occasionally, when looking to the extreme side, the eyes will develop a rhythmic motion called end-point nystagmus. **Nystagmus** is a rhythmic movement of the eyes with an abnormal slow drifting away from fixation and rapid return. With end-point nystagmus, there is a quick motion in the direction of the gaze followed by a

Eye Examination

- Six cardinal gaze positions
- Pupils (size, equality, reactivity)
- Nystagmus
- Visual field (peripheral vision)
- Visual acuity
- Symmetry of gaze
- Foreign objects/corneal abrasion
- Surrounding bone and soft tissue
- Hyphema

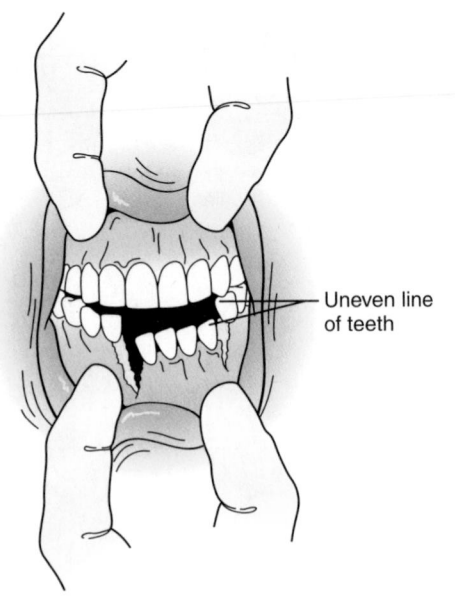

Uneven line of teeth

Figure 2-38

Malocclusion of teeth may be associated with fracture of mandible or maxilla.

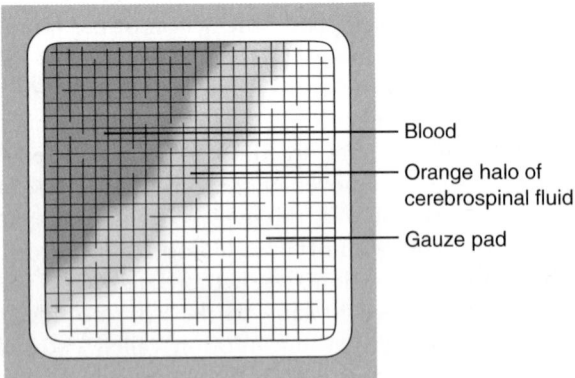

Blood

Orange halo of cerebrospinal fluid

Gauze pad

Figure 2-39

An orange halo will form around the blood on a gauze pad if cerebrospinal fluid is present.

slow return. This test differentiates end-point nystagmus from pathological nystagmus, in which there is a quick movement of the eyes in the same direction regardless of gaze. Pathological nystagmus exists in the region of full binocular vision, not just at the periphery. Cerebellar nystagmus is greater when the eyes are deviated toward the side of the lesion.

While testing the cardinal positions, the examiner should also watch for lid lag. Normally, the upper lid covers the top of the iris, rising when the patient looks up and quickly lowering as the eye lowers. With lid lag, the upper lid delays lowering as the eye lowers.

Peripheral vision, or the visual field (peripheral limits of vision), can be tested with the confrontation test (Figure 2-43). The patient is asked to cover the right eye while the examiner covers his or her own left eye, so that the open eyes of the examiner and of the patient are directly opposite each other. While the examiner and the patient look into each other's eye, the examiner fully extends his or her right arm to the side, midway between the patient and the examiner, and then moves it toward them with the fingers waving. The patient tells the examiner when he or she first sees the moving fingers. The examiner then compares the patient's response with the time or distance at which the examiner first noted the fingers. The test is then repeated to the other side.

The nasal, temporal, superior, and inferior fields should all be tested in a similar fashion. The visual field should describe angles of 60° nasally, 90° temporally, 50° superiorly, and 70° inferiorly. Double simultaneous testing may also be performed. This method uses two stimuli (e.g., moving fingers) that are simultaneously presented in the right and left visual fields, and the patient is asked which finger is moving. Normally, the patient should say "both," without hesitation. With any loss of vision field (i.e., if the patient is unable to see in the same visual fields as before), the patient must be referred for further examination.

The eyelids should be everted to look at the underside of the eyelid and to give a clearer view of the globe, especially if the patient complains of a foreign body. The upper eyelid may be everted with the use of a special lid retractor or a cotton swab (Figure 2-44). The patient is asked to look down and to the right and then down and to the left while the superior aspect of the eye is examined. The examiner can check the inferior aspect of the eye and its conjunctival lining by carefully pulling the lower eyelid downward and gently holding it against the bony orbit. Next, the patient is asked to look up and to the right and then up and to the left while the inferior aspect of the eye is examined. These two techniques may also be used to look for a contact lens that has migrated away from the cornea.

Both eyelids should be checked for laceration. Lacerations in the area of the lacrimal gland are especially important to detect because, if they are not looked after

Table 2-20

Muscles of the Face

	Action	Cranial Nerve
Muscles of the Mouth		
Orbicularis oris	Compresses lips against anterior teeth, closes mouth, protrudes lips	VII (Zygomatic, buccal, and mandibular branches)
Depressor anguli oris	Depresses angle of mouth	VII (Buccal and mandibular branches)
Levator anguli oris	Elevates angle of mouth	VII (Zygomatic and buccal branches)
Zygomaticus major	Draws angle of mouth upward and back	VII (Zygomatic and buccal branches)
Risorius	Draws angle of mouth laterally	VII (Zygomatic and buccal branches)
Muscle of the Lips		
Levator labii superioris	Elevates upper lip, flares nostril	VII (Zygomatic and buccal branches)
Muscle of the Cheek		
Buccinator	Compresses cheeks against molar teeth; sucking and blowing	VII (Buccal branches)
Muscle of the Chin		
Mentalis	Puckers skin of chin, protrudes lower lip	VII (Mandibular branches)
Muscle of the Nose		
Nasalis	Compresses nostrils / Dilates or flares nostrils	VII (Zygomatic and buccal branches)
Muscle of the Eye		
Orbicularis oculi	Closes eye forcefully / Closes eye gently / Squeezes lubricating tears against eyeball	VII (Temporal and zygomatic branches)
Muscles of the Forehead		
Procerus	Transverse wrinkling of bridge of nose	VII (Temporal and zygomatic branches)
Corrugator	Vertical wrinkling of bridge of nose	VII (Temporal branches)
Frontalis	Pulls scalp upward and back	VII (Temporal branches)

Adapted from Liebgott B: *The anatomical basis of dentistry*, pp. 242–243, St. Louis, 1986, Mosby.

properly, the tearing function of the lacrimal gland may be lost (Figure 2-45).

The reaction of the pupils to light should then be tested. First, the light in the room is dimmed. The pupils dilate in a dark environment or with a long focal distance and constrict in a light environment or with a short focal distance. The examiner shines a pen light directly into one of the patient's eyes for approximately 5 seconds (Figure 2-46). Normally, constriction of the pupil occurs, followed by slight dilation. The pupillary reaction is classified as brisk (normal), sluggish, nonreactive, or fixed. An oval or slightly oval pupil or one that is fixed and dilated indicates increased intracranial pressure. The fixation and dilation of both pupils is a terminal sign of anoxia and ischemia to the brain. If the dilation is significant, an injury to the optic nerve may be suspected. If both pupils are midsize, midposition, and nonreactive, midbrain damage is usually indicated. In a fully conscious, alert patient who has sustained a blow near the eye, a dilated, fixed pupil usually implies injury to the ciliary nerves of the eye rather than brain injury. The other eye is tested similarly, and the results are compared.

Normally, both pupils constrict when a light is shined in one eye. The reaction of the eye being tested is called the **direct light reflex;** the reaction of the other pupil is called the **consensual light reflex.** This reaction is brisker in the young and people with blue eyes.[35] If the optic nerve is damaged, the affected pupil constricts in response to light in the opposite eye (consensual) and

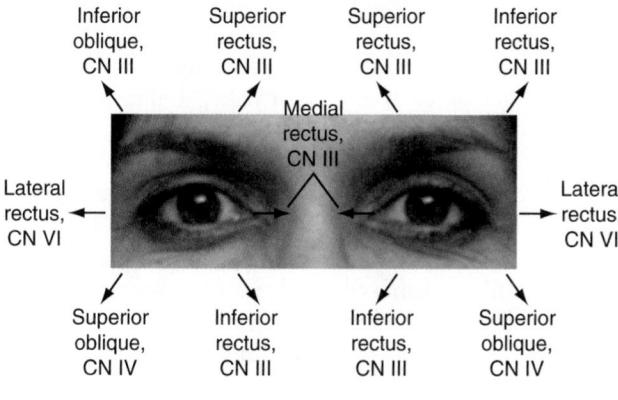

Figure 2-40

The six cardinal fields of gaze, showing eye muscles and cranial nerves (CN) involved in the movement.

Figure 2-41

Blowout fracture of the orbital floor. The dashed line indicates normal position of the globe. The inferior oblique and inferior rectus muscles are "caught" in the fracture site, preventing the eye from returning to its normal position. (Modified from Paton D and Goldberg MF: *Management of ocular injuries*, p. 63, Philadelphia, 1976, WB Saunders.)

Figure 2-42

Fresh blowout fracture of left orbit with limitation of upward *(top)* and downward *(bottom)* movements of the left eye. (Modified from Paton D and Goldberg MF: *Management of ocular injuries*, p. 65, Philadelphia, 1976, WB Saunders.)

dilates in response to light shined into it (direct). If the oculomotor nerve is affected, the affected pupil is fixed and dilated and does not respond to light, either directly or consensually. If the pupils do not react, it is an indication of injury to the oculomotor nerve and its connections or of injury to the head. The eye also appears laterally displaced owing to paresis of the medial rectus muscle.

Figure 2-43

Confrontation eye test.

The pupil is then tested for constriction to accommodation. The patient is asked to look at a distant object and then at a test object—a pencil or the examiner's finger held 10 cm (4 inches) from the bridge of the nose. The pupils dilate when the patient looks at a far object and constrict when the patient focuses on the near object. The eyes also adduct (go "cross-eyed") when the patient looks at the close object. These actions are called the **accommodation-convergence** reflex.[35] When looking at distant objects, the eyes should be parallel. Deviation or lack of parallelism is called **strabismus** and indicates weakness of one of the extraocular muscles or lack of neural coordination.[55]

When inspected under normal overhead light, the lens of the eye should be transparent. Shining a light on the lens may cause it to appear gray or yellow. The cornea should be smooth and clear. If the patient has extreme pain in the corneal area, a corneal abrasion should be suspected (Figure 2-47). An appropriate specialist may test for corneal abrasion by using a fluorescein strip and a slit lamp. The cornea should be crystal clear when it is viewed, and the iris details should match those of the other eye.

To check for depth of the anterior chamber of the eye or a narrow corneal angle, the examiner shines a light obliquely across each eye. Normally, it illuminates the entire iris. If the corneal angle is narrow because of a shallow anterior chamber, the examiner will be able to see a crescent-shaped shadow on the side of the iris away from the light (Figure 2-48). This finding indicates an anatomical predisposition to narrow-angled glaucoma.

To test for **symmetry of gaze,** the examiner aims a light source approximately 60 cm (24 inches) from the patient while standing directly in front of the patient and holding the light distant enough to prevent convergence of the patient's gaze. The patient is asked to stare at the light. The dots of reflected light on the two corneas should be in the same relative location (Figure

Figure 2-44

Eversion of the eyelid. **A,** Grasping eyelash. **B,** Putting moistened cotton-tipped applicator over eyelid. **C,** Everting eyelid over the cotton-tipped applicator.

2-49). When one eye does not look directly at the light, the reflected dot of light moves to the side opposite the deviation. For example, if the eye deviates medially, the reflection appears more laterally placed than in the other eye. The examiner can approximate the angle of deviation by noting the position of the reflection. Each millimeter of displacement in the reflection represents approximately 7° of ocular deviation. To bring out a mild deviation, the

Figure 2-45

A lower lid laceration *(arrow)*. (From Pashby TJ and Pashby RC: Treatment of sports eye injuries. In Schneider RC et al, editors: *Sports injuries: mechanisms, prevention and treatment*, p. 576, Baltimore, 1985, Williams & Wilkins.)

examiner may use a cover-uncover test (Figure 2-50). The patient looks at a specific point, such as the bridge of the examiner's nose. One of the patient's eyes is then covered with a card. Normally, the uncovered eye will not move. If it moves, it was not straight before the other eye was covered. The other eye is then tested in a similar fashion.

Visual acuity is tested using a vision chart. Visual acuity is the ability of the eye to perceive fine detail, for example, when reading. If a standard eye wall chart is not available, a pocket visual acuity card may be used. This pocket card is usually viewed at a distance of 35 to 36 cm (14 inches). As with the wall chart, the patient is asked to examine the smallest line possible. If neither eye chart is available, any printed material may be used. A patient who wears glasses or contact lenses should be tested both without and with the corrective lenses. The test is done quickly so the patient cannot memorize the chart. Visual acuity is recorded as a fraction in which the numerator indicates the distance of the patient from the chart (e.g., 20 ft) and the denominator indicates the distance at which the normal eye can read the line. Thus, 20/100 means the patient can read at 20 ft what the average person can read at 100 ft. The smaller the fraction, the worse the myopia (nearsightedness). Patients with corrected vision of less than 20/40 should be referred to the appropriate specialist.[35] Intraocular examination with an ophthalmoscope, if available, may reveal lens, vitreous, or retinal damage.

A

B

Figure 2-46
Testing the pupils for reaction to light. **A,** Light shining in eye.
B, Light shining away from eye.

Examination of the Nose[31–34]

Patency of the nasal passages can be determined by occluding one of the patient's nostrils by pushing a finger against the side of the nostril. The patient is then asked to breathe in and out of the opposite nostril with the mouth closed. The process is repeated on the other side. Normally, no sound is heard, and the patient can breathe easily through the open nostril.

Nasal Examination

- Patency
- Nasal cavities
- Sinuses
- Fracture
- Nasal discharge (bloody, straw-colored, clear)

A

B

Figure 2-47
Corneal abrasion. **A,** Without fluorescein. **B,** With fluorescein.
(From Torg JS: *Athletic injuries to the head, neck and face*, p. 262,
Philadelphia, 1982, Lea & Febiger.)

If available, a nasal speculum and light may be used to inspect the nasal cavity. The nasal mucosa and turbinates can be inspected for color, foreign bodies, and abnormal masses (e.g., polyp). The nasal septum should be in midline and straight and is normally thicker anteriorly than posteriorly. If the nasal cavities are asymmetric, it may indicate a deviated septum. If the patient demonstrates a septal hematoma, it must be treated fairly quickly, because the hematoma may cause excessive pressure on the septum, making it avascular. This avascularity can result in a "saddle nose" deformity owing to necrosis and absorption of the underlying cartilage (Figure 2-51).

Illumination of the frontal and maxillary sinuses may be performed if sinus tenderness is present or infection is suspected. The examination must be performed in a completely darkened room. To illuminate the maxillary sinuses, the examiner places the light source lateral to the patient's nose just beneath the medial aspect of the eye. The examiner then looks through the patient's open mouth for illumination of the hard palate. To illuminate the frontal sinuses, the examiner places the light source against the medial aspect of each supraorbital rim. The examiner looks for a dim red glow as light is transmitted just below the eyebrow. The sinuses usually show differing degrees of illumination. The absence of a glow indicates either that the sinus is filled with secretions or that it has never developed.

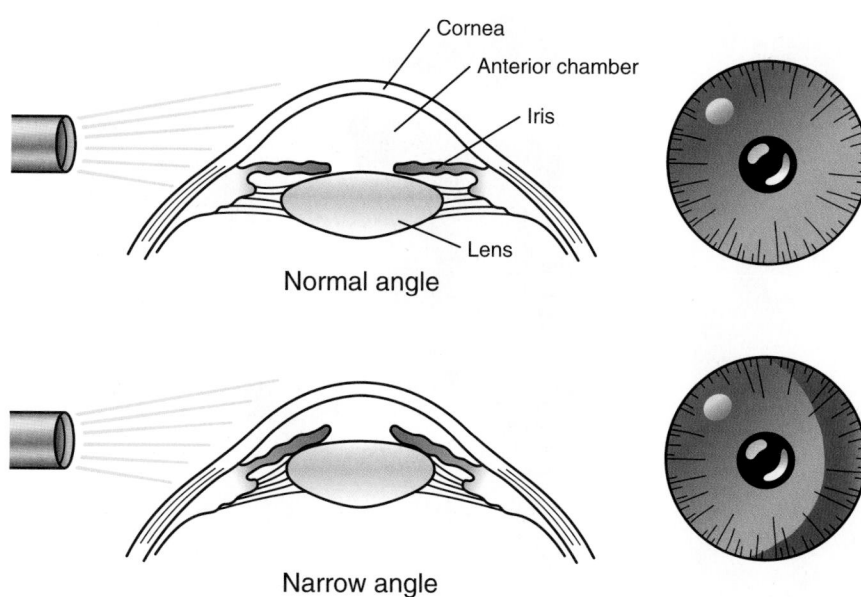

Figure 2-48
Normal and narrow corneal angle (depth of anterior chamber). (Modified from Swartz HM: *Textbook of physical diagnosis*, p. 144, Philadelphia, 1989, WB Saunders.)

Figure 2-49
Symmetry of gaze. Note white "dots" of light on pupils.

Examination of the Teeth[31–34]

The examiner should observe the teeth to see if they are in normal position and whether any teeth are missing, chipped, or depressed (see Figure 2-23). Using the gloved index finger and thumb, the examiner applies mild pressure to each tooth, pressing inward toward the tongue and outward toward the lips. Normally, a small amount of movement is observed. If a tooth is loose, excessive movement or increased pain or numbness relative to other teeth indicates a positive test. A tooth that has been avulsed may be cleansed with warm water and reinserted into the socket. The patient is then referred to the appropriate specialist.

Tooth Examination
• Number of teeth
• Position of teeth
• Movement of teeth
• Condition of teeth
• Condition of gums

Examination of the Ear[30–34]

Examination of the ear deals primarily with whether the patient is able to hear. Several tests may be used to examine hearing.

Ear Examination
• Tenderness (exterior and interior)
• Ear discharge (bloody, straw-colored, clear)
• Hearing
• Balance

Whispered Voice Test. The patient's response to the examiner's whispered voice can be used to determine hearing ability. The examiner masks the hearing in

Figure 2-50
Cover-uncover test for mild ocular deviation. As patient gazes at a specific point **(A)**, examiner covers one eye and looks for movement in uncovered eye **(B)**.

Figure 2-51
"Saddle nose" deformity *(arrow)* that occurred as a result of loss of septal cartilage support secondary to septal hematoma and abscess. (From Handler SD: Diagnosis and management of maxillofacial injuries. In Torg, JS, editor: *Athletic injuries to the head, neck and face*, p. 232, Philadelphia, 1982, Lea & Febiger.)

the examiner gradually increases his or her volume until the patient responds appropriately. The procedure is repeated in the other ear. The patient should be able to hear whispered words in each ear at a distance of 30 to 60 cm (12 to 24 inches) and respond correctly at least 50% of the time.[30,31]

Ticking Watch Test. The ticking watch test uses a nonelectric ticking watch to test high-frequency hearing. The examiner positions the watch approximately 15 cm (6 inches) from the ear to be tested, slowly moving it toward the ear. The patient then indicates when he or she hears the ticking sound. The distance can be measured and will give some idea of the patient's ability to hear high-frequency sound.[30,31]

Weber Test. The examiner places the base of a vibrating tuning fork on the midline vertex of the patient's head. The patient should hear the sound equally well in both ears (Figures 2-52 and 2-53). If the patient hears better in one ear (i.e., the sound is lateralized), the patient is asked to identify which ear hears the sound better. To test the reliability of the patient's response, the examiner repeats the procedure while occluding one ear with a finger and asks the patient which ear hears the sound better. It should be heard better in the occluded ear.[30,31]

one of the patient's ears by placing a finger gently in the patient's ear canal. Standing approximately 30 to 60 cm (12 to 24 inches) away from the patient, the examiner whispers one- or two-syllable words and asks the patient to repeat them. If the patient has difficulty,

A   **B**   **C**

Figure 2-52

The Weber test. **A,** When a vibrating tuning fork is placed on the center of the forehead, the sound is heard in the center without lateralization to either side (normal response). **B,** In the presence of a conductive hearing loss, the sound is heard on the side of the conductive loss. **C,** In the presence of sensorineural loss, the sound is better heard on the opposite (unaffected) side.

Weber (away from the lesion)

Air >> bone   Rinne (air >> bone)

30 cm   13 cm

Watch tick   Watch tick
Finger twitching   Finger twitching

SENSORINEURAL LOSS

Weber (to the left)

Air >> bone   Rinne (air < bone)

30 cm   13 cm

Watch tick   Watch tick
Finger twitching   Finger twitching

CONDUCTIVE LOSS

Tuning fork > 512cos   Weber (midline)
Rinne (air >> bone)

Air >> bone

30 cm   13 cm

Watch tick
Finger twitching
Whispered voice

NORMAL

Figure 2-53

Bedside hearing tests and results with sensorineural or conductive loss in left ear and with normal hearing.

Rinne Test. The Rinne test is performed by placing the base of the vibrating tuning fork against the patient's mastoid bone. The examiner counts or times the interval with a watch. The patient tells the examiner when he or she no longer hears the sound, and the examiner notes the number of seconds. The examiner then quickly positions a still-vibrating tine 1 to 2 cm (0.5 to 0.8 inch) from the auditory canal and asks patient to indicate when he or she no longer hears the sound. The examiner then compares the number of seconds the sound was heard by bone conduction and by air conduction. The counting or timing of the interval between the two sounds determines the length of time that sound is heard by air conduction (see Figure 2-53). Air-conducted sound should be heard twice as long as bone-conducted sound. For example, if bone conduction is heard for 15 seconds, the air conduction should be heard for 30 seconds.[30-32]

Schwabach Test. This test compares the patient's and examiner's hearing by bone conduction. The examiner alternately places the vibrating tuning fork against the patient's mastoid process and against the examiner's mastoid bone until one of them no longer hears a sound. The examiner and patient should hear the sound for equal amounts of time.[30,31]

Conductive hearing loss implies that the patient experiences a reduction of all sounds rather than difficulty in interpreting sounds. **Sensorineural or perceptual** hearing loss indicates that the patient has difficulty interpreting the sounds.

To examine the internal structure of the ear, the examiner may use an otoscope, if one is available. In this case, the examiner would observe the canal as well as the eardrum (tympanic membrane), noting any blockage, excessive wax, swelling, redness, transparency (usually pearly gray), bulging, retraction, or perforation of the eardrum.

Special Tests

Examiners perform only those special tests that they think will have value. For example, the tests for expanding intracranial lesions would not be performed with a facial injury unless an associated injury to the brain or other neurological tissues is suspected. The reliability, validity, specificity and sensitivity of some special/diagnostic tests used in the head and face are outlined in Appendix 2-1.

Tests for Expanding Intracranial Lesions

For each of these tests, the patient must be able to stand normally when the eyes are open.

Neurological Control Test—Upper Limb. The examiner asks the patient to stand with his or her arms forward flexed 90° and eyes closed. The patient holds this position for approximately 30 seconds. If the examiner notes that one arm tends to move or drift outward and downward, the test is considered positive for an expanding intracranial lesion on the side opposite the side with the drift.

Neurological Control Test—Lower Limb. The examiner asks the patient to sit on the edge of a table or in a chair with his or her legs extended in front and not touching the ground. The patient closes his or her eyes for approximately 20 to 30 seconds. If the examiner notes that one leg tends to move or drift, the test is considered positive for an expanding intracranial lesion on the side opposite that with the drift.

Romberg Test. The examiner asks the patient to stand with feet together and arms by the sides with the eyes open. The examiner notes whether the patient has any problem with balance. The patient then closes his or her eyes for at least 20 seconds, and the examiner notes any differences. A positive Romberg test is elicited if the patient sways or falls to one side when the eyes are closed, and this reaction indicates an expanding intracranial lesion, possible disease of the spinal cord posterior columns, or proprioceptive problems.

Walk or Stand in Tandem Test. Patients with expanding intracranial lesions demonstrate increasing difficulty in walking in tandem ("walking the line") or standing in tandem (one foot in front of other). Standing in tandem is more difficult to perform than walking in tandem.

Tests for Coordination

Finger-to-Nose Test. The patient stands or sits with the eyes open and brings the index finger to the nose. The test is repeated with the eyes closed. Both arms are tested several times with increasing speed. Normally, the tests should be accomplished easily, smoothly, and quickly with the eyes open and closed.

Finger-Thumb Test. The patient touches each finger with the thumb of the same hand. The normal or uninjured side is tested first, followed by the injured side. The examiner compares the two sides for coordination and timing.

Hand "Flip" Test. The patient touches the back of the opposite, stationary hand with the anterior aspect of the fingers, flips the test hand over, and touches the opposite hand with the posterior aspect of the fingers. The movement is repeated several times, with both sides being tested. The examiner compares the two sides for coordination and speed.

Finger Drumming Test. The patient to drums the index and middle finger of one hand up and down as quickly as possible on the back of the other hand. The test is repeated with the opposite hand. The examiner compares the two sides for coordination and speed.

Hand-Thigh Test. The patient pats his or her thigh with the hand as quickly as possible. The uninjured side is tested first. The patient may be asked to supinate and pronate the hand between each hand-thigh contact to make the test more complex. The examiner watches for speed and coordination and compares the two sides.

Past Pointing Test. The patient and examiner face each other. The examiner holds up both index fingers approximately 15 cm (6 inches) apart. The patient is asked to lift the arms over the head and then bring the arms down to touch the patient's index fingers to the examiner's index fingers (Figure 2-54). The test is repeated with the patient's eyes closed. Normally, the test can be performed without difficulty. Patients with

Figure 2-54
Past pointing. (Redrawn from Reilly BM: *Practical strategies in outpatient medicine*, p. 195, Philadelphia, 1991, WB Saunders.)

given by pressure. The patient then tells the examiner which way the digit moved.

Proprioceptive Space Test. With the patient's eyes closed, the examiner places one of the patient's hands or feet in a selected position in space. The patient then imitates that position with the other limb or to find the hand or foot with the other limb. True proprioceptive loss causes the patient to be unable to properly position or to find the normal limb with the limb that has proprioceptive loss.

Past Pointing Test. The test is performed as described under Tests for Coordination.

Reflexes and Cutaneous Distribution

With a head injury patient, deep tendon reflexes (see Table 1-28) should be tested. Accentuation of one or more of the reflexes may indicate trauma to the brain on the opposite side. Pathological reflexes (see Table 1-30) may also be altered with a head injury.

The **corneal reflex** (trigeminal nerve, cranial nerve V) is used to test for damage or dysfunction to the pons. In some cases, the patient may look to one side to avoid involuntary blinking. The examiner touches the cornea (not the eyelashes or conjunctiva) with a small, fine point of cotton (Figure 2-55). The normal response is a bilateral blink, because the reflex arc connects both facial nerve nuclei. If the reflex is absent, the test is considered positive.

vestibular disease have problems with past pointing. The test may also be used to test proprioception.

Heel-to-Knee Test. The patient, who is lying supine with the eyes open, takes the heel of one foot and touches the opposite knee with the heel and then slides the heel down the shin. The test is repeated with the eyes closed, and both legs are tested. The test can be repeated several times with increasing speed, with the examiner noting any differences in coordination or the presence of tremor. Normally, the test should be accomplished easily, smoothly, and quickly with the eyes open and closed.

Tests for Proprioception

Proprioceptive Finger-Nose Test. The patient keeps the eyes closed. The examiner lightly touches one of the patient's fingers and asks the patient to touch the patient's nose with that finger. The examiner then touches another finger on the other hand, and the patient again touches the nose. Patients with proprioceptive loss have difficulty doing the test without visual input.

Proprioceptive Movement Test. With the patient's eyes closed, the examiner moves the patient's finger or toe up or down by grasping it on the sides to lessen clues

Figure 2-55
Test of corneal reflex.

The **gag reflex** may be tested using a tongue depressor that is inserted into the posterior pharynx and depressed toward the hypopharynx. The reflex tests cranial nerves IX and X, and its absence in a trauma setting may indicate caudal brain stem dysfunction.

Consensual light reflex may be tested by shining a light into one eye. This action causes the lighted pupil to constrict. If there is normal communication between the two oculomotor nerves, the nonlighted pupil also constricts.

The **jaw reflex** is usually tested only if the temporomandibular joint or cervical spine is being examined.

The examiner should check the sensation of the head and face, keeping in mind the differences in dermatome and sensory nerve distributions (Figure 2-56). Lip anesthesia or paresthesia is often seen in patients with mandibular fracture.

Nerve Injuries of the Head and Face

Bell's palsy involves paralysis of the facial nerve (cranial nerve VII) and usually occurs where the nerve emerges from the stylomastoid foramen. Pressure in the foramen caused by inflammation or trauma affects the nerve and therefore the muscles of the face (occipitofrontalis, corrugator, orbicularis oculi, and the nose and mouth muscles) on one side. The inflammation may result from a middle ear infection, viral infection, chilling of the face, or tumor. The observable result is smoothing of the face on the affected side owing to loss of muscle action, the eye on the affected side remaining open, and

the lower eyelid sagging. The patient is unable to wink, whistle, purse the lips, or wrinkle the forehead. Speech sounds, especially those requiring pursing of the lips, are affected, resulting in slurred speech. The mouth droops, and it and the nose may deviate to the opposite side, especially in longstanding cases, of which there are remarkably few (90% of patients recover completely within 2 to 8 weeks). Facial sensation on the affected side is lost, and taste sensation is sometimes lost as well. The House-Brackmann Facial Nerve Grading System (Table 2-21) may be used to grade the level of facial nerve involvement.[56]

Joint Play Movements

Because no articular joints are involved in the assessment of the head and face, there are no joint play movements to test.

Palpation

During palpation of the head and face, the examiner should note any tenderness, deformity, crepitus, or other signs and symptoms that may indicate the source of pathology. The examiner should note the texture of the skin and surrounding bony and soft tissues. Normally, the patient is palpated in the sitting or supine position, beginning with the skull and moving from anterior to posterior, to the face, and finally to the lateral and posterior structures of the head.

The skull is palpated by a gentle rotary movement of the fingers, progressing systematically from front to back. Normally, the skin of the skull moves freely and has no tenderness, swelling, or depressions.

The temporal area and temporalis muscle should be laterally palpated for tenderness and deformity. The external ear or auricle and the periauricular area should also be palpated for tenderness or lacerations.

The occiput should be palpated posteriorly for tenderness. The presence of **Battle's sign** should be noted, if observed, because this signals a possible basilar skull fracture.

The face is palpated beginning superiorly and working inferiorly in a systematic manner. Like the skull, the forehead is palpated by gentle rotary movements of the fingers, feeling the movement of the skin and the occipitofrontalis muscle underneath. Normally, the skin of the forehead moves freely and is smooth and even with no tender areas. The examiner then palpates around the eye socket or orbital rim, moving over the eyebrow and supraorbital rims, around the lateral side of the eye, and along the zygomatic arch to the infraorbital rims, looking for deformity, crepitus, tenderness, and lacerations (Figure 2-57, *A* and *B*).

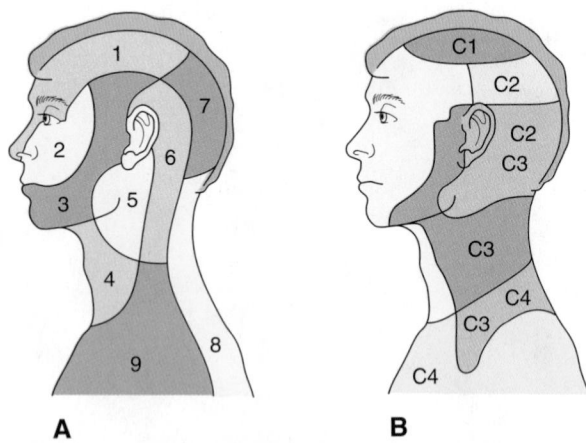

Figure 2-56

A, Sensory nerve distribution of the head, neck and face. (1) Ophthalmic nerve. (2) Maxillary nerve. (3) Mandibular nerve. (4) Transverse cutaneous nerve of neck (C2-C3). (5) Greater auricular nerve (C2-C3). (6) Lesser auricular nerve (C2). (7) Greater occipital nerve (C2-C3). (8) Cervical dorsal rami (C3-C5). (9) Suprascapular nerve (C5-C6). **B,** Dermatome pattern of the head, neck, and face. Note the overlap of C3.

Table 2-21

House-Brackmann Facial Nerve Grading System

Parameter	Grade I	Grade II	Grade III	Grade IV	Grade V	Grade VI
Overall appearance	Normal	Slight weakness on close inspection	Obvious but not disfiguring difference between both sides	Obvious weakness or disfiguring asymmetry	Only barely perceptible motion	No movement
At rest	Normal symmetry and tone	Normal symmetry and tone	Normal symmetry and tone	Normal symmetry and tone	Asymmetry	Asymmetry
Forehead movement	Normal function	Moderate-to-good function	Slight-to-moderate function	None	None	None
Eyelid closure	Normal closure	Complete closure with minimum effort	Complete closure with effort	Incomplete closure	Incomplete closure	No movement
Mouth	Normal and symmetric	Slight asymmetry	Slight asymmetry with maximum effort	Asymmetry with maximum effort	Slight movement	No movement
Synkinesis (involuntary movement), contracture and/or hemifacial spasm	None	May have very slight synkinesis; no contracture or hemifacial spasm	Noticeable but not severe synkinesis contracture and/or hemifacial spasm	Synkinesis, contracture and/or asymmetrical facial spasm disfiguring leading to severe enough to interfere with function	Synkinesis, contracture and/or hemifacial spasm usually absent but disfiguring present	Disfiguring present

Modifed from Dutton M. *Orthopedic examination, evaluation and intervention,* p.1130, New York, 2004, McGraw Hill. Adapted From House JW and Brackmann DE: Facial nerve grading system, *Otolaryngol Head Neck Surg* 93:146–147, 1985.

A   B

Figure 2-57 ▬▬▬

Palpation of the face. **A,** Upper orbital rim. **B,** Lower orbital rim.

(Continued)

Figure 2-57 cont'd
Palpation of the face. **C,** Nose. **D,** Mandible. **E,** Maxilla.

The orbicularis oculi muscles surround the orbit, and the medial side of the orbital rim and nose are then palpated for tenderness, deformity, and fracture. The nasal bones, including the lateral and alar cartilage, are palpated for any crepitus or deviation (Figure 2-57, C). The septum should be inspected to see if it has widened, possibly indicating a septal hematoma, which often occurs with a fracture. It should also be determined whether the patient can breathe through the nose or smell.

The frontal and maxillary sinuses should be inspected for swelling. To palpate the frontal sinuses, the examiner uses the thumbs to press up under the bony brow on each side of the nose (Figure 2-58, *A*). The examiner then presses under the zygomatic processes using either the thumbs or index and middle fingers to palpate the maxillary sinuses (Figure 2-58, *B*). No tenderness or swelling over the soft tissue should be present. The sinus areas may also be percussed to detect tenderness. A light tap directly over each sinus with the index finger can be used to detect tenderness.

The examiner then moves inferiorly to palpate the jaw. The examiner palpates the mandible along its entire length, noting any tenderness, crepitus, or deformity. The examiner, using a rubber glove, may also palpate along the mandible interiorly, noting any tenderness or pain (Figure 2-57, *D*). The outside hand may be used to stabilize the jaw during this procedure. The mandible may also be tapped with a finger along its length to see if signs of tenderness are elicited. The muscles of the cheek (buccinator) and mouth (orbicularis oris) should be palpated at the same time.

The maxilla may be palpated in a similar fashion, both internally and externally, noting position of the teeth, tenderness, and any deformity (Figure 2-57, *E*). The examiner may grasp the teeth anteriorly to see if the teeth and mandible or maxilla move in relation to the rest of the face, which may indicate a Le Fort fracture (Figure 2-59).

The trachea should be palpated for midline position. The examiner places a thumb along each side

Figure 2-58

A, Palpation of frontal sinuses. *B*, Palpation of maxillary sinuses.

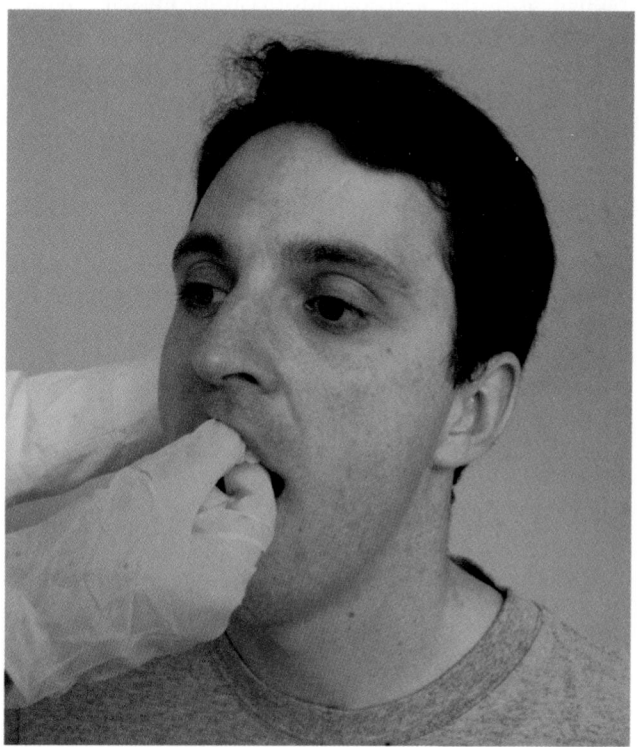

Figure 2-59

Palpation of maxillary fracture with anteroposterior rocking motion.

Figure 2-60

Incomplete fracture of angle of mandible on the left side *(arrows)*. **A,** Anteroposterior view. **B,** Lateral view.
(From O'Donoghue DH: *Treatment of injuries to athletes*, p. 114, Philadelphia, 1984, WB Saunders.)

of the trachea, comparing the spaces between the trachea and the sternocleidomastoid muscle, which should be symmetric. The hyoid bone and the thyroid and cricoid cartilages should be identified. Normally, they are smooth and nontender and move when the patient swallows.

Diagnostic Imaging

Plain Film Radiography

Anteroposterior view. The examiner should note the normal bone contours, looking for fractures of the various bones (Figures 2-60 through 2-62).

Lateral view. The examiner should again note bony contours, looking for the possibility of fractures (Figures 2-60 and 2-63).

Computed Tomography

Computed tomography scans help to differentiate between bone and soft tissue and give a more precise view of fractures (Figures 2-64 and 2-65).

Magnetic Resonance Imaging

Magnetic resonance imaging is especially useful for demonstrating lesions of the soft tissues of the head and face and for differentiating between bone and soft tissue (Figures 2-66 and 2-67).

Figure 2-61

Anteroposterior skull radiograph showing a depressed parietal skull fracture *(large arrow)* with multiple bony fragments into the brain *(small arrows)*. (From Albright JP et al: Head and neck injuries in sports. In Scott WN et al, editors: *Principles of sports medicine*, p. 53, Baltimore, 1984, Williams & Wilkins.)

Figure 2-62
Plain posteroanterior view showing blowout fracture of the orbit
(arrows). (From Paton D and Goldberg MF: *Management of ocular
injuries*, p. 70, Philadelphia, 1976, WB Saunders.)

Figure 2-63
Lateral radiograph of the nasal bones demonstrating a nasal fracture
(arrow). (From Torg JS: *Athletic injuries to the head, neck and face*,
p. 229, Philadelphia, 1982, Lea & Febiger.)

Figure 2-64
Axial computed tomogram of orbital blowout fracture showing fracture of the orbit (1) with orbital contents
herniated into the maxillary sinus. (From Sinn DP and Karas ND: Radiographic evaluation of facial injuries.
In Fonseca RJ and Walker RV, editors: *Oral and maxillofacial trauma*, Philadelphia, 1991, WB Saunders.)

Figure 2-65
The computed tomographic scan is ideal for condylar fractures as seen in the right condyle. (From Bruce R and Fonseca RJ: Mandibular fractures. In Fonseca RJ and Walker RV, editors: *Oral and maxillofacial trauma*, p. 389, Philadelphia, 1991, WB Saunders.)

A   **B**

Figure 2-66
Magnetic resonance images showing blowout fracture. Sagittal (**A**) and coronal (**B**) T1-weighted scans demonstrate a blowout fracture of the right orbit with depression of the orbital floor *(white arrows)* into the superior maxillary sinus. The inferior rectus muscle *(long arrow)* is clearly identified and is not entrapped by the floor fracture. (From Harms SE: The orbit. In Edelman RR and Hesselink JR, editors: *Clinical magnetic resonance imaging*, p. 619, Philadelphia, 1990, WB Saunders.)

Figure 2-67

T1-weighted axial magnetic resonance images of the head and brain at two levels. PICA, posterior inferior cerebellar artery. (From Greenberg JJ et al: Brain: indications, techniques, and atlas. In Edelman RR and Hesselink JR, editors: *Clinical magnetic resonance imaging*, p. 384, Philadelphia, 1990, WB Saunders.)

Précis of the Head and Face Assessment*

History (sitting)
Observation (sitting)
Examination* (sitting)
Head injury
Neural watch
Glasgow Coma Scale
Concussion
Memory tests
Headache
Expanding intracranial lesion
Proprioception
Coordination
Head injury card
Facial injury
Bone and soft tissue contours
Fractures
Cranial nerves
Facial muscles
Eye injury
Six cardinal gaze positions
Pupils (size, equality, reactivity)
Visual field (peripheral vision)
Visual acuity
Symmetry of gaze
Hyphema
Foreign objects, corneal abrasion
Nystagmus
Surrounding bone and soft tissue
Nasal injury
Patency

Nasal cavities
Sinuses
Fracture
Nose discharge (bloody, straw-colored, clear)
Tooth injury
Number of teeth
Position of teeth
Movement of teeth
Condition of teeth
Condition of gums
Ear injury
Tenderness or pain
Ear discharge (bloody, straw colored, clear)
Hearing tests
Balance
Special tests
Tests for expanding intracranial lesions
Tests for coordination
Tests for proprioception
Reflexes and cutaneous distribution
Palpation
Diagnostic imaging

---

*When examining the head and face, if only one area has been injured (e.g., the nose), then only that area needs to be examined, provided the examiner is certain that adjacent structures have not also been injured. After any examination, the patient should be warned of the possibility that symptoms may exacerbate as a result of the assessment.

Case Studies

When doing these case studies, the examiner should list the appropriate questions to be asked and why they are being asked, identify what to look for and why, and specify what things should be tested and why. Depending on the patient's answers (and the examiner should consider different responses), several possible causes of the patient's problem may become evident (examples are given in parentheses). A differential diagnosis chart should be made up (see Table 2-22 as an example). The examiner can then decide how different diagnoses may affect the treatment plan.

1. A 27-year-old man was playing football. He received a "knee to the head," rendering him unconscious for approximately 3 minutes. How would you differentiate between a first-time, fourth-degree concussion and an expanding intracranial lesion?

2. A 13-year-old boy received an elbow in the nose and cheek while play-wrestling. The nose is crooked and painful and bled after the injury, and the cheek is sore. Describe your assessment plan for this patient (nasal fracture versus zygoma fracture).

3. A 23-year-old woman was in an automobile accident. She was a passenger in the front seat and was not wearing a seat belt. The car in which she was riding hit another car, which had run a red light. The woman's face hit the dashboard, and she received a severe facial injury. Describe your assessment plan for this patient (Le Fort fracture versus mandibular fracture).

4. An 83-year-old man tripped in the bathroom and hit his chin against the bathtub, knocking himself unconscious. Describe your assessment plan for this patient (cervical spine lesion versus mandibular fracture).

5. An 18-year-old woman was playing squash. She was not wearing eye protectors and was hit in the eye with the ball. Describe your assessment plan for this patient (ruptured globe versus blowout fracture).

6. A 15-year-old boy was playing field hockey. He was not wearing a mouth guard and was hit in

Continued

Case Studies—cont'd

the mouth and jaw by the ball. There was a large amount of blood. Describe your assessment plan for this patient (tooth fracture versus mandible fracture).

7. A 16-year-old male wrestler comes to you complaining of ear pain. He has just finished a match, which he lost. Describe your assessment

plan for this patient (cauliflower ear versus external otitis).

8. A 17-year-old female basketball player comes to you complaining of eye pain. She says she received a "finger in the eye" when she went up to get the ball. Describe your assessment plan for this patient (hyphema versus corneal abrasion).

Table 2-22

Differential Diagnosis of 4° Concussion and Intracranial Lesion

Sign or Symptom	4° Concussion	Intracranial Lesion
Confusion	Yes, but should improve with time	Will have increased confusion with time
Amnesia	Posttraumatic, retrograde	Not usually
Loss of consciousness	Yes, but recovers	Lucid interval varies
Tinnitus	Severe	Not a factor
Dizziness	Severe, but improves	May get worse
Headache	Often	Severe
Nystagmus or irregular eye movements	Not usually	Possible
Pupil inequality	Not usually	Possible early; present later
Irregular respiration	No	Possible early; present later
Slowing of heart	No	Possible early; present later
Intractable vomiting	Not usually	Possible
Lateralization	No	Yes
Coordination affected	Yes, but improves	Yes, and gets worse
Seizure	Not usually	Possible early; probable late
Personality change	Possible	Possible

References

To enhance this text and add value for the reader, all references have been incorporated into a CD-ROM that is provided with this text. The reader can view the reference source and access it online whenever possible. There are a total of 69 cited and other general references for this chapter.

APPENDIX 2-1

Reliability, Validity, Specificity and Sensitivity of Special/Diagnostic Tests Used in the Head and Face

CALORIC TEST

Sensitivity

- To recognize presence of spontaneous and positional nystagmus warm monothermal test 97%, cool monothermal test 89%[57]

FINGER DRUMMING TEST

Reliability

- Interrater r = 0.67[58]

FINGER-TO-NOSE TEST

Reliability	Validity
• Intrarater dymetria k = 0.54, tremor k = 0.18, Time of execution ICC = 0.97[59] • Interrater dymetria k = 0.36, tremor k = 0.26, Time of execution ICC = 0.91[59] • Interrater kinetic tremor: for starting position specify k = 0.37–0.64, no starting position specified k = 0.4–0.57, arm 90 degrees of abduction and elbow extended k = 0.38–0.66, arm 90 degrees of abduction touching nose for 5 sec k = 0.33–0.64[60] • Intention tremor: for starting position specify k = 0.67–0.83, no starting position specified k = 0.63–0.84, arm 90 degrees of abduction and elbow extended k = 0.55–0.87, arm 90 degrees of abduction touching nose for 5 sec k = 0.61–0.83[60]	• Correlation with coin pick up r = 0.77, pouring water r = 0.70–0.84, pick up phone r = 0.70–0.84[60]

GLASGOW COMA SCALE

Reliability	Validity
• Test-retest k = 0.39–0.80[61] • Test-retest k = 0.72, interrater k = 0.64 (severe commitment k = 0.59, minor commitment k = 0.69)[62] • Test-retest: experienced nurses reliability coefficient = 0.94, new graduates reliability coefficient = 0.94, student nurses reliability coefficient = 0.86[63] • Test-retest: eye opened r = 0.89, best motor response r = 0.85, best verbal response r = 0.97[64] • Interrater: eye r = 0.75, k = 0.72, verbal r = 0.66, k = 0.48, motor r = 0.81, k = 0.63, total r = 0.86, k = 0.40[65]	• Correlation with a videotape and discussion within a group of experts p = 0.000[61]

ONE LEG STANCE TEST

Reliability

- Interrater: eyes open ICC = 0.99, eyes closed ICC = 0.99[66]
- Test-retest: eyes open ICC = 0.90, eyes closed ICC = 0.74[66]

RINNE TEST

Sensitivity

- 72.9% using a force of 72.9% (accuracy is 76%)[67]

ROMBERG TEST

Reliability	Validity
• Between morning and afternoon p > 0.84, five consecutive days p > 0.78[68] • Interrater: eyes open ICC = 0.99, eyes closed ICC = 0.99[66] • Test retest: eyes open ICC = 0.90, eyes closed ICC = 0.76[66]	• Association with sway speed r = 0.46[69]

SIT-TO-STAND

Reliability

- Interrater ICC = 0.98[66]
- Test-retest ICC = 0.92[66]

CERVICAL SPINE

Examination of the cervical spine involves determining whether the injury or pathology occurs in the cervical spine or in a portion of the upper limb. Cyriax[1] called this assessment the **scanning examination.** In the initial assessment of a patient who complains of pain in the neck and/or upper limb, this procedure is always carried out unless the examiner is absolutely sure of the location of the lesion. If the injury is in the neck, the scanning examination is definitely called for to rule out neurological involvement. After the lesion site has been determined, a more detailed assessment of the affected area is performed if it is outside the cervical spine.

Because many conditions affecting the cervical spine can be manifested in other parts of the body, the cervical spine is a complicated area to assess properly, and adequate time must be allowed to ensure that as many causes or problems are examined as possible.

Applied Anatomy

The cervical spine consists of several pairs of joints. It is an area in which stability has been sacrificed for mobility, making the cervical spine particularly vulnerable to injury because it sits between a heavy head and a stable thoracic spine and ribs. The cervical spine is divided into two areas—the **cervicoencephalic** for the upper cervical spine and the **cervicobrachial** for the lower cervical spine. The cervicoencephalic or cervicocranial region (C0-C2) shows the relationship between the cervical spine and the occiput, and injuries in this region have the potential of involving the brain, brainstem and spinal cord (Figure 3-1).[2,3] Injuries in this area lead to symptoms of headache, fatigue, vertigo, poor concentration, hypertonia of sympathetic nervous system, and irritability.

In addition, there may be cognitive dysfunction, cranial nerve dysfunction, and sympathetic system dysfunction.[2,3]

The **atlanto-occipital joints** (C0-C1) are the two uppermost joints. The principal motion of these two joints is flexion-extension (15° to 20°), or nodding of the head. Side flexion is approximately 10°, whereas rotation is negligible. The **atlas** (C1) has no vertebral body as such. During development, the vertebral body of C1 evolves into the **odontoid process,** which is part of C2. The atlanto-occipital joints are ellipsoid and act in unison. Along with the atlanto-axial joints, these joints are the most complex articulations of the axial skeleton.

There are several ligaments that stabilize the atlanto-occipital joints. Anteriorly and posteriorly are the atlanto-occipital membranes. The anterior membrane is strengthened by the anterior longitudinal ligament. The posterior membrane replaces the ligamentum flavum between the atlas and occiput. The tectorial membrane, which is a broad band covering the dens and its ligaments, is found within the vertebral canal and is a continuation of the posterior longitudinal ligament. The alar ligaments are two strong rounded cords found on each side of the upper dens passing upwards and laterally to attach on the medial sides of the occipital condyles. The alar ligaments limit flexion and rotation and play a major role in stabilizing C1 and C2, especially in rotation.[4]

The **atlanto-axial joints** (C1-C2) constitute the most mobile articulations of the spine. Flexion-extension is approximately 10°, and side flexion is approximately 5°. Rotation, which is approximately 50°, is the primary movement of these joints. With rotation, there is a decrease in height of the cervical spine at this level as the vertebrae approximate because of the shape of the facet joints. The odontoid process of C2 acts as a

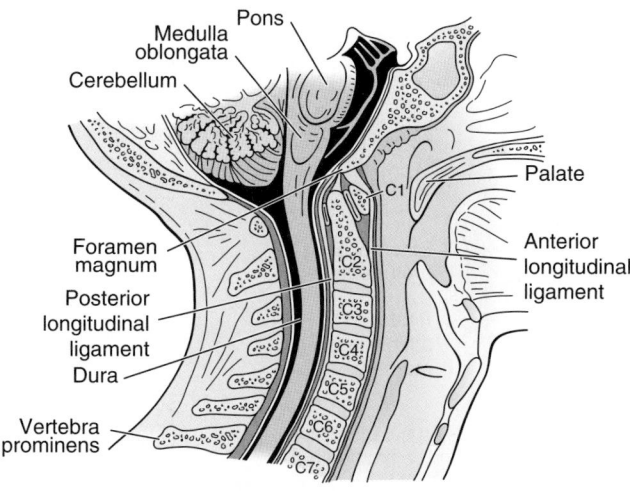

Figure 3-1

This sagittal view of the cervical spine shows the relations among the brain stem, the medulla oblongata, the foramen magnum, the spinal canal, and the cervical spine. The lower portion of the medulla is outside and below the foramen; therefore, with subluxation of the atlas on the axis, compression of the brain stem can occur through pressure of the odontoid against the upper spinal cord and the lower medulla. Note that the anterior arch of the atlas is only millimeters from the pharynx. (Redrawn from Bland JH: *Disorders of the cervical spine*, p. 47, Philadelphia, 1994, W.B. Saunders.)

pivot point for the rotation. This middle, or median, joint is classified as a **pivot (trochoidal) joint.** The lateral atlanto-axial, or facet, joints are classified as **plane joints.** Generally, if a person can talk and chew, there is probably some motion occurring at C1-C2. At the atlanto-axial joints, the main supporting ligament is the transverse ligament of the atlas, which holds the dens of the axis against the anterior arch of the atlas. It is this

ligament that weakens or ruptures in rheumatoid arthritis. As the ligament crosses the dens, there are two projections off the ligament, one going superiorly to the occiput and one inferiorly to the axis. The ligament and the projections form a cross, and the three parts taken together are called the cruciform ligament of the atlas (Figure 3-2).

The vertebral artery—part of the vertebrobasilar system that passes through the transverse processes of the cervical vertebrae usually starting at C6 but entering as high as C4—supplies 20% of the blood supply to the brain (primarily the hindbrain) along with the internal carotid artery (80%) (Figure 3-3).[5,6] In its path, the vertebral artery lies close to the facet joints and vertebral body where it may be compressed by osteophyte formation or injury to the facet joint. In addition, in older individuals, atherosclerotic changes and other vascular risk factors (e.g., hypertension, high fat or cholesterol levels, diabetes, smoking) may contribute to altered blood flow in the arteries.[7] The vertebral and internal carotid arteries are stressed primarily by rotation, extension, and traction movements, but other movements may also stretch the artery.[8-10] Rotation and extension of as little as 20° have been shown to significantly decrease vertebral artery blood flow.[11,12] The greatest stresses are placed on the vertebral arteries in four places: where it enters the transverse process of C6, within the bony canals of the vertebral transverse processes, between C1 and C2, and between C1 and the entry of the arteries into the skull.[13,14] These latter two areas have the greatest potential for problems (e.g., thrombosis, dissection, stroke) related to treatment and their concomitant stress on the vertebral arteries.[15] Dutton[13] reports that the most common mechanism for non-penetrating injury to the vertebral artery is neck extension, with or without side flexion or rotation.[16,17] Given

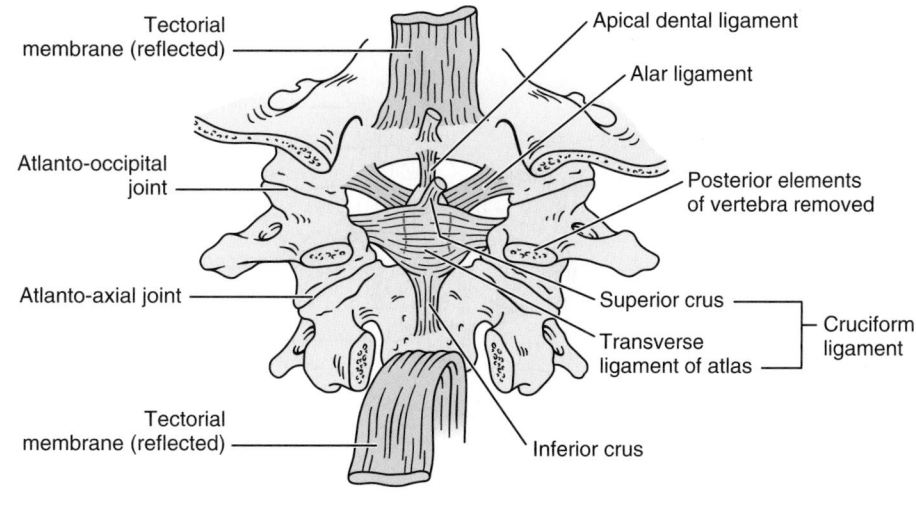

Figure 3-2

Ligaments of the upper cervical spine. **A,** Posterior deep view.

(Continued)

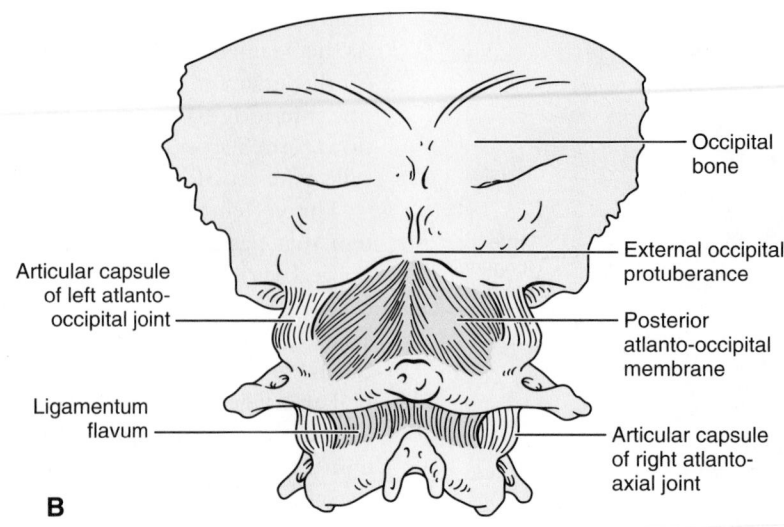

Occipital bone

Articular capsule of left atlanto-occipital joint

External occipital protuberance

Posterior atlanto-occipital membrane

Ligamentum flavum

Articular capsule of right atlanto-axial joint

B

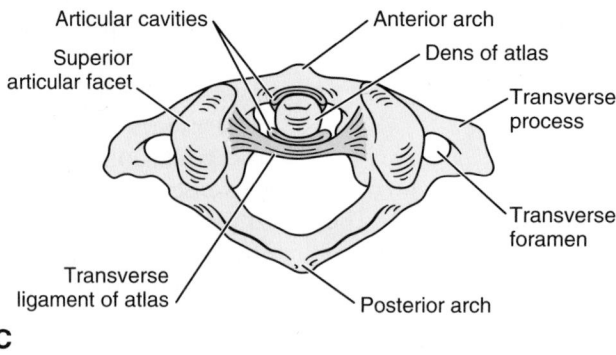

Articular cavities

Superior articular facet

Anterior arch

Dens of atlas

Transverse process

Transverse foramen

Transverse ligament of atlas

Posterior arch

C

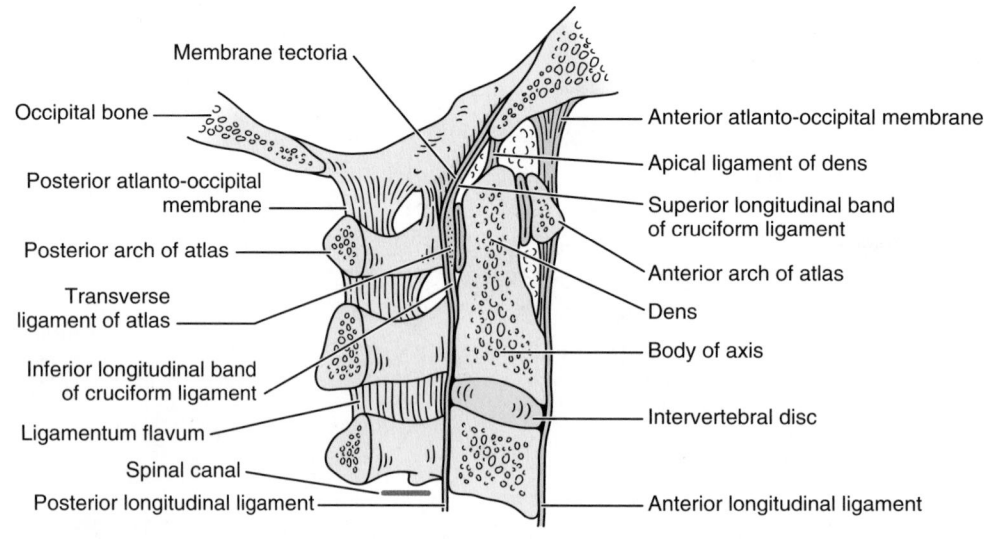

Membrane tectoria

Occipital bone

Posterior atlanto-occipital membrane

Posterior arch of atlas

Transverse ligament of atlas

Inferior longitudinal band of cruciform ligament

Ligamentum flavum

Spinal canal

Posterior longitudinal ligament

Anterior atlanto-occipital membrane

Apical ligament of dens

Superior longitudinal band of cruciform ligament

Anterior arch of atlas

Dens

Body of axis

Intervertebral disc

Anterior longitudinal ligament

D

Figure 3-2 cont'd
B, Posterior superficial view. **C,** Superior view. **D,** Lateral view.

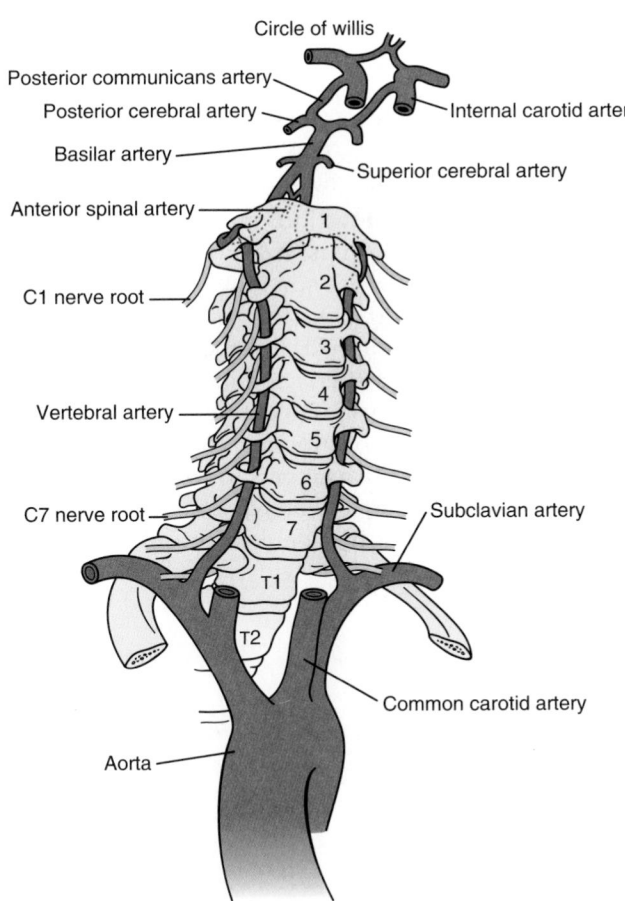

Figure 3-3

Anterolateral drawing of the course of the vertebral artery from C6 to C1 through the bony rings of the foramina transversaria. Note the double U-turn the artery makes from C2 to C1 and the posterior course around the lateral mass of the atlas. (Modified from Bland JH, Nakano KK: Neck pain. In Kelley WN et al, editors: *Textbook of rheumatology,* 1st ed. Philadelphia, 1981, W.B. Saunders.)

Figure 3-4

Cervical spine-plane of facet joints. **A,** Lateral view. **B,** Superior view.

the type of injury possible, symptoms may be delayed.[18,19] Symptoms related to the vertebral artery include vertigo, nausea, tinnitus, "drop attacks" (falling without fainting), visual disturbances, or, in rare cases, stroke or death.

The lower cervical spine (C3-C7) is called the *cervicobrachial area,* since pain in this area is commonly referred into the upper extremity.[2,3] Pathology in this region leads to neck pain alone, arm pain alone, or both neck and arm pain. Thus, symptoms include neck and/or arm pain, headaches, restricted ROM, paresthesia, altered myotomes and dermatomes, and radicular signs. Cognitive dysfunction and cranial nerve dysfunction are not commonly symptoms of injuries in this area although sympathetic dysfunction may be. Injury to both areas, if severe enough, may result in psychosocial issues.

There are **14 facet (apophyseal) joints** in the cervical spine (C1-C7). The upper four facet joints in the two upper thoracic vertebrae (T1-T2) are often included in the examination of the cervical spine. The superior facets of the cervical spine face upward, backward, and medially; the inferior facets face downward, forward, and laterally (Figure 3-4). This plane facilitates flexion and extension, but it prevents simple rotation or side flexion without both occurring to some degree together. This is called a **coupled movement** with rotation and side flexion both occurring with either movement.[20] Ishii et al.[21,22] reported that between C0 and C2, as well as C7 and T1, the two movements occur in opposite directions while between C2 and C7, they occur in the same direction. These joints move primarily by gliding and are classified as **synovial (diarthrodial)** joints. The capsules are lax to allow sufficient movement. At the same time, they provide support and a check-rein type of restriction at end range. The greatest flexion-extension of the facet joints occurs between C5 and C6; however, there is almost as much movement at C4-C5 and C6-C7. Because of this mobility, degeneration is more likely to be seen at these levels. The neutral or resting position of the cervical spine is slightly extended. The close packed position of the facet joints is complete extension.

Cervical Spine	
Resting position:	Slight extension
Close packed position:	Full extension
Capsular pattern:	Side flexion and rotation equally limited, extension

The **recurrent meningeal** or **sinuvertebral nerve** innervates the anterior dura sac, the posterior annulus fibrosus, and the posterior longitudinal ligament. The facet joints are innervated by the medial branch of the dorsal primary rami.[23] For C3-C7, the main ligaments are the anterior longitudinal ligament, the posterior longitudinal ligament, the ligamentum flavum, and the supraspinal and interspinal ligaments (Figure 3-5). There are also ligaments between the transverse processes (intertransverse ligaments), but in the cervical spine, they are rudimentary.

Some anatomists[24-27] refer to the costal or uncovertebral processes as **uncinate joints** or **joints of Luschka** (Figure 3-6). These structures were described by von Luschka in 1858. The uncus gives a "saddle" form to the upper aspect of the cervical vertebra, which is more pronounced posterolaterally; it has the effect of limiting side flexion. Extending from the uncus is a "joint" that appears to form because of a weakness in the annulus fibrosus. The portion of the vertebra above, which "articulates" or conforms to the uncus, is called the *échancrure,* or notch. Notches are found from C3 to T1, but according to most authors,[24-27] they are not seen until age 6 to 9 years and are not fully developed until 18 years of age. There is some controversy as to whether they should be classified as real joints because some authors believe they are the result of degeneration of the intervertebral disc.

The **intervertebral discs** make up approximately 25% of the height of the cervical spine. No disc is found between the atlas and the occiput (C0-C1) or between the atlas and the axis (C1-C2). It is the discs rather than the vertebrae that give the cervical spine its lordotic shape (Figure 3-7). The **nucleus pulposus** functions as a buffer to axial compression in distributing compressive forces, whereas the **annulus fibrosus** acts to withstand tension within the disc. The intervertebral disc has some innervation on the periphery of the annulus fibrosus.[28,29]

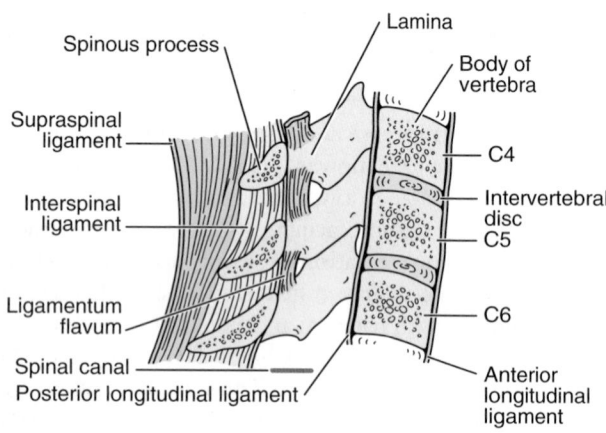

Figure 3-5
Median section of C4-C6 vertebrae to illustrate the intervertebral disc and the ligaments of the cervical spine.

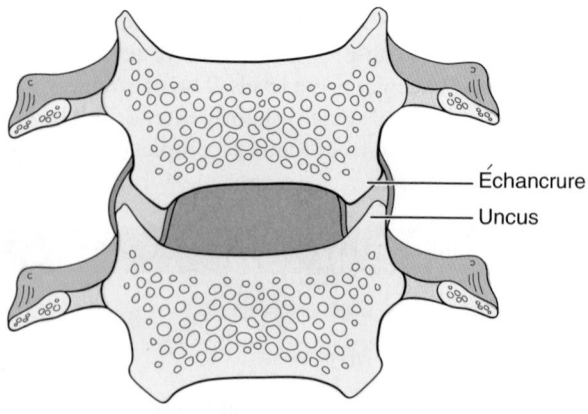

Figure 3-6
Joints of Luschka.

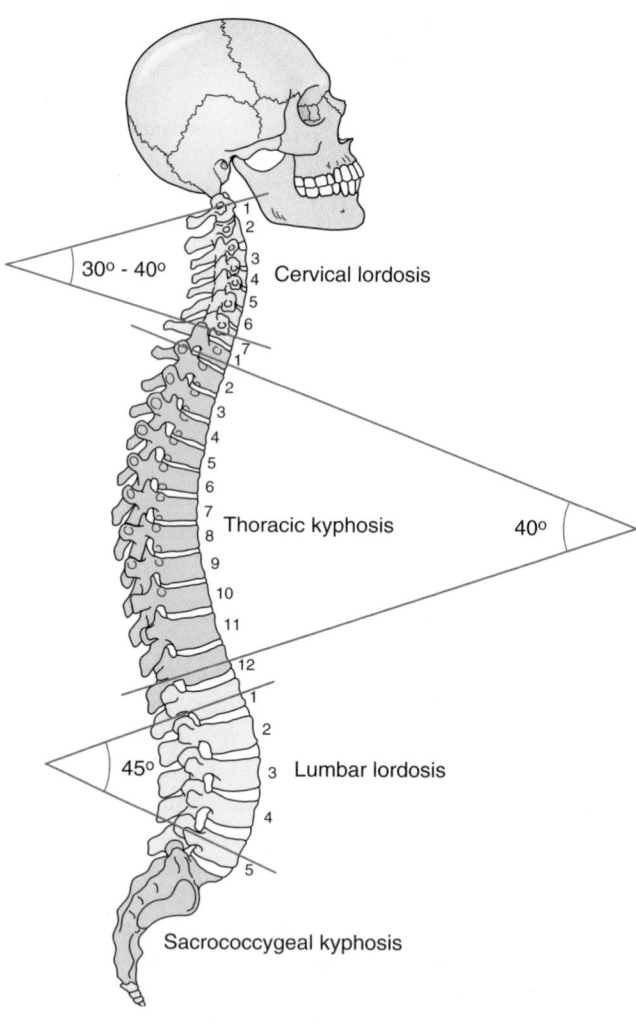

Figure 3-7
The normal sagittal plane curvatures across the regions of the vertebral column. The curvatures represent the normal resting postures of the region. (Modified from Neumann DA: *Kinesiology of the musculoskeletal system—foundations for physical rehabilitation*, p. 276, St Louis, 2002, Mosby.)

There are seven vertebrae in the cervical spine, with the body of each vertebra (except C1) supporting the weight of those above it. The facet joints may bear some of the weight of the vertebrae above, but this weight is minimal if the normal lordotic posture is maintained. However, even this slight amount of weight bearing can lead to spondylitic changes in these joints. The outer ring of the vertebral body is made of cortical bone, and the inner part is made of cancellous bone covered with the cartilaginous end plate. The vertebral arch protects the spinal cord while the spinous processes, most of which are bifid in the cervical spine, provide for attachment of muscles. The transverse processes have basically the same function. In the cervical spine, the transverse processes are made up of two parts: the anterior portion that provides the foramen for the vertebral body, and the posterior portion containing the two articular facets (see Figure 3-4, *B*). In the cervical spine, the spinous processes are at the level of the facet joints of the same vertebra. Generally, the spinous process is considered to be absent or at least rudimentary on C1. This is why the first palpable vertebra descending from the external occiput protuberance is the spinous process of C2.

Although there are seven cervical vertebrae, there are eight **cervical nerve roots.** This difference occurs because there is a nerve root exiting between the occiput and C1 that is designated the C1 nerve root. In the cervical spine, each nerve root is named for the vertebra below it. As an example, C5 nerve root exists between the C4 and C5 vertebrae (Figure 3-8). In the rest of the spine, each nerve

root is named for the vertebra above; the L4 nerve root, for example, exists between the L4 and L5 vertebrae. The switch in naming of the nerve roots from the one below to the one above is made between the C7 and T1 vertebrae. The nerve root between these two vertebrae is called C8, accounting for the fact that there are eight cervical nerve roots and only seven cervical vertebrae.

Patient History

In addition to the questions listed under Patient History in Chapter 1, the examiner should obtain the following information from the patient.

1. *What is the patient's age?* Spondylosis is often seen in persons 25 years of age or older, and it is present in 60% of those older than 45 years and 85% of those older than 65 years of age. Symptoms of osteoarthritis do not usually appear until a person is 60 years of age or older (Table 3-1).

2. *How severe are the symptoms?* Table 3-2 outlines many of the signs and symptoms that may arise from cervical spine pathology.[30] Watkins[31] provided a severity scale for neurological injury in football that can be used as a guideline for injury severity involving the cervical spine, especially if one is contemplating allowing the patient to return to activity (Figure 3-9). A combined score (A+B) of 4 is considered a mild episode, 4 to 7 is a moderate episode, and 8 to 10 is a severe episode. This scale can be combined with radiologic information on canal size (score C) to give a general determination of the possibility of symptoms returning if the patient returns to activity. In this case, a score of 6 (A+B+C) indicates minimum risk, 6 to 10 is moderate risk, and 10 to 15 is severe risk. Watkins[31] also points out that extenuating factors such as age of patient, level of activity, and risk versus benefit also play a role and, although not included in the score, must be considered.

3. *What was the mechanism of injury?* Was trauma, stretching, or overuse involved? Was the patient moving when the injury occurred? These questions help determine the type and severity of injury. For example, trauma may cause a whiplash type (acceleration) injury or whiplash associated disorder (WAD) (Table 3-3),[32] stretching may lead to "burners," overuse or sustained postures may result in thoracic outlet symptoms, and a report of an insidious onset in someone older than 55 years of age may indicate cervical spondylosis. Was the patient hit from the side, front, or behind? Did the patient see the accident coming? "Burners" or "stingers" typically occur from a blow to part of the brachial plexus or from stretching or compression of the brachial plexus (Table 3-4; Figure 3-10). The answers to these questions help the examiner determine how the injury occurred, the tissues injured, and the severity of the injuries.

Figure 3-8
Anterior view of cervical spine showing nerve roots. Note how each cervical nerve root is numbered for the vertebra below it.

Table 3-1

Differential Diagnosis of Cervical Spondylosis, Spinal Stenosis, and Disc Herniation

	Cervical Spondylosis	Cervical Spinal Stenosis	Cervical Disc Herniation*
Pain	Unilateral	May be unilateral or bilateral	May be unilateral (most common) or bilateral
Distribution of pain	Into affected dermatomes	Usually several dermatomes affected	Into affected dermatomes
Pain on extension	Increases	Increases	May increase (most common)
Pain on flexion	Decreases	Decreases	May increase or decrease (most common)
Pain relieved by rest	No	Yes	No
Age group affected	60% of those >45 yr 85% of those >65 yr	11–70 yr Most common: 30–60 yr	17–60 yr
Instability	Possible	No	No
Levels commonly affected	C5-C6, C6-C7	Varies	C5-C6
Onset	Slow	Slow (may be combined with spondylosis or disc herniation)	Sudden
Diagnostic imaging	Diagnostic	Diagnostic	Diagnostic (be sure clinical signs support)

* Posterolateral protusion.

Table 3-2

Signs and Symptoms Arising from Cervical Spine Pathology

Signs	Symptoms
Falling	Pain
Tender scalp	Headache
Tender bones	Dizziness
Anesthesia	Vertigo
Hyperesthesia	Paresthesia
Dysesthesia	Fatigue
Atrophy	Insomnia
Upper extremity weakness	"Restless arms and legs"
Asymmetry	Cough
Sweating or lack of sweating	Sneeze
Nystagmus	Nausea
Tender muscles	Diarrhea
Fasciculation	Threatened faint
Pathologic gait	Visual disturbance
Transient loss of hearing, consciousness, sight	Auditory disturbance
	Arm and leg pain and ache
Drop attack	Stiff neck
Ataxia	Torticollis
Spastic gait	Gait disturbance
Reflex changes	Poor balance
	Speech disturbance
	Muscle twitch
	Depressed mood
	Tinnitus
	Diplopia

(Modified from Bland JH: *Disorders of the cervical spine.* p. 161, Philadelphia, 1994, W.B. Saunders.)

4. *What is the patient's usual activity or pastime?* Do any particular activities or postures bother the patient? What type of work does the patient do? Are there any positions that the patient holds for long periods (e.g., when sewing, typing, or working at a desk)? Does the patient wear glasses? If so, are they bifocals or trifocals? Upper cervical symptoms may result from excessive nodding as the patient tries to focus through the correct part of the glasses. Cervicothoracic (lower cervical/upper thoracic spine) joint problems are often painful when activities that require push-and-pull motion, such as lawn mowing, sawing, and cleaning windows, are performed. What movements bother the patient? For example, extension can aggravate symptoms in patients with radicular signs and symptoms.[33]

5. *Did the head strike anything, or did the patient lose consciousness?* If the injury was caused by a motor vehicle accident, it is important to know whether the patient was wearing a seat belt, the type of seat belt (lap or shoulder), and whether the patient saw the accident coming. These questions give some idea of the severity and mechanisms of injury. If the patient was unconscious or unsteady, the character of each episode of altered consciousness should be noted (see Chapter 2).

6. *Did the symptoms come on right away?* Bone pain usually occurs immediately, but muscle or ligamentous pain can either come on immediately (e.g., a tear) or occur several hours or days later (e.g., stretching caused by a motor vehicle accident). Seventy percent of whiplash patients reported immediate symptom occurrence

Watkins' Severity Scale for Neurological Deficit

Grade	Neurological Deficit
1	Unilateral arm numbness or dysesthesia; loss of strength
2	Bilateral upper extremity loss of motor and sensory function
3	Ipsilateral arm, leg, and trunk loss of motor and sensory function
4	Transient quadriparesis (temporary sensory loss in all 4 limbs)
5	Transient quadriplegia (temporary motor loss in all 4 limbs)

Score:_____ (A)

Grade	Time Symptoms Present
1	Less than 5 minutes
2	Less than 1 hour
3	less than 24 hours
4	Less than 1 week
5	Greater than 1 week

Score:_____ (B)

Severity Score: A + B = _____
(≤4: mild episode; 4–7: moderate episode; 8–10: severe episode)

Grade	Central Canal Diameter
1	>12 mm
2	Between 10–12
3	10 mm
4	8–10 mm
5	<8 mm

Score:_____ (C)

Return to Activity Score: A + B + C = _____
(≤6: minimum risk; 6–10: moderate risk; 10–15: severe risk)

Figure 3-9
Watkins' Severity Scale for Neurological Deficit. (Data from Watkins RG: Neck injuries in football. In Watkins RG, editor: *The spine in sports*, p. 327, St. Louis, 1996, Mosby-Year Book.)

while the rest reported delayed symptoms.[30,34–38] How long have the symptoms been present? Myofascial pain syndromes demonstrate generalized aching and at least three trigger points, which have lasted for at least 3 months, with no history of trauma.[39]

7. *What are the sites and boundaries of the pain?* Have the patient point to the location or locations of the pain. Symptoms do not go down the arm for a C4 nerve root injury or for nerve roots above that level. **Cervical radiculopathy,** or injury to the nerve roots in the cervical spine, presents primarily with unilateral motor and sensory symptoms into the upper limb, with muscle weakness (myotome), sensory alteration (dermatome), reflex hypoactivity, and sometimes focal activity being the primary signs.[40–43] Acute radiculopa-thies are commonly associated with disc herniations whereas chronic types are more related to spondylo-sis.[41] Disc herniations in the cervical spine commonly cause severe neck pain that may radiate into the shoulder, scapula and/or arm, limit ROM, and an increase in pain on coughing, sneezing, jarring, or straining.[38] **Cervical myelopathy,** or injury to the spinal cord itself, is more likely to present with spastic weakness, paresthesia, and possible incoordination in one or both lower limbs, as well as proprioceptive and/or sphincter dysfunction (Tables 3-5 and 3-6).[44]

8. *Is there any radiation of pain?* It is helpful to correlate this answer with dermatome and sensory peripheral nerve findings when performing sensation testing and palpation later in the examination.

Table 3-3

The Quebec Severity Classification of Whiplash Associated Disorders (WADs)

Grade	Clinical Presentation
0	No neck symptoms, no physical sign(s)
1	No physical sign(s), neck pain, stiffness, or tenderness only, neck complaints predominate, normal ROM, normal reflexes, dermatomes and myotomes
2	Neck symptoms (pain, stiffness) and musculoskeletal sign(s) such as decreased range of motion and point tenderness, soft tissue complaints (pain, stiffness) into shoulders and back, normal reflexes, dermatomes, myotomes
3	Neck symptoms (pain, stiffness, restricted ROM) and neurological sign(s) such as decreased or absence of deep tendon reflexes, weakness (positive myotomes) and sensory (positive dermatome) deficits, x-ray shows no fracture, CT/MRI may show nerve involvement, possible disc lesion
4	Neck symptoms (pain, stiffness, restricted ROM) with fracture or dislocation, and objective neurological signs, possible spinal cord signs

Modified from Spitzer WO et al.: Scientific monograph of the Quebec Task Force on Whiplash-Associated Disorders: redefining "whiplash" and its management, *Spine* 20:8S-58S, 1995.

Is the pain deep? Superficial? Shooting? Burning? Aching? For example, when an athlete experiences a "burner," the sensation is a lightning-like, burning pain into the shoulder and arm, followed by a period of heaviness or loss of function in the arm. Figure 3-11 shows the radiation of pain with facet (apophyseal) joint pathology.[45]

9. *Is the pain affected by laughing? Coughing? Sneezing? Straining?* If so, an increase in intrathoracic or intra-abdominal pressure may be contributing to the problem.

10. *Does the patient have any headaches? If so, where? How frequently do they occur?* For example, do they occur every day, two times per day, two days per week, one day per month?[46] How intense are they? How long do they last? Are they affected by medication and, if so, by how much medication and what kind? Are there any precipitating factors (e.g., food, stress, posture)? See Tables 2-9, 2-10, and 2-11, which indicate the influence of time of day, body position, headache location, and type of pain on diagnosis of the type of headache the patient may have. Table 2-12 outlines the salient features of some of the more common headaches. Craniovertebral joint dysfunction commonly is accompanied by headaches. For example, C1 headaches occur at the base and top of the head, whereas C2 headaches are referred to the temporal area.

Table 3-4

Differential Diagnosis of Cervical Nerve Root and Brachial Plexus Lesion

	Cervical Nerve Root Lesion	Brachial Plexus Lesion
Cause	Disc herniation Stenosis Osteophytes Swelling with trauma Spondylosis	Stretching of cervical spine Compression of cervical spine Depression of shoulder
Contributing factors	Congenital defects	Thoracic outlet syndrome
Pain	Sharp, burning in affected dermatomes	Sharp, burning in all or most of arm dermatomes, pain in trapezius
Paresthesia	Numbness, pins and needles in affected dermatomes	Numbness, pins and needles in all or most arm dermatomes (more ambiguous distribution)
Tenderness	Over affected area of posterior cervical spine	Over affected area of brachial plexus or lateral to cervical spine
Range of motion	Decreased	Decreased but usually returns rather quickly
Weakness	Transient paralysis usually Myotome may be affected	Transient muscle weakness Myotomes affected
Deep tendon reflexes	Affected nerve root may be depressed	May be depressed
Provocative test	Side flexion, rotation and extension with compression increase symptoms Cervical traction decreases symptoms Upper limb tension tests positive	Side flexion with compression (same side) or stretch (opposite side) may increase symptoms Upper limb tension tests may be positive

Signs of Headaches Having a Cervical Origin

- Occipital or suboccipital component to headache
- Neck movement alters headache
- Painful limitation of neck movements
- Abnormal head or neck posture
- Suboccipital or nuchal tenderness
- Abnormal mobility at C0-C1
- Sensory abnormalities in the occipital and suboccipital areas

11. *Does a position change alter the headache or pain?* If so, which positions increase or decrease the pain? The patient may state that the pain and referred symptoms are decreased or relieved by placing the hand or arm of the affected side on top of the head. This is called **Bakody's sign,** and it is usually indicative of problems in the C4 or C5 area.[47,48]

12. *Is paresthesia (a "pins and needles" feeling) present?* This sensation occurs if pressure is applied to the nerve

Figure 3-10

Mechanism of injury for brachial plexus (burner or stinger) pathology.

Table 3-5

Signs and Symptoms in Cervical Myelopathy

Motor Changes	Sensory Changes
Initial symptoms (predominantly lower limbs)	Headache and head pain
Spastic paraparesis	Neck, eye, ear, throat, or sinus pain
Stiffness and heaviness, scuffing of the toe, difficulty climbing stairs	Sensory symptoms in the pharynx and larynx
Weakness, spasms, cramps, easy fatigability	Paroxysmal hoarseness and aphonia
Decreased power, especially of flexors (dorsiflexors of ankles and toes; flexors of hips)	Rotary vertigo
Hyperreflexia of knee and ankle jerks, with clonus	Tinnitus synchronous with pulse or continuous whistling noises
Positive Babinski's sign, extensor hypertonia	Deafness
Decreased or absent superficial abdominal and cremasteric reflexes	Oculovisual changes (e.g., blurring, photophobia, scintillating scotomata, diplopia, homonymous hemianopsia, and nystagmus)
Drop foot, crural monoplegia	Autonomic disturbance (e.g., sweating, flushing, rhinorrhea, salivation, lacrimation, nausea, and vomiting)
Later symptoms (in order of occurrence)	Weakness in one or both legs, drop attacks with or without loss of consciousness
Various combinations of upper and lower limb involvement	Numbness on one or both sides of the body
Mixed picture of upper and lower motoneuron dysfunction	Dysphagia or dysarthria
Atrophy, weakness, hypotonia, hyper-reflexia to hyporeflexia, and absent deep tendon reflexes	Myoclonic jerks
	Hiccups
	Respiratory changes (e.g., Cheyne-Stokes respiration, Biot's respiration, or ataxic respiration)

Modified from Bland JH: *Disorders of the cervical spine*, pp. 215–216, Philadelphia, 1994, W.B. Saunders.

Table 3-6

Differential Diagnosis of Neurological Disorders of the Cervical Spine and Upper Limb

Cervical Radiculopathy (Nerve Root Lesion)	Cervical Myelopathy	Brachial Plexus Lesion (Plexopathy)	Burner (Transient Brachial Plexus Lesion)	Peripheral Nerve (Upper Limb)
Arm pain in dermatome distribution	Hand numbness, head pain, hoarseness, vertigo, tinnitus, deafness	Pain more localized to shoulder and neck (sometimes face)	Temporary pain in dermatome	No pain
Pain increased by extension and rotation or side flexion	Extension, rotation, and side flexion may all cause pain	Pain on compression of brachial plexus	Pain on compression or stretch of brachial plexus	No pain early; if contracture occurs (late), pain on stretching
Pain may be relieved by putting hand on head (C5,6)	Arm positions have no effect on pain	Arm positions have no effect on pain*	Arm positions have no effect on pain*	Arm positions have no effect on pain*
Sensation (dermatome) affected	Sensation affected, abnormal pattern	Sensation (dermatome) affected	Sensation (dermatome) affected	Peripheral nerve sensation affected
Gait not affected	Wide-based gait, drop attacks, ataxia; proprioception affected	Gait not affected	Gait not affected	Gait not affected
Altered hand function	Loss of hand function	Loss of arm function	Loss of function temporary	Loss of function of muscles supplied by nerve
Bowel and bladder not affected	Possible loss of bowel and bladder control	Bowel and bladder not affected	Bowel and bladder not affected	Bowel and bladder not affected
Weakness in myotome but no spasticity	Spastic paresis (especially in lower limb early, upper limb affected later)	Weakness in myotome	Temporary weakness in myotome	Weakness of muscles supplied by nerve
DTR hypoactive	Lower limb DTR hyperactive / Upper limb DTR hyperactive	DTR hypoactive	DTR not affected	DTR may be decreased
Negative pathological reflex	Positive pathological reflex	Negative pathological reflex	Negative pathological reflex	Negative pathological reflex
Negative superficial reflex	Decreased superficial reflex	Negative superficial reflex	Negative superficial reflex	Negative superficial reflex
Gait not affected	Gait affected	Gait not affected	Gait not affected	Gait not affected
Atrophy (late sign), hard to detect early	Atrophy	Atrophy	Atrophy possible	Atrophy (not usually with neuropraxia)

DTR, Deep tendon reflexes.

*Except in neurotension test positions.

root. It may become evident if pressure is relieved from a nerve trunk. Numbness and/or paresthesia in the hands or legs and deteriorating hand function all may relate to cervical myelopathy (see Table 3-5).

13. *Does the patient experience any tingling in the extremities?* Are the symptoms bilateral? Bilateral symptoms usually indicate either systemic disorders (e.g., diabetes, alcohol abuse) that are causing neuropathies or central space–occupying lesions.

14. *Are there any lower limb symptoms?* This finding may indicate a severe problem affecting the spinal cord

(myelopathy; see Table 3-5). These symptoms may include numbness, paresthesia, stumbling, difficulty walking, and lack of balance or agility. All of these symptoms could indicate cervical myelopathy. Likewise, signs of sphincter (bowel or bladder) or sexual dysfunction may be related to cervical myelopathy.

15. *Does the patient have any difficulty walking? Does the patient have problems with balance?* Does the patient stumble when walking, have trouble walking in the dark, or walk with feet wide apart? Positive responses may indicate a cervical myelopathy. Abnormality of the

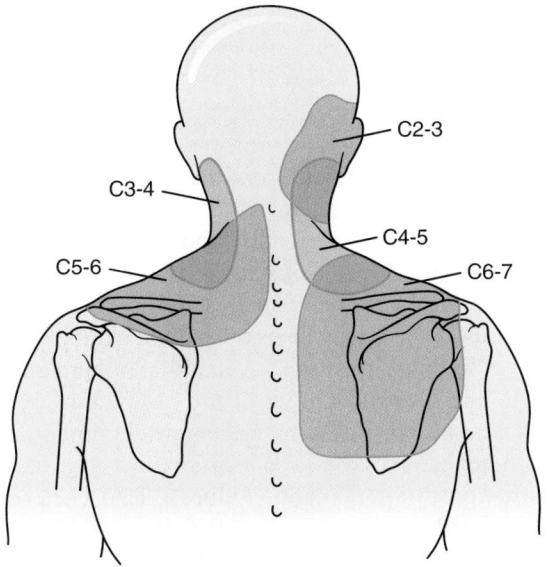

Figure 3-11

Referred pain patterns suggested with pathology of the apophyseal joints. (Redrawn from Porterfield JA, DeRosa C: *Mechanical neck pain—perspective in functional anatomy*, p.104, Philadelphia, 1995, W.B. Saunders. Adapted from Dwyer A, April C, Bogduk N: Cervical zygapophyseal joint pain patterns, *Spine* 15:453–457, 1990.)

Table 3-7

Signs and Symptoms of Vertebrobasilar Artery Insufficiency*

Dizziness
Giddiness
Drop attacks
Syncope
Stroke
Diplopia, blurred vision
Visual hallucination
Tinnitus (ringing in the ears)
Flushing
Sweating
Lacrimation (tearing)
Rhinorrhea (runny nose)
Scotomata (visual defect in defined area of eye[s])
Hiccups
Myotonic jerks
Tremor and rigidity
Disorientation
Vertigo
Photophobia (sensitivity to light)
Numbness and tingling
Quadriparesis
Dysphagia (difficulty swallowing)
Dysarthria (difficulty articulating)
Photopsia (sensation of flashing lights)
Visual anosognosia (unawareness of visual defect)
Nystagmus
Ataxia

Modified from Bland JH: *Disorders of the cervical spine*, p. 217, Philadelphia, 1994, W.B. Saunders.

*These paraspinal symptoms result mainly from rotation and extension of the neck, although they sometimes occur during flexion. The spectrum of neurologic symptoms and signs is as broad as that of the structures potentially involved. In a complex, bizarre, and poorly explained neurologic syndrome, vertebrobasilar artery insufficiency should be suspected.

cranial nerves combined with gait alterations may indicate systemic neurological dysfunction.[49]

16. *Does the patient experience dizziness, faintness, or seizures?* What is the degree, frequency, and duration of the dizziness? Is it associated with certain head positions or body positions? Semicircular canal problems or vertebral artery problems (Table 3-7) can lead to dizziness. Dizziness from a vertebral artery problem is commonly associated with other symptoms. Falling with no provocation while remaining conscious is sometimes called a **drop attack**.[50] Has the patient experienced any visual disturbances? Disturbances such as diplopia (double vision), nystagmus ("dancing eyes"), scotomas (depressed visual field), and loss of acuity may indicate severity of injury, neurological injury, and sometimes increased intracranial pressure (see Chapter 2).[47]

17. *Does the patient exhibit or complain of any sympathetic symptoms?* There may be injury to the cranial nerves or the sympathetic nervous system, which lies in the soft tissues of the neck anterior and lateral to the cervical vertebrae. The cranial nerves and their functions are shown in Table 2-1. Severe injuries (e.g., acceleration/whiplash type) can lead to hypertonia of the sympathetic nervous system.[2] Some of the sympathetic signs and symptoms the examiner may elicit are "ringing" in the ears (tinnitus), dizziness, blurred vision, photophobia, rhinorrhea, sweating, lacrimation, and loss of strength.

18. *Is the condition improving? Worsening? Staying the same?* The answers to these questions give the examiner some indication of the condition's progress.

19. *Which activities aggravate the problem? Which activities ease the problem?* Are there any head or neck positions that the patient finds particularly bothersome? These positions should be noted. For example, does reading (flexed cervical spine) bother the patient? If symptoms are not varied by a change in position, the problem is not likely to be mechanical in origin. Lesions of C3, C4, and C5 may affect the diaphragm and thereby affect breathing.

20. *Does the patient complain of any restrictions when performing movements?* If so, which movements are restricted? It is important that the patient not demonstrate the movements at this stage; the actual movements will be done during the examination.

21. *Is the patient a mouth breather?* Mouth breathing encourages forward head posture and increases activity of accessory respiratory muscles.

22. *Is there any difficulty in swallowing (dysphagia), or have there been any voice changes?* Such a change may be caused by neurological problems, mechanical pressure, or muscle incoordination. Pain on swallowing may indicate soft-tissue swelling in the throat, vertebral subluxation, osteophyte projection, or disc protrusion into the esophagus or pharynx. In addition, swallowing becomes more difficult and the voice becomes weaker as the neck is extended.

23. *What can be learned about the patient's sleeping position?* Is there any problem sleeping? How many pillows does the patient use, and what type are they (e.g., feather, foam, buckwheat)? Foam pillows tend to retain their shape and have more "bounce"; they do not offer as much support as a good feather or buckwheat pillow. What type of mattress does the patient use (e.g., hard, soft)? Does the patient "hug" the pillow or abduct the arms when sleeping? These positions can increase the stress on the lower cervical nerve roots.

24. *Does the patient display any cognitive dysfunction?* If a possible head injury is suspected, the clinician should also consider testing for mental status (see Chapter 2).

Observation

For a proper observation, the patient must be suitably undressed. However, the examiner should also watch the patient as he or she enters the examination room, and before or while he or she undresses. The spontaneous movements of these activities can be very helpful in determining the patient's problems. For example, can the patient easily move the head when undressing? A male patient should wear only shorts, and a female patient should wear a bra and shorts for this part of the assessment. In some cases, the bra may have to be removed to determine whether there are any problems such as thoracic outlet syndrome, thoracic symptoms being referred to the cervical spine, or functional restriction of movement of the ribs. The examiner should note the willingness of the patient to move and the patterns of movement demonstrated. Facial expression of the patient can often give the examiner an indication of the amount of pain the patient is experiencing.

The patient may be seated or standing. Usually, a standing posture is best because the posture of the whole body can be observed (see Chapter 15). Abnormalities in one area frequently affect another area. For example, excessive lumbar lordosis may cause a "poking" chin to compensate for the lumbar deformity and to maintain the body's center of gravity. In the cervical spine region, the examiner should note the following:

Head and Neck Posture. Is the head in the midline and does the patient have a normal lordotic curvature (30°–40°) (Figure 3-12; see Figure 3-7)? This curvature along with the other spinal curvatures in the lower spine provides a shock absorption mechanism for the spine and helps the body maintain its centre of gravity.[51] From the front, the chin should be in line with the sternum (manubrium) and from the side, the ears should be in line with the shoulder and the forehead vertical. Is there evidence of torticollis (congenital or acquired) (Figure 3-13), Klippel-Feil syndrome (congenital fusion of some cervical vertebra, usually C3-C5) (Figure 3-14), or other neck deformity? Does the patient exhibit a poking chin or a "military posture?" A habitual poking chin can result in adaptive shortening of the occipital muscles. It also causes the cervical spine to change alignment resulting in increased stress of the facet joints and posterior discs and other posterior elements (Figure 3-15). The position may also lead to weaknesses of the deep neck flexors.[52] Janda[53] described a cervical **"upper crossed syndrome"** to show the effect of a "poking chin" posture on the muscles. With this syndrome, the deep neck flexors are weak, as are the rhomboids, serratus anterior, and often the lower trapezius. Opposite these weak muscles are tight pectoralis major and minor, along with upper trapezius and levator scapulae (Figure 3-16). Does the head sit in the middle of the shoulders? Is the head tilted or rotated to one side or the other, indicating possible torticollis? Does this posture appear to be habitual (in other words, does the patient always go back to this posture)? Habitual posture may result from postural compensation, weak muscles, hearing loss, temporomandibular joint problems, or wearing of bifocals or trifocals. The trapezius neck line should be equal on both sides. Head and neck posture should be checked with the patient sitting and then standing, and any differences should be noted.

Shoulder Levels. Usually the shoulder on the dominant side will be slightly lower than that on the nondominant side. With injury, the injured side may be elevated to provide protection (e.g., upper trapezius and/or levator scapulae) or because of muscle spasm. Rounded shoulders may be the result of or the cause of a poking chin. Rounding also causes the scapulae to protract, the humerus to medially rotate, and the anterior structures of the shoulder to tighten.

Muscle Spasm or Any Asymmetry. Is there any atrophy of the deltoid muscle (axillary nerve palsy) or torticollis (muscle spasm, tightness, or prominence of the sternocleidomastoid muscle)? (See Figure 3-13.)

Facial Expression. The examiner should observe the patient's facial expression as the patient moves from position to position, makes different movements, and explains the problem. Such observation should give the examiner an idea of how much the patient is subjectively suffering.

Bony and Soft-Tissue Contours. If the cervical spine is injured, the head tends to be tilted and rotated away from the pain, and the face is tilted upward. If the patient

A   **B**   **C**

Figure 3-12

Observation views of head and neck. **A,** Anterior view. **B,** Posterior view. **C,** Lateral or side view. With normal posture, the ear should be in line with the shoulder and the forehead vertical. Note that this model is a "chin poker" with the head sitting anteriorly.

Figure 3-13

Example of congenital torticollis showing prominent sternocleidomastoid muscle on the right. (From Gartland JJ: *Fundamentals of orthopedics*, p. 279, Philadelphia, 1987, W.B. Saunders.)

is hysterical, the head tends to be tilted and rotated toward the pain, and the face is tilted down.

Evidence of Ischemia in Either Upper Limb. The examiner should note any altered coloration of the skin, ulcers, or vein distention as evidence of upper limb ischemia.

Normal Sitting Posture. The nose should be in line with the manubrium and xiphoid process of the sternum. From the side, the ear lobe should be in line with the acromion process and the high point on the iliac crest for proper postural alignment. The normal curve of the cervical spine is a lordotic type of curve. Referred pain from conditions such as spondylosis tends to occur in the shoulder and arm rather than the neck.

Examination

A complete examination of the cervical spine must be performed, including the neck and both upper limbs. Many of the symptoms that occur in an upper limb originate from the neck. Unless there is a history of definite trauma to a peripheral joint, an upper limb scanning examination must be performed to rule out problems within the neck.

Figure 3-14

Klippel-Feil syndrome in a 12-year-old boy. Clinical appearance of the patient. **A,** Anterior view.
B, Posterior view. **C,** Lateral view. Note the short neck with the head appearing to sit directly on the thorax.
Anteroposterior (**D**) and lateral (**E,** extension; **F,** flexion) roentgenograms of the cervical spine. Note the
failure of segmentation and the fusion into a homogeneous mass of bone of the four lower cervical vertebrae.
(From Tachdjian MO: *Pediatric orthopedics,* p. 77, Philadelphia, 1972, W.B. Saunders.)

Active Movements

The first movements that are carried out are the active movements of the cervical spine, with the patient in the sitting position. The examiner is looking for differences in range of movement and in the patient's willingness to do the movement. The range of motion (ROM) taking place in this phase is the summation of all movements of the entire cervical spine, not just at one level. This combined movement allows for greater mobility in the cervical spine while still providing a firm support for the trunk and appendages. The ROM available in the cervical spine is the result of many factors, such as the flexibility of the intervertebral discs, the shape and inclination

of the articular processes of the facet joints, and the slight laxity of the ligaments and joint capsules. Female patients tend to have a greater active range of motion than males, except in flexion, but the differences are not great. The range available decreases with age, except rotation at C1-C2, which may increase.[54,55]

The movements should be done in a particular order so that the most painful movements are done last and no residual pain is carried over from the previous movement.[1] If the patient has complained of pain on specific movements in the history, these movements are done last. In the very acute cervical spine, only some movements—those that give the most information—are performed in order to avoid undue exacerbation of symptoms.

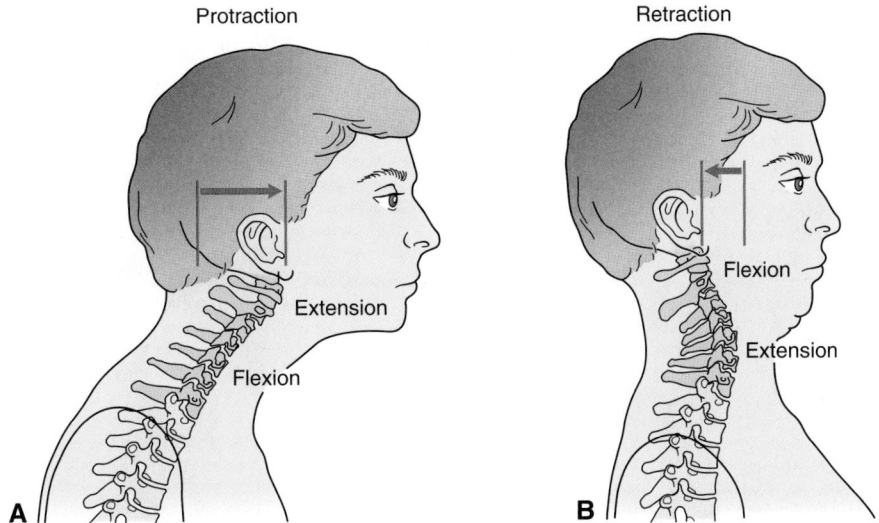

Protraction   Retraction

Figure 3-15

Protraction and retraction of the cranium. **A,** During protraction of the cranium, the lower-to-mid cervical spine flexes as the upper craniocervical region extends. **B,** During retraction of the cranium, in contract, the lower-to-mid cervical spine extends as the upper craniocervical region flexes. Note the change in distance between the C1-C2 spinous processes during the two movements. (Modified from Neumann DA: *Kinesiology of the musculoskeletal system—foundations for physical rehabilitation,* p. 284, St Louis, 2002, C.V. Mosby.)

Active Movements of the Cervical Spine

- Flexion
- Extension
- Side flexion left and right
- Rotation left and right
- Combined movements (if necessary)
- Repetitive movements (if necessary)
- Sustained positions (if necessary)

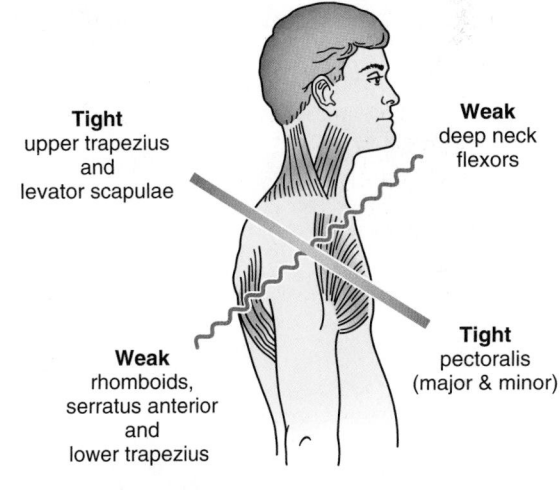

Figure 3-16

Upper crossed syndrome.

While the patient performs the active movements, the examiner looks for limitation of movement and possible reasons for pain, spasm, stiffness, or blocking. As the patient reaches the full range of active movement, passive **overpressure** may be applied very carefully, but only if the movement appears to be full and not too painful (see passive movement in later discussion). The overpressure helps the examiner to test the end feel of the movement as well as differentiating between physiological (active) end range and anatomical (passive) end range. The examiner must be careful when applying overpressure to rotation or any combination of rotation, side flexion, and extension.[8] In these positions, the vertebral artery is often compressed, which can lead to a decrease in blood supply to the brain. Should this occur, the patient may complain of dizziness or feel faint. If the patient exhibits these symptoms, the examiner must use extreme care during these movements, the rest of the assessment, and treatment.

The examiner can differentiate between movement in the upper and lower cervical spine. During flexion, **nodding** occurs in the upper cervical spine, whereas **flexion** occurs in the lower cervical spine. If the nodding movement does not occur, it indicates restriction of movement in the upper cervical spine; if flexion does not occur, it indicates restriction of motion in the lower cervical spine. Movement can occur between C1 and C2 without affecting the other vertebrae, but this is not true with other cervical vertebrae. In other words, for C2 to C7, if one vertebra moves, the ones adjacent to it will also move. Thus, the active movements in the cervical spine can be divided into two parts: those testing the upper cervical spine (C0-C2) and those involving the rest of the cervical spine (C2-C7) (Figure 3-17). Table 3-8 gives the approximate ROMs in the different parts of the cervical spine.[56]

Figure 3-17

Active movements of the cervical spine. **A,** Anterior nodding (upper cervical spine). **B,** Flexion. **C,** Extension. **D,** Posterior nodding (upper cervical spine). **E,** Side flexion. **F,** Rotation.

Table 3-8

Approximate Range of Motion for the Three Planes of Movement for the Joints of the Craniocervical Region*

Joint or Region	Flexion and Extension (Sagittal Plane, Degrees)	Axial Rotation (Horizontal Plane, Degrees)	Lateral Flexion (Frontal Plane, Degrees)
Atlanto-occipital joint	Flexion: 5 Extension: 10 Total: 15	Negligible	About 5
Atlanto-axial joint complex	Flexion: 5 Extension: 10 Total: 15	40–45	Negligible
Intracervical region (C2–7)	Flexion: 35 Extension: 70 Total: 105	45	35
Total across craniocervical region	Flexion: 45–50 Extension: 85 Total: 130–135	90	About 40

(From Neumann DA: *Kinesiology of the musculoskeletal system—foundations for physical rehabilitation*, p. 278, St Louis, 2002, C.V. Mosby.)
*The horizontal and frontal plane motions are to one side only. Data are compiled from multiple sources and subject to large intersubject variations.

Flexion

To test flexion movement in the upper cervical spine, the patient is asked to nod or place the chin on the Adam's apple. Normally this movement is pain free. Positive symptoms (e.g., tingling in feet, electric shock sensation down the neck [Lhermitte's sign], severe pain, nausea, cord signs) all indicate severe pathology (e.g., meningitis, tumor, dens fracture).[13] While the patient is flexing (nodding) the head, the examiner can palpate the relative movement between the mastoid and transverse process of C1 on each side comparing both sides for hypomobility or hypermobility between C0 and C1.[13] Likewise, the examiner can palpate the posterior arch of C1 and the lamina of C2 during the nodding movement to compare the relative movement.[13] For flexion, or forward bending, of the lower cervical spine, the maximum ROM is 80° to 90°. The extreme of ROM is normally found when the chin is able to reach the chest with the mouth closed; however, up to two finger widths between chin and chest is considered normal. If the deep neck flexors are weak, the sternocleidomastoid muscles will initiate the flexion movement, causing the jaw to lead the movement, not the nose, since the sternocleidomastoid muscles will cause the chin to initially elevate before flexion occurs.[46,57,58] In flexion, the intervertebral disc widens posteriorly and narrows anteriorly. The intervertebral foramen is 20% to 30% larger on flexion than on extension. The vertebrae shift forward in flexion and backward in extension (Figures 3-18 and 3-19). Also, the mastoid process moves away from the C1 transverse process on flexion and extension. As the patient forward flexes, the examiner should look for a posterior bulging of the spinous process of the axis (C2). This bulging may result from forward subluxation of the atlas, which allows the spinous process of the axis to become more prominent. If this sign appears, the examiner should exercise **extreme caution** during the remainder of the cervical assessment. To verify the subluxation, the Sharp-Purser test (see under Special Tests) may be performed, but only with extreme care.

Extension

To test extension in the upper cervical spine, the patient is asked to lift the chin up without moving the neck. The examiner can lift the occiput at the same time. If serious symptoms arise (e.g., tingling in the feet, loss of balance, drop attack), it is suggestive of spinal cord compression or vertebrobasilar dysfunction.[13] Extension, or backward bending of the cervical spine, is normally limited to 70°. Because there is no anatomic block to stop movement going past this position, problems often result from whiplash or cervical strain. Normally, there is sufficient extension to allow the plane of the nose and forehead to be nearly horizontal. When the head is held in extension, the atlas tilts upward, resulting in posterior compression between the atlas and occiput.

Side Flexion

Side, or lateral, flexion is approximately 20° to 45° to the right and left (Figure 3-20). As the patient does the movement, the examiner can palpate adjacent transverse processes on the convex side to determine relative movement at each level. When the patient does the movement, the examiner should ensure that the ear moves toward the shoulder and not the shoulder toward the ear.

Rotation

Normally, rotation is 70° to 90° right and left, and the chin does not quite reach the plane of the shoulder (Figure 3-21). Rotation and side flexion always occur together (coupled movement) but not necessarily in the

Figure 3-18
Kinematics of craniocervical flexion. **A,** Atlanto-occipital joint. **B,** Atlanto-axial joint complex. **C,** Intracervical region (C2-C7). Note in **C** that flexion slackens the anterior longitudinal ligament and increases the space between the adjacent laminae and spinous processes. Elongated and taut tissues are indicated by thin black arrows; slackened tissue is indicated by a wavy black arrow. (Modified from Neumann DA: *Kinesiology of the musculoskeletal system—foundations for physical rehabilitation*, p. 281, St Louis, 2002, C.V. Mosby.)

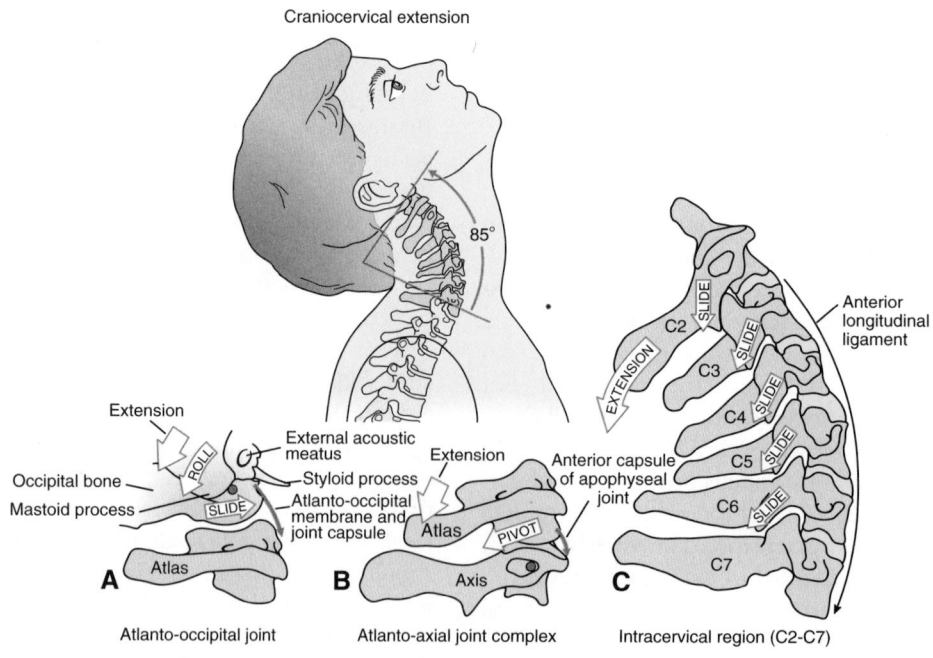

Figure 3-19
Kinematics of craniocervical extension. **A,** Atlanto-occipital joint. **B,** Atlanto-axial joint complex. **C,** Intracervical region (C2-C7). Elongated and taut tissues are indicated by thin black arrows. (Modified from Neumann DA: *Kinesiology of the musculoskeletal system—foundations for physical rehabilitation*, p. 280, St Louis, 2002, C.V. Mosby.)

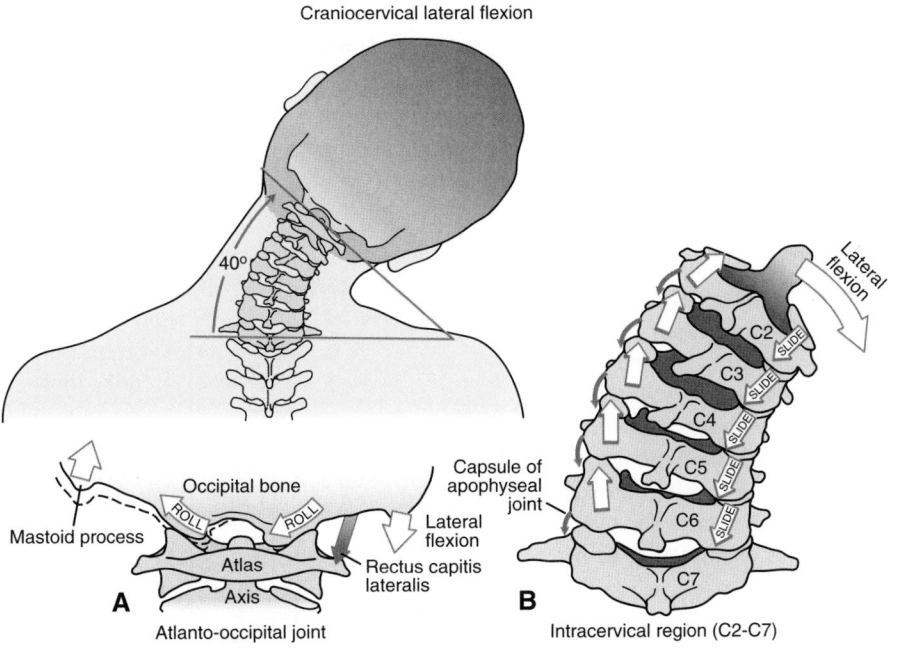

Figure 3-20
Kinematics of craniocervical lateral flexion. **A,** Atlanto-occipital joint. The primary function of the rectus capitis lateralis is to laterally flex this joint. Note the slight compression and distraction of the joint surfaces. **B,** Intracervical region (C2-C7). Note the ipsilateral coupling pattern between axial rotation and lateral flexion. Elongated and taut tissue is indicated by thin black arrows. (Modified from Neumann DA: *Kinesiology of the musculoskeletal system—foundations for physical rehabilitation,* p. 286, St Louis, 2002, C.V. Mosby.)

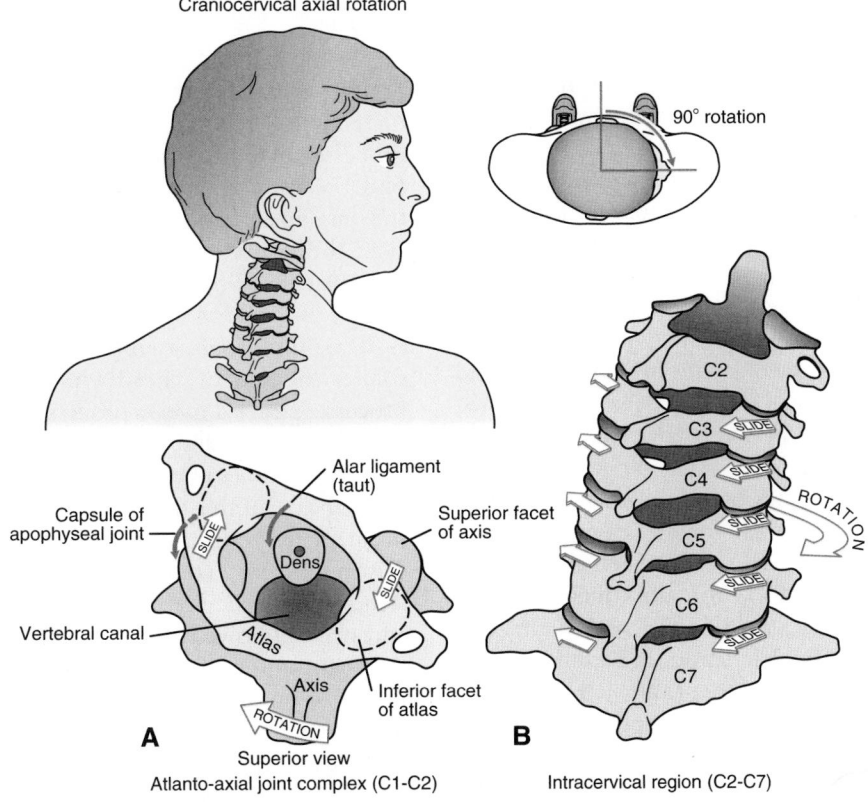

Figure 3-21
Kinematics of craniocervical axial rotation. **A,** Atlanto-axial joint complex. **B,** Intracervical region (C2-C7). (Modified from Neumann DA: *Kinesiology of the musculoskeletal system—foundations for physical rehabilitation,* p. 285, St Louis, 2002, C.V. Mosby.)

same direction.[20,21] This combined movement, which may or may not be visible in a given patient, occurs because of the shape of the articular surfaces of the facet joints; this shape is coronally oblique. Most of the rotation occurs between C1 and C2. If the patient can rotate 40° to 50°, then it is unlikely that the C1/C2 articulation is at fault.[13] If, however, side flexion occurs early to allow full motion, C1-C2 is probably involved.[13]

If, in the history, the patient has complained that **repetitive movements** or **sustained postures** have caused problems, not only should the specific movements be performed, but they should be either repeated several times or sustained to see if the symptoms are exacerbated. If a patient has complained in the history that a movement in other than a cardinal plane or a **combined movement** (e.g., side flexion, rotation, and extension combined) exacerbates the symptoms, then these movements should be performed as well. Table 3-9 outlines examples of movement restrictions and possible causes.

Passive Movements

If the patient does not have full ROM or the examiner has not applied overpressure to determine the end feel of the movement, the patient should be asked to lie in a supine position. The examiner then passively tests flexion, extension, side flexion, and rotation, as in the active movements. The passive ROM with the patient supine is normally greater than the active and passive ROM with the patient sitting. For example, in sitting, active side flexion is about 45°, whereas in supine lying, passive side flexion is 75° to 80°, with the examiner often able to take the ear to the shoulder. This increased range in the supine position results from relaxation of the muscles that, in sitting, are trying to hold the head up against gravity. For the cervical spine, therefore, passive movements with overpressure should be performed along with active movements. Active movements with overpressure at end of range do not give a true impression of end feel for the cervical spine. During passive movements, the examiner can palpate between adjacent vertebra to feel the relative amount of movement on each side. For flexion, the examiner palpates between the mastoid process and the transverse process for movement between C0 and C1 (Figure 3-22, *A*) and between the arch of C1 and spinous process of C2 for movement between C1 and C2 (Figure 3-22, *B*). For the rest of the cervical spine and upper thoracic spine, the examiner can palpate between the spinous processes at each level while passively and progressively flexing the spine. To feel the movement, the examiner will find that as one works down the spine from C2 to C7, more flexion is required to feel the movement (Figure 3-22, *C*). Movement at each segment during side flexion and rotation may be felt by palpating the adjacent transverse processes on each

Table 3-9

Movement Restriction and Possible Causes

Movement Restriction	Possible Causes

Extension and right side bending	Right extension hypomobility
	    Left flexor muscle tightness
	    Anterior capsular adhesions
	    Right subluxation
	    Right small disc protrusion

Flexion and right side bending	Left flexion hypomobility
	    Left extensor muscle tightness
	    Left posterior capsular
	      adhesions
	    Left subluxation

Extension and right side bending restriction greater than extension and left side bending	Left capsular pattern (arthritis, arthrosis)
Flexion and right side bending restriction equal to extension and left side flexion	Left arthrofibrosis (very hard capsular end-feel)
Side bending in neutral, flexion, and extension	Uncovertebral hypomobility or anomaly

(From Dutton M: *Orthopedic examination, evaluation and intervention*, p. 1050, New York, 2004, McGraw Hill.)

side while doing the movement (Figure 3-23). To test rotation between the occiput and C1, the examiner holds the patient's head in position and palpates the transverse processes of C1 (Figure 3-24). The examiner must first find the mastoid process on each side and then move the fingers inferiorly and anteriorly until a hard bump (i.e., the transverse process of C1) is palpated on each side (usually below the ear lobe and just behind the jaw). Palpation in the area of the C1 transverse process is generally painful, so care must be taken. The examiner then rotates the patient's head while palpating the transverse processes; the transverse process on the side to which the head is rotated will seem to disappear (bottom one) while the other side (top one) seems to be accentuated in the normal case. If this disappearance/accentuation does not occur, there is restriction of movement between C0 and C1 on that side. To test rotation at C1-C2, the examiner stands beside the seated patient and side bends the head and neck, followed by rotation to the opposite side. As the rotation is performed, the examiner palpates the relative position of the C1 and C2 transverse processes as the head is rotated. To limit side flexion to a specific segment, as the examiner side flexes the head, the examiner applies an opposing translation force in the opposite direction to the passive movement to limit movement below that being tested.[13] With all of these movements, the end feel should be a solid tissue stretch.

Figure 3-22
Testing passive movement in the cervical spine. **A,** Position testing for occipito-atlantal joint. **B,** Position testing for atlanto-axial joint. **C,** Flexion testing of C2-T1.

Passive Movements of the Cervical Spine and Normal End Feel

- Flexion (tissue stretch)
- Extension (tissue stretch)
- Side flexion right and left (tissue stretch)
- Rotation right and left (tissue stretch)

If the passive movements with overpressure are normal and pain free, the examiner may, with great care, test other positions. For the flexion-rotation test, the patient lies supine while the examiner flexes the neck fully and, while holding this position, passively rotates the head as far as possible within comfort limits.[59] Hall and Robinson[59] report significant restriction in rotation in patients complaining of cervicogenic headache indicating C1-C2 segmental dysfunction. The quadrant position is

Figure 3-23
Testing passive movement in the cervical spine. **A,** Side flexion. **B,** Rotation.

Figure 3-24
Left rotation of the occiput on C1. Note the index finger palpating the right transverse process of C1.

pathology (radicular signs), apophyseal joint involvement (localized pain), or vertebral artery involvement (dizziness, nausea).[46]

In addition to the passive movements of the whole cervical spine, physiological movements between each pair of vertebrae may be performed. These are called **passive physiological intervertebral movements (PPIVMs)**. By stabilizing or blocking the movement of one vertebra (usually the distal one) and then passively moving the head through the different physiological movements (e.g., flexion, extension, side flexion, rotation), each segment can be tested. Needless to say, the amount of movement of each segment will be considerably less than the whole.[61]

Passive movements are performed to determine the end feel of each movement. This may give the examiner an idea of the pathology involved. The normal **end feels** of the cervical spine motions are tissue stretch for all four movements. As with active movements, the most painful movements are done last. The examiner should also note whether a **capsular pattern** (i.e., side flexion and rotation equally limited; extension less limited) is present. Overpressure may be used to test the entire spine (Figure 3-25, *A*) by testing it at the end of the ROM, or proper positioning may be used to test different parts of the cervical spine.[62] For example, end feel for movement of the lower cervical spine into extension is tested with minimal extension and the head pushed directly posterior (Figure 3-25, *C*), whereas the upper

end-range extension, side flexion, and rotation, a position that increases the vulnerability of anterior, posterior, and lateral tissues of the neck, including the vertebral artery.[60] If overpressure is applied in the quadrant position and symptoms result, it is highly suggestive of nerve root cervical spine is tested by "nodding" the head into extension and pushing posteriorly at an approximate 45° angle (Figure 3-25, B).[63]

Resisted Isometric Movements

The same movements that were done actively (flexion, extension, side flexion, and rotation) are then tested isometrically. It is better for the examiner to place the patient in the resting position and then say, "Don't let me move you," rather than to tell the patient, "Contract the muscle as hard as possible." In this way, the examiner ensures that the movement is as isometric as possible and that a minimal amount of movement occurs (Figure 3-26). The examiner should ensure that these movements are done with the cervical spine in the neutral position and that painful movements are done last. Neck flexion tests cranial nerve XI and the C1 and C2 myotomes as well as muscle strength or state. By using Table 3-10 and looking at the various combinations of muscles that cause

the movement (Figure 3-27), the examiner is often able to decide which muscle is at fault. If, in the history, the patient has complained that certain loaded or combined movements (those movements giving resistance other than gravity) are painful, the examiner should not hesitate to carefully test these movements isometrically to better ascertain the problem. If a neurological injury is suspected, the examiner must carefully assess for muscle weakness to determine the structures injured. If a severe neuropraxia or axonotmesis has occurred, there may be residual weakness even though muscle atrophy may not be evident.

Resisted Isometric Movements of the Cervical Spine

- Flexion
- Extension
- Side flexion right and left
- Rotation right and left

A

B

C

Figure 3-25
A, Overpressure to the whole cervical spine. **B,** Overpressure to the upper cervical spine. **C,** Overpressure to the low cervical spine. Clinician must differentiate between temporomandibular joint symptoms and cervical symptoms.

Figure 3-26

Positioning for resisted isometric movement. **A,** Flexion. Note slight flexion of neck before giving resistance.
B, Extension. Note slight flexion of neck before giving resistance. **C,** Side flexion (left side flexion shown).
D, Rotation (left rotation shown).

Scanning Examination

Peripheral Joint Scan

After the resisted isometric movements to the cervical spine have been completed, a peripheral joint scanning examination is performed to rule out obvious pathology in the extremities and to note areas that may need

more detailed assessment.[1] The following joints are scanned bilaterally:

Temporomandibular Joints. The examiner checks the movement of the joints by placing the index or little fingers in the patient's ears (Figure 3-28). The pulp aspect of the finger is placed forward to feel for equality of movement of the condyles of the temporomandibular joints and for

Peripheral Joint Scanning Examination

Temporomandibular joints	Open mouth
	Closed mouth
Shoulder joints	Elevation through abduction
	Elevation through forward flexion
	Elevation through plane of scapula (SCAPTION)
	Apley scratch test (right and left)
	Rotation in 90° abduction
Elbow joints	Flexion
	Extension
	Supination
	Pronation
Wrist and hand joints	Flexion
	Extension
	Abduction
	Adduction
	Opposition of thumb and little finger

clicking or grinding as well as to ensure that the ears are clear. Pain or tenderness, especially on closing the mandible, usually indicates posterior capsulitis. As the patient opens the mouth, the condyle normally moves forward. To open the mouth fully, the condyle must rotate and translate equally bilaterally. If this does not occur, mouth opening will be limited and/or deviation of the mandible will occur (see Chapter 4). The examiner should observe the patient as he or she opens and closes the mouth and should watch for any deviation during the movement.

Shoulder Girdle. The examiner quickly scans this complex of joints (glenohumeral, acromioclavicular, sternoclavicular and "scapulothoracic" joint) by asking the patient to actively elevate each arm through abduction, followed by active elevation through forward flexion and elevation through the plane of the scapula (SCAPTION). In addition, the examiner quickly tests medial and lateral rotation of each shoulder with the arm at the side and with the arm abducted to 90°. Any pattern of restriction should be noted. If the patient is able to reach full abduction without difficulty or pain, the examiner may decide that there is no problem with the shoulder complex (see Chapter 5).

Elbow Joints. The elbow joints are actively moved through flexion, extension, supination, and pronation. Any restriction of movement or abnormal signs and symptoms should be noted, because they may be indicative of pathology (see Chapter 6).

Wrist and Hand. The patient actively performs flexion, extension, and radial and ulnar deviation of the wrist. Active movements (flexion, extension, abduction, adduction, and opposition) are performed for the fingers and thumb. These actions can be accomplished by having the patient make a fist and then spread the fingers and thumb

wide. Again, any alteration in signs and symptoms or restriction of motion should be noted (see Chapter 7).

Myotomes

Having completed the peripheral joint scanning examination, the examiner should then determine muscle power and possible neurological weakness originating from the nerve roots in the cervical spine by testing the myotomes (Table 3-11 and Figure 3-29). Myotomes are tested by resisted isometric contractions with the joint at or near the resting position. As with the resisted isometric movements previously mentioned, the examiner should position the seated patient and say, "Don't let me move you," so that an isometric contraction is obtained.

The contraction should be held for **at least 5 seconds** so that weakness, if any, can be noted. Where applicable, both sides are tested at the same time to provide a comparison. If possible, the examiner must not apply pressure over the joints, because this action may mask symptoms if the joints are tender.

To test neck flexion (C1-C2 myotome), the patient's head should be slightly flexed. The examiner applies pressure to the forehead while stabilizing the trunk with a hand between the scapulae (see Figure 3-29, A). The examiner should ensure the neck does not extend when applying pressure to the forehead. To test neck side flexion (C3 myotome and cranial nerve XI), the examiner places one hand above the patient's ear and applies a side flexion force while stabilizing the trunk with the other hand on the opposite shoulder (see Figure 3-29, B). Both right and left side flexion must be tested.

The examiner then asks the patient to elevate the shoulders (C4 myotome and CN XI) to about half of full elevation. The examiner applies a downward force on both of the patient's shoulders while the patient attempts to hold them in position (see Figure 3-29, C). The examiner should ensure that the patient is not "bracing" the arms against the thighs if testing is done while sitting.

To test shoulder abduction (C5 myotome), the examiner asks the patient to elevate the arms to about 75° to 80° in the scapular plane with the elbows flexed to 90° and the forearms pronated or in neutral (see Figure 3-29, D).

Cervical Myotomes

- Neck flexion: C1-C2
- Neck side flexion: C3 and CN XI
- Shoulder elevation: C4 and CN XI
- Shoulder abduction/shoulder lateral rotation: C5
- Elbow flexion and/or wrist extension: C6
- Elbow extension and/or wrist flexion: C7
- Thumb extension and/or ulnar deviation: C8
- Abduction and/or adduction of hand intrinsics: T1

Table 3-10

Muscles of the Cervical Spine: Their Actions and Nerve Supply

Action	Muscles Acting	Nerve Supply
Forward flexion of head	1. Rectus capitis anterior	C1-C2
	2. Rectus capitis lateralis	C1-C2
	3. Longus capitis	C1-C3
	4. Hyoid muscles	Inferior alveolar
		Facial
		Hypoglossal
		Ansa cervicalis
	5. Obliquus capitis superior	C1
	6. Sternocleidomastoid (if head in neutral or flexion)	Accessory, C2
Extension of head	1. Splenius capitis	C4-C6
	2. Semispinalis capitis	C1-C8
	3. Longissimus capitis	C6-C8
	4. Spinalis capitis	C6-C8
	5. Trapezius	Accessory, C3-C4
	6. Rectus capitis posterior minor	C1
	7. Rectus capitis posterior major	C1
	8. Obliquus capitis superior	C1
	9. Obliquus capitis inferior	C1
	10. Sternocleidomastoid (if head in some extension)	Accessory, C2
Rotation of head (muscles on one side contract)	1. Trapezius (face moves to opposite side)	Accessory, C3, C4
	2. Splenius capitis (face moves to the same side)	C4-C6
	3. Longissimus capitis (face moves to same side)	C6-C8
	4. Semispinalis capitis (face moves to same side)	C1-C8
	5. Obliquus capitis inferior (face moves to same side)	C1
	6. Sternocleidomastoid (face moves to opposite side)	Accessory, C2
Side flexion of head	1. Trapezius	Accessory, C3-C4
	2. Splenius capitis	C4-C6
	3. Longissimus capitis	C6-C8
	4. Semispinalis capitis	C1-C8
	5. Obliquus capitis inferior	C1
	6. Rectus capitis lateralis	C1-C2
	7. Longus capitis	C1-C3
	8. Sternocleidomastoid	Accessory, C2
Flexion of neck	1. Longus colli	C2-C6
	2. Scalenus anterior	C4-C6
	3. Scalenus medius	C3-C8
	4. Scalenus posterior	C6-C8
	5. Infrahyoid muscles	Ansa cervicalis
		Hypoglossal
	6. Suprahyoid muscles	Inferior alveolar
		Facial
		C1
Extension of neck	1. Splenius cervicis	C6-C8
	2. Semispinalis cervicis	C1-C8
	3. Longissimus cervicis	C6-C8
	4. Levator scapulae	C3-C4
		Dorsal scapular
	5. Iliocostalis cervicis	C6-C8
	6. Spinalis cervicis	C6-C8
	7. Multifidus	C1-C8
	8. Interspinalis cervicis	C1-C8

Continued

Action	Muscles Acting	Nerve Supply
	9. Trapezius	Accessory
	10. Rectus capitis posterior major	C3-C4
	11. Rotatores brevis	C1
	12. Rotatores longi	C1-C8
Side flexion of neck	1. Levator scapulae	C1-C8
		Dorsal scapular
	2. Splenius cervicis	C4-C6
	3. Iliocostalis cervicis	C6-C8
	4. Longissimus cervicis	C6-C8
	5. Semispinalis cervicis	C1-C8
	6. Multifidus	C1-C8
	7. Intertransversarii	C1-C8
	8. Scaleni	C3-C8
	9. Sternocleidomastoid	Accessory, C2
	10. Obliquus capitis inferior	C1
	11. Rotatores breves	C1-C8
	12. Rotatores longi	C1-C8
	13. Longus colli	C2-C6
Rotation* of neck (muscles on one side contract)	1. Levator scapulae (face moves to same side)	C3–C4
		Dorsal scapular
	2. Splenius cervicis (face moves to same side)	C4–C6
	3. Iliocostalis cervicis (face moves to same side)	C6–C8
	4. Longissimus cervicis (face moves to same side)	C6–C8
	5. Semispinalis cervicis (face moves to same side)	C1–C8
	6. Multifidus (face moves to opposite side)	C1–C8
	7. Intertransversarii (face moves to same side)	C1–C8
	8. Scaleni (face moves to opposite side)	C3–C8
	9. Sternocleidomastoid (face moves to opposite side)	Accessory, C2
	10. Obliquus capitis inferior (face moves to same side)	C1
	11. Rotatores brevis (face moves to same side)	C1–C8
	12. Rotatores longi (face moves to same side)	C1–C8

*Occurs in conjunction with side flexion owing to direction of facet joints.

The examiner applies a downward force on the humerus while the patient attempts to hold the arms in position. To prevent rotation, the examiner places his or her forearms over the patient's forearms while applying pressure to the humerus.

To test elbow flexion and extension, the examiner asks the patient to put the arms by the sides, with the elbows flexed to 90° and forearms in neutral. The examiner applies a downward isometric force (see Figure 3-29, E) to the forearms to test the elbow flexors (C6 myotome) and an upward isometric force (see Figure 3-29, G) to test the elbow extensors (C7 myotome). For testing of wrist movements (extension, flexion, ulnar deviation) the patient's arms are by the side; elbows at 90°; forearms pronated; and wrists, hands, and fingers in neutral. The examiner applies a downward force (see Figure 3-29, F) to the hands to test wrist extension (C6 myotome), and an upward force (see Figure 3-29, H) to test wrist flexion (C7 myotome). To apply a lateral force (radial deviation) to test ulnar deviation (C8 myotome), the clinician stabilizes the patient's forearm with one hand and applies a radial deviation force to the side of the hand.

In the test for thumb extension (C8 myotome), the patient extends the thumb just short of full range of motion (see Figure 3-29, I). The examiner applies an isometric force to bring the thumbs into flexion. To test hand intrinsics (T1 myotome), the patient squeezes a piece of paper between the fingers while the examiner tries to pull it away; the patient may squeeze the examiner's fingers, or the patient may abduct the fingers slightly with the examiner isometrically adducting them (see Figure 3-29, J).

Sensory Scanning Examination

The examiner then tests sensation by doing a **sensory scanning examination.** This "sensory scan" is accomplished by running relaxed hands over the patient's head (sides and back); down over the shoulders, upper chest, and back; and down the arms, being sure to cover all

Figure 3-27

Anatomic relations of the lower cervical spine. *1,* Splenius capitis. *2,* Splenius cervicis. *3,* Semispinalis cervicis and capitis. *4,* Multifidus and rotatores. *5,* Longissimus capitis. *6,* Longissimus cervicis. *7,* Levator scapulae. *8,* Scalenus posterior. *9,* Scalenus medius. *10,* Scalenus anterior. *11,* Sternocleidomastoid. *12,* Trapezius.

aspects of the arm. If any difference is noted between the sides in this "sensation scan," the examiner may then use a pinwheel, pin, cotton batting, or brush (or a combination of these) to map out the exact area of sensory difference and to determine if any sensory difference is due to a nerve root (see later section on reflexes and cutaneous distribution), peripheral nerve, or some other neurological deficit. The sensory scanning examination may also include the testing of reflexes, especially the deep tendon reflexes, to test for upper and lower neuron pathology and pathological reflexes for upper motor neuron pathology, and the performance of selected neurodynamic tests (e.g., upper limb tension test, slump test) if peripheral nerve irritability is suspected.

Functional Assessment

If, in the history, the patient has complained of functional difficulties or the examiner suspects some functional impairment, a series of functional tests or movements may be performed to determine the patient's functional capacity, keeping in mind the patient's age and health. These tests may include activities of daily living such as the following:

Breathing. Normal, unlabored breathing should be seen with the mouth closed. There should be no gulping or gasping.

Figure 3-28

Testing temporomandibular joints.

> ### Functional Assessment of the Cervical Spine
>
> • Activities of daily living
> • Numerical scoring table (if desired)

Table 3-11

Myotomes of the Upper Limb

Nerve Root	Test Action	Muscles*
C1-C2	Neck flexion	Rectus lateralis, rectus capitis anterior, longus capitis, longus coli, longus cervicis, sternocleidomastoid
C3	Neck side flexion	Longus capitis, longus cervicis, trapezius, scalenus medius
C4	Shoulder elevation	Diaphragm, trapezius, levator scapulae, scalenus anterior, scalenus medius
C5	Shoulder abduction	Rhomboid major and minor, deltoid, supraspinatus, infraspinatus, teres minor, biceps, scalenus anterior and medius
C6	Elbow flexion and wrist extension	Serratus anterior, latissimus dorsi, subscapularis, teres major, pectoralis major (clavicular head), biceps, coracobrachialis, brachialis, brachioradialis, supinator, extensor carpi radialis longus, scalenus anterior, medius and posterior
C7	Elbow extension and wrist flexion	Serratus anterior, latissimus dorsi, pectoralis major (sternal head), pectoralis minor, triceps, pronator teres, flexor carpi radialis, flexor digitorum superficialis, extensor carpi radialis longus, extensor carpi radialis brevis, extensor digitorum, extensor digiti minimi, scalenus medius and posterior
C8	Thumb extension and ulnar deviation	Pectoralis major (sternal head), pectoralis minor, triceps, flexor digitorum superficialis, flexor digitorum profundus, flexor pollicis longus, pronator quadratus, flexor carpi ulnaris, abductor pollicis longus, extensor pollicis longus, extensor pollicis brevis, extensor indicis, abductor pollicis brevis, flexor pollicis brevis, opponens pollicis, scalenus medius and posterior
T1	Hand intrinsics	Flexor digitorum profundus, intrinsic muscles of the hand (except extensor pollicis brevis), flexor pollicis brevis, opponens pollicis

*Muscles listed may be supplied by additional nerve roots; only primary nerve root sources are listed.

A   **B**   **C**

Figure 3-29

Positioning to test myotomes. **A,** Neck flexion (C1, C2). **B,** Neck side flexion to the left (C3). **C,** Shoulder elevation (C4).

Continued

Figure 3-29 cont'd
D, Shoulder abduction (C5). **E,** Elbow flexion (C6). **F,** Wrist extension (C6). **G,** Elbow extension (C7). **H,** Wrist flexion (C7). **I,** Thumb extension (C8). **J,** Finger abduction (T1).

Table 3-12

Functional Strength Testing of the Cervical Spine

Starting Position	Action	Functional Test*
Supine lying	Lift head, keeping chin tucked in (neck flexion)	6–8 repetitions: functional 3–5 repetitions: functionally fair 1–2 repetitions: functionally poor 0 repetitions: nonfunctional
Prone lying	Lift head backward (neck extension)	Hold 20–25 seconds: functional Hold 10–19 seconds: functionally fair Hold 1–9 seconds: functionally poor Hold 0 seconds: nonfunctional
Side lying (pillows under head so head is not side flexed)	Lift head sideways away from pillow (neck side flexion) (must be repeated for other side)	Hold 20–25 seconds: functional Hold 10–19 seconds: functionally fair Hold 1–9 seconds: functionally poor Hold 0 seconds: nonfunctional
Supine lying	Lift head off bed and rotate to one side, keeping head off bed or pillow (neck rotation) (must be repeated both ways)	Hold 20–25 seconds: functional Hold 10–19 seconds: functionally fair Hold 1–9 seconds: functionally poor Hold 0 seconds: nonfunctional

Adapted from Palmer ML, Epler M: *Clinical assessment procedures in physical therapy*, pp. 181–182, Philadelphia, 1990, J.B. Lippincott.
*Younger patients should be able to do the most repetitions and for the longest time; with age, time and repetitions decrease.

Swallowing. This is a complex movement involving muscles of the lips, tongue, jaw, soft palate, pharynx, and larynx as well as the suprahyoid and infrahyoid muscles.

Looking Up at the Ceiling. At least 40° to 50° of neck extension is usually necessary for everyday activities. If this range is not available, the patient will bend the back or the knees, or both, to obtain the desired range.

Looking Down at Belt Buckle or Shoe Laces. At least 60° to 70° of neck flexion is necessary. If this range is not available, the patient will flex the back to complete the task.

Shoulder Check. At least 60° to 70° of cervical rotation is necessary. If this range is not available, the patient will rotate the trunk to accomplish this task.

Tuck Chin In. This action produces upper cervical flexion with lower cervical extension.[63]

Poke Chin Out. This action produces upper cervical extension with lower cervical flexion.[63]

Neck Strength. In athletes, neck strength should be approximately 30% of body weight to decrease chance of injury.[64]

Paresthesia. Paresthesia, especially referred to the hands, may make cooking and handling utensils particularly difficult or even dangerous.

Table 3-12 lists functional strength tests that can give the examiner some indication of the patient's functional strength capacity. For flexion, if the jaw juts forward at the beginning of the movement, it indicates an imbalance pattern of strong sternocleidomastoid and weak deep neck reflexors.[13] Vernon and Mior[65] have developed a numerical scoring functional test called the neck disability index (Figure 3-30), which is a modification of the Oswestry low back pain index.[66] This index and similar tests (e.g., Bournemouth Questionnaire [Figure 3-31]) can be used to detect change in patients over time.[67,68]

Special Tests

There are several special tests that may be performed if the examiner believes they are relevant. Some of these tests should always be performed (e.g., instability tests, vertebral artery tests), especially if treatment is to be given to the upper cervical spine; while others should be performed only if the examiner wants to use them as confirming tests. Some tests are provocative and should only be used if the examiner wants to cause symptoms. Other tests relieve symptoms and are used when the symptoms are present. The reliability of many of these tests commonly depends on the experience and skill of the examiner.[69,70] The reliability, validity, specificity, and sensitivity of some special/diagnostic tests used in the cervical spine are outlined in Appendix 3-1.

Special Tests Commonly Performed on Cervical Spine

- Foraminal compression (Spurling's) test
- Distraction test
- Upper limb tension test
- Shoulder abduction test
- Vertebral artery (cervical quadrant) test

Neck Disability Index

This questionnaire has been designed to give the doctor information as to how your neck pain has affected your ability to manage in everyday life. Please answer every section and mark in each section only the ONE box which applies to you. We realize you may consider that two of the statements in any one section relate to you, but please just mark the box which most closely describes your problem.

Section 1 — Pain Intensity

- [ ] I have no pain at the moment. (0)
- [ ] The pain is very mild at the moment. (1)
- [ ] The pain is moderate at the moment. (2)
- [ ] The pain is fairly severe at the moment. (3)
- [ ] The pain is very severe at the moment. (4)
- [ ] The pain is the worst imaginable at the moment. (5)

Section 2 — Personal Care (Washing, Dressing, etc.)

- [ ] I can look after myself normally without causing extra pain. (0)
- [ ] I can look after myself normally but it causes extra pain. (1)
- [ ] It is painful to look after myself and I am slow and careful. (2)
- [ ] I need some help but manage most of my personal care. (3)
- [ ] I need help every day in most aspects of self care. (4)
- [ ] I do not get dressed, I wash with difficulty and stay in bed. (5)

Section 3 — Lifting

- [ ] I can lift heavy weights without extra pain. (0)
- [ ] I can lift heavy weights but it gives extra pain. (1)
- [ ] Pain prevents me from lifting heavy weights off the floor, but I can manage if they are conveniently positioned, for example on a table. (2)
- [ ] Pain prevents me from lifting heavy weights, but I can manage light to medium weights if they are conveniently positioned. (3)
- [ ] I can lift very light weights. (4)
- [ ] I cannot lift or carry anything at all. (5)

Section 4 — Reading

- [ ] I can read as much as I want to with no pain in my neck. (0)
- [ ] I can read as much as I want to with slight pain in my neck. (1)
- [ ] I can read as much as I want with moderate pain in my neck. (2)
- [ ] I cannot read as much as I want because of moderate pain in my neck. (3)
- [ ] I can hardly read at all because of severe pain in my neck. (4)
- [ ] I cannot read at all. (5)

Section 5 — Headaches

- [ ] I have no headaches at all. (0)
- [ ] I have slight headaches that come infrequently. (1)
- [ ] I have moderate headaches which come infrequently. (2)
- [ ] I have moderate headaches which come frequently. (3)
- [ ] I have severe headaches which come frequently. (4)
- [ ] I have headaches almost all the time. (5)

Section 6 — Concentration

- [ ] I can concentrate fully when I want to with no difficulty. (0)
- [ ] I can concentrate fully when I want to with slight difficulty. (1)
- [ ] I have a fair degree of difficulty in concentrating when I want to. (2)
- [ ] I have a lot of difficulty in concentrating when I want to. (3)
- [ ] I have a great deal of difficulty in concentrating when I want to. (4)
- [ ] I cannot concentrate at all. (5)

Section 7 — Work

- [ ] I can do as much work as I want to. (0)
- [ ] I can do my usual work, but no more. (1)
- [ ] I can do most of my usual work, but no more. (2)
- [ ] I cannot do my usual work. (3)
- [ ] I can hardly do any work at all. (4)
- [ ] I cannot do any work at all. (5)

Section 8 — Driving

- [ ] I can drive my car without any neck pain. (0)
- [ ] I can drive my car as long as I want with slight pain in my neck. (1)
- [ ] I can drive my car as long as I want with moderate pain in my neck. (2)
- [ ] I cannot drive my car as long as I want because of moderate pain in my neck. (3)
- [ ] I can hardly drive at all because of severe pain in my neck. (4)
- [ ] I cannot drive my car at all. (5)

Section 9 — Sleeping

- [ ] I have no trouble sleeping. (0)
- [ ] My sleep is slightly disturbed (less than 1 hr. sleepless). (1)
- [ ] My sleep is mildly disturbed (1–2 hrs. sleepless). (2)
- [ ] My sleep is moderately disturbed (2–3 hrs. sleepless). (3)
- [ ] My sleep is greatly disturbed (3–5 hrs. sleepless). (4)
- [ ] My sleep is completely disturbed (5–7 hrs. sleepless). (5)

Section 10 — Recreation

- [ ] I am able to engage in all my recreation activities with no neck pain at all. (0)
- [ ] I am able to engage in all my recreation activities, with some pain in my neck. (1)
- [ ] I am able to engage in most, but not all, of my usual recreation activities because of pain in my neck. (2)
- [ ] I am able to engage in a few of my usual recreation activities because of pain in my neck. (3)
- [ ] I can hardly do any recreation activities because of pain in my neck. (4)
- [ ] I cannot do any recreation activities at all. (5)

Scores (out of 50):   0–4 No disability
5–14 Mild disability
15–24 Moderate disability
25–34 Severe disability
>35 Complete disability

Figure 3-30

Neck disability index. (Modified from Vernon H, Mior S: The neck disability index: a study of reliability and validity, *J Manip Physiol Ther* 14:411, 1991.)

The following scales have been designed to find out about your neck pain and how it is affecting you. Please answer ALL the scales by circling ONE number on EACH scale that best describes how you feel:

1. Over the past week, on average how would you rate your neck pain?

No pain   Worst pain possible

0   1   2   3   4   5   6   7   8   9   10

2. Over the past week, how much has your neck pain interfered with your daily activities (housework, washing, dressing, lifting, reading, driving)?

No interference   Unable to carry out activities

0   1   2   3   4   5   6   7   8   9   10

3. Over the past week, how much has your neck pain interfered with your ability to take part in recreational, social, and family activities?

No interference   Unable to carry out activities

0   1   2   3   4   5   6   7   8   9   10

4. Over the past week, how anxious (tense, uptight, irritable, difficulty in cocentrating/relaxing) have you been feeling?

Not at all anxious   Extremely anxious

0   1   2   3   4   5   6   7   8   9   10

5. Over the past week, how depressed (down-in-the-dumps, sad, in low spirits, pessimistic, unhappy) have you been feeling?

Not at all depressed   Extremely depressed

0   1   2   3   4   5   6   7   8   9   10

6. Over the past week, how have you felt your work (both inside and outside the home) has affected (or would affect) your neck pain?

Have made it no worse   Have made it much worse

0   1   2   3   4   5   6   7   8   9   10

7. Over the past week, how much have you been able to control (reduce/help) your neck pain on your own?

Completely control it   No control whatsoever

0   1   2   3   4   5   6   7   8   9   10

Figure 3-31

Global dimensions of the Neck Bournemouth Questionnaire. (From Bolton JE, Humphreys BK: The Bournemouth Questionnaire: A short-form comprehensive outcome measure. II Psychometric properties in neck pain patients, *J Manip Physiol Ther* 25:148, 2002.)

Tests for Neurological Symptoms

Foraminal Compression (Spurling's) Test.[71] This test is performed if, in the history, the patient has complained of nerve root symptoms, which at the time of examination are diminished or absent. This test is designed to provoke symptoms. The patient bends or side flexes the head to the unaffected side first, followed by the affected side (Figure 3-32). The examiner carefully presses straight down on the head. Bradley and colleagues[49] advocate doing this test in three stages, each of which is increasingly provocative; if symptoms are produced, one does not proceed to the next stage. The first stage involves compression with the head in neutral. The second stage involves compression with the head in extension, and the final stage is with the head in extension and rotation to the unaffected side, then to the side of complaint, with compression. The third part of the test

more closely follows the test as described by Spurling.[71] A test result is classified as positive if pain radiates into the arm toward which the head is side flexed during compression; this indicates pressure on a nerve root (cervical radiculitis). **Radiculitis** implies pain in the dermatomal distribution of the nerve root affected.[49] Neck pain with no radiation into the shoulder or arm does not constitute a positive test. The dermatome distribution of the pain and altered sensation can give some indication as to which nerve root is involved. The test positions narrow the intervertebral foramen so that the following conditions may lead to symptoms: stenosis; cervical spondylosis; osteophytes; trophic, arthritic or inflamed facet joints; or herniated disc, which also narrow the foramen; or even vertebral fractures. If the pain is felt in the opposite side to which the head is taken, it is called a **reverse Spurling's sign** and is indicative of muscle spasm in conditions such as tension myalgia and WADs.[72]

A very similar test is called the **maximum cervical compression test**. With this test, the patient side flexes the head and then rotates it to the same side. The test is repeated to the other side. A positive test is indicated if pain radiates into the arm.[29] If the head is taken into extension (as well as side flexion and rotation) and compression is applied, the intervertebral foramina close maximally to the side of movement and symptoms are accentuated. Pain on the concave side indicates nerve root or facet joint pathology, whereas pain on the convex side indicates muscle strain (Figure 3-33).[73] This second position may also compress the vertebral artery. If one is testing the vertebral artery, the position should be held for 20 to 30 seconds to elicit symptoms (e.g., dizziness, nystagmus, feeling faint, nausea) that would indicate compression of the vertebral artery.

Jackson's Compression Test. This test is also a modification of the foraminal compression test. The patient rotates the head to one side. The examiner then carefully presses straight down on the head (Figure 3-34). The test is repeated with the head rotated to the other side. The test is positive if pain radiates into the arm, indicating pressure on a nerve root. The pain distribution (dermatome) can give some indication of which nerve root is affected.[47]

Distraction Test. The distraction test is used for patients who have complained of radicular symptoms in the history and show radicular signs during the examination. It is used to alleviate symptoms. To perform the distraction test, the examiner places one hand under the patient's chin and the other hand around the occiput, then slowly lifts the patient's head (Figure 3-35)—in effect, applying traction to the cervical spine. The test is classified as positive if the pain is relieved or decreased when the head is lifted or distracted, indicating pressure on nerve roots that has been relieved. This test may also be used to check radicular signs referred to the shoulder complex

Figure 3-32
Foraminal compression test. Patient flexes head to one side *(1)*, and examiner presses straight down on head *(2)*.

Figure 3-34
Jackson's compression test.

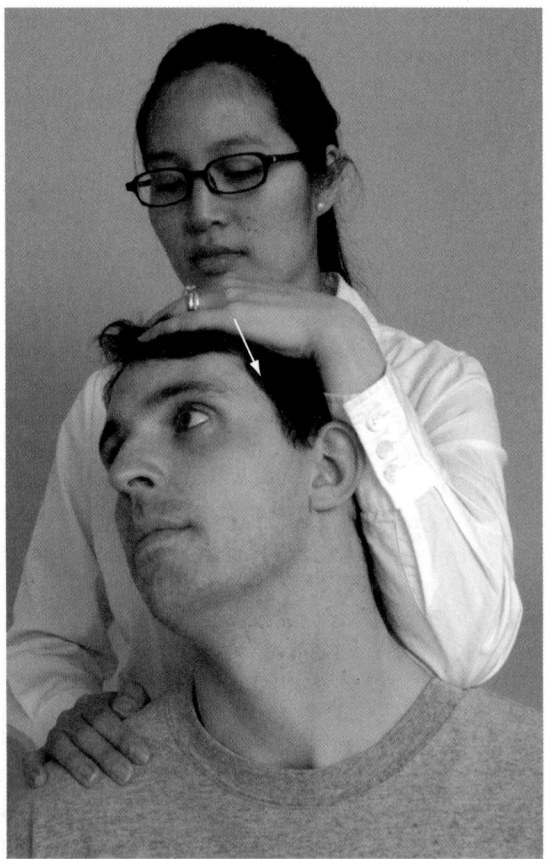

Figure 3-33
Maximum cervical compression test.

anteriorly or posteriorly. If the patient abducts the arms while traction is applied, the symptoms are often further relieved or lessened in the shoulder, especially if C4 or C5 nerve roots are involved. In this case, the test would still be indicative of nerve root pressure in the cervical spine, not shoulder pathology. Increased pain on distraction may be the result of muscle spasm, ligament sprain, muscle strain, dural irritability, or disc herniation.[13]

Upper Limb Tension Tests (Brachial Plexus Tension or Elvey Test). The upper limb tension tests (ULTT) are equivalent to the straight leg raise (SLR) test in the lumbar spine. They are tension tests designed to put stress on the neurological structures of the upper limb, although, in truth, stress is put on all the tissues of the upper limb. The neurological tissue is differentiated by what is defined as sensitizing tests (e.g., neck flexion with the SLR test). This test, first described by Elvey,[62] has since been divided into four tests (Table 3-13). Modification of the position of the shoulder, elbow, forearm, wrist, and fingers places greater stress on specific nerves (nerve bias).[74]

Each test begins by testing the good side first and positioning the shoulder, followed by the forearm, wrist, fingers, and last, because of its large ROM, the elbow. Each phase is added until symptoms are produced. To further "sensitize" the test, side flexion of the cervical spine may be performed.[62,73] Symptoms are more easily aggravated into the upper limb than the lower limb when doing tension tests,[74,75] and if the neurological signs are worsening or in the acute phase, or if a cauda equina or spinal cord lesion is present, these stress tests are contraindicated.[74]

When positioning the shoulder, it is essential that a constant depression force be applied to the shoulder girdle so that, even with abduction, the shoulder girdle remains depressed. If the shoulder is not held depressed, the test is less likely to work. While the shoulder girdle is depressed, the glenohumeral joint is taken to the appropriate abduction position (110° or 10°, depending on

Figure 3-35
Distraction test.

the test), and the forearm, wrist, and fingers are taken to their appropriate end-of-range position; for example, in ULTT2 the wrist is in full extension (Figure 3-36). Elbow extension stresses the radial and median nerves, whereas flexion stresses the ulnar nerve. Wrist and finger extension stresses the median and ulnar nerve while releasing stress on the radial nerve.[74] If required (ULTT2, 3, and 4), the glenohumeral joint is appropriately rotated and held. The elbow position is often not performed until last because the large elbow ROM is easiest to measure when recording available range to show improvement over time. As the elbow is taken toward its extreme (end-of-range) position, symptoms

are usually felt.[75] Some of these symptoms are normal (Table 3-14), and some are pathological. If symptoms are minimal or no symptoms appear, the head and cervical spine are taken into contralateral side flexion. This final movement is sometimes referred to as a **sensitizing test.** This sensitizing test may be within or near the test limb (e.g., neck side flexion in ULTT), or it may be in another quadrant (e.g., right ULTT and right SLR).

The tests are designed to stress tissues. Although they stress the neurological tissues, they also stress some contractile and inert tissues. Differentiation among the types of tissues depends on the signs and symptoms presented (Table 3-15).

Finally, although specific ULTTs are described, if the patient describes neurological symptoms when doing functional movements (e.g., getting wallet out of back pocket) these movements should also be tested by positioning the limb and taking the joints toward their end range.

Evans[48] described a modification of the ULTT that he called the **brachial plexus tension test.** The sitting patient abducts the arms with the elbows extended, stopping just short of the onset of symptoms. The patient laterally rotates the shoulder just short of symptoms, and the examiner then holds this position. Finally, the patient flexes the elbows so that the hands lie behind the head (Figure 3-37). Reproduction of radicular symptoms with elbow flexion is considered a positive test. This test is similar to ULTT4 and stresses primarily the ulnar nerve and the C8 and T1 nerve roots.

Evans[48] outlined a second similar test. The seated patient abducts the arm to 90° with the elbow fully flexed. The arm is extended at the shoulder and then the elbow is extended (Figure 3-38). If radicular pain results, the test is positive **(Bikele's sign).** This test in reality is a modification of the ULTT4 done actively.

Table 3-13

Upper Limb Tension Tests Showing Order of Joint Positioning and Nerve Bias

	ULTT1	ULTT2	ULTT3	ULTT4
Shoulder	Depression and abduction (110°)	Depression and abduction (10°)	Depression and abduction (10°)	Depression and abduction (10°–90°), hand to ear
Elbow	Extension	Extension	Extension	Flexion
Forearm	Supination	Supination	Pronation	Supination
Wrist	Extension	Extension	Flexion and ulnar deviation	Extension and radial deviation
Fingers and thumb	Extension	Extension	Flexion	Extension
Shoulder	—	Lateral rotation	Medial rotation	Lateral rotation
Cervical spine	Contralateral side flexion	Contralateral side flexion	Contralateral side flexion	Contralateral side flexion
Nerve bias	Median nerve, anterior interosseous nerve, C5, C6, C7	Median nerve, musculocutaneous nerve, axillary nerve	Radial nerve	Ulnar nerve, C8 and T1 nerve roots

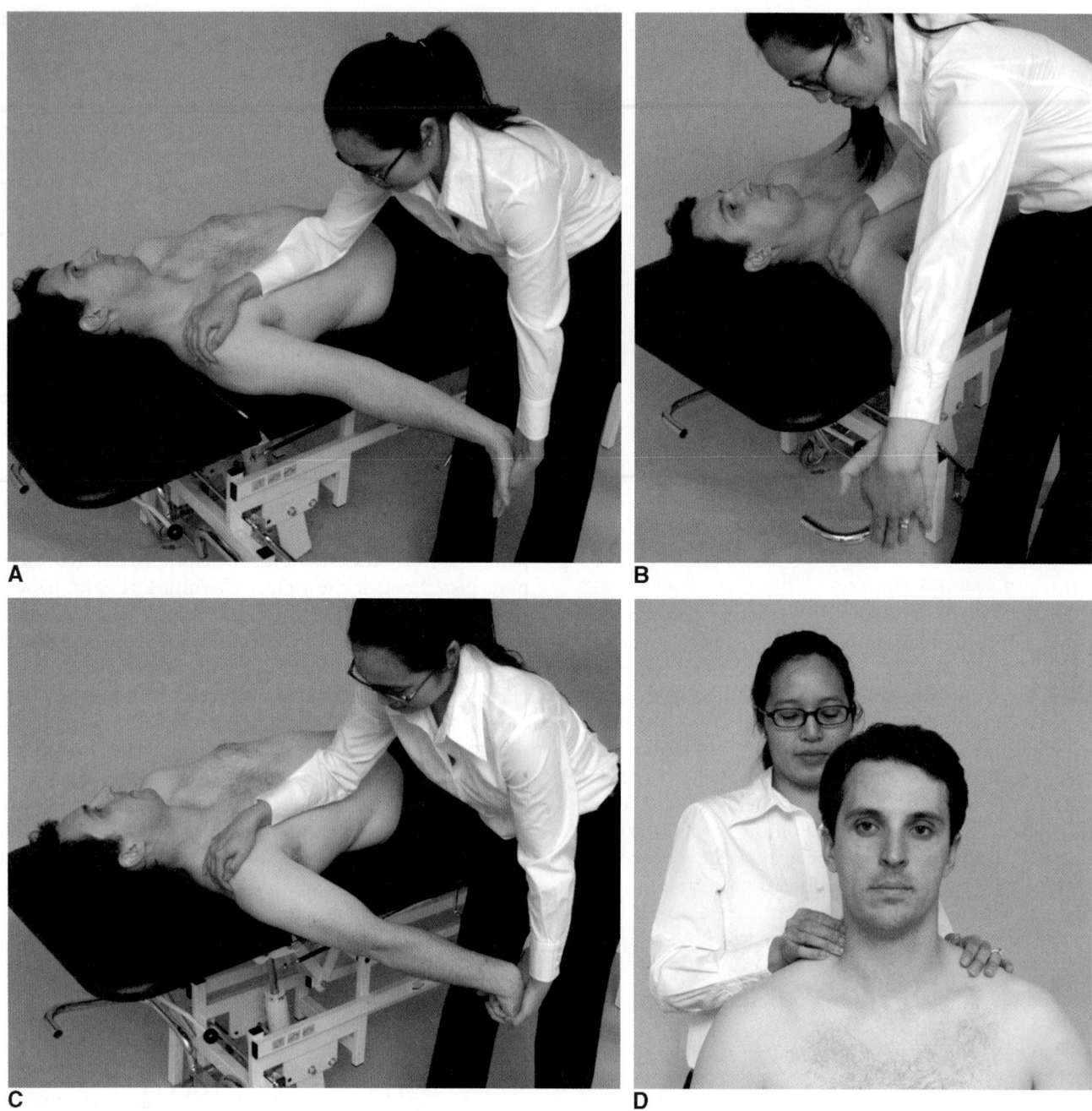

Figure 3-36
Upper limb tension tests (Elvey tests). **A,** ULTT1. **B,** ULTT2. **C,** ULTT3. **D,** ULTT4.

Shoulder Depression Test. This test may be used to evaluate for brachial plexus lesions (see Table 3-6), since the test position is the mechanism of injury for these lesions, plexopathies, and radiculopathies. With brachial plexus lesions, more than one nerve root is commonly affected. The examiner side flexes the patient's head to one side (e.g., the left) while applying a downward pressure on the opposite shoulder (e.g., the right) (Figure 3-39). If the pain is increased, it indicates irritation or compression of the nerve roots or foraminal encroachments such as osteophytes in the area on the side being compressed, or adhesions around the dural sleeves of the nerve and adjacent joint capsule or a hypomobile joint capsule on the side being stretched. Differentiation is by the dermatome (and possibly myotome) distribution of symptoms.

Shoulder Abduction (Relief) Test. This test is used to test for radicular symptoms, especially those involving the C4 or C5 nerve roots. The patient is sitting or lying down,

Table 3-14

Upper Limb Tension Test: Normal and Pathological Signs and Symptoms

Normal (Negative)	Pathological (Positive)
Deep ache or stretch in cubital fossa (99%)	Production of patient's symptoms (most important feature)
Deep ache or stretch into anterior and radial aspect of forearm and radial aspect of hand (80%)	A sensitizing test in the ipsilateral quadrant alters the symptoms
Tingling to the fingers supplied by appropriate nerve (nerve bias)	Different symptoms between right and left (contralateral quadrant)
Stretch in anterior shoulder area	
Above responses increased with contralateral cervical side flexion (90%)	
Above responses decreased with ipsilateral cervical side flexion (70%)	

Adapted from Butler DS: *Mobilisation of the nervous system,* Melbourne, 1991, Churchill Livingstone.

and the examiner passively or the patient actively elevates the arm through abduction, so that the hand or forearm rests on top of the head (Figure 3-40).[47,76] A decrease in or relief of symptoms indicates a cervical extradural compression problem such as a herniated disc, epidural vein compression, or nerve root compression, usually in the C4-C5 or C5-C6 area. Differentiation is by the dermatome (and possible myotome) distribution of the symptoms. This finding is also called **Bakody's sign**.[48] Abduction of the arm decreases the length of the neurological pathway and decreases the pressure on the lower nerve roots.[76,77] If the pain increases with the positioning of the arm, it implies that pressure is increasing in the interscalene triangle.[48]

Scalene Cramp Test.[39] The patient sits and rotates the head to the affected side and pulls the chin down into the hollow above the clavicle by flexing the cervical spine. If pain increases, it is usually in the trigger points of the scalenes toward which the head rotates. Radicular signs may indicate plexopathy or thoracic outlet symptoms.

Valsalva Test. This test is used to determine the effect of increased pressure on the spinal cord. The examiner asks the patient to take a deep breath and hold it while bearing down, as if moving the bowels. A positive test is indicated by increased pain, which may be caused by increased intrathecal pressure. This increased pressure within the spinal cord usually results from a space-occupying lesion, such as a herniated disc, a tumor, stenosis, or osteophytes. Test results are very subjective. The test should be performed with care and caution because the patient may become dizzy and pass out during the test or shortly afterward if the procedure blocks the blood supply to the brain.

Tinel's Sign for Brachial Plexus Lesions.[78] The patient sits with the neck slightly side flexed. The examiner taps the area of the brachial plexus (Figure 3-41) with a finger along the nerve trunks in such a way that the different nerve roots are tested. Pure local pain implies that there is an underlying cervical plexus lesion. A positive Tinel's sign (tingling sensation in the distribution of a nerve) means the lesion is anatomically intact and some recovery is occurring. If pain is elicited in the distribution of a peripheral nerve, the sign is positive for a neuroma and indicates a disruption of the continuity of the nerve.

Brachial Plexus Compression Test.[79] The examiner applies firm compression to the brachial plexus by squeezing the plexus under the thumb or fingers (Figure 3-42). Pain at the site is not diagnostic; the test is positive only if pain radiates into the shoulder or upper extremity. It is positive for mechanical cervical lesions having a mechanical component.

Tests for Upper Motor Neuron Lesions (Cervical Myelopathy)

Romberg's Test. For Romberg's test, the patient is standing and is asked to close the eyes. The position is held for 20 to 30 seconds. If the body begins to sway excessively or the patient loses balance, the test is considered positive for an upper motor neuron lesion.

Table 3-15

Differential Diagnosis of Contractile, Inert, and Nervous Tissue Based on Stretch or Tension

	Contractile Tissue	Inert Tissue (Ligament)	Neurogenic Tissue
Pain	Cramping, dull ache	Dull→sharp	Burning, bright, lightning-like
Tingling	No	No	Yes
Constancy	Intermittent	Intermittent	Longer symptom duration
Dermatome pattern	No	No	Yes (if nerve root pathological)
Peripheral nerve sensory distribution	No	No	Yes (if peripheral nerve or nerve root is affected)
Resistance to stretch	Muscle spasm	Boggy, hard capsular	Soft tissue stretch

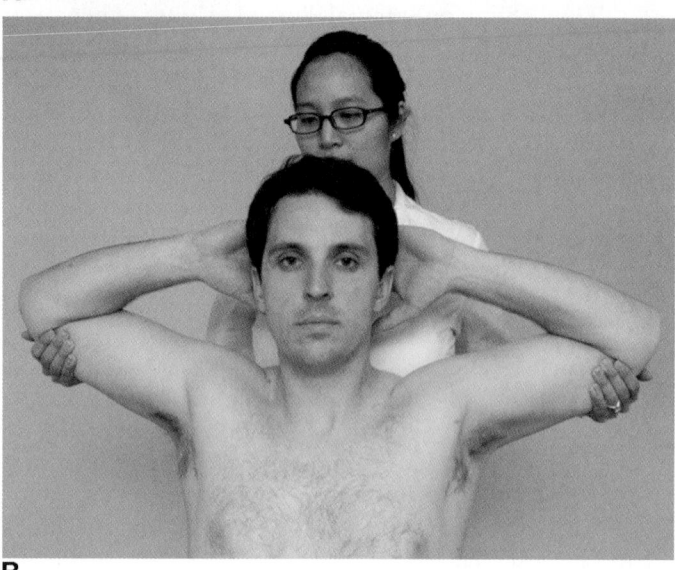

Figure 3-37

Brachial plexus tension test. **A,** The patient abducts and then laterally rotates the arms until symptoms are felt; the patient then lowers the arms until symptoms disappear and the examiner holds the patient's arms in the position. **B,** While the shoulders are held in position, the patient flexes the elbows and places the hands behind the head. A positive test is indicated by return of symptoms.

Lhermitte's Sign. This is a test for the spinal cord itself and a possible upper motor neuron lesion. The patient is in the long leg sitting position on the examining table. The examiner passively flexes the patient's head and one hip simultaneously, with the leg kept straight (Figure 3-43). A positive test occurs if there is a sharp, electric shock-like pain down the spine and into the upper or lower limbs; it indicates dural or meningeal irritation in the spine or possible cervical myelopathy.[48] Coughing or sneezing may produce similar results. The test is similar to a combination of the Brudzinski test and the SLR test (see Chapter 9). If the patient actively flexes the head to the chest while in the supine lying position, the test is called the **Soto-Hall test**. If the hips are flexed to 135°, greater traction is placed on the spinal cord.[47]

Tests for Vascular Signs (Vascular "Clearing" Tests)

Vertebral and internal carotid artery testing is an important component of the cervical spine assessment in cases where end range mobilization and manipulation treatment techniques are contemplated, especially if the techniques involve a rotary component (greater than 45°) and the upper cervical spine (C0-C3).[80–82] The vertebral artery is especially vulnerable to injury as it transitions from its protective area in the foramen transversarium within the cervical spine transverse processes, then looping before it enters the cranial vault behind the first vertebra. Vertebrobasilar insufficiency leads to ischemic symptoms from the pons, medulla, and cerebellum (see Figure 3-1).[83] Grant,[80] Rivett et al,[84] Magarey et al,[83] and Thiel and Rix[85] have reported that the vertebral artery

Figure 3-38
Bikele's sign. A, The arm is abducted to 90° with the elbow fully flexed. **B,** The arm and then the elbow are extended.

tests have not been conclusively proven to be effective in indicating stretching and occlusion of the vertebral artery but do say that the tests should be performed to decrease the risk of potentially catastrophic complications when doing end range mobilization or manipulation, especially of the upper cervical spine. Table 3-16 outlines vertebral and internal carotid artery signs and symptoms associated with pathology. Although the following text discusses many vertebral artery tests, not all of them have to be performed. However, it is imperative that the patient be tested in the position in which the treatment will be given and held in that position for

at least 10 to 30 seconds, especially if the technique is an end range technique or involves the upper cervical spine.[6,86–88] Any of the signs and symptoms that indicate vertebral-basilar artery problems would indicate the treatment should not be given. When doing more than one test, 10 seconds should elapse between each test to ensure there are no latent symptoms from the previous test. It is recommended that if mobilization or manipulation of the cervical spine is contemplated, the clinician should follow the Australian Physiotherapy Association's Protocol for Pre-manipulative Testing of the Cervical Spine.[89] If, when performing the vertebral

Figure 3-39
Shoulder depression test.

Figure 3-41
Tinel's sign for brachial plexus lesions. Dots indicate percussion points.

Figure 3-40
Shoulder abduction (Bakody's) test.

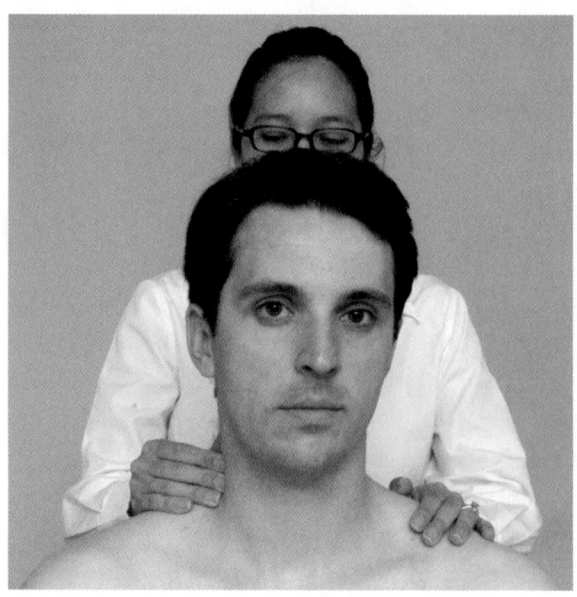

Figure 3-42
Maneuver to compress and squeeze the brachial plexus.

artery tests, or if in the history, the patient complains of signs and symptoms that may be related to the vertebral artery, care should be taken when mobilizing the upper cervical spine.[81,90,91]

These tests are often more effective if performed with the patient sitting because the blood must flow against gravity and there is a restriction caused by the passive movement. However, the supine position allows greater passive range of movement.[92] Movements to the right tend to have more effect on the left vertebral artery, and movements to the left tend to have more effect on the right artery.

Figure 3-43
Lhermitte's sign. **A,** Patient in long sitting. **B,** Examiner flexes patient's head and hip simultaneously.

Signs and Symptoms That May Indicate Possible Vertebral-Basilar Artery Problems[80,83]

- Dizziness/Vertigo
- Dysphagia (difficulty swallowing)
- Drop attacks
- Malaise and nausea
- Vomiting
- Unsteadiness in walking, incoordination
- Visual disturbances
- Severe headaches
- Weakness in extremities
- Sensory changes in face or body
- Dysarthria (difficulty with speech)
- Unconsciousness, disorientation, lightheadedness
- Hearing difficulties
- Facial paralysis

NOTE: Similar symptoms may be seen with other conditions (e.g., benign paroxysmal positional vertigo, head injury, epilepsy, ear disease.)[13]

Vertebral Artery (Cervical Quadrant) Test. With the patient supine, the examiner passively takes the patient's head and neck into extension and side flexion (Figure 3-44).[93] After this movement is achieved, the examiner rotates the patient's neck to the same side and holds it for approximately 30 seconds. A positive test provokes referring symptoms if the opposite artery is affected. This test must be done with care. If dizziness or nystagmus occurs, it is an indication that the vertebral arteries are being compressed. The **DeKleyn-Nieuwenhuyse test**[94] performs a similar function but involves extension and rotation instead of extension and side flexion. Both tests may also be used to assess nerve root compression in the lower cervical spine. To test the upper cervical spine, the examiner "pokes" the patient's chin and follows with extension, side flexion, and rotation.

Static Vertebral Artery Tests. The examiner may test the following passive movements with the patient supine or sitting, as advocated by Grant,[95] watching for eye nystagmus and complaints by the patient of dizziness, lightheadedness, or visual disturbances. Each of these tests is increasingly provocative; if symptoms occur with the first test, there is no need to progress to the next test.

In the sitting position:
1. Sustained full neck and head extension
2. Sustained full neck and head rotation, right and left (if this movement causes symptoms, it is sometimes called a positive **Barre-Lieou sign**)[48]
3. Sustained full neck and head rotation with extension right and left (**DeKleyn's test**)[48]
4. Provocative movement position*
5. Quick head movement into provocative position*

Table 3-16

Vascular Pathology Signs and Symptoms Related to the Vertebral and Internal Carotid Arteries

Factors to Consider when Assessing Cervical Vascular Problems	Vascular Risk Factors
Risk factors Position testing (especially rotation and extension) Cranial nerve examination Eye examination Cognitive function Blood pressure examination "Headache like no other"	Hypertension Hypercholesterolemia (high cholesterol) Hyperlipidemia (high fat) Hyperhomocysteinemia (hardening of the arteries) Diabetes mellitus General clotting disorders Infection Smoking Direct vessel trauma Iatrogenic causes (surgery, medical interventions)
Vertebral Artery Non-Ischemic (Local) Signs and Symptoms	**Internal Carotid Non-Ischemic (Local) Signs and Symptoms**
Ipsilateral posterior neck pain Occipital headache C5-C6 cervical root impairment (rare)	Head/neck pain Homer's syndrome: a rare condition caused by injury to the sympathetic nerves of the face it involves a collection of symptoms including sinking of the eyeball into the face (enophthalmia), small (constricted) pupils (miosis), ptosis (drooping eyelid), anhidrosis (facial dryness) Pulsatile tinnitus Cranial nerve palsies (most commonly CN IX to XII) Ipsilateral carotid bruit (less common) Scalp tenderness (less common) Neck swelling (less common) CN VI palsy (less common) Orbital pain (less common)
Vertebral Artery Ischemic Signs and Symptoms	**Internal Carotid Artery Ischemic Signs and Symptoms**
"Headache like no other" Ipsilateral posterior upper cervical pain Occipital headache Hindbrain transient ischemic attack: dizziness, diplopia, dysarthria, dysphagia, drop attacks, nausea, nystagmus, facial numbness, ataxia, vomiting, hoarseness, loss of short-term memory, weakness, hypotonia/limb weakness (arm or leg), anhidrosis (lack of facial sweating), hearing disturbances, malaise, perioral dysthesia, photophobia, papillary changes, clumsiness, and agitation Hindbrain stroke: Wallenberg's syndrome (a neurological condition caused by a stroke in the vertebral or posterior inferior cerebral artery of the brainstem); symptoms include difficulty swallowing, hoarseness, dizziness, nausea and vomiting, rapid involuntary movements of the eyes (nystagmus), and problems with balance and gait coordination	Ipsilateral frontal temporal headache (clusterlike, thunderclap, migraine without aura, or simply "different from previous headaches") Upper/middle and anterolateral cervical pain, facial pain and sensitivity (carotidynia) Transient ischemic attack (TIA) Ischemic stroke Retinal infarction Amaurosis fugax (transient episodic blindness caused by decreased blood flow to the retina)

Data from Kerry R, Taylor AJ: Cervical artery dysfunction assessment and manual therapy, *Man Ther* 11:243–253, 2006.

6. Quick repeated head movement into provocative position*
7. Head still, sustained trunk movement left and right (10–30 seconds)
8. Head still, repeated trunk movement left and right

*Provocative position implies movement into the position that provokes symptoms.

In supine position:

1. Sustained full neck and head extension
2. Sustained full neck and head rotation left and right
3. Sustained full neck and head rotation with extension eft and right (if combined with side flexion, it is called the **Hallpike maneuver**[48]). Extension combined with rotation has been found to be the position most likely to occlude the vertebral artery.[80]

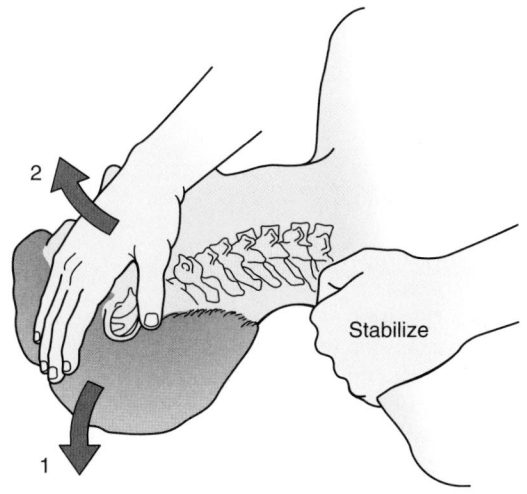

Figure 3-44
Vertebral artery (cervical quadrant) test. Examiner passively moves patient's head and neck into extension and side flexion (1), then rotation (2), holding for 30 seconds.

Table 3-17

Relationship of Head Position to Blood Flow to Head and Neurological Function

Head Position	Blood Flow	Neurological Space
Neutral	Normal	Normal
Flexion	Normal	Normal
Extension	Usually normal	Decreased
Side flexion	Slight decrease in ipsilateral artery	Decrease on ipsilateral side
	Normal in contralateral artery	Increase on contralateral side
Rotation	Slight decrease in ipsilateral artery	Decrease on ipsilateral side
	Significant decrease in contralateral artery	Increase on contralateral side
Extension and rotation	Bilateral decrease, greater in contralateral artery	Bilateral decrease, greater on ipsilateral side
Flexion and rotation	Bilateral decrease	Decrease on ipsilateral side
		Increase on contralateral side

4. Unilateral posteroanterior oscillation (Maitland's grade IV) of C1-C2 facet joints (prone lying) with head rotated left and right
5. Simulated mobilization and manipulation position

Each position should be held for at least 10 to 30 seconds unless symptoms are evoked. Extension in isolation is more likely to test the patency of the intervertebral foramen, whereas rotation and side flexion or, especially, rotation and extension are more likely to test the vertebral artery (Table 3-17).[10] If symptoms are evoked, care should be taken concerning any treatment to follow.

Aspinall[96] advocated the use of a progressive series of clinical tests to evaluate the vertebral artery. With these tests, the examiner progressively moves from the lower cervical spine and lower vertebral artery to the upper cervical spine and upper vertebral artery where it is more vulnerable to pathology. Table 3-18 demonstrates Aspinall's progressive clinical tests for the vertebral arteries.

Hautant's Test.[48,97] This test has two parts and is used to differentiate dizziness or vertigo caused by articular problems from that caused by vascular problems. The patient sits and forward flexes both arms to 90° (Figure 3-45). The eyes are then closed. The examiner watches for any loss of arm position. If the arms move, the cause is nonvascular. The patient is then asked to rotate, or extend and rotate, the neck; this position is held while the eyes are again closed. If wavering of the arms occurs, the dysfunction is caused by vascular impairment to the brain. Each position should be held for 10 to 30 seconds.

Barre's Test.[94] The patient stands with the shoulders forward flexed to 90°, elbows straight and forearms supinated, palms up and eyes closed, holding the position for 10 to 20 seconds. The test is considered positive if one arm slowly falls with simultaneous forearm pronation. The cause is thought to be diminished blood flow to the brain stem. This test is identical to the first part of Hautant's test.

Underburg's Test.[48] The patient stands with the shoulders forward flexed to 90°, elbows straight and forearms supinated. The patient then closes the eyes and marches in place while holding the extended and rotated head to one side. The test is repeated with head movement to the opposite side. The test is considered positive if there is dropping of the arms, loss of balance, or pronation of the hands; a positive result indicates decreased blood supply to the brain.

Naffziger's Test.[48,98] The patient is seated and the examiner stands behind the patient with his or her fingers over the patient's jugular veins (Figure 3-46). The examiner compresses the veins for 30 seconds (Naffziger recommended 10 minutes!) and then asks the patient to cough. Pain may indicate a nerve root problem or space-occupying lesion (e.g., tumor). If lightheadedness or similar symptoms occur with compression of the jugular veins, the test should be terminated.

Tests for Vertigo and Dizziness

Temperature (Caloric) Test. The examiner alternately applies hot and cold test tubes several times just behind the patient's ears on the side of the head; each side is done in turn. A positive test is associated with the inducement of vertigo, which indicates inner ear problems.

Dizziness Test. The patient sits and the examiner grasps the patient's head. The examiner actively rotates the

Table 3-18

Aspinall's Progressive Clinical Tests for Vertebral Artery Pathology

Vertebral Artery Area	Position		Test
	Sitting	**Lying**	
Area 1 (lower cervical spine)	X		Active cervical rotation
Area 2 (middle cervical spine)	X		Active cervical rotation
	X	X	Passive cervical rotation
	X		Active cervical extension
	X	X	Passive cervical extension
	X	X	Passive cervical extension with rotation
	X		Passive segmental extension with rotation
	X	X	Passive cervical flexion
	X	X	Cervical flexion with traction
		X	Accessory oscillatory anterior/posterior movement—transverse processes C2-C7 in combined extension and rotation
		X	Sustained manipulation position
Area 3 (upper cervical spine)	X		Active cervical rotation
	X	X	Passive cervical rotation
	X		Active cervical extension
	X	X	Passive cervical extension
	X	X	Passive cervical rotation with extension
	X	X	Cervical rotation with extension and traction
	X		Cervical rotation with flexion
		X	Accessory oscillatory anterior/posterior movement—transverse processes C1-C2 in combined rotation and extension
		X	Sustained manipulation position

From Aspinall W: Clinical testing for the craniovertebral hypermobility syndrome, *J Orthop Sports Phys Ther* 12:180–181, 1989.

A   **B**

Figure 3-45

Positioning for Hautant's test. **A,** Forward flexion of both arms to 90°. **B,** Rotation and extension of neck with arms forward flexed to 90°.

Figure 3-46
Naffziger's test (compression of jugular veins).

Tests for Cervical Instability (Instability "Clearing" Tests)

Instability in the cervical spine is most commonly the result of ligament damage (e.g., transverse ligament, alar ligaments), bone or joint damage (e.g., fracture or dislocation) or weak muscles (e.g., deep flexors or extensors). The instability may be the result of chronic arthritic conditions (e.g., rheumatoid arthritis), trauma, long-term corticosteroid use, congenital malformations, Down syndrome, and osteoporosis.[13] One commonly should have a high level of suspicion of instability if in the history, the patient complains of instability, a lump in the throat, lip paresthesia, severe headache (especially with movement), muscle spasm, nausea, or vomiting.[13]

Sharp-Purser Test. This test should be performed *with extreme caution*. It is a test to determine subluxation of the atlas on the axis (Figure 3-47). If the transverse ligament that maintains the position of the odontoid process relative to C1 (Figure 3-48) is torn, C1 will translate forward (sublux) on C2 on flexion. Thus, the examiner may find the patient reticent to do forward flexion if the

patient's head as far as possible to the right and then to the left, holding the head at the extreme of motion for a short time (10–30 seconds) while the shoulders remain stationary. The patient's head is then returned to neutral. Next, the patient's shoulders are actively rotated as far to the right as possible, held for 10 to 30 seconds, and then to the left as far as possible, and held for 10 to 30 seconds while keeping the head facing straight ahead. If the patient experiences dizziness in both cases, the problem lies in the vertebral arteries, because in both cases the vertebral artery may be "kinked," decreasing the blood flow. If the patient experiences dizziness only when the head is rotated, the problem lies within the semicircular canals of the inner ear.

Fitz-Ritson[99] advocates a modification of this test. For the first part of the test, he advocates that the examiner hold the shoulders still while the patient rapidly rotates the head left and right with eyes closed. If vertigo results, the problem is in the vestibular nuclei or muscles and joints of the cervical spine. In addition, patients may lose their balance, veer to one side, or possibly vomit. The second stage is the same as previously mentioned, except that the eyes are closed. If vertigo is experienced this time, Fitz-Ritson believes that the problem is in the cervical spine because the vestibular apparatus is not being moved.

Signs and Symptoms of Cervical Instability

- Severe muscle spasm
- Patient does not want to move head (especially into flexion)
- Lump in throat
- Lip or facial paresthesia
- Severe headache
- Dizziness
- Nausea
- Vomiting
- Soft end feel
- Nystagmus
- Pupil changes

Cervical Spine Instability Clearing Tests*

- Sharp-Purser test
- Transverse ligament stress test
- Pettman's distraction test
- Anterior shear test
- Lateral shear test
- Lateral flexion alar ligament stress test
- Rotational alar ligament stress test

*These tests should be performed if the examiner anticipates doing mobilization (especially end range techniques) or manipulation techniques to the cervical spine, especially the upper cervical spine. If instability is present, mobilization and/or manipulation should **NOT** be performed.

Figure 3-47
Subluxation of the atlas on neck flexion. Note the bulge in the posterior neck caused by the forward subluxation of the atlas, bringing the spinous process of the axis into prominence beneath the skin *(arrow)*. (Courtesy Harold S. Robinson, M.D., Vancouver, British Columbia.)

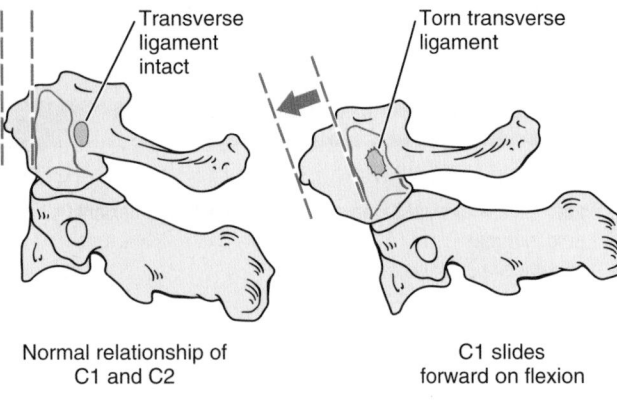

Figure 3-48
Forward translation of C1 on C2 on flexion as a result of torn transverse ligament.

Figure 3-49
The Sharp-Purser test for subluxation of the atlas on the axis.

aspect of the atlas (Figure 3-50). Normally, no movement or symptoms are perceived by the patient. For the test to be positive, the patient should feel a lump in the throat as the atlas moves toward the esophagus; this is indicative of hypermobility at the atlantoaxial articulation.

Transverse Ligament Stress Test.[97,101] The patient lies supine with the examiner supporting the occiput with the palms and the third, fourth, and fifth fingers. The examiner places the index fingers in the space between

transverse ligament has been damaged. The examiner places one hand over the patient's forehead while the thumb of the other hand is placed over the spinous process of the axis to stabilize it (Figure 3-49). The patient is asked to slowly flex the head; while this is occurring, the examiner presses backward with the palm. A positive test is indicated if the examiner feels the head slide backward during the movement. The slide backward indicates that the subluxation of the atlas has been reduced, and the slide may be accompanied by a "clunk."

Aspinall[100] advocates use of an additional test if the Sharp-Purser test is negative. The patient is placed in supine. The examiner stabilizes the occiput on the atlas in flexion and holds the occiput in this flexed position. The examiner then applies an anteriorly directed force to the posterior

Figure 3-50
Aspinall's transverse ligament test.

the patient's occiput and C2 spinous process so that the fingertips are overlying the neural arch of C1. The head and C1 are then carefully lifted anteriorly together, allowing no flexion or extension (Figure 3-51). This anterior shear is normally resisted by the transverse ligament (Figure 3-52). The position is held for 10 to 20 seconds to see whether symptoms occur, indicating a positive test. Positive symptoms include soft end feel; muscle spasm; dizziness; nausea; paresthesia of the lip, face, or limb; nystagmus; or a lump sensation in the throat. The test indicates hypermobility at the atlantoaxial articulation.

Pettman's Distraction Test.[101] This test is used to test the tectorial membrane. The patient lies supine with the head in neutral. The examiner applies gentle traction to the head. Provided no symptoms are produced, the patient's head is lifted forward, flexing the spine, and traction is reapplied. If the patient complains of symptoms such as pain, or paresthesia in the second position, then the test is considered positive for a lax tectorial membrane (Figure 3-53).

Anterior Shear or Sagittal Stress Test.[50,101] This test is designed to test the integrity of the supporting ligamentous and capsular tissues of the cervical spine. It is similar to the PACVP testing in the joint play section. The patient lies supine with the head in neutral resting on the bed. The examiner applies an anteriorly directed force through the posterior arch of C1 or the spinous processes of C2 to T1 or bilaterally through the lamina of each vertebral body. In each case, the normal end feel is tissue stretch with an abrupt stop (Figure 3-54). Positive signs, especially when the upper cervical spine is tested,

Figure 3-51

Testing the transverse ligament of C1. Examiner's hands support head and C1.

include nystagmus, pupil changes, dizziness, soft end feel, nausea, facial or lip paresthesia, and a lump sensation in the throat.[50]

Lateral (Transverse) Shear Test.[97,101] This test is used to determine instability of the atlantoaxial articulation caused by odontoid dysplasia. The patient lies supine with the head supported. The examiner places the radial side of the second metacarpophalangeal (MCP) joint of one hand against the transverse process of the atlas and the MCP joint of the other hand against the opposite transverse process of the axis. The examiner's hands are then carefully pushed together, causing a shear of one bone on the other (Figure 3-55). Normally, minimal motion and no symptoms (cord or vascular) are produced. Because

Figure 3-52

Relationship of C1 to C2 and the position of the transverse ligament.

Figure 3-53

Pettman's distraction test. **A,** First position. **B,** Second (flexed) position.

Figure 3-54

Anterior sagittal stress test.

Lateral Flexion Alar Ligament Stress Test.[70,97,101] The patient lies supine with the head in the physiological neutral position while the examiner stabilizes the axis with a wide pinch grip around the spinous process and lamina (Figure 3-56). The examiner then attempts to side flex the head and axis. Normally, if the ligament is intact, minimal side flexion occurs, with a strong capsular end feel and a solid stop.

Rotational Alar Ligament Stress Test.[101] The patient is positioned in sitting. The examiner grips the lamina and spinous process of C2 between the finger and thumb. While stabilizing C2, the examiner passively rotates the patient's head left or right moving to the "no symptom" side first. If more than 20° to 30° rotation is possible without C2 moving, it is indicative of injury to the contralateral alar ligament especially if the lateral flexion alar stress test is positive in the same direction. If the excessive motion is in the opposite direction for both tests, the instability is due to an increase in the neutral zone in the joint (Figure 3-57).

this test is normally painful because of the compression of soft tissues against the bone, the patient should be warned beforehand that pain is a normal sensation to be expected. The test can also be used to test other levels of the cervical spine (i.e., C2–C7).

Transverse process

Figure 3-55

A, Atlantoaxial lateral shear test. **B,** Metacarpophalangeal joints against transverse processes.

Figure 3-56

Lateral flexion alar ligament stress test. Examiner attempts to side flex the patient's head while stabilizing the axis.

Tests for Cervical Muscle Strength

Craniocervical Flexion Test.[102–104] The patient lies supine in crook lying so the forehead and chin are parallel to the bed (horizontal), placing the craniocervical and cervical spine in mid position. The head is supported on a folded towel and an inflatable pressure sensor is positioned behind the neck and below the occiput (Figure 3-58). The inflatable bladder is inflated just enough to fill the space between the bed and the neck with no pressure felt on the neck. The patient is then asked to slowly nod the chin toward the sternum and to maintain end range for 10 seconds. This movement should increase the pressure reading by 10 mmHg. To test endurance, the test may be repeated 10 times. Inability to do the test or to increase the pressure indicates weakness of the deep cervical flexors.

Tests for First Rib Mobility

Although the first rib would normally be included with assessment of the thoracic spine, the examiner should always test for mobility of the first rib when examining the cervical spine, especially if side flexion is limited and there is pain or tenderness in the area of the first rib or T1.

For the first test, the patient lies supine while fully supported. The examiner palpates the first rib bilaterally lateral to T1 and places his or her fingers along the path of the patient's ribs just posterior to the clavicles (Figure 3-59). While palpating the ribs, the examiner notes the movement of both first ribs as the patient takes a deep breath in and out, and any asymmetry is noted. The examiner then palpates one first rib and side flexes the head to the opposite side until the rib is felt to move up. The range of neck side flexion is noted. The side flexion is then repeated to the opposite side, and results from

Figure 3-57

Rotational alar ligament stress test. While the examiner grips the lamina of C2, the patient's head is rotated left and right with the other hand.

Figure 3-58

Craniocervical flexion test.

Figure 3-59

Testing mobility of the first rib (anterior aspect).

the two sides are compared. Asymmetry may be caused by hypomobility of the first rib or tightness of the scalene muscles on the same side.

For the second test, the patient lies prone, and the examiner again palpates the first rib (Figure 3-60). Using the thumb, reinforced by the other thumb, the examiner pushes the rib caudally, noting the amount of movement, end feel, and presence of pain. The other first rib is tested in a similar fashion, and the two sides are compared. Normally, a firm tissue stretch is felt with no pain, except possibly where the examiner's thumbs are compressing soft tissue against the rib.

Tests for Thoracic Outlet Syndrome

See Special Tests in Chapter 5.

Figure 3-60

Testing mobility of the first rib (posterior aspect).

Reflexes and Cutaneous Distribution

If the examiner suspects neurological involvement during the assessment, reflex testing and cutaneous sensation should be tested. For the cervical spine, the following reflexes should be checked for differences between the two sides, as shown in Figure 3-61: biceps (C5-C6), the brachioradialis (C5-C6), the triceps (C7-C8), and the jaw jerk (cranial nerve V). Bland[30] felt the jaw jerk was a useful diagnostic test. A normal (negative) jaw jerk combined with positive (exaggerated) tendon reflexes in the upper limb suggested the lesion was below the foramen magnum. If both reflexes were abnormal, then the lesion is above the pons.

Common Reflexes Checked in Cervical Spine Assessment

- Biceps (C5, C6)
- Triceps (C7, C8)
- Hoffmann's sign (if upper motor neuron lesion suspected)

The reflexes are tested with a reflex hammer. The examiner tests the biceps and jaw jerk reflexes by placing his or her thumb over the patient's biceps tendon or at midpoint of the chin and then tapping the thumbnail with the reflex hammer to elicit the reflex. The jaw reflex may also be tested with a tongue depressor (see Figure 3-61, *B*). The examiner holds the tongue depressor firmly against the lower teeth while the patient relaxes the jaw and then strikes the tongue depressor with the reflex hammer. The brachioradialis and triceps reflexes are tested by directly tapping the tendon or muscle.

If an upper motor neuron lesion is suspected, the pathological reflexes (e.g., **Babinski's reflex**) should be checked (see Table 1-30). **Hoffmann's sign** is the upper limb equivalent of the Babinski test. To test for Hoffmann's sign, the examiner holds the patient's middle finger and briskly flicks the distal phalanx. A positive sign is noted if the interphalangeal joint of the thumb of the same hand flexes. Denno and Meadows[105] advocated a dynamic Hoffmann's sign. The patient is asked to repeatedly flex and extend the head, and then the test is performed as described previously. Denno and Meadows believed that the dynamic test shows positive results earlier than the static or normal Hoffmann's sign. Because an upper motor neuron lesion affects both the upper and lower limb, initially unilaterally and at later stages bilaterally, Babinski's test may be performed if desired. Clonus, most easily seen by sudden dorsiflexion of the ankle resulting in four or five reflex twitches of the plantar flexors, is also a sign of an upper motor neuron lesion.[106]

The examiner then checks the **dermatome pattern** of the various nerve roots as well as the **sensory distribution** of the peripheral nerves (Figures 3-62 and 3-63) using a sensation scan (see previous discussion). Dermatomes vary from person to person and overlap a great deal, and the diagrams shown are estimations only. For example, C5 dermatome may stop distally on the radial side of the arm at the elbow, forearm, or wrist. Cervical radiculopathies may also show modified patterns. Levine et al[41] point out that about 45% of patients have modified patterns and do not follow strict dermatome patterns. Classically, these patients also have referred pain into the trapezius and periscapular area posteriorly, and some will have pain into the breast area anteriorly.

Because of the spinal cord and associated nerve roots and their relation to the other bony and soft tissues in the cervical spine, referred pain is a relatively common experience in lesions of the cervical spine. Within the cervical

Figure 3-61

Testing of upper limb reflexes. **A,** Jaw. **B,** Jaw (tongue depressor method). **C,** Brachioradialis. **D,** Biceps.

Continued

E

Figure 3-61 cont'd
E, Triceps.

spine, the intervertebral discs, facet joints, and other bony and soft tissues may refer pain to other segments of the neck (dermatomes) or to the head, the shoulder, the scapular area, and the whole of the upper limb (Figures 3-64 and 3-65).[39,54] Table 3-19 shows the muscles of the cervical spine and their referral of pain.

Brachial Plexus Injuries of the Cervical Spine[107,108]

Erb-Duchenne Paralysis. This paralysis is an upper brachial plexus injury involving injury to the upper nerve roots (C5, C6) as a result of compression or stretching. The injury frequently occurs at Erb's point. With

Figure 3-62
Sensory nerve distribution of the head, neck, and face. *1,* Ophthalmic nerve. *2,* Maxillary nerve. *3,* Mandibular nerve. *4,* Transverse cutaneous nerve of neck (C2-C3). *5,* Greater auricular nerve (C2-C3). *6,* Lesser auricular nerve (C2). *7,* Greater occipital nerve (C2-C3). *8,* Cervical dorsal rami (C3-C5). *9,* Suprascapular nerve (C5-C6).

this injury, it is primarily the muscles of the shoulder region and elbow that are affected; the muscles of the hand (especially the intrinsic muscles) are not involved. However, sensation over the radial surfaces of the forearm and hand and the deltoid area are affected.

Klumpke (Dejerine-Klumpke) Paralysis. This injury involves the lower brachial plexus and results from compression or stretching of the lower nerve roots (C8, T1). Atrophy and weakness are evident in the muscles of the forearm and hand as well as in the triceps. The obvious changes are in the distal aspects of the upper limb. The resultant injury is a functionless hand. Sensory loss occurs primarily on the ulnar side of the forearm and hand.

Brachial Plexus Birth Palsy.[109] These injuries to the brachial plexus occur in 0.1% to 0.4% of births with the majority showing full recovery within 2 months. Those infants who have not recovered within 3 months are at considerable risk to decreased strength and range of motion in the upper limb.

Burners and Stingers.[110,111] These are transient injuries to the brachial plexus, which may be the result of trauma (see Figure 3-10) combined with factors such as stenosis or a degenerative disc (spondylosis). Recurrent burners are not associated with more severe neck injury, but their effect on the nerve may be cumulative.[110]

Joint Play Movements

The joint play movements that are carried out in the cervical spine may be general movements (called *passive intervertebral movements [PIVMs]*) that involve the entire cervical spine (first four below) or specific movements

Figure 3-63
Dermatomes of the cervical spine.

isolated to one segment. As the joint play movements are performed, the examiner should note any decreased ROM, pain, or difference in end feel.

Side Glide. The examiner holds the patient's head and moves it from side to side, keeping the head parallel to the shoulders (Figure 3-66).[112]

Anterior and Posterior Glide. The examiner holds the patient's head with one hand around the occiput and one hand around the chin, taking care to ensure that the patient is not choked.[63] The examiner then draws

Joint Play Movements of the Cervical Spine

- Side glide of the cervical spine (general)
- Anterior glide of the cervical spine (general)
- Posterior glide of the cervical spine (general)
- Traction glide of the cervical spine (general)
- Rotation of the occiput on C1 (specific)
- Posteroanterior central vertebral pressure (specific)
- Posteroanterior unilateral vertebral pressure (specific)
- Transverse vertebral pressure (specific)

Figure 3-64
Referral of symptoms from the cervical spine to areas of the spine, head, shoulder girdle, and upper limb.

the head forward in the same plane as the shoulders for anterior glide (Figure 3-67) and posteriorly for posterior glide. While doing these movements, the examiner must prevent flexion and extension of the head.

Traction Glide. The examiner places one hand around the patient's chin and the other hand on the occiput.[64] Traction is then applied in a straight longitudinal direction, with the majority of the pull being through the occiput (Figure 3-68).

Vertebral Pressures. For the last three joint play movements (Figure 3-69), the patient lies prone with the forehead resting on the back of the hands.[93] These techniques are specific to each vertebra and are applied to each vertebra in turn, or at least to the ones that the examination has indicated may be affected by pathology. They are sometimes called **passive accessory intervertebral movements (PAIVMs)**.[61] The examiner palpates the spinous processes of the cervical spine, starting at the C2 spinous process and working downward to the T2 spinous process. The positions of the examiner's hands, fingers, and thumbs in performing **posteroanterior central vertebral pressures (PACVPs)** are shown in Figure 3-69, *A*. Pressure is then applied through the examiner's thumbs pushing carefully from the shoulders, and the vertebra is pushed forward. The examiner must take care to apply pressure slowly, with

carefully controlled movements, in order to "feel" the movement, which in reality is minimal. This "springing test" may be repeated several times to determine the quality of the movement and the end feel. End range can be determined by feeling the adjacent spinous process (above or below). When the adjacent spinous process begins to move, the end range of the vertebra to which the PACVP is being applied has been reached.

For **posteroanterior unilateral vertebral pressure (PAUVP)**, the examiner's fingers move laterally away from the tip of the spinous process so that the thumbs rest on the lamina or transverse process, about 2 to 3 cm (1–1.5 inches) lateral to the spinous process of the cervical or thoracic vertebra (see Figure 3-69, *B*). Anterior springing pressure is applied as in the central pressure technique. This pressure causes a minimal rotation of the vertebral body. If one was to palpate the spinous process while doing the technique, the spinous process would be felt to move to the side the pressure is applied. Similarly, end range can be determined by feeling the adjacent spinous process (above or below). When the adjacent spinous process begins to rotate, the end range of the vertebra to which the PAUVP is being applied has been reached. Both sides should be done and compared.

For **transverse vertebral pressure**, the examiner's thumbs are placed along the side of the spinous process of the cervical or thoracic spine (see Figure 3-69, *C*). The examiner then applies a transverse springing pressure to the side of the spinous process, feeling for the quality of movement. This pressure also causes rotation of the vertebral body, and end range can be determined by feeling for rotation of the adjacent spinous process.

Palpation

If, after completing the examination of the cervical spine, the examiner decides the problem is in another joint, palpation should be delayed until that joint is completely examined. However, during palpation of the cervical spine, the examiner should note any tenderness, trigger points, muscle spasm, or other signs and symptoms that may indicate the source of the pathology. Pain provocation and landmark location has been found to have the greatest intrarater reliability with palpation.[113] As with any palpation, the examiner should note the texture of the skin and surrounding bony and soft tissues on the posterior, lateral, and anterior aspects of the neck. Usually, palpation is performed with the patient supine so that maximum relaxation of the neck muscles is possible. However, the examiner may palpate with the patient sitting (patient resting the head on forearms that are resting on something at shoulder height) or lying prone (on a table with a face hole) if it is more comfortable for the patient.

To palpate the posterior structures, the examiner stands at the patient's head behind the patient. With the patient

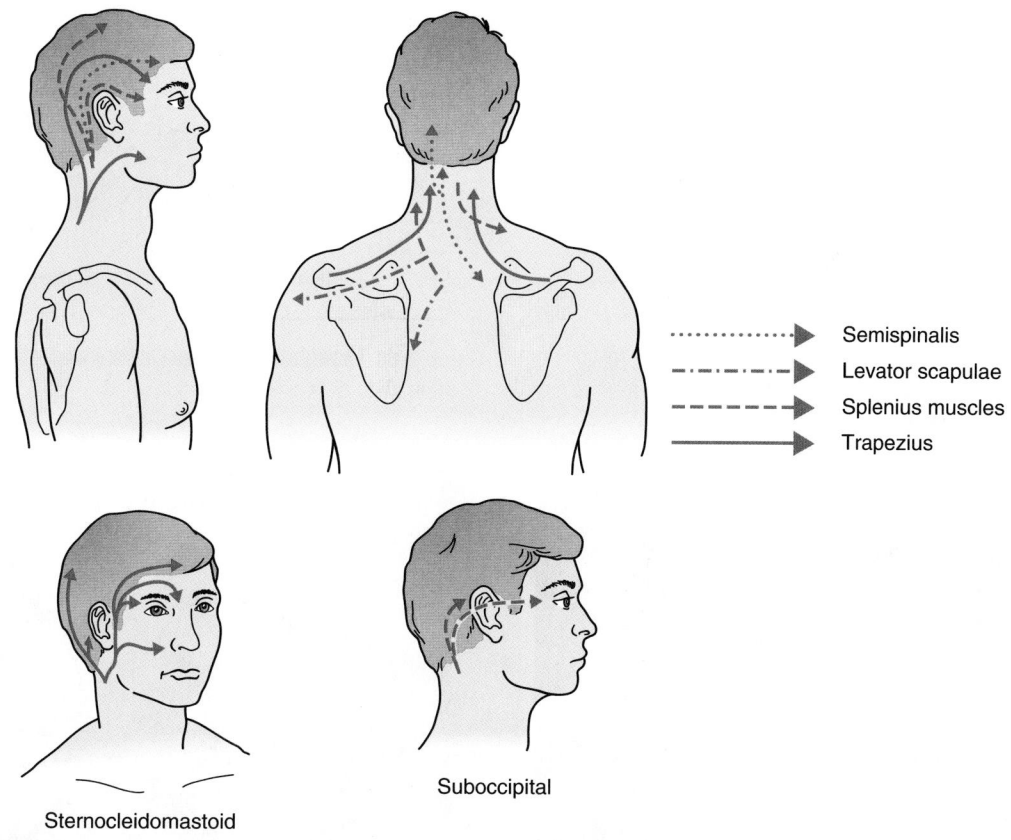

	Semispinalis
	Levator scapulae
	Splenius muscles
	Trapezius

Sternocleidomastoid

Suboccipital

Figure 3-65
Muscles and their referred pain patterns. Diagram shows primarily one side.

Table 3-19

Muscles of the Cervical Spine and Their Referral of Pain

Muscle	Referral Pattern
Trapezius	Right and left occiput, lateral aspect of head above ear to behind eye, tip of jaw Spinous processes to medial border of scapula and along spine of scapula; may also refer to lateral aspect of upper arm
Sternocleidomastoid	Back and top of head, front of ear over forehead to medial aspect of eye; cheek Behind ear, ear to forehead
Splenius capitis	Top of head
Splenius cervicis	Posterior neck and shoulder angle, side of head to eye
Semispinalis cervicis	Back of head
Semispinalis capitis	Band around head at level of forehead
Multifidus	Occiput to posterior neck and shoulder angle to base of spine of scapula
Suboccipital	Lateral aspect of head to eye
Scalenes	Medial border of scapula and anterior chest down posterolateral aspect of arm to anterolateral and posterolateral aspect of hand

Figure 3-66
Side glide of the cervical spine. Glide to the right is illustrated.

Figure 3-67
Anterior glide of the cervical spine.

Figure 3-68
Traction glide of the cervical spine.

A

B

C

Figure 3-69
Vertebral pressures to the cervical spine. **A,** Posteroanterior central vertebral pressure on tip of spinous process. **B,** Posteroanterior unilateral vertebral pressure on posterior aspect of transverse process. **C,** Transverse vertebral pressure on side of spinous process.

lying supine, the patient's head is "cupped" in the examiner's hand while the examiner palpates with the fingers of both hands. For the lateral and anterior structures, the examiner stands at the patient's side. If the examiner suspects that the problem is in the cervical spine, palpation is done on the following structures (Figure 3-70).

Posterior Aspect

External Occipital Protuberance. The protuberance may be found in the posterior midline. The examiner palpates the posterior skull in midline and moves caudally until coming to a point where the fingers "dip" inward. The part of the bone just before the dip is the external occipital protuberance. The inion, or "bump of knowledge," is the most obvious point on the external occipital protuberance and lies in the midline of the occiput.

Spinous Processes and Facet Joints of Cervical Vertebrae. The spinous processes of C2, C6, and C7 are the most obvious. If the examiner palpates the occiput of the skull and descends in the midline, the C2 spinous process will be palpated as the first bump. The next spinous processes that are most obvious are C6 and C7, although C3, C4, and C5 can be differentiated with careful palpation and by flexing the spine. The examiner can differentiate between C6 and C7 by passively flexing and extending the patient's neck. With this movement, the C6 spinous process moves in and out and the C7 spinous process remains stationary. The movements between the spinous processes of C2 through C7 or T1 may be palpated by feeling between each set of spinous processes. While palpating between the spinous processes, the examiner can use the opposite hand or his/her chest to push the head into nodding flexion and releasing, causing the cervical spine to flex and extend; the palpating finger will feel the movement between the two spinous processes and tension (when flexing)

in the interspinous and supraspinous ligaments. Relative movement between the cervical vertebrae can then be determined (i.e., hypomobility, normal movement, or hypermobility).[63] The facet joint may be palpated 1.3 to 2.5 cm (0.5–1 inch) lateral to the spinous process. Usually the facet joints are not felt as distinct structures but rather as a hard bony mass under the fingers. The muscles in the adjacent area may be palpated for tenderness, swelling, and other signs of pathology. Careful palpation should also include the suboccipital structures.

Mastoid Processes (Below and Behind Ear Lobe). If the examiner palpates the skull following the posterior aspect of the ear, there will be a point on the skull at which the finger again dips inward. The point just before the dip is the mastoid process.

Lateral Aspect

Transverse Processes of Cervical Vertebrae. The C1 transverse process is the easiest to palpate. The examiner first palpates the mastoid process and then moves inferiorly and slightly anteriorly until a hard bump is felt. If the examiner applies slight pressure to the bump, the patient should say it feels uncomfortable. These bumps are the transverse processes of C1. If the examiner rotates the patient's head while palpating the transverse processes of C1, the uppermost transverse process will protrude farther and the lower one will seem to disappear. If this does not occur, the segment is hypomobile. The other transverse processes may be palpated if the musculature is sufficiently relaxed. After the C1 transverse process has been located, the examiner moves caudally, feeling for similar bumps. Normally, the bumps are not directly inferior but rather follow the lordotic path of the cervical vertebrae under the sternocleidomastoid muscle. These structures are situated more anteriorly than one might suspect (see Figure 3-70). During flexion, the space between the mastoid and the transverse processes increases. On extension, it decreases. On side flexion, the mastoid and transverse processes approach one another on the side to which the head is side flexed and separate on the other side.[63]

Lymph Nodes and Carotid Arteries. The lymph nodes are palpable only if they are swollen. The nodes lie along the line of the sternocleidomastoid muscle. The carotid pulse may be palpated in the midportion of the neck, between the sternocleidomastoid muscle and the trachea. The examiner should determine whether the pulse is normal and equal on both sides.

Temporomandibular Joints, Mandible, and Parotid Glands. The temporomandibular joints may be palpated anterior to the external ear. The examiner may either palpate directly over the joint or place the little or index finger (pulp forward) in the external ear to feel for movement in the joint. The examiner can then move the fingers along the length of the mandible, feeling for any abnormalities. The angle of the mandible is at the level of the

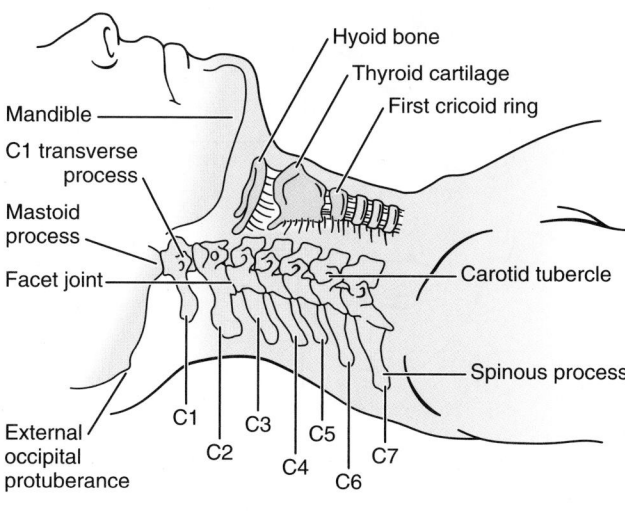

Figure 3-70
Palpation landmarks of the cervical spine.

C2 vertebra. Normally, the parotid gland is not palpable because it lies over the angle of the mandible. If it is swollen, however, it is palpable as a soft, boggy structure.

Anterior Aspect

Hyoid Bone, Thyroid CartilagLe, and First Cricoid Ring. The hyoid bone may be palpated as part of the superior part of the trachea above the thyroid cartilage anterior to the C2-C3 vertebrae. The thyroid cartilage lies anterior to the C4-C5 vertebrae. With the neck in a neutral position, the thyroid cartilage can be moved easily. In extension, it is tight and crepitations may be felt. Adjacent to the cartilage is the thyroid gland, which the examiner should palpate. If the gland is abnormal, it will be tender and enlarged. The cricoid ring is the first part of the trachea and lies above the site for an emergency tracheostomy. The ring moves when the patient swallows. Rough palpation of the ring may cause the patient to gag. While palpating the hyoid bone, the examiner should ask the patient to swallow; normally, the bone should move and cause no pain. The cricoid ring and thyroid cartilage also move when palpated as the patient swallows.

Paranasal Sinuses. Returning to the face, the examiner should palpate the paranasal sinuses (frontal and maxillary) for signs of tenderness and swelling (Figure 3-71).

First Three Ribs. The examiner palpates the manubrium sternum and, moving the fingers laterally, follows the path of the first three ribs posteriorly, feeling whether one rib is protruded more than the others. The examiner should palpate the ribs individually and with care, because it is difficult to palpate the ribs as they pass under the clavicle. The patient should be asked to breathe in and out deeply a few times so that the examiner can compare the movements of the ribs during breathing. Normally, there is equal mobility on both sides. The first rib is more prone to pathology than the second and third ribs and can refer pain to the neck and/or shoulder.

Supraclavicular Fossa. The examiner can palpate the supraclavicular fossa, which is superior to the clavicle. Normally, the fossa is a smooth indentation. The examiner should palpate for swelling after trauma (possible fractured clavicle), abnormal soft tissue (possible swollen glands), and abnormal bony tissue (possible cervical rib). In addition, the examiner should palpate the sternocleidomastoid muscle along its length for signs of pathology, especially in cases of torticollis.

Diagnostic Imaging

Imaging techniques should primarily be performed as an adjunct to the clinical examination. The appearance of many degenerative changes or anatomical or congenital variations is relatively high in the cervical spine, and many of the changes have no relationship with the patient's complaints.[114]

Figure 3-71

Paranasal sinuses. Radiograph (**A**) and illustration (**B**) of frontal and maxillary sinuses.

Plain Film Radiography

Normally, a standard set of x-rays for the cervical spine is made up of an anteroposterior view, a lateral view, and an open or odontoid ("through-the-mouth") view. Other views are included if other pathologies are suspected. In cases of trauma and an alert and stable patient, the Canadian C-Spine Rule[115] may be used to determine if diagnostic imaging is required (Figure 3-72).

Anteroposterior View. The examiner should look for or note the following (Figures 3-73 and 3-74): the shape of the vertebrae, the presence of any lateral wedging or osteophytes, the disc space, and the presence of a cervical rib. Frontal alignment should also be ascertained.

For Alert (Glasgow Coma Scale Score = 15) and Stable Trauma Patients Where Cervical Spine (C-Spine) Injury is a Concern

1. Any High-Risk Factor That Mandates Radiography?

Age ≥65 Years
or
Dangerous Mechanism*
or
Paresthesias in Extremities

↓ No

2. Any Low-Risk Factor That Allows Safe Assessment of Range of Motion?

Simple Rear-end MVC†
or
Sitting Position in ED
or
Ambulatory at Any Time
or
Delayed Onset of Neck Pain‡
or
Absence of Midline C-Spine Tenderness

↓ Yes

3. Able to Actively Rotate Neck? 45° Left and Right

Yes → Radiography
No → Radiography
Unable → Radiography

Able → No Radiography

*Dangerous Mechanism:
• Fall from ≥1 Meter/5 Stairs
• Axial Load to Head, eg, Diving
• MVC High Speed (>100 km/hr), Rollover, Ejection
• Motorized Recreational Vehicles
• Bicycle Collision

† Simple Rear-end MVC Excludes:
• Pushed into Oncoming Traffic
• Hit by Bus/Large Truck
• Rollover
• Hit by High-Speed Vehicle

‡ Delayed:
• Not immediate Onset of Neck Pain

MVC indicates motor vehicle collision; ED, emergency department.

Figure 3-72

The Canadian C-Spine Rule. (From Stiell IG et al: The Canadian C-spine rule for radiography in alert and stable trauma patients, *JAMA* 286[15]:1846, 2001.)

Lateral View. Lateral views of the cervical spine give the greatest amount of radiological information. The examiner should look for or note the following (Figures 3-75 to 3-78).

1. Normal or abnormal curvature. The curvature may be highly variable, because 20% to 40% of normal spines have a straight or slightly kyphotic curve in neutral.[116] McAviney et al[117] reported the normal lordosis in the cervical spine as 30° to 40° (see Figure 3-7) when measuring the lines intersecting the posterior aspects of the vertebral bodies of C2 and C7. They felt patients with a lordosis of less than 20° were more likely to experience cervicogenic symptoms. Are the "lines" of the vertebrae normal? The line joining the anterior portion of the vertebral bodies (anterior vertebral line) should form a smooth, unbroken arc from C2 to C7 (see Figure 3-76). Similar lines should be seen for the posterior vertebral bodies (posterior vertebral line), which form the anterior aspect of the spinal canal, and the posterior aspect of the spinal canal (posterior canal line). Disruption of any of these lines would be an indication of instability possibly caused by ligamentous injury.

2. "Kinking" of the cervical spine. Kinking may be indicative of a subluxation or dislocation in the cervical spine.

3. General shape of the vertebrae. Is there any fusion, collapse, or wedging? The examiner should count the vertebrae, because x-ray films do not always show C7 or T1, and it is essential that they be visualized for a proper radiological examination.

4. Displacement. Do the vertebrae sit in normal alignment with one another (Figures 3-79 and 3-80)?

5. Disc space. Is it normal? Narrow? Narrowing may indicate cervical spondylosis.

6. Lipping at the vertebral edges (see Figures 3-75, *A* and 3-76). Lipping indicates degeneration.

7. Osteophytes (see Figures 3-75, *A* and 3-76). Osteophytes indicate degeneration or abnormal movement (instability).

8. Normally, the ratio of the spinal canal diameter to the vertebral body diameter (Torg ratio) in the cervical spine is 1. If this ratio is less than 0.8, it is an indication of possible cervical stenosis.[44,118–121] This comparison is shown in Figure 3-77 (ratio AB:BC). Cantu[119] points out that this measurement is a static measurement and may not apply to stenosis that occurs during movement of the cervical spine.

9. Prevertebral soft-tissue width. Measured at the level of the anteroinferior border of the C3 vertebra, this width is normally 7 mm.[122] Edema or hemorrhage is suspected if the space is wider than 7 mm. The retropharyngeal space, lying between the anterior border of the vertebral body and the posterior border of the pharyngeal air shadow, should be 2 to 5 mm in width at C3. From C4 to C7, the space is called the *retrotracheal space* and should be 18 to 22 mm in width (see Figure 3-77).

Figure 3-73
Anteroposterior films of the cervical spine. **A,** Normal spine. **B,** Cervical rib.

Figure 3-74
Diagram of structures seen on anteroposterior cervical spine film.

Figure 3-75
Lateral radiograph of the cervical spine. **A,** Normal curve showing osteophytic lipping. **B,** Cervical spine in flexion. **C,** Cervical spine in extension.

10. Subluxation of the facets.
11. Abnormal soft-tissue shadows.
12. Forward shifting of C1 on C2. This finding indicates instability between C1 and C2. Normally, the joint space between the odontoid process and the anterior arch of the atlas (sometimes called the *atlas-dens index [ADI]*) does not exceed 2.5 to 3 mm in the adult.
13. Instability. Instability is present when more than 3.5 mm of horizontal displacement of one vertebra occurs in relation to the adjacent vertebra (see Figure 3-79).

Open or Odontoid ("Through-the-Mouth") View. This anteroposterior view enables the examiner to determine the state of the odontoid process of C2 and its relation with C1 (Figure 3-81; see Figure 3-80). It may also show the atlanto-occipital and atlantoaxial joints.

Oblique View. This view provides information on the neural foramen and posterior elements of the cervical spine. The examiner should look for or note the following (Figures 3-82 and 3-83):
1. Lipping of the joints of Luschka (osteophytes)

Figure 3-76

X-ray films of a 68-year-old man with multiple radiologic signs of cervical osteoarthritis *(arrows)*. **A,** The cervical spine in flexion, which is very limited. Note that the atlas tips up, as compared with that in **B.** All intervertebral disc spaces below C2-C3 are very narrow. Anterior and posterior osteophytes are apparent *(arrows)*. The spine extends very little in **B** and is quite straight in **A** (i.e., no significant flexion). (From Bland JH: *Disorders of the cervical spine*, p. 213, Philadelphia, 1994, W.B. Saunders).

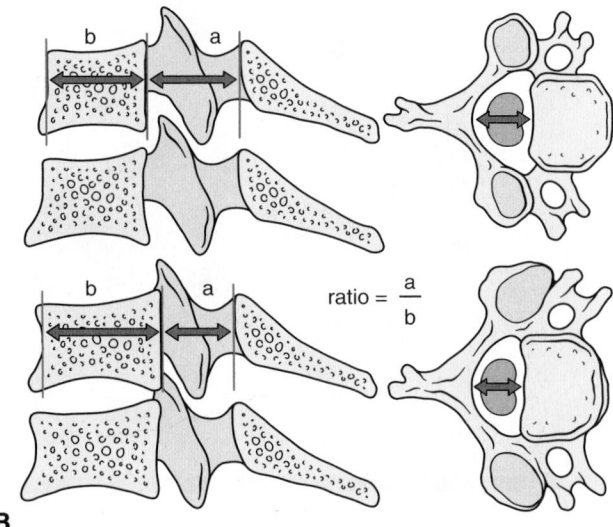

Figure 3-77

A, Normal cervical spine. Lateral projection. Note the alignment and appearance of the facet joints: *A,* anterior vertebral line; *B,* posterior vertebral line; *C,* posterior canal line. Retropharyngeal space *(between top arrows)* should not exceed 5 mm. Retrotracheal space *(between bottom arrows)* should not exceed 22 mm. **B,** The Torg ratio is calculated by dividing the shortest distance between the posterior vertebral body and the spinolaminar line *(a)* by the vertebral body width *(b)*. (**A,** Modified from Forrester DM, Brown JC: *The radiology of joint disease*, p. 408, Philadelphia, 1987, W.B. Saunders, **B,** Redrawn from McAlindon RJ: On field evaluation and management of head and neck injured athletes, *Clin Sports Med* 21:10, 2002. Adapted from Torg JS, Pavlov H: Cervical spinal stenosis with cord neurapraxia and transient quadriplegia, *Clin Sports Med* 6:115–133, 1987; with permission.)

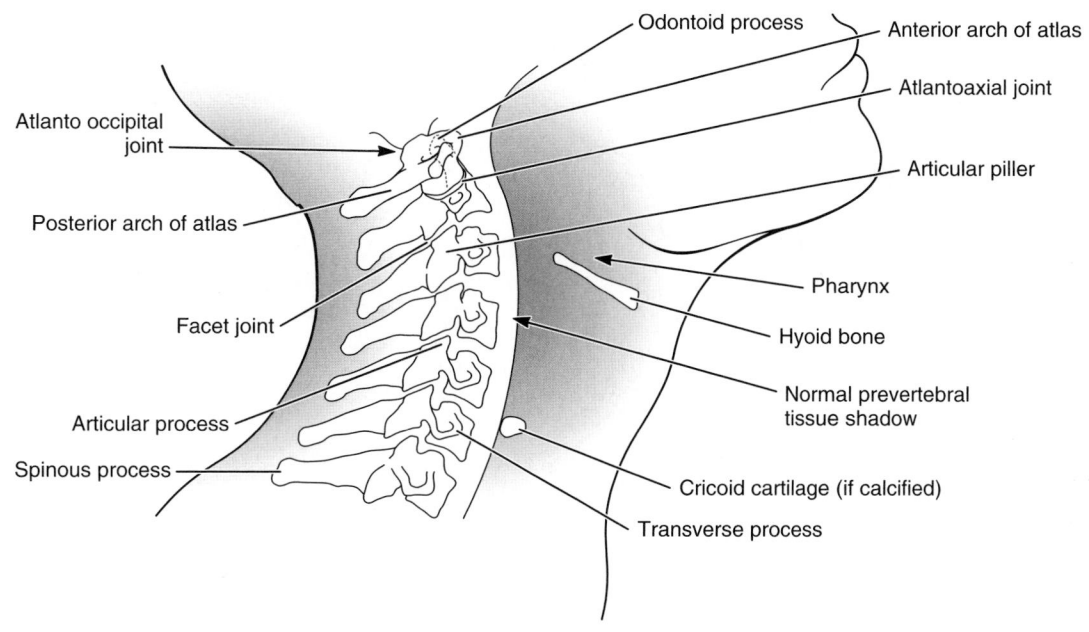

Figure 3-78
Diagram of structures seen on lateral film of the cervical spine.

Figure 3-79
Atlantoaxial subluxation. Flexion view shows abnormal widening of the atlantoaxial space *(arrow)*, which measures 4 mm. (From Resnick D, Kransdorf MJ: *Bone and joint imaging*, p 883, Philadelphia, 2005, Saunders.)

2. Overriding of the facet joints (subluxation, spondylosis)
3. Facet joints and intervertebral foramen (see Figure 3-83)

Pillar View. This special view is used to evaluate the lateral masses of the cervical spine and especially the facet joints (Figure 3-84). It is usually reserved for patients with suspected facet fractures.[123]

Computed Tomography

Computed tomography (CT) helps to delineate the bone and soft-tissue anatomy of the cervical spine in cross section and can show, for example, a disc prolapse. It also shows the true size and extent of osteophytes better than do plain x-rays (Figure 3-85). CT scans are especially useful for showing bone fragments in the spinal canal after a fracture and bony defects in the vertebral bodies and neural arches. CT scans may be combined with myelography to outline the spinal cord and nerve roots inside the thecal sac (Figure 3-86). CT scans are used only after conventional radiographs have been taken and a need for them is shown.

Myelography

Myelograms are the modality of choice with brachial plexus avulsions, either Erb-Duchenne paralysis (C5 and C6) or Klumpke's paralysis (C7, C8, and T1). They may also be used to demonstrate narrowing in the intervertebral foramen and cervical spinal stenosis. They may be used to outline the contour of the thecal sac, nerve roots, and spinal cord (Figure 3-87).

Magnetic Resonance Imaging

This noninvasive technique can differentiate between various soft tissues and bone (Figures 3-88 and 3-89). Because it shows differences based on water content, magnetic resonance imaging (MRI) can differentiate between the nucleus pulposus and the annulus fibro-

Figure 3-80

Cervicobasilar junction: normal osseous relationships. **A,** Chamberlain's line is drawn from the posterior margin of the hard palate to the posterior border of the foramen magnum. The odontoid process normally does not extend more than 5 mm above this line. **B,** The bimastoid line (lower line), connecting the tips of the mastoids, is normally within 2 mm of the odontoid tip. The digastric line (upper line), connecting the digastric muscle fossae, is normally located above the odontoid process. **C,** The basilar angle, which normally exceeds 140°, is formed by the angle of intersection of two lines—one drawn from the nasion to the tuberculum sellae, and the second drawn from the tuberculum sellae to the anterior edge of the foramen magnum. **D,** The atlanto-occipital joint angle, constructed on frontal tomograms by the intersection of two lines drawn along the axes of these articulations, is normally not greater than 150°. (From Resnick D, Kransdorf MJ: *Bone and joint imaging*, p 37, Philadelphia, 2005, Saunders.)

Occipital condyle

Atlanta-occipital joint

Odontoid process

Joint space between C1–C2

C2 superior articular process

Spinous process of C2

Figure 3-81

Through-the-mouth radiograph.

Figure 3-82
Abnormal x-ray findings on oblique view. Note loss of normal curve; narrowing at C4, C5, and C6; osteophytes and lipping of C4, C5, and C6; and encroachment on intervertebral foramen at C4-C5, C5-C6, and C6-C7.

Figure 3-83
Oblique radiograph of the cervical spine showing intervertebral foramen and facet joints. Severe lipping in lower cervical spine and spondylosis are also evident.

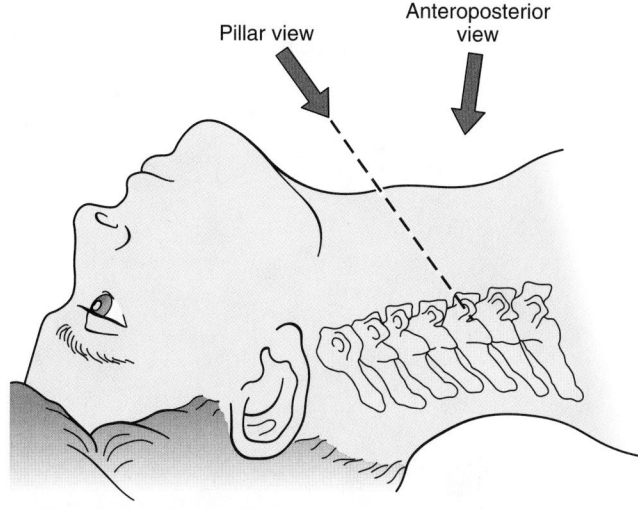

Figure 3-84
Diagram of pillar view showing orientation of facet joints.

sus. MRI may be used to reveal disc protrusions, but it has been reported that patients showing these lesions are often asymptomatic, highlighting the fact that diagnostic imaging abnormalities should be considered only in relation to the history and clinical examination.[124] An MRI allows visualization of the nerve roots, spinal cord, and thecal sac as well as the bone and bone marrow. It is also used to identify postoperative scarring and disc herniation.[125] Magnetic resonance angiography is also useful for determining the patency and status of the vertebral artery.[126–128]

Figure 3-85
Foraminal stenosis caused by hypertrophic facet arthropathy and by spondylosis. Metrizamide-enhanced computed tomography scan through C5-C foramina details the markedly overgrown facet *(white arrow)* and the bony "bar," or spondylotic spurring *(black arrows).* The right foramen is almost occluded by abnormal bone. (From Dorwart RH, LaMasters DL: Application of computed tomographic scanning of the cervical spine, *Orthop Clin North Am* 16:386, 1985.)

Figure 3-86

Postcontrast computed tomogram showing normally patent neural foramen at the C6–7 level on the left side *(open arrow)*. The nerve root sleeve fills with contrast medium and enters the neural foramen. On the right side *(closed arrow)*, there is no evidence of filling of the nerve root sleeve within the neural foramen as a result of lateral C6-C disc herniation. (From Bell GR, Ross JS: Diagnosis of nerve root compression: myelography, computed tomography, and MRI, *Orthop Clin North Am* 23:410, 1992.)

Figure 3-87

Myelogram of cervical spine.

Figure 3-88

Magnetic resonance image of the cervical and upper thoracic spine. Sagittal view *(left)*, with close-up of cervical spine *(right)*. (From Foreman SM, Croft AC: *Whiplash injuries: the cervical acceleration/deceleration syndrome*, p. 126, Baltimore, 1988, Williams & Wilkins.)

Figure 3-89
Posterior disc displacement: MR imaging findings. Sagittal
T2-weighted (TR/TE, 2608/96) fast spin echo MR image reveals an
extruded paracentral disc of low signal intensity at the C6-C7 spinal
level. (From Resnick D, Kransdorf MJ: *Bone and joint imaging*,
p 415, Philadelphia, 2005, Saunders. Courtesy D. Goodwin, MD,
Hanover, NH.)

Figure 3-90
Xeroradiograph of cervical spine (lateral view). Arrow indicates
calcified mass. (From Forrester DM, Brown JC: *The radiology of joint
disease*, p. 420, Philadelphia, 1987, W.B. Saunders.)

Xeroradiography
Xeroradiography helps to delineate bone and soft tissue by enhancing the interfaces between tissues (Figure
3-90).

Précis of the Cervical Spine Assessment*

History
Observation (standing or sitting)
Examination (sitting)
  Active movements
    Flexion
    Extension
    Side flexion (right and left)
    Rotation (right and left)
    Combined movements (if necessary)
    Repetitive movements (if necessary)
    Sustained positions (if necessary)
  Resisted isometric movements (as in active movements)
  Scanning examination
    Peripheral joint
    Temporomandibular joints (open mouth and
      closed mouth)
    Shoulder girdle (elevation through abduction,
      elevation through forward flexion, elevation
      through plane of scapula, medial and lateral
      rotation with arm at side; medial and lateral
      rotation at 90° abduction)
    Elbow (flexion, extension, supination, pronation)
    Wrist (flexion, extension, radial, and ulnar deviation)
    Fingers and thumb (flexion, extension,
      abduction, adduction)
    Myotomes
    Neck flexion (C1,C2)
    Neck side flexion (C3)
    Shoulder elevation (C4)
    Shoulder abduction (C5)
    Elbow flexion (C6) and/or extension (C7)
    Wrist flexion (C7) and/or extension (C6)
    Thumb extension (C8) and/or ulnar deviation
      (C8)
    Hand intrinsics (abduction or adduction) (T1)
    Sensory Scanning Examination
  Special tests
    Foraminal compression (Spurling's) test
    Distraction test
    Shoulder abduction test
    Vertebral artery tests
  Reflexes and cutaneous distribution
    Biceps (C5-C6)
    Triceps (C7-C8)
    Hoffmann's sign (or Babinski's test)
    Sensory scan

Examination, supine
  Passive movements
    Flexion
    Extension
    Side flexion
    Rotation
  Special tests
    Upper limb tension test
    Vertebral artery tests

NOTE 1: *The following tests should be performed if
the* examiner anticipates treating the patient by
mobilization or manipulation. In this case, they are
called **clearing tests** *for treatment.*
Vertebral artery tests (supine or sitting)
Sharp-Purser test (sitting)
Pettman's distraction test (supine)
Anterior shear test (supine)
Transverse ligament stress test (supine)
Lateral shear test (supine)
Lateral flexion alar ligament stress test (supine)

NOTE 2: *If any of the above tests are positive, mobilization*
or manipulation should only be performed **with
extreme care** *and the level exhibiting the positive signs*
should be stabilized during the treatment.

Joint play movements
  Side glide of cervical spine
  Anterior glide of cervical spine
  Posterior glide of cervical spine
  Traction glide of cervical spine
  Rotation of occiput on C1
  Palpation
Examination, prone
  Joint play movements
    Posteroanterior central vertebral pressure
    Posteroanterior unilateral vertebral pressure
    Transverse vertebral pressure
  Palpation
  Diagnostic imaging
After any examination, the patient should be warned of the
  possibility of exacerbation of symptoms as a result of
  the assessment.

*The précis is shown in an order that limits the amount of moving
that the patient has to do but ensures that all necessary structures
are tested.

Case Studies

When doing these case studies, the examiner should list the appropriate questions to be asked and why they are being asked,
what to look for and why, and what things should be tested and why. Depending on the answers of the patient (and the examiner
should consider different responses), several possible causes of the patient's problems may become evident (examples are given in
parentheses). A differential diagnosis chart should be made up (see Table 3-20 as an example). The examiner can then decide how
different diagnoses may affect the treatment plan.

1. A 2-month-old baby is brought to you by a concerned parent. The child does not move the head
properly, and the sternocleidomastoid muscle on the
left side is prominent. Describe your assessment plan
before beginning treatment (congenital torticollis
versus Klippel-Feil syndrome).

2. A 54-year-old man comes to you complaining of
neck stiffness, especially on rising; sometimes he has

Continued

Case Studies—cont'd

numbness into his left arm. Describe your assessment plan (cervical spondylosis versus subacromial bursitis).

3. An 18-year-old male football player comes to you complaining of a "dead arm" after a tackle he made 2 days ago. Although he can now move the left arm, it still does not feel right. Describe your assessment plan (brachial plexus lesion versus acromioclavicular sprain).

4. A 23-year-old woman comes to you after a motor vehicle accident. Her car was hit from behind while stopped for a red light. She could tell the accident was going to occur because she could see in the rearview mirror that the car behind her was not going to be able to stop. The car that hit her was going 50 kph (30 mph), and skid marks were visible for only 5 m from the location of her car. Describe your assessment plan (cervical sprain versus cervical facet syndrome).

5. A woman comes to you complaining of persistent headaches that last for days at a time. She is 35 years old and has recently lost her job. She complains that she sometimes sees flashing lights and cannot stand having anyone around her when the pain is very bad. Describe your assessment plan for this patient (migraine versus tension headache).

6. A 26-year-old man comes to you complaining of pain in his neck. The pain was evident yesterday when he got up and has not decreased significantly since then. He thinks that he may have "slept wrong." There is no previous history of trauma. Describe your

assessment plan for this patient (acquired torticollis versus cervical disc lesion).

7. A 75-year-old woman comes to you complaining primarily of neck pain but also of stiffness. She exhibits a dowager's hump. There is no history of trauma. Describe your assessment plan for this patient (osteoporosis versus cervical spondylosis).

8. A 47-year-old man comes to you complaining of elbow and neck pain. There is no recent history of trauma, but he remembers being in a motor vehicle accident 19 years ago. He now works at a desk all day. Describe your assessment for this patient (cervical spondylosis versus tennis elbow versus double-crush injury).

9. A 16-year-old boy comes to you with a complaint of having hurt his neck. While "fooling" with some friends at the lake, he ran away from them and dove into the water to get away. The top of his head hit the bottom, and he felt a burning pain. The pain decreased as he came out of the water, but he still has a residual ache. Describe your plan for this patient (cervical fracture versus cervical sprain).

10. A 14-year-old girl comes to you complaining of neck pain. She has long hair. She states that when she "whipped" her hair out of her eyes, which she has done many times before, she felt a sudden pain in her neck. Although the pain intensity has decreased, it is still there, and she cannot fully move her neck. Describe your assessment plan for this patient (cervical sprain versus acquired torticollis).

Table 3-20
Differential Diagnosis of Cervical Facet Syndrome, Cervical Nerve Root Lesion, and Thoracic Outlet Syndrome

Signs and Symptoms	Facet Syndrome	Cervical Nerve Root	Thoracic Outlet Syndrome
Pain referral	Possible	Yes	Possible
Pain on hyperextension and rotation	Yes (often without increased referral of symptoms)	Yes with increased symptoms	No
Spine stiffness	Yes	Possible	Possible
Paresthesia	No	Yes	Possible
Reflexes	Not affected	May be affected	May be affected
Muscle spasm	Yes	Yes	Yes
Tension tests	May or may not be positive	Positive	May be positive
Pallor and coolness	No	No	Possible
Muscle weakness	No	Possible	Not early (later small hand muscles)
Muscle fatigue and cramps	No	No	Possible

References

To enhance this text and add value for the reader, all references have been incorporated into a CD-ROM that is provided with this text. The reader can view the reference source and access it online whenever possible. There are a total of 142 cited and other general references for this chapter.

Reliability, Validity, Specificity and Sensitivity of Special/Diagnostic Tests Used in the Cervical Spine

BRACHIAL PLEXUS TENSION TEST

Reliability	Validity
• Test retest ICC = 0.83 SEM = 16.8[129]	• Discriminant validity cardiac group × musculoskeletal group (p < .001) The cardiac normally have more nerve commitment and on the study they had significant smaller angles[129]

CERVICAL ROTATION LATERAL FLEXION TEST

Reliability	Validity
• Interrater for the position of the first rib k=1[130]	• Correlation with radiologic findings k = 0.84[130]

DISTRACTION TEST

Reliability	Specificity	Sensitivity	Odds Ratio
• k = 0.88[131]	• 100% for neurologic and radiologic signs[132]	• 26% for radicular sign, 32% for neurologic sign, 40% for radiologic sign, 43% for neurologic and radiologic sign[132]	• Positive likelihood ratios for neurologic and radiologic sign 43, negative likelihood ratios for neurologic and radiologic sign 0.57

EXTENSION ROTATION TEST FOR LEFT VERTEBRAL ARTERY

Specificity	Sensitivity	Odds Ratio
• 67%[133]	• 0%[133]	• Positive likelihood ratios 0, negative likelihood ratios 1.49

EXTENSION ROTATION TEST FOR RIGHT VERTEBRAL ARTERY

Specificity	Sensitivity	Odds Ratio
• 86%[133]	• 0%[133]	• Positive likelihood ratios 0, negative likelihood ratios 1.16

FORAMINAL COMPRESSION (SPURLING'S) TEST

Specificity	Sensitivity	Odds Ratio
• 92%[134] • 100% for radicular pain, 92% for neurologic and radiologic signs[132]	• 77%[134] • 28% for radicular symptom, 26% for neurologic sign, 36% for radiologic sign, 40% for neurologic and radiologic sign[132]	• Positive likelihood ratios 9.62, negative likelihood ratios 0.25 • Positive likelihood ratios neurologic and radiologic signs 5, negative likelihood ratios for neurologic and radiologic signs 0.65

NECK DISABILITY INDEX

Reliability	Validity	Specificity	Sensitivity	Odds Ratio
• Test-retest r = 0.89[65] • Test-retest ICC = 0.68[135]	• Internal consistency Cronbach's alpha 0.80, correlation with McGill pain questionnaire r = 0.7, VAS 0.6[65]	• 59%[135]	• 52%[135]	• Positive likelihood ratio 1.27, negative likelihood ratios 0.81

PALPATION OF THE CONGENITAL BLOCK

Reliability	Specificity	Sensitivity	Odds Ratio
• All blocks k = 0.67, C2-C3 K = 0.76, C5-C6 k = 0.46[136]	• All blocks 98%, C2-C3 98%, C5-C6 91%[136]	• All blocks 74%, C2-C3 78%, C5-C6 55%[136]	• Positive likelihood ratios for all blocks 37, for C2-C3 39, for C5-C6 6.11 • Negative likelihood ratios for all blocks 0.26, for C2-C3 0.22, for C5-C6 0.49

PATIENT SPECIFIC FUNCTIONAL SCALE

Reliability	Specificity	Sensitivity	Odds Ratio
• Test-retest ICC = 0.82[135]	• 100%[135]	• 95%[135]	• Positive likelihood ratio 95, negative likelihood ratio 0.05

SF-12 (FOR CERVICAL SPONDYLOTIC MYELOPATHY)

Reliability	Validity	Responsiveness
• Chronbach's alpha for physical component 0.77, for mental component 0.77[137]	• Correlation with SF-36 r > 0.92[137]	• Effect size for physical component 0.64, for mental component 0.75[137]

SF-36 (FOR CERVICAL SPONDYLOTIC MYELOPATHY)

Reliability	Validity	Responsiveness
• Chronbach's alpha for physical component 0.93, for mental component 0.89[137]	• Correlation with SF-12 r > 0.92[137]	• Effect size for physical component 0.73, for mental component 0.80[137]

SHARP-PURSER TEST

Specificity	Sensitivity	Odds Ratio
• 96%[138]	• 69%[138]	• Positive likelihood ratios 17.25, negative likelihood ratios 0.32

SHOULDER ABDUCTION TEST

Specificity	Sensitivity	Odds Ratio
• 100% for neurologic signs, 80% for radiologic signs[132]	• 31% for radicular symptom, 36% for neurologic sign, 38% for radiologic sign, 43% for neurologic and radiologic sign[132]	• Positive likelihood ratios for radiologic signs 1.90 • Negative likelihood ratios for neurologic signs 0.64, for radiologic signs 0.77

SPURLING A TEST

Reliability	Specificity	Sensitivity	Odds Ratio
• k = 0.60[131]	• 50%[131]	• 86%[131]	• Positive likelihood ratios 1.72, negative likelihood ratios 0.28

SPURLING B TEST

Reliability	Specificity	Sensitivity	Odds Ratio
• k = 0.62[131]	• 74%[131]	• 50%[131]	• Positive likelihood ratios 1.92, negative likelihood ratios 0.67

Continued

APPENDIX 3-1—cont'd

ULTT A

Reliability	Specificity	Sensitivity	Odds Ratio
• k=0.76[131]	• 22%[131]	• 97%[131]	• Positive likelihood ratios 1.24, negative likelihood ratios 0.14

ULTT B

Reliability	Specificity	Sensitivity	Odds Ratio
• k=0.83[131]	• 33%[131]	• 72%[131]	• Positive likelihood ratios 1.07, negative likelihood ratios 0.85

UPPER LIMB TENSION TEST (BRACHIAL COMPRESSION)

Reliability	Validity	Specificity	Sensitivity	Odds Ratio
• Radial for cervical neutral and first pain ICC=0.93 SEM=3.88, cervical neutral strong pain ICC=0.96 SEM=2.19, cervical side flexion first pain ICC=0.94 SEM=4.03, cervical side flexion strong pain ICC=0.88 SEM=4.65[139] • Median nerve intrarater symptomatic group ICC=0.98 SEM 2.8, asymptomatic group ICC=0.97 SEM=3.5[140]	• In vitro study using "buckle" force transducers in the nerve. ULTT for median nerve caused more tension on median nerve in comparison to the others $p<.001$, for radial nerve caused more tension on radial nerve tension on radial nerve compared with ulnar $p<.001$ but not compared with median nerve[141] • The test of ulnar nerve had no significant differences between nerves[141] • When tensioning the nerve on neck using flexion and rotation, the tests caused more tension in the intended nerve when compared with the other two tests[141]	• Median 94%[134]	• Median 77%[134]	• Positive likelihood ratios 12.83, negative likelihood ratios 0.24

VALSALVA TEST

Reliability	Specificity	Sensitivity	Odds Ratio
• k=0.69[131]	• 94%[131]	• 22%[131]	• Positive likelihood ratios 3.66, negative likelihood ratios 0.83

VERTEBRAL ARTERY TEST

Reliability	Validity
• Interrater k=0.90[84]	• There was a significant relationship between mean Doppler frequency and the cervical spine position $p<.01$[142] • Test hypothesis there is no difference between positions for vertebral artery: peak flow for negative group $p=.015$, positive group $p=.001$, end diastolic flow negative group $p=.08$, positive group $p=.25$, R peak flow for negative group $p=.0003$, positive group $p=.0001$, end diastolic flow negative group $p=.03$, positive group $p=.0003$[84]

TEMPOROMANDIBULAR JOINT

The temporomandibular joints are two of the most frequently used joints in the body, but they probably receive the least amount of attention. Without these joints, we would be severely hindered when talking, eating, yawning, kissing, or sucking. In any examination of the head and neck, the temporomandibular joints should be included. Temporomandibular disorders (TMDs) consist of several complex multifactorial ailments involving many interrelating factors including psychosocial issues.[1-3] Three cardinal features of TMD are orofacial pain, restricted jaw motion, and joint noise.[1] Much of the work in this chapter has been developed from the teachings of Rocabado.[4]

Applied Anatomy

The temporomandibular joint is a synovial, condylar, modified ovoid and hinge-type joint with fibrocartilaginous surfaces rather than hyaline cartilage[5] and an articular disc; this disc completely divides each joint into two cavities (Figure 4-1). Both joints, one on each side of the jaw, must be considered together in any examination. Along with the teeth, these joints are considered to be a "trijoint complex."

Gliding, translation, or **sliding movement** occurs in the upper cavity of the temporomandibular joint, whereas **rotation** or **hinge movement** occurs in the lower cavity (Figure 4-2). Rotation occurs from the beginning to the midrange of movement. The upper head of the lateral pterygoid muscle draws the disc, or **meniscus,** anteriorly and prepares for condylar rotation during movement. The rotation occurs through the two condylar heads between the articular disc and the condyle. In addition, the disc provides congruent contours and lubrication for the joint. Gliding, which occurs as a second movement, is a translatory movement of the condyle and disc along the slope of the articular eminence. Both gliding and rotation are essential for full opening and closing of the mouth (Figure 4-3). The capsule of the temporomandibular joints is thin and loose. In the resting position, the mouth is slightly open, the lips are together, and the teeth are not in contact but slightly apart. In the close packed position, the teeth are tightly clenched, and the heads of the condyles are in the posterior aspect of the joint. **Centric occlusion** is the relation of the jaw and teeth when there is maximum contact of the teeth, and it is the position assumed by the jaw in swallowing. The position in which the teeth are fully interdigitated is called the **median occlusal position.**[6]

Temporomandibular Joints	
Resting position:	Mouth slightly open, lips together, teeth not in contact
Close packed position:	Teeth tightly clenched
Capsular pattern:	Limitation of mouth opening

The temporomandibular joints actively displace only anteriorly and slightly laterally. When the mouth is opening, the condyles of the joint rest on the disc in the articular eminences, and any sudden movement, such as a yawn, may displace one or both condyles forward. As the mandible moves forward on opening, the disc moves medially and posteriorly until the collateral ligaments and lateral pterygoid stop its movement. The disc is then "seated" on the head of the mandible, and both

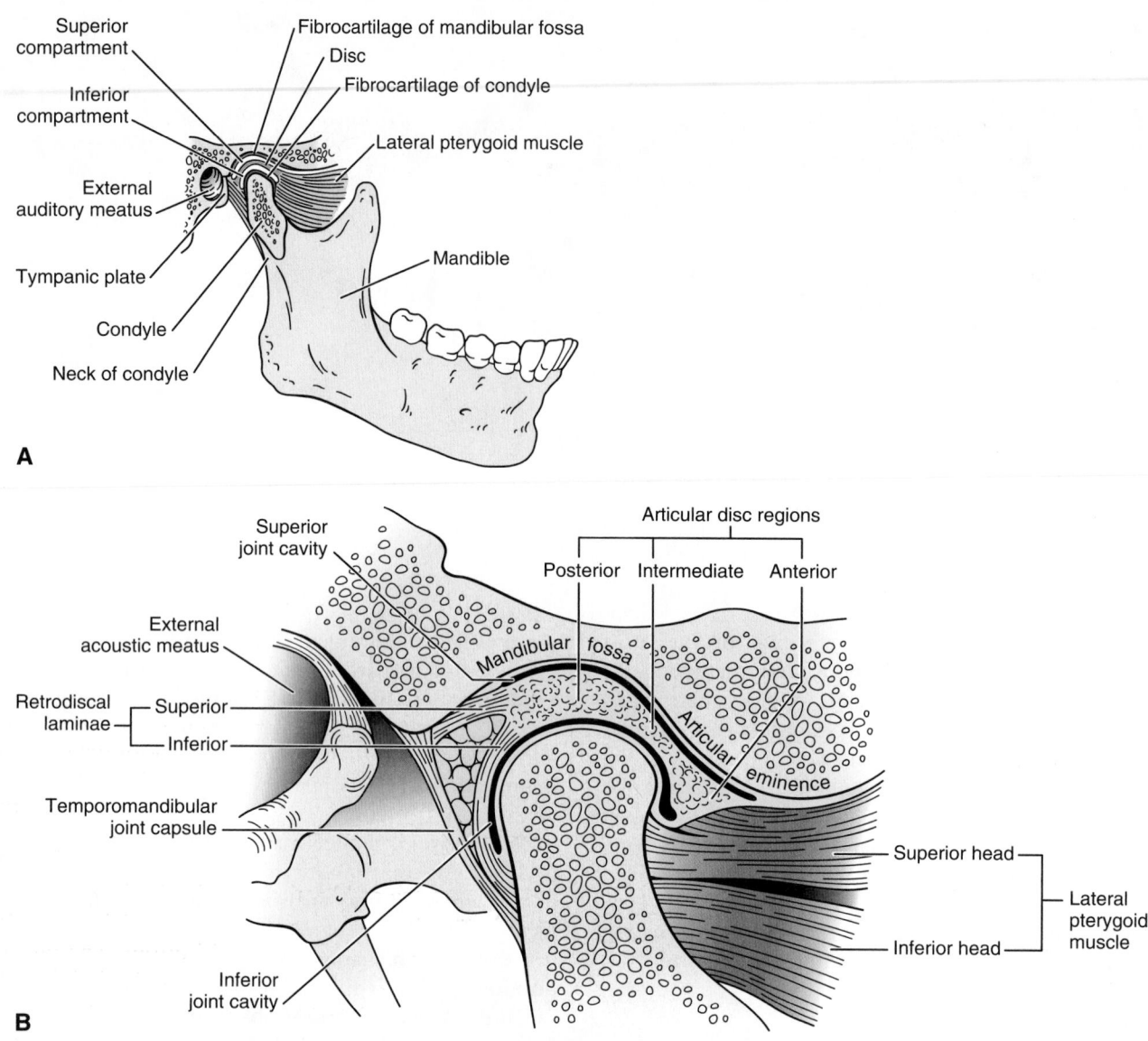

A, The temporomandibular joint. **B,** Close up of temporomandibular joint. (**B,** Redrawn from Neumann DA: *Kinesiology of the musculoskeletal system—foundations for physical rehabilitation,* p. 357, St Louis, 2002, C.V. Mosby.)

Figure 4-1

disc and mandible move forward to full opening. If this "seating" of the disc does not occur, full range of motion at the temporomandibular joint is limited. In the first phase, mainly rotation occurs, primarily in the inferior joint space. In the second phase, in which the mandible and disc move together, mainly translation occurs in the superior joint space.[7]

The hyoid bone, found in the anterior throat region, is sometimes referred to as the skeleton of the tongue.[6] It serves as an attachment for the extrinsic tongue muscles and infrahyoid muscles and, by so doing, provides reciprocal stabilization during swallowing and through its muscle

attachments can affect cervical and even shoulder function. Figure 4-4 outlines the effect of a forward head posture and the relation to the hyoid bone and related muscles.

The temporomandibular joints are innervated by branches of the auriculotemporal and masseteric branches of the mandibular nerve. The disc is innervated along its periphery but is aneural and avascular in its intermediate (force-bearing) zone.

The **temporomandibular,** or **lateral, ligament** restrains movement of the lower jaw and prevents compression of the tissues behind the condyle. In reality, this collateral ligament is a thickening in the joint capsule.

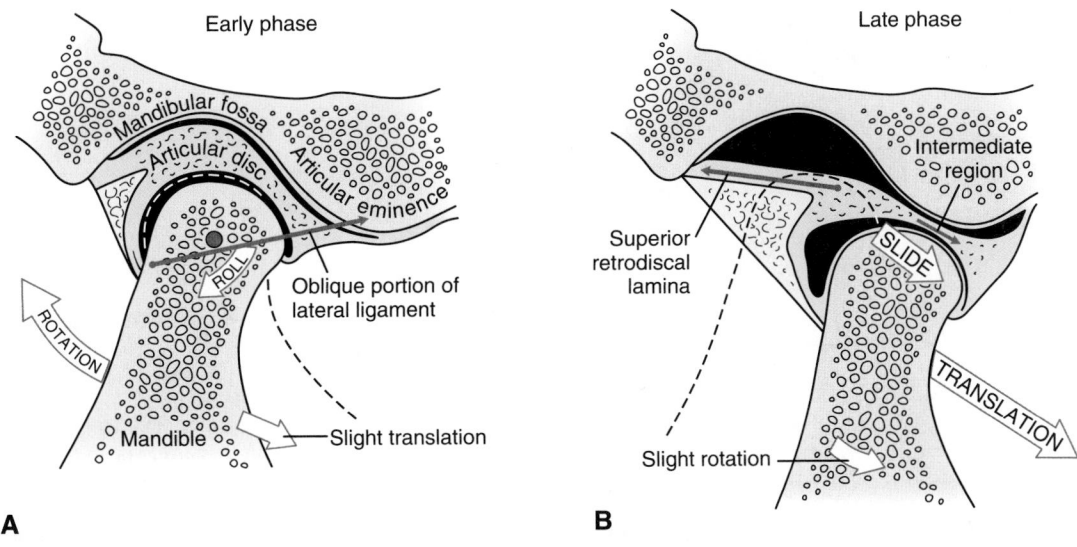

Early phase

Late phase

Mandibular fossa

Articular disc

Articular eminence

ROLL

ROTATION

Oblique portion of lateral ligament

Slight translation

Mandible

A

Intermediate region

Superior retrodiscal lamina

SLIDE

TRANSLATION

Slight rotation

B

Figure 4-2

Arthrokinematics of opening the mouth: **A,** Early phase. **B,** Late phase. (Modified from Neumann DA: *Kinesiology of the musculoskeletal system— foundations for physical rehabilitation,* p. 360, St Louis, 2002, C.V. Mosby.)

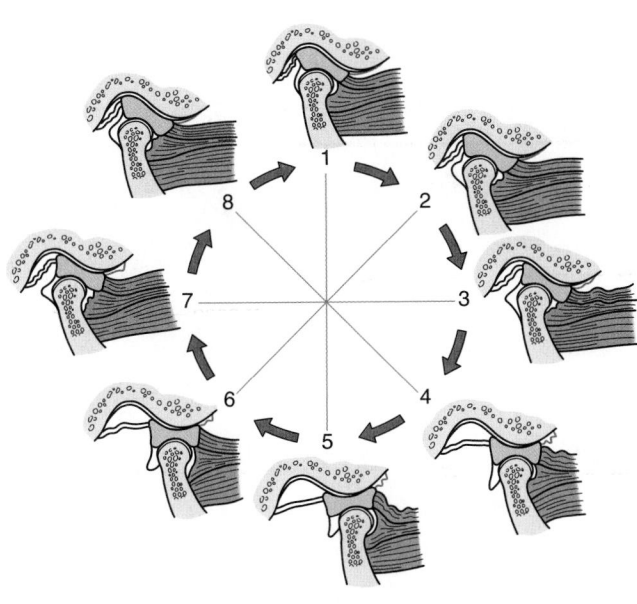

1 2 3 4 5 6 7 8

Figure 4-3

Normal functional movement of the condyle and disc during the full range of opening and closing. Note that the disc is rotated posteriorly on the condyle as the condyle is translated out of the fossa. The closing movement is the exact opposite of the opening movement.

The **sphenomandibular** and **stylomandibular ligaments** act as "guiding" restraints to keep the condyle, disc, and temporal bone firmly opposed. The stylomandibular ligament is a specialized band of deep cerebral fascia with thickening of the parotid fascia.

In the human, there are 20 deciduous, or temporary ("baby"), teeth and 32 permanent teeth (Figure 4-5).

The temporary teeth are shed between the ages of 6 and 13 years. In the adult, the incisors are the front teeth (four maxillary and four mandibular), with the maxillary incisors being larger than the mandibular incisors. The incisors are designed to cut food. The canine teeth (two maxillary and two mandibular) are the longest permanent teeth and are designed to cut and tear food. The premolars crush and break down the food for digestion; usually they have two cusps. There are eight premolars in all, two on each side, top and bottom. The final set of teeth are the molars, which crush and grind food for digestion. They have four or five cusps, and there are two or three on each side, top and bottom (total 8–12). The third molars are called *wisdom teeth.* Missing teeth, abnormal tooth eruption, malocclusion, or dental caries (decay) may lead to problems of the temporomandibular joint. By convention, the teeth are divided into four quadrants—the upper left, the upper right, the lower left, and the lower right quadrants (Figure 4-6).

Patient History

In addition to the questions listed under Patient History in Chapter 1, the examiner should obtain the following information from the patient.[8,9]

1. *Is there pain or restriction on opening or closing of the mouth?* Pain in the fully opened position (e.g., pain associated with opening to bite an apple, yawning) is probably caused by an extra-articular problem, whereas pain associated with biting firm objects (e.g., nuts, raw fruit and vegetables) is probably caused by an intra-articular problem.[10] Limited opening may be

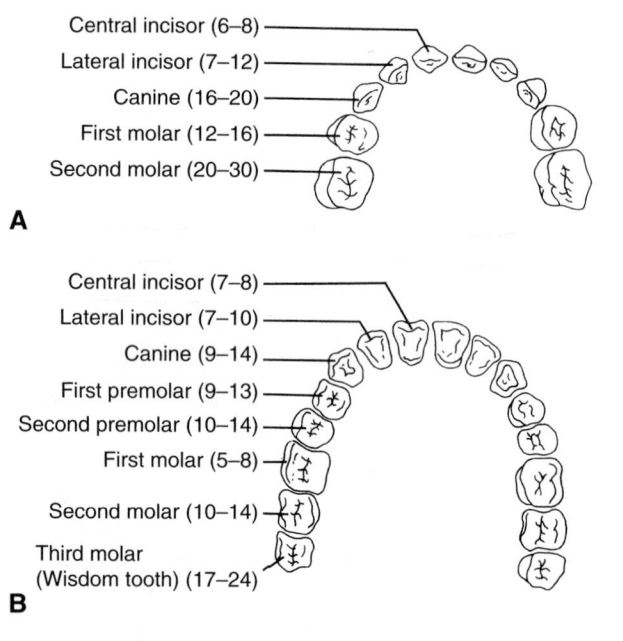

Figure 4-4

A forward head posture shows one mechanism by which passive tension in selected suprahyoid and infrahyoid muscles alter the resting posture of the mandible. The mandible is pulled inferiorly and posteriorly, changing the position of the condyle within the temporomandibular joint. Note the interrelationship to the cervical spine and shoulder. (Modified from Neumann DA: *Kinesiology of the musculoskeletal system—foundations for physical rehabilitation,* p. 366, St Louis, 2002, C.V. Mosby.)

Figure 4-5

Teeth in a child (**A**) and in an adult (**B**). Numbers indicate age (in months for a child, in years for an adult) at which teeth erupt.

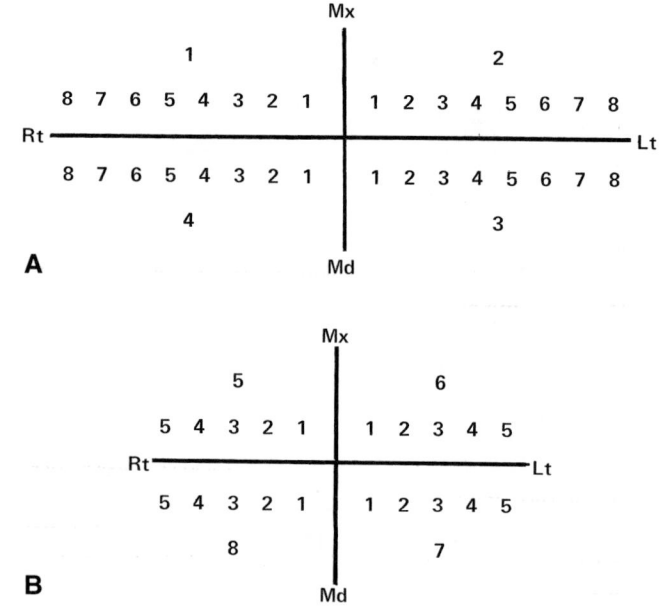

Figure 4-6

Numeric symbols for dentition in an adult (**A**) and in a child (**B**). (From Liebgott B: *The Anatomical basis of dentistry,* St Louis, 1986, C.V. Mosby.)

due to the disc displaced anteriorly, inert tissue tightness, or muscle spasm. Restriction can lead to anxiety in patients because of its effect on everyday activities (e.g., eating, talking).[3]

2. *Is there pain on eating? Does the patient chew on the right? Left? Both sides equally?* Loss of molars or worn dentures can lead to loss of vertical dimension, which can make chewing painful. **Vertical dimension** is the distance between any two arbitrary points on the face, one of these points being above and the other below the mouth, usually in midline. Often, chewing on one side is the result of malocclusion.[10]

3. *What movements of the jaw cause pain? Do the symptoms change over a 24-hour period?* The examiner should watch the patient's jaw movement while the patient is talking. A history of stiffness on waking with pain on function that disappears as the day goes on suggests osteoarthritis.[11]

4. *Do any of these actions cause pain or discomfort: Yawning? Biting? Chewing? Swallowing? Speaking? Shouting?* If so, where? All of these actions cause movement, compression, and/or stretching of the soft tissues of the temporomandibular joints.

5. *Does the patient breathe through the nose or the mouth?* Normal breathing is through the nose with the lips closed and no "air gulping." If the patient is a "mouth breather," the tongue does not sit in the proper position against the palate. In the young, if the tongue does not push against the palate, developmental abnormalities may occur, because the tongue normally provides internal pressure to shape the mouth. The buccinator and orbicularis oris muscle complex provides external pressure to counterbalance the internal pressure of the tongue. Loss of normal neck balance often results in the individual's becoming a mouth breather and an upper respiratory breather, making greater use of the accessory muscles of respiration. Conditions such as adenoids, tonsils, and upper respiratory tract infections may cause the same problem.

6. *Has the patient complained of any* **crepitus** *or* **clicking**? Normally, the condyles of the temporomandibular joint slide out of the concavity and onto the rim of the disc. Clicking is the result of abnormal motion of the disc and mandible. Early clicking implies a developing dysfunction while late clicking is more likely to mean a chronic problem. Clicking may occur when the condyle slides back off the rim into the center (Figure 4-7).[12] If the disc sticks or is bunched slightly, opening causes the condyle to move abruptly over the disc and into its normal position, resulting in a single click (see Figure 4-7).[13] There may be a partial anterior displacement (subluxation) or dislocation of the disc, which the condyle must override to reach its normal position when the mouth is fully open (Figure 4-8). This override may also cause a click. Similarly, a click may occur if the disc is displaced anteriorly and/or medially, causing the condyle to override the posterior rim of the disc later than normal during mouth opening. This is referred to as *disc displacement with reduction.* If clicking occurs in both directions, it is called **reciprocal clicking** (Figure 4-9). The opening click occurs somewhere during the opening or protrusive path, and the click indicates the condyle is slipping over the thicker posterior border of the disc to its position in the thinner middle or intermediate zone. The closing (reciprocal) click occurs near the end of the closing or retrusive path as the pull of the superior lateral pterygoid muscle causes the disc to slip more anteriorly and the condyle to move over its posterior border.

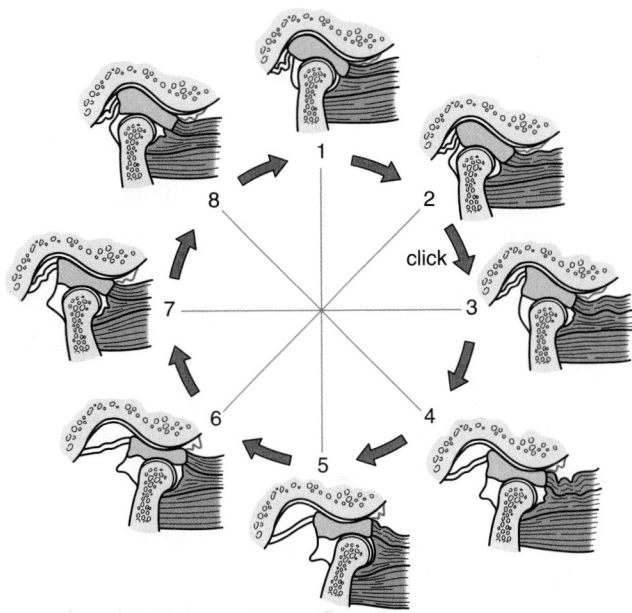

Figure 4-7

Single click. Between positions 2 and 3, a click is felt as the condyle moves across the posterior border into the intermediate zone of the disc. Normal condyle-disc function occurs during the remaining opening and closing movement. In the closed joint position *(1)*, the disc is again displaced forward (and medially) by activity of the superior lateral pterygoid muscle.

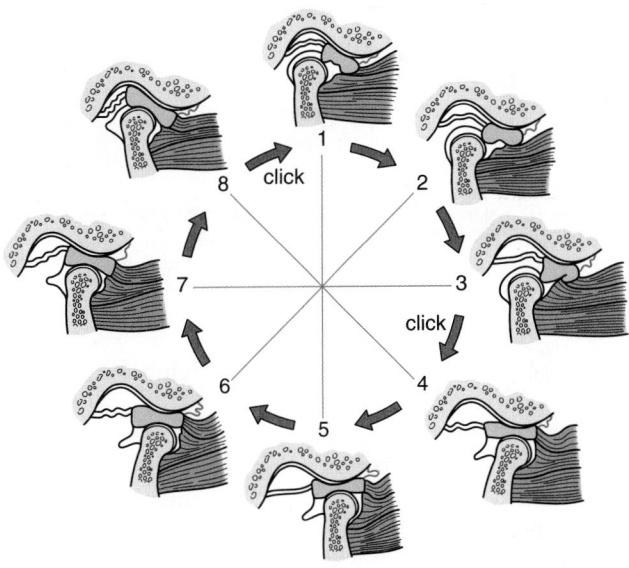

Figure 4-8

Functional dislocation of the disc with reduction. During opening, the condyle passes over the posterior border of the disc into the intermediate area of the disc, thus reducing the dislocated disc.

Clicks may also be caused by adhesions (Figure 4-10), especially in people who clench their teeth (bruxism). These "adhesive" clicks occur in isolation, after the period of clenching.[14] If adhesions occur in the superior or inferior joint space, translation or rotation

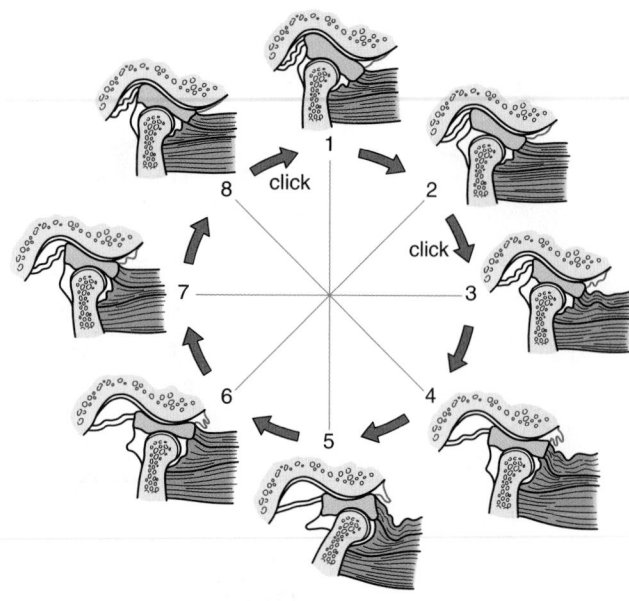

Figure 4-9

Reciprocal click. Between positions 2 and 3, a click is felt as the condyle moves across the posterior border of the disc. Normal condyle-disc function occurs during the remaining opening and closing movement until the closed joint position is approached. A second click is heard as the condyle once again moves from the intermediate zone to the posterior border of the disc between positions 8 and 1.

Figure 4-10

A, Adhesion in the superior joint space. **B,** The presence of the adhesion limits the joint to rotation only. **C,** If the adhesion is freed, normal translation can occur.

will be limited. This presents as a temporary closed lock, which then opens with a click.

If the articular eminence is abnormally developed (i.e., short, steep posterior slope or long, flat anterior slope), the maximum anterior movement of the disc may be reached before maximum translation of the condyle has occurred. As the condyle overrides the disc, a loud crack is heard, and the condyle-disc leaps or jogs (subluxes) forward.[14]

"Soft" or "popping" clicks that are sometimes heard in normal joints are caused by ligament movement, articular surface separation, or sucking of loose tissue behind the condyle as it moves forward. These clicks usually result from muscle incoordination. "Hard" or "cracking" clicks are more likely to indicate joint pathology or joint surface defects. Soft crepitus (like rubbing knuckles together) is a sound that sometimes

occurs in symptomless joints and is not necessarily an indication of pathology.[15] Hard crepitus (like a footstep on gravel) is indicative of arthritic changes in the joints. The clicking may be caused by uncoordinated muscle action of the lateral pterygoid muscles, a tear or perforation in the disc, osteoarthrosis, or occlusal imbalance. Normally, the upper head of the lateral pterygoid muscle pulls the disc forward. If the disc does not move first, the condyle clicks over the disc as it is pulled forward by the lower head of the lateral pterygoid muscle. Iglarsh and Snyder-Mackler[7] have divided disc displacement into four stages (Table 4-1).

7. *Has the mouth or jaw ever locked?* Locking may imply that the mouth does not fully open or it does not fully close and is often related to problems of the disc or joint degeneration. Locking is usually preceded by reciprocal clicking. If the jaw has locked in the closed position, the locking is probably caused by a disc, with the condyle being posterior or anteromedial to the disc. Even if translation is blocked (e.g., "locked" disc), the mandible can still open 30 mm by rotation. If there is functional dislocation of the disc with reduction (see Figure 4-8), the disc is usually positioned anteromedially, and opening is limited. The patient complains that the jaw "catches" sometimes, so the locking occurs only occasionally and, at those times, opening is limited. If there is functional anterior dislocation of the disc without reduction, a **closed lock** occurs. Closed lock implies there has been anterior and/ or medial displacement of the disc, so that the disc does not return to its normal position during the entire movement of the condyle. In this case, opening is limited to about 25 mm, the mandible deviates to the affected side (Figure 4-11), and lateral movement to the uninvolved side is reduced.[14] If locking occurs in the open position,

Table 4-1

Temporomandibular Disc Dysfunction

Stage	Characteristics
Stage 1	Disc slightly anterior and medial on mandibular condyle
	Inconsistent click (may or may not be present)
	Mild or no pain
Stage 2	Disc anterior and medial
	Reciprocal click present (early on opening, late on closing)
	Severe consistent pain
Stage 3	Reciprocal consistent click present (later on opening, earlier on closing)
	Most painful stage
Stage 4	Click rare (disc no longer relocates)
	No pain

Data from Iglarsh ZA, Snyder-Mackler L: Temporomandibular joint and the cervical spine. *In* Richardson JK, Iglarsh ZA (eds): *Clinical orthopedic physical therapy*, Philadelphia, 1994, WB Saunders.

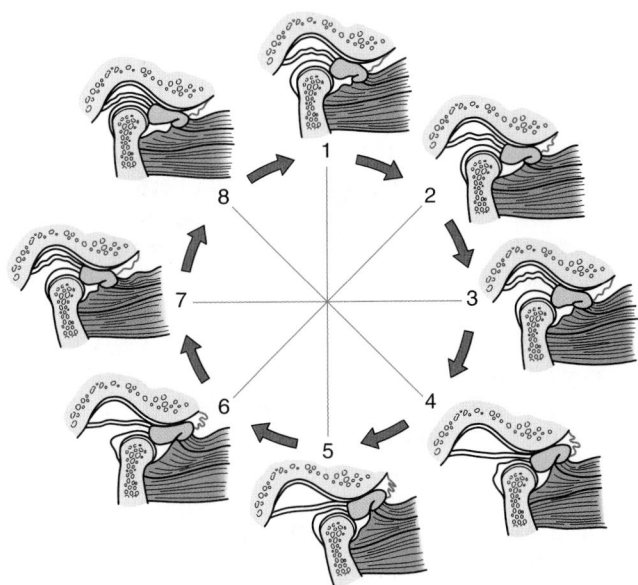

Figure 4-11

Closed lock. The condyle never assumes a normal relation to the disc but instead causes the disc to move forward ahead of it. This condition limits the distance the condyle can translate forward.

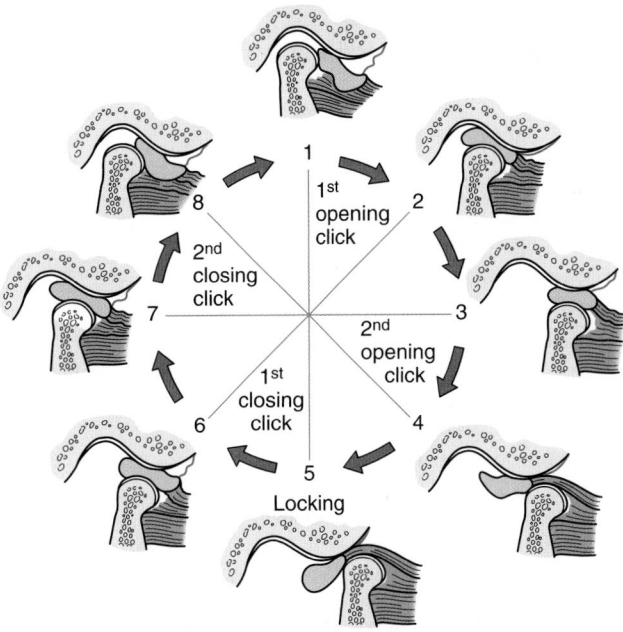

Figure 4-12

Open lock (disc incoordination). *1,* The disc always stays in anterior position with the jaw closed. *1–4,* Disc is displaced posterior to the condyle with one or two opening clicks. *5–6,* The disc disturbs jaw closing after maximum opening. *6-1,* The disc is again displaced to anterior position from the posterior with one or two clicks.

Figure 4-13

Normally the maxillary anterior teeth overlap the mandibular anterior teeth almost half the length of the mandibular crowns. (From Okeson JP: *Management of temporomandibular disorders and occlusion,* p. 84, St Louis, 1998, C.V. Mosby.)

it is probably caused by subluxation of the joint or possibly by posterior disc displacement (see Figure 4-11). With an **open lock,** there are two clicks on opening, when the condyle moves over the posterior rim of the disc and then when it moves over the anterior rim of the disc, and two clicks on closing. If, after the second click occurs on opening, the disc lies posterior to the condyle, it may not allow the condyle to slide back (Figure 4-12).[16] If the condyle dislocates outside the fossa, it is a true dislocation with open lock; the patient cannot close the mouth, and the dislocation must be reduced.[16]

8. *Does the patient have any habits such as smoking pipes, using a cigarette holder, leaning on the chin, chewing gum, biting the nails, chewing hair, pursing and chewing lips, continually moving the mouth, or any other nervous habits?* All these activities place additional stress on the temporomandibular joints.

9. *Does the patient grind the teeth or hold them tightly?* **Bruxism** is the forced clenching and grinding of the teeth, especially during sleep. This may lead to facial, jaw, or tooth pain, or headaches in the morning along with muscle hypertrophy. If the front teeth are in contact and the back ones are not, facial and temporomandibular pain may develop as a result of malocclusion. Normally, the upper teeth cover the upper one third of the bottom teeth (Figure 4-13).

10. *Does there appear to be any related psychosocial problems?* Temporomandibular dysfunction is often accompanied by related psychosocial issues.[1,17] Table 4-2 outlines psychosocial factors that may affect the temporomandibular joint.

11. *Are any teeth missing?* If so, which ones and how many? The presence or absence of teeth and their relation to one another must be noted on a table similar to the one shown in Figure 4-6. Their presence or absence can have an effect on the temporomandibular joints and their muscles. If some teeth are missing, others may deviate to fill in the space, altering the occlusion.

12. *Are any teeth painful or sensitive?* This finding may be indicative of dental caries or abscess. Tooth pain may lead to incorrect biting when chewing, which puts abnormal stresses on the temporomandibular joints.

13. *Does the patient have any difficulty swallowing?* Does the patient swallow normally or gulp? What happens

Table 4-2
Checklist of Psychological and Behavioral Factors*

1. Clinically significant anxiety or depression
2. Evidence of drug abuse
3. Repeated failures with conventional therapies
4. Evidence of secondary gain
5. Major life events (e.g., new job, marriage or divorce, death)
6. Pain duration greater than 6 months
7. History of possible stress-related disorders
8. Inconsistency in response to drugs
9. Inconsistent, inappropriate, and vague reports of pain, or both
10. Overdramatization of symptoms
11. Symptoms that vary with life events

(From McNeill C et al: Temporomandibular disorders: diagnosis, management, education and research, *J Am Dent Assoc* 120:259, 1990.)
*Note: The first two factors are the most significant and warrant further evaluation by a mental health professional; factors 3–6 need at least one more factor for consideration of referral; and factors 7–11 require three or more factors for consideration of referral to a mental health professional.

to the tongue when the patient swallows? Does it move normally, anteriorly, or laterally? Is there any evidence of tongue thrust or thumb sucking? For example, the facial nerve (cranial nerve VII) and the trigeminal nerve (cranial nerve V), which control facial expression and mastication and contribute to speech, also control anterior lip seal. If lip seal is weakened, the teeth may move anteriorly, an action that would be accentuated in "tongue thrusters." The normal resting position of the tongue is against the anterior palate (Figure 4-14). It is the position in which one would place the tongue to make a "clicking" sound.

14. *Are there any ear problems such as hearing loss, ringing in the ears, blocking of the ears, earache, or dizziness?* Symptoms such as these may be caused by inner ear, cervical spine, or temporomandibular joint problems.

15. *Does the patient have any habitual head postures?* For example, holding the telephone between the ear and the shoulder compacts the temporomandibular joint on that side. Reading or listening to someone while leaning one hand against the jaw has the same effect.

16. *Has the patient noticed any voice changes?* Changes may be caused by muscle spasm.

17. *Does the patient have headaches?* If so, where? Temporomandibular joint problems can refer pain to the head. Is there any history of infection or swollen glands?

18. *Does the patient ever feel dizzy or faint?*

19. *Has the patient ever worn a dental splint?* If so, when? For how long?

20. *Has the patient ever been seen by a dentist?* A periodontist (a dentist who specializes in the study of tissues around the teeth and diseases of these tissues)? An orthodontist (a dentist who specializes in correction and prevention of irregularities of the teeth)? An endodontist (a dentist who specializes in the treatment of diseases of the tooth pulp, root canal, and periapical areas)? If so, why did the patient see the specialist, and what was done?

Observation

When assessing the temporomandibular joints, the examiner must also assess the posture of the cervical spine and head. For example, it is necessary that the head be "balanced" on the cervical spine and be in proper postural alignment.

1. Is the face symmetrical horizontally and vertically, and are facial proportions normal (Figure 4-15)? The examiner should check the eyebrows, eyes, nose, ears, and corners of

A, Normal resting position of the tongue. Tongue position cannot be seen because of teeth. Upper and lower teeth are not in contact. **B,** Mouth opened to show tongue against upper anterior palate. This would not be considered the normal resting position because the mouth is open too much.

Figure 4-14

A   B

Figure 4-15

Facial symmetry. Look for symmetry both vertically and horizontally. Also note the changes in symmetry occurring with no smile (**A**) and smile (**B**).

the mouth for symmetry on both horizontal and vertical planes. Horizontally, the face of an adult is divided into thirds (Figure 4-16); this demonstrates normal vertical dimension. Usually the upper and lower teeth are used to measure vertical dimension. The horizontal bipupital, otic, and occlusive lines should be parallel to each other (Figure 4-17). Loss of teeth on one side can lead to convergence in which at least two of the lines may converge because the jaw line is short on one side relative to the other. A quick way to measure the vertical dimension is to measure from the lateral edge of the eye to the corner of the mouth and from the nose to the chin (Figure 4-18). Normally, the two measurements are equal. If the second measurement is smaller than the first by 1 mm or more, there has been a loss of vertical dimension, which may have resulted from loss of teeth, overbite, or temporomandibular joint dysfunction. In children, elderly persons, and those with massive tooth loss, the lower third of the face is not well developed (lack of teeth) or has recessed (Figure 4-19). As the teeth grow, the lower third develops into its normal proportion. The examiner should notice whether there is any paralysis, which could be indicated by **ptosis** (drooping of an eyelid) or by drooping of the mouth on one side (Bell's palsy).

2. The examiner should note whether the teeth are normally aligned or there is any crossbite, underbite, or overbite (Figure 4-20). With **crossbite,** the teeth of the mandible are lateral to the upper (maxillary) teeth on one side and medial on the opposite side. There is abnormal interdigitation of the teeth. With anterior crossbite, the

Figure 4-18

A quick measurement of vertical dimension. Normally, the distance from the lateral edge of the eye to the corner of the mouth equals the distance from nose to point of chin.

Figure 4-16

Divisions of the face (vertical dimension).

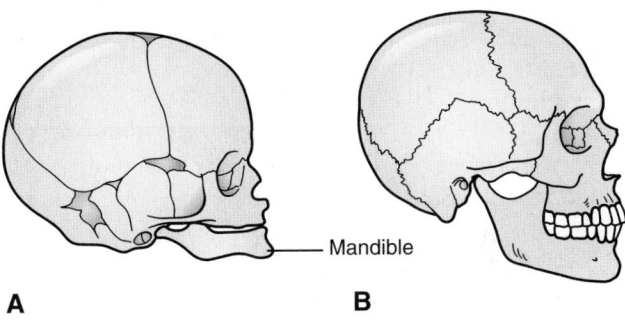

A   B

Figure 4-19

Human skull at birth (**A**) and in the adult (**B**). Note the difference brought about by development of the teeth and lower jaw in the adult.

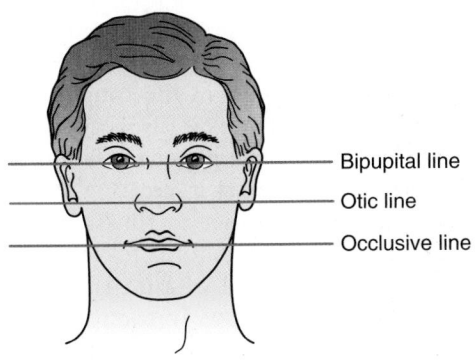

Figure 4-17

Normally, bipupital, otic, and occlusive lines are parallel.

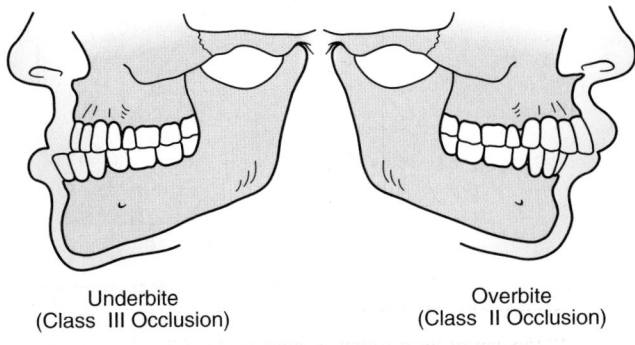

Underbite   Overbite
(Class III Occlusion)   (Class II Occlusion)

Figure 4-20

Underbite and overbite.

lower incisors are ahead of the upper incisors. With posterior crossbite, there is a transverse abnormal relation of the teeth. In **underbite,** the mandibular teeth are unilaterally, bilaterally, or in pairs in **buccoversion** (i.e., they lie anterior to the maxillary teeth). In **overbite,** the anterior maxillary incisors extend below the anterior mandibular incisors when the jaw is in centric occlusion. A small amount of overbite (2–3 mm) anteriorly is the most common position of the teeth. This is because the maxillary arch is slightly longer than the mandibular arch. **Overjet** (Figure 4-21) is the distance that the maxillary incisors close over the mandibular incisors when the mouth is closed. This distance is normally 2 to 3 mm. **Occlusal interference** refers to premature teeth contact, which tends to deflect the jaw laterally and/or anteriorly.[18] Any orthodontic appliances or false teeth present should also be evaluated for fit and possible sore spots.

3. The examiner should note whether there is any **malocclusion** that may result in a faulty bite. Malocclusion may be a major factor in the development of disc problems of the temporomandibular joints. Occlusion occurs when the teeth are in contact and the mouth is closed. Malocclusion is defined as any deviation from normal occlusion. Class I occlusion refers to the normal anteroposterior relation of the maxillary teeth to mandibular teeth. A slight modification with only the incisors affected

and overjet slightly larger is sometimes classified as a Class I malocclusion. Class II malocclusion (overbite) occurs when the mandibular teeth are positioned posterior to their normal position relative to the maxillary teeth. This malocclusion deformity involves all the teeth, including the molars. The designation Class II Division 1 malocclusion (also called large overjet or **horizontal overlap**) indicates that the maxillary incisors demonstrate significant overjet. Class II Division 2 malocclusion (also called deep overbite or **vertical overlap**) implies that overjet is not significant but that there is overbite and lateral flaring of the lateral maxillary incisors.[19] Class III malocclusion (i.e., underbite) occurs when the mandibular teeth are positioned anterior to their normal position relative to the maxillary teeth. If maxillary and mandibular teeth are on the same vertical plane, a Class III malocclusion would be present.

4. What is the facial profile? The orthognathic profile is the normal, "straight-jawed" form. With this facial profile, a vertical line dropped perpendicular to the bipupital line would touch the upper and lower lips and the tip of the chin. In a person with a retrognathic profile, the chin would lie behind the vertical line and the person would be said to have a "receding chin." With the prognathic profile, the chin would be in front of the vertical line and the person would have a protruded or "strong" chin (Figure 4-22).[19]

5. The examiner should note whether the patient demonstrates normal bony and soft-tissue contours. When the patient bites down, do the masseter muscles bulge as they normally should? Hypertrophy caused by overuse may lead to abnormal wear of the teeth. When looking at the soft tissues, it is important to note symmetry. The upper lip should normally cover two thirds of the maxillary teeth at rest. If it does not, the lip is said to be short.[7] If the lip can be drawn over the upper teeth, however, the upper lip is said to be functional and no treatment is necessary. The lower lip normally covers the mandibular teeth and, when the mouth is closed, part of the maxillary teeth.

6. Is the patient able to move the tongue properly? Can the patient move the tongue up to and against the palate? Can the tongue be protruded or rolled? Is the patient able to "click" the tongue? **Tongue thrusting** refers to forward movement of the tongue, usually to push against the lower teeth; it also occurs when the tongue is pushed against the upper teeth and the lower teeth are closed firmly against it, creating an oral seal.[20] Tongue thrusters find it easier to thrust the tongue if the head is protruded. Therefore, to test for tongue thrusting, the patient's head posture is corrected and the patient is asked to swallow. In the tongue thruster, swallowing causes the tongue to move forward resulting in protrusion of the head. Tongue thrusting may be due to hyperactivity of the masticatory muscles. When

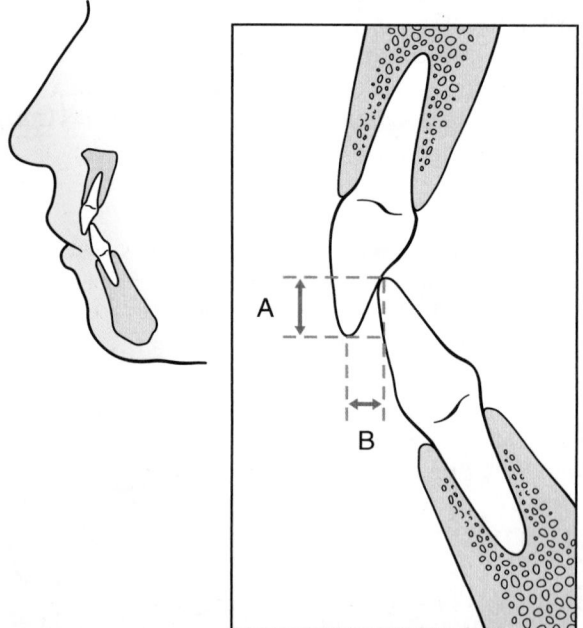

Figure 4-21

Overlap of maxillary anterior teeth. **A,** Vertical overlap (overbite). **B,** Horizontal overlap (overjet). (Redrawn from Friedman MH, Weisberg J: The temporomandibular joint. *In* Gould JA [ed]: *Orthopedics and sports physical therapy,* p. 578, St Louis, 1990, C.V. Mosby.)

Orthognathic

Retrognathic

Prognathic

Figure 4-22
Facial profiles.

one swallows, the hyoid bone should move up and down quickly. If it moves only upward and slowly, and the suboccipital muscles posteriorly contract, it is suggestive of a tongue thrust.[21]

7. Where does the tongue rest? Is the tongue bitten frequently? Does the tongue have any scalloping or ridges? Does the patient swallow normally? Do the lips part when swallowing? What is the tongue position when swallowing? Do the facial muscles tighten on swallowing? All of these factors give the examiner some idea of the mobility of the structures of the mouth and jaw and their neurological mechanisms.

Examination

The examiner must remember that many problems of the temporomandibular joints may be the result of or related to problems in the cervical spine or teeth. Therefore, the cervical spine is at least partially included in any temporomandibular assessment.

Active Movements

With the patient in the sitting position, the examiner watches the active movements, noting whether they deviate from what would be considered normal range of motion and whether the patient is willing to do the movement. The patient is first asked to carry out active movements of the cervical spine. The most painful movements, if any, should be done last.

Active Movements of the Cervical Spine
• Flexion • Extension • Side flexion left and right • Rotation left and right • Combined movements (if necessary) • Repetitive movements (if necessary) • Sustained positions (if necessary)

During flexion of the neck, the mandible moves up and forward, and the posterior structures of the neck become tight. During extension, the mandible moves down and back and the anterior structures of the neck become tight. The examiner should note whether the patient can flex and extend the neck while keeping the mouth closed or whether the patient must open the mouth to do these movements. The patient should be asked to place a fist under the chin and then open the mouth while keeping the fist in place and the lower jaw against it. If the mouth opens in this way, movement of the neck into extension is occurring because the head is rotating backwards on the temporomandibular condyles. This test movement would be especially important if the patient subjectively feels that there is a loss of neck extension. With side flexion of the neck to the right, maximum occlusion occurs on the right. Side flexion and rotation of the neck occur to the same side, so that if these movements are carried out to the right, maximum occlusion also occurs to the right.

Having observed the neck movements, the examiner goes on to note the active movements of the temporomandibular joints. The movements of the mandible can be measured with a millimeter ruler, depth gauge, or Vernier calipers. When using the ruler, the examiner should pick a midline point from which to measure opening and lateral deviation.[22] This same ruler can be used to measure protrusion and retrusion.

Active Movements of the Temporomandibular Joints
• Opening of the mouth • Closing of the mouth • Protrusion of the mandible • Lateral deviation of the mandible right and left

Opening and Closing of the Mouth

With opening and closing of the mouth, the normal arc of movement of the jaw is smooth and unbroken; that is, both temporomandibular joints are working in unison with no asymmetry or sideways movement, and both joints are bilaterally rotating and translating equally. Any alteration may cause or indicate potential problems in the temporomandibular joints. To observe any asymmetries, opening and closing of the mouth must be done slowly. The first phase of opening is rotation, which can be tested by having the patient open the mouth as widely as possible while maintaining the tongue against the roof (hard palate) of the mouth. Usually this movement causes minimal pain and occurs even in the presence of acute temporomandibular dysfunction. The second phase of opening is translation and rotation as the condyles move along the slope of the eminence. This phase begins when the tongue loses contact with the roof of the mouth.[2] Most of the clicking sensations occur during this phase.

Normally, the mandible should open and close in a straight line (Figures 4-23 and 4-24), provided the bilateral action of the muscles is equal and the inert tissues have normal pliability. If deviation occurs to the left on opening (see Figure 4-23), (a C-type curve) or to the right (a reverse C-type curve), hypomobility is evident toward the side of the deviation caused either by a displaced disc without reduction or unilateral muscle hypomobility[9]; if the deviation is an S-type or reverse S-type curve, the problem is probably muscular imbalance or medial displacement as the condyle "walks around" the disc on the affected side.[9] The chin deviates toward the affected side, usually because of spasm of the pterygoid or masseter muscles or an obstruction in the joint. Early deviation on opening is usually caused by muscle spasm,

Figure 4-24

Active opening of mouth. **A,** Anteroposterior view. **B,** Side view.

whereas late deviation on opening is usually a result of capsulitis or a tight capsule. Pain or tenderness, especially on closing, indicates posterior capsulitis.

The examiner should then determine whether the patient's mouth can functionally be opened. The **functional or full active opening** is determined by having the patient try to place two or three flexed proximal interphalangeal joints within the mouth opening (Figure 4-25).[23] This opening should be approximately 35 to 55 mm.[3] Normally, only about 25 to 35 mm of opening is needed for everyday activity. If the patient has pain on opening, the examiner should also measure the amount of opening to the point of pain and compare this distance with functional opening.[8] If the space is less than this, the temporomandibular joints are said to

NORMAL OPENING   ABNORMAL OPENING   ABNORMAL CLOSED

Figure 4-23

Mandibular motion.

Figure 4-25
Functional opening "knuckle" test.

be hypomobile. Kropmans et al[24] have pointed out that for treatment, at least 6 mm of change has to be seen to be a detectable difference when doing more than one measurement or to determine the effect of treatment.

As the mouth opens, the examiner should palpate the external auditory meatus with the index or little finger (fleshy part anterior). The patient is then asked to close the mouth. When the examiner first feels the condyle touch the finger, the temporomandibular joints are in the resting position. This resting position of the temporomandibular joints is called the **freeway space,** or **interocclusal space.** The freeway space is the potential space or vertical distance that is found between the teeth when the mandible is in the resting position. To determine the freeway space, the examiner marks a point on the chin and a point vertically above on the upper lip below the nose. The patient closes the mouth into centric occlusion, and the distance between the two points is measured. Then the patient is asked to say three simple words (e.g., "boy, boy, boy") and then maintain this position of the jaw without moving. The distance between the two points is measured again. The difference between the two measurements is the freeway space.[18] Normally, the space between the front teeth at this point is 2 to 4 mm.

If rotation does not occur at the temporomandibular joint, the mouth cannot open fully. There may be gliding at the temporomandibular joint, but rotation has not occurred. If translation (gliding) does not occur, the mandible may still open up to 30 mm as a result of rotation. Normally, when the mouth opens, the disc moves forward approximately 7 mm, and the condyle moves forward approximately 14 mm.[25]

If clicking (see 6. under History) occurs on opening, the examiner should ask the patient to open the mouth with the jaw protruded and retruded. If the clicking is eliminated with protrusion and accentuated with retrusion, it is likely the problem is an anterior disc displacement with reduction.[26] Anterior disc displacement without reduction cannot be determined as confidently.[27]

Protrusion of the Mandible

The examiner asks the patient to protrude or jut the lower jaw out past the upper teeth. The patient should be able to do this without difficulty. The normal movement is >7 mm, measured from the resting position to the protruded position.[3] The normal values vary depending on the degree of overbite (greater movement) or underbite (less movement).

Retrusion of the Mandible

The examiner asks the patient to retrude or pull the lower jaw in or back as far as possible. In full retention or centric relation, the temporomandibular joint is in a close packed position. The normal movement is 3 to 4 mm.[10]

Lateral Deviation or Excursion of the Mandible

For lateral deviation, the teeth are slightly disoccluded and the patient moves the mandible laterally, first to one side and then to the other. With the joints in the resting position, two points are picked on the upper and lower teeth that are at the same level. When the mandible is laterally deviated, the two points, which have moved apart, are measured, giving the amount of lateral deviation. The normal lateral deviation is 10 to 15 mm.[3] During lateral deviation, the opposite condyle moves forward, down, and toward the motion side. The condyle on the motion side (e.g., left condyle on left lateral deviation) remains relatively stationary and becomes more prominent.[10] Any lateral deviation from the normal opening position or abnormal protrusion to one side indicates that the lateral pterygoid, masseter, or temporalis muscle, the disc, or the lateral ligament on the opposite side is affected.

When charting any changes, the examiner should note the type of opening deviation as well as the functional opening and any lateral deviation (Figure 4-26).

Mandibular Measurement

Next, the examiner should measure the mandible from the posterior aspect of the temporomandibular joint to the notch of the chin (Figure 4-27). Both sides are measured and compared for equality (the normal distance is 10–12 cm). Any difference indicates a developmental problem or structural change leading to left or right convergence; the patient may not be able to obtain balancing in the midline.

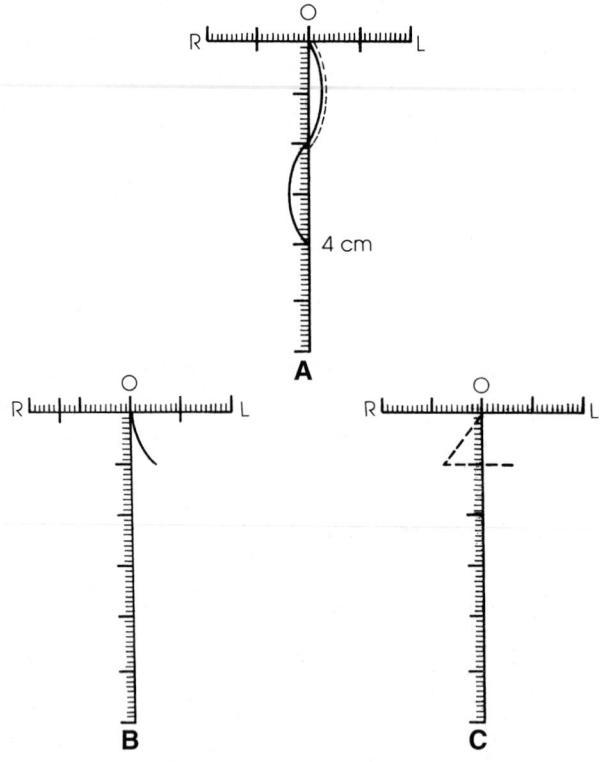

Figure 4-26

Charting temporomandibular motion. **A,** Deviation to both right *(R)* and left *(L)* on opening; maximum opening, 4 cm; lateral deviation equal (1 cm each direction); protrusion on functional opening *(dashed lines)*. **B,** Capsule-ligamentous pattern; opening limited to 1 cm; lateral deviation greater to R than L; deviation to L on opening. **C,** Protrusion is 1 cm; lateral deviation to R on protrusion (indicates weak lateral pterygoid on opposite side).

Figure 4-27

Measurement of the mandible.

Swallowing and Tongue Position

The patient is asked to relax and then swallow. The patient is asked to leave the tongue in the position it assumed when swallowing occurred. The examiner, wearing rubber gloves, then separates the lips and notes the position of the tongue (between teeth? at upper anterior palate?).[18]

Cranial Nerve Testing

If injury to the cranial nerves is suspected, the cranial nerves should be tested.

Cranial Nerve Testing	
CN I:	Smell coffee or some similar substance with eyes closed
CN II (optic nerve):	Read something with one eye closed
CN III, IV, VI:	Eye movements; note any ptosis
CN V (trigeminal nerve):	Contract muscles of mastication (masseter and temporalis)
CN VII (facial nerve):	Move eyebrows up and down, purse lips, show teeth. This cranial nerve is the most commonly injured one. If the patient is unable to whistle or wink or close an eye on one side, the symptoms may be indicative of Bell's palsy (paralysis of the facial nerve).
CN VIII (auditory nerve):	Eyes closed; talk to patient and have him or her repeat what was said
CN IX:	Have patient swallow
CN X (vagus nerve):	Have patient swallow
CN XI (spinal accessory):	Have patient contract sternomastoid
CN XII:	Have patient stick out tongue, move it to right and left

Passive Movements

Very seldom are passive movements carried out for the temporomandibular joints except when the examiner is attempting to determine the end feel of the joints. The amount of passive opening (full passive stretch) may also be measured and compared with functional opening amount.[8] The normal end feel of these joints is tissue stretch on opening and teeth contact ("bone to bone") on closing. When the teeth are in maximum contact, the horizontal overjet is sometimes measured. The overjet is the horizontal distance from the edge of the upper central incisors to the lower central incisors (see Figure 4-21). If the lower teeth extend over the upper teeth, this malocclusion condition is called an underbite. Overbite is the vertical overlap of the teeth.

Normal End Feel at the Temporomandibular Joints

- Opening: Tissue stretch
- Closing: Bone to bone

Resisted Isometric Movements

Resisted isometric movements of the temporomandibular joints are relatively difficult to test. The jaw should be in the resting position. The examiner applies firm but gentle resistance to the joints and asks the patient to hold the position, saying "Don't let me move you."

Resisted Isometric Movements of the Temporomandibular Joints

- Depression (opening)
- Occlusion (closing)
- Lateral deviation left and right

1. Opening of the mouth (depression). This movement may be tested by applying resistance at the chin or, using a rubber glove, over the teeth with one hand while the other hand rests behind the head or neck or over the forehead to stabilize the head (Figure 4-28, *A*; Table 4-3).
2. Closing of the mouth (elevation or occlusion). One hand is placed over the back of the head or neck to stabilize the head while the other hand is placed under the chin of the patient's slightly open mouth to resist the movement (see Figure 4-28, *B*). In a second method, the examiner uses a rubber glove and places two fingers over the patient's lower teeth (mandible) to resist the movement (see Figure 4-28, *C*).
3. Lateral deviation of the jaw. One of the examiner's hands is placed over the side of the head above the temporomandibular joint to stabilize the head. The other hand is placed along the jaw of the patient's slightly open mouth, and the patient pushes out against it (see Figure 4-28, *D*). Both sides are tested individually.

Functional Assessment

After the basic movements of the temporomandibular joints have been tested, the examiner should test functional activities or activities of daily living involving the use of the temporomandibular joints. These activities include chewing, swallowing, coughing, talking, and blowing. If the patient complains of pain while eating, the examiner can ask the patient to bite down on a tongue depressor held between the teeth in different positions to see if the compressive movement is painful in the teeth or temporomandibular joint. Biting down on one side stresses the temporomandibular joint on the opposite side.[6]

Special Tests

There are no routine special tests for the temporomandibular joints. The **Chvostek test** may be used to determine whether there is pathology involving the seventh cranial (facial) nerve (Figure 4-29). The examiner taps the parotid gland overlying the masseter muscle. If the facial muscles twitch, the test is considered positive.

If the patient is suffering from a facial nerve injury (Bell's palsy), the examiner may use the facial nerve grading system (see Table 2-21) developed by the American Academy of Otolaryngology.[8]

The examiner can listen to (auscultate) the temporomandibular joints during movement (Figure 4-30). The movements "listened to" include opening and closing of the mouth, lateral deviation of the mandible to the right and left, and mandibular protrusion. Normally, a sound would be heard only on occlusion. This is a single, solid sound, not a "slipping" sound. A slipping sound could occur if the teeth are not "hitting" simultaneously. The most common joint noise is reciprocal clicking (see Figure 4-9), which occurs when the mouth opens and when it closes. The clicking is clinical evidence that the condyle is slipping over the disc and then self-reducing. The opening click results when the condyle slips under the posterior aspect of the disc (reduces) or slips anterior to the disc (subluxes) on opening. The second click, which is quieter, occurs when the condyle slips posterior to the disc (subluxes) or into its proper position and reduces. A single click may occur if the condyle gets caught behind the disc on opening (see Figure 4-7) or if the condyle slips behind the disc on closing. On opening, the later the click occurs, the more anterior lies the disc. The later the opening click, the more the disc is displaced anteriorly and the more likely it is to lock. A closing click is usually caused by loosening of the structures attaching the disc to the condyle. Clicking is more likely to occur in hypermobile joints.[28,29]

Grating noise (crepitus) is usually indicative of degenerative joint disease or a perforation in the disc. Painful crepitus usually means that the disc has eroded, the condyle bone and temporal bone are rubbing together, and much of the fibrocartilage has been lost. While the examiner is listening, each movement should be done four or five times to ensure a correct diagnosis.

The reliability, validity, specificity, and sensitivity of some special/diagnostic tests used in the temporomandibular joint are outlined in Appendix 4-1.

Figure 4-28

Resisted isometric movements for the muscles controlling the temporomandibular joint. **A,** Opening of the mouth (depression). **B,** Closing of the mouth (elevation or occlusion). **C,** Closing of the mouth (alternative method). **D,** Lateral deviation of the jaw.

Table 4-3

Muscles of the Temporomandibular Joint: Their Actions and Nerve Supply

Action	Muscles Acting	Nerve Supply
Opening of mouth (depression of mandible)	1. Lateral (external) pterygoid	Mandibular (CN V)
	2. Mylohyoid*	Inferior alveolar (CN V)
	3. Geniohyoid*	Hypoglossal (CN XII)
	4. Digastric*	Inferior alveolar (CN V)
		Facial (CN VII)
Closing of mouth (elevation of mandible or occlusion)	1. Masseter	Mandibular (CN V)
	2. Temporalis	Mandibular (CN V)
	3. Medial (internal) pterygoid	Mandibular (CN V)
Protrusion of mandible	1. Lateral (external) pterygoid	Mandibular (CN V)
	2. Medial (internal) pterygoid	Mandibular (CN V)
	3. Masseter*	Mandibular (CN V)
	4. Mylohyoid*	Inferior alveolar (CN V)
	5. Geniohyoid*	Hypoglossal (CN XII)
	6. Digastric*	Inferior alveolar (CN V)
		Facial (CN VII)
	7. Stylohyoid*	Facial (CN VII)
	8. Temporalis (anterior fibers)*	Mandibular (CN V)
Retraction of mandible	1. Temporalis (posterior fibers)	Mandibular (CN V)
	2. Masseter*	Mandibular (CN V)
	3. Digastric*	Inferior alveolar (CN V)
		Facial (CN VII)
	4. Stylohyoid*	Inferior alveolar (CN VII)
	5. Mylohyoid*	Inferior alveolar (CN V)
	6. Geniohyoid*	Hypoglossal (CN XII)
Lateral deviation of mandible	1. Lateral (external) pterygoid (ipsilateral muscle)	Mandibular (CN V)
	2. Medial (internal) pterygoid (contralateral muscle)	Mandibular (CN V)
	3. Temporalis*	Mandibular (CN V)
	4. Masseter*	Mandibular (CN V)

CN, Cranial nerve.
*Act only when assistance is required.

Figure 4-29
Chvostek test.

Reflexes and Cutaneous Distribution

The reflex of the temporomandibular joints is called the **jaw reflex.** The examiner's thumb is placed on the chin of the patient with the patient's mouth relaxed and open in the resting position. The patient is asked to close the eyes. If this is not done, the patient commonly tenses as he or she sees the reflex hammer being swung toward the examiner's thumb or the tongue depressor and the test does not work. The examiner then taps the thumbnail with a neurological hammer (Figure 4-31, *A*). The jaw reflex may also be tested by using a tongue depressor (Figure 4-31, *B*). The examiner holds the tongue depressor firmly against the bottom teeth; while the patient relaxes the jaw muscles, the examiner taps the tongue depressor with the reflex hammer. The reflex closes the mouth and is a test of cranial nerve V.

The examiner must be aware of the dermatome patterns for the head and neck (Figure 4-32) as well as the sensory

Figure 4-30
Auscultation of the left temporomandibular joint.

A   **B**

Figure 4-31
Testing of the jaw reflex. **A,** Hitting examiner's thumb. **B,** Hitting tongue depressor.

nerve distribution of the peripheral nerves (see Figure 3-62). Pain may be referred from the temporomandibular joint to the teeth, neck, or head, and vice versa (Figure 4-33). Table 4-4 shows the muscles of the temporomandibular joint and their referral of pain.

Joint Play Movements

The joint play movements of the temporomandibular joints are then tested. Pain on performing these tests may indicate articular problems or pathology to the retrodiscal tissues.[30]

Figure 4-32
Dermatomes of the head.

Longitudinal Cephalad and Anterior Glide. Wearing rubber gloves, the examiner places the thumb on the patient's lower teeth inside the mouth with the index finger on the mandible outside the mouth. The mandible is then distracted by pushing down with the thumb and pulling down and forward with the index finger while the other fingers push against the chin, acting as a pivot point. The examiner should feel the tissue stretch of the joint. Each joint is done individually while the other hand and arm stabilize the head (Figure 4-34, *A*).

Lateral Glide of the Mandible. The patient lies supine with the mouth slightly open and the mandible relaxed. The examiner places the thumb inside the mouth along the medial side of the mandible and teeth. By pushing the thumb laterally, the mandible glides laterally.[21] Each joint is done individually (Figure 4-34, *B*).

Medial Glide of the Mandible. The patient is in side lying with the mandible relaxed. The examiner places the thumb (or overlapping thumbs) over the lateral aspect of the mandibular condyle outside the mouth

and applies a medial pressure to the condyle, gliding the condyle medially.[21] Each joint is done individually (Figure 4-34, *C*).

Posterior Glide of the Mandible. The patient is in side lying with the mandible relaxed. The examiner places the thumb (or overlapping thumbs) over the anterior aspect of the mandibular condyle outside the mouth and applies a posterior pressure to the condyle, gliding the condyle posteriorly.[21] Each joint is done individually (Figure 4-34, *D*).

Palpation

To palpate the **temporomandibular joints**, the examiner places the fingers (padded part anteriorly) in the patient's external auditory canals and asks the patient to actively open and close the mouth. As this is being done, the examiner determines whether both sides are moving simultaneously and whether the movement is smooth. If the patient feels pain on closing, the posterior capsule is usually involved.

The examiner then places the index fingers over the mandibular condyles and feels for elicited pain or tenderness on opening and closing of the mouth. The examiner

Figure 4-33
Referred pain patterns to and from the temporomandibular joint in the teeth, head, and neck.

Table 4-4

Temporomandibular Muscles and Referral of Pain

Muscle	Referral Pattern
Masseter	Cheek, mandible to forehead or ear
Temporalis	Maxilla to forehead and side of head above ear
Medial pterygoid	Posterior mandible to temporomandibular joint
Lateral pterygoid	Cheek to temporomandibular joint
Digastric	Lateral cervical spine to posterolateral skull
Occipitofrontal	Above eye, over eyelid, and up over lateral aspect of skull

Figure 4-34

Joint play of the temporomandibular joints when each side is tested individually. **A,** Longitudinal cephalad and anterior glide. **B,** Lateral glide of the mandible. Examiner pushes mandible laterally. **C,** Medial glide of the mandible. Examiner pushes mandible medially while palpating temporomandibular joint with other thumb. **D,** Posterior glide of the mandible. Examiner pushes mandible posteriorly while palpating temporomandibular joint with other thumb.

may also palpate the medial pterygoid, the medial and lower border of the inferior head of the lateral pterygoid, the temporalis and its tendon, and the masseter muscles and any other soft tissues for tenderness or indications of pathology (Figure 4-35). This procedure is followed by palpation of the following structures.

Mandible. The examiner palpates the mandible along its entire length, feeling for any differences between the left and right sides. As the examiner moves along the superior aspect of the angle of the mandible, the fingers pass over the parotid gland. Normally, the gland is not palpable, but with pathology (e.g., mumps), the site feels "boggy" rather than having the normal hard and bony feel.

Teeth. The examiner should note the position, absence, or tenderness of the teeth. The examiner wears

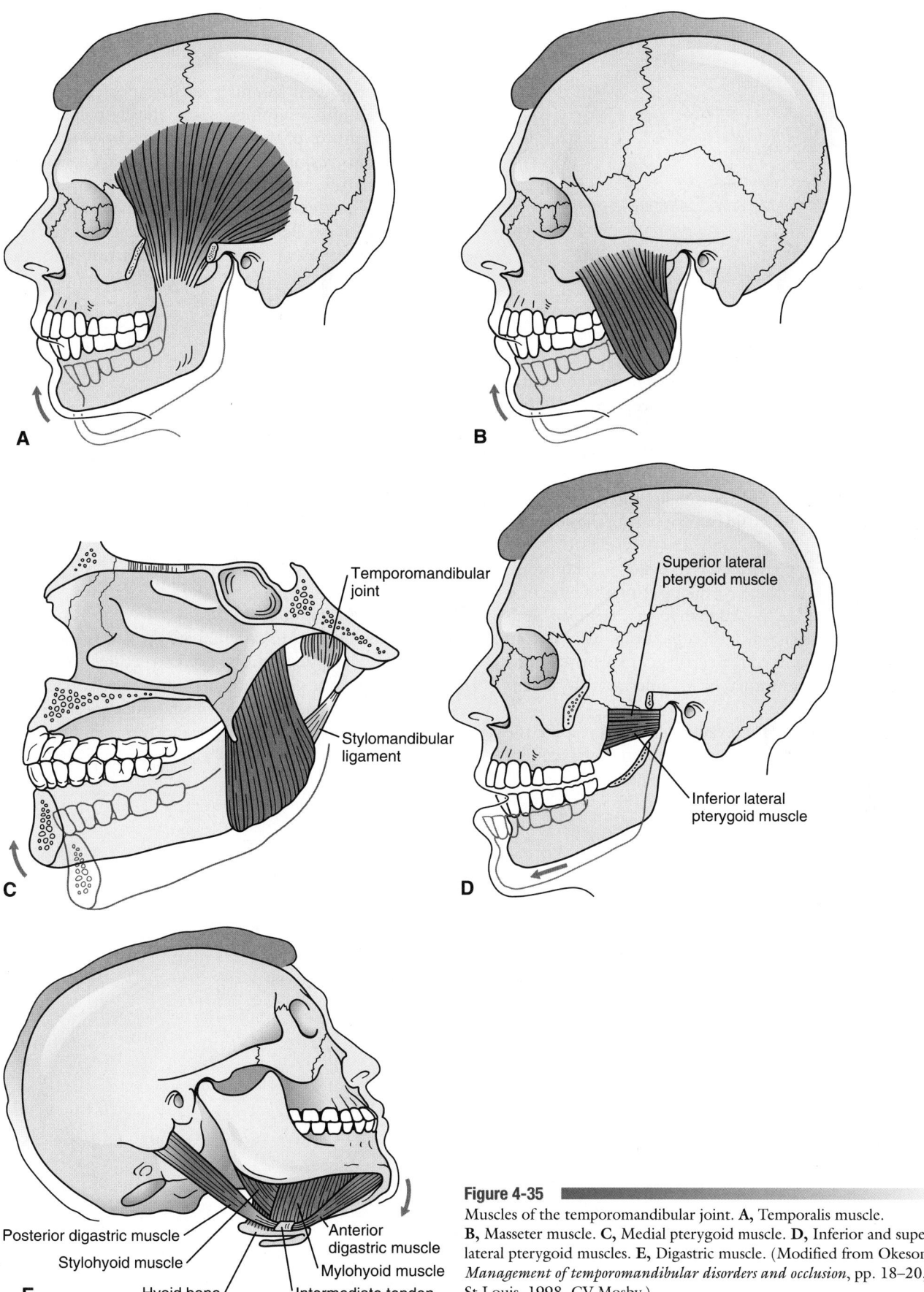

Figure 4-35

Muscles of the temporomandibular joint. **A,** Temporalis muscle.
B, Masseter muscle. **C,** Medial pterygoid muscle. **D,** Inferior and superior
lateral pterygoid muscles. **E,** Digastric muscle. (Modified from Okeson JP:
Management of temporomandibular disorders and occlusion, pp. 18–20, 22,
St Louis, 1998, CV Mosby.)

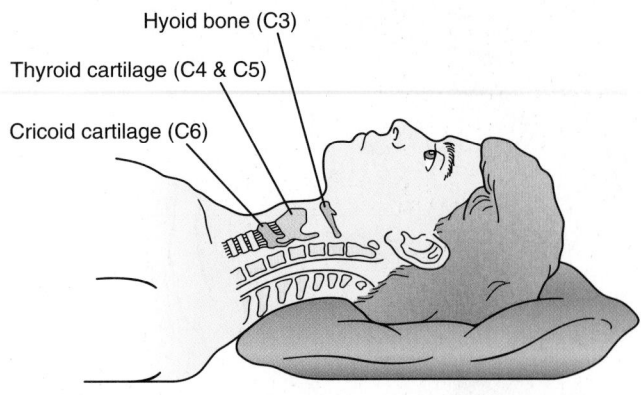

Hyoid bone (C3)

Thyroid cartilage (C4 & C5)

Cricoid cartilage (C6)

Figure 4-36

Position of hyoid bone, thyroid cartilage, and cricoid cartilage.

a rubber glove and palpates inside the patient's mouth. At the same time, the interior cheek region and gums may be palpated for pathology.

Hyoid Bone (Anterior to C2-C3 Vertebrae). While palpating the hyoid bone (Figure 4-36), the examiner asks the patient to swallow. Normally, the bone moves and causes no pain. The hyoid bone is part of the superior trachea.

Thyroid Cartilage (Anterior to C4-C5 Vertebrae). While the neck is in the neutral position, the thyroid cartilage can be easily moved; while in extension, it is tight and the examiner may feel crepitations. The thyroid gland, which is adjacent to the cartilage, may be palpated at the same time. If abnormal or inflamed, it will be tender and enlarged.

Mastoid Processes. The examiner should palpate the skull, following the posterior aspect of the ear. The examiner

will come to a point on the skull where the finger dips inward. The point just before the dip is the mastoid process (see Figure 3-70).

Cervical Spine. Beginning on the posterior aspect at the occiput, the examiner systematically palpates the posterior structures of the neck (spinous processes, facet joints, and muscles of the suboccipital region), working from the head toward the shoulders. On the lateral aspect, the transverse processes of the vertebrae, the lymph nodes (palpable only if swollen), and the muscles should be palpated for tenderness. A more detailed description of the palpation of these structures is given in Chapter 3.

Diagnostic Imaging

Plain Film Radiography

On the anteroposterior view, the examiner should look for condylar shape and normal contours. On the lateral view, the examiner should look for condylar shape and contours, position of condylar heads in the opened and closed positions (Figure 4-37), amount of condylar movement (closed versus open), and relation of temporomandibular joint to other bony structures of the skull and cervical spine (Figure 4-38).

Magnetic Resonance Imaging

This technique is used to differentiate the soft tissue of the joint, mainly the disc, from the bony structures and therefore has become the gold standard for testing the reliability of clinical findings in the temporomandibular joint.[31] It has the advantage of using nonionizing radiation (Figures 4-39 and 4-40).

Condyle

External auditory meatus

Neck of condyle

Mastoid air cells

Articular eminence

A

Mandibular fossa

Articular eminence

External auditory meatus

Mastoid air cells

Condyle

Neck of condyle

B

Figure 4-37

Radiographs of the right temporomandibular joint. **A,** Mouth closed. **B,** Mouth open. (From Liebgott B: *The anatomical basis of dentistry*, p. 295, St Louis, 1986, C.V. Mosby, Courtesy of Dr. Friedman.)

Figure 4-38

Lateral radiograph of the skull, left temporomandibular joint, and cervical spine.

Figure 4-39

Acute temporomandibular joint lock from a nonreducing displaced disc. **A,** T1-weighted sagittal spin echo MR image with the mouth closed shows the dislocated disc *(arrow)* anterior to the condyle. **B,** With attempted mouth opening, no appreciable anterior translation of the condyle occurs, but the disc folds on itself in the thin intermediate zone because of increased pressure from the condyle. The normal biconcave configuration of the disc and the normal intradiscal signal intensity are maintained *(arrow)*. (From Resnick D, Kransdorf MJ: *Bone and joint imaging*, p. 516, Philadelphia, 2005, W.B. Saunders.)

Figure 4-40

MR imaging of the temporomandibular joint (TMJ). **A,** T1-weighted sagittal spin echo MR image of a normal TMJ. View with the mouth closed shows high signal intensity from the condylar marrow *(C)* and articular eminence *(E)*. Surrounding cortical bone is devoid of signal. The disc, of low signal intensity, is interposed between the condyle and the fossa; the intermediate zone articulates with the condyle and eminence where they are most closely apposed. The *solid arrow* points to the anterior band and the *open arrow* to the posterior band of the disc. **B,** Sagittal gradient echo MR image used for fast (pseudodynamic) scanning shows a normal position of the disc with the mouth closed. Marrow becomes low in signal intensity with this sequence, and fluid in the inferior joint space becomes bright *(arrows)*; the disc remains low in signal intensity. *C,* Condyle; *E,* eminence.

Figure 4-40

Continued **C,** Sagittal gradient image of a normal TMJ with the mouth open. The intermediate zone of the disc maintains its position between the condyle *(C)* and the eminence *(E)*, whereas the posterior band slides posterior to the condyle *(arrow)*. **D,** T1-weighted sagittal spin echo MR image in a patient with clicking and pain demonstrates internal derangement, with both the anterior *(solid arrow)* and posterior *(open arrow)* bands of the disc displaced anteriorly relative to the condyle *(C)*. (From Resnick D, Kransdorf MJ: *Bone and joint imaging*, p. 509, Philadelphia, 2005, W.B. Saunders.)

Précis of the Temporomandibular Joint Assessment*

History
Observation
Examination

Active movements

Neck flexion
Neck extension
Neck side flexion (left and right)
Neck rotation (left and right)
Extend neck by opening mouth
Assess functional opening
Assess freeway space
Open mouth
Closed mouth (occlusion)
Measure protrusion of mandible
Measure retrusion of mandible
Measure lateral deviation of mandible
   (left and right)

Measure mandibular length
Swallowing and tongue position
Cranial nerve testing (if necessary)
Passive movements (as in active movements, if necessary)
Resisted isometric movements

Open mouth
Closed mouth (occlusion)
Lateral deviation of jaw

Special tests
Reflexes and cutaneous distribution
Joint play movements
Palpation
Diagnostic imaging

---

*Usually the entire assessment is done with the patient sitting. After any examination, the patient should be warned of the possibility of exacerbation of symptoms as a result of the assessment.

Case Studies

When doing these case studies, the examiner should list the appropriate questions to be asked and why they are being asked, what to look for and why, and what things should be tested and why. Depending on the answers of the patient (and the examiner should consider different responses), several possible causes of the patient's problem may become evident (examples are given in parentheses). A differential diagnosis chart should be made up (see Table 4-5 as an example). The examiner can then decide how different diagnoses may affect the treatment plan.

1. A 49-year-old woman comes to you complaining of neck and left temporomandibular joint pain. The pain is worse when she eats, especially if she chews on the left. Describe your assessment plan for this patient (cervical spondylosis versus temporomandibular dysfunction; see Table 4-5).

2. A 33-year-old woman comes to you complaining of pain and clicking when opening her mouth, especially when the mouth is open wide. She states that there is a small click on closing but minimal pain. Describe your assessment plan for this patient (temporomandibular joint arthritis versus temporomandibular disc dysfunction).

3. An 18-year-old male hockey player comes to you stating that he was hit in the jaw while playing. He is in severe pain and has difficulty speaking. Describe your assessment plan for this patient (cervical sprain versus temporomandibular joint dysfunction).

4. A 35-year-old man comes to you with his jaw locked open. Describe your assessment plan for this patient (temporomandibular disc dysfunction versus temporomandibular arthritis).

5. A 42-year-old woman comes to you complaining of jaw pain and headaches. She slipped on some wet stairs 3 days ago and fell, hitting her chin on the stairs. Describe your assessment plan for this patient (temporomandibular joint dysfunction versus head injury).

6. A 27-year-old nervous woman with long hair comes to you complaining of jaw pain. She has recently had a new dental plate installed. Describe your assessment plan for this patient (cervical sprain versus temporomandibular joint dysfunction).

Table 4-5

Differential Diagnosis of Cervical Spondylosis and Temporomandibular Joint (TMJ) Dysfunction

	Cervical Spondylosis	TMJ Dysfunction
History	Insidious onset	Insidious onset
	May complain of referred pain into shoulder, arm, or head	May be related to biting something hard
	Stiff neck	Pain may be referred to neck or head
Observation	Muscle guarding of neck muscles	Minimal or no muscle guarding
Active movements	Cervical spine movements limited	Cervical movements may be limited if they compress or stress TMJ
	TMJ movements normal	TMJ movements may or may not be painful but range of motion is altered
Passive movements	Restricted	Restricted
	May have altered end feel: muscle spasm or bone-to-bone	
Resisted isometric movements	Relatively normal	Normal
	Myotomes may be affected	
Special tests	Spurling's test may be positive	None
	Distraction test may be positive	
Reflexes and cutaneous distribution	Deep tendon reflexes may be hyporeflexic	No effect
	See history for referred pain	See history for referred pain

References

To enhance this text and add value for the reader, all references have been incorporated into a CD-ROM that is provided with this text. The reader can view the reference source and access it online whenever possible. There are a total of 31 cited and other general references for this chapter.

APPENDIX 4-1

RELIABILITY, VALIDITY, SPECIFICITY, AND SENSITIVITY OF SPECIAL/DIAGNOSTIC TESTS USED IN THE TEMPOROMANDIBULAR JOINT

CDC/TMD CRITERIA

Specificity	Sensitivity	Odds Ratio
• Absence of internal derangement 85%, internal derangement type I 21%[31]	• Absence of internal derangement 25%, internal derangement type I 85%[31]	• Positive likelihood ratio for absence of internal derangement 1.66, for internal derangement type I 1.07 • Negative likelihood ratio for absence of internal derangement 0.88, for internal derangement type I 0.19

CLICKING AND ELIMINATION TEST

Specificity	Sensitivity	Odds Ratio
• For anterior disk displacement 79.2%[26]	• For anterior disk displacement 75.7%[26]	• Positive likelihood ratio 3.64, negative likelihood ratio 0.31

CLICKING AND MANIPULATION TEST

Specificity	Sensitivity	Odds Ratio
• For anterior disk displacement 79.8%[26]	• For anterior disk displacement 67.6%[26]	• Positive likelihood ratio 3.45, negative likelihood ratio 0.41

CLICKING TEST

Specificity	Sensitivity	Odds Ratio
• For anterior disk displacement 89%[26]	• For anterior disk displacement 85.7%[26]	• Positive likelihood ratio 7.79, negative likelihood ratio 0.16

CREPITATION

Specificity	Sensitivity	Odds Ratio
• For anterior disk displacement 15.6%[27]	• For anterior disk displacement 15.6%[27]	• Positive likelihood ratio 0.18, negative likelihood ratio 5.41

DEFLECTION

Specificity	Sensitivity	Odds Ratio
• For anterior disk displacement 27%[27]	• For anterior disk displacement 27%[27]	• Positive likelihood ratio 0.37, negative likelihood ratio 2.70

ELIMINATION TEST

Specificity	Sensitivity	Odds Ratio
• For anterior disk displacement 50%[26]	• For anterior disk displacement 88.4%[26]	• Positive likelihood ratio 1.77, negative likelihood ratio 0.23

HISTORY OF CLICKING

Specificity	Sensitivity	Odds Ratio
• For anterior disk displacement 96.7%[27]	• For anterior disk displacement 58%[27]	• Positive likelihood ratio 17.57, negative likelihood ratio 0.43

Continued

APPENDIX 4-1—cont'd

LIMITED OPENING

Specificity	Sensitivity	Odds Ratio
• For anterior disk displacement 83.6%[27]	• For anterior disk displacement 43.3%[27]	• Positive likelihood ratio 2.62, negative likelihood ratio 0.68

LIMITED TRANSLATION

Specificity	Sensitivity	Odds Ratio
• For anterior disk displacement 77.8%[27]	• For anterior disk displacement 77.8%[27]	• Positive likelihood ratio 3.50, negative likelihood ratio 0.28

MANIPULATION TEST

Specificity	Sensitivity	Odds Ratio
• For anterior disk displacement 79.8%[26]	• For anterior disk displacement 79.8%[26]	• Positive likelihood ratio 3.99, negative likelihood ratio 0.25

MAXIMAL MOUTH OPENING

Reliability

• Interrater r=0.9 and intrarater r=0.9 (minimal detectable difference 6 mm)[24]

TMJ PAIN

Specificity	Sensitivity	Odds Ratio
• For anterior disk displacement 59.1%[27]	• For anterior disk displacement 59.1%[27]	• Positive likelihood ratio 1.44, negative likelihood ratio 0.69

CHAPTER 5

SHOULDER

The prerequisite to any treatment of a patient with pain in the shoulder region is a precise and comprehensive picture of the signs and symptoms as they present during the assessment and as they existed until that time. This knowledge ensures that the techniques used will suit the condition and that the degree of success will be estimated against this background. Shoulder pain can be caused by intrinsic disease of the shoulder joints or pathology in the periarticular structures, or it may originate from the cervical spine, chest, or visceral structures. Pathology is commonly related to the level of activity, and age can play a significant role. The shoulder complex is difficult to assess because of its many structures (most of which are located in a small area), its many movements, and the many lesions that can occur either inside or outside the joints. Influences such as referred pain from the cervical spine and the possibility of more than one lesion being present at one time, as well as the difficulty in deciding what weight to give to each response, make the examination even more difficult to understand. Assessment of the shoulder region often necessitates an evaluation of the cervical spine (see Chapter 3) to rule out referred symptoms, and the examiner must be prepared to include the cervical spine and its scanning examination in any shoulder assessment.

Applied Anatomy

The **glenohumeral joint** is a multiaxial, ball-and-socket, synovial joint that depends primarily on the muscles and ligaments rather than bones for its support, stability, and integrity.[1] Thus, the assessment of the muscles and ligaments/capsule can play a major role in the assessment of the shoulder. The **labrum,** which is the ring of fibrocartilage, surrounds and deepens the glenoid cavity of the scapula about 50%.[2] Only part of the humeral head is in contact with the glenoid at any one time. This joint has three axes and three degrees of freedom. The resting position of the glenohumeral joint is 55° of abduction and 30° of horizontal adduction. The close packed position of the joint is full abduction and lateral rotation. When relaxed, the humerus sits centered in the glenoid cavity; with contraction of the rotator cuff muscles, it is pushed or translated anteriorly, posteriorly, inferiorly, superiorly, or in any combination of these movements. This movement is small, but if it does not occur, full movement is impossible. The glenoid in the resting position has a 5° superior tilt or inclination and a 7° retroversion (slight medial rotation). The angle between the humeral neck and shaft is about 130°, and the humeral head is retroverted 30° to 40° relative to the line joining the epicondyle.[3]

The rotator cuff muscles play an integral role in shoulder movement. Their positioning on the humerus may be visualized by "cupping" the shoulder with the thumb anteriorly, as shown in Figure 5-1. The biceps tendon (Figure 5-2) runs between the thumb and index finger just anterior to the index finger. The rotator cuff controls osteokinematic and arthrokinematic motion of the humeral head in the glenoid and along with the biceps depresses the humeral head during movements into elevation.

The primary ligaments of the glenohumeral joint—the superior, middle, and inferior glenohumeral ligaments—play an important role in stabilizing the shoulder.[3,4] The superior glenohumeral ligament's primary role is limiting

- Subscapularis muscle
- Supraspinatus muscle
- Infraspinatus muscle
- Teres minor muscle

Figure 5-1

Positioning of the rotator cuff with thumb over subscapularis, index finger over supraspinatus, middle finger over infraspinatus, and ring finger over teres minor.

inferior translation in adduction. It also restrains anterior translation and lateral rotation up to 45° abduction. The middle glenohumeral ligament, which is absent in 30% of the population, limits lateral rotation between 45° and 90° abduction. The inferior glenohumeral ligament is the most important of the three ligaments. It has an anterior and posterior band with a thin "pouch" in between so it acts much like a hammock or sling. It supports the humeral head above 90° abduction, limiting inferior translation while the anterior band tightens on lateral rotation and the posterior band tightens on medial

rotation.[5] Excessive lateral rotation as seen in throwing may lead to stretching of the anterior portion of the ligament (and capsule), thereby increasing glenohumeral laxity.[6] The coracohumeral ligament primarily limits inferior translation and helps limit lateral rotation below 60° abduction. This ligament is found in the **rotator interval** between the anterior border of the supraspinatus tendon and the superior border of the subscapularis tendon, thus the ligament unites the two tendons anteriorly (Figure 5-3).[7,8] See Table 5-1 for structures limiting movement in different degrees of abduction.[5,9] The coracoacromial ligament forms an arch over the humeral head acting as a block to superior translation.[10] The transverse humeral ligament forms a roof over the bicipital groove to hold the long head of biceps tendon within the groove. The capsular pattern of the glenohumeral joint is lateral rotation most limited, followed by abduction and medial rotation. Branches of the posterior cord of the brachial plexus and the suprascapular, axillary, and lateral pectoral nerves innervate the joint.

Glenohumeral Joint

Resting position:	40–55° abduction, 30° horizontal adduction (scapular plane)
Close packed position:	Full abduction, lateral rotation
Capsular pattern:	Lateral rotation, abduction, medial rotation

The **acromioclavicular joint** is a plane synovial joint that augments the range of motion (ROM) of the humerus in the glenoid (Figure 5-4). The bones making up this joint are the acromion process of the scapula and the lateral end of the clavicle. The joint has three degrees of freedom. The capsule, which is fibrous, surrounds the joint.

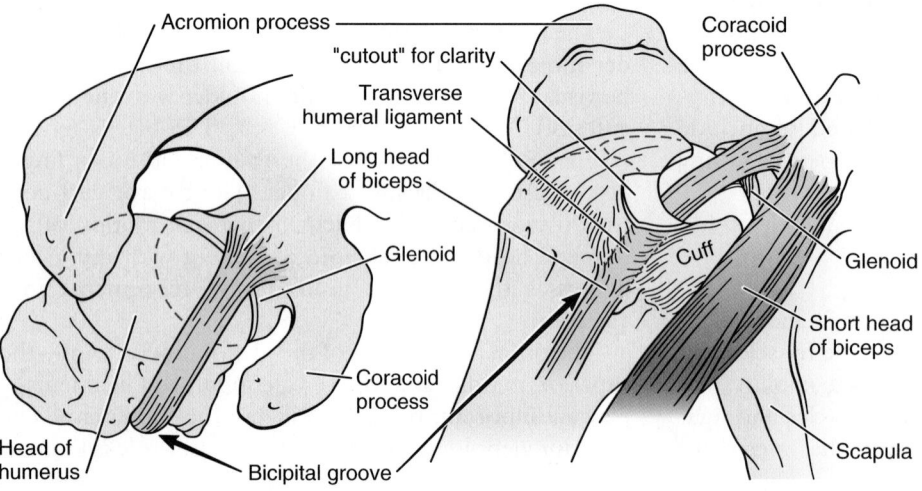

- Acromion process
- "cutout" for clarity
- Transverse humeral ligament
- Long head of biceps
- Glenoid
- Coracoid process
- Head of humerus
- Bicipital groove
- Coracoid process
- Cuff
- Glenoid
- Short head of biceps
- Scapula

Figure 5-2

The biceps apparatus.

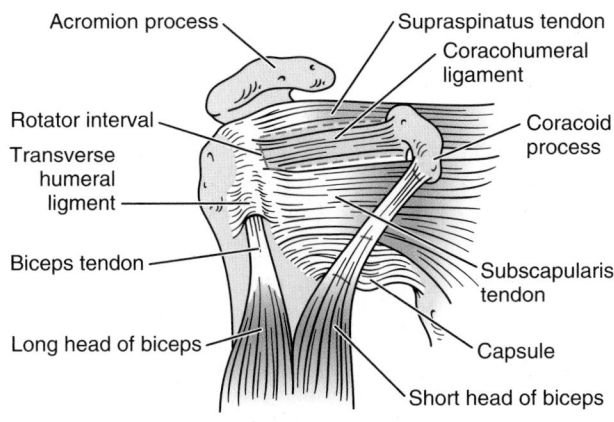

Figure 5-3

Rotator interval showing the relationship between the supraspinatus tendon, subscapularis tendon, and the coracohumeral ligament.

An articular disc may be found within the joint. Rarely does the disc separate the acromion and clavicular articular surfaces. This joint depends on ligaments for its strength. The acromioclavicular ligaments surround the joint and are commonly the first ligaments injured when the joint is stressed. The coracoclavicular ligament is the primary support of the acromioclavicular joint. It has two portions: the conoid and trapezoid parts. If a step deformity occurs, this ligament has been torn. In the resting position of the joint, the arm rests by the side in the normal standing position. In the close packed position of the acromioclavicular joint, the arm is abducted to 90°. The indication of a capsular pattern in the joint is pain at the extreme ROM, especially in horizontal adduction (cross-flexion) and full elevation. This joint is innervated by branches of the suprascapular and lateral pectoral nerve.

Acromioclavicular Joint	
Resting position:	Arm by side
Close packed position:	90° abduction
Capsular pattern:	Pain at extremes of range of motion, especially horizontal adduction and full elevation

Table 5-1

Structures Limiting Movement in Different Degrees of Abduction

Angle of Abduction	Lateral Rotation	Neutral	Medial Rotation
0°	Superior G-H ligament Anterior capsule	Coracohumeral ligament Superior G-H ligament Capsule (anterior and posterior) Supraspinatus	Posterior capsule
0–45° (note 30°–45° abduction in scapular plane [resting position]—maximum looseness of shoulder)	Coracohumeral ligament Superior G-H ligament Anterior capsule	Middle G-H ligament Posterior capsule Subscapularis Infraspinatus Teres minor	Posterior capsule
45°–60°	Middle G-H ligament Coracohumeral ligament Inferior G-H ligament (anterior band) Anterior capsule	Middle G-H ligament Inferior G-H ligament (especially anterior portion) Subscapularis Infraspinatus Teres minor	Inferior G-H ligament (posterior band) Posterior capsule
60°–90°	Inferior G-H ligament (anterior band) Anterior capsule	Inferior G-H ligament (especially posterior portion) Middle G-H ligament	Inferior G-H ligament (posterior band) Posterior capsule
90°–120°	Inferior G-H ligament (anterior band) Anterior capsule	Inferior G-H ligament	Inferior G-H ligament (posterior band) Posterior capsule
120°–180°	Inferior G-H ligament (anterior band) Anterior capsule	Inferior G-H ligament	Inferior G-H ligament (posterior band) Posterior capsule

Data from Curl LA, Warren RF: Glenohumeral joint stability: selective cutting studies on the static capsular restraints, *Clin Orthop Relat Res* 330:54–65, 1996; and Peat M, Culham E: Functional anatomy of the shoulder complex. In Andrews JR, Wilk KE, editors: *The athlete's shoulder,* New York, 1994, Churchill Livingstone.

G-H = Glenohumeral.

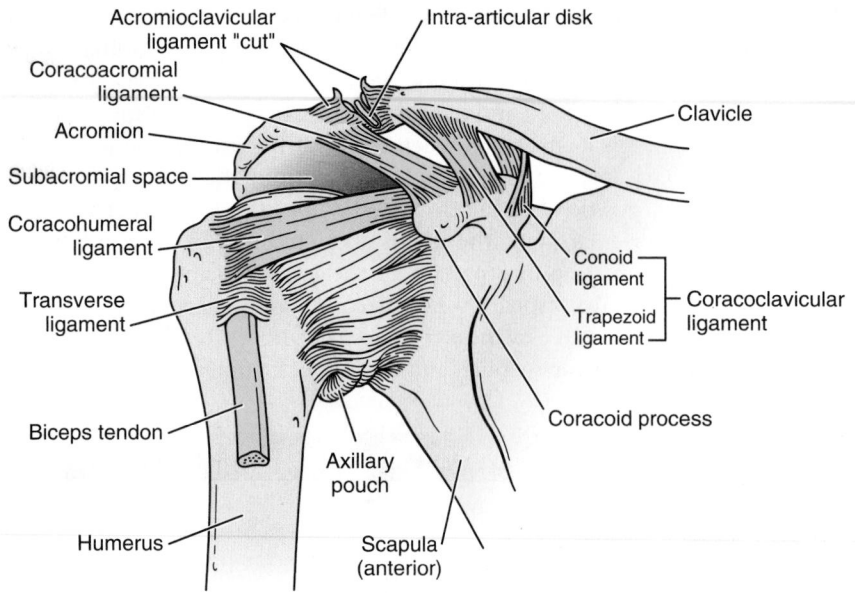

Figure 5-4

Anterior view of the right glenohumeral and acromioclavicular joints. Note the subacromial space or supraspinatus outlet located between the top of the humeral head and the underside of the acromion. (Modified from Neumann DA: *Kinesiology of the musculoskeletal system: foundations for physical rehabilitation,* p. 107, St. Louis, 2002, Mosby.)

The **sternoclavicular joint,** along with the acromioclavicular joint, enables the humerus in the glenoid to move through a full 180° of abduction (Figure 5-5). It is a saddle-shaped synovial joint with three degrees of freedom and is made up of the medial end of the clavicle, the manubrium sternum, and the cartilage of the first rib. It is the joint that joins the appendicular skeleton to the axial skeleton.[11] There is a substantial disc between the two bony joint surfaces, and the capsule is thicker anteriorly than posteriorly. The disc separates the articular surfaces of the clavicle and sternum and adds significant strength to the joint because of attachments, thereby preventing medial displacement of the clavicle. Like the acromioclavicular joint, the joint depends on ligaments for its strength. The ligaments of the sternoclavicular joint include the anterior and posterior sternoclavicular ligaments, which support the joint anteriorly and posteriorly, the interclavicular ligament, and the costoclavicular

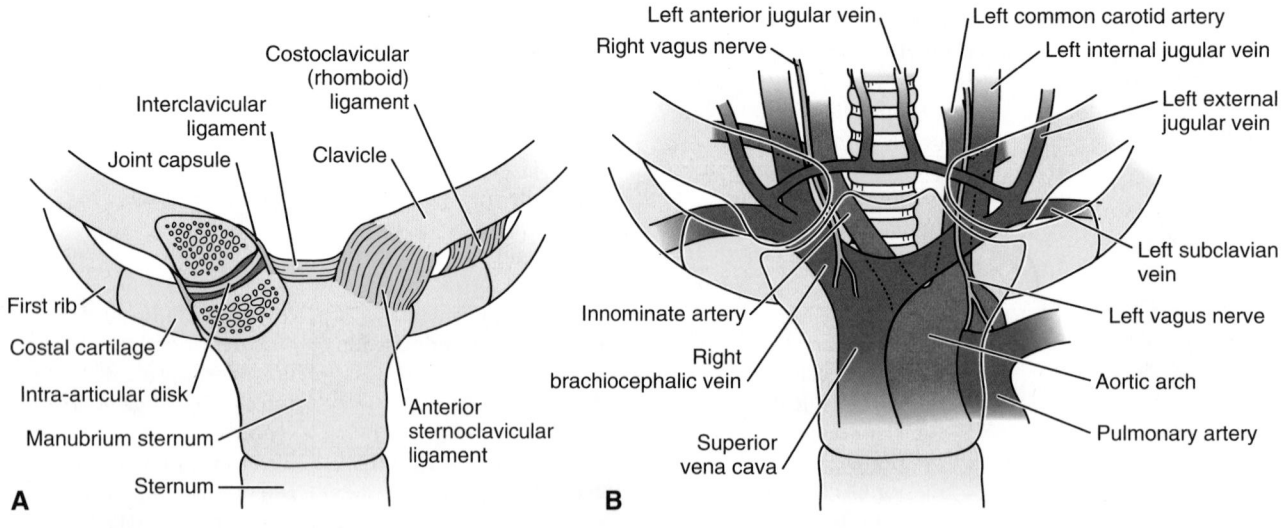

Figure 5-5

A, Bony and ligamentous anatomy of the sternoclavicular joint. The major supporting structures include the anterior capsule, the posterior capsule, the interclavicular ligament, the costoclavicular (rhomboid) ligament, and the intra-articular disk and ligament. **B,** Retrosternal anatomy. Note the proximity of the sternoclavicular joint to the trachea, aortic arch, and brachiocephalic vein. (Redrawn from Higginbotham TO, Kuhn JE: Atraumatic disorders of the sternoclavicular joint, *J Am Acad Ortho Surg* 13:139, 2005.)

ligament running from the clavicle to the first rib and its costal cartilage. This is the main ligament maintaining the integrity of the sternoclavicular joint. The movements possible at this joint and at the acromioclavicular joint are elevation, depression, protrusion, retraction, and rotation. The close packed position of the sternoclavicular joint is full or maximum rotation of the clavicle, which occurs when the upper arm is in full elevation. The resting position and capsular pattern are the same as with the acromioclavicular joint. The joint is innervated by branches of the anterior supraclavicular nerve and the nerve to the subclavius muscle. Major vessels and the trachea lie close behind the sternum and the sternoclavicular joint (see Figure 5-5, *B*).[11]

Sternoclavicular Joint	
Resting position:	Arm at side
Close packed position:	Full elevation and protraction
Capsular pattern:	Pain at extremes of range of motion, especially horizontal adduction and full elevation

Although the **scapulothoracic joint** is not a true joint, it functions as an integral part of the shoulder complex and must be considered in any assessment because a stable scapula enables the rest of the shoulder to function correctly. Some texts call this structure the scapulocostal joint. This "joint" consists of the body of the scapula and the muscles covering the posterior chest wall. The muscles acting on the scapula help to control its movements. The medial border of the scapula is not parallel with the spinous processes but is angled about 3° away (top to bottom), and the scapula lies 20° to 30° forward relative to the sagittal plane.[3] Because it is not a true joint, it does not have a capsular pattern nor a close packed position. The resting position of this joint is the same as for the acromioclavicular joint. The scapula extends from the level of T2 spinous process to T7 or T9 spinous process, depending on the size of the scapula. Because the scapula acts as a stable base for the rotator cuff muscles, the muscles controlling its movements must be strong and balanced because the joint funnels the forces of the trunk and legs into the arm.[12]

Patient History

In addition to the questions listed under Patient History in Chapter 1, the examiner should obtain the following information from the patient.[13] Most commonly, the patient complains of pain, especially on movement, restricted motion, or shoulder instability.

1. *What is the patient's age?* Many problems of the shoulder can be age related. For example, rotator cuff degeneration usually occurs in patients who are between 40 and 60 years of age. Rotator cuff tears, though, can occur at any age.[14] Primary impingement due to degeneration and weakness is usually seen in patients older than 35, whereas secondary impingement due to instability caused by weakness in the scapular or humeral control muscles is more common in people in their late teens or 20s especially those involved in vigorous overhead activities such as swimmers or pitchers in baseball.[15] Calcium deposits may occur between the ages of 20 and 40.[16] Chondrosarcomas may be seen in those older than 30 years of age, whereas frozen shoulder is seen in persons between the ages of 45 and 60 years if it results from causes other than trauma (Tables 5-2 and 5-3). Frozen shoulder due to trauma can occur at any age but is more common with increased age.

2. *Does the patient support the upper limb in a protected position (Figure 5-6) or hesitate to move it?* This action could mean that one of the joints of the shoulder complex is unstable or that there is an acute problem in the shoulder. In some cases, patients with lax shoulders will ask, "What happens when I do this?" In effect, the patient is subluxing the shoulder (Figure 5-7). This may or may not be pathological, but it is a sign of voluntary instability in which the patient uses his or her muscles to sublux the humerus in the glenoid, stressing the labrum and inert tissues.

3. *If there was an injury, what exactly was the mechanism of injury?* Did the patient fall on an outstretched hand (a "FOOSH" injury), which could indicate a fracture or dislocation of the glenohumeral joint? Did the patient fall on or receive a blow to the tip of the shoulder, or did the patient land on the elbow, driving the humerus up against the acromion? This finding may indicate an acromioclavicular dislocation or subluxation.[17] Does the shoulder feel unstable or feel like it is "coming out" during movement? Does the arm "go dead" when doing activity? "Going dead" implies the patient cannot use the arm functionally because of pain and a subjective feeling of unease when using the arm.[18] Patients with instability may appear normal on clinical examination, especially if shoulder muscles are not fatigued. Many overuse injuries are more evident immediately after the patient does repeated activity.[19] This may indicate gross or anatomical instability, as in recurrent shoulder dislocation, subluxation, or subtle translational instability. The spectrum of instability varies from gross or anatomical instability—the TUBS type (**T**raumatic onset, **U**nidirectional anterior with a **B**ankart lesion responding to **S**urgery) to a more subtle translational instability—the AMBRI type (**A**traumatic cause, **M**ultidirectional with **B**ilateral

Table 5-2

Differential Diagnosis of Rotator Cuff Degeneration, Frozen Shoulder, Atraumatic Instability, and Cervical Spondylosis

	Rotator Cuff Lesions	Frozen Shoulder	Atraumatic Instability	Cervical Spondylosis
History	Age 30–50 years Pain and weakness after eccentric load	Age 45+ (insidious type) Insidious onset or after trauma or surgery Functional restriction of lateral rotation, abduction, and medial rotation	Age 10–35 years Pain and instability with activity No history of trauma	Age 50+ years Acute or chronic
Observation	Normal bone and soft tissue outlines Protective shoulder hike may be seen	Normal bone and soft-tissue outlines	Normal bone and soft-tissue outlines	Minimal or no cervical spine movement Torticollis may be present
Active movement	Weakness of abduction or rotation, or both Crepitus may be present	Restricted ROM Shoulder hiking	Full or excessive ROM	Limited ROM with pain
Passive movement	Pain if impingement occurs	Limited ROM, especially in lateral rotation, abduction, and medial rotation (capsular pattern)	Normal or excessive ROM	Limited ROM (symptoms may be exacerbated)
Resisted isometric movement	Pain and weakness on abduction and lateral rotation	Normal, when arm by side	Normal	Normal, except if nerve root compressed Myotome may be affected
Special tests	Drop-arm test positive Empty can test positive	None	Load and shift test positive Apprehension test positive Relocation test positive Augmentation tests positive	Spurling's test positive Distraction test positive ULTT positive Shoulder abduction test positive
Sensory function and reflexes	Not affected	Not affected		Dermatomes affected Reflexes affected
Palpation	Tender over rotator cuff	Not painful unless capsule is stretched	Anterior or posterior pain	Tender over appropriate vertebra or facet
Diagnostic imaging	Radiography: upward displacement of humeral head; acromial spurring MRI diagnostic	Radiography: negative Arthrography: decreased capsular size	Negative	Radiography: narrowing osteophytes

MRI = magnetic resonance imaging; ROM = range of motion; ULTT = upper limb tension test.

shoulder findings with **R**ehabilitation as appropriate treatment and, rarely, **I**nferior capsular shift surgery).

4. *Are there any movements or positions that cause the patient pain or symptoms?* If so, which ones? The examiner must keep in mind that cervical spine movements may cause pain in the shoulder. Persons who

have had recurrent dislocations of the shoulder may find that any movement involving lateral rotation bothers them, because this movement is involved in anterior dislocations of the shoulder. Recurrent dislocators may sometimes show pain at extreme of medial rotation when the humeral head is "tightened"

Table 5-3

Differential Diagnosis of Shoulder Pathology

Pathology	Symptoms
External primary impingement (stage I)	Intermittent mild pain with overhead activities Over age 35
External primary impingement (stage II)	Mild to moderate pain with overhead activities or strenuous activities
External primary impingement (stage III)	Pain at rest or with activities Night pain may occur Scapular or rotator cuff weakness is noted
Rotator cuff tears (full thickness)	Classic night pain Weakness noted predominantly in abduction and lateral rotators Loss of motion
Adhesive capsulitis (idiopathic frozen shoulder)	Inability to perform activities of daily living owing to loss of motion Loss of motion may be perceived as weakness
Anterior instability (with or without external secondary impingement)	Apprehension to mechanical shifting limits activities Slipping, popping, or sliding may present as suitable instability Apprehension usually associated with horizontal abduction and lateral rotation Anterior or posterior pain may be present Weak scapular stabilizers
Posterior instability	Slipping or popping of the humerus out the back This may be associated with forward flexion and medial rotation while the shoulder is under a compressive load
Multidirectional instability	Looseness of shoulder in all directions This may be most pronounced while carrying luggage or turning over while asleep Pain may or may not be present

Modified from Maughon TS, Andrews JR: The subjective evaluation of the shoulder in the athlete. In Andrews JR, Wilk KE, editors: *The athlete's shoulder,* p. 36, New York, 1994, Churchill-Livingstone.

Figure 5-6

Patient supports the upper limb in protected position.

Figure 5-7

Voluntary instability. Note how the patient uses her muscles to sublux the humerus in the glenoid.

against the anterior glenoid. Excessive abduction and lateral rotation may lead to dead-arm syndrome in which the patient feels a sudden paralyzing pain and weakness in the shoulder.[18] This finding often indicates altered shoulder mechanics commonly involving a tight posterior capsule, altered arthrokinematics of the glenohumeral joint, and scapular dyskinesia.[18] In throwers, the condition may be referred to as a SICK scapula (malposition of **S**capula, prominence of **I**nferior medial border of scapula, **C**oracoid pain and malposition, and scapular dys**K**inesia).[20] If the patient complains of pain during specific phases of pitching (for example, during the late cocking and acceleration phases), anterior instability should be considered even in the presence of minimal clinical signs.[21] Commonly, instability and secondary impingement occur together. Secondary impingement implies that although impingement signs are present, they result from a primary problem somewhere else, commonly in the scapular or humeral control or stabilizer muscles. Stability of the shoulder depends on both dynamic stabilizers (the muscles) and static stabilizers (e.g., the capsule, labrum).[5] Night pain and resting pain are often related to rotator cuff tears and, on occasion, to tumors; activity-related pain usually signifies paratenonitis. Arthritis pain commonly shows, at least initially, at the extremes of motion. Acromioclavicular pain is especially evident at greater than 90° of abduction and tends to be localized to the joint. Similarly, sternoclavicular pain is localized to the joint and increases on horizontal adduction.

5. *What is the extent and behavior of the patient's pain?* For example, deep, boring, toothache-like pain in the neck, shoulder region, or both may indicate **thoracic outlet syndrome** (Figure 5-8) or acute brachial plexus neuropathy. Strains of the rotator cuff usually cause dull, toothache-like pain that is worse at night, whereas acute calcific tendinitis usually causes a hot, burning type of pain. Sprain of the first or second rib from direct trauma or sudden contraction of the scaleni may mimic an acute impingement or rotator cuff injury.[22]

6. *Are there any activities that cause or increase the pain?* For example, bicipital paratenonitis or tendinosis[23] are often seen in skiers and may result from holding on to a ski tow; in cross-country skiing, it may result from poling (using the pole for propulsion). Paratenonitis is inflammation of the paratenon of the tendon. The paratenon is the outer covering of the tendon whether or not it is lined with synovium. Tendinosis is actual degeneration of the tendon itself. With chronic overuse, tendinosis is more likely than paratenonitis[23,24] (Table 5-4; see Table 1-18). Elite swimmers may train for more than 15,000 m daily, which can lead to stress overload (repetitive microtrauma) of the structures

of the shoulder. Does throwing or reaching alter the pain? If so, what positions cause pain or discomfort? These questions may indicate which structures are injured.

7. *Do any positions relieve the pain?* Patients with nerve root pain may find that elevating the arm over the head relieves symptoms. For a patient with instability or inflammatory conditions, lifting the arm over the head usually exacerbates shoulder problems.

8. *What is the patient unable to do functionally?* Is the patient able to talk or swallow? Is the patient hoarse? These signs could indicate an injury to the sternoclavicular joint (if there is swelling) or a posterior dislocation of the joint because pressure is being applied to the trachea.

9. *How long has the problem bothered the patient?* For example, an idiopathic frozen shoulder goes through three stages: the condition becomes progressively worse, plateaus, and then progressively improves, with each stage lasting 3 to 5 months.[25,26]

10. *Is there any indication of muscle spasm, deformity, bruising, wasting, paresthesia, or numbness?*[27] These findings can help the examiner determine the acuteness of the condition and, potentially, the structures injured.

11. *Does the patient complain of weakness and heaviness in the limb after activity?* Does the limb tire easily? These findings may indicate vascular involvement. Are there any venous symptoms, such as swelling or stiffness, which may extend all the way to the fingers? Are there any arterial symptoms, such as coolness or pallor in the upper limb? These complaints may result from pressure on an artery, a vein, or both. An example is thoracic outlet syndrome (see Figure 5-8), in which pressure may be applied to the vascular or neurological structures as they enter the upper limb in three locations: at the scalene triangle, at the costoclavicular space, and under the pectoralis minor and the coracoid process.[28,29] Excessive repetitive demands placed on the shoulder, such as those seen in pitching, may lead to thoracic outlet syndrome, axillary artery occlusion, effort thrombosis, or pressure in the quadrilateral space. (The quadrilateral space has as its boundaries the medial border of the humerus laterally, the lateral border of the long head of triceps medially, the inferior border of teres minor, and the superior border of teres major.)[30]

12. *Is there any indication of nerve injury?* The examiner should evaluate the nerves and the muscles supplied by the nerves to determine possible nerve injury. Any history of weakness, numbness, or paresthesia may indicate nerve injury (Table 5-5). For example, the suprascapular nerve may be injured as it passes through the suprascapular notch under the transverse scapular ligament, leading to atrophy

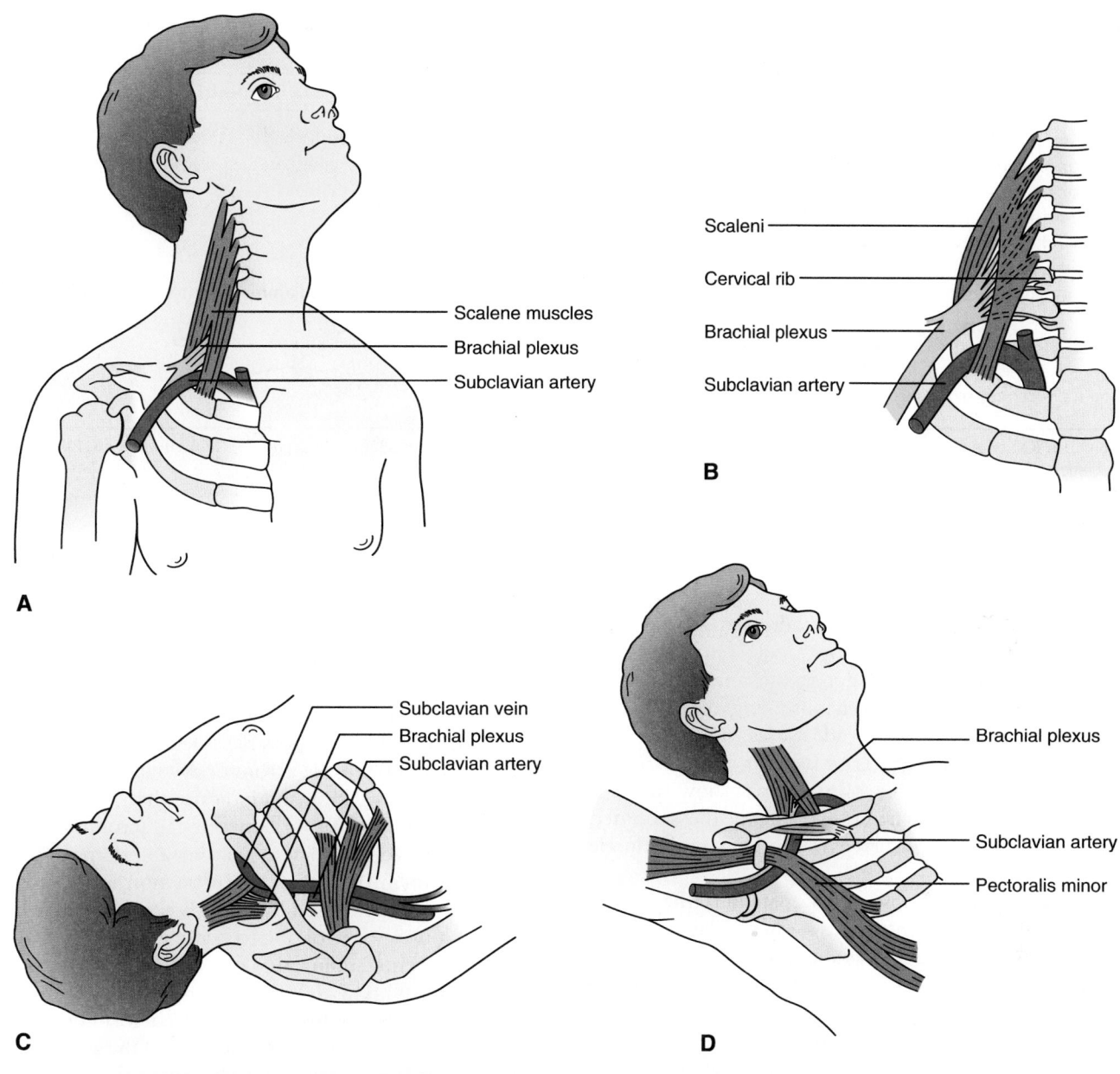

Scalene muscles
Brachial plexus
Subclavian artery

A

Scaleni
Cervical rib
Brachial plexus
Subclavian artery

B

Subclavian vein
Brachial plexus
Subclavian artery

C

Brachial plexus
Subclavian artery
Pectoralis minor

D

Figure 5-8

Location and causes of thoracic outlet syndrome. **A,** Scalenus anterior syndrome. **B,** Cervical rib syndrome. **C,** Costoclavicular space syndrome. **D,** Hyperabduction syndrome (abduction, extension, and lateral rotation).

and paralysis of the supraspinatus and infraspinatus muscles. The examiner should listen to the history carefully, because this condition could mimic a third-degree (rupture) strain of the supraspinatus tendon. Another potential nerve injury is one to the axillary (circumflex) nerve (Figure 5-9) or musculocutaneous nerve (Figure 5-10) after dislocation of the glenohumeral joint. With an axillary nerve injury, the deltoid muscle and the teres minor muscle are atrophied and weak or paralyzed. The radial nerve (see Figure 5-9) is sometimes injured as it winds around the posterior

aspect of the shaft of the humerus. The injury frequently occurs when the humeral shaft is fractured. If the nerve is damaged in this location, the extensors of the elbow, wrist, and fingers are affected, and an altered sensation occurs in the radial nerve sensory distribution.

13. *Which hand is dominant?* Often the dominant shoulder is lower than the nondominant shoulder and the ROM may not be the same for both. Usually, the dominant shoulder shows greater muscularity and often less ROM.

Table 5-4

Implications of the Diagnosis of Tendinosis Compared with Tendinitis

Trait	Overuse Tendinosis	Overuse Tendinitis
Prevalence	Common	Rare
Time for recovery, early presentation	6–10 weeks	Several days to 2 weeks
Time for full recovery, chronic presentation	3–6 months	4–6 weeks
Likelihood of full recovery to sport from chronic symptoms	~80%	99%
Focus of conservative therapy	Encouragement of collagen-synthesis maturation and strength	Anti-inflammatory modalities and drugs
Role of surgery	Excise abnormal tissue	Not known
Prognosis for surgery	70–85%	95%
Time for recovery from surgery	4–6 months	3–4 weeks

From Khan KM et al: Overuse tendinosis, not tendonitis. Part 1: a new paradigm for a difficult clinical problem, *Phys Sportsmed* 28:43, 2000. Reproduced with permission of McGraw-Hill.

Observation

The patient must be suitably undressed so that the examiner can observe the bony and soft-tissue contours of both shoulders and determine whether they are normal and symmetric. When observing the shoulder, the examiner looks at the head, the cervical spine, the thorax (especially the posterior aspect), and the entire upper limb. The hand, for example, may show vasomotor changes that result from problems in the shoulder, including shiny skin, hair loss, swelling, and muscle atrophy.

It is important to observe the patient as he or she removes clothes from the upper body and later replaces them. For example, does the patient undress the affected arm last or dress it first? This pattern indicates that the patient is limiting the movement of the arm as much as possible, signifying possible pathology. The patient's actions give some indication of functional restriction, pain, or weakness in the upper limb.

Anterior View

When looking at the patient from the anterior view (Figure 5-11, *A*), the examiner should begin by ensuring that the head and neck are in the midline of the body and observing their relation to the shoulders. A forward head posture is often associated with rounded shoulders, a medially rotated humerus and a protracted scapula resulting in the humeral head translating anteriorly, a tight posterior capsule, tightness of the pectoral, upper trapezius, and levator scapulae muscles, and weakness of the lower scapular stabilizers and deep neck flexors.[31] While observing the shoulder, the examiner should look for the possibility of a **step deformity** (Figure 5-12, *A*). Such a deformity may be caused by an acromioclavicular

dislocation, with the distal end of the clavicle lying superior to the acromion process. Seen at rest, a step deformity indicates both the acromioclavicular and coracoclavicular ligaments have been torn. The deformity may be accentuated by asking the patient to horizontally adduct the arm or to medially rotate the shoulder and bring the hand up the back as high as possible. Occasionally, swelling is evident anterior to the acromioclavicular joint. This is called the **Fountain sign** and indicates that degeneration has caused communication between the acromioclavicular joint and swollen subacromial bursa underneath.[32] If a **sulcus deformity** appears when traction is applied to the arm, it may be caused by multidirectional instability or loss of muscle control due to nerve injury or a stroke, leading to inferior subluxation of the glenohumeral joint (Figure 5-12, *C*). This deformity is lateral to the acromion and should not be confused with a step deformity. This is also referred to as a **sulcus sign** because of the appearance of a sulcus or groove below the acromion process (Figure 5-12, *B*). Flattening of the normally round deltoid muscle area may indicate an anterior dislocation of the glenohumeral joint or paralysis of the deltoid muscle (Figure 5-13). With an anterior dislocation, note also how the arm is held abducted because of the location of the humeral head below the glenoid. If the examiner palpated in the axilla, he or she would feel the head of the humerus. The examiner should note any abnormal bumps or malalignment in the bones that may indicate past injury, such as a healed fracture of the clavicle.

In most people, the dominant side is lower than the nondominant side. This difference may be caused by the extra use of the dominant side, which stretches the ligaments, joint capsules, and muscles, allowing the arm to sag slightly. Tennis players[33] and others who stretch their upper limbs in a reaching action show even greater

Table 5-5

Peripheral Nerve Injuries (Neuropathy) about the Shoulder

Affected Nerve (Root)	Muscle Weakness	Sensory Alteration	Reflexes Affected	Mechanism of Injury
Suprascapular nerve (C5–C6)	Supraspinatus, infraspinatus (arm lateral rotation)	Top of shoulder from clavicle to spine of scapula Pain in posterior shoulder radiating into arm	None	Compression in suprascapular notch Stretch into scapular protraction plus horizontal adduction Compression in spinoglenoid notch Direct blow Space occupying lesion (e.g., ganglion)
Axillary (circumflex) nerve (posterior cord; C5–C6)	Deltoid, teres minor (arm abduction)	Deltoid area Anterior shoulder pain	None	Anterior glenohumeral dislocation or fracture of surgical neck of humerus Forced abduction Surgery for instability
Radial nerve (C5–C8, T1)	Triceps, wrist extensors, finger extensors (shoulder, wrist, and hand extension)	Dorsum of hand	Triceps	Fracture humeral shaft Pressure (e.g., crutch palsy)
Long thoracic nerve (C5–C6, [C7])	Serratus anterior (scapular control)			Direct blow Traction Compression against internal chest wall (backpack injury) Heavy effort above shoulder height Repetitive strain
Musculocutaneous nerve (C5–C7)	Coracobrachialis, biceps, brachialis (elbow flexion)	Lateral aspect of forearm	Biceps	Compression Muscle hypertrophy Direct blow Fracture (clavicle and humerus) Dislocation (anterior) Surgery (Putti-Platt, Bankart)
Spinal accessory nerve (cranial nerve XI; C3–C4)	Trapezius (shoulder elevation)	Brachial plexus symptoms possible because of drooping of shoulder Shoulder aching	None	Direct blow Traction (shoulder depression and neck rotation to opposite side) Biopsy
Subscapular nerve (posterior cord; C5–C6)	Subscapularis, teres major (medial rotation)	None	None	Direct blow Traction
Dorsal scapular nerve (C5)	Levator scapulae, rhomboid major, rhomboid minor (scapular retraction and elevation)	None	None	Direct blow Compression
Lateral pectoral nerve (C5–C6)	Pectoralis major, pectoralis minor	None	None	Direct blow
Thoracodorsal nerve (C6–C7, [C8])	Latissimus dorsi	None	None	Direct blow Compression
Supraclavicular nerve	—	Mild clavicular pain Sensory loss over anterior shoulder	None	Compression

differences along with gross hypertrophy of the muscles on the dominant side (Figure 5-14). If the patient is protective of the shoulder, however, it may appear that the injured shoulder, whether dominant or nondominant, is higher than the normal side (see Figure 5-6).

The examiner notes whether the patient is able to assume the normal functional position for the shoulder, which is in the scapular plane with 60° of abduction and the arm in neutral or no rotation. In this position, or with the arm abducted to 90°, rupture or congenital absence

Figure 5-9
Motor distribution of the radial and axillary nerves.

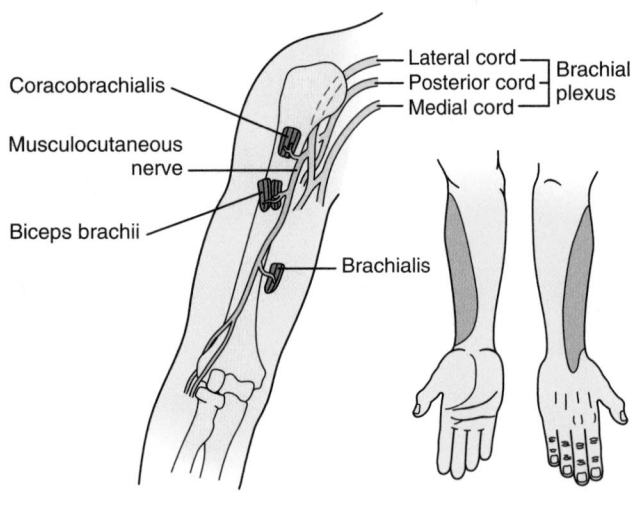

Figure 5-10
Motor and sensory distribution of musculocutaneous nerve.

of the pectoralis major may be evident (Figure 5-15).[34] Rupture of the pectoralis major is often accompanied by a tearing sensation and pop along with weakness, painful limitation of movement, and ecchymosis.[34] If the patient's arm is medially rotated from this position to bring the hand into midline, the biceps tendon is forced against the lesser tuberosity of the medial wall of the bicipital (intertubercular) groove. If this position is maintained for long periods, there may be increased wear of the biceps tendon, which can lead to bicipital tendinitis or paratenonitis. If the arm is horizontally adducted while it is medially rotated, anterior pain indicates impingement symptoms (Hawkins-Kennedy test—see special tests). The width and depth of the bicipital groove may vary (Figure 5-16), possibly leading to problems if the shoulder is overused. Especially wide or deep grooves lead to the greatest problems. The wide grooves tend to allow the tendon too much lateral movement, leading to inflammation of the paratenon (paratenonitis)[23]; the deep grooves tend to be too narrow, compressing the tendon, especially if it becomes inflamed.[35]

Posterior View

When viewing the patient from behind (see Figure 5-11, B), the examiner again notes bony and soft-tissue contours and body alignment. For example, atrophy of the upper trapezius may indicate spinal accessory nerve palsy, whereas atrophy of supraspinatus or infraspinatus may indicate supraspinous nerve palsy.[36] The spines of the

Figure 5-11
Views of the shoulder. **A,** Anterior. **B,** Posterior. **C,** Side.

Figure 5-12
A, Step deformity resulting from acromioclavicular dislocation. **B,** Sulcus sign for shoulder instability.
C, Subluxation of glenohumeral joint following a stroke (paralysis of deltoid muscle). (**B** from Warren RF:
Subluxation of the shoulder in athletes, *Clin Sports Med* 2:339, 1983.)

scapulae, which begin medially at the level of the third (T3) thoracic vertebra, should be at the same angle. The scapula itself should extend from the T2 or T3 spinous process to the T7 or T9 spinous process of the thoracic vertebrae. Sobush and associates developed a method for measuring the scapular position called the **Lennie test.**[37]

In this test, they measured from the spinous processes horizontally to three scapular positions: the medial aspect of the most superior point (superior angle), the root of the spine of the scapula, and the inferior angle (Figure 5-17).[37] If the scapula is sitting lower than normal against the chest wall, the superior medial border of the scapula

Figure 5-13

Subcoracoid dislocation of the shoulder. Note the prominent acromion, the arm held away from the side, and the flat deltoid. (From McLaughlin HL: *Trauma,* p. 246, Philadelphia, 1959, WB Saunders.)

may "washboard" over the ribs, causing a snapping or clunking sound **(snapping scapula)** during abduction and adduction.[38-42] The inferior angles of the scapulae should be equidistant from the spine.

Kibler et al. divided scapular dysfunction or dyskinesia into four patterns.[43] Type I shows the inferior medial border being prominent at rest and the inferior angle tilts dorsally with movement (scapular tilt), while the acromion tilts anteriorly over the top of the thorax. It may be seen at rest or during concentric or eccentric movement. If the inferior border tilts away from the chest wall, it may indicate the presence of weak muscles (e.g., lower trapezius, latissimus dorsi, serratus anterior) or a tight pectoralis minor or major pulling or tilting the scapula forward from above.[20] Type II is the classic winging of the scapula with the whole medial border of the scapula being prominent and lifting away from the posterior chest wall both statically and dynamically (Figure 5-18). It too may be seen at rest or during eccentric or concentric movements. This deformity may indicate the presence of a SLAP (Superior Labrum Anterior and Posterior [to the biceps])lesion weakness of the serratus anterior, rhomboids, lower, middle and upper trapezius, a long thoracic nerve problem or tight humeral rotators.[20] Type III is illustrated by the superior border of the scapula being elevated at rest and during movement; a shoulder shrug initiates the movement and there is minimal winging. This deformity is seen with active movement and may result from overactivity of the levator scapula and

upper trapezius along with imbalance of the upper and lower trapezius force couple (Figure 5-19). It is associated with impingement and rotator cuff lesions.[20] In the type IV pattern, both scapulae are symmetrical at rest and during motion; they rotate symmetrically upward with the inferior angles rotating laterally away from midline (rotary winging). It is seen during movement and may indicate the scapular control muscles are not stabilizing the scapula.

Dynamic winging (i.e., winging with movement) may be caused by a lesion of the long thoracic nerve affecting serratus anterior, trapezius palsy (spinal accessory nerve), rhomboid weakness, multidirectional instability, voluntary action, or a painful shoulder resulting in splinting of the glenohumeral joint, which in turn causes reverse scapulohumeral rhythm.[44] This splinting of the glenohumeral joint leads to reverse origin-insertion of the rotator cuff muscles so that instead of moving the humerus as they normally would, they work in reverse fashion and move the scapula. Commonly, with pathology, the scapular control muscles are weak and cannot counteract this action, resulting in protraction of the scapula and dynamic winging. The two other common causes of dynamic winging—long thoracic nerve palsy and spinal accessory nerve palsy—cause different scapula positioning and different winging patterns. Spinal accessory nerve palsy causes the scapula to depress and move laterally, with the inferior angle rotated laterally. If the trapezius is weak or paralyzed, the winging of the scapula occurs before 90° abduction, and there is little winging on forward flexion.[45] Long thoracic nerve palsy causes the scapula to elevate and move medially, with the inferior angle rotating medially (Figure 5-20).[46,47] If the serratus anterior is weak or paralyzed, the winging of the scapula occurs on abduction and forward flexion (especially with a "punch out" forward against resistance) (see Figure 5-18).[45,48] Radiculopathies at C3, C4 (trapezius), C5 (rhomboids), and C7 (serratus anterior, rhomboids) can also cause winging.[49,50]

Static winging (i.e., winging occurring at rest) is usually caused by a structural deformity of the scapula, clavicle, spine, or ribs.[51]

Sprengel's deformity, which is a congenitally high or undescended scapula (Figure 5-21), is the most common congenital deformity of the shoulder complex.[52-54] With this deformity, the scapular muscles are poorly developed or are replaced by a fibrous band. The condition may be unilateral or bilateral, and the range of the shoulder abduction decreases, although functional disability may be slight. Usually, the scapula is smaller than normal and is medially rotated.

The shoulder muscles may be accentuated by having the patient place the hands on the hips and contract the muscles. The examiner should check closely for wasting in the

A

B

C

Figure 5-14
Depressed right shoulder in a right-dominant individual—in this case, a tennis player. **A,** Hypertrophy of playing shoulder muscles. **B,** With muscles relaxed, the distance between spinous processes and medial border of scapula is widened on the right. **C,** Depressed shoulder.
(From Priest JD, Nagel DA: Tennis shoulder, *Am J Sports Med* 4:33, 1976.)

Figure 5-15
Congenital absence of sternal head of pectoralis major. Note fascial cord (*arrow*).

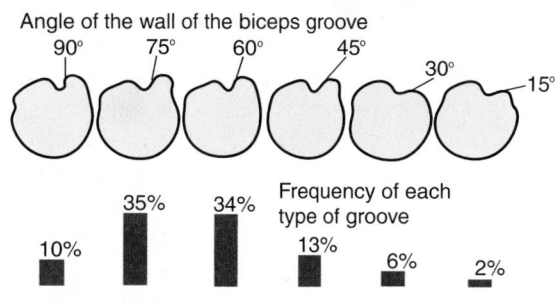

Figure 5-16
Different shapes of the bicipital groove. (Adapted from Hitchcock HH, Bechtol CO: Painful shoulder: observation on the role of the tendon of the long head of the biceps brachii in its causation, *J Bone Joint Surg Am* 30:267, 1948.)

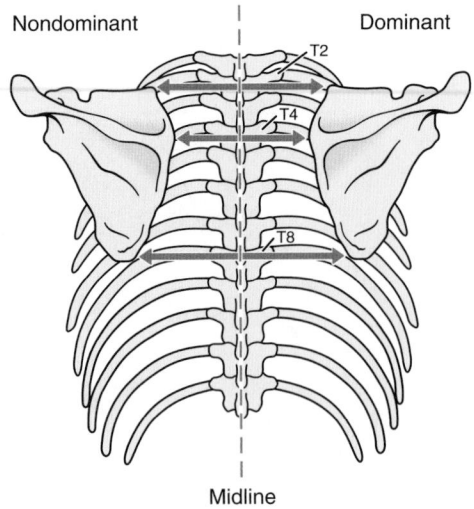

Nondominant   Dominant

T2

T4

T8

Midline

Figure 5-17

Lennie test. Measurements are taken at three positions on the scapula, and dominant and nondominant sides are compared.

supraspinatus and infraspinatus muscles (suprascapular nerve palsy), in the serratus anterior muscle (long thoracic nerve palsy), and in the trapezius muscle (spinal accessory nerve palsy), all of which can lead to winging of the scapula.

Examination

Because assessment of the shoulder may include an assessment of the cervical spine, the examination can be an extensive one. If the examiner has any doubt as to the location of the lesion, a cervical spine assessment

(see Chapter 3) should be performed. In addition, the examiner must remember that the arm, of which the shoulder is an integral part, may act as an open kinetic chain when the hand is free to move or as a closed kinetic chain when the hand is fixed to some relatively immovable object. For example, scapular instability may be evident in closed kinetic chain when the arm is fixed and the rotator cuff muscles work in reverse order (reverse origin-insertion; for example, the insertion of the muscles into the humerus becomes the stable part because the arm is fixed whereas the scapula becomes the mobile part and is more likely to move) (Figure 5-22). It may also be evident in open kinetic chain, especially during high-speed movements when the scapula needs to be stabilized (e.g., when hitting a ball) or when the scapular muscles should be working eccentrically to slow or stop a movement (i.e., they are unable to do so because of weakness). In open kinetic chain, the scapula acts as the base or origin of the muscles, whereas the insertion into the humerus is more mobile. Knowledge of muscle balance and muscle force couples becomes imperative in determining a diagnosis. For example, the legs, pelvis, and trunk act as force generators, whereas the shoulder acts as a funnel and force regulator with the arm acting as the force delivery system.[20] These **kinetic chains** and the intricate and complex interplay of the components of the kinetic chain have different effects on the shoulder. Eating, reaching, and dressing are considered open kinetic chain activities, whereas crutch walking and pushing up from a chair are considered closed kinetic chain movements.

As with any assessment, the examiner is comparing one side of the body with the other. This comparison is necessary because of individual differences among normal people.

A   B   C

Figure 5-18

Winging of the scapula. **A,** The shoulders at rest. **B,** Winging apparent when the patient is pushing forward. **C,** Winging when attempting full abduction. (From Foo CL, Swann M: Isolated paralysis of the serratus anterior: a report of 20 cases, *J Bone Joint Surg Br* 65:554, 1983.)

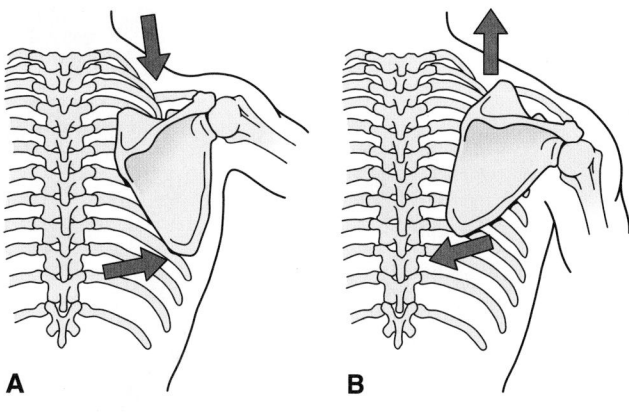

Figure 5-20

Scapular movement resulting in scapular winging caused by trapezius palsy (**A**) and serratus anterior palsy (**B**).

An understanding of the **force couples** acting on the shoulder complex and the necessity of balancing the muscle strength and endurance of these muscles is especially important when assessing the shoulder.[55] Force couples are groups of counteracting muscles that show obvious action when a movement is loaded or done quickly.[56] With a particular movement, one group of muscles (the agonists) acts concentrically whereas the other group (the antagonists) acts eccentrically in a controlled, harmonized fashion to produce smooth movement. In addition, these muscles may work by cocontraction or coactivation to provide a stabilizing effect and joint control. Table 5-6 gives examples of some of the force couples acting about the shoulder.

Active elevation through abduction is normally 170° to 180°. The extreme of the ROM occurs when the arm is abducted and lies against the ear on the same side of

Figure 5-19

Imbalance pattern of the upper and lower trapezius. Note overdevelopment of upper trapezius and lower trapezius working to prevent rotary winging.

Active Movements

The first movements to be examined are the active movements. These movements are usually done in such a way that the painful movements are performed last so pain does not carry over to the next movement. It is also essential to be able to differentiate between scapular movement and glenohumeral movements when watching active movements because scapular movement often compensates for restricted glenohumeral movement leading to weak and often lengthened scapular control muscles.

Active Movements of the Shoulder Complex

- Elevation through abduction (170° to 180°)
- Elevation through forward flexion (160° to 180°)
- Elevation through the plane of the scapula (170° to 180°)
- Lateral (external) rotation (80° to 90°)
- Medial (internal) rotation (60° to 100°)
- Extension (50° to 60°)
- Adduction (50° to 75°)
- Horizontal adduction/abduction (cross-flexion/cross-extension; 130°)
- Circumduction (200°)
- Scapular protraction
- Scapular retraction
- Combined movements (if necessary)
- Repetitive movements (if necessary)
- Sustained positions (if necessary)

Figure 5-21

Diagram (**A**) and photograph (**B**) of child with Sprengel's deformity. Note elevated shoulder and poorly developed scapula on the left. (**A** modified from Gartland JJ: *Fundamentals of orthopaedics*, p. 73, Philadelphia, 1979, WB Saunders. **B** courtesy of Dr. Roshen Irani.)

Figure 5-22

The pathomechanics of "classic winging" of the scapula. **A,** Winging of the right scapula caused by marked weakness of the right serratus anterior. The winging is exaggerated when resistance is applied against a shoulder abduction effort. Note how the stabilization occurs where the examiner's hand is offering resistance. Instead of the arm moving, the scapula moves because its stabilizing muscles are weak. **B,** Kinesiologic analysis of the winging scapula. Without an adequate upward rotation force from the serratus anterior *(fading arrow),* the scapula becomes unstable and cannot resist the pull of the deltoid. Subsequently, the force of the deltoid *(bidirectional arrow)* causes the scapula to downwardly rotate and the glenohumeral joint to partially abduct (reverse origin-insertion). (From Neumann DA: *Kinesiology of the musculoskeletal system: foundations for physical rehabilitation,* p. 107, St. Louis, 2002, Mosby.)

the head (Figure 5-23). As the patient elevates the upper extremity by abducting the shoulder, the examiner should note whether a **painful arc** is present (Figure 5-24).[57] A painful arc may be caused by subacromial bursitis, calcium deposits, or a peritenonitis or tendinosis[23,24] of the rotator cuff muscles. The pain results from pinching of

inflamed or tender structures under the acromion process and the coracoacromial ligament. Initially, the structures are not pinched under the acromion process, so the patient is able to abduct the arm 45° to 60° with little difficulty. As the patient abducts further (60° to 120°), the structures (e.g., subacromial bursa, rotator cuff tendon

Table 5-6

Force Couples about the Shoulder

Movement	Agonist/ Stabilizer	Antagonist/ Stabilizer
Protraction (scapula)	Serratus anterior* Pectoralis major[†] and minor[†]	Trapezius Rhomboids
Retraction (scapula)	Trapezius Rhomboids	Serratus anterior* Pectoralis major[†] and minor[†]
Elevation (scapula)	Upper trapezius[†] Levator scapulae[†]	Serratus anterior* Lower trapezius*
Depression (scapula)	Serratus anterior* Lower trapezius*	Upper trapezius[†] Levator scapulae[†]
Lateral rotation (upward rotation of inferior angle of scapula)	Trapezius (upper[†] and lower* fibers) Serratus anterior*	Levator scapulae[†] Rhomboids Pectoralis minor[†]
Medial rotation (downward rotation of inferior angle of scapula)	Levator scapulae[†] Rhomboids Pectoralis minor[†]	Trapezius (upper[†] and lower* fibers) Serratus anterior*
Scapular stabilization	Upper trapezius[†] Lower trapezius* Rhomboids	Serratus anterior*
Abduction (humerus)	Deltoid	Supraspinatus
Medial rotation (humerus)	Subscapularis[†] Pectoralis major[†] Latissimus dorsi Anterior deltoid	Infraspinatus* Teres minor Posterior deltoid
Lateral rotation (humerus)	Infraspinatus Teres minor Posterior deltoid	Subscapularis[†] Pectoralis major[†] Latissimus dorsi Anterior deltoid

*Muscles prone to weakness.
[†]Muscles prone to tightness.

insertions especially supraspinatus) become pinched and the patient is often unable to abduct fully because of pain. If full abduction is possible, however, the pain diminishes after approximately 120° because the pinched soft tissues have passed under the acromion process and are no longer being pinched. Often, the pain is greater going up (against gravity) than coming down, and there is more pain on active abduction than on passive abduction. If the movement is very painful, the patient often elevates the arm through forward flexion or hikes the shoulder using upper trapezius and levator scapulae in an attempt to decrease the pain. In some cases, retracting the scapula so that the space under the coracoacromial space is slightly enlarged may decrease pain. A second painful arc in the shoulder may be seen during the same

abduction movement. This painful arc (see Figure 5-24) occurs toward the end of abduction, in the last 10° to 20° of elevation, and is caused by pathology in the acromioclavicular joint or by a positive impingement test. In the case of the acromioclavicular joint lesion, the pain tends to be localized to the joint. With the impingement syndrome, the pain is usually found in the anterior shoulder region. Table 5-7 presents the signs and symptoms of three types of painful arc in the shoulder, with the superior type being the most common. The arc of pain may be present also during elevation through forward flexion and scaption, although the pain is usually less severe on these movements. The interconnection of the subacromial, subcoracoid, and subscapularis bursae with each other and with the glenohumeral joint capsule often produces a broad area of signs and symptoms, which may result in a painful arc.

When examining the movement of elevation through abduction, the examiner must take time to observe **scapulohumeral rhythm** of the shoulder complex (Figure 5-25), both anteriorly and posteriorly.[58–60] That is, during 180° of abduction, there is roughly a 2:1 ratio of movement of the humerus to the scapula, with 120° of movement occurring at the glenohumeral joint and 60° at the scapulothoracic joint; one should be aware, however, that there is a great deal of variability among individuals and may depend on the speed of movement,[61] and authors do not totally agree on the exact amounts of each movement.[59,60,62] Although all authors concede that there is more movement in the glenohumeral joint than in the scapulothoracic joint, Davies and Dickoff-Hoffman believe the ratio is greater, at least to 120° of abduction,[63] whereas Poppen and Walker[64] and others[7,65] believe the ratio is less (5:4 or 3:2) after 30° of abduction. During this total simultaneous movement at the four joints, there are three phases; the reader should understand that others will give values of the amount of each movement that vary from those noted here.

Scapulohumeral Rhythm		
Phase 1:	Humerus	30° abduction
	Scapula	minimal movement (setting phase)
	Clavicle	0°–5° elevation
Phase 2:	Humerus	40° abduction
	Scapula	20° rotation, minimal protraction or elevation
	Clavicle	15° elevation
Phase 3:	Humerus	60° abduction, 90° lateral rotation
	Scapula	30° rotation
	Clavicle	30°–50° posterior rotation, up to 15° elevation

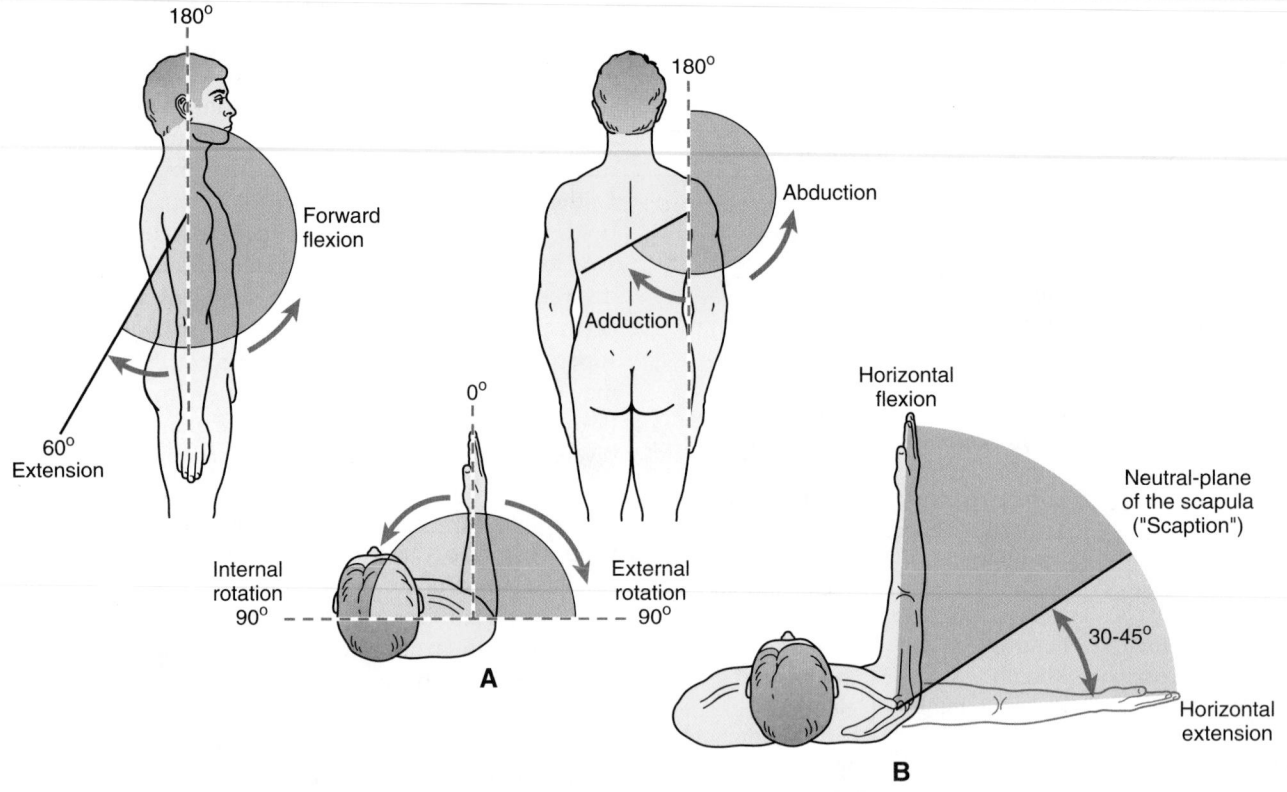

Figure 5-23

Movement in the shoulder complex. **A,** Range of motion of the shoulder. **B,** Axes of arm elevation. (Adapted from Perry J: Anatomy and biomechanics of the shoulder in throwing, swimming, gymnastics, and tennis, *Clin Sports Med* 2:255, 1983.)

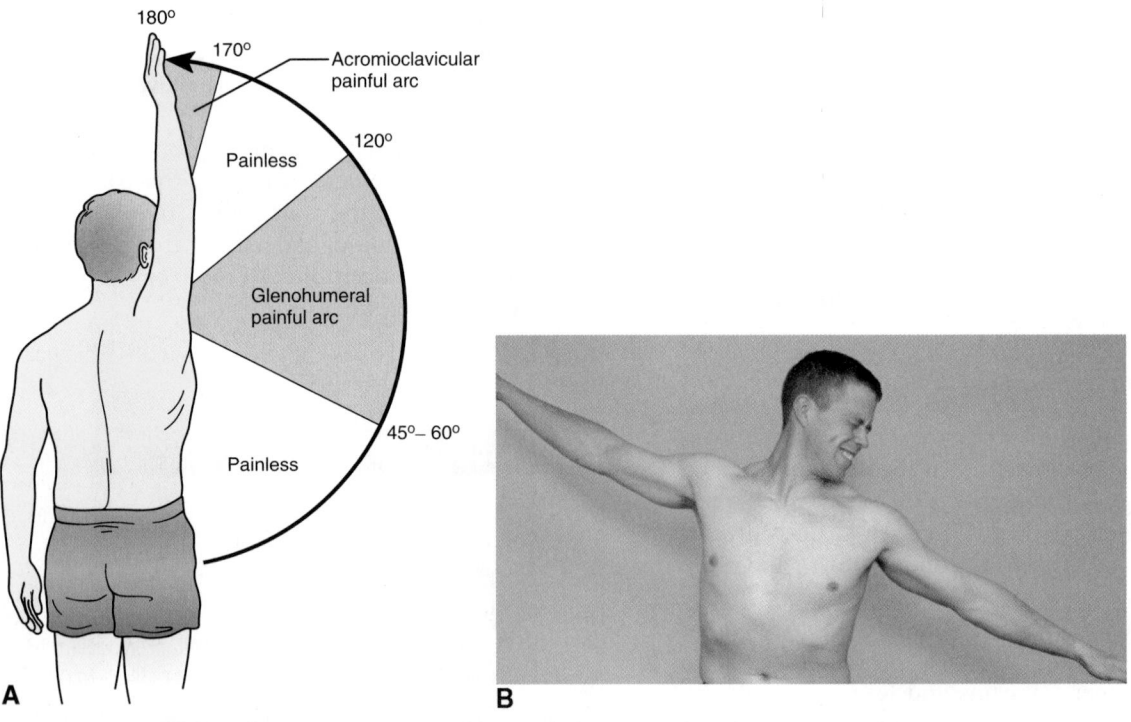

Figure 5-24

Painful arc in the shoulder. **A,** Painful arc of the glenohumeral joint. In the case of acromioclavicular joint problems only, the range of 170° to 180° would elicit pain. **B,** Note the impingement causing pain on the right at approximately 85°. (**A** modified from Hawkins RJ, Hobeika PE: Impingement syndrome in the athletic shoulder, *Clin Sports Med* 2:391, 1983.)

Table 5-7

Classification of Glenohumeral Painful Arcs

	Anterior	Posterior	Superior
Night pain	Yes	Yes	Maybe
Age	50+	50+	40+
Sex ratio	F > M	F > M	M > F
Aggravated by	Lateral rotation and abduction	Medial rotation and abduction	Abduction
Tenderness	Lesser tuberosity	Posterior aspect of greater tuberosity	Greater tuberosity
Acromioclavicular joint involvement	No	No	Often
Calcification (if present)	Supraspinatus, infraspinatus, and/or subscapularis	Supraspinatus and/or infraspinatus	Supraspinatus and/or subscapularis
Third-degree strain biceps brachii (long head)	No	No	Occasional
Prognosis	Good	Very good	Poor (without surgery)

From Kessel L, Watson M: The painful arc syndrome, *J Bone Joint Surg Br* 59:166, 1977.

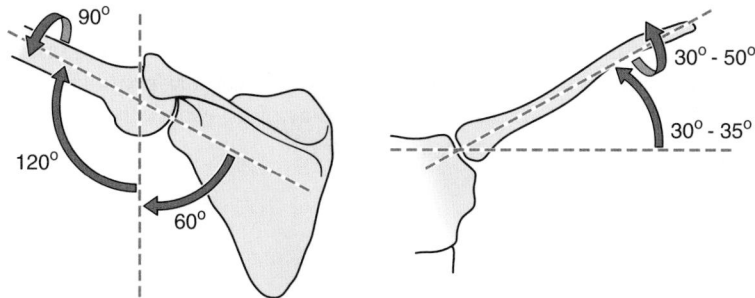

Figure 5-25

Movement of the scapula, humerus, and clavicle during scapulohumeral rhythm.

1. In the first phase of 30° of elevation through abduction, the scapula is said to be "setting." This setting phase means that the scapula may rotate slightly in, rotate slightly out, or not move at all.[48] Thus, there is no 2:1 ratio of movement during this phase. The angle between the scapular spine and the clavicle may also increase up to 5° by elevating at the sternoclavicular and acromioclavicular joints,[58] but this depends on whether the scapula moves during this phase. The clavicle rotates minimally during this stage.

2. During the next 60° of elevation (second phase), the scapula rotates about 20°, and the humerus elevates 40° with minimal protraction or elevation of the scapula.[58] Thus, there is a 2:1 ratio of scapulohumeral movement. During phase 2, the clavicle elevates because of the scapular rotation,[7,58] but the clavicle still does not rotate or does so minimally. During the second and third phase, the rotation of the scapula (total: 60°) is possible because there is 20° of motion at the acromioclavicular joint and 40° at the sternoclavicular joint.

3. During the final 90° of motion (third phase), the 2:1 ratio of scapulohumeral movement continues, and the angle between the scapular spine and the clavicle increases an additional 10°. Thus, the scapula continues to rotate and now begins to elevate. The amount of protraction continues to be minimal when the abduction movement is performed. It is in this stage that the clavicle rotates posteriorly 30° to 50° on a long axis and elevates up to a further 15°.[7] Also, during this final stage, the humerus laterally rotates 90°, so that the greater tuberosity of the humerus avoids the acromion process.

In the unstable shoulder, scapulohumeral rhythm is commonly altered because of incorrect dynamic functioning of the scapular or humeral stabilizers or both.[66] This may be related to incorrect arthrokinematics at the glenohumeral joint, so the examiner must be sure to check for normal joint play and the presence of hypomobile structures that could lead to these abnormal motions.[66]

Kibler pointed out that it is important to watch the movement especially of the scapula in both the ascending and descending phases of abduction.[67] Commonly, weakness of the scapular control muscles is more evident during descent, and an instability jog, hitch, or jump may occur when the patient loses control of the scapula.

The speed of abduction may also have an effect on the ratio.[68] Therefore, it is more important to look for asymmetry between the injured and the good sides than to be concerned with the actual degrees of movement occurring at each joint. That being said, if the clavicle does not rotate and elevate, elevation through abduction at the glenohumeral joint is limited to 120°.[58] If the glenohumeral joint does not move, elevation through abduction is limited to 60°, which occurs totally in the scapulothoracic joint. If there is no lateral rotation of the humerus during abduction, the total movement available is 120°, 60° of which occurs at the glenohumeral joint and 60° of which occurs at the scapulothoracic articulation.[7] The normal end of ROM is reached when there is contact of a surgical neck of humerus with the acromion process. **Reverse scapulohumeral rhythm** (Figure 5-26) means that the scapula moves more than the humerus. This occurs in conditions such as frozen shoulder. The patient appears to "hike" the entire shoulder complex rather than produce a smooth coordinated abduction movement.

Active elevation through forward flexion is normally 160° to 180°, and at the extreme of the ROM, the arm is in the same position as for active elevation through abduction. Active elevation (170° to 180°) through the plane of the scapula (30° to 45° of forward flexion),

termed **scaption,** is the most natural and functional motion of elevation (see Figure 5-23). Elevation in this position is sometimes called neutral elevation. The exact angle is determined by the contour of the chest wall on which the scapula rests. Often, movement into elevation is less painful in this position than elevation through abduction in which the glenohumeral joint is actually in extension, or elevation in forward flexion. Movement in the plane of the scapula puts less stress on the capsule and surrounding musculature and is the position in which most of the functions of daily activity are commonly performed. Strength testing in this plane also gives higher values. Patients with weakness spontaneously choose this plane when elevating the arm.[69,70] During scaption elevation, scapulohumeral rhythm is similar to that of abduction although there is greater individual variability. The three phases are similar, but there are differences. For example, in scaption elevation, there is little or no lateral rotation of the head of the humerus in the third phase.[65] Also, the total elevation in scaption is about 170°, with scapular rotation being about 65° and humeral abduction about 105°; although there is slightly more scapular rotation in scaption, this difference again may result from individual variation.[65] More scapular protraction is likely to occur in scaption elevation, especially in elevation through forward flexion.

Figure 5-26
Reverse scapulohumeral rhythm (notice shoulder hiking) and excessive scapular movement. Examples include frozen shoulder (**A**) or tear of rotator cuff (**B**). (**B** from Beetham WP, Polley HF, Slocum CH et al: *Physical examination of the joints,* p. 41, Philadelphia, 1965, WB Saunders.)

Active lateral rotation is normally 80° to 90° but may be greater in some athletes such as gymnasts and baseball pitchers. Care must be taken when applying overpressure with this movement, because it could lead to anterior dislocation of the glenohumeral joint, especially in those with recurrent dislocation problems. If glenohumeral lateral rotation is limited, the patient will compensate by retracting the scapula.

Active medial rotation is normally 60° to 100°. This is usually assessed by measuring the height of the "hitchhiking" thumb (thumb in extension) reaching up the patient's back. Common reference points include the greater trochanter, buttock, waist, and spinous processes, with T5 to T10 representing the normal degree of medial rotation.[71] When doing the test in this fashion, the examiner must be aware that, in reality, the range measured is not that of the glenohumeral joint alone. In fact, much of the range is gained by winging the scapula. In the presence of tight medial glenohumeral motion, greater winging and protraction of the scapula occurs. Doing the rotation testing in 90° abduction, if the patient can achieve this position, will give a clearer indication of true glenohumeral joint medial and lateral rotation. Rotation is measured when the scapula starts to move. If rotation is tested in 90° abduction and crepitus is present on rotation, it indicates abrasion of torn tendon margins against the coracoacromial arch and is called the **"abrasion sign."**[38]

It is important to compare medial and lateral rotation, especially in active people who use their dominant arm at extremes of motion and under high load situations. It is important to note any **glenohumeral internal (medial) rotation deficit (GIRD),**[18] which is the difference in medial rotation between the patient's two shoulders. Normally, the difference should be within 20°.[18] This may also be compared with the **glenohumeral external (lateral) rotation gain (GERG).** If the GIRD/GERG ratio is greater than 1, the patient will probably develop shoulder problems.[20]

Active extension is normally 50° to 60°. The examiner must ensure that the movement is in the shoulder and not in the spine because some patients may flex the spine or bend forward, giving the appearance of increased shoulder extension. Similarly, retraction of the scapula increases the appearance of glenohumeral extension. Weakness of full extension commonly implies weakness of the posterior deltoid in one arm and is sometimes called the **swallow tail sign** as both arms do not extend the same amount either because of injury to the muscle itself or to the axillary nerve.[72]

Adduction is normally 50° to 75° if the arm is brought in front of the body. Horizontal adduction, or cross-flexion, is normally 130°. To accomplish this movement, the patient first abducts the arm to 90° and then moves the arm across the front of the body. Horizontal abduction, or cross-extension, is approximately 45°. After abduct-

ing the arm to 90°, the patient moves the straight arm in a backward direction. In both cases, the examiner should watch the relative amount of scapular movement between the normal and pathological sides. If movement is limited in the glenohumeral joint, greater scapular movement occurs. Circumduction is normally approximately 200° and involves taking the arm in a circle in the vertical plane.

In addition to the above movements, several of which involve movement of the humerus and scapula, the patient should actively perform two distinct movements of the scapulae: scapular retraction and scapular protraction (Figure 5-27). For scapular retraction, the examiner asks the patient to squeeze the shoulder blades (scapula) together. Normally, the medial borders of the scapula remain parallel to the spine but move toward the spine with the soft tissue bunching up between the scapula (see Figure 5-27, *B*). Ideally, the patient should be able to do this movement without excessive contraction of the upper trapezius muscles. For scapular protraction, the patient tries to bring the shoulders together anteriorly so the scapula move away from midline with the inferior angle of the scapula commonly moving laterally more than the superior angle so some lateral rotation of the inferior angle occurs (see Figure 5-27, *C*). This protraction/retraction cycle may cause a clicking or snapping near the inferior angle or supramedial corner, which is sometimes called a **snapping scapula,** caused by the scapula rubbing over the underlying ribs.[41]

Injury to the individual muscles can affect several movements. For example, if the serratus anterior muscle is weak or paralyzed, the scapula "wings" away from the thorax on

A

Figure 5-27 ▬▬▬▬
A, Resting position.

Continued

Figure 5-27 cont'd
B, Scapular retraction. **C,** Scapular protraction.

its medial border. It also assists upper rotation of the scapula during abduction. Injury to the muscle or its nerve may therefore limit abduction. In fact, loss or weakness of serratus anterior affects all shoulder movements because scapular stabilization is lost.[56] Similarly, weakness of the lower trapezius muscle can alter scapular mechanics resulting in anterior secondary impingement. Many of the tests for these muscles are described in the Special Tests section.

When observing these movements, the examiner may ask the patient to perform them in combination, especially if the history has indicated that combined movements are bothersome. For example, **Apley's scratch test** combines medial rotation with adduction, and lateral rotation with abduction (Figure 5-28). This method may decrease the time required to do the assessment. In addition, by having the patient do the combined movements, the examiner gains some idea of the functional capacity of the patient. For example, abduction combined with flexion and lateral rotation or adduction combined with extension and medial rotation is needed to comb the hair, to zip a back zipper, or to reach for a wallet in a back pocket. However, the examiner must take care to notice which movements are restricted and which ones are not, because several movements are performed at the same time. Some examiners prefer doing the same motion in both arms at the same time: neck reach (abduction, flexion, and lateral rotation at the glenohumeral joint) and back reach (adduction, extension, and medial rotation at the glenohumeral joint). Some believe this method makes comparison easier (Figure 5-29).[32] Often, the dominant shoulder shows greater

Figure 5-28
Apley's scratch test. **A,** The right arm is in lateral rotation, flexion and abduction, and the left arm is in medial rotation, extension, and adduction.

B

A

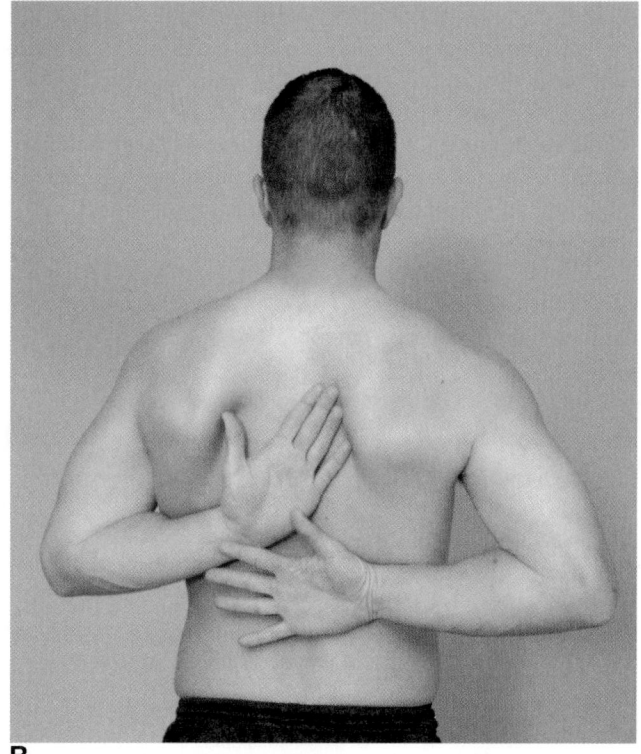

B

Figure 5-28 cont'd
B, The left arm is in lateral rotation, flexion and abduction, and the right arm is in medial rotation, extension and adduction. Note the difference in medial rotation and scapular winging in the right arm compared to the left arm in **A.**

Figure 5-29
A, Neck reach. **B,** Back reach.

restriction than the nondominant shoulder, even in normal people. An exception would be patients who continually use their arms at the extremes of motion (e.g., baseball pitchers). Because of the extra range of motion developed over time doing the activity, the dominant arm may show greater range of motion. However, the examiner must always be aware that shoulder movements include movements of the scapula and clavicle as well as the glenohumeral joint and that many of the perceived glenohumeral joint problems are, in reality, scapular muscle control problems, which may secondarily lead to glenohumeral joint problems, especially in people under 40 years of age. If, in the history, the patient has complained that shoulder movements in certain postures are painful or that sustained or repetitive movements increase symptoms, the examiner should consider having the patient hold a sustained arm position (10 to 60 seconds) or do the movements repetitively (10 to 20 repetitions). Ideally, these repeated movements should be performed at the speed and with the load that the patient was using when the symptoms were elicited. Thus, the volleyball player should do the spiking motion in which he or she jumps up to hit the imaginary ball.

Capsular tightness, although commonly tested during passive movement, can affect active movement by limiting some or all movements in the glenohumeral joint with compensating excessive movement of the scapula. Just as a frozen shoulder can affect all movements, selected tightness due to particular pathologies may affect only part of the capsule. For example, with anterior shoulder instability, posterior capsular tightness is a common finding combined with weak lower trapezius and serratus anterior muscles. Table 5-8 shows common selected capsular tightness and states their effect on movement.

Likewise, muscle tightness can affect both active and passive movement. For example, with anterior shoulder instability, the following muscles may be found to be tight: subscapularis, pectoralis minor and major, latissimus dorsi, upper trapezius, levator scapulae, sternocleidomastoid, scalenes, and rectus capitus. Weak muscles include serratus anterior, middle and lower trapezius, infraspinatus, teres minor, posterior deltoid, rhomboids, longus colli, and longus capitus.[41]

The biceps tendon does not move in the bicipital groove during movement; rather, the humerus moves over the fixed tendon. From adduction to full elevation of abduction, a given point in the groove moves along the tendon at least 4 cm. If the examiner wants to keep excursion of the bicipital groove along the biceps tendon to a minimum, the arm should be elevated with the humerus in medial rotation; elevating the arm with the humerus laterally rotated causes maximum excursion of the bicipital groove along the biceps tendon. Patients who have deltoid or supraspinatus pathology sometimes use this laterally rotated position because lateral rotation allows the biceps tendon to be used as a shoulder abductor in a "cheating" movement.

As the patient does the various movements, the examiner watches to see whether the components of the shoulder complex move in normal, coordinated sequence and whether the patient exhibits any apprehension when doing a movement. With **anterior instability** of the shoulder, the shoulder girdle often droops, and excessive scapulothoracic movement may occur on abduction. With **posterior instability,** horizontal adduction (cross-flexion) may cause excessive scapulothoracic movement. Any apprehension on movement suggests the possibility of instability. The examiner should also watch for **winging of the scapula** on active movements. Winging of the medial border of the scapula indicates injury to the serratus anterior muscle or the long thoracic nerve; rotary winging of the scapula or scapular tilt indicates upper trapezius pathology or injury to the spinal accessory nerve (cranial nerve XI; Table 5-9).[36,71,73] Scapular tilt (inferior angle of scapula moves away from rib cage) may also be caused by weak lower trapezius or a tight pectoralis minor. In some cases, it may be necessary to load the appropriate muscle isometrically (hold the contraction for 10 to 15 seconds) to demonstrate abnormal scapular stability. It has been reported that application of a resistance to adduction at 30° and at 60° of shoulder abduction is the best way to show scapular winging.[71] Eccentric loading of the shoulder in different positions, especially into horizontal adduction, may also demonstrate winging or loss of scapular control. Weakness of the scapular control muscles often leads to overactivity of the rotator cuff and biceps muscle leading to overuse pathology in those structures.

Causes of Scapular Imbalance Patterns

Increased protraction:	Tight pectoralis minor Weak/lengthened lower trapezius Weak/lengthened serratus anterior
Increased depression:	Weak upper trapezius
Loss of scapular stabilization:	Early/excessive protraction Early/excessive lateral rotation of scapula Early/excessive elevation of scapula Tight lateral rotators Secondary impingement

---

Humeral Movement Faults

Superior humeral translation:	Scapular downward rotators are predominating
Anterior humeral translation:	Weak subscapularis and teres major; tight infraspinatus, teres minor
Inferior humeral translation:	Weak upward scapular rotators; poor glenohumeral rotation timing
Decreased lateral rotation:	Short pectoralis major and/or latissimus dorsi
Excessive scapular retraction during lateral rotation:	Tight anterior capsule; tight medial rotators; poor scapulothoracic muscle control

---

Indications of Loss of Scapular Control

- Scapula protracting along chest wall, especially under load
- Early contraction of upper trapezius on abduction, especially under load
- Increased work of rotator cuff and biceps, especially with closed chain activity (reverse origin-insertion)
- Altered scapulohumeral rhythm

Table 5-8

Capsular Tightness: Its Effect and Resulting Humeral Head Translation

Where	Effect (Signs and Symptoms)	Resulting Translation
Posterior	Cross flexion decreased Medial rotation decreased Flexion (end range) decreased Decreased posterior glide Impingement signs in medial rotation Weak external rotators Weak scapular stabilizers	Anterior (with medical rotation)
Posteroinferior	Elevation anteriorly Medial rotation of elevated arm decreased Horizontal adduction decreased	Superior Anterosuperior Anterosuperior
Posterosuperior	Medial rotation limited	Anterosuperior
Anterosuperior	Flexion (end range) decreased Extension (end range) decreased Lateral rotation decreased Horizontal extension decreased Abduction (end range) decreased Decreased posteroinferior glide Impingement in medial rotation and cross flexion Increased night pain Weak rotator cuff May have positive ULTT Biceps tests may be positive	Posterior (with lateral rotation)
Anteroinferior	Abduction decreased Extension decreased Lateral rotation decreased Horizontal extension decreased Increased posterior glide	Posterior (with lateral rotation of elevated arm)

Data from Matsen FA et al: *Practice evaluation and management of the shoulder,* Philadelphia, 1994, WB Saunders.

Scapular Winging Faults

On concentric elevation:	Long/weak serratus anterior
On eccentric forward flexion:	Overactive rotator cuff; underactive scapular control muscles
Tilting of inferior angle:	Tight pectoralis minor; weak lower trapezius

If the scapula appears to wing, the examiner asks the patient to forward flex the shoulder to 90°. The examiner then pushes the straight arm toward the patient's body while the patient resists. If there is weakness of the upper or lower trapezius muscle, the serratus anterior muscle, or the nerves supplying these muscles, their inability to contract will cause the scapula to wing. Another way to test winging of the scapula is to have the patient stand and lean against the wall. The examiner then asks the patient to do a pushup away from the wall while the examiner watches for winging (see Figure 5-18; Figure 5-30, *A*). Similarly,

Table 5-9

Winging of the Scapula: Dynamic Causes and Effects

Cause	Effect (Signs and Symptoms)
Trapezius or spinal accessory nerve lesion	Inability to shrug shoulder
Serratus anterior or long thoracic nerve lesion	Difficulty elevating arm above 120°
Strain of rhomboids	Difficulty pushing elbow back against resistance (with hand on hip)
Muscle imbalance or contractures	Winging of upper margin of scapula on adduction and lateral rotation

asking the patient to do a floor pushup may demonstrate this winging (Figure 5-30, *B*). The patient should be tested in a relaxed starting position and be asked to do the pushup. Sometimes the winging is visible at rest only (static winging), sometimes during rest and activity, and sometimes only with the activity (dynamic winging).

Figure 5-30

Scapular winging is demonstrated by having the patient push against a wall (unilateral weakness) (**A**) or the floor (bilateral weakness) (**B**) with both arms forward flexed to 90°. (**A** from McClusky CM: Classification and diagnosis of glenohumeral instability in athletes, *Sports Med Arthro Rev* 8:163, 2000.)

Injury to other nerves in the shoulder region must not be overlooked (Table 5-10). As previously mentioned, damage to the suprascapular nerve may affect both the supraspinatus and infraspinatus muscles or it may affect

Table 5-10

Signs and Symptoms of Possible Peripheral Nerve Involvement

Spinal accessory nerve	Inability to abduct arm beyond 90°
	Pain in shoulder on abduction
Long thoracic nerve	Pain on flexing fully extended arm
	Inability to flex fully extended arm
	Winging starts at 90° forward flexion
Suprascapular nerve	Increased pain on forward shoulder flexion
	Shoulder weakness (partial loss of humeral control)
	Pain increases with scapular abduction
	Pain increases with cervical rotation to opposite side
Axillary (circumflex) nerve	Inability to abduct arm with neutral rotation
Musculocutaneous nerve	Weak elbow flexion with forearm supinated

only the infraspinatus, depending on where the pathology lies (see Figure 5-136), whereas injury to the musculocutaneous nerve can lead to paralysis of the coracobrachialis, biceps, and brachialis muscles. These changes affect elbow flexion and supination and forward flexion of the shoulder. There is also a loss of the biceps reflex. Injury to the axillary (circumflex) nerve leads to paralysis of the deltoid and teres minor muscles, affecting abduction and lateral rotation of the shoulder. There is also a sensory loss over the deltoid insertion area. Damage to the radial nerve affects all of the extensor muscles of the upper limb, including the triceps. Triceps paralysis may be overlooked when examining the shoulder unless arm extension is attempted along with elbow extension against gravity. Both of these movements are affected in high radial nerve palsy, although some triceps function may remain (e.g., in radial nerve palsy after a humeral shaft fracture).

Passive Movements

If the ROM is not full during the active movements and the examiner is unable to test the end feel, the examiner should perform all passive movements of the shoulder to determine the end feel, and any restriction should be noted. Such testing would show the presence of a capsular pattern.

> **Passive Movements of the Shoulder Complex and Normal End Feel**
>
> - Elevation through forward flexion of the arm (tissue stretch)
> - Elevation through abduction of the arm (bone-to-bone or tissue stretch)
> - Elevation through abduction of the glenohumeral joint only (bone-to-bone or tissue stretch)
> - Lateral rotation of the arm (tissue stretch)
> - Medial rotation of the arm (tissue stretch)
> - Extension of the arm (tissue stretch)
> - Adduction of the arm (tissue approximation)
> - Horizontal adduction (tissue stretch or approximation) and abduction of the arm (tissue stretch)
> - Quadrant test

The end feel of capsular tightness is different from the tissue stretch end feel of muscle tightness.[74] Capsular tightness has a more hard elastic feel to it, and it usually occurs earlier in the ROM. If one is unsure of the end feel, the examiner can ask the patient to contract the muscles acting in the opposite direction 10% to 20% of maximum voluntary contraction (MVC) and then relax. The examiner then attempts to move the limb further into range. If the range increases, the problem was muscular not capsular.

If the problem is capsular, capsular tightness should be measured. To measure posterior capsular tightness, the patient, suitably undressed (no shirt for males; bra for females), is placed in the side lying position with the test arm uppermost (the normal side is tested first) about 6 inches (15 cm) from the edge of the examining table.[75] The patient's hips and knees are flexed for stability. Both acromion processes should be perpendicular to the examining table, with the spine in neutral. The examiner stands in front of the patient and holds the patient's arm above the epicondyles of the elbow. The patient's arm is abducted to 90° with one hand while maintaining the shoulder in neutral rotation. With the other hand, the examiner stabilizes the lateral border of the scapula in the retracted position (Figure 5-31). While the scapular position is maintained, the examiner carefully horizontally adducts the arm until the movement ceases, the scapula begins to move, or rotation of the humerus occurs. The angle from the vertical to the arm indicates the passive ROM available. If the pathological side has less ROM and the end feel is capsular, capsular tightness is present. This capsular tightness should correlate well with decreased medial rotation provided the scapula is not allowed to move in compensation.[75,76]

Particular attention must be paid to passive medial and lateral rotation if the examiner suspects a problem with the glenohumeral joint capsule. Excessive scapular movement may be seen as compensation for a tight glenohumeral joint. **Subcoracoid bursitis** may limit full lateral rotation, and **subacromial bursitis** may limit full abduction because of compression or pinching of these structures. If lateral rotation of the shoulder is limited, the examiner should check forearm supination with the arm forward flexed to 90°. Patients who have a posterior dislocation at the glenohumeral joint exhibit restricted lateral rotation of the shoulder and limited supination in forward flexion **(Rowe sign).**[77] Even if overpressure has been applied on active movement, it is still necessary for the examiner to perform elevation through abduction of the glenohumeral joint only (Figure 5-32) and the quadrant test.

The examiner performs passive elevation through abduction or scaption of the glenohumeral joint with the clavicle and scapula fixed to determine the amount of abduction in the glenohumeral joint alone. This can give an indication of capsular tightness or subacromial space pathology.[32] Normally, this movement should be up to 120°, although Gagey and Gagey[78] have stated that anything greater than 105° indicates laxity in the inferior glenohumeral ligament.

A **B**

Figure 5-31

Testing for posterior capsular tightness. **A,** Starting position for the posterior shoulder flexibility measurement with the subject positioned correctly on his side. **B,** Maximum passive ROM of the posterior shoulder tissues. Note the scapular stabilization with the torso perpendicular to the examining table. As soon as the scapula begins to move, the examiner stops.

Figure 5-32
Passive abduction of the glenohumeral joint.

The rotation of the humerus in the quadrant position demonstrates Codman's "pivotal paradox"[70,79] and MacConaill's[80] conjunct rotation (rotation that automatically or subconsciously occurs with movement) in diadochal movement (a succession of two or more distinct movements). For example, if the arm, with the elbow flexed, is laterally rotated when the arm is at the side and then abducted in the coronal plane to 180°, the shoulder will be in 90° of medial rotation even though no apparent rotation has occurred. The path traced by the humerus during the quadrant test, in which the humerus moves forward at approximately 120° of abduction, is the unconscious rotation occurring at the glenohumeral joint. Thus, the quadrant test is designed to demonstrate whether the automatic or subconscious rotation is occurring during movement. The examiner should not only feel the movement but also determine the quality of the movement and the amount of anterior humeral movement. This test and the following locked quadrant test assess one area or quadrant of the 200° of circumduction. It is the quadrant of the circumduction movement in which the humerus must rotate to allow full pain-free movement. Although both of these tests should normally be pain free, the examiner should be aware that they place a high level of stress on the soft tissues of the glenohumeral joint, and discomfort should not be misinterpreted as pathological pain. If movement is painful and restricted, the tests indicate early stages of shoulder pathology.[81]

To test the **quadrant position**,[82,83] the examiner stabilizes the scapula and clavicle by placing the forearm under the patient's scapula on the side to be tested and extending the hand over the shoulder to hold the trapezius muscle and prevent shoulder shrugging (Figure 5-33). To test

A

B

Figure 5-33
Quadrant position. **A,** Adduction test. **B,** Abduction test (locked quadrant).

the position, the upper limb is elevated to rest alongside the patient's head with the shoulder laterally rotated. The patient's shoulder is then adducted. Because adduction occurs on the coronal plane, a point (the quadrant position) is reached at which the arm moves forward slightly from the coronal plane. At approximately 60° of adduction (from the arm beside the head), this position of maximum forward movement occurs (i.e., at about 120° of abduction) even if a backward pressure is applied. As the shoulder is further adducted, the arm falls back to the previous coronal plane. The quadrant position indicates the position at which the arm has medially rotated during its descent to the patient's side.

The quadrant position also may be found by abducting the medially rotated shoulder while maintaining extension. In this case, the quadrant position is reached (at approximately 120° of abduction) when the shoulder no longer abducts because it is prevented from laterally rotating by the catching of the greater tuberosity in the subacromial space. This position is referred to as the **locked quadrant position**.[83] If the arm is allowed to move forward, lateral rotation occurs and full abduction can be achieved.

The capsular pattern of the shoulder is lateral rotation showing the greatest restriction, followed by abduction and medial rotation. Each of these movements normally has a tissue-stretch end feel. Other movements may be limited, but not in the same order and not with as much restriction. Early capsular patterns may exhibit only limitations of lateral rotation or possibly lateral rotation and abduction. Finding of limitation, but not in the order described, indicates a noncapsular pattern.

Resisted Isometric Movements

Having completed the active and passive movements, which are done while the patient is standing, sitting, or lying supine (in the case of quadrant test), the patient lies supine to do the resisted isometric movements (Figure 5-34). The disadvantage of this position is that the examiner cannot observe the stabilization of the scapula during the testing. Normally, the scapula should not move during isometric testing. Scapular protraction, winging, or tilting during isometric testing would indicate weakness of the scapular control muscles. Although all the muscles around the shoulder can be tested in supine lying, it has been advocated that the muscles should be tested in more than one position (for example, different amounts of abduction or forward flexion) to determine the mechanical effect of the contraction in different situations. If, in the history, the patient complained of pain in one or more positions, these positions should be tested as well. If the initial position causes pain, other positions (e.g., position of injury, position of mechanical advantage) may be tried to further differentiate the specific contractile tissue that has been injured. During the active movements, the examiner should have noted which movements caused discomfort or pain so that this information can be correlated with that obtained from resisted isometric movements. By carefully noting which movements cause pain on isometric testing, the examiner should be able to determine which muscle or muscles are at fault (Table 5-11). For example, if the patient experiences pain primarily on medial rotation but also on abduction and adduction, the examiner would suspect a problem in the subscapularis muscle, because the other muscles involved in these actions were found to be pain free in other movements. To do the initial resisted isometric tests, the examiner positions the patient's arm at the side with the elbow flexed to 90°. The muscles of the shoulder are then tested isometrically with the examiner positioning the patient and saying, "Don't let me move you."

Resisted Isometric Movements of the Shoulder Complex

- Forward flexion of the shoulder
- Extension of the shoulder
- Adduction of the shoulder
- Abduction of the shoulder
- Medial rotation of the shoulder
- Lateral rotation of the shoulder
- Flexion of the elbow
- Extension of the elbow

Resisted isometric elbow flexion and extension must be performed, because some of the muscles (e.g., biceps, triceps) act over the elbow as well as the shoulder. The examiner should watch for the possibility of a third-degree strain (rupture) of the long head of biceps tendon ("Popeye muscle") when testing isometric elbow flexion (Figure 5-35).

During testing, the examiner will find differences in the relative strengths of the various muscle groups around the shoulder. The relative percentages for isometric testing will be altered for tests at faster speeds and tests in different planes. If, in the history, the patient complained that concentric, eccentric, or econcentric (biceps and triceps) movements were painful or caused symptoms, these movements should also be tested, with loading or no loading, as required.

Figure 5-34
Positioning of the patient for resisted isometric movements.

Table 5-11

Muscles about the Shoulder: Their Actions, Nerve Supply, and Nerve Root Derivation

Action	Muscles Acting	Nerve Supply	Nerve Root Derivation Retraction
Forward flexion	1. Deltoid (anterior fibers)	Axillary (circumflex)	C5–C6 (posterior cord)
	2. Pectoralis major (clavicular fibers)	Lateral pectoral	C5–C6 (lateral cord)
	3. Coracobrachialis	Musculocutaneous	C5–C7 (lateral cord)
	4. Biceps (when strong contraction required)	Musculocutaneous	C5–C7 (lateral cord)
Extension	1. Deltoid (posterior fibers)	Axillary (circumflex)	C5–C6 (posterior cord)
	2. Teres major	Subscapular	C5–C6 (posterior cord)
	3. Teres minor	Axillary (circumflex)	C5–C6 (posterior cord)
	4. Latissimus dorsi	Thoracodorsal	C6–C8 (posterior cord)
	5. Pectoralis major (sternocostal fibers)	Lateral pectoral	C5–C6 (lateral cord)
		Medial pectoral	C8, T1 (medial cord)
	6. Triceps (long head)	Radial	C5–C8, T1 (posterior cord)
Horizontal adduction	1. Pectoralis major	Lateral pectoral	C5–C6 (lateral cord)
	2. Deltoid (anterior fibers)	Axillary (circumflex)	C5–C6 (posterior cord)
Horizontal abduction	1. Deltoid (posterior fibers)	Axillary (circumflex)	C5–C6 (posterior cord)
	2. Teres major	Subscapular	C5–C6 (posterior cord)
	3. Teres minor	Axillary (circumflex)	C5–C6 (brachial plexus trunk)
	4. Infraspinatus	Suprascapular	C5–C6 (brachial plexus trunk)
Abduction	1. Deltoid	Axillary (circumflex)	C5–C6 (posterior cord)
	2. Supraspinatus	Suprascapular	C5–C6 (brachial plexus trunk)
	3. Infraspinatus	Suprascapular	C5–C6 (brachial plexus trunk)
	4. Subscapularis	Subscapular	C5–C6 (posterior cord)
	5. Teres minor	Axillary (circumflex)	C5–C6 (posterior cord)
	6. Long head of biceps (if arm laterally rotated first, trick movement)	Musculocutaneous	C5–C7 (lateral cord)
Adduction	1. Pectoralis major	Lateral pectoral	C5–C6 (lateral cord)
	2. Latissimus dorsi	Thoracodorsal	C6–C8 (posterior cord)
	3. Teres major	Subscapular	C5–C6 (posterior cord)
	4. Subscapularis	Subscapular	C5–C6 (posterior cord)
Medial rotation	1. Pectoralis major	Lateral pectoral	C5–C6 (lateral cord)
	2. Deltoid (anterior fibers)	Axillary (circumflex)	C5–C6 (posterior cord)
	3. Latissimus dorsi	Thoracodorsal	C6–C8 (posterior cord)
	4. Teres major	Subscapular	C5–C6 (posterior cord)
	5. Subscapularis (when arm is by side)	Subscapular	C5–C6 (posterior cord)
Lateral rotation	1. Infraspinatus	Suprascapular	C5–C6 (brachial plexus trunk)
	2. Deltoid (posterior fibers)	Axillary (circumflex)	C5–C6 (posterior cord)
	3. Teres minor	Axillary (circumflex)	C5–C6 (posterior cord)
Elevation of scapula	1. Trapezius (upper fibers)	Accessory	Cranial nerve XI
		C3–C4 nerve roots	C3–C4
	2. Levator scapulae	C3–C4 nerve roots	C3–C4
		Dorsal scapular	C5
	3. Rhomboid major	Dorsal scapular	(C4), C5
	4. Rhomboid minor	Dorsal scapular	(C4), C5
Depression of scapula	1. Serratus anterior	Long thoracic	C5–C6, (C7)
	2. Pectoralis major	Lateral pectoral	C5–C6 (lateral cord)
	3. Pectoralis minor	Medial pectoral	C8, T1 (medial cord)
	4. Latissimus dorsi	Thoracodorsal	C6–C8 (posterior cord)
	5. Trapezius (lower fibers)	Accessory	Cranial nerve XI
		C3–C4 nerve roots	C3–C4
Protraction (forward movement) of scapula	1. Serratus anterior	Long thoracic	C5–C6, (C7)
	2. Pectoralis major	Lateral pectoral	C5–C6 (lateral cord)
	3. Pectoralis minor	Medial pectoral	C8, T1 (medial cord)
	4. Latissimus dorsi	Thoracodorsal	C6–C8 (posterior cord)

Table 5-11—Cont'd

Action	Muscles Acting	Nerve Supply	Nerve Root Derivation Retraction
Retraction (backward movement) of scapula	1. Trapezius	Accessory	Cranial nerve XI
	2. Rhomboid major	Dorsal scapular	(C4), C5
	3. Rhomboid minor	Dorsal scapular	(C4), C5
Lateral (upward) rotation of inferior angle of scapula	1. Trapezius (upper and lower fibers)	Accessory C3–C4 nerve roots	Cranial nerve XI C3–C4
	2. Serratus anterior	Long thoracic	C5–C6, (C7)
Medial (downward) rotation of inferior angle of scapula	1. Levator scapulae	C3–C4 nerve roots	C3–C4
	2. Rhomboid major	Dorsal scapular	C5
	3. Rhomboid minor	Dorsal scapular	(C4), C5
	4. Pectoralis minor	Dorsal scapular Medial pectoral	(C4), C5 C8, T1 (medial cord)
Flexion of elbow	1. Brachialis	Musculocutaneous	C5–C6, (C7)
	2. Biceps brachii	Musculocutaneous	C5–C5
	3. Brachioradialis	Radial	C5–C6, (C7)
	4. Pronator teres	Median	C6–C7
	5. Flexor carpi ulnaris	Ulnar	C7–C8
Extension of elbow	1. Triceps	Radial	C6–C8
	2. Anconeus	Radial	C7–C8, (T1)

Relative Isometric Muscle Strengths

- Abduction should be 50% to 70% of adduction
- Forward flexion should be 50% to 60% of adduction
- Medial rotation should be 45% to 50% of adduction
- Lateral rotation should be 65% to 70% of medial rotation
- Forward flexion should be 50% to 60% of extension
- Horizontal adduction should be 70% to 80% of horizontal abduction

Functional Assessment

The shoulder complex plays an integral role in the activities of daily living, sometimes acting as part of an open kinetic chain and sometimes acting as part of a closed kinetic chain. Assessment of function plays an important part of the shoulder evaluation.[84] Limitation of function can greatly affect the patient. For example, placing the hand behind the head (e.g., to comb the hair) requires full lateral rotation, whereas placing the hand in the small of the back (e.g., to get a wallet out of a back pocket or undo a bra) requires full medial rotation. Matsen and colleagues have listed the functional ROM necessary to do some of the functional activities of daily living[38] (Table 5-12).

The functional assessment may be based on activities of daily living, work, or recreation, because these activities are of most concern to the patient (Figure 5-36),[85,86] or it may be based on numerical scoring charts (Figures 5-37 to 5-40 are examples), which are derived from clinical measures as well as functional measures. Some numerical

Figure 5-35
Rupture of the long head of the biceps brachii caused by the patient's awkward catch of partner in gymnastics. Bunching of muscle is attended by complete loss of function of the long head. (From O'Donoghue DH: *Treatment of injuries to athletes,* ed 4, p 53, Philadelphia, 1984, WB Saunders.)

Table 5-12

Range of Motion Necessary at the Shoulder to Do Certain Activities of Daily Living

Activity	Range of Motion	Activity	Range of Motion
Eating	70°–100° horizontal adduction* 45°–60° abduction	Hand behind head	10°–15° horizontal adduction* 110°–125° forward flexion 90° lateral rotation
Combing hair	30°–70° horizontal adduction* 105°–120° abduction 90° lateral rotation	Put something on shelf	70°–80° horizontal adduction* 70°–80° forward flexion 45° lateral rotation
Reach perineum	75°–90° horizontal abduction 30°–45° abduction 90°+ medial rotation	Wash opposite shoulder	60°–90° forward flexion 60°–120° horizontal adduction*
Tuck in shirt	50°–60° horizontal abduction 55°–65° abduction 90° medial rotation		

Adapted from Matsen FA et al: *Practical evaluation and management of the shoulder,* pp. 20, 24, Philadelphia, 1994, WB Saunders.
*Horizontal adduction is from 0° to 90° of abduction.

Please indicate with an "X" how often you performed each activity in your healthiest and most active state, in the past year.

	Never or less than once a month	Once a month	Once a week	More than once a week	Daily
Carrying objects 8 pounds or heavier by hand (such as a bag of groceries)					
Handling objects overhead					
Weight lifting or weight training with arms					
Swinging motion (as in hitting a tennis ball, golf ball, baseball, or similar object)					
Lifting objects 25 pounds or heavier (such as 3 gallons of water) NOT INCLUDING WEIGHT LIFTING					

For each of the following questions, please circle the letter that best describes your participation in that particular activity.

1) Do you participate in contact sports (such as, but not limited to, American football, rugby, soccer, basketball, wrestling, boxing, lacrosse, martial arts, etc)?

   A   No
   B   Yes, without organized officiating
   C   Yes, with organized officiating
   D   Yes, at a professional level (i.e., paid to play)

2) Do you participate in sports that involve hard overhand throwing (such as baseball, cricket, or quarterback in American football), overhead serving (such as tennis or volleyball), or lap/distance swimming?

   A   No
   B   Yes, without organized officiating
   C   Yes, with organized officiating
   D   Yes, at a professional level (i.e., paid to play)

Figure 5-36

Shoulder activity scale. It includes five numerically scored items and two alpha scored items. (From Brophy RH et al: Measurement of shoulder activity level, *Clin Orthop Relat Res* 439:105, 2005.)

Athletic Shoulder Outcome Rating Scale

Name _____ Age _____ Sex _____

Dominant Hand (R) _____ (L) _____ (Ambidextrous) _____

Date of Examination _____ Position Played _____

Surgeon _____ Years Played _____

Type of Sport _____ Prior Injury _____

Activity Level

1) Professional (major league)
2) Professional (minor league)
3) College
4) High school
5) Recreational (full time)
6) Recreational (occasionally)

Diagnosis

1) Anterior instability
2) Posterior instability
3) Multidirectional instability
4) Recurrent dislocations
5) Impingement syndrome
6) Acromioclavicular separation
7) Acromioclavicular arthrosis
8) Rotator cuff repair (partial)
9) Rotator cuff tear (complete)
10) Biceps tendon rupture
11) Calcific tendinitis
12) Fracture

Subjective (90 Points)

I. Pain

	Points
No pain with competition	10
Pain after competing only	8
Pain while competing	6
Pain preventing competing	4
Pain with ADLs	2
Pain at rest	0

II. Strength/Endurance

	Points
No weakness, normal competition fatigue	10
Weakness after competition, early competition fatigue	8
Weakness during competition, abnormal competition fatigue	6
Weakness or fatigue preventing competition	4
Weakness or fatigue with ADLs	2
Weakness or fatigue preventing ADLs	0

III. Stability

	Points
No looseness during competition	10
Recurrent subluxations while competing	8
Dead-arm syndrome while competing	6
Recurrent subluxations prevent competition	4
Recurrent subluxations during ADLs	2
Dislocation	0

IV. Intensity

	Points
Preinjury versus postinjury hours of competition (100%)	10
Preinjury versus postinjury hours of competition (less than 75%)	8
Preinjury versus postinjury hours of competition (less than 50%)	6
Preinjury versus postinjury hours of competition (less than 25%)	4
Preinjury and postinjury hours of ADLs (100%)	2
Preinjury and postinjury hours of ADLs (less than 50%)	0

V. Performance

	Points
At the same level, same proficiency	50
At the same level, decreased proficiency	40
At the same level, decreased proficiency, not acceptable to athlete	30
Decreased level with acceptable proficiency at that level	20
Decreased level, unacceptable proficiency	10
Cannot compete, had to switch sport	0

Objective (10 Points)

Range of Motion

	Points
Normal external rotation at 90°−90° position; normal elevation	10
Less than 5° loss of external rotation; normal elevation	8
Less than 10° loss of external rotation; normal elevation	6
Less than 15° loss of external rotation; normal elevation	4
Less than 20° loss of external rotation; normal elevation	2
Greater than 20° loss of external rotation, or any loss of elevation	0

Overall Results

Excellent:	90–100 points
Good:	70–89 points
Fair:	50–69 points
Poor:	Less than 50 points

Figure 5-37

Athletic shoulder outcome rating scale. (From Tibone JE, Bradley JP: Evaluation of treatment outcomes for the athlete's shoulder. In Matsen FA, Fu FH, Hawkins RJ, editors: *The shoulder: a balance of mobility and stability,* pp. 526–527, Rosemont, Ill, 1993, American Academy of Orthopedic Surgeons.)

evaluation scales are designed for specific populations, such as athletes (see Figure 5-37), or specific injuries, such as instability (see Figures 5-38 and 5-40). Other shoulder rating scales are also available.[87-95] When using numerical scoring charts, the examiner should not place total reliance on the scores, because most of these charts are based primarily on the examiner's clinical measures and not the patient's subjective functional, hoped-for outcome, which is the patient's primary concern.[96,97] Probably the most functional numerical shoulder tests from a patient's perspective are the **simple shoulder test** (Figure 5-41) developed by Lippitt, Matsen, and associates,[38,98] the **Disabilities of the Arm, Shoulder and Hand (DASH) Test** by Hudak et al.[99] (Figure 5-42), and the **Penn Shoulder Score** by Leggin et al.[100,101] Table 5-13 provides the examiner with a method of determining the patient's functional shoulder strength and endurance. This table is based on the general population and would not indicate a true functional reading of athletes or persons who do heavy work involving the shoulders. For athletes or those applying significant load to their shoulders while forward flexed, the **one-arm hop test** has been developed (Figure 5-43). To do this test, the patient assumes the pushup position, balancing on one arm. The patient then hops up onto a 10-cm (4-inch) step and then back to the floor. The hop is repeated five times and the time noted. The patient starts with the good arm and then uses the injured arm, and the two times are compared. Provided the patient is trained, completing this action in less than 10 seconds is considered normal.[102]

Burkhart et al. felt it was important to test core stability (i.e., testing kinetic chain function) and flexibility when assessing the shoulder to ensure the proper transfer of forces from the legs to the trunk and the shoulder as part

---

Walch-Duplay Rating Sheet for Anterior Instability of the Shoulder

Family Name: _____ First name: _____ Date: _____

Sport

(1) Type of Sport Practiced

    C = competition
    L = leisure (spare time)
    N = not practicing a sport

(2) Type of Sport

0 = no sport	
1 = risk free	athletics, rowing, fencing, swimming, breaststroke, underwater diving, voluntary gymnastics, cross-country skiing, shooting, sailing.
2 = with contact	martial arts, cycling, motorcycling or biking, scrambling, soccer, rugby, waterskiing, downhill skiing, parachute jumping, horse riding.
3 = with cocking of the arm	climbing, weight lifting, shot-putting, swimming overarm and butterfly, pole vaulting, figure skating, canoeing, golf, hockey, tennis, baseball.
4 = with blocked cocking or "high risk"	basketball, handball, volleyball, hang gliding, kayaking, water polo, javelin throwing, judo, karate, wrestling, sky diving, wind surfing, diving, ice hockey, acrobatics, gymnastics (floor, using apparatus).

(3) Side

    D = dominant
    d = nondominant

(4) Functional Score of the Shoulder (100 points) with respect to

resuming sport	25 points
stability	25 points
pain	25 points
mobility	25 points

Figure 5-38 ▬▬▬▬▬

Walch-Duplay rating sheet for anterior instability of the shoulder. (From Walch G: *Directions for the use of the quotation of anterior instabilities of the shoulder,* Abstracts of the First Open Congress of the European Society of Surgery of the Shoulder and Elbow, pp. 51–55, 1987, Paris.)

Walch-Duplay Rating Sheet for Anterior Instability of the Shoulder

Daily Activity

Return to the same level in the same sport * No discomfort	+25 points
Decrease of level in the same sport practiced * Slight discomfort in forceful movements	+15 points
Change in sport * Slight discomfort during simple movements	+10 points
Decrease of level and change, or stop sport * Severe discomfort	0 points

Stability

No apprehension	+25 points
Persistent apprehension	+15 points
Feeling of instability	0 points
True recurrence	−25 points

Pain

No pain or pain during certain climatic conditions	+25 points
Pain during forceful movements or when tired	+15 points
Pain during daily life	0 points

Mobility

Pure frontal abduction against a wall: symmetric Internal rotation (IR) limited to less than three vertebrae External rotation (ER) at 90° abduction limited to less than 10% of the opposite side	+25 points
Pure frontal abduction against a wall <150° IR: limited to less than three vertebrae ER: limited to less than 30% of the opposite side	+15 points
Pure frontal abduction against a wall <120° IR: limited to less than six vertebrae ER: limited to less than 50% of the opposite side	+5 points
Pure frontal abduction against a wall <90° IR: limited to more than six vertebrae ER: limited to more than 50% of the opposite side	0 points

Total points _____

Overall Functional Result

Excellent:	**91 to 100 points**
Good:	**76 to 90 points**
Medium:	**51 to 75 points**
Poor:	**50 points or less**

* Criterion if the patient did not participate in sports before the operation

Figure 5-38 cont'd

American Shoulder and Elbow Surgeons' Shoulder Evaluation Form

Name _____ Hosp # _____ Date _____ Shoulder: R / L

I. Pain: (5 = none, 4 = slight, 3 = after unusual activity, 2 = moderate, 1 = marked, 0 = complete disability, NA = not available) _____

II. Motion:

A. Patient Sitting
  1. Active total elevation of arm: _____ degrees*
  2. Passive internal rotation:
     (Circle segment of posterior anatomy reached by thumb)
     (Note if reach restricted by limited elbow flexion)

1 = Less than trochanter	5 = L5	9 = L1	13 = T9	17 = T5
2 = Trochanter	6 = L4	10 = T12	14 = T8	18 = T4
3 = Gluteal	7 = L3	11 = T11	15 = T7	19 = T3
4 = Sacrum	8 = L2	12 = T10	16 = T6	20 = T2
				21 = T1

  3. Active external rotation with arm at side: _____ degrees
  4. Active external rotation at 90° abduction: _____ degrees
     (Enter "NA" if cannot achieve 90° of abduction)

B. Patient Supine

  1. Passive total elevation of arm: _____ degrees*

  2. Passive external rotation with arm at side: _____ degrees

* Total elevation of arm measured by viewing patient from side and using goniometer to determine angle between *arm* and *thorax*.

III. Strength: (5 = normal, 4 = good, 3 = fair, 2 = poor, 1 = trace, 0 = paralysis)

A. Anterior deltoid _____   C. External rotation _____

B. Middle deltoid _____   D. Internal rotation _____

IV. Stability: (5 = normal, 4 = apprehension, 3 = rare subluxation, 2 = recurrent subluxation, 1 = recurrent dislocation, 0 = fixed dislocation, NA = not available)

A. Anterior _____   B. Posterior _____   C. Inferior _____

V. Function: (4 = normal, 3 = mild compromise, 2 = difficulty, 1 = with aid, 0 = unable, NA = not available)

A. Use back pocket	_____	I. Sleep on affected side	_____
B. Perineal care	_____	J. Pulling	_____
C. Wash opposite axilla	_____	K. Use hand overhead	_____
D. Eat with utensil	_____	L. Throwing	_____
E. Comb hair	_____	M. Lifting	_____
F. Use hand with arm at shoulder level	_____	N. Do usual work (specify _____)	_____
G. Carry 10–15 lb with arm at side	_____	O. Do usual sport (specify _____)	_____
H. Dress	_____		

VI. Patient Response: (3 = much better, 2 = better, 1 = same, 0 = worse, NA = not available/applicable) _____

Figure 5-39

American Shoulder and Elbow Surgeons' shoulder evaluation form. (Courtesy of the American Shoulder and Elbow Surgeons.)

12-Item Shoulder Instability Questionnaire

Item	Scoring Categories
1. During the last six months, how many times has your shoulder slipped out of joint (or dislocated?)	1 Not al all in 6 months 2 1 or 2 times in 6 months 3 1 or 2 times per month 4 1 or 2 times per week 5 More often than 1 or 2 times/week
2. During the last three months, have you had any trouble (or worry) dressing because of your shoulder?	1 No trouble at all 2 Slight trouble or worry 3 Moderate trouble or worry 4 Extreme difficulty 5 Impossible to do
3. During the last three months, how would you describe the worst pain you have had from your shoulder?	1 None 2 Mild ache 3 Moderate 4 Severe 5 Unbearable
4. During the last three months, how much has the problem with your shoulder interfered with your usual work (including school or college work, or housework)?	1 Not at all 2 A little bit 3 Moderately 4 Greatly 5 Totally
5. During the last three months, have you avoided any activities due to worry about your shoulder – feared that it might slip out of joint?	1 Not at all 2 Very occasionally 3 Some days 4 Most days or more than one activity 5 Every day or many activities
6. During the last three months, has the problem with your shoulder prevented you from doing things that are important to you?	1 No, not at all 2 Very occasionally 3 Some days 4 Most days or more than one activity 5 Every day or many activities
7. During the last three months, how much has the problem with your shoulder interfered with your social life (including sexual activity – if applicable)?	1 Not at all 2 Occasionally 3 Some days 4 Most days 5 Every day
8. During the last four weeks, how much has the problem with your shoulder interfered with your sporting activities or hobbies?	1 Not at all 2 A little/occasionally 3 Some of the time 4 Most of the time 5 All of the time

Figure 5-40

The 12-item shoulder instability questionnaire. (Modified from Dawson J, Fitzpatrick R, Carr A: The assessment of shoulder instability: the development and validation of a questionnaire, *J Bone Joint Surg Br* 81:422, 1999.)

Continued

Item	Scoring Categories
9. During the last four weeks, how often has your shoulder been 'on your mind' – how often have you thought about it?	1 Never, or only if someone asks 2 Occasionally 3 Some days 4 Most days 5 Every day
10. During the last four weeks, how much has the problem with your shoulder interfered with your ability or willingness to lift heavy objects?	1 Not at all 2 Occasionally 3 Some days 4 Most days 5 Every day
11. During the last four weeks, how would you describe the pain which you usually had from your shoulder?	1 None 2 Very mild 3 Mild 4 Moderate 5 Severe
12. During the last four weeks, have you avoided lying in certain positions in bed at night, because of your shoulder?	1 No nights 2 Only 1 or 2 nights 3 Some nights 4 Most nights 5 Every night

TOTAL SCORE: _____   Maximum score: 60   Minimum score: 12

Figure 5-40 cont'd ▬▬▬▬▬

of the kinetic chain.[20] They advocated testing one-legged stance (no Trendelenburg), one-legged squat (stable pelvis), one-legged step up and step down (stable pelvis), normal hip medial rotation bilaterally, and strength of hip abductors, trunk flexors, and abdominal muscles.

Special Tests

Special tests are often used in shoulder examinations to confirm findings or a tentative diagnosis. The examiner must be proficient in those tests that he or she decides to use. Proficiency increases the reliability of the findings, although the reliability of some of the tests has been questioned.[103] The reliability, validity, specificity, and sensitivity of some diagnostic/special tests used in the shoulder are outlined in Appendix 5-1. Depending on the history, some tests are compulsory, and others may be used as confirming or excluding tests. As with all passive tests, results are more likely to be positive in the presence of pathology when the muscles are relaxed, the patient is supported, and there is minimal or no muscle spasm.

Instability and Pseudolaxity Impingement

Anterior shoulder pain is commonly seen in patients young and old complaining of shoulder pain and dysfunction. In the older patient (40-plus years old), mechanical impingement occurs because of degenerative changes to the rotator cuff, the acromion process, the coracoid process, and the anterior tissues from stress overload resulting in impingement. In this case, impingement is the primary problem (thus the term **primary impingement**). It may be intrinsic because of rotator cuff degeneration or extrinsic because of the shape of the acromion and degeneration of the coracoacromial ligament.[104]

In the young patient (15 to 35 years old), anterior shoulder pain is primarily caused by problems with muscle dynamics with an upset in the normal force couple action leading to muscle imbalance and abnormal movement patterns at both the glenohumeral joint and the scapulothoracic articulation. These altered muscle dynamics lead to symptoms of anterior impingement (thus the term **secondary impingement**). The impingement signs are a secondary result of altered muscle dynamics in the scapula or glenohumeral joint.[104]

	Last	First	M.I.		

Name: _____ Date: __ / __ / __ Age: _____

Street/Apt #	City	State	Zip Code

Address: _____ Occupation: _____

Home	Business		Relative

Phone: (___) ___ - ___   (___) ___ - ___   (___) ___ - ___

Circle one	*Circle one*
Dominant Hand: Right / Left / Ambidextrous	Shoulder Evaluated: Right / Left

Answer Each Question Below by Checking "Yes" or "No"

Response

	Yes	No

1. Is your shoulder comfortable with your arm at rest by your side? ☐ ☐ 1

2. Does your shoulder allow you to sleep comfortably? ☐ ☐ 2

3. Can you reach the small of your back to tuck in your shirt with your hand? ☐ ☐ 3

4. Can you place your hand behind your head with the elbow straight out to the side? ☐ ☐ 4

5. Can you place a coin on a shelf at the level of your shoulder without bending your elbow? ☐ ☐ 5

6. Can you lift one pound (a full pint container) to the level of your shoulder without bending your elbow? ☐ ☐ 6

7. Can you lift eight pounds (a full gallon container) to the level of your shoulder without bending your elbow? ☐ ☐ 7

8. Can you carry twenty pounds at your side with the affected extremity? ☐ ☐ 8

9. Do you think you can toss a softball underhand ten yards with the affected extremity? ☐ ☐ 9

10. Do you think you can toss a softball overhand twenty yards with the affected extremity? ☐ ☐ 10

11. Can you wash the back of your opposite shoulder with the affected extremity? ☐ ☐ 11

12. Would your shoulder allow you to work full-time at your regular job? ☐ ☐ 12

Office Use Only

Diagnosis: DJD RA AVN IMP RCT FS TUBS AMBRII Other: _____

Dx Confirmed? _____ Pt# _____ Physician _____

SST: Initial / Pre-op / Follow-up: 6 mon 1 yr 18 mon 2 yr 3 yr 4 yr 5 yr Other: _____

Initial SST Date: __/__/__ Rx: _____ Surgery Date: __/__/__

Figure 5-41
Simple shoulder test questionnaire form. (From Lippitt SB et al: A practical tool for evaluating function: the simple shoulder test. In Matsen FA et al, editors: *The shoulder: a balance of mobility and stability,* p 514, Rosemont, Ill, 1993, American Academy of Orthopedic Surgeons.)

Please rate your ability to do the following activities in the last week by circling the number below the appropriate response.

	No Difficulty	Mild Difficulty	Moderate Difficulty	Severe Difficulty	Unable
1. Open a tight or new jar.	1	2	3	4	5
2. Write.	1	2	3	4	5
3. Turn a key.	1	2	3	4	5
4. Prepare a meal.	1	2	3	4	5
5. Push open a heavy door.	1	2	3	4	5
6. Place an object on a shelf above your head.	1	2	3	4	5
7. Do heavy household chores (e.g., wash walls, wash floors).	1	2	3	4	5
8. Garden or do yard work.	1	2	3	4	5
9. Make a bed.	1	2	3	4	5
10. Carry a shopping bag or briefcase.	1	2	3	4	5
11. Carry a heavy object (over 10 lbs).	1	2	3	4	5
12. Change a light bulb overhead.	1	2	3	4	5
13. Wash or blow dry your hair.	1	2	3	4	5
14. Wash your back.	1	2	3	4	5
15. Put on a pullover sweater.	1	2	3	4	5
16. Use a knife to cut food.	1	2	3	4	5
17. Recreational activities which require little effort (e.g., cardplaying, knitting, etc.).	1	2	3	4	5
18. Recreational activities in which you take some force or impact through your arm, shoulder or hand (e.g., golf, hammering, tennis, etc.).	1	2	3	4	5
19. Recreational activities in which you move your arm freely (e.g., playing frisbee, badminton, etc.).	1	2	3	4	5
20. Manage transportation needs (getting from one place to another).	1	2	3	4	5
21. Sexual activities.	1	2	3	4	5

DISABILITIES OF THE ARM, SHOULDER, AND HAND

	Not at All	Slightly	Moderately	Quite a Bit	Extremely
22. During the past week, *to what extent* has your arm, shoulder, or hand problem interfered with your normal social activities with family, friends, neighbors or groups? (*circle number*)	1	2	3	4	5

	Not Limited At All	Slightly Limited	Moderately Limited	Very Limited	Unable
23. During the past week, were you limited in your work or other regular daily activities as a result of your arm, shoulder or hand problem? (*circle number*)	1	2	3	4	5

Please rate the severity of the following symptoms in the last week. (*circle number*)

	None	Mild	Moderate	Severe	Extreme
24. Arm, shoulder, or hand pain.	1	2	3	4	5
25. Arm, shoulder, or hand pain when you performed any specific activity.	1	2	3	4	5
26. Tingling (pins and needles) in your arm, shoulder, or hand.	1	2	3	4	5
27. Weakness in your arm, shoulder, or hand.	1	2	3	4	5
28. Stiffness in your arm, shoulder, or hand.	1	2	3	4	5

Figure 5-42

The DASH Questionnaire. (From Dutton M: *Orthopedic examination, evaluation and intervention,* pp. 449–450, New York, 2004, McGraw-Hill.)

Continued

DISABILITIES OF THE ARM, SHOULDER, AND HAND

	No Difficulty	Mild Difficulty	Moderate Difficulty	Severe Difficulty	So Much Difficulty That I Can't Sleep
29. During the past week, how much difficulty have you had sleeping because of the pain in your arm, shoulder or hand? (*circle number*)	1	2	3	4	5

	Strongly Disagree	Disagree	Neither Agree nor Disagree	Agree	Strongly Agree
30. I feel less capable, less confident or less useful because of my arm, shoulder, or hand problem. (*circle number*)	1	2	3	4	5

Scoring DASH function/symptoms: Add up circled responses (item 1–30); subtract 30; divide by 1.20 = DASH score.
SPORTS/PERFORMING ARTS MODULE (Optional)

The following questions relate to the impact of your arm, shoulder, or hand problem on playing *your musical instrument or sport*. If you play more than one sport or instrument (or play both), please answer with respect to that activity which is most important.

Please indicate the sport or instrument which is most important to you: _____

☐ I do not play a sport or an instrument. (You may skip this section.)

Please circle the number that best describes your physical ability in the past week. Did you have any difficulty:

	No Difficulty	Mild Difficulty	Moderate Difficulty	Severe Difficulty	Unable
1. Using your usual technique for playing your instrument or sport?	1	2	3	4	5
2. Playing your musical instrument or sport because of arm, shoulder, or hand pain?	1	2	3	4	5
3. Playing your musical instrument or sport as well as you would like?	1	2	3	4	5
4. Spending your usual amount of time practicing or playing your instrument or sport?	1	2	3	4	5

WORK MODULE (Optional)

The following questions ask about the impact of your arm, shoulder, or hand problem on your ability to work (including homemakers if that is your main work role)

☐ I do not work. (You may skip this section.)

Please circle the number that best describes your physical ability in the past week. Did you have any difficulty:

	No Difficulty	Mild Difficulty	Moderate Difficulty	Severe Difficulty	Unable
1. Using your usual technique for your work?	1	2	3	4	5
2. Doing your usual work because of arm, shoulder, or hand pain?	1	2	3	4	5
3. Doing your work as well as you would like?	1	2	3	4	5
4. Spending your usual amount of time doing your work?	1	2	3	4	5

Figure 5-42 cont'd �\blacksquare

Table 5-13

Functional Testing of the Shoulder

Starting Position	Action	Function Test*
Sitting	Forward flex arm to 90°	Lift 4 to 5 lb weight: Functional Lift 1 to 3 lb weight: Functionally fair Lift arm weight: Functionally poor Cannot lift arm: Nonfunctional
Sitting	Shoulder extension	Lift 4 to 5 lb weight: Functional Lift 1 to 3 lb weight: Functionally fair Lift arm weight: Functionally poor Cannot lift arm: Nonfunctional
Side lying (may be done in sitting with pulley)	Shoulder medial rotation	Lift 4 to 5 lb weight: Functional Lift 1 to 3 lb weight: Functionally fair Lift arm weight: Functionally poor Cannot lift arm: Nonfunctional
Side lying (may be done in sitting with pulley)	Shoulder lateral rotation	Lift 4 to 5 lb weight: Functional Lift 1 to 3 lb weight: Functionally fair Lift arm weight: Functionally poor Cannot lift arm: Nonfunctional
Sitting	Shoulder abduction	Lift 4 to 5 lb weight: Functional Lift 1 to 3 lb weight: Functionally fair Lift arm weight: Functionally poor Cannot lift arm: Nonfunctional
Sitting	Shoulder adduction (using wall pulley)	Lift 4 to 5 lb weight: Functional Lift 1 to 3 lb weight: Functionally fair Lift arm weight: Functionally poor Cannot lift arm: Nonfunctional
Sitting	Shoulder elevation (shoulder shrug)	Five to six repetitions: Functional Three to four repetitions: Functionally fair One to two repetitions: Functionally poor Zero repetitions: Nonfunctional
Sitting	Sitting pushup (shoulder dysfunction)	Five to six repetitions: Functional Three to four repetitions: Functionally fair One to two repetitions: Functionally poor Zero repetitions: Nonfunctional

Data from Palmer ML, Epler M: *Clinical assessment procedures in physical therapy,* pp. 68–73, Philadelphia, 1990, JB Lippincott.

*Younger, more fit patients should easily be able to do more than the values given for these tests. A comparison between the good side and the injured side gives the examiner some idea about the patient's functional strength capacity.

A   B

Figure 5-43

One-arm hop test. **A,** Start position. **B,** End position.

Special Tests Commonly Performed on the Shoulder

Instability, anterior:	Load and shift test
	Crank (apprehension) and relocation test
Instability, posterior:	Load and shift test
	Posterior apprehension test
	Norwood test
Instability, inferior (multidirectional):	Sulcus sign
	Feagan test
Impingement tests:	Neer test
	Hawkins-Kennedy test
	Posterior internal impingement test
Labral lesions:	Clunk test (Bankart)
	Anterior slide test (Bankart/SLAP)
	Active compression test of O'Brien (SLAP)
	Biceps tension test (SLAP)
Scapular stability tests:	Lateral scapular-slide tests
	Wall/floor pushup
	Scapular retraction test
Muscle tendon pathology:	Speed's test
	Yergason's test
	Empty can test
	Lift-off sign
	Lag or "spring back" tests (subscapularis [medial rotation] and infraspinatus/teres minor [lateral rotation])
	Trapezius weakness
	Serratus anterior weakness
	Pectoralis major and minor tightness
Neurological involvement:	Upper limb tension tests
Thoracic outlet syndromes:	Roos test (EAST)

As secondary impingement is primarily a problem with muscle dynamics, it commonly presents in conjunction with instability, either of the scapula or at the glenohumeral joint. A hypermobile or lax joint does not imply instability.[105] Laxity implies that there is a certain amount of nonpathological "looseness" in a joint so that ROM is greater in one or more directions and the shoulder complex functions normally. It is usually found bilaterally. Instability implies the patient is unable to control or stabilize a joint during motion or in a static position either because static restraints have been injured (as would be noted in an anterior dislocation with tearing of the capsule and labrum, also called gross or anatomical instability) or because the muscles controlling the joint are weak or the force couples are unbalanced (also called translational instability).[106]

Both primary and second impingements occur anteriorly (thus the term *anterior primary* or *anterior secondary*

impingement). As the areas of impingement are in the supraspinatus outlet area, they are also called **outlet impingement syndromes**.[31]

Jobe and colleagues believed that impingement and instability often occur together in throwing athletes and, based on that assumption, developed the following classification:[21,107]

Grade I. Pure impingement with no instability (often seen in older patients)

Grade II. Secondary impingement and instability caused by chronic capsular and labral microtrauma

Grade III. Secondary impingement and instability caused by generalized hypermobility or laxity

Grade IV. Primary instability with no impingement

In this classification, secondary impingement implies the impingement occurs secondarily and that the main problem is instability.

A third type of impingement is termed **internal impingement** or nonoutlet impingement. This type of impingement is found posteriorly rather than anteriorly, mostly in overhead athletes. It involves contact of the undersurface of the rotator cuff (primarily supraspinatus and infraspinatus) with the posterosuperior glenoid labrum when the arm is abducted to 90° and laterally rotated fully.[104,108–112]

If the history indicates instability, then at least one test each for anterior, posterior, and multidirectional instability should be performed. Also, because of the interrelation of impingement and instability, tests for both should be applied if the history indicates that either condition may be present.[113]

It is important when looking at shoulder instability to realize that instability includes a spectrum of conditions from gross or anatomical instability seen with the TUBS lesion to translational instability (muscle weakness) seen with AMBRI lesions[38] (Table 5-14). Burkhart et al. also included **pseudolaxity**,[18] which includes altered glenohumeral arthrokinematics because of the presence of a SLAP lesion, a tight posteroinferior capsule, and often scapular dyskinesia. They felt the apparent increased anterior laxity resulted from the decreased cam effect in the glenohumeral joint combined with functional lengthening of the anteroinferior capsule and glenohumeral ligament.[18] A posterosuperior SLAP lesion allows laxity on the opposite side (circle concept of instability).[18] With the instability tests, the examiner is trying to duplicate the patient's symptoms as well as feel for abnormal movement. Therefore, a response of "That's what my shoulder feels like when it bothers me" is much more significant than the degree of laxity or translation found.[38]

Tests for Anterior Shoulder Instability

Load and Shift Test[71,114]. This test is designed to check primarily atraumatic instability problems of the glenohumeral joint. The patient sits with no back support

Table 5-14

Differential Diagnosis of Shoulder Instability (AMBRI) versus Traumatic Anterior Dislocation (TUBS)

	Shoulder Instability	Traumatic Anterior Dislocation
History	Feeling of shoulder slippage with pain Feeling of insecurity when doing specific activities No history of injury	Arm elevated and laterally rotated relative to body Feeling of insecurity when in specific position (of dislocation) Recurrent episodes of apprehension
Observation	Normal	Normal (if reduced) (if not, loss of rounding of deltoid caused by anterior dislocation)
Active movement	Normal ROM May be abnormal or painful at activity speed	Apprehension and decreased ROM in abduction and lateral rotation
Passive movement	Normal ROM Pain at extreme of ROM possible	Muscle guarding and decreased ROM in apprehension position
Resisted isometric movement	Normal in test position May be weak in provocative position	Pain into abduction and lateral rotation
Special tests	Load and shift test is positive	Apprehension positive Augmentation positive Relocation positive
Reflexes and cutaneous distribution	Normal reflexes and sensation	Reflexes normal Sensation normal, unless axillary or musculocutaneous nerve is injured
Palpation	Normal	Anterior shoulder is tender
Diagnostic imaging	Normal	Normal, unless still dislocated; defect possible

ROM = range of motion.

and with the hand of the test arm resting on the thigh. Ideally, the patient should be sitting in a properly aligned posture (i.e., ear lobe, tip of acromion, and high point of iliac crest in a straight line). If the patient slouches forward, the scapula protracts causing the humeral head to translate anteriorly in the glenoid and narrows the subacromial space.[115] For best results, the muscles about the shoulder should be as relaxed as possible. The examiner stands or sits slightly behind the patient and stabilizes the shoulder with one hand over the clavicle and scapula (Figure 5-44, A). With the other hand, the examiner grasps the head of the humerus with the thumb over the posterior humeral head and the fingers over the anterior humeral head (Figure 5-44, B). The examiner runs the fingers along the anterior humerus and the thumb along the posterior humerus to feel where the humerus is seated relative to the glenoid (Figure 5-45). If the fingers "dip in" anteriorly as they move medially, but the thumb does not, it indicates the humeral head is sitting anteriorly. Normally, the humeral head feels a bit more anteriorly (i.e., the "dip" is slightly greater anteriorly) when it is properly "seated" in the glenoid. Protraction of the scapula causes the glenoid head to shift anteriorly in the glenoid. The examiner must be careful with the finger

and thumb placement. In the presence of anterior or posterior pathology, finger and thumb placement may cause pain. The humerus is then gently pushed anteriorly or posteriorly (most common) in the glenoid if necessary to seat it properly in the glenoid fossa.[113] The seating places the head of the humerus in its normal position relative to the glenoid.[32] This is the "load" portion of the test. If the load is not applied (as is the case in the anterior drawer test), there is no "normal" or standard starting position for the test. The examiner then pushes the humeral head anteriorly (anterior instability) or posteriorly (posterior instability), noting the amount of translation and end feel. This is the "shift" portion of the test.

With anterior translation, if the head is not centered, posterior translation will be greater than anterior translation, giving a false negative test. If the head is properly centered first, however, with anterior instability present, anterior translation will be possible but posterior translation will be virtually absent because of the tight posterior capsule that accompanies a positive anterior instability. Differences between affected and normal sides should be compared in terms of the amount of translation and the ease with which it occurs. This comparison, along with reproduction of the patient's symptoms, is often

A   **B**

Figure 5-44

A, Load and shift test in sitting starting position. Note that the humerus is loaded or "centered" in the glenoid to begin. Examiner then shifts humerus anteriorly or posteriorly. **B,** Line drawing showing position of examiner's hands in relation to bones of patient's shoulder. Notice that examiner's left thumb holds the spine of the scapula for stability.

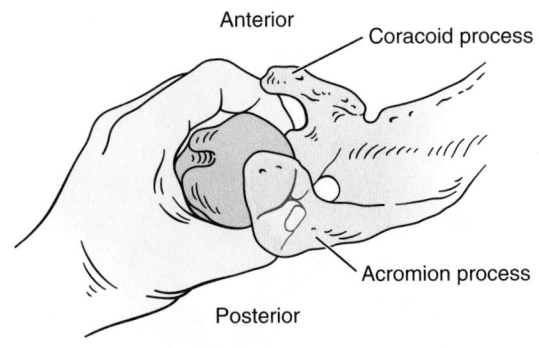

Anterior

Coracoid process

Acromion process

Posterior

Figure 5-45

Superior view of the shoulder showing palpation of the anterior and posterior glenohumeral joint to ensure the humeral head is centered in the glenoid.

considered more important than the amount of movement obtained. If the patient has multidirectional instability, both anterior and posterior translation may be excessive on the affected side compared with the normal side. The test may also be done with the patient in supine lying position.

Translation of 25% or less, of the humeral head diameter anteriorly, is considered normal, although results vary among patients.[116,117] Generally, anterior translation is less than posterior translation, although some authors disagree with this and say that anterior and posterior translation are virtually equal.[118,119] Sauers et al.[119] and Ellenbecker et al.[120] stated that hand dominance does not affect the amount of translation, but Lintner et al[121] disagreed saying that the nondominant shoulder shows more translation. Hawkins and Mohtadi,[114] Silliman and Hawkins,[113] and Altchek et al.[122] advocated a three-grade system for anterior translation (Figure 5-46). These authors feel that the head normally translates 0% to 25% of the diameter of the humeral head. Up to 50% of humeral head translation, with the head riding up to the glenoid rim and spontaneous reduction, is considered grade I. For grade II, the humeral head has more than 50% translation; the head feels as though it is riding over the glenoid rim but spontaneously reduces. Normal hypermobile shoulders may show grade II translation in any direction.[121] Grade III implies that the humeral head rides over the glenoid rim and does not spontaneously reduce. For posterior translation, translation of 50% of the diameter of the humeral head is considered normal, although results vary among patients.[116] Thus, normally, one would expect greater posterior translation than anterior translation when doing the test. However, all authors do not support this view.

The load and shift test may also be done in supine lying position.[123] To test anterior translation, the patient's arm is taken to 45° to 60° scaption (abduction in the plane of the scapula) and in neutral rotation by the examiner holding the forearm near the wrist (Figure 5-47). The

Figure 5-46

Grades of anterior glenohumeral translation.

examiner then places the other hand around the patient's upper arm near the deltoid insertion with the thumb anterior and the fingers posterior feeling the movement of the humeral head in the glenoid while applying an anterior or anteroinferior translation force (with the fingers) or a posterior translation force (with the thumb). Ideally, the humerus should be "loaded" in the glenoid before starting the test. With the hand holding the forearm, the examiner controls the arm position and applies an axial load to the humerus. During the translation movements with the thumb or fingers, the scapula should not move. As the anterior or anteroinferior translation force is applied, the examiner, using the other hand (the one holding the forearm) incrementally, laterally rotates the humerus (see Figure 5-47, *B*). This causes greater involvement of the anterior band of the inferior glenohumeral ligament, which, if intact, will limit movement so the amount of anterior translation decreases as lateral rotation increases. To test posterior translation (posterior instability), the arm is placed in scaption with 45° to 60° of lateral rotation (Figure 5-48). In this case, the thumb pushes the humerus posteriorly.[123,124] Incrementally, while applying the posterior translation, the examiner

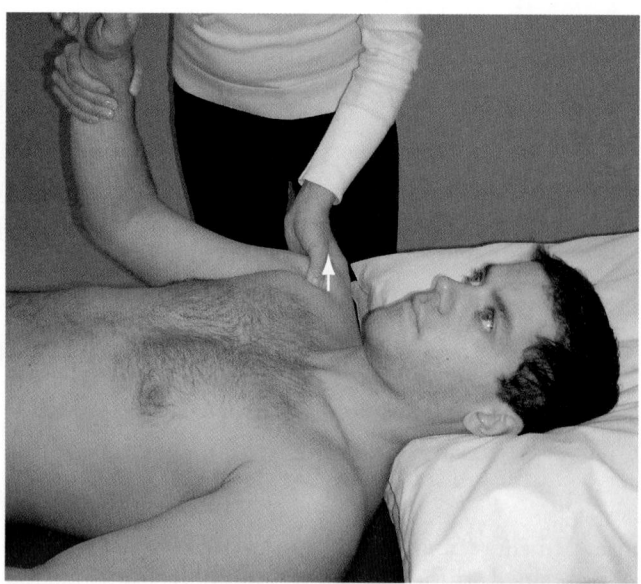

A   B

Figure 5-47

A, Initial position for load and shift test for anterior instability testing of the shoulder in supine lying position. The examiner's hand grasps the patient's upper arm with the fingers posterior. The examiner's arm positions the patient's arm and controls its rotation. The arm is placed in the plane of the scapula, abducted 45° to 60°, and maintained in 0° of rotation. The examiner's arm places an axial load to the patient's arm through the humerus. The examiner's fingers then shift the humeral head anteriorly, and anteroinferiorly over the glenoid rim. **B,** The second position for the load and shift test for anterior stability is as described in **A** for the initial position, except that the arm is progressively laterally rotated in 10° to 20° increments while the anterior dislocation force is alternatively applied and released.

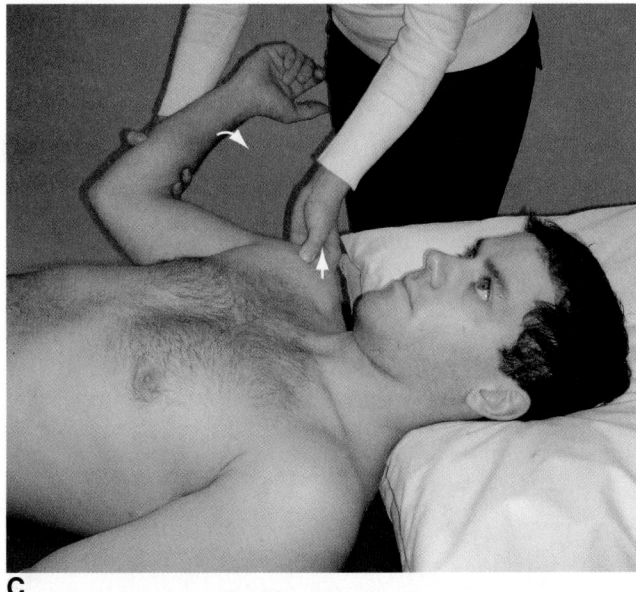

C

Figure 5-47 cont'd ▬▬▬▬▬

C, The examiner quantifies the degree of lateral rotation required to reduce the translation from grade 3 or 2 to grade 1. The examiner compares the normal and abnormal shoulders for this difference in translation with the humeral rotation. The degree of rotation required to reduce the translation is an indicator of the functional laxity of the anterior inferior capsular ligaments.

Figure 5-48 ▬▬▬▬▬

Load and shift test for posterior instability testing of the shoulder in supine lying position. The patient is supine on the examining table. The arm is brought into approximately 90° of forward elevation in the plane of the scapula. A posteriorly directed force is applied to the humerus with the arm in varying degrees of lateral rotation.

medially rotates the arm. Medial rotation causes the posterior band of the inferior glenohumeral ligament and the posteroinferior capsule to become increasingly tight so that posterior translation decreases as medial rotation increases.

Apprehension (Crank) Test for Anterior Shoulder Dislocation. This test is primarily designed to check for traumatic instability problems causing gross or anatomical instability of the shoulder, although the relocation portion of the test is sometimes used to differentiate between instability and impingement. The examiner abducts the arm to 90° and laterally rotates the patient's shoulder slowly (Figure 5-49). By placing a hand under the glenohumeral joint to act as a fulcrum (Figure 5-50), the apprehension test becomes the **fulcrum test**.[125] Kvitne and Jobe recommended applying a mild anteriorly directed force to the posterior humeral head when in the test position to see if apprehension or pain increases (Figure 5-51).[21] If posterior pain increases, this indicates posterior internal impingement.[112] Hamner et al. suggested that if posterior superior internal impingement is suspected, the relocation test should be done in 110° and 120° of abduction.[126] Translation of the humeral head in the glenoid is less than with other tests, provided the joint is normal, because the test is taking the joint into the close packed position.[116] A positive test is indicated when the patient looks or feels apprehensive or alarmed and resists further motion. Thus, the patient's apprehension is greater than the complaint of pain (i.e., apprehension predominates). The patient may also state that the feeling resembles what it felt like when the shoulder was dislocated. It is imperative that this test be done slowly. If the test is done too quickly, the humerus may dislocate. Hawkins and Bokor noted that the examiner should observe the amount of lateral rotation that exists when the patient becomes apprehensive and compare the range with the uninjured side.[127]

If the examiner then applies a posterior translation stress to the head of the humerus or the arm (**relocation test**), the patient will commonly lose the apprehension, any pain that is present commonly decreases, and further lateral rotation is possible before the apprehension or pain returns (see Figures 5-51, *A*, and 5-51, *C*). This relocation is sometimes referred to as the **Fowler sign** or **test** or the **Jobe relocation test**. The test is considered positive if pain decreases during the maneuver, even if there was no apprehension.[114,128] If the patient's symptoms decrease or are eliminated when doing the relocation test, the diagnosis is glenohumeral instability, subluxation, dislocation, or impingement. If apprehension predominated when doing the crank test and disappears with the relocation test, the diagnosis is glenohumeral instability, subluxation, or dislocation. If pain predominated when doing the crank test and disappears with the relocation test, the diagnosis

Figure 5-49
Anterior apprehension (crank) test.

Figure 5-50
Fulcrum test with left fist pushing head of humerus anteriorly.

is pseudolaxity or anterior instability either at the glenohumeral joint or scapulothoracic joint with secondary impingement or a posterior SLAP lesion.[129] The relocation test does not alter the pain for patients with primary impingement.[21,107,130] If, when doing the relocation test posteriorly, posterior pain decreases, it is a positive test for posterior internal impingement.[112,131] If the arm is released (**anterior release** or **"surprise" test** [see Figure 5-51, *D*]) in the newly acquired range, pain and forward translation of the head are noted in positive tests.[113,128,132] The resulting pain from this release procedure may be caused by anterior shoulder instability, labral lesion (Bankart lesion or SLAP lesion—superior labrum, anterior posterior), or bicipital peritenonitis or tendinosus. Most commonly, it is related to anterior

instability because the pain is temporarily produced by the anterior translation.[132] It has also been reported to cause pain in older patients with rotator cuff pathology and no instability.[133] This release maneuver should be done with care because it often causes apprehension and distrust on the part of the patient and it could cause a dislocation, especially in patients who have had recurrent dislocations. For most patients, therefore, when doing the relocation test, lateral rotation should be released before the posterior stress is released.

The crank test may be modified to test lateral rotation at different degrees of abduction, depending on the history and mechanism of injury.[123] The Rockwood test described next is simply a modification of the crank test.

modification of crank test - for traumatic

Rockwood Test for Anterior Instability[134]. The examiner stands behind the seated patient. With the arm at the patient's side, the examiner laterally rotates the shoulder. The arm is abducted to 45°, and passive lateral rotation is repeated. The same procedure is repeated at 90° and 120° (Figure 5-52). These different positions are performed because the stabilizers of the shoulder vary as the angle of abduction changes (see Table 5-1). For the test to be positive, the patient must show marked apprehension with posterior pain when the arm is tested at 90°. At 45° and 120°, the patient shows some uneasiness and some pain; at 0°, there is rarely apprehension.

Similarly, the Rowe and fulcrum tests stress the anterior shoulder structures. They are more likely to bring on apprehension sooner, because they stress the anterior structures sooner (i.e., the examiner pushes the head of the humerus forward). In effect, they are the opposite of the relocation test; they are therefore called **augmentation tests.** _?.

Rowe Test for Anterior Instability[135]. The patient lies supine and places the hand behind the head. The examiner places one hand (clenched fist) against the posterior humeral head and pushes up while extending the arm slightly (Figure 5-53). This part is similar to the fulcrum test. A look of apprehension or pain indicates a positive test for anterior instability. If a clunk or grinding sound may indicate a torn anterior labrum (see clunk test under "Tests for Labral Tears").

A **B**

Figure 5-51

Crank and relocation test. **A,** Abduction and lateral rotation (crank test). **B,** Abduction and lateral rotation combined with anterior translation of humerus, which may cause anterior subluxation or posterior joint pain.

Continued

C

D

Figure 5-51 cont'd
C, Abduction and lateral rotation combined with posterior translation of the humerus (relocation test).
D, Surprise test.

The following anterior instability tests are modifications of the anterior load and shift test in that they are designed to cause anterior translation of the head of the humerus in the glenoid. As with the load and shift test, the examiner can determine or grade the amount of anterior translation. Therefore, these tests can be used as substitutes for the load and shift test.

Prone Anterior Instability Test[136]. The patient lies prone. The examiner abducts the patient's arm to 90° and laterally rotates it 90°. While holding this position with one hand at the elbow, the examiner places the other hand over the humeral head and pushes it forward (Figure 5-54). A reproduction of the patient's symptoms indicates a positive test for anterior instability.

Andrews' Anterior Instability Test[136]. The patient lies supine with the shoulder abducted 130° and laterally rotated 90°. The examiner stabilizes the elbow and distal humerus with one hand and uses the other hand to grasp the humeral head and lift it forward (Figure 5-55). A reproduction of the patient's symptoms gives a positive test for anterior instability. If the examiner hears a clunk, an anterior labral tear may be present.

Anterior Drawer Test of the Shoulder[137]. The patient lies supine. The examiner places the hand of the affected shoulder in the examiner's axilla, holding the patient's hand with the arm so that the patient remains relaxed. The shoulder to be tested is abducted between 80° and 120°, forward flexed up to 20°, and

Figure 5-52
Rockwood test for anterior instability. **A,** Arm at side. **B,** Arm at 45°. **C,** Arm at 90°. **D,** Arm at 120°.

laterally rotated up to 30°. The examiner then stabilizes the patient's scapula with the opposite hand, pushing the spine of the scapula forward with the index and middle fingers. The examiner's thumb exerts counterpressure on the patient's coracoid process. Using the arm that is holding the patient's hand, the examiner places his or her hand around the patient's relaxed upper arm and draws the humerus forward. The movement may be accompanied by a click, by patient apprehension, or both. The amount of movement available is compared with that of the normal side. A positive test indicates anterior instability (Figure 5-56), depending on the amount of anterior translation. The click may indicate a labral tear or slippage of the humeral head over the glenoid rim.

Protzman Test for Anterior Instability[138]**.** The patient is sitting. The examiner abducts the patient's arm to 90° and supports the arm against the examiner's hip so that the patient's shoulder muscles are relaxed. The examiner palpates the anterior aspect of the head of the humerus with the fingers of one hand deep in the patient's axilla while the fingers of the other hand are placed over the posterior aspect of the humeral head. The examiner then pushes the humeral head anteriorly and inferiorly (Figure 5-57). If this movement causes pain and if palpation indicates abnormal anteroinferior movement, the test is positive for anterior instability. Normally, anterior translation should be no more than 25% of the diameter of the humeral head.[139] A click may sometimes be

Figure 5-53
Rowe test for anterior instability.

Figure 5-55
Andrews' anterior instability test.

Figure 5-54
Prone anterior instability test. Examiner stabilizes the arm in 90°
abduction and lateral rotation and then pushes anteriorly on the
humerus.

Figure 5-56
Anterior drawer test of the shoulder.

palpated as the humeral head slides over the glenoid rim.
The test may also be done with the patient in the supine
lying position with the elbow supported on a pillow.

Anterior Instability Test (Leffert's Test)[140]**.** The
examiner stands behind the shoulder being examined
while the patient sits. The examiner places his or her near
hand over the shoulder so that the index finger is over
the head of the humerus anteriorly and the middle finger
is over the coracoid process. The thumb is placed over

the posterior humeral head. The examiner's other hand
grasps the patient's wrist and carefully abducts and laterally rotates the arm (Figure 5-58). If, on movement of
the arm, the finger palpating the anterior humeral head
moves forward, the test is said to be positive for anterior
instability. Normally, the two fingers remain in the same
plane. With a positive test, when the arm is returned to
the starting position, the index finger returns to the starting position as the humeral head glides backward.

Dugas' Test[141]**.** This test is used if an unreduced
anterior shoulder dislocation is suspected. The patient
is asked to place the hand on the opposite shoulder and
then attempt to lower the elbow to the chest. With an
anterior dislocation, this is not possible, and pain in

Figure 5-57

Protzman test for anterior instability (posterior view).

the shoulder results. If the pain is only over the acromioclavicular joint, problems in that joint should be suspected.

Tests for Posterior Shoulder Instability

Load and Shift Test. This test is described under anterior shoulder instability.

Posterior Apprehension or Stress Test[124,142]. The patient is in a supine lying or sitting position. The examiner elevates the patient's shoulder in the plane of the scapula to 90° while stabilizing the scapula with the other hand (Figure 5-59). The examiner then applies a posterior force on the patient's elbow. While applying the axial load, the examiner horizontally adducts and medially rotates the arm. A positive result is indicated by a look of apprehension or alarm on the patient's face and the patient's resistance to further motion or the reproduction of the patient's symptoms. Pagnani and Warren reported that pain production is more likely than

A

B

C

Figure 5-58

Anterior instability test. **A,** Side view. **B,** Superior view. With the patient's arm by the side, the examiner's fingers are in the same plane. **C,** With a positive test, on abduction and lateral rotation, the index and middle fingers are no longer in the same plane. (Adapted from Leffert RD, Gumbery G: The relationship between dead arm syndrome and thoracic outlet syndrome, *Clin Orthop Relat Res* 223: 22-23, 1987.

A   **B**

Figure 5-59

Posterior apprehension test. **A,** Supine. **B,** Sitting medially rotated and adducted.

apprehension in a positive test.[143] They reported that with atraumatic multidirectional (inferior) instability, the test is negative. If the test is done with the patient in the sitting position, the scapula must be stabilized. A positive test indicates a posterior instability or dislocation of the humerus. The test should also be performed with the arm in 90° of abduction. The examiner palpates the head of the humerus with one hand while the other hand pushes the head of the humerus posteriorly. Translation of 50% of the humeral head diameter or less is considered normal, although results vary among patients.[116] If the humeral head moves posteriorly more than 50% of its diameter (Figure 5-60), posterior instability is evident.[139] The movement may be accompanied by a clunk as the humeral head passes over the glenoid rim.

Norwood Stress Test for Posterior Instability[144]. The patient lies supine with the shoulder abducted 60° to 100° and laterally rotated 90° and with the elbow flexed to 90° so that the arm is horizontal. The examiner stabilizes the scapula with one hand, palpating the posterior humeral head with the fingers, and stabilizes the upper limb by holding the forearm and elbow at the

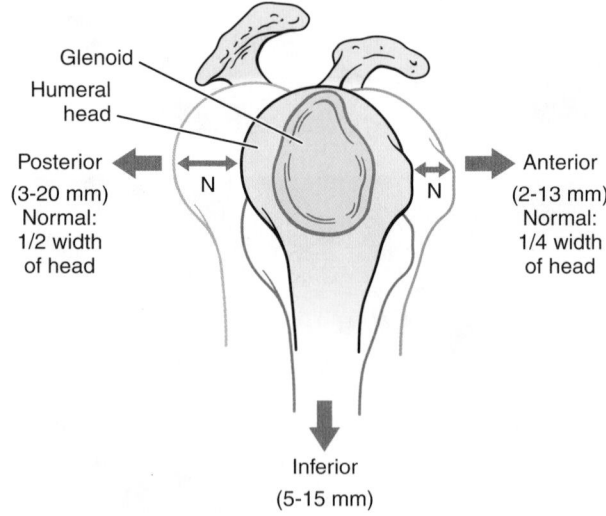

Figure 5-60

Normal translation movement of humeral head in glenoid. (Redrawn from Harryman DT et al: Laxity of the normal glenohumeral joint: A quantitative in vivo assessment, *J Shoulder Elbow Surg* 1:73, 1992.)

elbow or wrist. The examiner then brings the arm into horizontal adduction to the forward flexed position. At the same time, the examiner feels the humeral head slide posteriorly with the fingers (Figure 5-61). Cofield and Irving recommend medially rotating the forearm approximately 20° after the forward flexion then pushing the elbow posteriorly to enhance the effect of the test.[145] Similarly, the thumb may push the humeral head posteriorly as horizontal adduction in forward flexion is carried out to enhance the effect making the test similar to the posterior apprehension test. A positive test is indicated if the humeral head slips posteriorly relative to the glenoid. Care must be taken because the test does not always cause apprehension before subluxation or dislocation. The patient confirms that the sensation felt is the same as that felt during activities. The arm is returned to the starting position, and the humeral head is felt to reduce. A clicking caused by the passage of the head over the glenoid rim may accompany either subluxation or reduction.

Push-Pull Test[125]. The patient lies supine. The examiner holds the patient's arm at the wrist, abducts the arm 90°, and forward flexes it 30°. The examiner places the other hand over the humerus close to the humeral head. The examiner then pulls up on the arm at the wrist while pushing down on the humerus with the other hand (Figure 5-62). Normally, 50% posterior translation can

be accomplished. If more than 50% posterior translation occurs or if the patient becomes apprehensive or pain results, the examiner should suspect posterior instability.[139]

Posterior Drawer Test of the Shoulder[137,146]. The patient lies supine. The examiner stands at the level of the shoulder and grasps the patient's proximal forearm with one hand, flexing the patient's elbow to 120° and the shoulder to between 80° and 120° of abduction and between 20° and 30° of forward flexion. With the other hand, the examiner stabilizes the scapula by placing the index and middle fingers on the spine of the scapula and the thumb on the coracoid process (the examining table partially stabilizes the scapula as well). The examiner then rotates the upper arm medially and forward flexes the shoulder to between 60° and 80° while taking the thumb of the other hand off the coracoid process and pushing the head of the humerus posteriorly. The head of the humerus can be felt by the index finger of the same hand (Figure 5-63). The test is usually pain free, but the patient may exhibit apprehension. A positive test indicates posterior instability and demonstrates significant posterior translation (>50% humeral head diameter).

Miniaci Test for Posterior Subluxation[147]. The patient lies supine with the shoulder off the edge of the examining table. The examiner uses one hand to flex

A   **B**

Figure 5-61

Norwood stress test for posterior shoulder instability. **A,** Arm is abducted 90°. **B,** Arm is horizontally adducted to the forward flexed position.

Figure 5-62
Push-pull test.

(70° to 90°), adduct, and medially rotate the arm while pushing the humerus posteriorly. The patient may become apprehensive during this maneuver, as these motions will cause the humerus to sublux posteriorly. With the other hand, the examiner palpates the anterior and posterior shoulder. The examiner then abducts and laterally rotates the arm, a clunk will be heard, and the humerus reduces (relocates), indicating a positive test (Figure 5-64).

Jerk Test[125,148,149]. The patient sits with the arm medially rotated and forward flexed to 90°. The examiner grasps the patient's elbow and axially loads the humerus in a proximal direction. While maintaining the axial loading, the examiner moves the arm horizontally (cross-flexion/horizontal adduction) across the body (Figure 5-65). A positive test for recurrent posterior instability is the production of a sudden jerk or clunk as the humeral head slides off (subluxes) the back of the glenoid (Figure 5-66). When the arm is returned

A

B

C　**D**

Figure 5-63
Posterior drawer test of the shoulder. **A,** and **B,** The test. **C,** and **D,** Superimposed view of bones involved in the test.

E   F

Figure 5-63 cont'd

E, and **F,** Radiographic images of the test. (From Gerber C, Ganz R: Clinical assessment of instability of the shoulder, *J Bone Joint Surg Br* 66:554, 1984.)

A

Figure 5-64

Miniaci test for posterior subluxation. **A,** To start, the examiner uses one hand to flex, adduct, and medially rotate the arm while pushing the humerus posteriorly. **B,** The arm is then abducted and laterally rotated while the examiner palpates for a clunk.

to the original 90° abduction position, a second jerk may be felt as the head reduces. Kim et al. reported that the positive signs also indicate a positive test for a posteroinferior labral tear.[148]

Circumduction Test[150]. The patient is in the standing position. The examiner stands behind the patient grasping the patient's forearm with the hand. The examiner begins circumduction by extending the patient's arm while maintaining slight abduction. As the circumduction continues into elevation, the arm is brought over the top and into the flexed and adducted position. As the arm moves into forward flexion and adduction from above, it is vulnerable to posterior subluxation if the patient is unstable posteriorly. If the examiner palpates the posterior aspect of the patient's shoulder as the arm moves downward in forward flexion and adduction, the humeral head will be felt to sublux posteriorly in a positive test, and the patient will say, "That's what it feels like when it bothers me" (Figure 5-67).

Figure 5-65
Jerk test.

Tests for Inferior and Multidirectional Shoulder Instability

It is believed that if a patient demonstrates inferior instability, multidirectional instability is also present. Therefore, the patient with inferior instability will also demonstrate anterior or posterior instability. The primary complaint of these patients is pain rather than instability, with symptoms most commonly in midrange. Transient neurological symptoms may also be present.[151]

Test for Inferior Shoulder Instability (Sulcus Sign)[125,137]. The patient stands with the arm by the side and shoulder muscles relaxed. The examiner grasps the patient's forearm below the elbow and pulls the arm distally (Figure 5-68). The presence of a **sulcus sign** (see Figure 5-68, *B*) may indicate inferior instability or glenohumeral laxity.[152] A bilateral sulcus sign is not as clinically significant as unilateral laxity on the affected side.[153] The sulcus sign with a feeling of subluxation is also clinically significant.[153] The sulcus sign may be graded by measuring from the inferior margin of the acromion to the humeral head. A +1 sulcus implies a distance of less than 1 cm; +2 sulcus, 1 to 2 cm; and +3 sulcus, more than 2 cm.

It has been reported that the best position to test for inferior instability is at 20° to 50° of abduction with neutral rotation. Also, rotation will cause the capsule to tighten anteriorly (lateral rotation) or posteriorly (medial rotation), and the sulcus distance decreases.[123] Thus, more than one position should be tested.[46,143,154] Depending on the history, the examiner should test the patient in the position in which the sensation of instability is reported.

A   **B**

Figure 5-66
Positive jerk test. **A,** Normal appearance of the shoulder before the patient performs a jerk test. **B,** With axial loading and movement of the arm horizontally across the body, the humeral head slides off the back of the glenoid, as demonstrated by the prominence in the anterior aspect of the patient's shoulder. This maneuver resulted in a sudden jerk and some discomfort. (From Matsen FA et al: Glenohumeral instability. In Rockwood CA, Matsen FA, editors: *The shoulder,* p 551, Philadelphia, 1990, WB Saunders.)

Figure 5-67

Circumduction test. **A,** Starting position. **B,** The flexed adducted position where the shoulder is vulnerable to posterior subluxation.

Figure 5-68

A, Test for inferior shoulder instability (sulcus test). **B,** Positive sulcus sign (*arrows*).

Feagin Test[134]. The Feagin test is a modification of the sulcus sign test with the arm abducted to 90° instead of being at the side. Some authors consider it to be the second part of the sulcus test.[153] The patient stands with the arm abducted to 90° and the elbow extended and resting on the top of the examiner's shoulder. The examiner's hands are clasped together over the patient's humerus, between the upper and middle thirds. The examiner pushes the humerus down and forward (Figure 5-69, *A*). The test may also be done with the patient in a sitting position. In this case, the examiner holds the patient's arm at the elbow (elbow straight) abducted to 90° with one hand and arm holding the arm against the examiner's body. The other hand is placed just lateral to the acromion over the humeral head. Ensuring the shoulder musculature is relaxed, the examiner pushes the head of the humerus down and forward (Figure 5-69, *B*). Doing the test this way often gives the

Figure 5-70

A 21-year-old woman whose shoulder could be dislocated inferiorly and anteriorly and subluxated posteriorly. Note sulcus *(arrow)* anteriorly. She was unable to carry books, reach overhead, or use the arm for activities such as tennis or swimming. There were associated episodes of numbness and weakness of the entire upper extremity that at times lasted for 1 or 2 days. (From Neer CS, Foster CR: Inferior capsular shift for involuntary inferior and multidirectional instability of the shoulder, *J Bone Joint Surg Am* 62:900, 1980.)

A

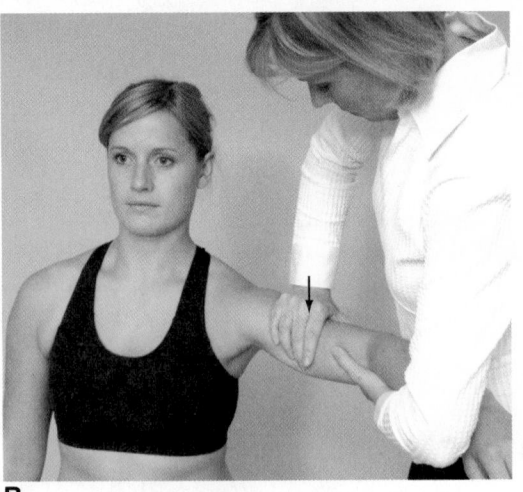

B

Figure 5-69

Feagin test. **A,** In standing. **B,** In sitting.

examiner greater control when doing the test. A sulcus may also be seen above the coracoid process (Figure 5-70). A look of apprehension on the patient's face indicates a positive test and the presence of anteroinferior instability. If both the sulcus sign and Feagin test are positive, it is a greater indication of multidirectional instability rather than just laxity. This test position also places more stress on the inferior glenohumeral ligament.

Rowe Test for Multidirectional Instability[135]. The patient stands forward flexed 45° at the waist with the arms relaxed and pointing at the floor. The examiner places one hand over the shoulder so that the index and middle fingers sit over the anterior aspect of the humeral head and the thumb sits over the posterior aspect of the humeral head. The examiner then pulls the arm down slightly (Figure 5-71). To test for anterior instability, the humeral head is pushed anteriorly with the thumb while the arm is extended 20° to 30° from the vertical position. To test for posterior instability, the humeral head is pushed posteriorly with the index and middle fingers while the arm is flexed 20° to 30° from the vertical position. For inferior instability, more traction is applied to the arm, and the sulcus sign is evident.

A B C

Figure 5-71
Rowe test for multidirectional instability. **A,** Testing for anterior instability. **B,** Testing for posterior instability. **C,** Testing for inferior instability.

Tests for Impingement

Anterior shoulder impingement, regardless of its cause (i.e., rotator cuff pathology, bicipital paratenonitis/tendinosis, scapular or humeral instability, labral pathology), results from structures being compressed in the anterior aspect of the humerus between the head of the humerus and the coracoid process under the acromion process (Figure 5-72).[155–158] Park et al. found that combining tests gave better results.[159] They found that the Hawkins-Kennedy test, the painful arc sign, and a positive infraspinatus test gave the best probability of impingement while the painful arc sign, drop arm test, and the infraspinatus test were best for full thickness rotator cuff tears.

Common Shoulder Impingement Tests

- Neer impingement test
- Hawkins-Kennedy impingement test
- Posterior internal impingement test

Neer Impingement Test[160]. The patient's arm is passively and forcibly fully elevated in the scapular plane with the arm medially rotated by the examiner. This passive stress causes = the greater tuberosity to jam against the anteroinferior border of the acromion (Figure 5-73).[161] The patient's face shows pain, reflecting a positive test result (Figure 5-74, *A*). The test indicates an overuse injury to the supraspinatus muscle and sometimes to the biceps tendon. If the test is positive when done with the arm laterally rotated, the examiner should check the acromioclavicular joint (**acromioclavicular differentiation test**).[162]

Hawkins-Kennedy Impingement Test[163]. The patient stands while the examiner forward flexes the arm to 90° and then forcibly medially rotates the shoulder (Figure 5-74, *B*). This movement pushes the supraspinatus tendon against the anterior surface[164] of the coracoacromial ligament and coracoid process.[161,165] The test may also be performed in different degrees of forward flexion (vertically "circling the shoulder") or horizontal adduction (horizontally "circling the shoulder"). Pain indicates a positive test for supraspinatus paratenonitis/tendinosis or secondary impingement.[23] McFarland et al. described the **coracoid impingment sign**,[166] which is the same as the Hawkins-Kennedy test but involves horizontally adducting the arm across the body 10° to 20° before doing the medial rotation (Figure 5-75). This is more likely to approximate the lesser tuberosity of the humerus and the coracoid process. The **Yocum test** is a modification of this test in which the patient's hand is placed on the opposite shoulder and the examiner elevates the elbow.[33,167]

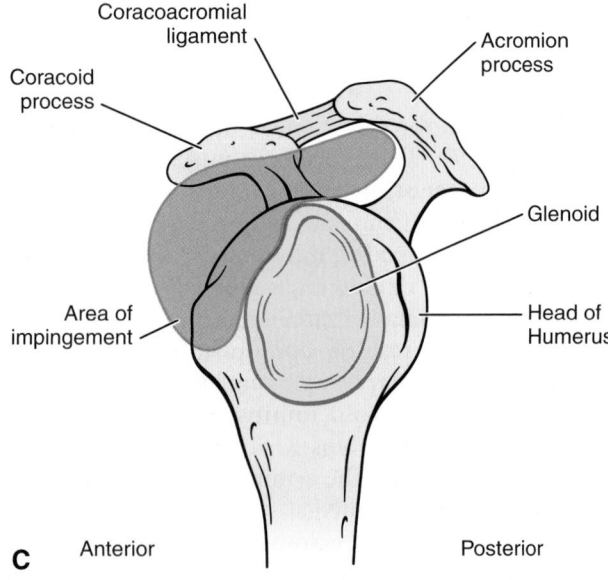

Figure 5-72

Impingement zone. **A,** Anterior view. **B,** Superior view. **C,** Lateral view.

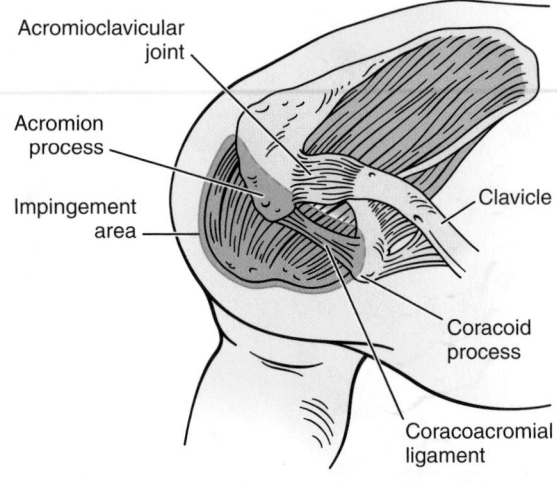

Figure 5-73

The functional arc of elevation of the proximal humerus is forward, as proposed by Neer. The greater tuberosity impinges against the anterior one third of the acromial surface. This critical area comprises the supraspinatus and bicipital tendons and the subacromial bursa.

Impingement Test[168]**.** The patient is seated. The examiner takes the arm to 90° abduction and full lateral rotation. This is the same position as for the apprehension test. However, if there is no history of possible traumatic subluxation or dislocation, the movement also can cause anterior translation of the humerus, resulting in secondary impingement of the rotator cuff. Therefore, a positive test indicates a grade II or III shoulder lesion based on Jobe's classification (see the previous discussion).[107] A positive test depends on production of the patient's symptoms, anterior or posterior shoulder pain, or both.

Branch et al. advocated testing the anterior capsule in a position of 30° to 40° abduction and 0° to 10° flexion.[169] Lateral rotation is then passively applied to stress the anterior capsule. To test the posterior capsule, they advocated placing the humerus in 60° to 70° abduction and 20° to 30° flexion, followed by passive medial rotation to stress the posterior capsule. By testing below 70° abduction, they felt impingement signs would be less.

Reverse Impingement Sign (Impingement Relief Test)[133]**.** This test is used if the patient has a positive painful arc or pain on lateral rotation. The patient lies supine. The examiner pushes the head of the humerus inferiorly as the arm is abducted or laterally rotated. Corso advocated doing the test in the standing position.[170] He also advocated an inferior glide of the humerus during abduction but suggested using a posteroinferior glide of the humeral head during forward

Figure 5-74

Impingement sign. **A,** A positive Neer impingement sign is present if pain and its resulting facial expression are produced when the examiner forcibly flexes the arm forward, jamming the greater tuberosity against the anteroinferior surface of the acromion. **B,** An alternative method (Hawkins-Kennedy impingement test) demonstrates the impingement sign by forcibly medially rotating the proximal humerus when the arm is forward flexed to 90°.

flexion. He advocated applying the glide just before the ROM where pain occurred on active movement. If the pain decreases or disappears when repeating the movements with the humeral head depressed, it is considered a positive test for mechanical impingement under the acromion (Figure 5-76).

Posterior Internal Impingement Test[39,131,171-173]. This type of impingement is found primarily in overhead athletes although it may be found in others who hold their arm in the vulnerable position. The impingement occurs when the rotator cuff impinges against the posterosuperior edge of the glenoid when the arm is abducted, extended, and laterally rotated (Figure 5-77). The result is of a "kissing" labral lesion posteriorly. The resulting impingement is between the rotator cuff and greater tuberosity on the one hand, and the posterior glenoid and labrum on the other. It often accompanies

anterior instability or pseudolaxity, and the deltoid activity increases to compensate for weakened rotator cuff muscles. The patient complains of pain posteriorly in late cocking and early acceleration phase of throwing. To perform the test, the patient is placed in the supine lying position. The examiner passively abducts the shoulder to 90°, with 15° to 20° forward flexion and maximum lateral rotation (Figure 5-78). The test is considered positive if it elicits localized pain in the posterior shoulder.[39]

Internal (Medial) Rotation Resistance Strength Test (IRRST)[174]. This test is a follow-up to a Neer test. The patient stands with the arm abducted to 90° and laterally rotated 80° to 85°. The examiner then applies an isometric resistance into lateral rotation followed by isometric resistance into medial (internal) rotation (Figure 5-79). The test is considered positive in a patient who has a positive impingement

Figure 5-75
The coracoid impingement sign with the test performed with the arm flexed 90°, adducted 10°, and internally rotated. The test is positive if it produces pain in the area of the coracoid.

test if the patient has good strength in lateral rotation but not medial rotation and indicates an internal impingement. If the patient exhibits more weakness on lateral rotation, it indicates a classic external anterior impingement.

Tests for Labral Tears

Injuries to the labrum are relatively common, especially in throwing athletes where the labrum plays a key role in glenohumeral stability.[20] In the young, the tensile strength of the labrum is less than the capsule, so it is more prone to injury when anterior stress (e.g., anterior dislocation) is applied to the glenohumeral joint.[175] The tear may be a **Bankart lesion**, in which the anteroinferior labrum is torn, or the superior labrum may have been injured, causing a **SLAP lesion** (superior labrum, anterior and posterior [to the biceps]) (Figure 5-80).[176–178] These injuries are classic examples of the **circle concept of instability.** This concept suggests that injury in one direction of the joint results in injury to structures on the other side of the joint. A Bankart lesion occurs most commonly with a traumatic anterior dislocation leading to anterior instability. In the right shoulder, for example, this injury results in the labrum being detached anywhere from the 3 o'clock to the 7 o'clock position resulting in both anterior and posterior structural injury (see Figure 5-80, *A*). Not only is the labrum torn, but the stability of the inferior glenohumeral ligament is lost.[179] The SLAP lesion has the labrum detaching (pulled or peeled depending on the mechanism) from the 10 o'clock to the 2 o'clock position (see Figure 5-80, *B*). The injury often results from a FOOSH injury, occurs during deceleration when throwing, or arises when sudden traction is applied to the biceps.[180,181] If the biceps tendon also detaches, the shoulder becomes unstable and the support of the superior glenohumeral ligament is lost. Snyder and colleagues have divided these SLAP lesions into four types:[182]

A **B** **C**

Figure 5-76
Reverse impingement sign (impingement relief test). **A,** In supine. **B,** In standing, doing test in abduction. **C,** In standing, doing test in forward flexion.

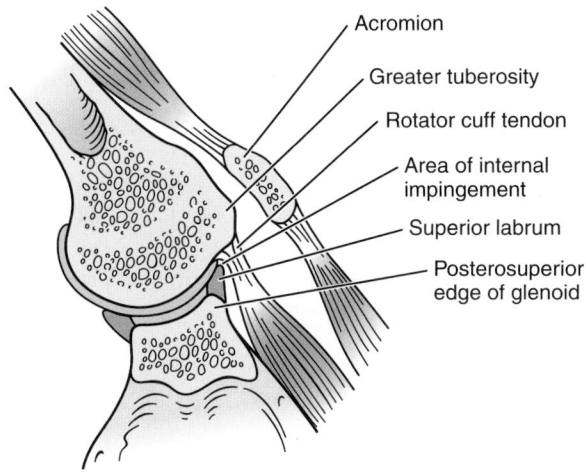

Figure 5-77
Area of posterior internal impingement.

A

B

Figure 5-79
Internal rotation resistance strength test. The patient is asked to maximally resist first external rotation and then internal rotation with the arm in 90° external rotation and 85° internal rotation.

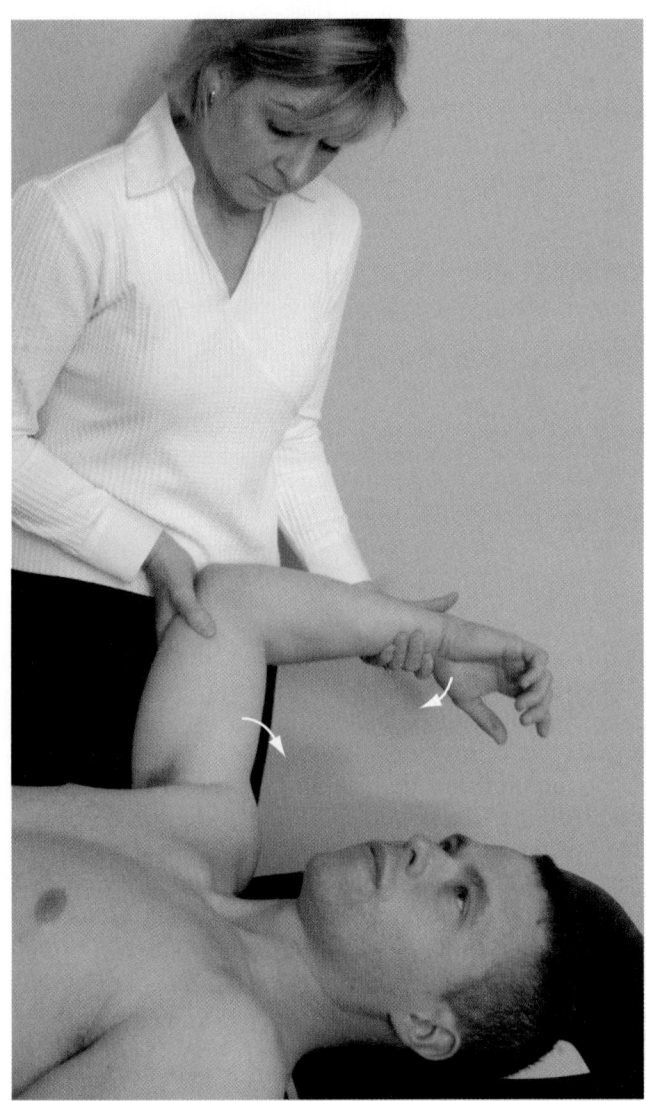

Figure 5-78
Posterior internal impingement test.

Type I. Superior labrum markedly frayed but attachments intact

Type II. Superior labrum has small tear and there is instability of the labral-biceps complex (most common)

Type III. Bucket-handle tear of labrum that may displace into joint; labral biceps attachment intact

Type IV. Bucket-handle tear of labrum that extends to biceps tendon, allowing tendon to sublux into joint

Parentis et al. felt that no single test could accurately diagnose a SLAP lesion.[183]

Clunk Test. The patient lies supine. The examiner places one hand on the posterior aspect of the shoulder over the humeral head. The examiner's other hand holds the humerus above the elbow. The examiner fully abducts the arm over the patient's head. The examiner then pushes anteriorly with the hand over the humeral head (a fist may be used to apply more anterior pressure) while the other hand rotates the humerus into

Figure 5-80
Labral lesions to the right shoulder. **A,** Bankart lesion. **B,** SLAP lesion.

lateral rotation (Figure 5-81). A clunk or grinding sound indicates both a positive test and a tear of the labrum.[184] The test may also cause apprehension if anterior instability is present. Walsh indicated that if the examiner follows these maneuvers with horizontal adduction that relocates the humerus, he or she may also hear a clunk or a click, indicating a tear of the labrum.[185]

The examiner may also position the arm in different amounts of abduction (vertically "circling the shoulder") and perform the test. This will stress different parts of the labrum.

Anterior Slide Test[186,187]. The patient is sitting with the hands on the waist, thumbs posterior. The examiner stands behind the patient and stabilizes the scapula and clavicle with one hand. With the other hand, the examiner applies an anterosuperior force at the elbow (Figure 5-82).

If the labrum is torn (SLAP lesion), the humeral head slides over the labrum with a pop or crack, and the patient complains of anterosuperior pain.

Active Compression Test of O'Brien[39,129,188]. This test is designed to detect SLAP (Type II) or superior labral lesions. The patient is placed in the standing position with the arm forward flexed to 90° and the elbow fully extended. The arm is then horizontally adducted 10° to 15° (starting position) and medially rotated so the thumb faces downward. The examiner stands behind the patient and applies a downward eccentric force to the arm (Figure 5-83). The arm is returned to the starting position and the palm is supinated, and the downward eccentric load is repeated. If pain or painful clicking is produced inside the shoulder (not over the acromiocla-vicular joint) in the first part of the test and eliminated or decreased in the second part, the test is considered

Figure 5-81
Clunk test.

positive for labral abnormalities. The test also "locks and loads" the acromioclavicular joint in medial rotation so the examiner must take care to differentiate between labral and acromioclavicular pathology.

Kim Test[148]. The patient sits with the back supported. The arm is abducted to 90° with the elbow supported in 90° flexion. The examiner's hand, while supporting the elbow and forearm, applies an axial compression force to the glenoid through the humerus. While maintaining the axial compression force, the arm is elevated diagonally upward using the same hand while the other hand applies a downward and backward force to the proximal

arm (Figure 5-84). A sudden onset of posterior shoulder pain and click indicates a positive test for a posteroinferior labral lesion.

Biceps Tension Test. This test determines whether a SLAP lesion is present. The patient, in standing, abducts and laterally rotates the arm to 90° with the elbow extended and forearm supinated. The examiner then applies an eccentric adduction force to the arm. A reproduction of the patient's symptoms is a positive test (Figure 5-85). The examiner should also do Speed's test (discussed later) to rule out biceps pathology.

Biceps Load Test[189]. This test is designed to check the integrity of the superior labrum. The patient is in the supine position with the shoulder abducted to 90° and laterally rotated, with the elbow flexed to 90° and the forearm supinated as it is for the apprehension or crank test. The examiner performs an apprehension test

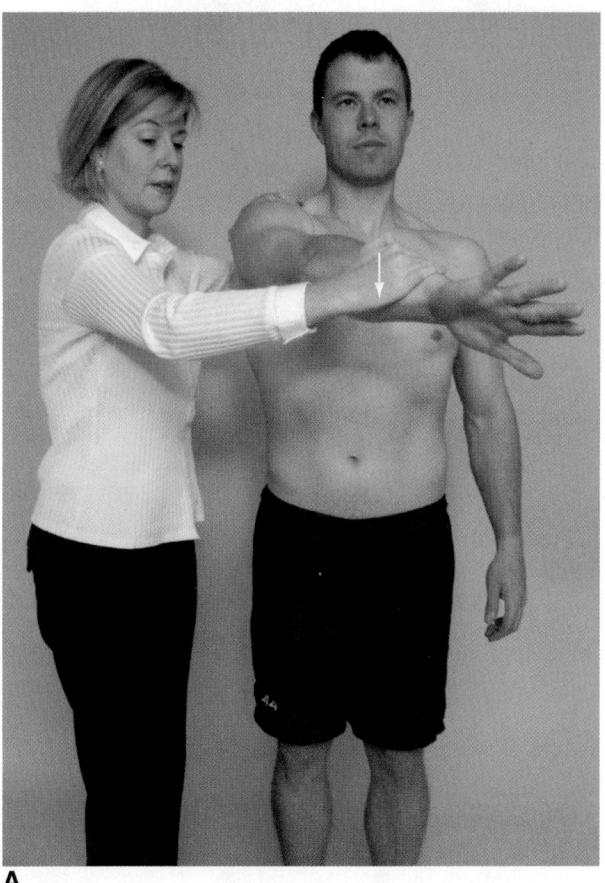

A

Figure 5-83
Active compression test of O'Brien. **A,** Position 1: The patient forward flexes the arm to 90° with the elbow extended and adducted 15° medial to the midline of the body and with the thumb pointed down. The examiner applies a downward force to the arm that the patient resists.

Continued

Figure 5-82
Anterior slide testing. Note the position of the examiner's hands and the patient's arms.

B

Figure 5-83 cont'd
B, Position 2: The test is performed with the arm in the same position, but the patient fully supinates the arm with the palm facing the ceiling. The same maneuver is repeated. The test is positive for a superior labral injury if pain is elicited in the first step and reduced or eliminated in the second step of this maneuver.

Figure 5-84
Kim test.

Figure 5-85
Biceps tension test. The patient's arm is abducted to 90° and laterally rotated. The examiner then applies an eccentric adduction force.

on the patient by taking the arm into full lateral rotation. If apprehension appears, the examiner stops lateral rotation and holds the position. The patient is then asked to flex the elbow against the examiner's resistance at the wrist. If apprehension decreases or the patient feels more comfortable, the test is negative for a SLAP lesion. If the apprehension remains the same or the shoulder becomes more painful, the test is considered positive (Figure 5-86).

SLAP Prehension Test[190]. The patient is in the sitting or standing position. The arm is abducted to 90° with the elbow extended and the forearm pronated (thumb down and shoulder medially rotated). The patient is then asked to horizontally adduct the arm. The movement is repeated with the forearm supinated

Figure 5-86
Biceps load test.

(thumb up and shoulder laterally rotated). If the patient feels pain in the bicipital groove in the first case (pronation) but the pain lessens or absent in the second case (supination), the test is considered positive for a SLAP lesion (Figure 5-87).

Labral Crank Test[191]. The patient is in the supine lying or sitting position. The examiner elevates the arm to 160° in the scapular plane. In this position, an axial load is applied to the humerus with one hand of the examiner while the other hand rotates the humerus medially and laterally. A positive test is indicated by pain on rotation, especially lateral rotation with or without a click or reproduction of the patient's symptoms (Figure 5-88).

Pain Provocation Test[192]. The patient is seated and the arm is abducted to between 90° and 100°, and the examiner laterally rotates the arm by holding the wrist (Figure 5-89). The forearm is taken into maximum supination and then maximum pronation. If pain is provoked only in the pronated position or if the pain is more severe in the pronated position, the test is considered positive for a superior (SLAP) tear. As with other superior labral tests, the biceps must be tested (Speed's test) to rule out biceps pathology causing the pain.

Compression Rotation Test[193]. The patient lies relaxed in supine position. The examiner grasps the arm and flexes the elbow with the arm abducted to about 20°. The examiner then pushes or compresses the humerus in the glenoid by pushing up on the elbow while the examiner's other hand rotates the humerus medially and laterally (Figure 5-90). If there is a snapping or catching sensation when the humeral head is felt, the test is positive for a labral tear (Bankart or SLAP lesion).

A

B

Figure 5-87

SLAP prehension test. **A,** Start position 1: Arm abducted to 90° with elbow extended and forearm pronated. The patient then horizontally adducts the arm. **B,** Start position 2: Same as position 1, but the forearm is supinated. The patient again horizontally adducts the arm. If position 1 is painful and position 2 is not, the test is considered positive.

A

B

Figure 5-88

Labral crank test. **A,** Crank test in sitting with lateral humeral rotation. **B,** Crank test in sitting with medial humeral rotation.

A

B

Figure 5-89

Pain provocation test. **A,** Test with forearm pronated. **B,** Test with forearm supinated.

Figure 5-90

Compression-rotation test.

Resisted Supination External Rotation Test[180]. This test is designed to check for SLAP lesions and is thought to re-create the peel-back mechanism of the superior labrum. The patient is placed in supine lying with the scapula near the edge of the bed. The examiner stands beside the patient holding the arm to be examined at the elbow and hand. The patient's arm is placed with the shoulder abducted to 90°, the elbow flexed to 65° to 70°, and the forearm is neutral or slight pronation. The patient is then asked to maximally supinate the hand while the examiner resists. While the patient continues to supinate against the examiner's resistance, the examiner laterally rotates the shoulder to end range (Figure 5-91). The test is considered positive if the patient has anterior or deep shoulder pain, clicking or catching in the shoulder, or reproduction of symptoms. It is considered negative if there is posterior shoulder pain, no pain, or apprehension.

Tests for Scapular Stability

For the muscles of the glenohumeral joint to work in a normal coordinated fashion, the scapula must be stabilized by its muscles to act as a firm base for the glenohumeral muscles. Thus, when doing these tests, the examiner is watching for movement patterns of the scapula as well as scapular dyskinesia.

"SICK" Scapula Signs and Symptoms[20]

- Insidious onset
- Prominence of inferior medial border of scapula
- Protraction of scapula
- Acromion less prominent
- Coracoid very tender to palpation
- Tight pectoralis minor
- Lack full forward flexion
- Tight short head of biceps

Lateral Scapular Slide Test[42,63,194]. This test determines the stability of the scapula during glenohumeral movements. The patient sits or stands with the arm resting at the side. The examiner measures the distance from the base of the spine of the scapula to the spinous process of T2 or T3 (most common), from the inferior angle of the scapula to the spinous process of T7-T9, or from T2 to the superior angle of the scapula. The patient is then tested holding two[194] (Figure 5-92) or four[63] other positions: 45° abduction (hands on waist, thumbs posteriorly),[63,194] 90° abduction with medial rotation,[63,194] 120° abduction,[63] and 150° abduction.[63] Davies and Dickoff-Hoffman[63] and Kibler[194] stated that in each position, the distance measured should not vary more than 1 to 1.5 cm

Figure 5-91

The resisted supination external rotation test. **A,** The examiner supports the limb in the starting position. The patient attempts to supinate his hand as the examiner resists. **B,** The shoulder is then gently externally rotated to the maximal point.

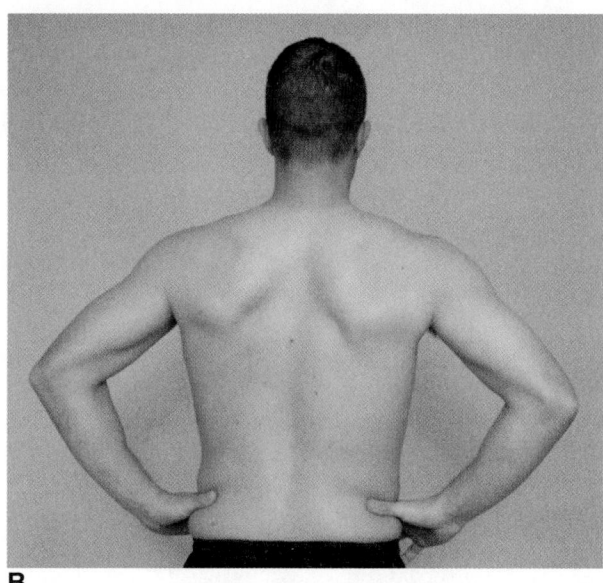

Figure 5-92

Lateral scapular slide test. The examiner measures from spinous process to scapula at level of base of spine of scapula (see arrows in **A**). **A,** Arms at side. **B,** Arms abducted, hands on waist, thumbs back.

Continued

(0.5 to 0.75 inch) from the original measure. However, there may be increased distances above 90° as the scapula rotates during scapulohumeral rhythm. Minimal protraction of the scapula should occur, however, during full elevation through abduction. It therefore is important to look for asymmetry of movement between left and right sides, as well as the amount of movement, when determining scapular stability.

The test may also be performed by loading the arm (providing resistance) at 45° and greater abduction **(scapular load test)** to see how the scapula stabilizes under dynamic load. This load may be applied anteriorly, posteriorly, inferiorly, or superiorly to the arm

C

Figure 5-92 cont'd
C, Arms abducted to 90°, thumbs down.

(Figure 5-93). Again, the scapula should not move more than 1.5 cm (0.75 inch). Odom and associates have stated that the test has poor reliability for differentiating normal and pathological shoulders.[195] However, loading the scapula, either by the weight of the arm or by applying a load to the arm, indicates the stabilizing ability of the scapular control muscles and whether abnormal winging or abnormal movement patterns occur.

Figure 5-93
Scapular load test in 45° abduction.

In the different positions, the examiner may test for scapular and humeral stability by performing an eccentric movement at the shoulder by pushing the arm forward **(eccentric hold test).** One arm is tested at a time. As the arm is pushed forward eccentrically, the examiner should watch the relative movement at the scapulothoracic joint (protraction) and the glenohumeral joint (horizontal adduction). Normally, slightly more movement (relatively) occurs at the glenohumeral joint. If instability due to muscle weakness exists at either joint, excessive movement will be evident at that joint relative to the other joint. In addition, the examiner should watch for winging of the scapula, which indicates scapular instability.

Wall Pushup Test[67,196]. The patient stands arms length from a wall. The patient is then asked to do a "wall pushup" 15 to 20 times (Figure 5-94). Any weakness of the scapular muscles or winging usually shows up with 5 to 10 pushups. For stronger or younger people, a normal pushup on the floor shows similar scapular changes, usually with fewer repetitions. Goldbeck and Davies have taken this test further in what they describe as a **closed kinetic chain upper extremity stability test.**[197] In this test, two markers (e.g., tape) are placed 91 cm (36 inches) apart. Patients assume the pushup position with one hand on each marker. When the examiner says "go," the subject moves one hand to touch the other and returns it to the original position and then does the same with the other hand, repeating the motions for 15 seconds. The examiner counts the number of touches or crossovers made in the allotted time. The test is repeated three times, and the average is the test score. This test is designed primarily for young, active patients.

Scapular Retraction Test[42,67,196,198]. The patient is in the standing position. The examiner, standing behind the patient, places the fingers of one hand over the clavicle with the heel of the hand over the spine of the scapula to stabilize the clavicle and scapula and to hold the scapula retracted. The examiner's other hand compresses the scapula against the chest wall (Figure 5-95). Holding the scapula in this position provides a firm stable base for the rotator cuff muscles, and often rotator cuff strength (if tested by a second examiner) will improve. The test may also be positive in patients with a positive relocation test. If scapular retraction decreases the pain, when the relocation test is performed, it indicates that the weak scapular stabilizers must be addressed in the treatment.[198] This test may also be done in supine. In patients with a SICK scapula, if the scapula is repositioned, forward flexion will improve.[20]

Scapular Isometric Pinch or Squeeze Test[67]. The patient is in a standing position and is asked to actively "pinch" or retract the scapulae together as hard as possible

Figure 5-95

Scapular retraction test. Examiner uses hands to stabilize clavicle and scapula.

and to hold the position for as long as possible (Figure 5-96). Normally, an individual can hold the contractions for 15 to 20 seconds with no burning pain or obvious muscle weakness. If burning pain occurs in less than 15 seconds, the scapular retractors are weak. When doing the test, the examiner must watch the patient carefully. Subconsciously, many patients will relax the contraction

A

B

C

Figure 5-94

Wall (**A**) and floor (**B**) pushup tests. **C,** Closed kinetic chain upper extremity stability test touching opposite hand.

A

Figure 5-96

Scapular isometric pinch test. **A,** Start position.

Continued

Figure 5-96 cont'd
B, Pinch position.

Figure 5-97
Scapular assistance test.

a slight amount, which is barely noticeable but allows the patient to hold the contraction in a comfort zone for longer periods with no burning.

Scapular Assistance Test[42,67,196,198]. This test evaluates scapular and acromial involvement in patients with impingement symptoms. The patient is in a standing position, and the examiner stands behind the patient. The examiner places the fingers of one hand over the clavicle with the heel of the hand over the spine of the scapula. This stabilizes the clavicle and scapula and holds the scapula retracted. The examiner's other hand holds the inferior angle of the scapula. As the patient actively abducts or forward flexes the arm, the examiner stabilizes and pushes the inferior medial border of the scapula up and laterally while keeping the scapula retracted. Decreased pain would be a positive test and would indicate that the scapular control muscles are weak as the assistance by the examiner simulates the activity of serratus anterior and lower trapezius during elevation (Figure 5-97).

Other Shoulder Joint Tests

Acromioclavicular Shear Test[139]. With the patient in the sitting position, the examiner cups his or her hands over the deltoid muscle, with one hand on the clavicle and one hand on the spine of the scapula. The examiner then squeezes the heels of the hands together

(Figure 5-98). Abnormal movement at the acromioclavicular joint indicates a positive test as well as acromioclavicular joint pathology.

Acromioclavicular Crossover, Crossbody, or Horizontal Adduction Test. The patient stands and reaches the hand across to the opposite shoulder. The examiner may also passively perform the test. With the patient in a sitting position, the examiner passively forward flexes

Figure 5-98
Acromioclavicular shear test.

the arm to 90° and then horizontally adducts the arm as far as possible (Figure 5-99).[32,162] If the patient feels localized pain over the acromioclavicular joint, the test is positive.[199-201] Localized pain in the sternoclavicular joint indicates that joint is at fault.

Ellman's Compression Rotation Test[202,203]. The patient lies on the unaffected side. The examiner compresses the humeral head into the glenoid while the patient rotates the shoulder medially and laterally. If the patient's symptoms are reproduced, glenohumeral arthritis is suspected (Figure 5-100).

Tests for Ligament Pathology

Crank Test (Also see under Tests for Anterior Shoulder Instability). The crank test may also be used to evaluate the different glenohumeral ligaments (Figure 5-101). For example, when the crank test is done with the arm by the side, primarily the superior glenohumeral ligament and capsule are being tested. At 45° to 60° abduction, the middle glenohumeral ligament, the coracohumeral ligament, the inferior glenohumeral ligament (anterior band), and anterior capsule are being tested. Over 90° abduction, the inferior glenohumeral

Figure 5-99
Acromioclavicular crossover, crossbody, or horizontal adduction test.

A

Figure 5-100
Ellman's compression-rotation test for glenohumeral arthritis.

B

Figure 5-101
Crank test used to test glenohumeral ligaments. **A,** Arm by the side—superior glenohumeral ligament tested. **B,** 45° to 60° abduction—middle glenohumeral ligament tested.

Continued

Figure 5-101 cont'd
C, Over 90° abduction—inferior glenohumeral ligament tested.

Figure 5-102
Posterior inferior ligament test. **A,** Anterior view. **B,** Posterior view.

ligament and anterior capsule are being tested (see Table 5-1).[204,205]

Posterior Inferior Glenohumeral Ligament Test[186]. Just as the crank test may be used to test the superior glenohumeral ligament, middle glenohumeral ligament, and the anterior portion of the inferior glenohumeral ligament, the posterior inferior glenohumeral test may be used to test the posterior portion of the inferior glenohumeral ligament. The patient sits while the examiner forward flexes the arm to between 80° and 90° and then horizontally adducts the arm 40° with medial rotation (Figure 5-102). While doing the movement, the examiner palpates the posteroinferior region of the glenoid. If the humerus protrudes or pain is felt in the area, the test is considered positive and indicates a lesion of the posterior portion of the inferior glenohumeral ligament. If movement (i.e., horizontal adduction) is restricted, it may also indicate a tight posterior capsule.

Coracoclavicular Ligament Test. The integrity of the conoid portion of the coracoclavicular ligament may be tested by placing the patient in a side lying position on the unaffected side with the hand resting against the lower back. The examiner stabilizes the clavicle while pulling the inferior angle of the scapula away from the chest wall. The trapezoid portion of the ligament may be tested from the same position. The examiner stabilizes the clavicle and pulls the medial border of the scapula away from the chest wall (Figure 5-103). Pain in either case in the area of the ligament (anteriorly under the clavicle between the outer one-third and inner two-thirds) constitutes a positive test.

Tests for Muscle or Tendon Pathology

Speed's Test (Biceps or Straight-Arm Test). The examiner resists shoulder forward flexion by the patient while the patient's forearm is first supinated, then pronated, and the elbow is completely extended.

Common Muscle and Tendon Pathology Tests

- Speed's test (biceps)
- Yergason's test (biceps)
- Empty can test (supraspinatus)
- Lift-off test (subscapularis)
- Lag or "spring back" tests (subscapularis—medial rotation; infraspinatus—lateral rotation)
- Trapezius weakness (three positions)
- Serratus anterior weakness
- Pectoralis major and minor tightness

The test may also be performed by forward flexing the patient's arm to 90° and then asking the patient to resist an eccentric movement into extension first with the arm supinated, then pronated (Figure 5-104). A positive test elicits increased tenderness in the bicipital groove especially with the arm supinated and is indicative of bicipital paratenonitis or tendinosis.[23] Speed's test is more effective than Yergason's test because the bone moves over more of the tendon during the Speed's test. It has been reported that this test may cause pain and will therefore be positive if a SLAP (type II) lesion is present.[164] If profound weakness is found on resisted supination, a severe second- or third-degree (rupture) strain of the distal biceps should be suspected.[206]

Yergason's Test. This test is primarily designed to check the ability of the transverse humeral ligament to hold the biceps tendon in the bicipital groove. With the patient's elbow flexed to 90° and stabilized against the thorax and with the forearm pronated, the examiner resists supination while the patient also laterally rotates the arm against resistance (Figure 5-105).[207] If the examiner palpates the biceps tendon in the bicipital groove during the supination and lateral rotation movement, the tendon will be felt to "pop out" of the groove if the transverse humeral ligament is torn. Tenderness in the bicipital groove alone without the dislocation may indicate bicipital paratenonitis/tendinosis.[23] This test is not as effective as Speed's test when testing the biceps tendon, because the bicipital groove moves only slightly over the tendon affecting only a small part of the tendon during the test and because biceps tendon pain tends to occur with motion or palpation rather than with tension.

Ludington's Test[208]. The patient clasps both hands on top of or behind the head, allowing the interlocking fingers to support the weight of the upper limbs (Figure 5-106). This action allows maximum relaxation of the biceps tendon in its resting position. The patient then alternately contracts and relaxes the biceps muscles. While the patient does the contractions and relaxations, the examiner palpates the biceps tendon, which will be felt on the uninvolved side but not on the affected side if the test result is positive. A positive result indicates that the long head of biceps tendon has ruptured.

A   **B**

Figure 5-103

Coracoclavicular ligament test. **A,** Conoid portion. **B,** Trapezoid portion.

Figure 5-104
Speed's test (biceps or straight-arm test).

Gilchrest's Sign[139,209]. While standing, the patient lifts a 2- to 3-kg (5- to 7-lb) weight over the head. The arm is laterally rotated fully and lowered to the side in the coronal plane. A positive test is indicated by discomfort or pain in the bicipital groove. A positive test indicates bicipital paratenonitis or tendinosis.[23] In some cases, an audible snap or pain may be felt at between 90° and 100° abduction.

Lippman's Test[210]. The patient sits or stands while the examiner holds the arm flexed to 90° with one hand. With the other hand, the examiner palpates the biceps tendon 7 to 8 cm (2.5 to 3 inches) below the glenohumeral joint and moves the biceps tendon from side to side in the bicipital groove. A sharp pain is a positive test and indicates bicipital paratenonitis or tendinosis.[23]

Heuter's Sign[209]. Normally, if elbow flexion is resisted when the arm is pronated, some supination occurs as the biceps attempts to help the brachialis muscle flex the elbow. This supination movement is called Heuter's sign. If it is absent, the distal biceps tendon has been disrupted.

Supraspinatus ("Empty Can" or Jobe) Test[211]. The patient's arm is abducted to 90° with neutral (no) rotation, and the examiner provides resistance to abduction. The shoulder is then medially rotated and angled forward 30° (empty can position) so that the patient's thumbs point toward the floor (Figure 5-107) in the plane of the scapula.

A

B

Figure 5-105
Yergason's test. **A,** Start position. **B,** End position.

Figure 5-106
Ludington's test.

Figure 5-107
Supraspinatus "empty can" test.

A

B

Figure 5-108
Drop-arm test. **A,** The patient abducts the arm to 90°. **B,** The patient tries to lower the arm slowly and is unable to do so; instead, the arm drops to his side. Examiner's hand illustrates the start position.

Others have said that testing the arm with the thumb up ("full can") is best for maximum contraction of supraspinatus.[212] Resistance to abduction is again given while the examiner looks for weakness or pain, reflecting a positive test result. A positive test result indicates a tear of the supraspinatus tendon or muscle, or neuropathy of the suprascapular nerve.

Drop-Arm (Codman's) Test. The examiner abducts the patient's shoulder to 90° and then asks the patient to slowly lower the arm to the side in the same arc of movement (Figure 5-108). A positive test is indicated if the patient is unable to return the arm to the side slowly or has severe pain when attempting to do so. A positive result indicates a tear in the rotator cuff complex.[213] A complete tear (3° strain) of the rotator cuff is more com-

mon in older patients (50+ years). In younger people, a partial tear (1° or 2° strain) is more likely to occur when the patient is abducting the arm and a strong downward, eccentric load is applied to the arm.

Abrasion Sign[38]. The patient sits and abducts the arm to 90° with the elbow flexed to 90°. The patient then medially and laterally rotates the arm at the shoulder. Normally, there are no signs and symptoms. If crepitus occurs, it is a sign that the rotator cuff tendons are frayed and are abrading against the under surfaces of the acromion process and the coracoacromial ligament.

Lift-Off Sign[212,214-217]. The patient stands and places the dorsum of the hand on the back pocket or against the midlumbar spine. Great subscapularis activity is shown with the second position (Figure 5-109).[218] The patient then lifts the hand away from the back. An inability to do so indicates a lesion of the subscapularis muscle. Abnormal motion in the scapula during the test may indicate scapular instability. If the patient is able to

Figure 5-109
Lift-off sign. **A,** Start position. **B,** Lift off position. **C,** Resistance to lift off provided by examiner. Examiner tests strength of subscapularis and watches positioning of scapula.

take the hand away from the back, the examiner should apply a load pushing the hand toward the back to test the strength of the subscapularis and to test how the scapula acts under dynamic loading. With a torn subscapularis tendon, passive (and active) lateral rotation increases.[215]

If the patient's hand is passively medially rotated as far as possible and the patient is asked to hold the position, it will be found that the hand moves toward the back (**subscapularis** or **medial rotation "spring back"** or **lag test**) because subscapularis cannot hold the position due to weakness or pain. This test is also called the **modified lift off test** (Figure 5-110).[215,219] A small lag between maximum passive medial rotation and active medial rotation implies a partial tear (1°, 2°) of subscapularis.[214] This modified test is reported to be more accurate in diagnosing rotator cuff tear.[220] The test may also be used to test the rhomboids. Medial border winging of the scapula during the test may indicate that the rhomboids are affected. Stefko et al. reported that maximum isolation of the subscapularis was achieved by placing the hand against the posteroinferior border of the scapula (**maximum medial rotation test**) and then attempting the lift off.[221] In the other positions for lift off, teres major, latissimus dorsi, posterior deltoid, or rhomboids may compensate for a weak subscapularis.

Abdominal Compression (Belly-Press) Test[214,217,222]**.** This test checks the subscapularis muscle, especially if the patient cannot medially rotate the shoulder enough to take it behind the back. The patient is in a standing position. The examiner places a hand on the abdomen so that the examiner can feel how much pressure the patient is applying to the abdomen. The patient places his or her hand of the shoulder being tested on the examiner's hand and pushes the hand as hard as he or she can into the stomach (medial shoulder rotation). While pushing the hand into the abdomen, the patient attempts to bring the elbow forward to the scapular plane causing greater medially shoulder rotation. If the patient is unable to maintain the pressure on the examiner's hand while moving the elbow forward or extends the shoulder, the test is positive for a tear of the subscapularis muscle (Figure 5-111).

Lateral Rotation Lag Sign (Infraspinatus "Spring Back" Test)[106]**.** The patient is seated or in standing position with the arm by the side and the elbow flexed to 90°. The examiner passively abducts the arm to 90° in the scapular plane, laterally rotates the shoulder to end range (some authors say 45°),[223] and asks the patient to hold it (Figure 5-112, *A*). For a positive test, the patient cannot hold the position and the hand springs back anteriorly toward midline, indicating infraspinatus and teres minor cannot hold the position due to weakness or pain (Figure 5-112, *B*).[216,224] The examiner will also find passive medial rotation will have increased on the affected side.

Figure 5-110

Subscapularis spring back or lag test. **A,** Start position. **B,** Patient is unable to hold the start position and hand springs back toward the lower back.

Figure 5-111

Abdominal compression test.

If the test is performed with the arm in 20° abduction or by the side in the scapular plane with the elbow at 90° and the shoulder laterally rotated, the examiner then takes the arm into maximum lateral rotation and asks the patient to hold the position (Figure 5-113, *A*). If the supraspinatus and infraspinatus are torn, the arm will medially rotate and spring back anteriorly indicating a positive test (Figure 5-113, *B*). This test has also been called the **ERLS test** (external [sic. lateral] rotation lag sign). Hertel et al. described a **drop sign** in which the patient is standing and abducts the arm to 90° with the elbow flexed to 90°.[220] The examiner maximally laterally rotates the arm, and the patient is asked to hold the position. If the arm falls or drops into medial rotation, the test is considered positive for tears to infraspinatus and supraspinatus and perhaps subscapularis (Figure 5-114).[166] If the patient is able to hold the position, the strength of infraspinatus can be graded as 3 or greater depending on the resistance to the examiner's medially rotated force.[223]

Hornblower's (Signe de Clairon) Sign[106,219,223]. This test, also called **Patte Test**, is designed to test the strength of teres minor. The patient is in a standing position. The examiner elevates the patient's arm to 90° in the scapular plane. The examiner then flexes the elbow to 90°, and the patient is asked to laterally rotate the shoulder against resistance.

A　　　　　　　　　　　　　　　　　**B**

Figure 5-112

Lateral rotation lag test to test the teres minor and infraspinatus. **A,** Arm is abducted 90°. **B,** Note how hand springs forward when released by examiner.

A positive test is indicated when the patient is unable to laterally rotate the arm and indicates a tear of teres minor.[225]

McClusky offered a second way to do the test.[106] The patient is standing with the arms by the side and then is asked to bring the hands to the mouth (Figure 5-115, *A*). With a massive posterior rotator cuff tear, the patient is unable to do this without abducting the arm first (Figure 5-115, *B*). This abduction with hands to the mouth is called **hornblower's sign**.

Infraspinatus Test. The patient stands with the arm at the side with the elbow at 90° and the humerus medially rotated to 45°. The examiner then applies a medial rotation force that the patient resists. Pain or the inability to resist medial rotation indicates a positive test for an infraspinatus strain (Figure 5-116).

Teres Minor Test. The patient lies prone and places the hand on the opposite posterior iliac crest. The patient is then asked to extend and adduct the medially rotated arm against resistance. Pain or weakness indicates a positive test for teres minor strain (Figure 5-117).

Trapezius Weakness[226]. The patient sits down and places the hands together over the head. The examiner stands behind the patient and pushes the elbows forward. Normally the three parts of the trapezius contract to stabilize the scapula (Figure 5-118, *A*). The upper trapezius can be tested separately by elevating the shoulder with the arm slightly abducted or to resisted shoulder abduction and head side flexion (Figure 5-118, *B*).[227,228] If the shoulder is elevated with the arm by the side, levator scapulae and rhomboids are more likely to be involved as well. The middle trapezius can be tested with the patient in a prone position with the arm abducted to 90° and laterally rotated. The test involves the examiner resisting horizontal extension of the arm watching for retraction of the scapula, which should normally occur (Figure 5-118, *C*).[227,228] If scapular protraction occurs, the middle fibers of trapezius are weak. To test the lower trapezius, the patient is in prone lying with arm abducted to 120° and the shoulder laterally rotated. The examiner applies resistance to diagonal extension and watches for scapular retraction that should normally occur

Figure 5-113
External rotation lag sign or drop test. **A,** Start position. **B,** Position in positive test.

Figure 5-114
The drop sign. **A,** The test is performed by the examiner placing the arm in 90° of abduction and maximum external rotation and asking the patient to hold the position. **B,** If the patient cannot hold this position, and the arm falls into internal rotation, the test is positive.

Figure 5-115
Hornblower's (Signe de Clairon) sign. **A,** Normal result. **B,** Positive test. Patient must abduct the arm to bring the hand to the mouth.

Figure 5-116
Infraspinatus test.

Figure 5-117
Teres minor test.

(Figure 5-118, *D*). If scapular protraction occurs, the lower trapezius is weak.[227] If the scapula is elevated more than normal, it may indicate a tight trapezius or the presence of cervical torticollis.

Serratus Anterior Weakness[226]. The patient is in a standing position and forward flexes the arm to 90°. The examiner applies a backward force to the arm (Figure 5-119). If serratus anterior is weak or paralyzed, the medial border of the scapula will wing (classic winging). The patient will also have difficulty abducting or forward flexing the arm above 90° with a weak serratus anterior, but it still may be possible with lower trapezius

compensation.[45] A similar finding may be accomplished by doing a wall or floor pushup.

Rhomboid Weakness[106,226]. The patient is in a prone lying position or sitting with the test arm behind the body so the hand is on the opposite side (opposite back pocket). The examiner places the index finger along and under the medial border of the scapula while asking the patient to push the shoulder forward slightly against resistance to relax the trapezius (Figure 5-120, *A*). The patient then is asked to raise the forearm and hand away from the body. If the rhomboids are normal, the thumb is pushed away from under the scapula (Figure 5-120, *B*).

Figure 5-118

Testing for trapezius weakness. **A,** All portions of triceps. **B,** Upper trapezius. **C,** Middle trapezius. **D,** Lower trapezius.

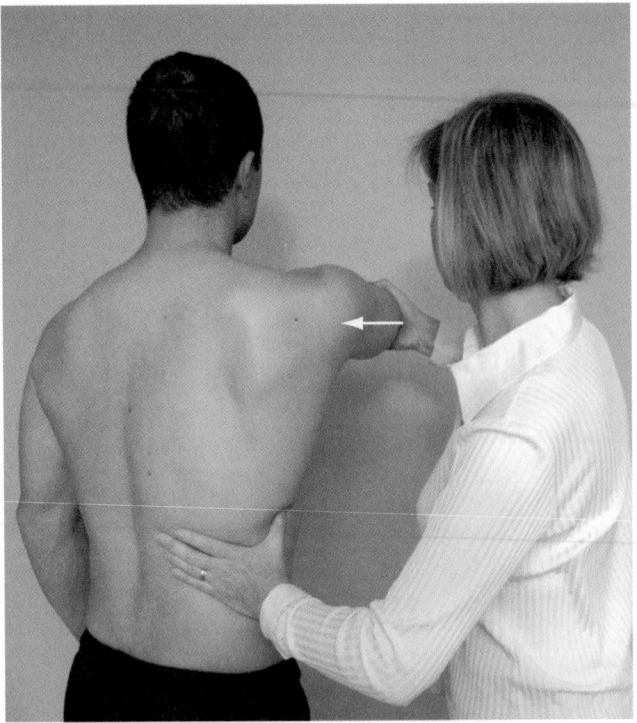

Figure 5-119
Testing for serratus anterior weakness. Punch out test: examiner applies a backward force.

Latissimus Dorsi Weakness[150]. The patient is in a standing position with the arms elevated in the plane of the scapula to 160°. Against resistance of the examiner, the patient is asked to medially rotate and extend the arm downward as if climbing a ladder (Figure 5-121).

Biceps Tightness. The patient lies supine with the shoulder in extension over the edge of the examining table with the elbow flexed and the forearm supinated. The examiner then extends the elbow, which would normally have a bone-to-bone end feel if the biceps is normal. If the biceps is tight, full elbow flexion will not occur and the end feel will be a muscular tissue stretch (Figure 5-122).[229]

Triceps Tightness. The patient is in a sitting position. The arm is fully elevated through forward flexion and lateral rotation. While stabilizing the humerus, the examiner flexes the elbow (see Figure 6-15, *B*).[229] Normally, the end feel would be soft tissue approximation. If the triceps is tight, elbow flexion will be limited and the end feel will be muscular tissue stretch.

Pectoralis Major Contracture Test. The patient lies supine and clasps the hands together behind the head. The arms are then lowered until the elbows touch the examining table (Figure 5-123, *A*). A positive test occurs if the elbows do not reach the table and indicates a tight pectoralis major muscle.

Pectoralis Minor Tightness. Pectoralis minor functions along with the rhomboids and levator scapulae to stabilize the scapula during arm extension. Tightness of the pectoralis minor can lead to increased scapular protraction and tilting of the inferior angle of the scapula posteriorly. Tightness of the pectoralis minor can be tested by having the patient in a supine lying position. The examiner places the heel of the hand over the coracoid process and pushes it toward the examining table (Figure 5-123, *B*). Normally, the posterior movement occurs with no discomfort to the patient, and the scapula lies flat against the table. However, if there is tightness (muscle tissue stretch)

A

B

Figure 5-120
Testing for rhomboid weakness. **A,** Start position. **B,** Test position.

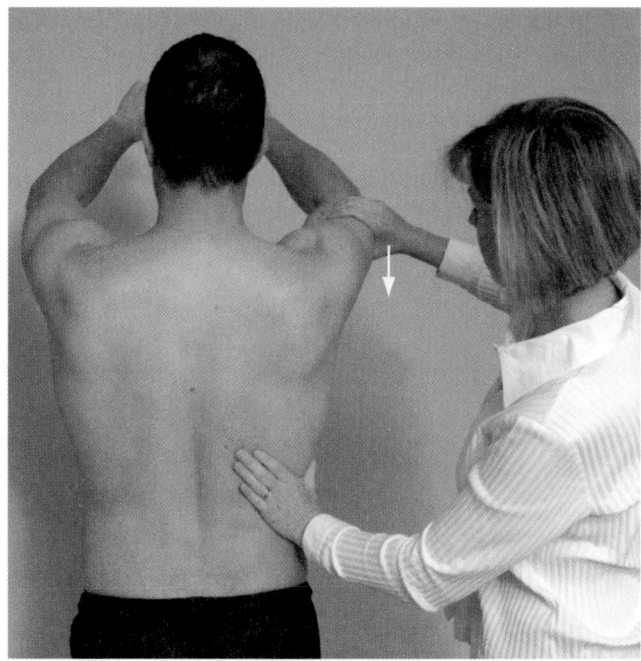

Figure 5-121
Testing for latissimus dorsi weakness.

Figure 5-122
Testing for biceps tightness.

A

B

Figure 5-123
Testing for tightness of (**A**) pectoralis major and (**B**) pectoralis minor. Examiner is testing end feel. Note position of examiner's hand on (**A**) humerus and (**B**) coracoid process.

over the pectoralis minor muscle during the posterior movement, the test would be considered positive.

Tightness of Latissimus Dorsi, Pectoralis Major, and Pectoralis Minor. The patient is placed in a supine lying position and is asked to fully elevate the arms through forward flexion. If the three muscles have normal length, the arms will extend to rest against the examining table. If the scapula does not lie flat against the table, it indicates that the pectoralis minor, pectoralis major, or latissimus dorsi is tight (the scapula remains protracted) (Figure 5-124).[227]

Tests for Neurological Function

Upper Limb Tension (Brachial Plexus Tension) Test[230]**.** This test is the upper limb equivalent of the straight leg raising test of the lower limb. It is used when the patient has presented with upper limb radicular signs or peripheral nerve symptoms. The patient is positioned to stress the neurological tissue entering the arm. The patient lies supine. The test may be performed by placing the joints of the upper limb in different positions to stress each of the neurological tissues differently.[231] There are, in effect, four upper limb tension tests (ULTT 1 to 4) (see Table 3-13 and

Figure 5-124
Testing for tightness of latissimus dorsi, pectoralis major, and pectoralis minor as a group.

of thoracic outlet syndrome is usually one of exclusion in which all other causes have been eliminated.[233-236] In fact, neurogenic signs are rare in thoracic outlet syndrome, and there is poor correlation between the vascular signs of the condition and neurological involvement. Thoracic outlet tests must not only decrease the pulse, they must also reproduce the patient's symptoms to be considered positive.[237] The tests do not show high reliability.

Common Tests for Thoracic Outlet Syndrome

- Roos test
- Wright test
- Costoclavicular syndrome test

Figure 3-36).[232] The key to performing the tests correctly is to ensure the shoulder is held in depression. If it is allowed to elevate, tension is taken off the neurological structures. Depending on the history, the examiner picks the ULTT that will stress the appropriate neurological tissue. Pain in the form of tingling or a stretch or ache in the cubital fossa indicates stretching of the dura mater in the cervical spine. The available range of passive movement at the elbow, when compared with the normal side, can indicate the restriction. Lateral or side flexion of the cervical spine to the opposite side can enhance the effect. If full ROM is not available in the shoulder, the test can still be performed by taking the shoulder to the point just short of pain in abduction and lateral rotation and performing the other maneuvers of the arm or by passively side flexing the cervical spine. The upper limb tension tests put tension on the upper limb neurological tissues even in normal individuals. Therefore, reproduction of the patient's symptoms, rather than stretching, constitutes a positive sign. This finding indicates the neurological tissue is being stressed but it does not tell the examiner where or why it is being stressed.

Tinel's Sign (at the Shoulder). The area of the brachial plexus above the clavicle in the area of the scalene triangle is tapped. A positive sign is indicated by a tingling sensation in one or more of the nerve roots.

Neurological Function Tests

- Upper limb tension tests

Tests for Thoracic Outlet Syndrome

Thoracic outlet syndromes may combine neurological and vascular signs, or the signs and symptoms of neurological deficit, restriction of arterial flow, or restriction of venous flow may be seen individually. For this reason, a diagnosis

With thoracic outlet tests that involve taking the pulse, the examiner must find the pulse before positioning the patient's arm or cervical spine. Because the pulse may be diminished even in a "normal" individual, it is more important to look for the reproduction of symptoms than for diminution of the pulse. Unless stated, the duration of these provocative tests should be no more than 1 to 2 minutes.[234]

Roos Test (EAST)[238]. The patient stands and abducts the arms to 90°, laterally rotates the shoulder, and flexes the elbows to 90° so that the elbows are slightly behind the frontal plane. The patient then opens and closes the hands slowly for 3 minutes (Figure 5-125). If the patient is unable to keep the arms in the starting position for 3 minutes or suffers ischemic pain, heaviness or profound weakness of the arm, or numbness and tingling of the hand during the 3 minutes, the test is considered positive

Figure 5-125
Roos test.

for thoracic outlet syndrome on the affected side. Minor fatigue and distress are considered negative tests. The test is sometimes called the **positive abduction and external rotation (AER) position test, the "hands up" test**, or the **elevated arm stress test (EAST)**.[238–241]

Wright Test or Maneuver. Wright advocated "hyperabducting" the arm so that the hand is brought over the head with the elbow and arm in the coronal plane with the shoulder laterally rotated (Figure 5-126, *A*).[242] He advocated doing the test in the sitting and then the supine positions. Having the patient take a breath or rotating or extending the head and neck may have an

additional effect. The pulse is palpated for differences. This test is used to detect compression in the costoclavicular space and is similar to the costoclavicular syndrome test described next.

Examiners have modified this test over time so that it has come to be described as follows. The examiner flexes the patient's elbow to 90° while the shoulder is extended horizontally and rotated laterally (Figure 5-126, *B*). The patient then rotates the head away from the test side. The examiner palpates the radial pulse, which becomes absent (disappears) when the head is rotated away from the test side. The test done in this

A **B**

Figure 5-126
A, Wright test. **B,** Modified Wright test or maneuver (Allen maneuver).

fashion has also been called the **Allen maneuver.** The pulse disappearance indicates a positive test result for thoracic outlet syndrome.

Costoclavicular Syndrome (Military Brace) Test. The examiner palpates the radial pulse and then draws the patient's shoulder down and back (Figure 5-127). A positive test is indicated by an absence of the pulse and implies possible thoracic outlet syndrome (costoclavicular syndrome). This test is particularly effective in patients who complain of symptoms while wearing a backpack or heavy coat.

Provocative Elevation Test[125]. The patient elevates both arms above the horizontal and is asked to rapidly open and close the hands 15 times. If fatigue, cramping, or tingling occurs during the test, the test is positive for vascular insufficiency and thoracic outlet syndrome. This test is a modification of the Roos test.

Shoulder Girdle Passive Elevation[133]. This test is used on patients who already present with symptoms. The patient sits and the examiner grasps the patient's arms from behind and passively elevates the shoulder girdle up and forward into full elevation (a passive bilateral shoulder shrug), and the position is held for 30 or more seconds (Figure 5-128). Arterial relief is evidenced by stronger pulse, skin color change (more pink), and increased hand temperature. Venous relief is shown by decreased cyanosis and venous engorgement. Neurological signs go from numbness to pins and needles or tingling as well as some pain as the ischemia to the nerve is released. This is referred to as a **release phenomenon.**

Adson Maneuver[243]. This test is probably one of the most common methods of testing for thoracic outlet syndrome reported in the literature. The examiner locates the radial pulse. The patient's head is rotated to face the test shoulder (Figure 5-129). The patient then extends the head while the examiner laterally rotates and extends the patient's shoulder. The patient is instructed to take a deep breath and hold it. A disappearance of the pulse indicates a positive test.

Halstead Maneuver. The examiner finds the radial pulse and applies a downward traction on the test extremity while the patient's neck is hyperextended and the head is rotated to the opposite side (Figure 5-130). Absence or disappearance of a pulse indicates a positive test for thoracic outlet syndrome.

Reflexes and Cutaneous Distribution

The reflexes in the shoulder region that are often assessed include the pectoralis major, clavicular portion (C5–

Figure 5-127
Costoclavicular syndrome test.

A

Figure 5-128
Shoulder girdle passive elevation. **A,** Start position.

B

Figure 5-128 cont'd
B, Relief position.

Figure 5-129
Adson maneuver.

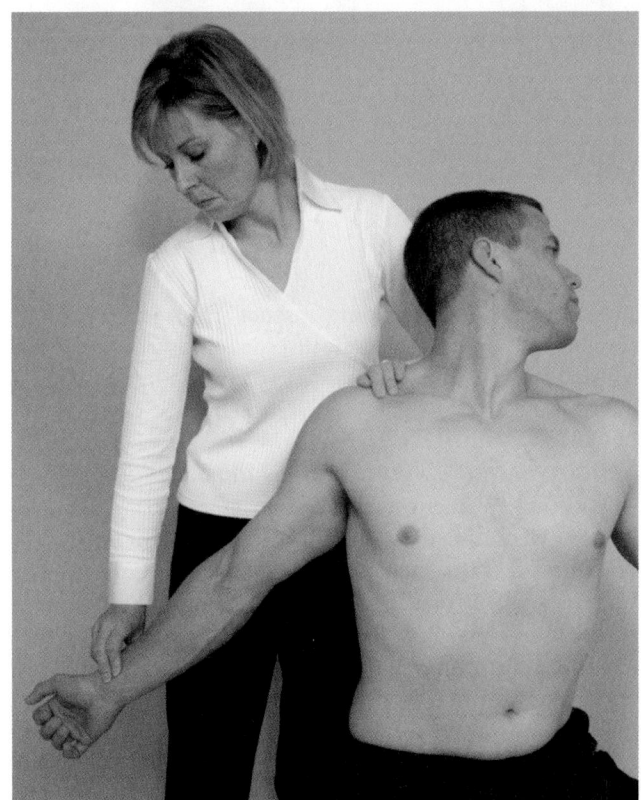

Figure 5-130
Halstead maneuver.

C6), sternocostal portion (C7–C8 and T1), the biceps (C5–C6), and the triceps (C7–C8) (Figure 5-131).

The examiner must be aware of the dermatome patterns of the nerve roots (Figure 5-132) as well as the cutaneous distribution of the peripheral nerves (Figure 5-133). Dermatomes vary from person to person, so the diagrams are estimations only. A scanning test for altered sensation is performed by running the relaxed hands and fingers over the neck, shoulders, and anterior and posterior chest area. Any difference in sensation between the two sides should be noted. These differences can be mapped more exactly using a pinwheel, a pin, a brush, or cotton batting. In this way, the examiner can use sensation to help differentiate between a peripheral nerve lesion and a nerve root lesion referred from the cervical spine.

True shoulder pain rarely extends below the elbow. Pain in the acromioclavicular or sternoclavicular joint tends to be localized to the affected joint and usually does not spread or radiate. Pain can be referred to the

Figure 5-131
Positioning to test the reflexes around the shoulder. **A,** Biceps.
B, Triceps. **C,** Pectoralis major.

shoulder and surrounding tissues from many structures,[244] including the cervical spine, elbow, lungs, heart, diaphragm, gallbladder, and spleen (Figure 5-134; Table 5-15).

Peripheral Nerve Injuries About the Shoulder

Axillary (Circumflex) Nerve (C5–C6). The axillary nerve is the most commonly injured nerve in the shoulder, and the most common cause of injury is anterior dislocation of the shoulder or fracture of the neck of the humerus.[245,246] The nerve injury may occur during the dislocation itself or during the reduction. Other traumatic events (e.g., fracture, bullet, or stab wounds) or brachial plexus injuries, compression (e.g., crutches), quadrilateral space entrapment (Figure 5-135) or shoulder surgery also may affect the axillary nerve.[247]

Motor loss (see Tables 5-5 and 5-10) includes an inability to abduct the arm (deltoid), although the patient

may attempt to laterally rotate the arm and use the long head of biceps to abduct the arm (trick movement). In some cases, a patient is asymptomatic, although he or she may demonstrate early fatigue with strenuous activities.[247] There is weakness of lateral rotation owing to the loss of teres minor.[247] The patient may attempt to use scapular movement (i.e., trapezius or serratus anterior) to compensate for the muscle loss (trick movement). Atrophy of the deltoid leads to loss of the lateral roundness (flattening) of the shoulder. Sensory loss is over the deltoid, with the main loss being a small, 2- to 3-cm (1-inch) circular area at the deltoid insertion (see Figure 5-9).

Suprascapular Nerve (C5–C6). The suprascapular nerve may be injured by a fall on the posterior shoulder, stretching, repeated microtrauma, or fracture of the scapula.[247] Commonly, the nerve is injured as it passes through the suprascapular notch under the transverse scapular (suprascapular) ligament or as it winds around

Figure 5-132
Dermatome pattern of the shoulder. Dermatomes on one side only are illustrated.

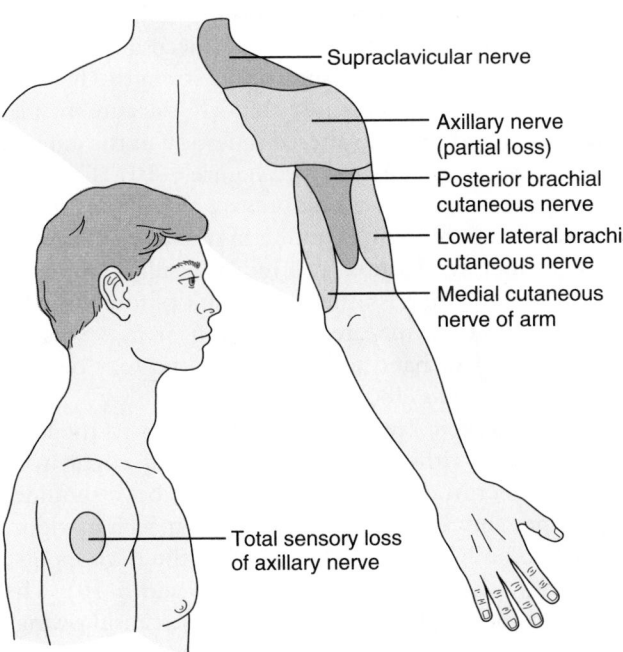

Figure 5-133
Cutaneous distribution of peripheral nerves around the shoulder.

Labels in Figure 5-133:
- Supraclavicular nerve
- Axillary nerve (partial loss)
- Posterior brachial cutaneous nerve
- Lower lateral brachial cutaneous nerve
- Medial cutaneous nerve of arm
- Total sensory loss of axillary nerve

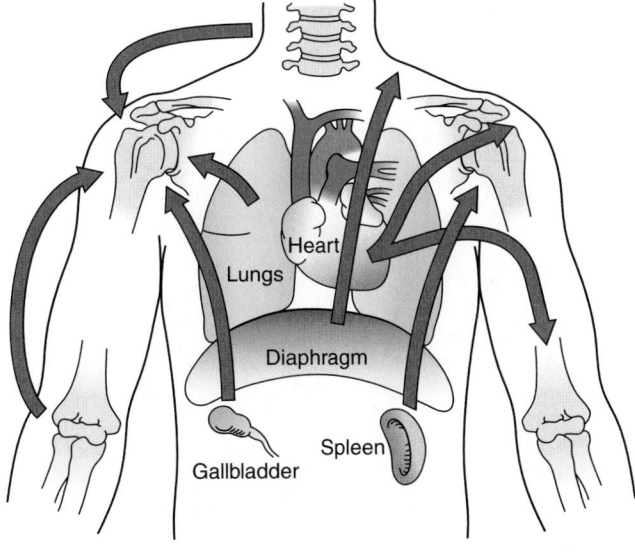

Figure 5-134
Structures referring pain to the shoulder.

Table 5-15

Shoulder Muscles and Referral of Pain

Muscle	Referral Pattern
Levator scapulae	Over muscle to posterior shoulder and along medial border of scapula
Latissimus dorsi	Interior angle of scapula up to posterior and anterior shoulder into posterior arm; may refer to area above iliac crest
Rhomboids	Medial border of scapula
Supraspinatus	Over shoulder cap and above spine of scapula; sometimes down lateral aspect of arm to proximal forearm
Infraspinatus	Anterolateral shoulder and medial border of scapula; may refer down lateral aspect of arm
Teres minor	Near deltoid insertion, up to shoulder cap, and down lateral arm to elbow
Subscapularis	Posterior shoulder to scapula and down posteromedial and anteromedial aspects of arm to elbow
Teres major	Shoulder cap down lateral aspect of arm to elbow
Deltoid	Over muscle and posterior glenoid area of shoulder
Coracobrachialis	Anterior shoulder and down posterior arm

the spine of the scapula under the spinoglenoid ligament (Figure 5-136).[44,247–252] Often, it is hard to distinguish from rotator cuff syndrome, so the history and mechanism of injury become important for differential diagnosis. Most commonly, the condition is seen in people who work with their arms overhead or in activities involving

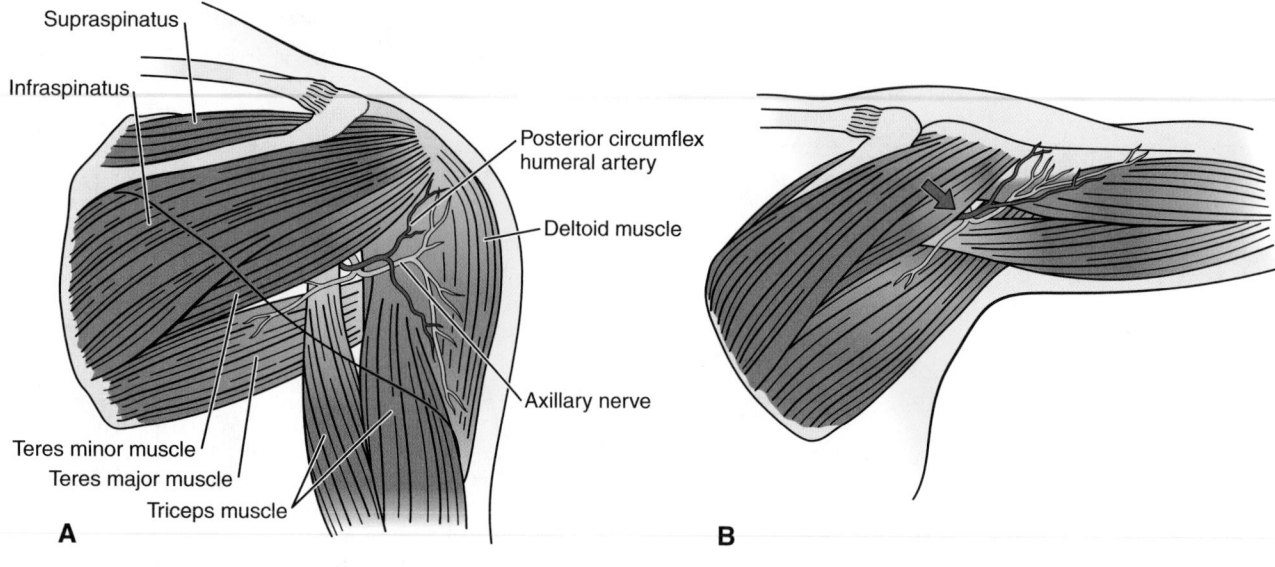

Supraspinatus

Infraspinatus

Posterior circumflex humeral artery

Deltoid muscle

Axillary nerve

Teres minor muscle
Teres major muscle
Triceps muscle

A

B

Figure 5-135

Quadrilateral space entrapment, posterior view of the shoulder. **A,** With the arm in adduction or at the side, there is no compression of the axillary nerve and posterior circumflex humeral artery. **B,** A mechanism of intermittent compression of the axillary nerve and posterior circumflex humeral artery as a result of shearing and closing down of the space by the teres major and teres minor. (Redrawn from Safran MR: Nerve injury about the shoulder in athletes. Part 1: suprascapular nerve and axillary nerve, *Am J Sports Med* 32:814, 2004.)

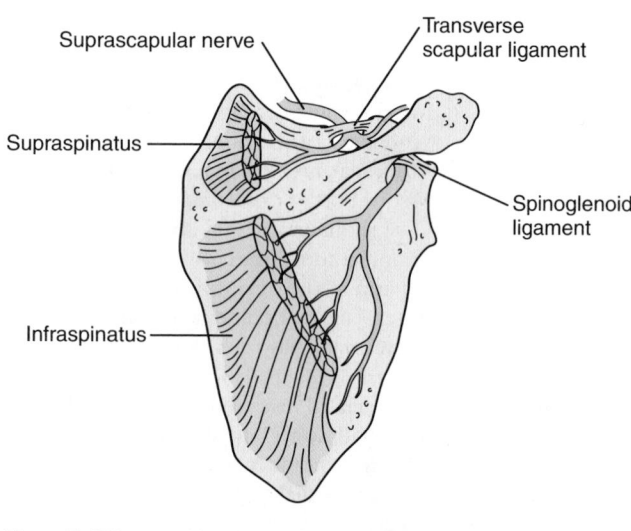

Suprascapular nerve

Transverse scapular ligament

Supraspinatus

Spinoglenoid ligament

Infraspinatus

Figure 5-136

Suprascapular nerve.

cocking and following through (e.g., volleyball spiking, pitching).[39,249,253,254]

Signs and symptoms include persistent rear shoulder pain and paralysis of the supraspinatus (suprascapular notch) and infraspinatus (suprascapular notch and spine of scapula), leading to decreased strength of abduction (supraspinatus) and lateral rotation (infraspinatus) of the shoulder. Wasting may also be evident in the muscles over the scapula.

Musculocutaneous Nerve (C5–C6). This nerve is not commonly injured, although it may be injured by trauma (e.g., humeral dislocation or fracture) or in conjunction with injury to the brachial plexus or adjacent axillary artery. Injury to this nerve (see Tables 5-5 and 5-10) results primarily in loss of elbow flexion (biceps and brachialis), shoulder forward flexion (biceps and coracobrachialis), and decreased supination strength (biceps). In addition, injury to its sensory branch, the antebrachial cutaneous nerve, leads to altered sensation in the anterolateral aspect of the forearm (see Figure 5-10). This sensory branch is sometimes compressed as it passes under the distal biceps tendon, resulting in **musculocutaneous nerve tunnel syndrome.** The injury results in sensory loss in the forearm; it is usually the result of forced elbow hyperextension or repeated pronation (e.g., excessive screwdriving, backhand tennis strokes) and may be misdiagnosed as tennis elbow.

Long Thoracic Nerve (C5–C8). Injury to the long thoracic nerve, although not common, may occur from repetitive microtrauma with heavy effort above shoulder height, pressure on the nerve from backpacking, vigorous upper limb activities[236] (e.g., shoveling, chopping, stretching), or wounds (see Tables 5-5 and 5-10). The result is paralysis of the serratus anterior, causing winging (medial border) of the scapula and pain and weakness on forward flexion of the extended arm.[39,45,48,56,245,246,250]

,[255,256]Abduction above 90° is difficult because of scapular winging. Stabilization of the scapula by the examiner enables the patient to further abduct the arm. Recovery time can be as long as 2 years.

Spinal Accessory Nerve (C3–C4). The spinal accessory nerve is vulnerable to traumatic injury as it passes the posterior triangle of the neck; injury spares the sternocleidomastoid muscles but affects the trapezius muscle. A common example would be abnormal pressure from a poorly fitting backpack (see Tables 5-5 and 5-10). Shoulder drooping (scapula is translated laterally and rotates downward) and scapular winging (medial superior portion) with medial rotation of the inferior angle, especially on abduction, may be evident, along with deepening of the supraclavicular fossa (asymmetric neck line) as a result of trapezius atrophy (Figure 5-137).[39,257,258] The patient has difficulty abducting the arm above 90°.[245] Interestingly, Safran reported that spinal accessory palsy results in scapular winging on abduction but not forward flexion.[236]

Joint Play Movements

Joint play movements are usually performed with the patient lying supine.[48,259] The examiner compares the amount of available movement and end feel on the affected side with the movement on the unaffected side and notes whether the movements affect the patient's symptoms.

To perform the backward joint play movement of the humerus, the examiner grasps the patient's upper limb, placing one hand over the anterior humeral head. The other hand is placed around the humerus above and near the elbow while the patient's hand is held against the examiner's thorax by the examiner's arm (Figure 5-138, *A*). The examiner then applies a backward force (similar

---

Joint Play Movements of the Shoulder Complex

- Backward glide of the humerus
- Forward glide of the humerus
- Lateral distraction of the humerus
- Caudal glide of the humerus (long arm traction)
- Backward glide of the humerus in abduction
- Lateral distraction of the humerus in abduction
- Anteroposterior and cephalocaudal movements of the clavicle at the acromioclavicular joint
- Anteroposterior and cephalocaudal movements of the clavicle at the sternoclavicular joint
- General movement of the scapula to determine mobility

A

B

Figure 5-137

Spinal accessory nerve palsy. A 17-year-old male patient with a 1-year history of shoulder pain. **A,** Winging of the superior medial angle of the scapula with abduction. A line drawn along the medial border of the normal left shoulder is to be compared with the symptomatic right shoulder. **B,** Forward elevation does not result in winging in this patient, differentiating spinal accessory nerve palsy winging from long thoracic nerve palsy winging. (From Safran MR: Nerve injury about the shoulder in athletes. Part 2: long thoracic nerve, spinal accessory nerve, burners/stingers, thoracic outlet syndrome, *Am J Sports Med* 32:1065, 2004.)

Figure 5-138

Joint play movements of the shoulder complex. **A,** Backward glide of the humerus. **B,** Forward glide of the humerus. **C,** Lateral distraction of the humerus. **D,** Long arm traction applied below elbow. **E,** Long arm traction applied above elbow. **F,** Backward glide of the humerus in abduction.

Figure 5-138 cont'd
G, Joint play of the acromioclavicular joint. **H,** Joint play of the sternoclavicular joint. **I,** General movement of
the scapula to determine mobility.

to a posterior shift), keeping the patient's arm parallel
to the body so that no rotation or torsion occurs at the
glenohumeral joint.

Forward joint play movement of the humerus is carried out in a similar fashion, with the examiner's hands
placed as shown in Figure 5-138, *B*. The examiner applies
an anterior force (anterior drawer), keeping the patient's
arm parallel to the body so that no rotation or torsion
occurs at the glenohumeral joint.

To apply a lateral distraction joint play movement to
the humerus, the examiner's hands are placed as shown
in Figure 5-138, *C*. A lateral distraction force is applied
to the glenohumeral joint, with the patient's arm kept
parallel to the body so that no rotation or torsion occurs
at the glenohumeral joint. The examiner must be careful to apply the lateral distraction force with the flat of
the hand, as one sometimes has a tendency, when apply-

ing a force, to turn the hand so the distraction is applied
through the side of the index finger. This is uncomfortable for the patient.

Caudal glide (long arm traction) joint play movement
is performed with the patient in the same supine position. The examiner grasps above the patient's wrist with
one hand and palpates with the other hand, below the
distal spine of the scapula posteriorly and below the distal clavicle anteriorly over the glenohumeral joint line
(Figure 5-138, *D*). The examiner then applies a traction
force to the shoulder while palpating to see whether the
head of the humerus drops down (moves distally) in the
glenoid cavity as it normally should. If the patient complains of pain in the elbow, the test may be done with the
hands positioned as in Figure 5-138, *E*.

The examiner then abducts the patient's arm to 90°,
grasping above the patient's wrist with one hand while

stabilizing the thorax with the other hand. The examiner applies a long arm traction force to determine joint play in this position.

With the patient's arm abducted to 90°, the examiner places one hand over the anterior humerus while stabilizing the patient's arm with the other hand and stabilizing the patient's hand against the thorax with the same arm. A backward force is then applied, keeping the patient's arm parallel to the body. This is a backward joint play movement of the humerus in abduction (Figure 5-138, *F*).

To assess the acromioclavicular and sternoclavicular joints (Figures 5-138, *G*, and 5-138, *H*, respectively), the examiner gently grasps the clavicle as close to the joint to be tested as possible and moves it in and out or up and down while palpating the joint with the other hand. Because the bone lies just under the skin, these techniques are uncomfortable for the patient where the examiner grasps the clavicle. The examiner should warn the patient before attempting this technique. A comparison of the amount of movement available is made between the two sides. Care should be taken not to squeeze the clavicle, as this too may cause pain.

For a determination of mobility of the scapula, the patient lies on one side to fixate the thorax with the arm relaxed and resting behind the low back (hand by opposite back pocket). The uppermost scapula is tested in this position. The examiner faces the patient, placing the lower hand along the medial border of the patient's scapula. The hand of the examiner's other arm holds the upper (cranial) dorsal surface of the patient's scapula. To relax the scapula further, the patient is asked to relax against the examiner and the examiner uses his or her body to push the patient's test shoulder posteriorly, retracting it to obtain a better hold on the scapula. By holding the scapula in this way, the examiner is able to move it medially, laterally, caudally, cranially, and away from the thorax (Figure 5-138, *I*).

Palpation

When palpating the shoulder complex, the examiner should note any muscle spasm, tenderness, abnormal bumps, or other signs and symptoms that may indicate the source of pathology. The examiner should perform palpation in a systematic manner, beginning with the anterior structures and working around to the posterior structures. Findings on the injured side should be compared with those on the unaffected side. Any differences between the two sides should be noted, because they may indicate the cause of the patient's problems.

Anterior Structures

The anterior structures of the shoulder may be palpated with the patient in the supine lying or sitting position (Figure 5-139, *A*).

Clavicle. The clavicle should be palpated along its full length for tenderness or abnormal bumps, such as callus formation after a fracture, and to ensure that it is in its resting position relative to the uninjured side. That is, it may be rotated anteriorly or posteriorly more than the unaffected side, or one end may be higher than that of the uninjured side, indicating a possible subluxation or dislocation at the sternoclavicular or acromioclavicular joint.

Sternoclavicular Joint. The sternoclavicular joint should be palpated for normal positioning in relation to the sternum and first rib. Palpation should also include the supporting ligaments and sternocleidomastoid muscle. Adjacent to the joint, the suprasternal notch may be palpated. From the notch, the examiner moves the fingers laterally and posteriorly to palpate the first rib. The examiner should apply slight caudal pressure to the first rib on both sides and note any difference. Spasm of the scalene muscles or pathology in the area may elevate the first rib on the affected side.

Acromioclavicular Joint. Like the sternoclavicular joint, the acromioclavicular joint should be palpated for normal positioning and tenderness. Likewise, supporting ligaments (acromioclavicular and coracoclavicular) and the trapezius, subclavius, and deltoid (anterior, middle, and posterior fibers) muscles should be palpated for tenderness and spasm.

Coracoid Process. The coracoid process may be palpated approximately 2.5 cm (1 inch) below the junction of the lateral one third and medial two thirds of the clavicle. The short head of biceps and coracobrachialis muscles originate from, and the pectoralis minor inserts into, this process. With a SICK scapula syndrome, the coracoid is often very tender.[20]

Sternum. In the midline of the chest, the examiner should palpate the three portions of the sternum (manubrium, body, and xiphoid process), noting any abnormality or tenderness.

Ribs and Costal Cartilage. Adjacent to the sternum, the examiner should palpate the sternocostal and costochondral articulations, noting any swelling, tenderness, or other abnormality. These "articulations" are sometimes sprained or subluxed, or a costochondritis (Tietze's syndrome) may be evident. The examiner should palpate the ribs as they extend around the chest wall, seeking any potential pathology and noting whether they are aligned with each other, or one protrudes more than the adjacent ones as sometimes occurs with anterior shoulder pathology.

Humerus and Rotator Cuff Muscles. Moving laterally from the chest and caudally from the acromion process, the examiner should palpate the humerus and its surrounding structures for potential pathology. The examiner first palpates the lateral tip of the acromion process and then moves inferiorly to the greater tuberosity of the humerus. The examiner should then laterally

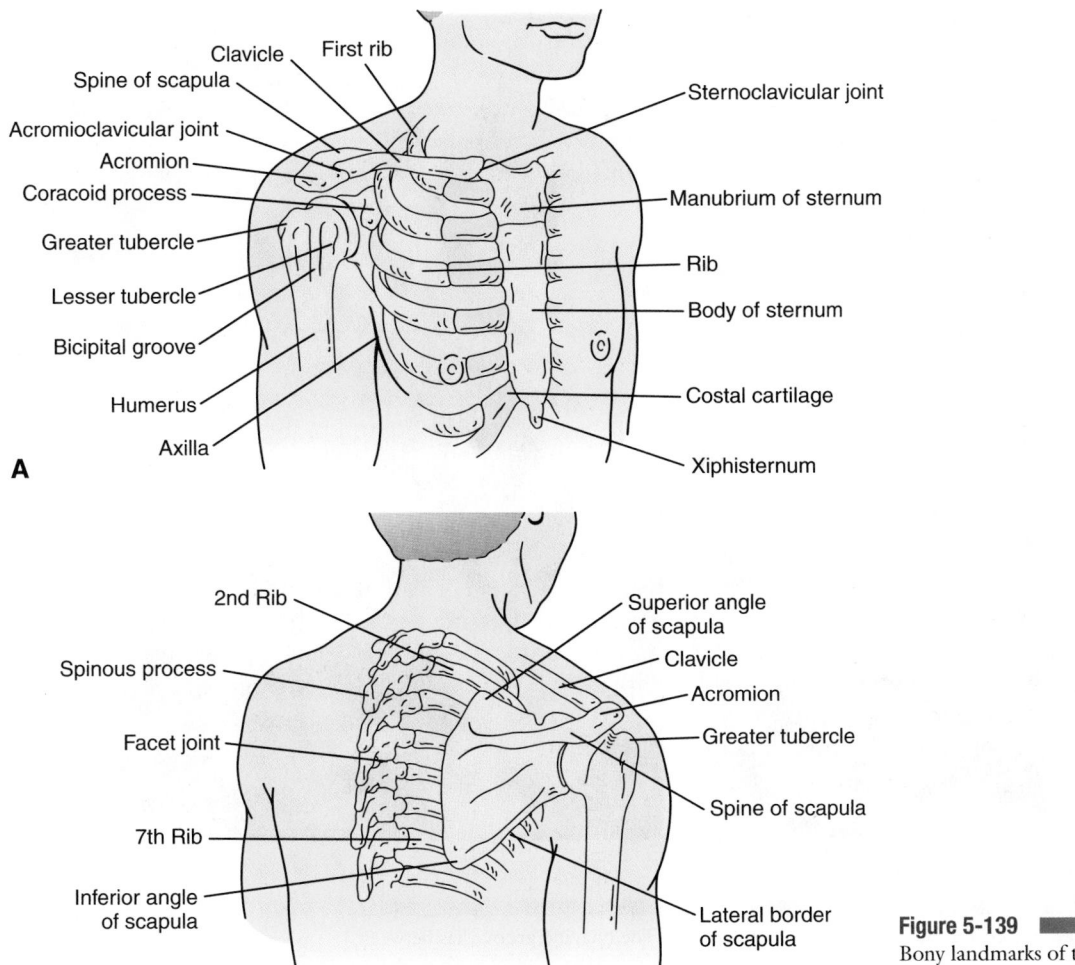

A

Clavicle
First rib
Spine of scapula
Acromioclavicular joint
Acromion
Coracoid process
Greater tubercle
Lesser tubercle
Bicipital groove
Humerus
Axilla

Sternoclavicular joint
Manubrium of sternum
Rib
Body of sternum
Costal cartilage
Xiphisternum

B

2nd Rib
Spinous process
Facet joint
7th Rib
Inferior angle of scapula

Superior angle of scapula
Clavicle
Acromion
Greater tubercle
Spine of scapula
Lateral border of scapula

Figure 5-139
Bony landmarks of the shoulder region. **A,** Anterior view. **B,** Posterior view.

rotate the humerus. During palpation, the long head of the biceps in the bicipital groove will slip under the fingers, followed by the lesser tuberosity of the humerus (Figure 5-140). As with all palpation, the testing should be done gently and carefully to prevent causing the patient undue pain. By rotating the humerus alternately laterally and medially, the smooth progression over the three structures is normally noted **(de Anquin test),** and the lesser tuberosity is felt at the level of the coracoid process. If the examiner then palpates along the lesser tuberosity and the lip of the bicipital groove, the fingers will rest on the tendon of the subscapularis muscle. The subscapularis may also be palpated in the triangle made up of the superior border of pectoralis major, the clavicle, and the medial border of the deltoid.[260] If the examiner places the thumb over the lesser tuberosity and "grips" the shoulder between the second, third, and fourth fingers as shown in Figure 5-1, the fingers will be over the insertion of the other three rotator cuff muscles: supraspinatus, infraspinatus, and teres minor. Moving laterally over the bicipital groove to its other lip, the examiner may palpate the insertion of the pectoralis major muscle.

The patient is then asked to further medially rotate the humerus so that the forearm rests behind the back, and the examiner palpates 2 cm inferior to the anterior aspect of the acromion process for the supraspinatus tendon. Any tenderness of the tendon should be noted. The examiner then passively abducts the patient's shoulder to between 80° and 90° and palpates the notch formed by the acromion and spine of the scapula with the clavicle. In the notch, the examiner is palpating the musculotendinous junction of the supraspinatus muscle.

The examiner should then palpate the head of the humerus and its relationship to the glenoid cavity. By placing the fingers over the anterior humeral head and the thumb over the posterior humeral head, the examiner then slides the fingers and thumbs medially (see Figure 5-45). As the humeral head is larger than the glenoid with only about 25% to 30% of the head in contact with the glenoid at any one time, the examiner's fingers and thumb will "dip in" as they approach the glenohumeral joint. This "dipping in" should be slightly greater anteriorly. If there is no dipping anteriorly or posteriorly, it means the humeral head is sitting further posteriorly or

Figure 5-140

Palpation around the shoulder. **A,** Greater tuberosity. **B,** Lesser tuberosity. The bicipital groove lies between these two landmarks.

anteriorly than it should. Once the examiner has found the glenohumeral joint (at the point of hardness after the "dip in"), he or she can palpate along the joint line superiorly and inferiorly on the anterior and posterior surface feeling for any pain or the presence of pathology (torn labrum, ligament, or capsule). The examiner can determine the joint line by medially and laterally rotating the humerus while palpating. The examiner should be able to differentiate the glenoid (does not move) from the humerus (rotates). As the technique is uncomfortable to the patient, the patient should be warned about possible discomfort, and the results should be compared with the normal side. With care, the examiner can palpate all of the glenoid edge except superiorly where the proximity of the acromion to the humerus does not allow it.

Axilla. With the shoulder slightly abducted (20° to 30°), the examiner palpates the structures of the axilla, latissimus dorsi muscle (posterior wall), pectoralis major muscle (anterior wall), serratus anterior muscle (medial wall), lymph nodes (palpable only if swollen), and brachial artery. The inferior glenohumeral joint and glenoid edge may also be palpated in the axilla. The patient is then asked to lie prone on the elbows (sphinx position) with the shoulders slightly laterally rotated and the elbow slightly adducted in relation to the shoulder. The examiner then palpates just inferior to the most lateral aspect of the scapula for the insertion of the infraspinatus muscle. Just distal to this insertion, the examiner may be able to palpate the insertion of the teres minor.

Posterior Structures

To complete the palpation, the patient may be either sitting or lying prone with the upper limb by the trunk (see Figure 5-139, *B*).

Spine of Scapula. From the acromion process the examiner moves his or her hands along the spine of the scapula, noting any tenderness or abnormality.

Scapula. The examiner follows the spine of the scapula to the medial border of the scapula and then follows the outline of the scapula, which normally extends from the spinous process of T2 to the spinous process of T9, depending on the size of the scapula. The superior angle lies at the level of the T2 spinous process. The base or root of the spine of the scapula lies between T3 and T4, and the inferior angle lies between T7 and T9. Along the medial border and spine of the scapula, the examiner can palpate the trapezius muscle (upper, middle, and lower parts) and the rhomboids. At the inferior angle, the latissimus dorsi may be palpated. The examiner then moves around the inferior angle of the scapula and along its lateral border. Against the lateral border and along the ribs, the serratus anterior can be palpated. Near the glenoid, long head of triceps, and teres minor may be palpated. After the borders of the scapula have been palpated, the posterior surface (supraspinatus and infraspinatus muscles) may be palpated for tenderness, atrophy, or spasm. By positioning the arm in forward flexion (60°), adduction and lateral rotation, infraspinatus and teres minor may be palpated just under and slightly inferior to the posterior aspect of the acromion.[260]

Spinous Processes of Lower Cervical and Thoracic Spine. In the midline, the examiner may palpate the cervical and thoracic spinous processes for any abnormality or tenderness. This is followed by palpation of the trapezius muscle.

Diagnostic Imaging

Diagnostic imaging is used in conjunction with a physical examination to determine a diagnosis. It should never be used in isolation, but any findings should be related to clinical signs to rule out false positive indications or age-related changes.[261–263]

Plain Film Radiography[264–266]

Anteroposterior View. This may be a true anterior-posterior view or a tilt view (Figure 5-141). A great deal of information can be obtained from either view (Figure 5-142).
1. The relation of the humerus to the glenoid cavity should be examined. The "empty glenoid" sign may recognize posterior dislocations. Normally, the radiograph shows overlapping shadows of the humerus and glenoid. With a posterior dislocation, this shadow is reduced or absent (Figure 5-143).[267]
2. The relation of the clavicle to the acromion process and the humerus to the glenoid should also be observed.
3. The examiner should determine whether the epiphyseal plate of the humeral head is present and, if so, whether it is normal.
4. The examiner should note whether there are any calcifications in any of the tendons (Figure 5-144), especially those of the supraspinatus or infraspinatus muscles, or fractures.[268,269]
5. The examiner should note the configuration of the undersurface of the acromion (see Figure 5-142, *D*; Figure 5-145)[270,271] and the presence of any subacromial spurs (Figure 5-146). The possible configurations are type I (flat [17%]), type II (curved [43%]), and type III (hooked [39%]). Hooked acromion is not seen in young people and is thought to be part of a degenerative process.

Routine A-P shoulder

Posterior glenoid rim

Anterior glenoid rim

Anterior and posterior glenoid rims superimposed

True A-P shoulder

45°

Figure 5-141

Positioning for the anteroposterior radiographic view.

Figure 5-142

Normal radiographic examination. **A,** Lateral rotation. The greater tuberosity (GT) is shown in profile.
The humeral head normally overlaps the glenoid on this view. The anterior *(black arrows)* and posterior
(arrowheads) glenoid margins are well shown and do not overlap because of the anterior tilt of the glenoid.
The anatomical *(black A)* and surgical *(S)* necks of the humerus are indicated. White A = acromion process;
CP = coracoid process. A vacuum phenomenon *(white arrow)* is present. **B,** Medial rotation. The overlap of
the greater tuberosity and the humeral head produces a rounded appearance of the proximal humerus. LT
= lesser tuberosity. A small exostosis is noted projecting from the humeral metaphysis. **C,** Posterior oblique.
The glenohumeral cartilage space is shown in profile with no overlap of the humerus and glenoid. **D,** Normal
scapular Y view. This true lateral view of the scapula (anterior oblique of the shoulder) shows the humeral head
centered over the glenoid *(arrows)*. A = acromion; C = clavicle; CP = coracoid process. **E,** Diagram of normal
scapular Y view.

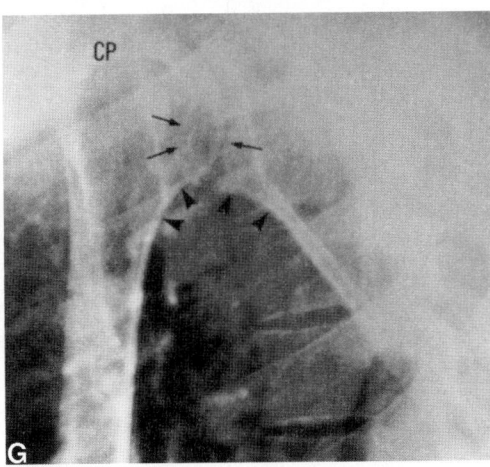

Figure 5-142 cont'd
F, Axillary view. A = acromion; ANT = anterior; C = clavicle; CP = coracoid process. **G,** Normal transthoracic view. The smooth arch formed by the inferior border of the scapula and the posterior aspect of the humerus is indicated *(arrowheads)*. A faint view of the coracoid process (CP) is shown. The margins of the glenoid are indicated *(arrows)*. This view is slightly oblique, allowing the glenoid to be shown more en face than usual. (From Weissman BNW, Sledge CB: *Orthopedic radiology,* p 219, Philadelphia, 1986, WB Saunders.)

6. Medial rotation of the humerus with this view may show a defect on the lateral aspect of the humeral head from recurrent dislocations. This defect is called a **Hill-Sachs lesion** (Figure 5-147) and may be classed as engaged or nonengaged.[272] Engaged implies the area of the lesion articulates with the glenoid when the arm is in abduction and lateral rotation.

7. The examiner should look at the acromiohumeral interval (the space between the acromion and the humerus) and see whether it is normal.[273] The normal interval is 7 to 14 mm (Figure 5-148). If this distance decreases, it may indicate rotator cuff tears.[274] Likewise, if the arm is medially rotated and the view shows the coracohumeral distance of less than 11 mm, this indicates impingement and rotator cuff pathology.[275]

8. A stress anteroposterior radiograph may be used to gap the injured acromioclavicular joint to see whether there has been a third-degree sprain or to show an inferior laxity at the glenohumeral joint (Figure 5-149). Equal weights of 9 kg (20 lb) are tied to each of the patient's hands to apply traction to the arms. If a third-degree acromioclavicular sprain has occurred, the coracoclavicular distance will increase and a step deformity will be evident.

Axillary Lateral View. This view shows the relation of the humeral head to the glenoid. It is used to diagnose anterior and posterior dislocations at the glenohumeral

Normal

Posterior dislocation

Figure 5-143
"Empty glenoid" sign of posterior dislocation on anteroposterior radiograph. The head of the humerus fills the glenoid in the normal radiograph *(left)*. With a posterior dislocation, the glenoid is "empty," especially in its anterior portion *(right)*. (From Magee DJ, Reid DC: Shoulder injuries. In Zachazewski JE et al, editors: *Athletic injuries and rehabilitation,* p 523, Philadelphia, 1996, WB Saunders.)

A   B

Figure 5-144

Calcific tendinitis—supraspinatus and infraspinatus. **A,** Lateral rotation view shows calcification projected over the base of the greater tuberosity *(white arrow)* and above the greater tuberosity *(open arrow)*. **B,** Medial rotation view projects the infraspinatus calcification *(white arrow)* in profile and documents its posterior location. The supraspinatus calcification *(open arrow)* is rotated medially and maintains its superior location. (From Weissman BNW, Sledge CB: *Orthopedic radiology,* p. 227, Philadelphia, 1986, WB Saunders.)

joint (Figure 5-150) and to look for avulsion fractures of the glenoid or a Hill-Sachs lesion. It does, however, require the patient to be able to abduct the arm 70° to 90°. This view is the best for observation of the acromio-clavicular joint. In addition, the examiner should note the relations of the glenoid cavity, humerus, scapula, and clavicle and any calcifications in the subscapularis, infra-spinatus, or teres minor muscles.

Figure 5-146

External subacromial impingement syndrome: route radiographic abnormalities. Frontal radiograph of the shoulder shows a large enthesophyte *(arrow)* extending from the anteroinferior portion of the acromion and associated with osteophytes at the acromioclavicular joint and in the inferior portion of the humeral head. (From Resnick D, Kransdorf MJ: *Bone and joint imaging,* p. 922, Philadelphia, 2005, WB Saunders.)

Figure 5-145

Acromion morphology.

Figure 5-147
Glenohumeral joint: Hill-Sachs lesion. In a patient with a previous anterior dislocation, an internal rotation view reveals the extent of the Hill-Sachs lesion *(arrowheads)*. (From Resnick D, Kransdorf MJ: *Bone and joint imaging*, p. 833, Philadelphia, WB 2005, Saunders.)

Figure 5-148
Acromiohumeral interval.

Figure 5-149
Stress radiograph for third-degree acromioclavicular sprain.
A, No stress. **B,** Stress. Note the increase in the distance between the coracoid process and the clavicle. **C,** Lateral view showing the complete separation.

Transscapular (Y) Lateral View. This view (Figure 5-151) shows the position of the humerus relative to the glenoid and the acromion and coracoid processes. This view is the true lateral view of the scapula (see Figure 5-142, *D*, and 5-142, *E*).

Stryker Notch View. For this view, the patient lies supine with the arm forward flexed and the hand on top of the head. The radiograph centers on the coracoid process. This view is used to assess a Hill-Sachs lesion (Figure 5-152) or a Bankart lesion.[276]

West Point View. The patient is positioned in a prone position (Figure 5-153). This projection gives a good view of the glenoid to delineate glenoid fractures.[277]

Figure 5-150
Axillary lateral view.

Figure 5-151
Positioning for transscapular (Y) lateral view.

Figure 5-152
A Stryker notch view demonstrates a notch in the posterolateral aspect of the humeral head, representing a large Hill-Sachs lesion.

Figure 5-153
Positioning patient for West Point axillary view. The beam (bottom left) is also angled downward to form an angle of 25° from the horizontal plane.

Arch View. This lateral view is used to determine the width and height of the subacromial arch. It helps the examiner determine the type of acromial arch (Figure 5-154).

Arthrography

An arthrogram of the shoulder is useful for delineating many of the soft tissues and recesses around the glenohumeral joint (Figures 5-155 and 5-156).[147,278-280] The joint can normally hold approximately 16 to 20 mL of solution. With adhesive capsulitis (idiopathic frozen shoulder), the amount the joint can hold may decrease to 5 to 10 mL. The arthrogram shows a decrease in the capacity of the joint and obliteration of the axillary fold. Also, there is an almost complete lack of filling of the subscapular bursa with adhesive capsulitis (Figure 5-157). Tearing of any structures, such as the supraspinatus tendon and rotator cuff, may result in extravasation of the radiopaque dye.[281]

Figure 5-154
Arch view of acromioclavicular joint. Notice the separation of the clavicle and acromion. The view also shows the relation of the humerus to the glenoid (Y view).

A

B

C

Figure 5-155
Normal single-contrast arthrogram. **A,** Lateral rotation. **B,** Medial rotation. A = axillary recess; S = subscapularis recess; *open arrows* = tendon of long head of biceps within biceps sheath. The humeral articular cartilage is coated with contrast medium *(white arrows)*. There is no contrast agent in the subacromial-subdeltoid bursa. The defect created by the glenoid labrum *(black arrows)* is shown. Filling of the subscapularis recess is often poor on lateral rotation views because of bursal compression by the subscapularis muscle. **C,** In the axillary view, the anterior *(single arrow)* and posterior *(double arrows)* glenoid labral margins are shown. The biceps tendon *(arrowheads)* is surrounded by contrast medium in the biceps tendon sheath. No contrast agent overlies the surgical neck of the humerus. (From Weissman BNW, Sledge CB: *Orthopedic radiology,* p. 222, Philadelphia, 1986, WB Saunders.)

A   B

Figure 5-156

Normal double-contrast arthrogram. Upright views of the patient with a sandbag suspended from the wrist, and the humerus in lateral rotation (**A**) and medial rotation (**B**) show the structures noted on single-contrast examination and allow better appreciation of the articular cartilages. (From Weissman BNW, Sledge CB: *Orthopedic radiology,* p. 222, Philadelphia, 1986, WB Saunders.)

A

Figure 5-157

Typical arthrographic picture in adhesive capsulitis. Note the absence of a dependent axillary fold and poor filling of the biceps. (From Neviaser JS: Arthrography of the shoulder joint: study of the findings of adhesive capsulitis of the shoulder, *J Bone Joint Surg Am* 44:1328, 1962.)

Figure 5-158

Tomogram and computed tomography scan of the glenoid labrum. **A,** Normal glenoid labrum on posterior oblique double-contrast arthrotomography. Tomographic section through the anterior margin of the glenoid in the posterior oblique position shows smooth articular cartilage on the humeral head *(black arrow)* and glenoid and a smooth contour to the glenoid labrum *(white arrow).*

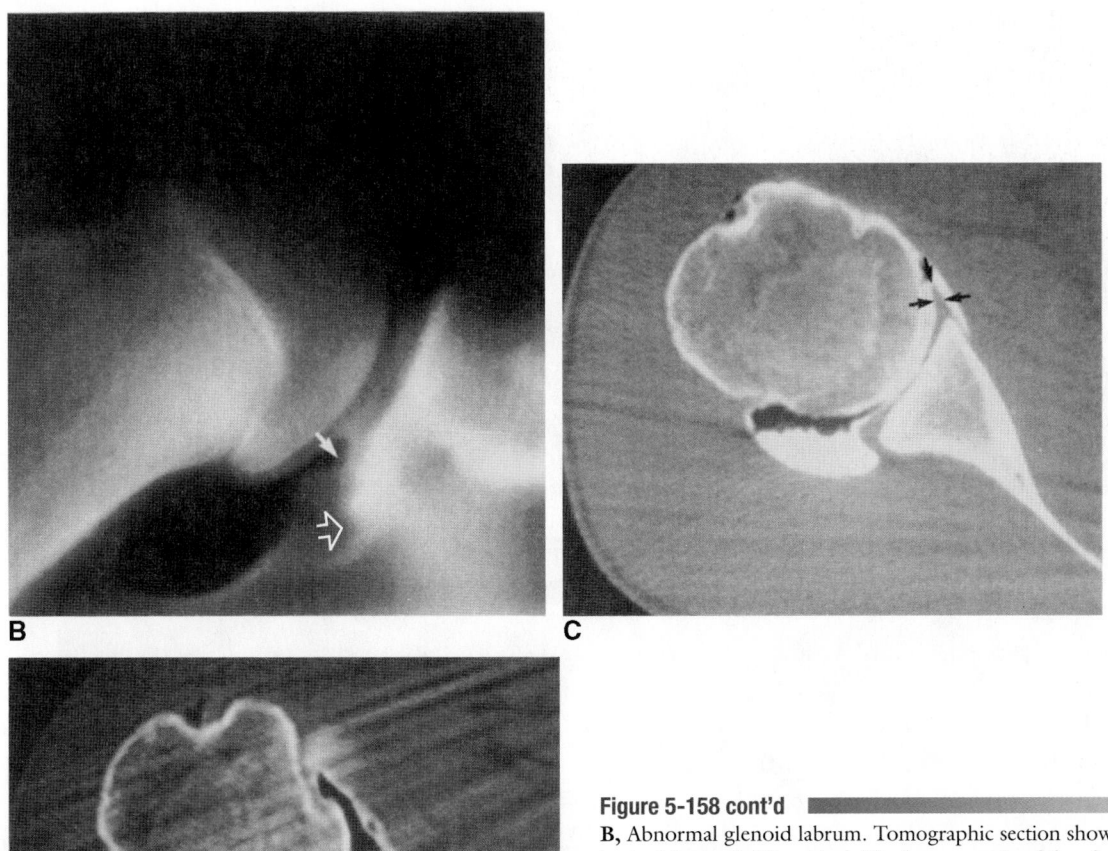

Figure 5-158 cont'd

B, Abnormal glenoid labrum. Tomographic section shows a triangular defect in the labrum *(white arrow)*. The bony margin of the glenoid is also irregular *(open arrow)*. The patient had suffered a single anterior dislocation. **C,** Normal glenoid labrum on computed tomography after double-contrast arthrography. The sharply pointed anterior *(arrows)* and slightly rounder posterior margins of the labrum are visible. **D,** Computed tomoarthrogram shows an absence of the anterior labrum and a loose body *(arrow)* posteriorly. (**B** courtesy of Dr. Ethan Braunstein, Brigham and Women's Hospital, Boston, Massachusetts; **C** and **D,** Courtesy of Dr. Arthur Newberg, Boston, Massachusetts. From Weissman BNW, Sledge CB: *Orthopedic radiology,* p 257, Philadelphia, 1986, WB Saunders.)

Ultrasonography

Diagnostic ultrasound is becoming a more frequently used device in the shoulder. It can be used to measure the acromiohumeral distance,[282] amount of laxity,[283,284] and for rotator cuff tears.[285]

Computed Tomography

Computed tomography, especially when combined with radiopaque dye (**computed tomoarthrogram,** or CTA), is effective in diagnosing bone and soft-tissue anomalies and injuries around the shoulder, including tears of the labrum (Figures 5-158, 5-159, and 5-160) and the rotator cuff.[274,286] This technique helps delineate capsular redundancy, glenoid rim abnormalities, and loose bodies.[269,287–289]

Magnetic Resonance Imaging

Magnetic resonance imaging (MRI) is proving to be useful in diagnosing soft-tissue injuries to the shoulder and has, in fact, become the method of choice for demonstrating soft-tissue abnormalities of the shoulder.[266,290–294] However, it is important that these abnormalities be correlated with clinical findings.[291] It is possible to differentiate bursitis, peritenonitis/tendinosis, muscle strains, especially with injuries to the rotator cuff.[295] It is also useful for differentially diagnosing causes of impingement and instability syndromes. Labral tears, Hill-Sachs lesions, glenoid irregularities, and the state of bone marrow can also be diagnosed in the shoulder with the use of MRI (Figures 5-161 through 5-167).[147,266,269,296–301] Magnetic resonance arthrography has been found to increase the sensitivity to detecting partial thickness tears.[295,302]

Angiography

In the case of thoracic outlet syndromes and other syndromes involving arterial impingement, angiograms are sometimes used to demonstrate blockage of the subclavian artery during certain moves (Figure 5-168).

Figure 5-159

Normal shoulder, computed arthrotomography. Normal anatomy is demonstrated by computed arthrotomographic sections at the level of the bicipital tendon origin **(A)**, the coracoid process **(B)**, the subscapularis tendon, **(C)** and the inferior joint level **(D).** Bt = bicipital tendon; H = humeral head; Co = coracoid process; G = glenoid process; GT = greater tuberosity; LT = lesser tuberosity; SuST = subscapularis tendon; AGL = anterior glenoid labrum; PGL = posterior glenoid labrum. (From De Lee JC, Drez D, editors: *Orthopedic sports medicine: principles and practice*, p. 721, Philadelphia, 1994, WB Saunders.)

Figure 5-160
Computed tomography scan of labral tear *(arrow)*.

Figure 5-161
T1-weighted axial magnetic resonance images from cranial (**A**) to caudal (**C**). D = deltoid muscle; SS = supraspinatus muscle; C = coracoid; H = humerus; SB = subscapularis muscle; G = glenoid of scapula; sdb = subdeltoid-subacromial bursa; IS = infraspinatus muscle; sbt = subscapularis tendon; al = anterior labrum; TM = teres minor muscle; pl = posterior labrum. (From Meyer SJF, Dalinka MK: Magnetic resonance imaging of the shoulder, *Orthop Clin North Am* 21:499, 1990.)

Figure 5-162

Shoulder impingement syndrome: subacromial enthesophyte. Sagittal oblique T1-weighted (TR/TE, 800/20) spin echo MR image shows the enthesophyte *(open arrow)*, which is intimate with the coracoacromial ligament *(solid arrow)* and supraspinatus tendon *(arrowhead)*. (From Resnick D, Kransdorf MJ: *Bone and joint imaging,* p. 375, Philadelphia, 2005, WB Saunders.)

Figure 5-163

Full-thickness rotator cuff tear: MR imaging. In the coronal oblique plane, intermediate-weighted (TR/TE, 2000/20) **(A)** and T2-weighted (TR/TE, 2000/80) **(B)** spin echo MR images show fluid in a gap *(solid arrow)* in the supraspinatus tendon; the fluid is of increased signal intensity in **B.** Also in **B,** note the increased signal intensity related to fluid in the glenohumeral joint *(open arrow)* and subdeltoid bursa *(arrowhead)*. Osteoarthritis of the acromioclavicular joint is evident. **C,** In the same patient, sagittal oblique T2-weighted (TR/TE, 2000/60) spin echo MR images show the site *(arrow)* of disruption of the supraspinatus tendon, which is of high signal intensity. (From Resnick D, Kransdorf MJ: *Bone and joint imaging,* p. 925, Philadelphia, 2005, WB Saunders.)

Figure 5-164

A, T1-weighted coronal image demonstrating mild thickening of the supraspinatus tendon with intermediate signal *(arrow)* present within the substance of the tendon. **B,** T2-weighted coronal image at the same level also demonstrating thickening of the tendon with intermediate signal *(arrow)* within the tendon. The presence of intermediate signal within the tendon is diagnostic of tendinopathy, whereas bright (fluid) signal within the tendon is diagnostic of a tear. **C,** A globular area of low signal abnormality *(arrow)* in the infraspinatus tendon and mild surrounding edema consistent with calcific bursitis. (From Sanders TG, Miller MD: A systematic approach to magnetic resonance imaging interpretation of sports medicine injuries of the shoulder, *Am J Sports Med* 33:1094, 2005.)

Figure 5-165

Rotator cuff tear. Criteria for diagnosing a rotator cuff tear on magnetic resonance (MR) imaging include the presence of fluid in the expected location of the tendon or retraction of the tendon. **A,** MR arthrogram of a partial-thickness articular surface tear of the supraspinatus tendon as contrast *(arrow)* extends into the substance of the tendon but not completely through the thickness of the tendon. **B,** Conventional T2-weighted coronal image. **C,** Sagittal image. Both **(B)** and **(C)** demonstrate fluid signal intensity *(arrows)* extending partially through the thickness of the tendon involving the bursal surface. **D,** An interstitial tear *(arrow)* of the supraspinatus tendon. Fluid signal intensity *(arrow)* is present within the substance of the tendon but does not extend to either the articular or bursal surface of the tendon. **E,** A full-thickness tear with bright fluid signal *(arrow)* extending all the way through the thickness of the tendon from top to bottom. **F,** A complete tear of the supraspinatus tendon extending from front to back, with approximately 3 cm of retraction of the musculotendinous junction *(arrow)*. (From Sanders TG, Miller MD: A systematic approach to magnetic resonance imaging interpretation of sports medicine injuries of the shoulder, *Am J Sports Med* 33:1094, 2005.)

Figure 5-166

Bankart lesions. **A,** Cartilage undermining *(arrows)* the anterior and posterior labrum. The articular cartilage is intermediate in signal intensity and smooth and tapering as it undermines the fibrocartilage of the glenoid labrum. This image should not be confused with a tear, which will be irregular in appearance and usually extends completely beneath the labrum. **B,** Marked irregularity and fraying *(arrow)* of the anteroinferior labrum. **C,** A displaced Bankart lesion *(arrow)*. **D,** T2-weighted coronal image through the level of the anterior labrum demonstrating an irregular fluid collection *(arrow)* located within a tear of the anterior labrum, between the labrum and the glenoid. This irregularity is referred to as the "double axillary pouch" sign and is very for an anterior labral tear. **E,** A minimally displaced Bankart fracture *(arrows)* through the inferior glenoid. **F,** Axial image with intra-articular contrast. **G,** Abduction external rotation image with intra-articular contrast. Both **F** and **G** demonstrate a small collection of contrast *(arrows)* extending partially beneath the anterior labrum, representing a nondisplaced Bankart (Perthes) lesion. **H,** A medialized Bankart lesion *(arrows)*. **I,** T2-weighted axial image through the superior aspect of the humeral head demonstrating a concavity *(arrow)* of the posterosuperior humeral head, representing a Hill-Sachs deformity. The humeral head should be round on the top three images, with no flattening or concavity. (From Sanders TG, Miller MD: A systematic approach to magnetic resonance imaging interpretation of sports medicine injuries of the shoulder, *Am J Sports Med* 33:1097, 2005.)

Figure 5-167

Superior labral anterior posterior (SLAP) tear. **A,** Fraying and irregularity *(arrow)* of the undersurface of the superior labrum, consistent with a SLAP tear. **B,** A linear area of high signal *(arrow)* extending into the substance of the superior labrum. The presence of any high signal within the substance of the superior labrum is diagnostic of a SLAP tear. **C,** Displacement *(arrow)* of the superior labrum away from the glenoid. This image represents a type II SLAP tear. **D,** A bucket-handle tear (type III SLAP tear) of the superior labrum, with the bucket-handle fragment *(arrow)* dangling in the superior joint. **E,** Axial image demonstrating an irregular collection of contrast extending into the biceps anchor consistent with a type IV SLAP tear, with involvement of the biceps anchor. (From Sanders TG, Miller MD: A systematic approach to magnetic resonance imaging interpretation of sports medicine injuries of the shoulder, *Am J Sports Med* 33:1096, 2005.)

A   **B**

Figure 5-168
Angiograms of the subclavian artery with the arm at rest (**A**) and abducted (**B**). Note complete obstruction of the subclavian artery in **B**. (From Brown C: Compressive, invasive referred pain to the shoulder, *Clin Orthop* 173:59, 1983.)

Précis of the Shoulder Assessment*

History (sitting)
Observation (sitting or standing)
Examination
   Active movements (sitting or standing)
      Elevation through forward flexion of the arm
      Elevation through abduction of the arm
      Elevation through the plane of the scapula (scaption)
      Medial rotation of the arm
      Lateral rotation of the arm
      Adduction of the arm
      Horizontal adduction and abduction of the arm
      Circumduction of the arm
   Passive movements (sitting)
      Elevation through abduction of the arm
      Elevation through forward flexion of the arm
      Elevation through abduction at the glenohumeral
         joint only
      Lateral rotation of the arm
      Medial rotation of the arm
      Extension of the arm
      Adduction of the arm
      Horizontal adduction and abduction of the arm
   Special tests (sitting or standing)
      Instability tests
         Load and shift test (anterior and posterior)
         Sulcus sign
         Feagin test
         Posterior apprehension test
      Impingement tests
         Neer test
         Hawkins-Kennedy test
         Posterior internal impingement test
      Labral tears
         Clunk test (Bankart)
         Anterior slide test (Bankart)

         Active compression test of O'Brien (SLAP)
         Biceps tension test (SLAP)
      Scapular stability
         Lateral scapular slide test
         Wall (floor) push up
      Muscle/tendon pathology
         Speed's test (biceps)
         Yergason's test (biceps)
         Empty can test (supraspinatus)
         Lift-off sign (subscapularis)
         Medial rotation "spring back" or lag test (subscapu-
            laris)
         Lateral rotation "spring back" or lag test (infraspina-
            tus/teres minor)
         Serratus anterior weakness
      Thoracic outlet tests
         Roos test
   Reflexes and cutaneous distribution (sitting)
      Reflexes
      Sensory scan
      Peripheral nerves
         Axillary nerve
         Suprascapular nerve
         Musculocutaneous nerve
         Long thoracic nerve
         Spinal accessory nerve
   Palpation (sitting)
   Resisted isometric movements (supine lying)
      Forward flexion of the shoulder
      Extension of the shoulder
      Abduction of the shoulder
      Adduction of the shoulder
      Medial rotation of the shoulder
      Lateral rotation of the shoulder
      Flexion of the elbow

Précis of the Shoulder Assessment*—cont'd

Extension of the elbow
Special tests (supine lying)
    Instability tests
        Crank (apprehension) and relocation tests (anterior)
        Norwood test (posterior)
        Push-pull test (posterior)
    Labral tears
        Clunk test
    Muscle/tendon pathology
        Trapezius weakness—3 positions (prone lying)
        Pectoralis minor tightness (supine lying)
        Pectoralis major tightness (supine lying)
    Neurological tests
        Upper limb tension tests
Joint play movements (supine lying)
    Backward glide of the humerus

Forward glide of the humerus
Lateral distraction of the humerus
Long arm traction
Backward glide of the humerus in abduction
Anteroposterior and cephalocaudal movements of the clavicle at the acromioclavicular joint
Anteroposterior and cephalocaudal movements of the clavicle at the sternoclavicular joint
General movement of the scapula to determine mobility
Diagnostic imaging

*The précis is shown in an order that limits the amount of movement that the patient has to do but ensures that all necessary structures are tested. After any examination, the patient should be warned of the possibility that symptoms may exacerbate as a result of the assessment.

Case Studies

When doing these case studies, the examiner should list the appropriate questions to ask the patient and should specify why they are being asked, what to look for and why, what things should be tested, and why. Depending on the patient's answers (and the examiner should consider numerous responses), several possible causes of the patient's problem may become evident (examples are given in parentheses). The examiner should prepare a differential diagnosis chart. He or she can then decide how different diagnoses may affect the treatment plan. For example, a 23-year-old man comes to the clinic complaining of shoulder pain. He says that 2 days earlier he was playing touch football. When his friend threw the ball, he reached for it, lost his balance, and fell on the tip of his shoulder but managed to hang onto the ball. How would you differentiate between acromioclavicular sprain and supraspinatus tendinitis? Table 5-16 demonstrates a differential diagnosis chart for the two conditions.

1. A 47-year-old man comes to you complaining of pain in the left shoulder. There is no history of overuse activity. The pain that occurs when he elevates his shoulder is referred to his neck and sometimes down the arm to his wrist. Describe your assessment plan for this patient (cervical spondylosis versus subacromial bursitis).

2. An 18-year-old woman recently had a Putti-Platt procedure for a recurring dislocation of the left shoulder. When you see her, her arm is still in a sling, but the surgeon wants you to begin treatment. Describe your assessment for this patient.

3. A 68-year-old woman comes to you complaining of pain and restricted ROM in the right shoulder. She tells you that 3 months earlier she slipped on a rug on a tile floor and landed on her elbow. Both her elbow and shoulder hurt at that time. Describe your assessment plan for this patient (olecranon bursitis versus adhesive capsulitis).

4. Parents bring their 5-year-old son in to see you. They state that he was running around the recreation room chasing a friend when he tripped over a stool and landed on his shoulder. He refuses to move his arm and is crying because the accident occurred only 2 hours earlier. Describe your assessment plan for this patient (clavicular fracture versus humeral epiphyseal injury).

5. A 35-year-old female master swimmer comes to you complaining of shoulder pain. She states she has been swimming approximately 2000 m per day in two training sessions; she recently increased her swimming from 1500 m per day to get ready for a competition in 3 weeks. Describe your assessment plan for this patient (subacromial bursitis versus biceps tendinitis).

6. A 20-year-old male tennis player comes to you complaining that when he serves the ball, his arm "goes dead." He has had this problem for 3 weeks but never before. He has increased his training during the past month. Describe your assessment plan for this patient (thoracic outlet syndrome versus brachial plexus lesion).

Continued

Case Studies–cont'd

7. A 15-year-old female competitive swimmer comes to you complaining of diffuse shoulder pain. She notices the problem most when she does the backstroke. She complains that her shoulder sometimes feels unstable when doing this stroke. Describe your assessment plan for this patient (anterior instability versus supraspinatus tendinitis).

8. A 48-year-old man comes to you complaining of neck and shoulder pain. He states that he has difficulty abducting his right arm. There is no history of trauma, but he remembers being in a car accident 10 years earlier. Describe your assessment plan for this patient (cervical spondylosis versus adhesive capsulitis).

Table 5-16

Differential Diagnosis of Acromioclavicular Joint Sprain and Supraspinatus Paratenonitis

	Acromioclavicular Joint Sprain	Supraspinatus Paratenonitis
Observation	Step deformity (third-degree)	Normal
Active movement	Pain especially at extreme of motion (horizontal adduction and full elevation especially painful)	Pain on active movement, especially of abduction
Passive movement	Pain on horizontal adduction and elevation Muscle spasm end feel at end of ROM possible	No pain except if impingement occurs
Resisted isometric movement	May have some pain if test causes stress on joint (e.g., abduction)	Pain on abduction May have some pain on stabilizing for other movements
Functional tests	Pain on extremes of movement	Pain on any abduction movement
Special tests	Acromioclavicular shear test painful	Empty can test positive Impingement tests positive
Reflexes and cutaneous distribution	Negative	Negative
Joint play	Acromioclavicular joint play movements painful	Negative
Palpation	Acromioclavicular joint painful	Supraspinatus tendon and insertion tender or painful

ROM = range of motion.

References

To enhance this text and add value for the reader, all references have been incorporated into a CD-ROM that is provided with this text. The reader can view the reference source and access it online whenever possible. There are a total of 331 cited and other general references for this chapter.

APPENDIX 5-1

RELIABILITY, VALIDITY, SPECIFICITY, AND SENSITIVITY OF SPECIAL/DIAGNOSTIC TESTS USED IN THE SHOULDER

AC RESISTED EXTENSION TEST

Specificity	Sensitivity	Odds Ratio
• Chronic acromioclavicular lesions 85%[303]	• Chronic acromioclavicular lesions 72%[303]	• Positive likelihood ratio 4.8, negative likelihood ratio 0.33

ACTIVE COMPRESSION TEST OF O'BRIEN

Specificity	Sensitivity	Odds Ratio
• For SLAP 47%, for any labral lesion including SLAP 73%[304] • For labral tear 31%[305] • Labral abnormality 98.5%, acromioclavicular joint abnormality 96.6%[187] • Unstable superior labral anterior posterior lesions 11.1%[180] • For labral tear 55%[306] • Chronic acromioclavicular lesions 95%[303]	• For SLAP 54%, for any labral lesion including SLAP 63%[304] • For labral tear 54%[305] • Labral abnormality 100%, acromioclavicular joint abnormality 100%[187] • Unstable superior labral anterior posterior lesions 77.8%[179] • For labral tear 47%[306] • Chronic acromioclavicular lesions 72%[303]	• Positive likelihood ratio for SLAP 1.02, any labral lesion 2.33; negative likelihood ratio for SLAP 0.98, any labral lesion 0.51 • Positive likelihood ratio 0.78, negative likelihood ratio 1.48 • Positive likelihood ratio for labral abnormality 66.66, acromioclavicular joint abnormality 0 • Positive likelihood ratio 0.87, negative likelihood ratio 1.90 • Positive likelihood ratio 1.04, negative likelihood ratio 0.96 • Positive likelihood ratio 14.4, negative likelihood ratio 0.29

AMERICAN SHOULDER AND ELBOW SURGEONS STANDARDIZED ASSESSMENT FORM (ASES)

Reliability	Validity	Specificity	Sensitivity	Responsiveness	Odds Ratio
• Total ICC = 0.84, pain ICC = 0.79, function ICC = 0.82[307] ICC = 0.96[308] • Test-retest overall ICC = 0.94[309]	• Internal consistency cronbach's alpha 0.86, convergent validity of ASES with (Penn score r = 0.78, SF-36 physical function score r = 0.41, SF-36 role physical score r = 0.33, SF-36 physical component summary r = 0.40) divergent validity SF-36 role emotional score r = 0.24, SF-36 mental health score r = 0.05, SF-36 mental component r = 0.15, discriminant validity higher scores of the ASES in patients with score "gotten much better" than those who had "gotten slightly better" p < 0.001 and between rating of the physiotherapist of the functional limitation of the patient p < 0.001[307]	• 75%[307]	• 91%[307]	• Total SRM = 1.54 effect size = 1.39, pain SRM = 1.08 effect size = 1.07, function SRM = 1.34 effect size = 1.24[307] • Shoulder instability effective size = 0.86, SRM = 0.93, rotator cuff disease effect size = 1.33, SRM 1.16, glenohumeral arthritis effect size = 1.74, SRM 1.11[309]	• Positive likelihood ratio 3.64, negative likelihood ratio 0.12

Continued

APPENDIX 5-1—cont'd

AMERICAN SHOULDER AND ELBOW SURGEONS STANDARDIZED ASSESSMENT FORM (ASES)—cont'd

Reliability	Validity	Specificity	Sensitivity	Responsiveness	Odds Ratio
	• Cronbach alpha for shoulder instability 0.61, rotator cuff disease 0.64, glenohumeral arthritis 0.62[309] • Content validity showed minimum floor and ceiling effects[309] • Criterion validity correlation with physical functioning $r = 0.57$ (p <0 .001), role physical activity $r = 0.32$ (p = 0.002), bodily pain $r = 0.58$ (p < 0.001), role emotional $r = -0.09$ (p = 0.49), mental health $r = -0.08$ (p = 0.67), vitality $r = 0.11$ (p = 0.27), social function $r = 0.10$ (p = 0.34)[309] • Construct validity: 23 hypotheses were constructed by consensus and showed to be true and significant (p < 0.05)[309]				

ANTERIOR APPREHENSION TEST

Specificity	Sensitivity	Odds Ratio
• For SLAP 63%, for any labral lesion including SLAP 87%[304]	• For SLAP 30%, for any labral lesion including SLAP 40%[304]	• Positive likelihood ratio for SLAP 0.81, for any labral lesion 3.08; negative likelihood ratio for SLAP 1.11, for any labral lesion 0.69

ANTERIOR RELEASE TEST

Reliability	Validity	Specificity	Sensitivity	Odds Ratio
• Interrater for pain ICC = 0.31, apprehension ICC = 0.63, pain or apprehension ICC = 0.45[310]	• Accuracy: 90.2%[311]	• 88.9%[311]	• 91.9%[311]	• Positive likelihood ratio 8.28, negative likelihood ratio 0.01

ANTERIOR SLIDE TEST

Specificity	Sensitivity	Odds Ratio
• Superior glenoid labral tear 91.5%[184] • Labral tear 84%[306]	• Superior glenoid labral tear 78.4%[184] • Labral tear 8%[306]	• Positive likelihood ratio 9.22, negative likelihood ratio 0.24 • Positive likelihood ratio 0.5, negative likelihood ratio 1.09

APPREHENSION (CRANK) TEST

Reliability	Specificity	Sensitivity	Odds Ratio
• Intrarater for amount of external rotation ICC = 0.95[312] • Interrater for: pain ICC = 0.31, apprehension ICC = 0.47, pain or apprehension ICC = 0.44[310]	• 98.91%[312]	• 52.78%[312]	• Positive likelihood ratio 48.42, negative likelihood ratio 0.48

AUGMENTATION TEST

Reliability

• Interrater for pain ICC 0.09, apprehension ICC = 0.48, pain or apprehension ICC = 0.33[310]

BICEPS LOAD TEST II FOR SLAP LESIONS

Specificity	Sensitivity	Odds Ratio
• 96.6%[313]	• 89.7[313]	• Positive likelihood ratio 26.38, negative likelihood ratio 0.11

COMBINATION FOR SLAP AND LABRAL LESIONS

Test	Reliability	Specificity	Sensitivity
• Jobe and O'Brien	• For any labral lesion including SLAP 91%[304]	• For any labral lesion including SLAP 41%[304]	• Positive likelihood ratio 4.55, negative likelihood ratio 0.65[304]
• Jobe and Apprehension	• For any labral lesion including SLAP 93%[304]	• For any labral lesion including SLAP 38%[304]	• Positive likelihood ratio 5.43, negative likelihood ratio 0.67[304]
• O'Brien and Apprehension	• For any labral lesion including SLAP 82%[304]	• For any labral lesion including SLAP 38%[304]	• Positive likelihood ratio 2.11, negative likelihood ratio 0.76[304]
• Jobe and O'Brien and Apprehension	• For any labral lesion including SLAP 91%[304]	• For any labral lesion including SLAP 34%[304]	• Positive likelihood ratio 3.78, negative likelihood ratio 0.72[304]
• Jobe or O'Brien	• For any labral lesion including SLAP 73%[304]	• For any labral lesion including SLAP 72%[304]	• Positive likelihood ratio 2.67, negative likelihood ratio 0.38[304]
• Jobe or Apprehension	• For any labral lesion including SLAP 80%[304]	• For any labral lesion including SLAP 47%[304]	• Positive likelihood ratio 2.35, negative likelihood ratio 0.66[304]
• O'Brien or Apprehension	• For any labral lesion including SLAP 73%[304]	• For any labral lesion including SLAP 72%[304]	• Positive likelihood ratio 2.67, negative likelihood ratio 0.38[304]
• Jobe or O'Brien or Apprehension	• For any labral lesion including SLAP 73%[304]	• For any labral lesion including SLAP 72%[304]	• Positive likelihood ratio 2.67, negative likelihood ratio 0.38[304]
• MRI and Crank	• For any labral lesion including SLAP 67%[304]	• For any labral lesion including SLAP 43%[304]	• Positive likelihood ratio 1.30, negative likelihood ratio 0.85[304]
• MRI and O'Brien	• For any labral lesion including SLAP 82%[304]	• For any labral lesion including SLAP 50%[304]	• Positive likelihood ratio 2.78, negative likelihood ratio 0.61[304]

COMPRESSION ROTATION TEST

Specificity	Sensitivity	Odds Ratio
• For labral tear 76%[306]	• For labral tear 24%[306]	• Positive likelihood ratio 1, negative likelihood ratio 1

Continued

APPENDIX 5-1—cont'd

CRANK TEST

Specificity	Sensitivity	Odds Ratio
• For labral tear 100%[192] • For SLAP 67%, for any labral lesion including SLAP 73%[304] • For labral tear 93%[191] • For labral tear 56%[305] • Unstable superior labral anterior posterior lesions 70%[180]	• For labral tear 83%[192] • For SLAP 39%, for any labral lesion including SLAP 40%[304] • For labral tear 91%[19] • For labral tear 46%[305] • Unstable superior labral anterior posterior lesions 34.6%[180]	• Positive likelihood ratio for SLAP 1.05, for any labral lesion 1.48; negative likelihood ratio for SLAP 0.91, for any labral lesion 0.82 • Positive likelihood ratio 13, negative likelihood ratio 0.10 • Positive likelihood ratio 1.04, negative likelihood ratio 0.96 • Positive likelihood ratio 1.15, negative likelihood ratio 0.93

CROSS BODY ADDUCTION TEST

Specificity	Sensitivity	Odds Ratio
• Tendinitis and bursitis 79.7%, partial tear 78.5%, full tear 80.8%, overall 82%[159] • Chronic acromioclavicular lesions 79%[303]	• Tendinitis and bursitis 25.4%, partial tear 16.7%, full tear 23.4%, overall 22.5%[159] • Chronic acromioclavicular lesions 77%[303]	• Positive likelihood ratio for tendinitis and bursitis 1.25, partial tear 0.78, full tear 1.22, overall 1.25; negative likelihood ratio for tendinitis and bursitis 0.94, partial tear 1.06, full tear 0.95, overall 0.95 • Positive likelihood ratio 3.67, negative likelihood ratio 0.29

DASH, DISABILITY OF THE ARM, SHOULDER, AND HEAD

Reliability	Validity	Responsiveness
• Test-retest ICC = 0.96 SEM = 4.6[314]	• Construct validity: people still working had less disability $p < 0.0001$, less disability in those who could do all they wanted $p < 0.0001$[314] • Concurrent validity with shoulder pain and disability index (pain) $r = 0.82$, (function) $r = 0.88$, Brigham questionnaire (symptoms) $r = 0.71$, (function) $r = 0.89$, pain severity $r = 0.72$, overall rating of problem $r = 0.71$, ability to function $r = 0.79$, ability to work $r = 0.76$[314] • Subjects with workers compensation benefits scored worse $p = 0.0047$[315]	• For observed change SRM = 0.78 effect size 0.59, rating problem as better SRM = 1.06 effect size 0.75, rating function as better SRM = 1.20 effect size 0.84[314]

DEPALMA'S CLASSIFICATION OF SHOULDER CALCIFIC TENDINITIS

Reliability
• Interrater k = 0.234, intrarater 0.332 < k < 0.57[316]

DROP ARM TEST

Specificity	Sensitivity	Odds Ratio
• 97.2%[317] • Tendinitis and bursitis 77.3%, partial tear 77.5%, full tear 87.5%, overall 26.9%[159] • Chronic acromioclavicular lesions 72%[303]	• 7.8%[317] • Tendinitis and bursitis 13.6%, partial tear 14.3%, full tear 34.9%, overall 88.4%[159] • Chronic acromioclavicular lesions 35%[303]	• Positive likelihood ratio 2.78, negative likelihood ratio 0.95 • Positive likelihood ratio for tendinitis and bursitis 0.60, partial tear 0.63, full tear 2.79, overall 1.21; negative likelihood ratio for tendinitis and bursitis 1.12, partial tear 1.10, full tear 0.74, overall 0.43 • Positive likelihood ratio 1.25, negative likelihood ratio 0.90

END FEEL OF SHOULDER EXTERNAL ROTATION

Reliability

• Intrarater k = 0.90, interrater k = 0.83[318]

END FEEL OF SHOULDER FULL ABDUCTION

Reliability

• Intrarater k = 0.86, interrater k = 0.44[318]

END FEEL OF SHOULDER GLENOHUMERAL ABDUCTION

Reliability

• Intrarater k = 0.63, interrater k = 0.1[318]

END FEEL OF SHOULDER HORIZONTAL ABDUCTION

Reliability

• Intrarater k = 1, interrater k = 0.75[318]

END FEEL OF SHOULDER INTERNAL ROTATION

Reliability

• Intrarater k = 0.89, interrater k = 0.43[318]

GROWER SIGN

Reliability

• k = 0[319]

HAWKINS TEST

Specificity	Sensitivity	Odds Ratio
• 25%[317] • Tendinitis and bursitis 44.5%, partial tear 44.4%, full tear 48.3%, overall 66.3%[158] • Chronic acromioclavicular lesions 45%[297] • Bursitis 44.3%, rotator cuff pathosis 42.6%, overall 60%[320]	• 92%[317] • Tendinitis and bursitis 75.5%, partial tear 75.4%, full tear 68.7%, overall 71.5%[158] • Chronic acromioclavicular lesions 47%[297] • Bursitis 91.7%, rotator cuff pathosis 87.5%, overall 88.9%[320]	• Positive likelihood ratio 1.23, negative likelihood ratio 0.32 • Positive likelihood ratio for tendinitis and bursitis 1.36, partial tear 1.36, full tear 1.33, overall 2.12; negative likelihood ratio for tendinitis and bursitis 0.55, partial tear 0.55, full tear 0.65, overall 0.43 • Positive likelihood ratio 0.85, negative likelihood ratio 1.78 • Positive likelihood ratio for bursitis 1.65, rotator cuff pathosis 1.52, overall 2.22; negative likelihood ratio for bursitis 0.19, rotator cuff pathosis 0.29, overall 0.18

Continued

APPENDIX 5-1—cont'd

HORIZONTAL ABDUCTION

Specificity	Sensitivity	Odds Ratio
• 27.7%[317]	• 82%[317]	• Positive likelihood ratio 1.13, negative likelihood ratio 0.65

INFRASPINATUS MUSCLE TEST

Specificity	Sensitivity	Odds Ratio
• Tendinitis and bursitis 68.9%, partial tear 69.1%, full tear 84%, overall 90.1%[159]	• Tendinitis and bursitis 25%, partial tear 19.4%, full tear 50.5%, overall 41.6%[159]	• Positive likelihood ratio for tendinitis and bursitis 0.80, partial tear 0.63, full tear 3.16, overall 4.20; negative likelihood ratio for tendinitis and bursitis 1.09, partial tear 1.17, full tear 0.59, overall 0.65

INSTABILITY CATCH

Reliability
• k = 0.25[319]

INTERNAL ROTATION RESISTANCE STRENGTH TEST/KIM TEST

Reliability	Specificity	Sensitivity	Odds Ratio
• k = 0.85[321] • Interrater reliability 0.91[148]	• 96%[321] • Labral lesion 94%[148]	• 88%[321] • Labral lesion 80%[148]	• Positive likelihood ratio 22, negative likelihood ratio 0.12 • Positive likelihood ratio 13.33, negative likelihood ratio 0.21

JERK TEST

Specificity	Sensitivity	Odds Ratio
• Labral lesion 98%[148]	• Labral lesion 73%[148]	• Positive likelihood ratio 36.5, negative likelihood ratio 0.27

LAG TEST

Validity	Specificity	Sensitivity
• A lag of 10 to 15 degrees was observed in all patients with complete rupture of the supraspinatus and infraspinatus, and 15 of 16 patients with infra, supra, and subscapularis[220]	• Internal rotation lag sign is as specific as lift off test $p = 1$, external rotation lag sign is as specific as the drop test and both are more specific than jobe test $p = 0.002$[220]	• Internal rotation lag sign more sensitive as lift off test $p = 0.002$, external rotation lag sign is more sensitive as the drop test $p < 0.001$ and less sensitive as the jobe test $p = 0.05$[220]

LATERAL SCAPULAR SLIDE TEST

Reliability	Specificity	Sensitivity	Odds Ratio
• Intrarater ICC = 0.75 SEM = 0.61 for subjects without shoulder impairments, ICC = 0.52 SEM = 0.78 for subjects with shoulder impairments[195]	• Bilateral difference greater than 1 cm position 1 = 48%, position 2 = 54%, position 3 = 56%; differences greater than 1.5 cm position 1 = 53%, position 2 = 58%, position 3 = 52%[195] • Equal or greater than 1.5 cm difference between right and left side with arm beside the boy 54.9%, with hand on the waist 57.7%, with arms abducted 90 degrees and internally rotated 35.2%, overall 26.7%[322]	• Bilateral difference greater than 1 cm position 1 = 35%, position 2 = 41%, position 3 = 43%; differences greater than 1.5 cm position 1 = 28%, position 2 = 50%, position 3 = 34%[195]	• Positive likelihood ratio for bilateral difference greater than 1 cm position 1 = 67%, position 2 = 0.89, position 3 = 0.98; differences greater than 1.5 cm position 1 = 0.59, position 2 = 1.19, position 3 = 0.71; negative likelihood ratio for bilateral difference greater than 1 cm position 1 = 1.35, position 2 = 1.09, position 3 = 1.02; differences greater than 1.5 cm position 1 = 1.36, position 2 = 0.86, position 3 = 1.27

LENNIE TEST

Reliability	Validity
• Interrater distance from: midline ICC > 0.66, angular position ICC > 0.64, scapular symmetry ICC = 0.74[37]	• Correlation with landmarks and radiographic measurements distance from: midline r > 0.69, angular position r > 0.43, scapular symmetry r = 0.62[37]

LOAD AND SHIFT TEST

Reliability

• Intrarater between grades of commitment: all grades k = 0.342, between grades I and II+ k = 0.529; interrater for all grades k = 0.091, between grades I and II k = 0.208 (when analyzing only grades I and II the end feel is excluded)
• Intrarater anterior ICC = 0.72, posterior ICC = 0.42, inferior ICC = 0.65, sulcus ICC = 0.60[310]
• Test-retest for dynamometer measurement r = 0.996[323]
• Test-retest with KT1000, dominant side ICC = 0.67, nondominant ICC = 0.76[324]

MR ARTHROGRAPHY FOR SLAP LESIONS

Reliability	Specificity	Sensitivity	Odds Ratio
• Interrater k = 0.77[325]	• 78%[325]	• 89%[325]	• Positive likelihood ratio 4.04, negative likelihood ratio 0.14

MRI FOR LABRAL TEAR

Specificity	Sensitivity	Odds Ratio
• 92%[305]	• 42%[305]	• Positive likelihood ratio 5.25, negative likelihood ratio 0.63

MRI FOR ROTATOR CUFF TEAR

Specificity	Sensitivity	Odds Ratio
• Complete and partial tear together 67%, partial tear 68%[326]	• Complete and partial tear together 100%, partial tear 100%[326]	• Positive likelihood ratio for complete and partial tear together 4.35, partial tear 3.12; negative likelihood ratio for complete and partial tear together 0, partial tear 0

Continued

APPENDIX 5-1—cont'd

NEER IMPINGEMENT TEST

Specificity	Sensitivity	Odds Ratio
• 30.5%[317] • Tendinitis and bursitis 49.2%, partial tear 47.5%, full tear 47.2%, overall 68.7%[159] • Chronic acromioclavicular lesions 41%[303] • Bursitis 47.5%, rotator cuff pathosis 50.8%, overall 62.5%[320]	• 88.7%[317] • Tendinitis and bursitis 85.7%, partial tear 75.4%, full tear 59.32%, overall 68%[159] • Chronic acromioclavicular lesions 57%[303] • Bursitis 75%, rotator cuff pathosis 83.3%, overall 77%[320]	• Positive likelihood ratio 1.27, negative likelihood ratio 0.37 • Positive likelihood ratio for tendinitis and bursitis 1.69, partial tear 1.44, full tear 1.12, overall 2.17; negative likelihood ratio for tendinitis and bursitis 0.29, partial tear 0.52, full tear 0.86, overall 0.46 • Positive likelihood ratio 0.96, negative likelihood ratio 1.05 • Positive likelihood ratio for bursitis 1.43, rotator cuff pathosis 1.69, overall 2.05; negative likelihood ratio for bursitis 0.53, rotator cuff pathosis 0.33, overall 0.37

PAINFUL ARC TEST

Reliability	Specificity	Sensitivity	Odds Ratio
• In flexion k = 0.69, on return from flexion k = 0.61[319]	• 80.5%[317] • 9.9%[327] • Tendinitis and bursitis 46.9%, partial tear 47%, full tear 61.8%, overall 81.1%[159] • Chronic acromioclavicular lesions 47%[303]	• 32.5%[317] • 97.5%[327] • Tendinitis and bursitis 70.6%, partial tear 67.4%, full tear 75.8%, overall 73.5%[159] • Chronic acromioclavicular lesions 50%[303]	• Positive likelihood ratio 1.67, negative likelihood ratio 0.84 • Positive likelihood ratio 1.08, negative likelihood ratio 0.25 • Positive likelihood ratio for tendinitis and bursitis 1.33, partial tear 1.27, full tear 1.98, overall 3.98; negative likelihood ratio for tendinitis and bursitis 0.63, partial tear 0.69, full tear 0.39, overall 0.33 • Positive likelihood ratio 0.94, negative likelihood ratio 1.06

PENN SHOULDER SCORE

Reliability	Validity	Responsiveness
• Test-retest overall ICC = 0.94, pain subscale ICC = 0.88 SEM = 3.8, satisfaction subscale ICC = 0.93 SEM = 1.3, function subscale ICC-0.93 SEM = 6.1[101]	• Cronbach alpha = 0.93, correlation with constant shoulder score r = 0.85, American Shoulder and Elbow Surgeons Shoulder Score = 0.87, correlation of each item with total score: pain r = 0.80, satisfaction r = 0.44, function r = 0.95[101]	• Effect size for overall score 1.01 SRM = 1.27, pain subscale 0.85 SRM = 0.95, satisfaction 1.19 SRM = 1.15, function 0.80 SRM = 1.09[101]

POSTERIOR SHEAR TEST

Reliability
• k = 0.35[319]

PRONE INSTABILITY TEST

Reliability
• k = 0.87[319]

RELOCATION, FOWLER, OR JOBE RELOCATION TEST

Reliability	Specificity	Sensitivity	Odds Ratio
• Intrarater for amount of external rotation ICC = 0.89[312] • Interrater for: pain ICC = 0.31, apprehension ICC = 0.71, pain or apprehension ICC = 0.44[310]	• 54.35%[312] • For SLAP 63%, for any labral lesion including SLAP 87%[304]	• 45.83%[312] • For SLAP 36%, for any labral lesion including SLAP 44%[304]	• Positive likelihood ratio 1, negative likelihood ratio 0.99 • Positive likelihood ratio for SLAP 0.97, for any labral lesion 3.38; negative likelihood ratio SLAP 1.01, for any labral lesion 0.64

RESISTED SUPINATION EXTERNAL ROTATION TEST

Specificity	Sensitivity	Odds Ratio
• Unstable superior labral anterior posterior lesions 81.8%[180]	• Unstable superior labral anterior posterior lesions 82.8%[180]	• Positive likelihood ratio 4.55, negative likelihood ratio 0.21

SHOULDER PAIN AND DISABILITY INDEX

Reliability
• ICC = 0.91[308]

SHOULDER SEVERITY INDEX

Reliability
• ICC = 0.97[308]

SIMPLE SHOULDER TEST

Reliability	Validity
• ICC = 0.99[308]	• Patients in work compensation performed worse on the test p = 0.0034[315]

SPEED'S TEST (BICEPS OR STRAIGHT-ARM TEST)

Validity	Specificity	Sensitivity	Odds Ratio
• Accuracy 56% (arthroscopy)[328]	• 55.5%[317] • 75% (arthroscopy as gold for biceps and SLAP)[328] • For SLAP 74%, for any labral lesion including SLAP 87%[304] • Tendinitis and bursitis 69.8%, partial tear 70.6%, full tear 75.3%, overall 83.3%[159] • Chronic acromioclavicular lesions 71%[303]	• 68.5%[317] • 44% (arthroscopy as gold for biceps and SLAP)[328] • For SLAP 9%, for any labral lesion including SLAP 18%[304] • Tendinitis and bursitis 33.3%, partial tear 33.3%, full tear 39.9%, overall 38.3%[159] • Chronic acromioclavicular lesions 24%[303]	• Positive likelihood ratio 1.54, negative likelihood ratio 0.57 • Positive likelihood ratio 1.76, negative likelihood ratio 0.75 • Positive likelihood ratio for SLAP 0.35, any labral lesion 1.38; negative likelihood ratio for SLAP 1.23, any labral lesion 0.94 • Positive likelihood ratio for tendinitis and bursitis 1.10, partial tear 1.13, full tear 1.61, overall 2.29; negative likelihood ratio for tendinitis and bursitis 0.95, partial tear 0.94, full tear 0.80, overall 0.74 • Positive likelihood ratio 0.83, negative likelihood ratio 1.07

SUBJECTIVE SHOULDER RATING SCALE

Reliability
• ICC = 0.71[308]

Continued

APPENDIX 5-1—cont'd

SUPRASPINATUS (EMPTY CAN OR JOBE) TEST

Reliability	Specificity	Sensitivity	Odds Ratio
• Measuring rotator cuff pathology - interrater k = 0.43[329]	• Partial thickness tears of the supraspinatus 54%, full thickness tear 70%, large and massive full thickness tears 70%[329] • Tendinitis and bursitis 6.9%, partial tear 67.8%, full tear 82.4%, overall 89.5%[159]	• Partial thickness tears of the supraspinatus 62%, full thickness tear 41%, large and massive full thickness tears 88%[329] • Tendinitis and bursitis 25%, partial tear 32.1%, full tear 52.6%, overall 44.1%[159]	• Positive likelihood ratio for partial thickness tears of the supraspinatus 1.35, full thickness tear 1.36, large and massive full thickness tears 2.93; negative likelihood ratio for partial thickness tears of the supraspinatus 0.70, full thickness tear 0.84, large and massive full thickness tears 0.17 • Positive likelihood ratio for tendinitis and bursitis 0.27, partial tear 1, full tear 2.99, overall 4.2; negative likelihood ratio for tendinitis and bursitis 10.87, partial tear 1, full tear 0.57, overall 0.62

SURPRISE TEST (ANTERIOR INSTABILITY)

Specificity	Sensitivity	Odds Ratio
• 98.91%[312]	• 63.89%[312]	• Positive likelihood ratio 58.61, negative likelihood ratio 0.36

ULTRASONOGRAPHY FOR ROTATOR CUFF TEAR

Specificity	Sensitivity	Odds Ratio
• Complete and partial tear together 67%, partial tear 80%[326]	• Complete and partial tear together 97%, partial tear 98%[326]	• Positive likelihood ratio for complete and partial tear together 2.94, partial tear 4.9; negative likelihood ratio for complete and partial tear together 0.04, partial tear 0.02

UPPER LIMB TENSION (BRACHIAL PLEXUS TENSION) TEST

Reliability

• Medial nerve: intrarater ICC > 0.88 SEM < 2.41, interrater ICC = 0.33 SEM = 6.35[330]

YERGASON'S TEST

Validity	Specificity	Sensitivity	Odds Ratio
• Accuracy 63%[328] EMG showed that the activity of the upper and lower subscapularis was significantly higher than the other muscles (p > 0.05)[331] • EMG showed that the subscapularis had a mean activation greater than 50% MMT; using a denervation anesthetic technique and a group of patients with detached subscapularis, they had the same EMG patter but were unable to perform the maximum internal rotation test (elevating the dorsum of the hand from the posterior-inferior border of the scapula)[221]	• 79% (arthroscopy for biceps and SLAP)[328] • For SLAP 96%, for any labral lesion including SLAP 93%[304]	• 37%[317] • 43% (arthroscopy for labral biceps and SLAP)[328] • For SLAP 12%, for any labral lesion including SLAP 9%[304]	• Positive likelihood ratio 2.05, negative likelihood ratio 0.72 • Positive likelihood ratio for SLAP 3, any labral lesion 1.28; negative likelihood ratio for SLAP 0.92, any labral lesion 0.98

ELBOW

The elbow's primary role in the upper limb complex is to help an individual position his or her hand in the appropriate location to perform its function. Once the shoulder has positioned the hand in a gross fashion, the elbow allows for adjustments in height and length of the limb, allowing one to position the hand correctly. In addition, the forearm rotates, in part at the elbow, to place the hand in the most effective position to perform its function.

Applied Anatomy

The elbow consists of a complex set of joints that require careful assessment for proper treatment. The treatment must be geared to the pathology of the condition, because the joint responds poorly to trauma, harsh treatment, or incorrect treatment.

Because they are closely related, the joints of the elbow complex make up a compound synovial joint, with injury to any one part affecting the other components as well (Figure 6-1). The elbow articulations are made up of the ulnohumeral joint and the radiohumeral joint. In addition, the complexity and intricate relation of the elbow articulations are further increased by the superior radioulnar joint, which has continuity with the elbow articulations. These three joints make up the **cubital** articulations. The capsule and joint cavity are continuous for all three joints. The combination of these joints allows two degrees of freedom at the elbow. The trochlear joint allows one degree of freedom (flexion-extension), and the radiohumeral and superior radioulnar joints allow the other degree of freedom (rotation).

The **ulnohumeral** or **trochlear joint** (see Figure 6-1) is found between the trochlea of the humerus and the trochlear notch of the ulna and is classified as a uniaxial hinge joint. The bones of this joint are shaped so that the axis of movement is not horizontal but instead passes downward and medially, going through an arc of movement. This position leads to the carrying angle at the elbow (Figure 6-2). The resting position of this joint is with the elbow flexed to 70° and the forearm supinated 10°. The neutral position (0°) is midway between supination and pronation in the thumb-up position (Figure 6-3). The capsular pattern is flexion more limited than extension, and the close packed position is extension with the forearm in supination. On full extension, the medial part of the olecranon process is not in contact with the trochlea; on full flexion, the lateral part of the olecranon process is not in contact with the trochlea. This change allows the side-to-side joint play movement necessary for supination and pronation. A small amount of rotation occurs at this joint. In early flexion, 5° of medial rotation occurs; in late flexion, 5° of lateral rotation occurs.

Ulnohumeral (Trochlear) Joint	
Resting position:	70° elbow flexion, 10° supination
Close packed position:	Extension with supination
Capsular pattern:	Flexion, extension

The **radiohumeral joint** is a uniaxial hinge joint between the capitulum of the humerus and the head of the radius (see Figure 6-1). The resting position is with the elbow fully extended and the forearm fully supinated. The close packed position of the joint is with the elbow flexed to 90° and the forearm supinated 5°. As with the trochlear joint, the capsular pattern is flexion more limited than extension.

361

Figure 6-1

Anterior view of the right elbow disarticulated to expose the ulnohumeral and radiohumeral joints. The margin of the proximal radioulnar joint is shown within the elbow's capsule.

Radiohumeral Joint

Resting position:	Full extension and full supination
Close packed position:	Elbow flexed to 90°, forearm supinated to 5°
Capsular pattern:	Flexion, extension, supination, pronation

The ulnohumeral and radiohumeral joints are supported medially by the **ulnar collateral ligament,** a fan-shaped structure, and laterally by the **radial collateral ligament,** a cordlike structure (Figure 6-4).[1] These ligaments, along with the ulnohumeral articulation, are the primary restraints to instability in the elbow.[2] The lateral (radial) collateral ligament is the primary restraint to posterolateral instability (most common instability), whereas the medial (ulnar) collateral ligament is the primary restraint to valgus instability.[2] The ulnar collateral ligament has three parts, which along with the flexor carpi ulnaris muscle form the **cubital** tunnel through which passes the ulnar nerve (see Figure 6-4). Any injury or blow to the area or injury that increases the carrying angle puts an abnormal stress on the nerve as it passes through the tunnel. This can lead to problems such as **tardy ulnar palsy,** the symptoms of which can occur many years after the original injury and may be caused by the "double crush" phenomena of a cubital tunnel problem combined with a cervical spine problem.

Figure 6-2

Carrying angle of the elbow.

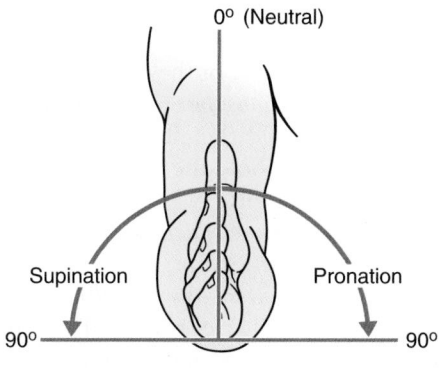

0° (Neutral)

Supination　　　Pronation

90°　　　　　　　90°

Figure 6-3

Figure 6-3
"Thumb-up" or neutral (zero) position between supination and pronation.

Superior Radioulnar Joint	
Resting position:	35° supination, 70° elbow flexion
Close packed position:	5° supination
Capsular pattern:	Equal limitation of supination and pronation

The three elbow articulations are innervated by branches from the musculocutaneous, median, ulnar, and radial nerves. The **middle radioulnar articulation** is not a true joint but is made up of the radius and ulna and the **interosseous membrane** between the two bones. The interosseous membrane is tense only midway between supination and pronation (neutral position). Although this "joint" is not part of the elbow joint complex, it is affected by injury to the elbow joints; conversely, injury to this area can affect the mechanics of the elbow articulations. The interosseous membrane prevents proximal displacement of the radius on the ulna. The displacement is most likely to occur with pushing movements. The **oblique cord** connects the radius and ulna, running from the lateral side of the **ulnar tuberosity** to the radius

The **superior radioulnar joint** is a uniaxial pivot joint. The head of the radius is held in proper relation to the ulna and humerus by the **annular ligament** (see Figures 6-1 and 6-4), which makes up four fifths of the joint.[3] The resting position of this joint is supination of 35° and elbow flexion of 70°. The close packed position is supination of 5°. The capsular pattern of this joint is equal limitation of supination and pronation.

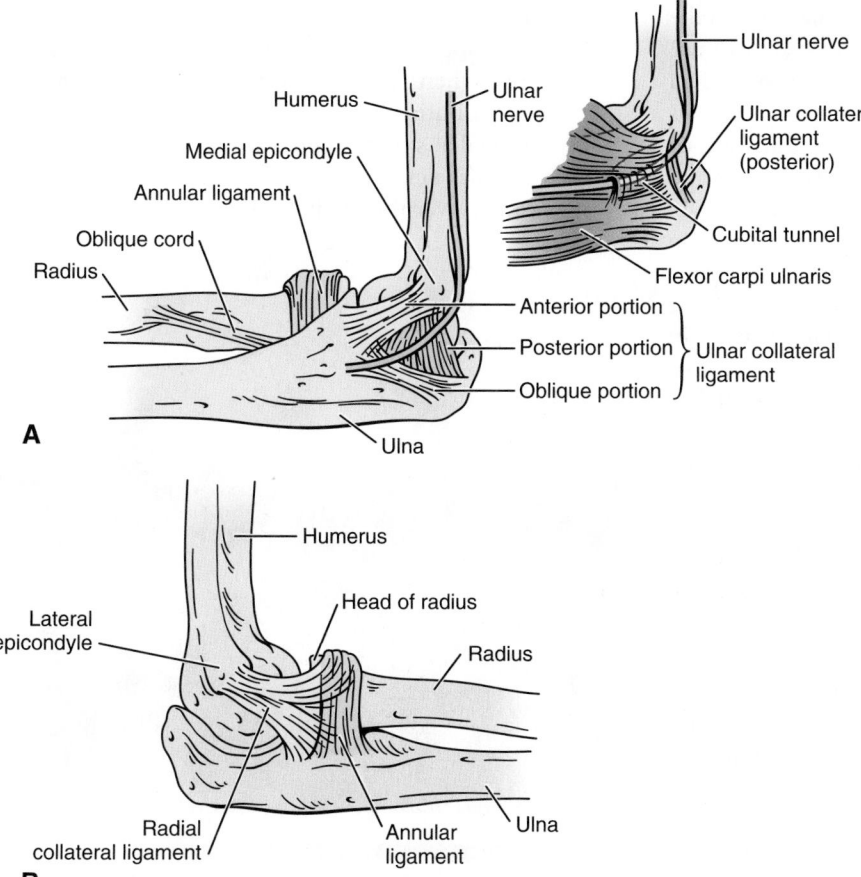

A

Humerus
Medial epicondyle
Annular ligament
Oblique cord
Radius

Ulnar nerve

Ulnar nerve
Ulnar collateral ligament (posterior)
Cubital tunnel
Flexor carpi ulnaris

Anterior portion
Posterior portion　} Ulnar collateral ligament
Oblique portion

Ulna

B

Humerus
Head of radius
Radius

Lateral epicondyle

Radial collateral ligament
Annular ligament
Ulna

Figure 6-4
Ligaments of the elbow. **A,** Ligaments on medial side of elbow. Note the passage of the ulnar nerve through the cubital tunnel.
B, Ligaments on the lateral side of elbow.

slightly below the **radial tuberosity**. Its fibers run at right angles to those of the interosseous membrane (see Figure 6-1). The cord assists in preventing displacement of the radius on the ulna, especially during movements involving pulling.

Patient History

In addition to the questions listed under Patient History in Chapter 1, the examiner should obtain the following information from the patient:

1. *How old is the patient? What is the patient's occupation?* Tennis elbow (lateral epicondylitis) problems usually occur in persons 35 years of age or older and in those who use a great deal of wrist flexion and extension in their occupations or activities, requiring wrist stabilization in slight extension (functional position). If the patient is a child who complains of pain in the elbow and lacks supination on examination, the examiner could suspect a dislocation of the head of the radius. This type of injury is often seen in young children. A parent may give the child a sharp "come-along" tug on the arm, or the child may trip while the parent is holding the hand, dislocating the head of the radius. Between the ages of 15 and 20, osteochondritis dissecans may be found.[4]

2. *What was the mechanism of injury?* Did the patient fall on the outstretched hand (FOOSH injury) or on the tip of the elbow? Were any repetitive activities involved? Does the patient's job involve any repetitive activities? Did the patient perform any unusual activities in the previous week? Did the patient feel a "pop" when throwing or doing other activity? If the pop was followed by pain and swelling on the medial side of the elbow, it may indicate an ulnar collateral ligament sprain.[5] Such questions help determine the structure injured and the degree of injury.

3. *How long has the patient had the problem? Does the condition come and go? What activities aggravate the problem?* Such questions indicate the seriousness of the condition and how much it bothers the patient.

4. *What are the details of the present pain and other symptoms?* What are the sites and boundaries of the pain? Is the pain radiating, does it ache, and is it worse at night? Aching pain over the lateral epicondyle that radiates may indicate a tennis elbow problem. Depending on the patient's age and past history, the examiner may want to consider referral of pain from the cervical spine or the possibility of a double crush neurological injury. Also, multiple joint diseases (e.g., rheumatoid arthritis, osteoarthritis) must be considered if the patient complains of pain in several joints.

5. *Are there any activities that increase or decrease the pain? Does pulling (traction), twisting (torque), or pushing (compression) alter the pain?* For example, writing, twisting motions of the arm (e.g., turning key, opening door), ironing, gripping, carrying, and leaning on forearm all stress the elbow.[6] Such questions may indicate the tissues being stressed or the tissues injured.

6. *Are there any positions that relieve the pain?* Patients often protectively hold the elbow to the side (in the resting position) and hold the wrist for support, especially in acute conditions.

7. *Is there any indication of deformity, bruising (Figure 6-5), wasting, or muscle spasm?*

8. *Are any movements impaired?* Which movements does the patient feel are restricted? If flexion or extension is limited, two joints may be involved, the ulnohumeral or the radiohumeral. If supination or pronation is problematic, any one of five joints could be involved: the radiohumeral, superior radioulnar at the elbow, middle radioulnar, inferior radioulnar, or ulnomeniscocarpal joints at the wrist.

9. *What is the patient unable to do functionally?* Which hand is dominant? Is the patient able to position the hand properly? Are abnormal movements of the upper limb complex necessary to position the hand? Questions such as these help the examiner determine how functionally limiting the condition is to the patient.

10. *What is the patient's usual activity or pastime? Have any of these activities been altered or increased in the past month?*

11. *Does the patient complain of any abnormal nerve distribution pain?* The examiner should note the presence and location of any tingling or numbness for reference when checking dermatomes and peripheral nerve distribution later in the examination. Snapping on the medial side may indicate recurrent dislocation of the radial nerve or the medial head of the triceps dislocating over the medial epicondyle.[4]

Figure 6-5
Bruising around elbow following dislocation (now reduced).

12. *Does the patient have a history of previous overuse injury or trauma?* This question is especially important in regard to the elbow because the ulnar nerve may be affected by tardy ulnar palsy.

Observation

The patient must be suitably undressed so that both arms are exposed to allow the examiner to compare the two sides. If the history indicates an insidious onset of elbow problems, the examiner should take the time to observe full body posture, especially the neck and shoulder areas, for possible referral of symptoms.

The examiner first places the patient's arm in the anatomical position to determine whether there is a normal **carrying angle**[7] (see Figure 6-2). It is the angle formed by the long axis of the humerus and the long axis of the ulna and is most evident when the elbow is straight and the forearm is fully supinated (Figure 6-6). In the adult, this would be a slight valgus deviation between the humerus and the ulna when the forearm is supinated and the elbow is extended. In males, the normal carrying angle is 5° to 10°; in females, it is 10° to 15°. If the carrying angle is more than 15°, it is called **cubitus valgus;** if it is less than 5° to 10°, it is called **cubitus varus** (Figure 6-7). Because of the shape of the humeral condyles that articulate with

Figure 6-6
Carrying angle. The carrying angle may be determined by noting the angle of intersection between a line connecting midpoints in the distal humerus and a line connecting midpoints in the proximal ulna.

the radius and ulna, the carrying angle changes linearly depending on the degree of extension or flexion. Cubitus valgus is greatest in extension. The angle decreases as the elbow flexes, reaching varus in full flexion.[8] If there has been a fracture or epiphyseal injury to the distal humerus and a cubitus varus results, a **gun stock deformity** may occur in full extension (Figure 6-8, see Figure 6-7).

If swelling exists, all three joints of the elbow complex are affected because they have a common capsule. Joint swelling is often most evident in the triangular space between the radial head, tip of olecranon, and lateral epicondyle (Figure 6-9). Swelling resulting from olecranon bursitis (student's elbow) is more discrete, being more sharply demarcated as a "goose egg" over the olecranon process (Figure 6-10). With swelling, the joint would be held in its resting position, with the elbow held in approximately 70° of flexion, because it is in the resting position that the joint has maximum volume.

The examiner should look for normal bony and soft-tissue contours anteriorly and posteriorly. Often, athletes such as pitchers, other throwers, and rodeo riders have a much larger forearm because of muscle and bone hypertrophy on the dominant side.

The examiner should note whether the patient can assume the normal position of function of the elbow (Figure 6-11). A normal functional position is 90° of flexion with the forearm midway between supination and pronation.[9] The forearm may also be considered to be in a functional position when slightly pronated, as in writing. From this position, forward flexion of the shoulder along with slightly more elbow flexion (up to 120°) enables the person to bring food to the mouth; supination of the forearm decreases the amount of shoulder flexion necessary to accomplish this. At 90° of elbow flexion, the olecranon process of the ulna and the medial and lateral epicondyles of the humerus normally form an isosceles triangle (Figure 6-12). When the arm is fully extended, the three points normally form a straight line.[10] The isosceles triangle is sometimes called the **triangle sign.** If there is a fracture, dislocation, or degeneration leading to loss of bone or cartilage, the distance between the apex and the base decreases and the isosceles triangle no longer exists. The triangle can be measured on x-ray films.[8]

Examination

If the history indicates an insidious onset of elbow symptoms, and if the patient has complained of weakness and pain, the examiner may consider performing an examination of the cervical spine, which includes the upper limb peripheral joint scanning examination and myotome testing. Because of the potential referral of symptoms from the cervical spine and the necessity of differentiating nerve root symptoms from peripheral nerve lesions, the consideration of including cervical assessment is essential.

A Normal carrying angle   **B** Excessive cubitus valgus   **C** Cubitus varus   **D** Gun stock deformity

Figure 6-7

A, The elbow's axis of rotation extends slightly, obliquely in a medial-lateral direction through the capitulum and the trochlea. Normal carrying angle of the elbow is shown with the forearm deviated laterally from the longitudinal axis of the humerus axis between 5° and 15°. **B,** Excessive cubitus valgus deformity is shown with the forearm deviated laterally 30°. **C,** Cubitus varus deformity is depicted with the forearm deviated medially –5°. **D,** Gunstock deformity with –15° medial deviation. (**A-C** redrawn from Neumann DA: *Kinesiology of the musculoskeletal system: foundations for physical rehabilitation,* p. 138, St. Louis, 2002, Mosby.)

Figure 6-8

Cubitus varus with "gun stock" deformity on the left arm. (From Regan WD, Morrey BF: The physical examination of the elbow. In Morrey BF, editor: *The elbow and its disorders,* ed 2, p. 74, Philadelphia, 1993, WB Saunders.)

Active Movements

The examination is performed with the patient in the sitting position. As always, active movements are done first, and it is important to remember that the most painful movements are done last. In addition, structures outside the joint may affect range of motion. For example, with lateral epicondylitis, the long extensors of the forearm are often found to be tight or shortened, so the position of the wrist and fingers may affect movement.

Active elbow flexion is 140° to 150°. Movement is usually stopped by contact of the forearm with the muscles of the arm.

Active elbow extension is 0°, although up to a 10° hyperextension may be exhibited, especially in women. This hyperextension is considered normal if it is equal on both sides and there is no history of trauma. Normally, the movement is arrested by the locking of the olecranon process of the ulna into the olecranon fossa of the humerus. In some cases, under violent compressive loads (e.g., gymnastics, weight lifting), the olecranon process may act as a pivot, resulting in posterior dislocation of the elbow. This mechanism of injury is more likely to occur in someone with elbows that normally hyperextend (Figure 6-13). Loss of elbow extension is a sensitive indicator of intra-articular pathology. It is the first movement lost after injury to the elbow and the first regained with

Figure 6-9
The triangular area in which intra-articular swelling is most evident in the elbow.

Radial collateral ligament

Olecranon bursitis

Annular ligament

A

B

Figure 6-10
A, Olecranon bursitis. **B,** Actual inflamed bursa. The orange color is from disinfectant applied before aspiration.

Figure 6-11
Position of most common function of the elbow—90° flexion, midway between supination and pronation.

Figure 6-12
Relation of the medial and lateral epicondyles and the olecranon at the elbow in extension *(left)* and flexion *(right)*.

healing. However, terminal flexion loss is more disabling than the same degree of terminal extension loss because of the need of flexion for many activities of daily living. Loss of either motion affects the area of reach of the hand, which in turn affects function.

Active Movements of the Elbow Complex

- Flexion of the elbow (140° to 150°)
- Extension of the elbow (0° to 10°)
- Supination of the forearm (90°)
- Pronation of the forearm (80° to 90°)
- Combined movements (if necessary)
- Repetitive movements (if necessary)
- Sustained positions (if necessary)

Figure 6-13
Normal elbow hyperextension.

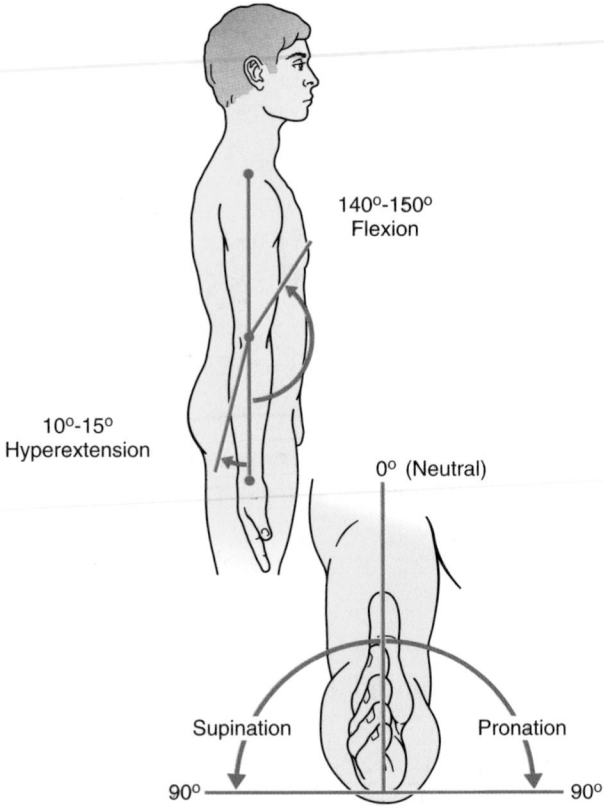

Figure 6-14
Range of motion at the elbow.

Active supination should be 90°, so that the palm faces up. The examiner should ensure that the shoulder is not adducted further in an attempt to give the appearance of increased supination or to compensate for a lack of sufficient supination (Figure 6-14).[11]

For active pronation, the range of motion (ROM) is approximately the same (80° to 90°), so that the palm faces down. The examiner should be sure that the patient does not abduct the shoulder in an attempt to increase the amount of pronation or to compensate for a lack of sufficient pronation.[11] However, for both supination and pronation, only about 75° of movement occurs in the forearm articulations. The remaining 15° is the result of wrist action.

If, in the history, the patient has complained that combined movements, repetitive movements, or sustained positions cause pain, these specific movements should be included in the active movement assessment. If the patient has difficulty or cannot complete a movement, but it is pain free, the examiner must consider a severe injury to the contractile tissue (rupture) or a neurological injury, and further testing is necessary.

Passive Movements

If the ROM is full on active movements, overpressure may be gently applied to test the end feel in each direction. If the movement is not full, passive movements should be carried out carefully to test the end feel and to test for a capsular pattern.

Passive Movements of the Elbow Complex and Normal End Feel

- Elbow flexion (tissue approximation)
- Elbow extension (bone to bone)
- Forearm supination (tissue stretch)
- Forearm pronation (tissue stretch)

It should be pointed out that although tissue approximation is the normal end feel of elbow flexion, in thin patients the end feel may be bone to bone as a result of the coronoid process hitting in the coronoid fossa. Likewise, in thin individuals, pronation may be bone to bone.

In addition to the end feel tests during passive movements, the examiner should note whether a capsular pattern is present. The capsular pattern for the elbow complex as a whole is more limitation of flexion than extension.

In some cases, the examiner may want to determine whether muscles crossing the elbow are tight. If the muscles are tight, the end feel will be a muscle stretch, and ROM at one of the joints that the muscle passes over will be restricted (usually the joint that is the last to be stretched). If the muscle is normal, the end feel will be the normal joint tissue stretch end feel and the ROM will be normal. To test biceps length (Figure 6-15, *A*), the patient is placed in supine with the shoulder to be tested off the edge of the bed. The shoulder is passively extended to end range and then the elbow is extended.[12] Normally, elbow extension should be the same as that seen with active movement.

To test triceps length (Figure 6-15, *B*), the patient is placed in sitting. The examiner passively forward flexes the arm to full elevation while the elbow is in extension. The elbow is then passively flexed.[9] Normally, elbow flexion should be similar to that seen with active movement.

To test the length of the long wrist extensors (as one would want to do with lateral epicondylitis), the patient is placed in supine lying with the elbow extended (Figure 6-15, *C*). The examiner passively flexes the fingers and then flexes the wrist.[12] Normally, wrist flexion and finger flexion should be the same as found with active movement.

To test the length of the long wrist flexors (Figure 6-15, *D*), the patient is placed in supine lying with the elbow extended. The examiner passively extends the fingers and then the wrist.[12] Normally, wrist extension and finger extension should be the same as that found with active movement.

Resisted Isometric Movements

For proper testing of the muscles of the elbow complex, the movement must be resisted and isometric. Muscle flexion power around the elbow is greatest in the range of 90° to 110° with the forearm supinated. At 45° and 135°, flexion power is only 75% of maximum.[9] Isometrically, research shows that men are two times stronger than women at the elbow; extension is 60% of flexion, and pronation is about 85% of supination.[13] To perform the resisted isometric tests, the patient is seated (Figure 6-16). If the examiner finds that a particular movement or movements cause pain, Table 6-1 can be used to help differentiate the cause. It is also necessary to carry out wrist extension and flexion, because a large number of muscles act over the wrist as well as the elbow.

Resisted Isometric Movements of the Elbow Complex

- Elbow flexion
- Elbow extension
- Supination
- Pronation
- Wrist flexion
- Wrist extension

A

B

Figure 6-15
Testing length of tight muscles. **A,** Biceps. **B,** Triceps.

Continued

Figure 6-15 cont'd
C, Long wrist extensors. **D,** Long wrist flexors.

Figure 6-16
Positioning for resisted isometric movements. **A,** Elbow extension. **B,** Elbow flexion.

Figure 6-16 cont'd
C, Forearm supination. **D,** Forearm pronation. **E,** Wrist flexion. **F,** Wrist extension.

If, in the history, the patient has complained that combined movements under load, repetitive movements under load, or sustained positions under load cause pain, the examiner should carefully examine these resisted isometric movements and positions as well, but only after the basic movements have been tested isometrically. For example, the biceps is a strong supinator and flexor of the elbow, but its ability to generate force depends on the position of the elbow. The biceps play a greater role in elbow flexion when the forearm is supinated than when

Table 6-1

Muscles about the Elbow: Their Actions, Nerve Supply, and Nerve Root Derivation

Action	Muscles Acting	Nerve Supply	Nerve Root Derivation
Flexion of elbow	1. Brachialis	Musculocutaneous	C5-C6, (C7)
	2. Biceps brachii	Musculocutaneous	C5-C6
	3. Brachioradialis	Radial	C5-C6, (C7)
	4. Pronator teres	Median	C6-C7
	5. Flexor carpi ulnaris	Ulnar	C7-C8
Extension of elbow	1. Triceps	Radial	C6-C8
	2. Anconeus	Radial	C7-C8, (T1)
Supination of forearm	1. Supinator	Posterior interosseous (Radial)	C5-C6
	2. Biceps brachii	Musculocutaneous	C5-C6
Pronation of forearm	1. Pronator quadratus	Anterior interosseous (Median)	C8, T1
	2. Pronator teres	Median	C6-C7
	3. Flexor carpi radialis	Median	C6-C7
Flexion of wrist	1. Flexor carpi radialis	Median	C6-C7
	2. Flexor carpi ulnaris	Ulnar	C7-C8
Extension of wrist	1. Extensor carpi radialis longus	Radial	C6-C7
	2. Extensor carpi radialis brevis	Posterior interosseous (Radial)	C7-C8
	3. Extensor carpi ulnaris	Posterior interosseous (Radial)	C7-C8

it is pronated. At 90° of elbow flexion, biceps makes its greatest contribution to supination.[14] If the history indicates that concentric, eccentric, or econcentric movements have caused symptoms, these movements should also be tested with load or no load, as required.

If the resisted isometric contraction is weak and pain free, the examiner must consider a major injury to the contractile tissue (third-degree strain) or neurological injury. For example, weakness of elbow flexion and supination may occur with a rupture of the distal biceps tendon, especially if these findings follow a sudden sharp pain in the antecubital fossa when an extension force is applied to the flexing elbow.[14] If there is no history of trauma, the most likely cause is neurological, either a nerve root or peripheral nerve lesion. By selectively testing the muscles and sensory distribution (Table 6-2) and by having a knowledge of nerve compression sites (see the section on reflexes and cutaneous distribution), the examiner should be able to determine the neurological tissue injured and where the injury has occurred.

Functional Assessment

When assessing the elbow, it is important to remember that the elbow is the middle portion of an integral upper limb kinetic chain. It allows the hand to be positioned in space; it helps stabilize the upper extremity for power and detailed work activities; and it provides power to the arm for lifting activities.[15] Motion in the elbow allows the hand to be positioned so that

daily functions can be performed easily. The full range of elbow movements is not necessary to perform these activities; most activities of daily living are performed at between 30° and 130° of flexion and between 50° of pronation and 50° of supination (Figures 6-17 and 6-18). To reach the head, approximately 140° of flexion is needed. The activities of combing or washing the hair, reaching a back zipper, and walking with crutches require a greater ROM. Activities such as pouring fluid, drinking from a container, cutting with a knife, reading a newspaper, and using a screwdriver require an adequate range of supination and pronation. Figures 6-19 and 6-20 show the ROM or arc of movement necessary to do certain activities or the ROM needed to touch parts of the body. Examiners must remember that elbow injuries may preclude lifting objects as light as a cup of coffee, owing to lifting mechanics. Because of the length of the lever arm of the forearm when the elbow is at 90°, loads at the hand are magnified 10-fold at the elbow.[16] Figure 6-21 is a numerical scoring assessment form that can be used to assess the elbow and includes an important functional component. Table 6-3 demonstrates functional tests of strength for the elbow.

Special Tests

An examiner should perform only those special tests that have relevance or will help to confirm the diagnosis. If the history has not indicated any trauma or repetitive movement that could be associated with problems, the examiner, depending on the age of the patient, may want

Table 6-2

Nerve Injuries about the Elbow

Nerve	Motor Loss	Sensory Loss	Functional Loss
Median nerve (C6-C8,T1)	Pronator teres Flexor carpi radialis Palmaris longus Flexor digitorum superficialis Flexor pollicis longus Lateral half of flexor digitorum profundus Pronator quadratus Thenar eminence Lateral two lumbricals	Palmar aspect of hand with thumb, index, middle, and lateral half of ring finger Dorsal aspect of distal third of index, middle, and lateral half of ring finger	Pronation weak or lost Weak wrist flexion and abduction Radial deviation at wrist lost Inability to oppose or flex thumb Weak thumb abduction Weak grip Weak or no pinch (ape hand deformity)
Anterior interosseous nerve (branch of median nerve)	Flexor pollicis longus Lateral half of flexor digitorum profundus Pronator quadratus Thenar eminence Lateral two lumbricals	None	Pronation weak especially at 90° elbow flexion Weak opposition and flexion of thumb Weak finger flexion Weak pinch (no tip-to-tip)
Ulnar nerve (C7-C8,T1)	Flexor carpi ulnaris Medial half of flexor digitorum profundus Palmaris brevis Hypothenar eminence Adductor pollicis Medial two lumbricals All interossei	Dorsal and palmar aspect of little and medial half of ring finger	Weak wrist flexion Loss of ulnar deviation at wrist Loss of distal flexion of little finger Loss of abduction and adduction of fingers Inability to extend second and third phalanges of little and ring fingers (benediction hand deformity) Loss of thumb adduction
Radial nerve (C5-8,T1)	Anconeus Brachioradialis Extensor carpi radialis longus and brevis Extensor digitorum Extensor pollicis longus and brevis Abductor pollicis longus Extensor carpi ulnaris Extensor indices Extensor digiti minimi	Dorsum of hand (lateral two thirds) Dorsum and lateral aspect of thumb Proximal two thirds of dorsum of index, middle, and half ring finger	Loss of supination Loss of wrist extension (wrist drop) Inability to grasp Inability to stabilize wrist Loss of finger extension Inability to abduct thumb
Posterior interosseous nerve (branch of radial nerve)	Extensor carpi radialis brevis Extensor digitorum Extensor pollicis longus and brevis Abductor pollicis longus Extensor carpi ulnaris Extensor indices Extensor digiti minimi	None	Weak wrist extension Weak finger extension Difficulty stabilizing wrist Difficulty with grasp Inability to abduct thumb

to include some of the nerve root compression tests (see Chapter 3) to rule out the possibility of referred symptoms from the cervical spine or the possibility of a "double crush" injury. The reliability, validity, specificity, and sensitivity of some of the diagnostic/special tests used in the elbow are outlined in Appendix 6-1.

Ligamentous (Instability) Tests

These tests are designed to test for valgus and varus instability in the elbow.

Ligamentous Valgus Instability Test. To test for valgus instability, the patient's arm is stabilized with one of the examiner's hands at the elbow and the other hand

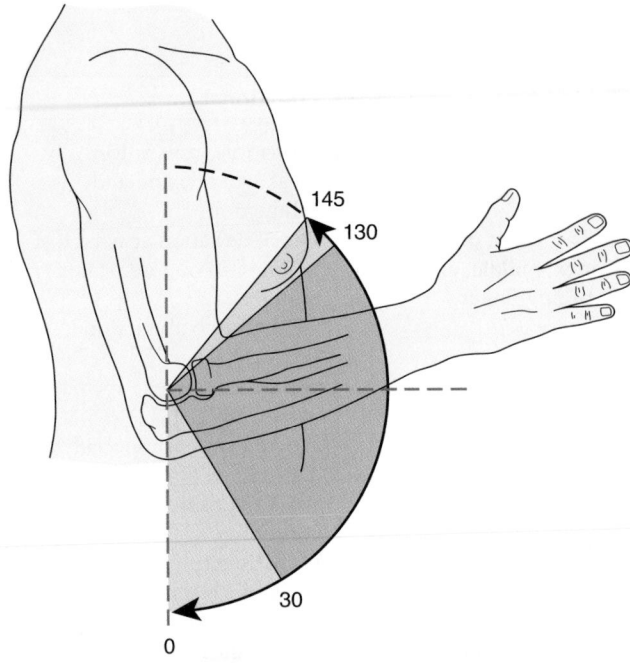

Figure 6-17

Normal range of elbow flexion is approximately 0° to 145°. However, the functional arc of motion is somewhat less, and most activities can be performed with flexion of 30° to 130°. (Redrawn from Regan WD, Morrey BF: The physical examination of the elbow. In Morrey BF, editor: *The elbow and its disorders,* ed 2, p. 81, Philadelphia, 1993, WB Saunders.)

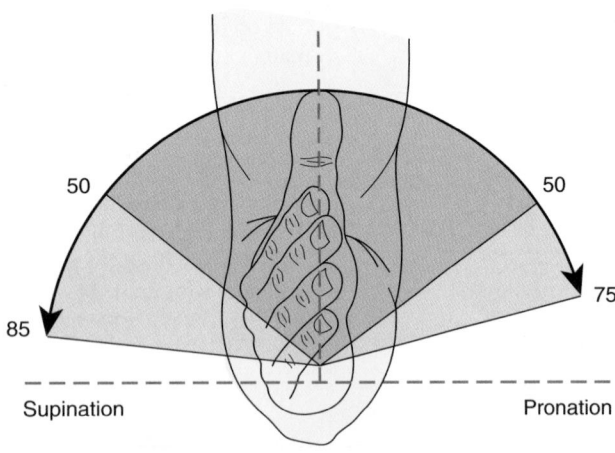

Figure 6-18

Pronation and supination motions average 75° and 85°, respectively. Most activities of daily living, however, can be accomplished with 50° of each motion. (Redrawn from Regan WD, Morrey BF: The physical examination of the elbow. In Morrey BF, editor: *The elbow and its disorders,* ed 2, p. 81, Philadelphia, 1993, WB Saunders.)

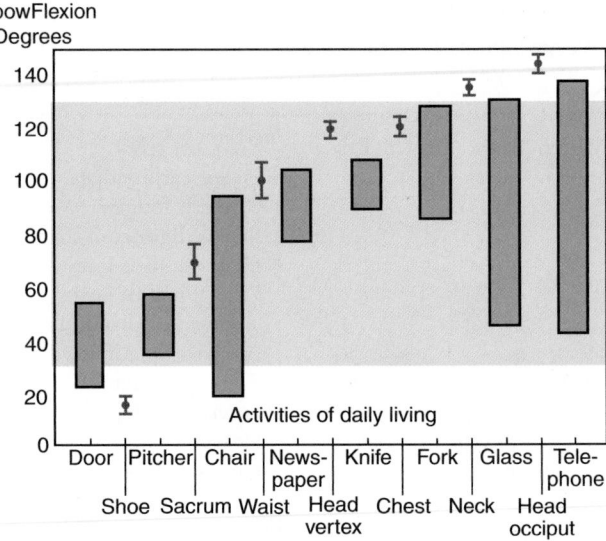

Figure 6-19

The arc and position of elbow flexion required to accomplish 15 daily activities. Most of these activities are accomplished within a flexion range of 30° to 130°. (Modified from Morrey BF et al: A biomechanical study of normal functional elbow motion, *J Bone Joint Surg Am* 63:873, 1981.)

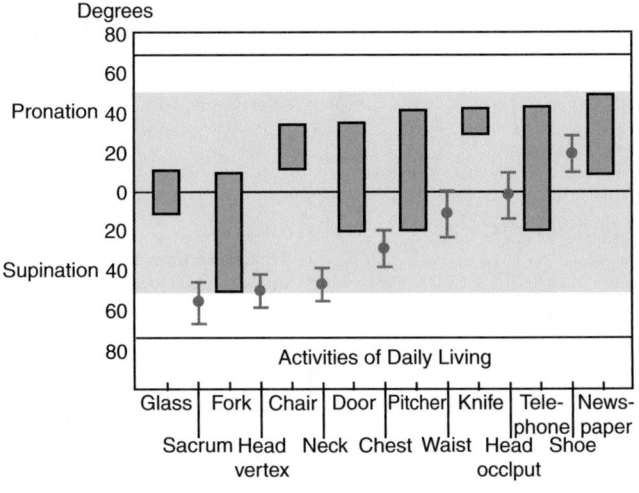

Figure 6-20

Fifteen activities of daily living accomplished with pronation and supination of up to 50° each. (Modified from Morrey BF, et al: A biomechanical study of normal functional elbow motion, *J Bone Joint Surg Am* 63:874, 1981.)

Special Tests Commonly Performed on the Elbow

- Ligamentous instability tests
- Lateral epicondylitis test (method 1 or 2)
- Elbow flexion test (ulnar nerve)
- Pinch grip test (median nerve and anterior interosseous nerve)

Elbow Evaluation

Name: _____ UH#: _____ Elbow: R/L

Procedure: _____ Date: _____ Dominant: R/L

Date of Exam (month/day/year)	/ /	/ /	/ /	/ /	/ /
Pain (maximum points) 5 = none (30); 4 = slight—with continuous activity, no medication (25); 3 = moderate—with occasional activity, some medication (15); 2 = moderately severe—much pain, frequent medication (10); 1 = severe—constant pain, markedly limited activity (5); 0 = complete disability (0)	_____ ( )				
Motion degrees (37 points maximum) Extension (8 pts max) Flexion (17 pts max) Pronation/Supination (pt) = 0.1 per degree—6 maximum	Extension _____°( ) Flexion _____°( ) Pronation _____°( ) Supination _____°( )				
Strength (15 points maximum) 5 = normal; 4 = good; 3 = fair; 2 = poor; 1 = trace; 0 = paralysis; NA = not available Flex. Ext. Pro. Sup. Normal 5 (5) (4) (3) (3) Good 4 (4) (3) (2) (2) Fair 3 (3) (2) (1) (1) Poor 2 (2) (1) (0) (0) Trace 1 (1) (0) (0) (0) None 0 (0) (0) (0) (0)	Extension _____( ) Flexion _____( ) Pronation _____( ) Supination _____( )				
Instability (6 points maximum) Ant./Post. Med./Lat. None 3 3 Mild <5 mm, <5° 2 2 Moderate <10 mm, <10° 1 1 Severe >10 mm, >10° 0 0	Ant./Post. _____ Med./Lat. _____				

Function (12 points maximum)
4 = normal (1); 3 = mild compromise (0.75); 2 = difficulty (0.5); 1 = with aid (0.25); 0 = unable (0); NA = not applicable
 	
(Index—multiply × 0.25)
1. Use back pocket
2. Rise from chair
3. Perineal care
4. Wash opposite axilla
5. Eat with utensil
6. Comb hair
7. Carry 10–15 pounds with arm at side
8. Dress
9. Pulling
10. Throwing
11. Do usual work
     Specify work:
12. Do usual sport
     Specify sport:
	_____( )
	_____( )
	_____( )
	_____( )
	_____( )
	_____( )
	_____( )
	_____( )
	_____( )
	_____( )
	_____( )
	
	_____( )				

Patient Response 3 = much better; 2 = better; 1 = same; 0 = worse; NA = not available/not applicable	_____				
Completed By: Name of Examiner					
Index Key: 95–100 = excellent; 80–95 = good; 50–80 = fair; <50 = poor	( )	( )	( )	( )	( )

Figure 6-21

Clinical elbow evaluation form that provides objective data and grading as well as functional information. The use of such a rating index in the clinical setting provides an objective means of comparing different treatment options. (From Morrey BF et al: Functional evaluation of the elbow. In Morrey BF, editor: *The elbow and its disorders,* pp. 88-89, Philadelphia, 1985, WB Saunders. Copyright Mayo Clinic Foundation, Rochester, MN.)

Table 6-3

Functional Testing of the Elbow

Starting Position	Action	Functional Test*
Sitting	Bring hand to mouth lifting weight (elbow flexion)	Lift 2.3-2.7 kg: Functional Lift 1.4-1.8 kg: Functionally fair Lift 0.5-0.9 kg: Functionally poor Lift 0 kg: Nonfunctional
Standing 90 cm from wall, leaning against wall	Push arms straight (elbow extension)	5-6 Repetitions: Functional 3-4 Repetitions: Functionally fair 1-2 Repetitions: Functionally poor 0 Repetitions: Nonfunctional
Standing, facing closed door	Open door starting with palm down (supination of arm)	5-6 Repetitions: Functional 3-4 Repetitions: Functionally fair 1-2 Repetitions: Functionally poor 0 Repetitions: Nonfunctional
Standing, facing closed door	Open door starting with palm up (pronation of arm)	5-6 Repetitions: Functional 3-4 Repetitions: Functionally fair 1-2 Repetitions: Functionally poor 0 Repetitions: Nonfunctional

Data from Palmer ML Epler M: *Clinical assessment procedures in physical therapy,* pp. 109-111, Philadelphia, 1990, JB Lippincott.
*Younger patients should be able to lift more (2.7-4.5 kg) more often (6-10 repetitions). With age, weight and repetitions will decrease.

placed above the patient's wrist. An abduction or valgus force at the distal forearm is applied to test the medial collateral ligament (valgus instability) while the ligament is palpated.[2] Regan and Morrey advocate doing the valgus stress test with the humerus in full lateral rotation.[16] The examiner should note any laxity, decreased mobility, or altered pain that may be present compared with the uninvolved elbow.

Moving Valgus Stress Test[2,17]. The patient lies supine or stands with the arm abducted and elbow flexed fully. While maintaining a valgus stress, the examiner quickly extends the patient's elbow. Reproduction of the patient's pain between 120° to 70° indicates a positive test and a partial tear of the medial collateral ligament (Figure 6-22).

Milking Manoeuver[2]. The patient sits with the elbow flexed to 90° or more and the forearm supinated.

Figure 6-22

A, The moving valgus stress test. **B,** Schematic representation of the moving valgus stress test. The shear range refers to the range of motion that causes pain while the elbow is being extended with valgus stress. The shear angle is the point that causes maximum pain. (**B** used with permission of the Mayo Foundation.)

Figure 6-23
"Milking" maneuver to test medial collateral ligament.

The examiner grasps the patient's thumb under the forearm and pulls it imparting a valgus stress to the elbow (Figure 6-23). Reproduction of symptoms indicates a positive test and a partial tear of the medial collateral ligament.

Ligamentous Varus Instability Test. With the patient's elbow slightly flexed (20° to 30°) and stabilized with the examiner's hand, an adduction or varus force is applied by the examiner to the distal forearm to test the lateral collateral ligament (varus instability) while the ligament is palpated (Figure 6-24). Normally, the examiner feels the ligament tense when stress is applied. Regan and Morrey advocated doing the varus stress test with the humerus in full medial rotation.[16] The examiner applies the force several times with increasing pressure while noting any alteration in pain or

ROM. If excessive laxity is found when doing the test, or a soft end feel is felt, it indicates injury to the ligament (1°, 2°, or 3° sprain) and may, especially with a 3° sprain, indicate posterolateral joint instability. Posterolateral elbow instability is the most common pattern of elbow instability in which there is displacement of the ulna (accompanied by the radius) on the humerus so the ulna supinates or laterally rotates away from or off the trochlea.[18]

Posterolateral Rotary Apprehension Test[2,18-22]. The patient lies supine with the arm to be tested overhead. The elbow is supinated at the wrist, and a valgus stress is applied to the elbow while the examiner flexes the elbow. This movement (between 20° and 30° flexion) and stress will cause the patient to be apprehensive that the elbow will dislocate while reproducing the patient's symptoms. In the conscious patient, actual subluxation is rare. A positive test indicates posterolateral rotary instability (Figure 6-25).

Lateral Pivot Shift Test of the Elbow[2,18]. The patient lies supine with the arm to be tested overhead. The examiner grasps the patient's wrist and forearm with the elbow extended and the forearm fully supinated.[21] The patient's elbow is then flexed while a valgus stress and axial compression is applied to the elbow while maintaining supination. This causes the radius (and ulna) to sublux off the humerus leading to a prominent radial head posterolaterally and a dimple between the radial head and capitellum (Figure 6-26, *A*).[2,21] If the examiner continues flexing the elbow, at about 40° to 70°, there is a sudden reduction (clunk) of the joint, which can be palpated and seen (Figure 6-26, *B*).[19] If the patient is unconscious,

A   **B**

Figure 6-24
Testing the collateral ligaments of the elbow. **A,** Lateral collateral ligament. **B,** Medial collateral ligament.

Figure 6-25
Posterolateral rotary apprehension test.

Figure 6-27
Posterolateral rotary drawer test.

subluxation and a clunk on reduction when the elbow is extended may occur, but these symptoms seldom present in the conscious patient.

Posterolateral Rotary Drawer Test[2]. The patient lies supine with the arm to be tested overhead and the elbow flexed 40° to 90° while the examiner holds the forearm and arm similar to doing a drawer test at the knee. As the humerus is stabilized, and the radius and ulna pushed posterolaterally, the radius and ulna will rotate around an intact medial collateral ligament indicating a tear of the lateral collateral ligament and posterolateral instability at the elbow (Figure 6-27).

Stand Up Test[2,4]. The patient is seated in a chair without arms. The patient is asked to push up on the seat with his or her hands with the forearms supinated into standing. If the patient's symptoms are reproduced, the test is positive for injury to the posterior band of the medial collateral ligament (Figure 6-28).

Figure 6-26
Posterolateral pivot-shift apprehension test of the elbow. **A,** The patient lies supine with the arm overhead. A mild supination force is applied to the forearm at the wrist. The patient's elbow is then flexed while a valgus stress and compression is applied to the elbow. **B,** If the examiner continues flexing the elbow at about 40° to 70°, subluxation and a clunk on reduction when the elbow is extended may occur, but usually only in the unconscious patient. **C,** Actual test with elbow positioned to resemble knee.

Figure 6-28
Standup test.

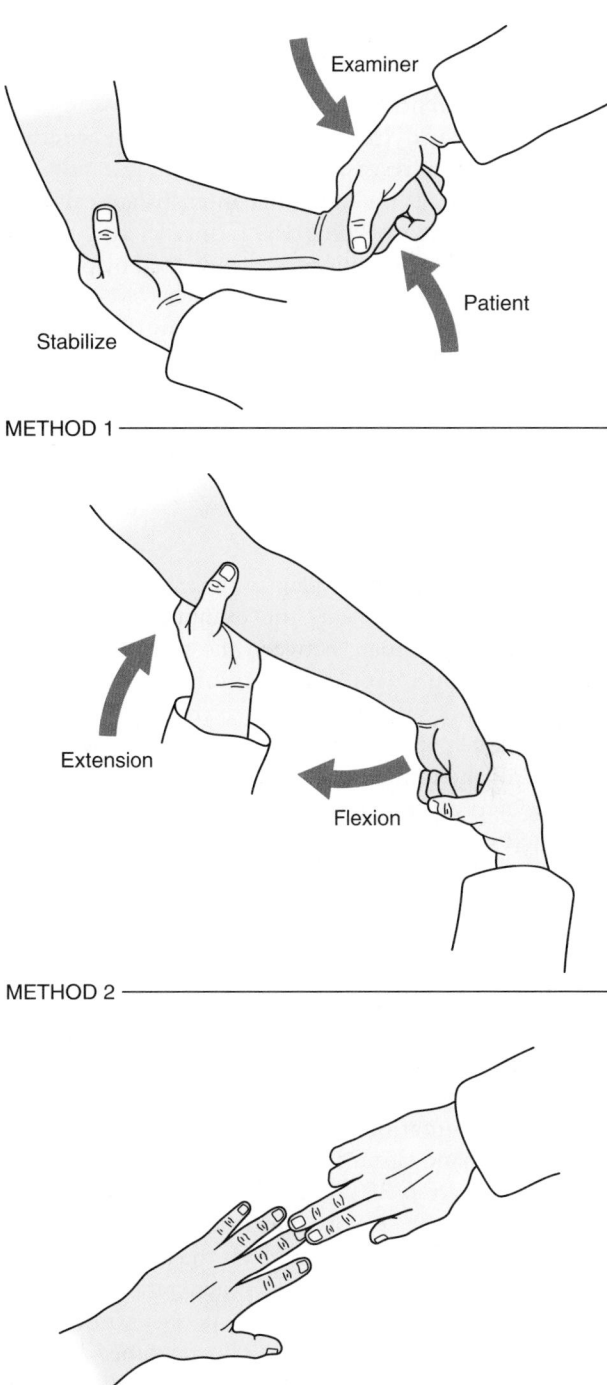

METHOD 1 ─────────────────

METHOD 2 ─────────────────

METHOD 3 ─────────────────

Figure 6-29
Tests for tennis elbow.

Tests for Epicondylitis

Chronic overuse injury to the extensor (tennis elbow or lateral epicondylitis) or flexor (golfer's elbow or medial epicondylitis) tendons at the elbow result from repeated microtrauma to the tendon leading to disruption and degeneration of the tendon's internal structure (tendinosus).[23] It appears to be a degenerative condition in which the tendon has failed to heal properly after repetitive microtrauma injury.[23,24]

When testing for epicondylitis, whether medial or lateral, the examiner must keep in mind that there may be referral of pain from the cervical spine or peripheral nerve involvement. If the epicondylitis does not respond to treatment, the examiner would be wise to check for neurological pathology.

Lateral Epicondylitis (Tennis Elbow or Cozen's) Test (Method 1). The patient's elbow is stabilized by the examiner's thumb, which rests on the patient's lateral epicondyle (Figure 6-29). The patient is then asked to actively make a fist, pronate the forearm, and radially deviate and extend the wrist while the examiner resists the motion. A sudden severe pain in the area of the lateral epicondyle of the humerus is a positive sign. The epicondyle may be palpated to indicate the origin of the pain.

Lateral Epicondylitis (Tennis Elbow or Mill's) Test (Method 2). While palpating the lateral epicondyle, the examiner passively pronates the patient's forearm, flexes the wrist fully, and extends the elbow (see Figure 6-29). Pain over the lateral epicondyle of the humerus indicates a positive test. This maneuver also puts stress on the radial nerve and, in the presence of compression of the radial nerve, causes symptoms similar to those of tennis elbow.[25] Electrodiagnostic studies help differentiate the two conditions.

Lateral Epicondylitis (Tennis Elbow) Test (Method 3). The examiner resists extension of the third digit of the hand distal to the proximal interphalangeal joint, stressing the extensor digitorum muscle and tendon (see Figure 6-29). A positive test is indicated by pain over the lateral epicondyle of the humerus.

Medial Epicondylitis (Golfer's Elbow) Test. While the examiner palpates the patient's medial epicondyle, the patient's forearm is passively supinated and the examiner extends the elbow and wrist. A positive sign is indicated by pain over the medial epicondyle of the humerus.

Tests for Joint Dysfunction

If the patient complains of pain in the elbow joint, especially on elbow movement, the examiner can perform two tests to differentiate between the radiohumeral and ulnohumeral joints. **To test the radiohumeral joint**, the examiner positions the elbow joint at the position of pain and then radially deviates the wrist to compress the radial head against the humerus. The production of pain would be considered a positive test. **To test the ulnohumeral joint**, the examiner again positions the elbow joint at the position of discomfort and causes compression of the ulnohumeral joint by ulnar deviation at the wrist.[6] Again, pain indicates a positive test.

Tests for Neurological Dysfunction

Tinel's Sign (at the Elbow). The area of the ulnar nerve in the groove (between the olecranon process and medial epicondyle) is tapped. A positive sign is indicated by a tingling sensation in the ulnar distribution of the forearm and hand distal to the point of compression of the nerve (Figure 6-30). The test indicates the point of regeneration of the sensory fibers of a nerve. The most distal point at which the patient feels the abnormal sensation represents the limit of nerve regeneration.

Wartenberg's Sign. The patient sits with his or her hands resting on the table. The examiner passively spreads the fingers apart and asks the patient to bring them together again. Inability to squeeze the little finger to the remainder of the hand indicates a positive test for ulnar neuropathy.[16]

Elbow Flexion Test. The patient is asked to fully flex the elbow with extension of the wrist and shoulder girdle abduction and depression[26,27] and to hold this position for 3 to 5 minutes (Figure 6-31). Tingling or paresthesia in the ulnar nerve distribution of the forearm and hand indicates a positive testi. The test helps to determine whether a cubital tunnel (ulnar nerve) syndrome is present.

Test for Pronator Teres Syndrome[16]. The patient sits with the elbow flexed to 90°. The examiner strongly

Figure 6-30
Tinel's sign at the elbow for the ulnar nerve.

Figure 6-31
Elbow flexion test for ulnar nerve pathology.

resists pronation as the elbow is extended. Tingling or paresthesia in the median nerve distribution in the forearm and hand indicates a positive test.

Pinch Grip Test. The patient is asked to pinch the tips of the index finger and thumb together. Normally, there should be a tip-to-tip pinch. If the patient is unable to pinch tip to tip and instead has an abnormal pulp-to-pulp pinch of the index finger and thumb, this is a positive sign for pathology to the anterior interosseous nerve, a branch of the median nerve (Figure 6-32). This finding may indicate an entrapment of the anterior interosseous nerve as it passes between the two heads of the pronator teres muscle.[28]

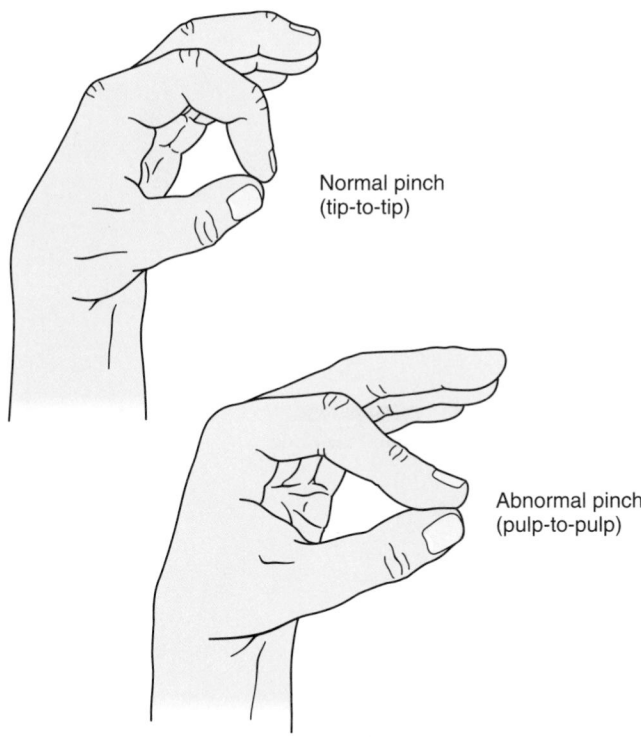

Figure 6-32
Normal tip-to-tip pinch compared with the abnormal pulp-to-pulp pinch seen in anterior interosseous nerve syndrome.

Reflexes and Cutaneous Distribution

The reflexes around the elbow that are often checked (Fig. 6-33) include the biceps (C5-C6), brachioradialis (C5-C6), and triceps (C7-C8). The examiner should also assess the dermatomes around the elbow and the cutaneous distribution of the various nerves, noting any difference (Figures 6-34 and 6-35). When looking at the dermatomes, the examiner should realize there is a great deal of variability in the distribution patterns. Except for T2 dermatome, which commonly ends at the elbow, all other dermatomes extend distally to the forearm, wrist, and hand; therefore, the elbow cannot be looked at in isolation when viewing dermatomes. Similarly, the peripheral nerves extend into the forearm, wrist, and hand, so testing for sensory loss must involve the whole upper limb, not just the elbow. Pain may be referred to the elbow and surrounding tissues from the neck (often mimicking tennis elbow), the shoulder, or the wrist (Figure 6-36; Table 6-4).

In the extremities, the neurological tissues (nerve roots and peripheral nerves) play a significant role in function. Injury, pinching, or stress to these structures can have dire consequences functionally for the patient. The next section is a review of the peripheral nerves and how and where they may be traumatized about the elbow.

A

B

C

Figure 6-33
Reflexes around the elbow. **A,** Biceps. **B,** Brachioradialis. **C,** Triceps.

Peripheral Nerve Injuries about the Elbow

Median Nerve (C6-C8, T1) In the elbow region, the median nerve proper can be injured by trauma (e.g., lacerations, fractures, dislocations), by systemic disease, and especially by compression and/or traction.[29,30]

Figure 6-34
Dermatomes around the elbow.

Anterior aspect

Posterior aspect

Figure 6-35
Sensory nerve distribution around the elbow. (*1*) Lower lateral cutaneous nerve of arm (radial). (*2*) Medial cutaneous nerve of arm. (*3*) Medial cutaneous nerve of forearm. (*4*) Lateral cutaneous nerve of forearm (musculocutaneous nerve). (*5*) Posterior cutaneous nerve of forearm (radial nerve).

The median nerve may also be pinched or compressed above the elbow as it passes under the **ligament of Struthers,** an anomalous structure found in approximately 1% of the population (Figure 6-37).[31] The ligament runs from an abnormal spur on the shaft of the humerus

Figure 6-36
Pain referred to the elbow.

Table 6-4
Elbow Muscles and Referral of Pain

Muscles	Referral Pattern
Biceps	Upper shoulder (bicipital groove) to anterior elbow
Brachialis	Anterior arm, elbow to lateral thenar eminence
Triceps	Posterior shoulder, arm, elbow, and forearm to medial two fingers, medial epicondyle
Brachioradialis	Lateral epicondyle, lateral forearm to posterior web space between thumb and index finger
Anconeus	Lateral epicondyle area
Supinator	Lateral epicondyle and posterior web space between thumb and index finger
Pronator teres	Anterior forearm to wrist and part of anterior thumb
Extensor carpi ulnaris	Medial wrist
Extensor carpi radialis brevis	Posterior forearm to posterior wrist
Extensor carpi radialis longus	Lateral epicondyle to posterolateral wrist
Extensor indices	Posterior forearm to appropriate digit
Palmaris longus	Anterior forearm to palm
Flexor digitorum superficialis	Palm to appropriate digit
Flexor carpi ulnaris	Anteromedial wrist
Flexor carpi radialis	Anteromedial wrist

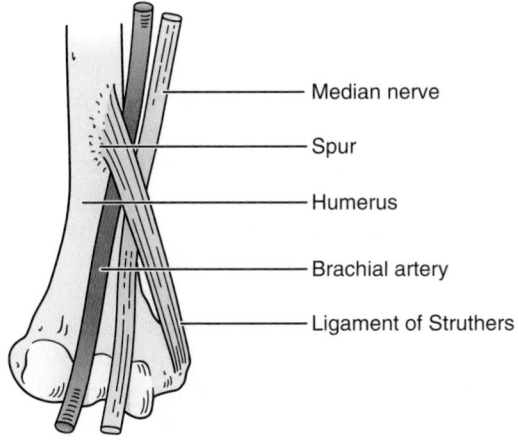

Figure 6-37
Compression of the median nerve by ligament of Struthers.

to the medial epicondyle of the humerus. Because the brachial artery sometimes accompanies the nerve through this tunnel, it may also be compressed, resulting in possible vascular as well as neurological symptoms. In this case, the neurological involvement would include weakness of the pronator teres muscle and of those muscles affected by the pronator syndrome (see later discussion). The condition may also be called the **humerus supracondylar process syndrome**. Pressure in the ligament of Struthers area leads to motor loss (see Table 6-2) and sensory loss (see Figure 7-72.) of the median nerve. Initially, the patient complains of pain and paresthesia in the elbow and forearm; abnormality of motor function is secondary. With time, however, motor function is also affected, with wrist and finger flexion as well as thumb movements being most affected.

A second area of compression of the median nerve as it passes through the elbow occurs where it passes through the two heads of pronator teres (**pronator** syndrome). In this case, the pronator teres remains normal, but the other muscles supplied by the median nerve (see Table 6-2) are affected, as is its sensory distribution. Pronation is possible, but weakness is evident as pronation is loaded. If the elbow is flexed to 90° and pronation is tested, there will be noticeable weakness because, in this position, the action of pronator teres is minimized.

Butlers and Singer reported four possible ways of eliciting median nerve symptoms if the nerve is suffering from pathology: resisted pronation with elbow and wrist flexion for 30 to 60 seconds; resisted elbow flexion and supination; resisted long finger flexion at the proximal interphalangeal joint; and direct pressure over the proximal aspect of pronator teres during pronation.[32] It is interesting to note that one of the tests is similar to Mill's test for lateral epicondylitis. The results should be compared with the good side, and production of the patient's symptoms is considered a positive test.

Anterior Interosseous Nerve. The anterior interosseous nerve, which is a branch of the median nerve, is sometimes pinched or entrapped as it passes between the two heads of the pronator teres muscle, leading to pain and functional impairment of flexor pollicis longus, the lateral half of the flexor digitorum profundus, and the pronator quadratus muscles. The condition is called **anterior interosseous nerve syndrome** or **Kiloh-Nevin syndrome** (Figure 6-38)[33,34] and is characterized by a pinch deformity (see Figure 6-32). The deformity results from the paralysis of the flexors of the index finger and thumb. This leads to extension of the distal interphalangeal joint of the index finger and the interphalangeal joint of the thumb. The

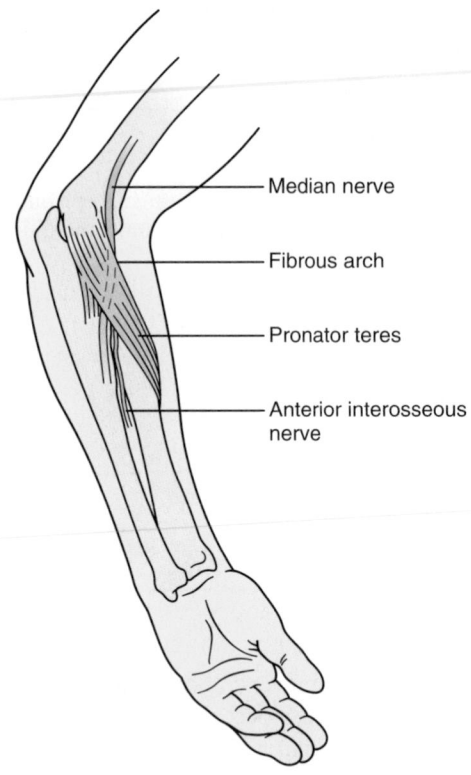

Figure 6-38
Anterior interosseous syndrome.

resulting pinch is pulp to pulp rather than tip to tip. It has been reported that the nerve may also be injured with a forearm fracture (Monteggia fracture).[35] With anterior interosseous syndrome, there is no sensory loss, because the anterior interosseous nerve is a motor nerve; signs and symptoms of the condition are related to motor function.

Ulnar Nerve (C7-C8, T1). In the elbow region, the ulnar nerve is most likely to be injured, compressed, or stretched in the **cubital tunnel** (see Figure 6-4).[31,36-40] In fact, it is a common entrapment neuropathy, second only to carpal tunnel syndrome. The ulnar nerve may be injured or compressed as a result of swelling (e.g., trauma, pregnancy), osteophytes, arthritic diseases, trauma, or repeated microtrauma. This tunnel, which is relatively long, can compress the nerve as the nerve passes through the tunnel or between the two heads of the flexor carpi ulnaris muscle. Compression is altered as the elbow moves from extension (decreased) to flexion (increased), causing traction on the nerve, and is further enhanced if a significant cubitus valgus is present.[41,42] Symptoms therefore are more likely to occur when the elbow is flexed. It is usually in the cubital tunnel area that the ulnar nerve is affected, leading to tardy ulnar palsy.

Tardy ulnar palsy implies that the symptoms of nerve injury come on long after the patient has been injured; this delayed reaction seems to be unique to the ulnar nerve.

Although most common in adults, it has been reported in children, and in children the delay has been up to 29 months.[43] In adults, the possibility of a double crush injury (at cervical spine and elbow) should always be considered.

Injury to the ulnar nerve in the cubital tunnel affects the flexor carpi ulnaris and the ulnar half of the flexor digitorum profundus in the forearm, the hypothenar eminence in the hand (flexor digiti minimi, abductor digiti minimi, opponens digiti minimi, and adductor pollicis), the interossei, and the third and fourth lumbricals (see Table 6-2). Although these muscles show weakness and atrophy over time, the earliest and most obvious symptoms are sensory, with pain and paresthesia in the medial elbow and forearm and paresthesia in the ulnar sensory distribution of the hand (see Figure 7-72).

Radial Nerve (C5-C8, T1). The radial nerve may be injured near the elbow if there is a fracture of the shaft of the humerus. The nerve may be damaged as it winds around behind the humerus in the radial groove. Injury may occur at the time of the fracture, or the nerve may get caught in the callus of fracture healing. Because the radial nerve supplies all of the extensor muscles of the arm, only the triceps is spared with this type of injury, and even it may show some weakness.

The major branch of the radial nerve in the forearm is the **posterior interosseous nerve,** which is given off in front of the lateral epicondyle of the humerus.[31,44] This branch may compress as it passes between the two heads of the supinator in the **arcade** or **canal of Frohse**, a fibrous arch in the supinator muscle occurring in 30% of the population (Figure 6-39). Compression leads to functional involvement of the forearm extensor muscles (see Table 6-2) and functional wrist drop, so the patient has difficulty or is unable to stabilize the wrist for proper hand function. Diagnosis of this condition is often delayed because there is no sensory deficit. This compression zone is one of five sites in the tunnel through which the radial nerve passes.

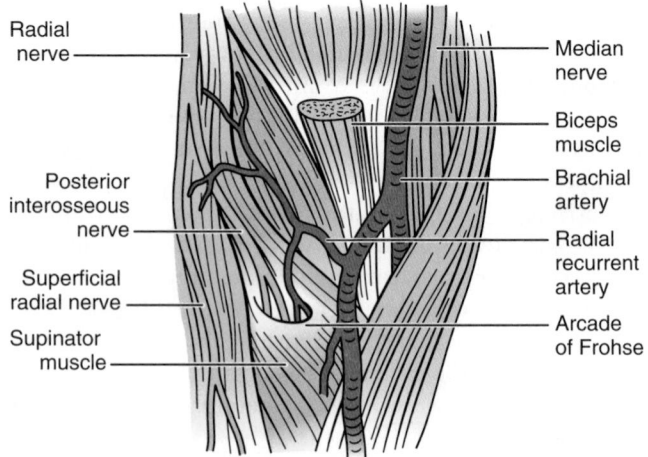

Figure 6-39
Canal or arcade of Frohse.

The nerve may also be compressed at the entrance to the tunnel anterior to the head of the radius, near where the nerve supplies brachioradialis and extensor carpi radialis longus, between the ulnar half of the tendon of extensor carpi radialis brevis and its fascia, and at the distal border of supinator.[45,46] This condition, sometimes called **radial tunnel syndrome,** may mimic tennis elbow.[25,45,47–50] If the patient has a persistent form of tennis elbow, a possible nerve lesion or cervical problem should be considered.

A third area of pathology is compression of the superficial branch of the radial nerve as it passes under the tendon of the brachioradialis. This branch is sensory only, and the patient complains primarily of nocturnal pain along the dorsum of the wrist, thumb, and web space. Trauma, a tight cast, or any swelling in the area may cause the compression. The condition is referred to as **cheiralgia paresthetica** or **Wartenberg's disease.**[39]

Joint Play Movements

When examining the joint play movements (Figure 6-40), the examiner must compare the injured side with the normal side.

Joint Play Movements of the Elbow Complex
• Radial deviation of the ulna and radius on the humerus • Ulnar deviation of the ulna and radius on the humerus • Distraction of the olecranon from the humerus in 90° of flexion • Anteroposterior glide of the radius on the humerus

Radial and ulnar deviations of the ulna and radius on the humerus are performed in a fashion similar to those in the collateral ligament tests but with less elbow flexion. The examiner stabilizes the patient's elbow by holding the patient's humerus firmly and places the other hand above the patient's wrist, abducting and adducting the forearm (see Figure 6-40, *A*). The patient's elbow is almost straight (extended) during the movement, and the end feel should be bone to bone.

To distract the olecranon from the humerus, the examiner flexes the patient's elbow to 90°. Wrapping both hands around the patient's forearm close to the elbow, the examiner then applies a distractive force at the elbow, ensuring that no torque is applied (see Figure 6-40, *B*). If the patient has a sore shoulder, counter force should be applied with one hand around the humerus.

To test anteroposterior glide of the radius on the humerus, the examiner stabilizes the patient's forearm. The patient's arm is held between the examiner's body and arm. The examiner places the thumb of his or her hand over the anterior radial head while the flexed index finger is over the posterior radial head. The examiner then pushes the radial head posteriorly with the thumb and anteriorly with the index finger (see Figure 6-40, *C*). Commonly, posterior movement is easier to obtain, with anterior movement, in normals, being the result of the radial head returning to its normal position with a tissue stretch end feel. This movement must be performed with care because it can be very painful as a result of pinching of the skin between the examiner's digits and the bone. In addition, pain may result from

A

B

Figure 6-40
Joint play movements of the elbow complex. **A,** Radial and ulnar deviation of the ulna on the humerus.
B, Distraction of the olecranon process from the humerus.

Continued

Figure 6-40 cont'd
C, Anteroposterior movement of the radius.

Figure 6-41
Joint play of the head of the radius (method 2). Anteroposterior (**A**) and posteroanterior (**B**) glide of the radius.

the force being applied even in the normal arm, so both sides must be compared.

The anterior and posterior glide of the radius may be tested in a slightly different way as well. To do anteroposterior glide of the head of the radius, the patient is placed in supine with the arm by the side. The examiner stands beside the patient, facing the patient's head, and holds the patient's arm slightly flexed by holding the hand between the examiner's thorax and elbow. The examiner places the thumbs over the head of the radius and carefully applies an anteroposterior pressure to the head of the radius feeling the amount of movement and end feel. To do posteroanterior glide, the patient is in supine lying with the arm at the side and the hand resting on the stomach. The examiner places the thumbs over the posterior aspect of the radial head and carefully applies a posteroanterior pressure (Figure 6-41).

Palpation

With the patient's arm relaxed, the examiner begins palpation on the anterior aspect of the elbow and moves to the medial aspect, the lateral aspect, and finally the posterior aspect (Figure 6-42). The patient may sit or lie supine, whichever is more comfortable. The joint line is located about 2 cm below an imaginary line joining the two epicondyles.[4] The examiner is looking for any tenderness, abnormality, change in temperature or in texture of the tissues, or abnormal bumps. As with all palpation, the injured side must be compared with the normal or uninjured side.

Anterior Aspect

Cubital Fossa. The fossa is bound by the pronator teres muscle medially, the brachioradialis muscle laterally, and an imaginary line joining the two epicondyles superiorly. Within the fossa, the biceps tendon and brachial artery may be palpated. After crossing the elbow joint, the **brachial artery** divides into two branches, the radial artery and the ulnar artery. The examiner must be aware of the brachial artery because it has the potential for being injured as a result of severe trauma at the elbow (e.g., fracture, dislocation). Trauma to this area may lead to compartment syndromes such as **Volkmann's ischemic contracture.** The median and musculocutaneous nerves are also found in the fossa, but they are not palpable. Pressure on the median nerve may cause symptoms in its cutaneous distribution.

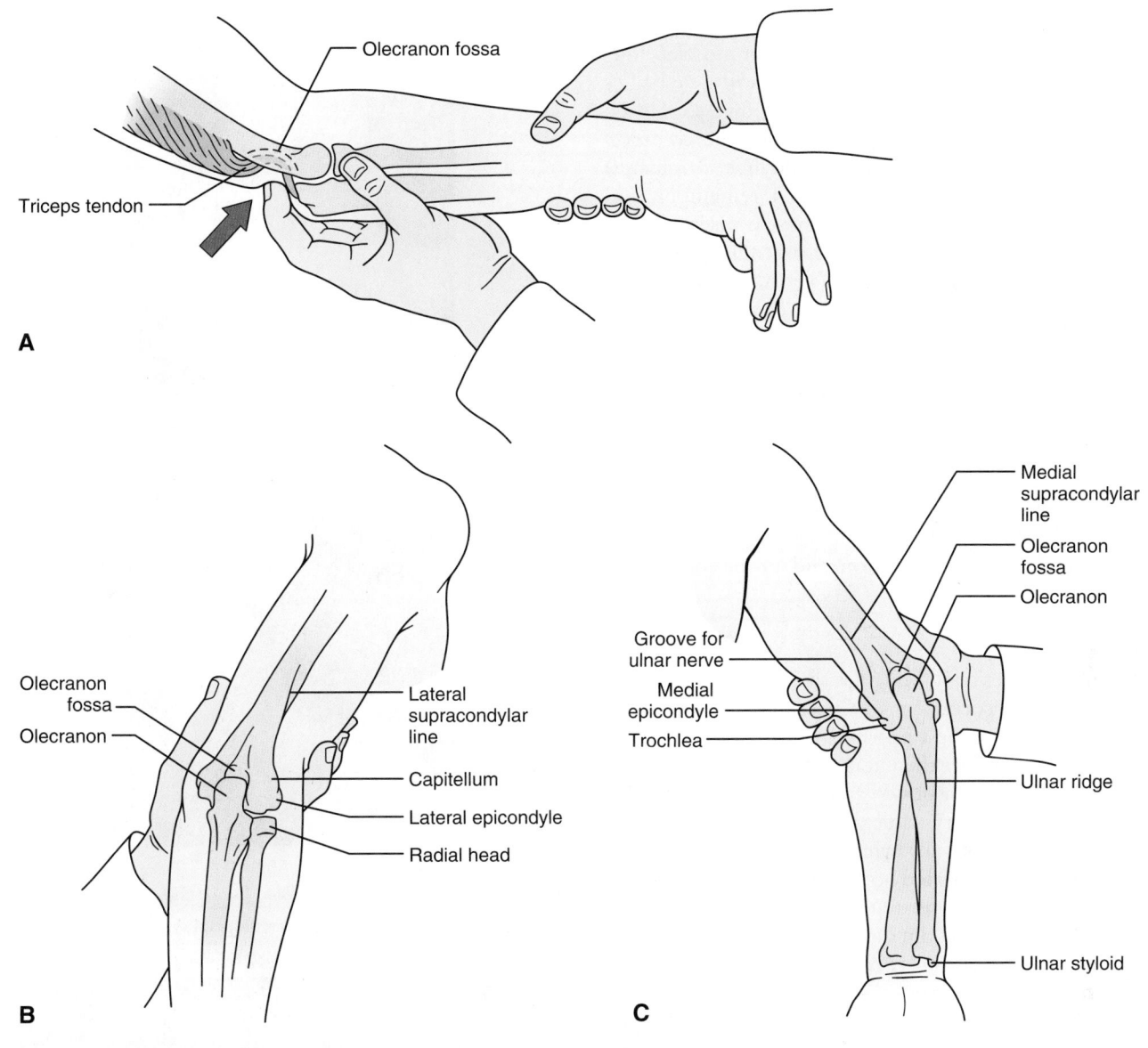

Figure 6-42
Palpation around the elbow. **A,** Olecranon fossa. **B,** Posterolateral aspect of the elbow. **C,** Posteromedial aspect of the elbow.

Coronoid Process and Head of Radius. Within the cubital fossa, if the examiner palpates carefully so as not to hurt the patient, the coronoid process of the ulna and the head of the radius may be palpated. Palpation of the radial head is facilitated by supination and pronation of the forearm. The examiner may palpate the head of the radius from the posterior aspect at the same time by placing the fingers over the head on the posterior aspect and the thumb over it on the anterior aspect. In addition to the muscles previously mentioned, the biceps and brachialis muscles may be palpated for potential abnormality.

Medial Aspect

Medial Epicondyle. Originating from the medial epicondyle are the **wrist flexor-forearm pronator** groups of muscles. Both the muscle bellies and their insertions into bone should be palpated. Tenderness over the epicondyle where the muscles insert is sometimes called golfer's elbow or tennis elbow of the medial epicondyle.

Medial (Ulnar) Collateral Ligament. This fan-shaped ligament may be palpated as it extends from the medial epicondyle to the medial margin of the coronoid process anteriorly and to the olecranon process posteriorly.

Ulnar Nerve. If the examiner moves posteriorly behind the medial epicondyle, the fingers will rest over the ulnar nerve in the cubital tunnel (proximal part). Usually, the nerve is not directly palpable, but pressure on the nerve often causes abnormal sensations in its cutaneous distribution. It is this nerve that is struck when someone hits his or her "funny bone."

Lateral Aspect

Lateral Epicondyle. The wrist extensor muscles originate from the lateral epicondyle, and their muscle bellies as well as their insertions into the epicondyle should be palpated. It is at this point of insertion of the common extensor tendon that lateral epicondylitis originates. When palpating, the examiner should remember that the extensor carpi radialis longus muscle inserts above the epicondyle along a short ridge extending from the epicondyle to the humeral shaft. The examiner palpates the brachioradialis and supinator muscles on the lateral aspect of the elbow at the same time.

Lateral (Radial) Collateral Ligament. This cordlike ligament may be palpated as it extends from the lateral epicondyle of the humerus to the annular ligament and lateral surface of the ulna.

Annular Ligament. Distal to the lateral epicondyle, the annular ligament and head of the radius may be palpated if this has not previously been done. The palpation is facilitated by supination and pronation of the forearm.

Posterior Aspect

Palpation of posterior structures is shown in Figure 6-42.

Olecranon Process and Olecranon Bursa. The olecranon process is best palpated with the elbow flexed to 90°. If the examiner then grasps the skin overlying the process, the olecranon bursa can be palpated. Normally, it just feels like slippery tissue as the skin is moved. The examiner should note any synovial thickening, swelling, or the presence of any **rice bodies**, which are small seeds of fragmented fibrous tissue that can act as further irritants to the bursa should it be affected.

Triceps Muscle. The triceps muscle, which inserts into the olecranon process, should be palpated both at its insertion and along its length for any signs of abnormality.

Diagnostic Imaging

Plain Film Radiography

Anteroposterior View. The examiner should note the relation of the epicondyles, trochlea, capitulum, radial head, radial tuberosity, coronoid process, and olecranon process (Figure 6-43). Any loose bodies, calcification, myositis ossificans, joint space narrowing, or osteophytes should be identified. If the patient is a young child, the examiner should check the epiphyseal plate to see if it is normal for each bone.

Lateral View. The examiner should note the relation of the epicondyles, trochlea, capitulum, radial head, radial tuberosity, coronoid process, and olecranon process. As with the anteroposterior view, any loose bodies, calcifications in or around the joint (Figure 6-44), myositis ossificans, dislocations (Figure 6-45), joint space

A

B

Figure 6-43 ▬▬▬▬▬
Posteroanterior (**A**) and lateral (**B**) radiographs of the elbow.

Figure 6-44 ▬▬▬▬▬
Excessive ossification *(arrow)* after dislocation of elbow treated by early active use. (From O'Donoghue DH: *Treatment of injuries to athletes,* ed 4, p. 232, Philadelphia, 1984, WB Saunders.)

Figure 6-45
Lateral film of a dislocated elbow, showing the lower end of the humerus resting on the ulna in front of the coronoid. Note fragmentation of the coronoid. (From O'Donoghue DH: *Treatment of injuries to athletes,* ed 4, p. 227, Philadelphia, 1984, WB Saunders.)

Figure 6-47
Cubital tunnel. The ulnar nerve *(asterisk)* lies in a tunnel bridged by the arcuate ligament *(dashed line),* which extends from the medial epicondyle to the olecranon process. LAT = lateral.

Figure 6-46
Coronoid process fracture with hemarthrosis. The posterior fat pad *(arrows)* is shown clearly on this lateral view with the arm flexed to 90°, indicating joint effusion. The anterior fat pad *(open arrow)* is clearly visible. There is a fracture of the coronoid process *(curved arrow)* and a loose body *(arrowhead).* (From Weissman BNW, Sledge CB: *Orthopedic radiology,* p. 179, Philadelphia, 1986, WB Saunders.)

narrowing, or osteophytes should be noted. The presence of the **fat pad** sign (Figure 6-46) occurs with elbow joint effusion and may indicate, for example, a fracture, acute rheumatoid arthritis, infection, or osteoid osteoma.[51] Plain radiographs may also be used to visualize the cubital tunnel (Figure 6-47) and to measure the carrying angle (see Figure 6-6).

Axial View. This view is taken with the elbow flexed to 45°. It shows the olecranon process and epicondyles. It is useful for showing osteophytes and loose bodies.[28]

Arthrography
Figure 6-48 illustrates the views seen in normal elbow arthrograms. With the advent of magnetic resonance imaging, this technique is seldom used today.

Magnetic Resonance Imaging
Magnetic resonance imaging (MRI) is used to differentiate bone and soft tissues. Because of its high soft-tissue contrast, MRI, a noninvasive technique, is able to discriminate among bone marrow, cartilage, tendons, nerves, and vessels without the use of a contrast medium (Figures 6-49 to 6-51).[52,53] The technique is used to demonstrate tendon ruptures, collateral ligament ruptures, cubital tunnel pathology, epicondylitis, and osteochondritis dissecans.[54-56]

Xerography
Figure 6-52 illustrates the detailed borders of the various structures around the elbow.

Figure 6-48

Normal elbow arthrogram. Anteroposterior **(A),** external oblique **(B),** and lateral **(C)** views in extension show the normal annular (*a*), anterior (*A*), and posterior (*P*) recesses. **D,** Lateral tomogram with the arm extended. The area of the trochlea that is devoid of cartilage *(arrow)* is shown. From Weissman BNW, Sledge CB: *Orthopedic radiology,* p. 178, Philadelphia, 1986, WB Saunders.)

Figure 6-49

Normal common extensor tendon and the medial collateral ligament (MCL). **A,** Oblique coronal T1-weighted A spine echo and fat-saturated proton density. **B,** Fast spin echo image demonstrates the normal, smooth, thin contour and low signal of the common extensor tendon (*long* arrow) and anterior bundle of the MCL (*short arrows*). (From Schenk M, Dalinka MK: Imaging of the elbow: an update, *Orthop Clin North Am* 28:519, 1997.)

Figure 6-50

Lateral epicondylitis tendinitis. Oblique coronal fat-saturated proton density **(A)** and T2-weighted **(B)** fast spin echo images. Focal calcification within the common extensor tendon *(white arrow)*. There is a moderately increased signal within the tendon, without fiber disruption. Note the edema in the peritendinous tissues *(black arrows)*, suggesting active inflammation. (From Schenk M, Dalinka MK: Imaging of the elbow: an update, *Orthop Clin North Am* 28:524, 1997.)

Figure 6-51

A and **B**, MCL tear. Surgically proven tear in an athlete who was injured 3 months before imaging and complained of persistent pain with throwing. Oblique coronal fat-saturated proton density image shows a complete tear of the anterior bundle at its distal attachment to the ulna *(long arrow)*. Note the lateral ulna collateral ligament inserting into the ulna *(short arrows)*. Also note the bright signal within the subcutaneous fat laterally *(open arrows)*, which is secondary to incomplete fat suppression and should not be mistaken for edema. Three-dimensional gradient echo image reformatted along the plane of the MCL also demonstrates the distal tear *(arrow)*. (From Schenk M, Dalinka MK: Imaging of the elbow: an update, *Orthop Clin North Am* 28:528, 1997.)

Figure 6-52

Xerogram of the elbow demonstrating the fat pads and supinator fat stripe resulting from subtle radial head fracture. (From Berquist TH: Diagnostic radiographic techniques of the elbow. In Morrey BF, editor: *The elbow and its disorders*, p. 106, Philadelphia, 1993, WB Saunders.)

Précis of the Elbow Assessment*

History
Observation
Examination
   Active movements
      Elbow flexion
      Elbow extension
      Supination
      Pronation
      Combined movements (if necessary)
      Repetitive movements (if necessary)
      Sustained positions (if necessary)
   Passive movements (as in active movements, if necessary)
   Resisted isometric movements
      Elbow flexion
      Elbow extension
      Supination
      Pronation
      Wrist flexion
      Wrist extension

Special tests
Reflexes and cutaneous distribution
   Reflexes
   Sensory scan
   Peripheral nerves
      Median nerve and branches
      Ulnar nerve
      Radial nerve and branches
Joint play movements
   Radial deviation of ulna and radius on humerus
   Ulnar deviation of ulna and radius on humerus
   Distraction of olecranon process on humerus in 90° of flexion
   Anteroposterior glide of radius on humerus
Palpation
Diagnostic imaging

---

*The entire assessment may be done with the patient in sitting position. After any examination, the patient should be warned of the possibility that symptoms may exacerbate as a result of the assessment.

Case Studies

When doing these case studies, the examiner should list the appropriate questions to ask the patient and should specify why they are being asked, what to look for and why, and what things should be tested and why. Depending on the patient's answers (and the examiner should consider numerous different responses), several possible causes of the patient's problem may become evident (examples are given in parentheses). The examiner should prepare a differential diagnosis chart (Table 6-5 is an example for question 1). The examiner can then decide how different diagnoses may affect the treatment plan.

1. A 24-year-old woman comes to you complaining of pain in her right elbow on the medial side. The pain sometimes extends into the forearm and is often accompanied by tingling into the little finger and half of the ring finger. The pain and paresthesia are particularly bothersome when she plays recreational volleyball, which she enjoys very much. Describe your assessment plan for this patient (ulnar neuritis versus medial epicondylitis).

Continued

Case Studies—cont'd

2. A 52-year-old man is referred to you with a history of right elbow pain. He complains of tenderness over the lateral epicondyle. He informs you that he has not done any repetitive forearm activity and does not play tennis. He has some restriction of neck movement. Describe your assessment plan for this patient (cervical spondylosis versus lateral epicondylitis).

3. A 26-year-old male football player is referred to you after surgery for a ruptured (third-degree strain) left biceps tendon at its insertion. His cast has been removed, and you have been asked to restore the patient to normal function. Describe your assessment plan for this patient.

4. Parents bring their 4-year-old daughter in to see you. They state that about 2 hours previously they were out shopping and the mother was holding the little girl's arm. The little girl tripped, and the mother "yanked" her up as she fell. The little girl started to cry and would not move her elbow. Describe your assessment plan for this patient (radial head dislocation versus ligamentous sprain).

5. A 46-year-old man comes to you complaining of diffuse left elbow pain. When he carries a briefcase for three or four blocks, his elbow becomes stiff and sore. When he picks up things with his left hand, the pain increases dramatically. Describe your assessment plan for this patient (lateral epicondylitis versus osteoarthritis).

6. A 31-year-old man comes to you complaining of posterior elbow pain. He says he banged his elbow on the table 10 days earlier, and he has had posterior swelling for 8 or 9 days. Describe your assessment plan for this patient (olecranon bursitis versus joint synovitis).

7. A 14-year-old female gymnast comes to you complaining of elbow pain. She explains she was doing a vault and bent her elbow backward, at which time she heard a snap. The injury occurred 1 hour earlier, and there is some swelling; she does not want to move the elbow. Describe your assessment plan for this patient (biceps tendon rupture versus epiphyseal fracture).

Table 6-5
Differential Diagnosis of Ulnar Neuritis and Medial Epicondylitis

	Ulnar Neuritis	**Medial Epicondylitis**
History	May follow repetitive activity May follow bumped elbow May follow previously injured elbow Pain in forearm and into ulnar distribution of hand	Usually follows repetitive activity Pain in forearm, may radiate to wrist
Observation	Normal	Normal
Active movements	Weakness of ulnar deviation Weakness of little and ring finger flexion	Slight pain on wrist flexion
Passive movements	Normal, or pain may come on with elbow flexion and wrist flexion	Normal, but pain may occur with elbow extension and wrist extension
Resisted isometric movements	Weakness of ulnar deviation Weakness of little and ring finger flexion	Pain on wrist extension with elbow extension Pain on supination and wrist and finger flexion Golfer's elbow test positive
Special tests Sensation	Tinel's sign positive Wartenberg's sign positive Elbow flexion test positive Paresthesia and pain in forearm, little finger, and half of ring finger	Pain in forearm, possibly to wrist

References

To enhance this text and add value for the reader, all references have been incorporated into a CD-ROM that is provided with this text. The reader can view the reference source and access it online whenever possible. There are a total of 57 cited and other general references for this chapter.

APPENDIX 6-1

RELIABILITY, VALIDITY, SPECIFICITY, AND SENSITIVITY OF SPECIAL/DIAGNOSTIC TESTS USED IN THE ELBOW

MOVING VALGUS STRESS TEST

Specificity	Sensitivity
75%[17]	100%[17]

PATIENT RELATED FOREARM EVALUATION QUESTIONNAIRE

Reliability

Test retest: pain section ICC = 0.87, function section ICC = 0.77, total ICC = 0.86[57]

FOREARM, WRIST, AND HAND

The hand and wrist are the most active and intricate parts of the upper extremity. Because of this, they are vulnerable to injury, which can lead to large functional difficulties, and they do not respond well to serious trauma. Their mobility is enhanced by a wide range of movement at the shoulder and complementary movement at the elbow. The 28 bones, numerous articulations, and 19 intrinsic and 20 extrinsic muscles of the wrist and hand provide a tremendous variability of movement. In addition to being an expressive organ of communication, the hand has a protective role and acts as both a motor and a sensory organ, providing information such as temperature, thickness, texture, depth, and shape as well as the motion of an object. It is this sensual acuity that enables the examiner to accurately examine and palpate during an assessment.

The assessment of the hand and wrist should be performed with two objectives in mind. First, the injury or lesion should be assessed as accurately as possible to ensure proper treatment. Second, the examiner should evaluate the remaining function to determine whether the patient will have any incapacity in everyday life.

Although the joints of the forearm, wrist, and hand are discussed separately, they do not act in isolation but rather as functional groups. The position of one joint influences the position and action of the other joints. For example, if the wrist is flexed, the interphalangeal joints do not fully flex, primarily because of passive insufficiency of the finger extensors and their tendons. Each articulation depends on balanced forces for proper positioning and control. If this balance or equilibrium is not present because of trauma, nerve injury, or other factors, the loss of counterbalancing forces results in deformities. In addition, the entire upper limb should be considered

a kinetic chain that enables the hand to be properly positioned. The actions of the shoulder, elbow, and wrist joints enable the hand to be placed on almost any area of the body.

Applied Anatomy

The **distal radioulnar joint** is a uniaxial pivot joint that has one degree of freedom.[1] Although the radius moves over the ulna, the ulna does not remain stationary. It moves back and laterally during pronation and forward and medially during supination. The resting position of the joint is 10° of supination, and the close packed position is 5° of supination. The capsular pattern of the distal radioulnar joint is full range of motion (ROM) with pain at the extreme of rotation.

Distal Radioulnar Joint	
Resting position:	10° of supination
Close packed position:	5° of supination
Capsular pattern:	Pain at extreme of rotation

The **radiocarpal (wrist) joint** is a biaxial ellipsoid joint.[1,2] The radius articulates with the scaphoid and lunate. The distal radius is not straight but is angled toward the ulna (15°–20°), and its posterior margin projects more distally to provide a "buttress effect."[3] The lunate and triquetrum also articulate with the triangular cartilaginous disc (triangular fibrocartilage complex [TFCC]) (Figures 7-1 and 7-2) and not the ulna.

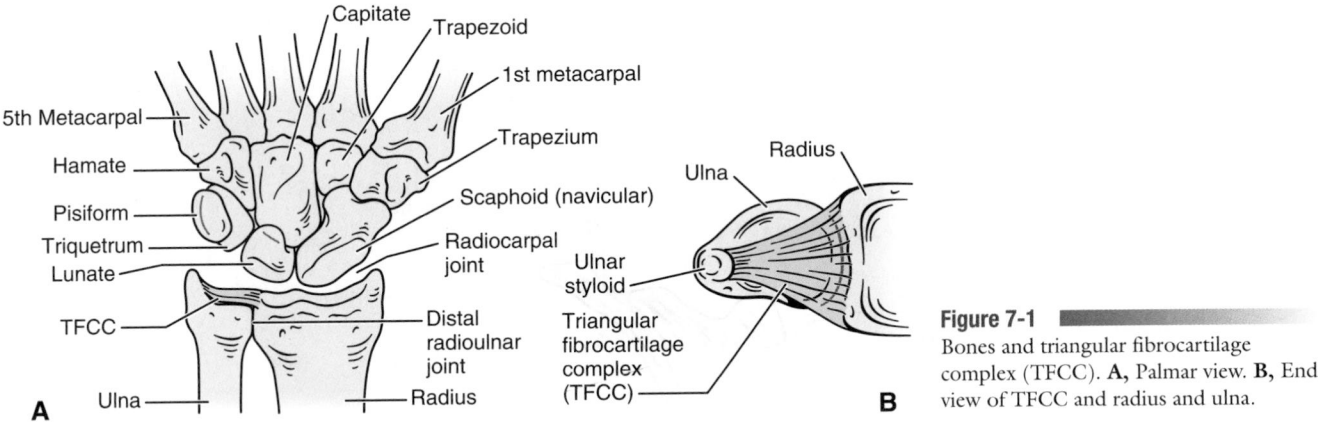

Figure 7-1
Bones and triangular fibrocartilage
complex (TFCC). **A,** Palmar view. **B,** End
view of TFCC and radius and ulna.

Figure 7-2
Articulations of the wrist: specific compartments. Ulnar limit of
the radiocarpal compartment (coronal section). Note the extent
of this compartment *(1)*, its relationship to the inferior radioulnar
compartment *(2)*, the intervening triangular fibrocartilage *(arrow)*,
and the prestyloid recess *(arrowhead)*, which is intimate with the ulnar
styloid(s). (From Resnick D, Kransdorf MJ: *Bone and joint imaging*,
p. 27, Philadelphia, 2005, W.B. Saunders.)

be damaged by forced extension and pronation. The
distal end of the radius is concave and the proximal row
of carpals is convex, but the curvatures are not equal.
The joint has two degrees of freedom, and the resting
position is neutral with slight ulnar deviation. The close
packed position is extension, and the capsular pattern is
equal limitation of flexion and extension.

Radiocarpal (Wrist) Joint

Resting position:	Neutral with slight ulnar deviation
Close packed position:	Extension
Capsular pattern:	Flexion and extension equally limited (works with midcarpal joints)

The disc extends from the ulnar side of the distal radius
and attaches to the ulna at the base of the ulnar styloid process. The disc adds stability to the wrist. It creates a close relation between the ulna and carpal bones
and binds together and stabilizes the distal ends of the
radius and ulna.[4,5] With the disc in place, the radius
bears 60% of the load and the ulna bears 40%. If the disc
is removed, the radius transmits 95% of the axial load
and the ulna transmits 5%.[6] Therefore, the cartilaginous
disc acts as a cushion for the wrist joint and as a major
stabilizer of the distal radioulnar joint.[3,7] The disc can

The stability of the carpals (wrist) is primarily maintained
by a complex configuration of ligaments (Figure 7-3).[8]
The ligaments stabilizing the scaphoid, lunate, and triquetrum are the most important.[9] Of these ligaments, the
radioscapholunate ligament is one of the most important
because it is commonly injured and, when intact, maintains
carpal stability.[10] This ligament is most likely to be injured
with a pronated FOOSH injury (wrist extension, ulnar
deviation and intercarpal supination).[9,11] Lunotriquetral
injuries are more likely to occur with wrist extension,
radial deviation, and intercarpal supination.[9] The palmar
ligaments are much stronger than the dorsal ligaments.
The palmar extrinsic ligaments control the movement of
the wrist and scaphoid with the radioscapholunate ligament acting as a sling for the scaphoid.[10] This ligament
along with the radiolunate ligament allows the scaphoid
to rotate around them, and both stabilize the scaphoid at
the extremes of motion.[10] On the ulnar side, the ligaments

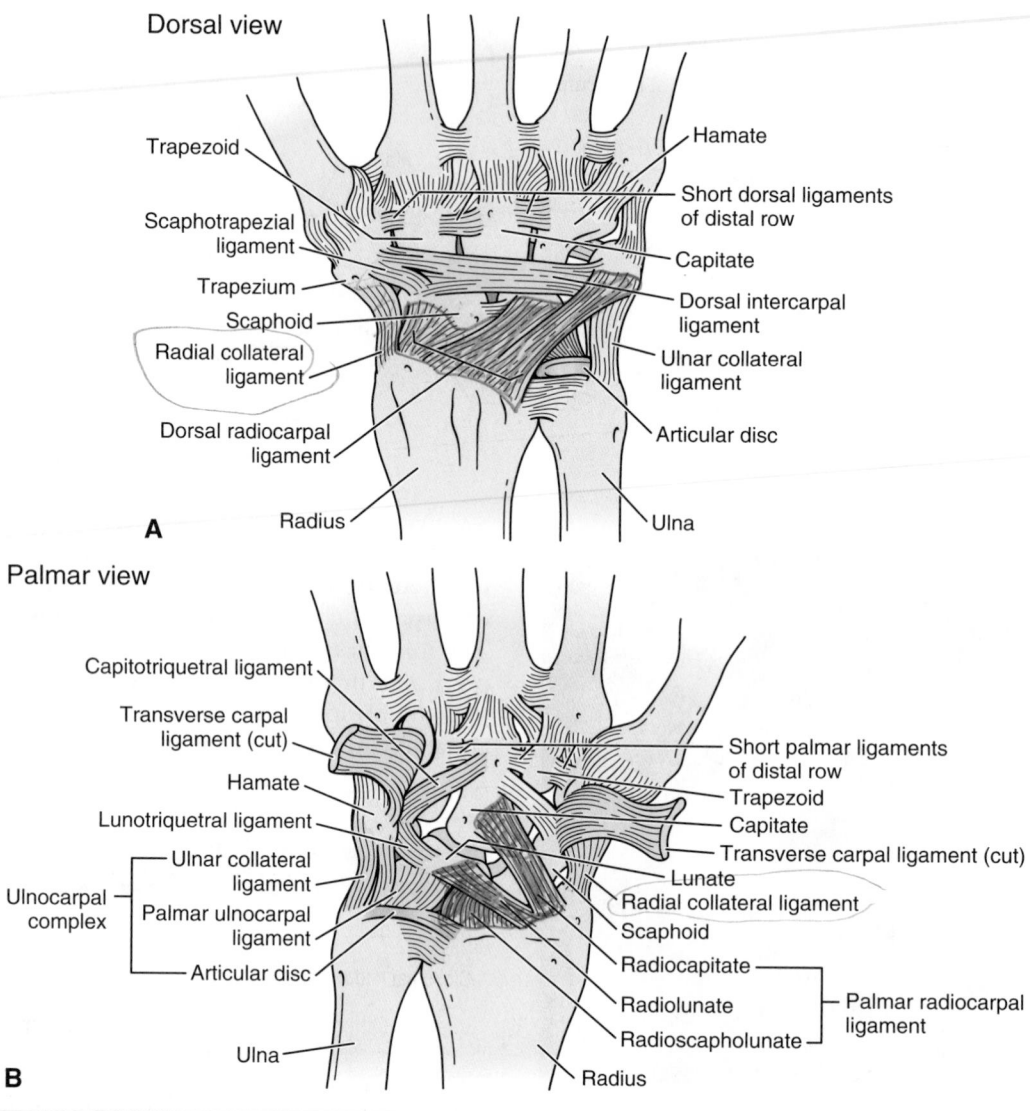

Dorsal view

Trapezoid
Scaphotrapezial ligament
Trapezium
Scaphoid
Radial collateral ligament
Dorsal radiocarpal ligament
Radius

Hamate
Short dorsal ligaments of distal row
Capitate
Dorsal intercarpal ligament
Ulnar collateral ligament
Articular disc
Ulna

A

Palmar view

Capitotriquetral ligament
Transverse carpal ligament (cut)
Hamate
Lunotriquetral ligament
Ulnocarpal complex
 — Ulnar collateral ligament
 — Palmar ulnocarpal ligament
 — Articular disc
Ulna

Short palmar ligaments of distal row
Trapezoid
Capitate
Transverse carpal ligament (cut)
Lunate
Radial collateral ligament
Scaphoid
Radiocapitate —
Radiolunate — Palmar radiocarpal ligament
Radioscapholunate —
Radius

B

Figure 7-3

Ligaments of the wrist. **A,** Dorsal aspect of the right wrist. **B,** Palmar aspect of the right wrist. The transverse carpal ligament has been cut and reflected to show the underlying ligaments. (Redrawn from Neumann DA: *Kinesiology of the musculoskeletal system—foundations for physical rehabilitation,* pp. 178–179, St Louis, 2002, C.V. Mosby.)

(palmar lunotriquetral, capitotriquetral, dorsal intercarpal, and the fibrocartilaginous disc) control the triquetrum.

The **intercarpal joints** include the joints between the individual bones of the proximal row of carpal bones (scaphoid, lunate, and triquetrum) and the joints between the individual bones of the distal row of carpal bones (trapezium, trapezoid, capitate, and hamate). Perilunate injuries involve the lunate and its relation with the other carpals as well as the radius and ulna.[12] They are bound together by small intercarpal ligaments (dorsal, palmar, and interosseous), which allow only a slight amount of gliding movement between the bones. The close packed position is extension, and the resting position is neutral

or slight flexion. The **pisotriquetral joint** is considered separately because the pisiform sits on the triquetrum and does not take a direct part in the other intercarpal movements.

Intercarpal Joints	
Resting position:	Neutral or slight flexion
Close packed position:	Extension
Capsular pattern:	None

The **midcarpal joints** form a compound articulation between the proximal and distal rows of carpal bones, with the exception of the pisiform bone. On the medial side, the scaphoid, lunate, and triquetrum articulate with the capitate and hamate, forming a compound sellar (saddle-shaped) joint. On the lateral aspect, the scaphoid articulates with the trapezoid and trapezium, forming another compound sellar joint. As with the intercarpal joints, these articulations are bound together by dorsal and palmar ligaments; however, there are no interosseous ligaments between the proximal and distal rows of bones. Therefore, greater movement exists at the midcarpal joints than between the individual bones of the two rows of the intercarpal joints. The close packed position of these joints is extension with ulnar deviation, and the resting position is neutral or slight flexion with ulnar deviation.

Midcarpal Joints

Resting position:	Neutral or slight flexion with ulnar deviation
Close packed position:	Extension with ulnar deviation
Capsular pattern:	Equal limitation of flexion and extension (works with radiocarpal joints)

At the thumb, the **carpometacarpal joint** is a sellar joint that has three degrees of freedom, whereas the second to fifth carpometacarpal joints are plane joints.[13] The capsular pattern of the carpometacarpal joint of the thumb is abduction most limited, followed by extension. The resting position is midway between abduction and adduction and midway between flexion and extension. The close packed position of the carpometacarpal joint of the thumb is full opposition. For the second to fifth carpometacarpal joints, the capsular pattern of restriction is equal limitation in all directions. The bones of these joints are held together by dorsal and palmar ligaments. In addition, the thumb articulation has a strong lateral ligament extending from the lateral side of the trapezium to the radial side of the base of the first metacarpal, and the medial four articulations have an interosseous ligament similar to that found in the carpal articulation.

The carpometacarpal articulations of the fingers allow only gliding movement. The second and third carpometacarpal joints tend to be relatively immobile and are the primary "stabilizing" joints of the hand, whereas the fourth and fifth joints are more mobile to allow the hand to adapt to different shaped objects during grasping. The carpometacarpal articulation of the thumb is unique in

Carpometacarpal Joints

Resting position:	Thumb, midway between abduction and adduction, and midway between flexion and extension Fingers, midway between flexion and extension
Close packed position:	Thumb, full opposition Fingers, full flexion
Capsular pattern:	Thumb, abduction, then extension Fingers, equal limitation in all directions

that it allows flexion, extension, abduction, adduction, rotation, and circumduction. It is able to do this because the articulation is saddle shaped. Because of the many movements possible at this joint, the thumb is able to adopt any position relative to the palmar aspect of the hand.[13]

The plane **intermetacarpal joints** have only a small amount of gliding movement between them and do not include the thumb articulation. They are bound together by palmar, dorsal, and interosseous ligaments.

The **metacarpophalangeal joints** are condyloid joints. The collateral ligaments of these joints are tight on flexion and relaxed on extension. These articulations are also bound by palmar ligaments and deep transverse metacarpal ligaments. The dorsal or extensor hood (Figure 7-4) reinforces the dorsal aspect of the metacarpophalangeal joints while volar plates reinforce the palmar aspect.[3] Each joint has two degrees of freedom. The first metacarpophalangeal joint has three degrees of freedom, thus facilitating the movement of the carpometacarpal joint of the thumb.[13] The close packed position of the first metacarpophalangeal joint is maximum opposition, and the close packed position for the second through the fifth metacarpophalangeal joints is maximum flexion.[14] The resting position of the metacarpophalangeal joints is slight flexion, whereas the capsular pattern is more limitation of flexion than extension.

Metacarpophalangeal Joints

Resting position:	Slight flexion
Close packed position:	Thumb, full opposition Fingers, full flexion
Capsular pattern:	Flexion, then extension

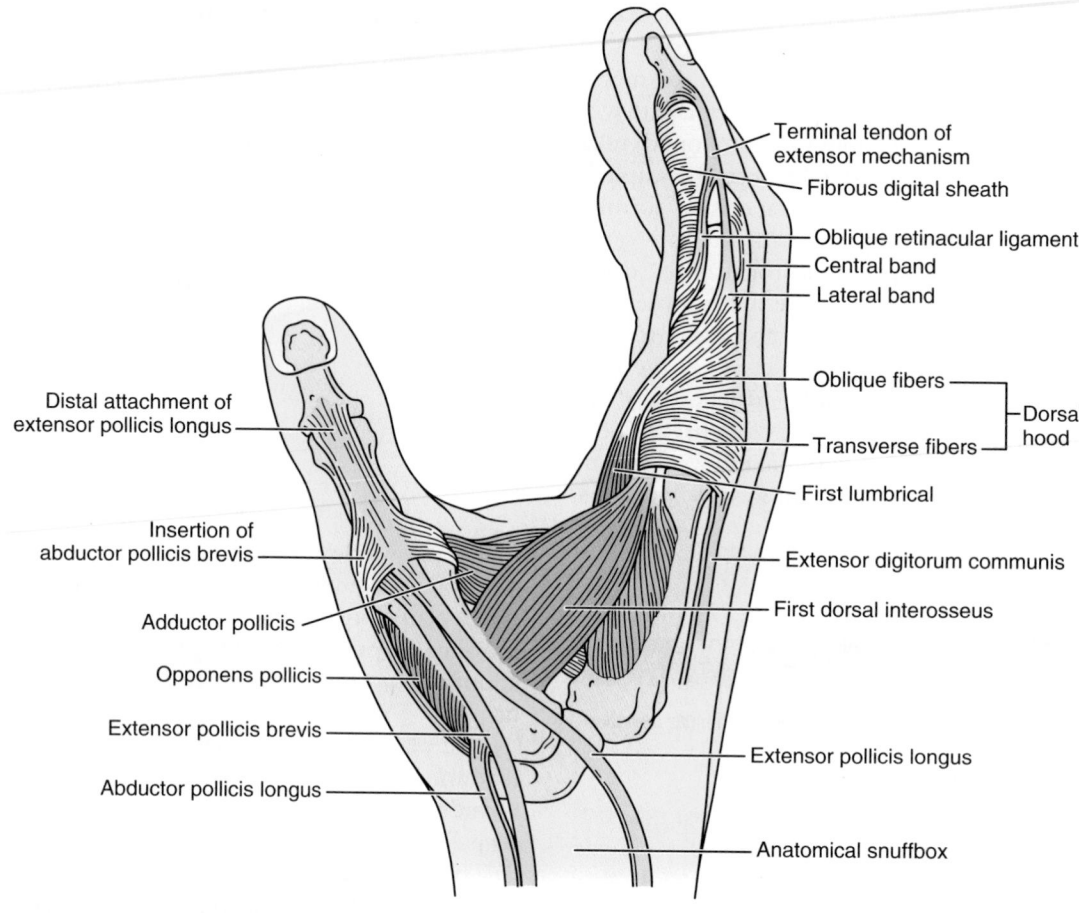

Figure 7-4

Radial (lateral) view of the muscles, tendons, and extensor mechanism including the dorsal hood of the right hand. (Redrawn from Neumann DA: *Kinesiology of the musculoskeletal system—foundations for physical rehabilitation,* St Louis, 2002, C.V. Mosby.)

The **interphalangeal joints** are uniaxial hinge joints, each having one degree of freedom. The close packed position of the proximal interphalangeal joints and distal interphalangeal joints is full extension; the resting position is slight flexion. The capsular pattern of these joints in flexion is more limited than extension. The bones of these joints are bound together by a fibrous capsule and by the palmar and collateral ligaments. During flexion, there is some rotation in these joints so that the pulp of the fingers faces more fully the pulp of the thumb. If the metacarpophalangeal joints and the proximal interphalangeal joints of the fingers are flexed, they converge toward the scaphoid tubercle (Figure 7-5). This is sometimes referred to as a **cascade sign**. If one or more fingers do not converge, it usually indicates trauma (e.g., fracture) to the digits that has altered their normal alignment.

Interphalangeal Joints	
Resting position:	Slight flexion
Close packed position:	Full extension
Capsular pattern:	Flexion, extension

Patient History

The assessment of the forearm, wrist, and hand often takes longer than that of other joints of the body because of the importance of the hand to everyday function and because of the many structures and joints involved.

In addition to the questions listed under Patient History in Chapter 1, the examiner should obtain the following information from the patient:

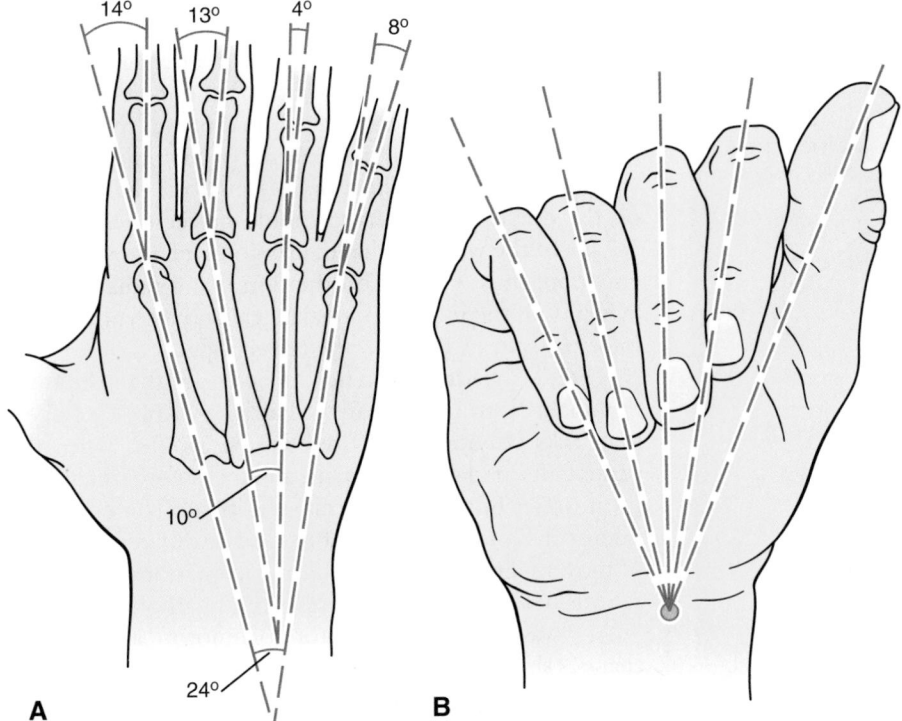

Figure 7-5
Alignment of the fingers. **A,** Normal physiological alignment. **B,** Oblique flexion of the last four digits. Only the index ray flexes toward the median axis. When the last four digits are flexed separately at the metacarpophalangeal and proximal interphalangeal joints, their axes converge toward the scaphoid tubercle. (Redrawn from Tubiana R: *The hand.* Philadelphia, pp. 22, 1981, W.B. Saunders 197.)

1. *What is the patient's age?* Certain conditions are more likely to occur at different ages. For example, arthritic changes are most commonly seen in patients who are older than 40 years of age.[15]

2. *What is the patient's occupation?* Certain occupations are more likely to affect the wrist and hand. For example, typists are more likely to suffer repetitive strain injuries, and automobile mechanics are more likely to suffer traumatic injuries.

3. *What was the mechanism of injury?*[15,16] For example, a fall on the outstretched hand (FOOSH) injury may lead to a lunate dislocation, Colles fracture, or scaphoid fracture, or extension of the fingers may cause dislocation of the fingers. A rotational force applied to the wrist or near it may lead to a Galeazzi fracture, which is a fracture of the radius and dislocation of the distal end of the ulna.

4. *What tasks is the patient able or unable to perform?* For example, is there any problem with buttoning, dressing, tying shoelaces, or any other everyday activity? This type of question gives an indication of the patient's functional limitations.

5. *When did the injury or onset occur, and how long has the patient been incapacitated?* These questions are not necessarily the same; for instance, a burn may occur at a certain time, but incapacity may not occur until hypertrophic scarring appears. The wrist is commonly injured by weight bearing (e.g., gymnastics), by rotational stress combined with ulnar deviation (e.g., hit-

ting a racquet), by twisting, and by impact loading (FOOSH injury).[16,17]

6. *Which hand is the patient's dominant hand?* The dominant hand is more likely to be injured, and the functional loss, at least initially, is greater.

7. *Has the patient injured the forearm, wrist, or hand previously?* Was it the same type of injury? Was the mechanism of injury the same? If so, how was it treated?

8. *Which part of the forearm, wrist, or hand is injured?* If the flexor tendons (which are round, have synovial sheaths, and have a longer excursion than the extensor tendons) are injured, they respond much more slowly to treatment than do extensor tendons (which are flat or ovoid). Within the hand, there is a surgical "no man's land" (Figure 7-6), which is a region between the distal palmar crease and the midportion of the middle phalanx of the fingers. Damage to the flexor tendons in this area require surgical repair and usually lead to the formation of adhesive bands that restrict gliding. In addition, the tendons may become ischemic, being replaced by scar tissue. Because of this, the prognosis after surgery in this area is poor.

Observation

While observing the patient and viewing the forearms, wrists, and hands from both the anterior and posterior aspects, the examiner should note the patient's willingness and ability to use the hand. Normally, when the hand

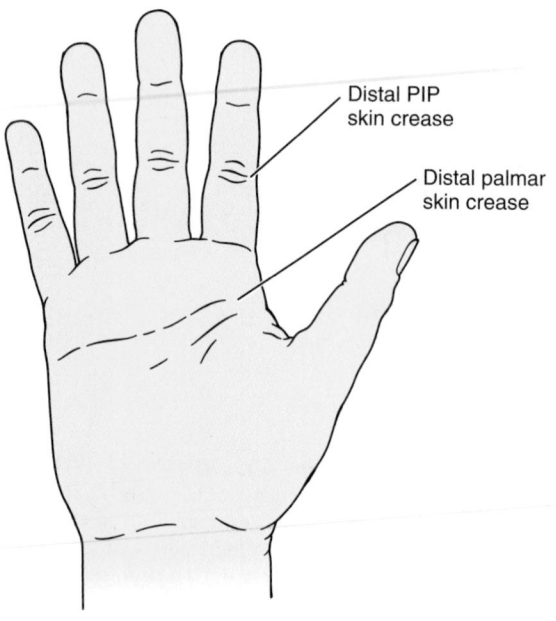

Distal PIP skin crease

Distal palmar skin crease

Figure 7-6

Surgical "no-man's land" (palmar view).

is in the resting position and the wrist is in the normal position, the fingers are progressively more flexed as one moves from the radial side of the hand to the ulnar side. Loss of this normal attitude may be caused by pathology affecting the hand, such as a lacerated tendon, or by a contracture such as Dupuytren's contracture.

The bone and soft-tissue contours of the forearm, wrist, and hand should be compared for both upper limbs, and any deviation should be noted. The cosmetic appearance of the hand is very important to some patients. The examiner should note the patient's reaction to the appearance of the hand and be prepared to provide a cosmetic evaluation. This evaluation should always be included with the more important functional assessment. The posture of the hand at rest often demonstrates common deformities.

Are the normal skin creases present? Skin creases occur because of movement at the various joints. The examiner should note any muscle wasting on the thenar eminence (median nerve), first dorsal interosseous muscle (C7 nerve root), or hypothenar eminence (ulnar nerve) that may be indicative of peripheral nerve or nerve root injury.

Any localized swellings (e.g., ganglion) that are seen on the dorsum of the hand should be recorded (Figure 7-7).[18] In the wrist and hand, effusion and synovial thickening are most evident on the dorsal and radial aspects. Swelling of the metacarpophalangeal and interphalangeal joints is most obvious on the dorsal aspect.

The dominant hand tends to be larger than the nondominant hand. If the patient has an area on the fingers that lacks sensation, this area will be avoided when the patient lifts or identifies objects, and the patient will instead use another finger with normal sensitivity. Therefore, the examiner should watch for abnormal or different patterns of movement, which may indicate adaptations or modifications necessitated by the presence of pathology.

Any vasomotor, sudomotor, pilomotor, and trophic changes should be recorded. These changes may be indicative of a peripheral nerve injury, peripheral vascular disease, diabetes mellitus, Raynaud's disease, or reflex neurovascular syndromes (also called complex regional pain syndrome, reflex sympathetic dystrophy, shoulder-hand syndrome, and Sudeck's atrophy). The changes seen could include loss of hair on the hand, brittle fingernails, increase or decrease in sweating of the palm, shiny skin, radiographic evidence of osteoporosis, or any difference in temperature between the two limbs. Table 7-1 illustrates vasomotor, sudomotor, pilomotor, and trophic changes that occur in the hand when sympathetic nerve function has been affected.

The examiner should note any hypertrophy of the fingers. Hypertrophy of the bone may be seen in Paget's disease, neurofibromatosis, or arteriovenous fistula.

The presence of Heberden's or Bouchard's nodes (Figure 7-8) should be recorded. Heberden's nodes appear on the dorsal surface of the distal interphalangeal

Figure 7-7

Ganglion or small cystic swelling on the dorsum of the right hand just distal to the wrist joint. (From Polley HF, Hunder GG: *Rheumatologic interviewing and physical examination of the joints*, p. 96, Philadelphia, 1978, W.B. Saunders.)

Table 7-1

Sympathetic Changes After Nerve Injury

Sympathetic Function	Feature	Early Changes	Late Changes
Vasomotor	Skin color	Rosy	Mottled or cyanotic
	Skin temperature	Warm	Cool
Sudomotor	Sweating	Dry skin	Dry or overly moist
Pilomotor	Gooseflesh response	Absent	Absent
Trophic	Skin texture	Soft, smooth	Smooth, nonelastic
	Soft-tissue atrophy	Slight	More pronounced, especially in finger pulps
	Nail changes	Blemishes	Curved in longitudinal and horizontal planes, "talonlike"
	Hair growth	May fall out or become longer and finer	May fall out or become longer and finer
	Rate of healing	Slowed	Slowed

From Callahan AD: Sensibility assessment for nerve lesions-in-continuity and nerve lacerations. *In* Mackin EJ, et al (eds): *Hunter-Mackin-Callahan rehabilitation of the hand and upper extremity,* p. 225, St Louis, 2002, Mosby.

A

B

C

Figure 7-8

A, Bouchard's nodes. **B,** Heberden's nodes. **C,** Degenerative joint disease (osteoarthritis) of both hands. Osteoarthritic enlargement of the distal interphalangeal joints (Heberden's nodes) and the proximal interphalangeal joints (Bouchard's nodes) is present. The metacarpophalangeal joints are not affected. (**C,** From Polley HF, Hunder GG: *Rheumatologic interviewing and physical examination of the joints,* p. 120, Philadelphia, 1978, W.B. Saunders.)

joints and are associated with osteoarthritis. Bouchard's nodes are on the dorsal surface of the proximal interphalangeal joints. They are often associated with gastrectasis and osteoarthritis.

Any ulcerations may indicate neurological or circulatory problems. Any alteration in the color of the limb with changes in position may indicate a circulatory problem.

The examiner should note any rotational or angulated deformities of the fingers, which may be indicative of previous fracture. The nail beds are normally parallel to one another. The fingers, when extended, are slightly rotated toward the thumb to aid pinch. Ulnar drift (Figure 7-9) may be seen in rheumatoid arthritis, owing to the shape of the metacarpophalangeal joints and the pull of the long tendons.

The presence of any wounds or scars should be noted because they may indicate recent surgery or past trauma. If wounds are present, are they new or old? Are they healing properly? Is the scar red (new) or white (old)? Is the scar mobile or adherent? Is it normal, hypertrophic, or keloid? Palmar scars may interfere with finger extension. Web space scars may interfere with finger separation and metacarpophalangeal joint flexion.

The examiner should take time to observe the fingernails. "Spoon-shaped" nails (Figure 7-10) are often the result of fungal infection, anemia, iron deficiency, long-term diabetes, local injury, developmental abnormality,

Figure 7-10
Spoon-shaped nails.

chemical irritants, or psoriasis. They may also be a congenital or hereditary trait. "Clubbed" nails (Figure 7-11) may result from hypertrophy of the underlying soft tissue or respiratory or cardiac problems such as chronic obstructive pulmonary disease, congenital heart defects, or cor pulmonale. Table 7-2 shows other pathological processes that may affect the fingernails.

Common Hand and Finger Deformities

Swan-Neck Deformity. This deformity usually involves only the fingers. There is flexion of the metacarpophalangeal and distal interphalangeal joints, but the real deformity is extension of the proximal interphalangeal joint. The condition is a result of contracture of the intrinsic muscles or tearing of the volar plate and is often seen in patients with rheumatoid arthritis or following trauma (Figure 7-12).

Boutonnière Deformity. Extension of the metacarpophalangeal and distal interphalangeal joints and flexion of the proximal interphalangeal joint (primary deformity) are seen with this deformity. The deformity is the result of a rupture of the central tendinous slip of the extensor hood and is most common after trauma or in rheumatoid arthritis (Figure 7-13).

Ulnar Drift. This deformity, which is commonly seen in patients with rheumatoid arthritis but can occur with other conditions, results in ulnar deviation of the digits because of weakening of the capsuloligamentous structures of the metacarpophalangeal joints and the accompanying "bowstring" effect of the extensor communis tendons (see Figure 7-9).

Extensor Plus Deformity. This deformity is caused by adhesions or shortening of the extensor communis

Figure 7-9
The most common deformities occurring in rheumatoid arthritis are ulnar drift and palmar subluxation at the metacarpophalangeal joints. Note swan-neck and boutonnière deformities present in digits. (From Swanson AB: Pathomechanics of deformities in hand and wrist. *In* Hunter J, Schneider LH, Mackin EJ, Callahan AD [eds]: *Rehabilitation of the hand: surgery and therapy*, p. 895, St Louis, 1990, C.V. Mosby.)

Figure 7-11

Clubbing of the distal interphalangeal joints and rounding of the nails in a patient with hypertrophic osteoarthropathy. **A,** Close-up side view of index finger. **B,** Dorsal aspect of both hands. (From Polley HF, Hunder GG: *Rheumatologic interviewing and physical examination of the joints,* p. 122, Philadelphia, 1978, W.B. Saunders.)

tendon proximal to the metacarpophalangeal joint. It results in the inability of the patient to simultaneously flex the metacarpophalangeal and proximal interphalangeal joints, although they may be flexed individually.

Claw Fingers. This deformity results from the loss of intrinsic muscle action and the overaction of the extrinsic (long) extensor muscles on the proximal phalanx of the fingers. The metacarpophalangeal joints are hyperextended, and the proximal and distal interphalangeal joints are flexed (Figure 7-14). If intrinsic function is lost, the hand is called an intrinsic minus hand. The normal cupping of the hand is lost, both the longitudinal and the transverse arches of the hand (Figure 7-15) disappear, and there is intrinsic muscle wasting. The deformity is most often caused by a combined median and ulnar nerve palsy.

Trigger Finger[19] Also known as digital tenovaginitis stenosans, this deformity is the result of a thickening of the flexor tendon sheath, which causes sticking of the tendon when the patient attempts to flex the finger.

A low-grade inflammation of the proximal fold of the flexor tendon leads to swelling and constriction (stenosis) in the digital flexor tendon. When the patient attempts to flex the finger, the tendon sticks, and the finger "lets go," often with a snap. As the condition worsens, eventually the finger will flex but not let go, and it will have to be passively extended. The condition is more likely to occur in middle-aged women, whereas "trigger thumb" is more common in young children. The condition usually occurs in the third or fourth finger. It is most often associated with rheumatoid arthritis and tends to be worse in the morning.

Ape Hand Deformity. Wasting of the thenar eminence of the hand occurs as a result of a median nerve palsy, and the thumb falls back in line with the fingers as a result of the pull of the extensor muscles. The patient is also unable to oppose or flex the thumb (Figure 7-16).

Bishop's Hand or Benediction Hand Deformity. Wasting of the hypothenar muscles of the hand, the interossei muscles, and the two medial lumbrical muscles

Table 7-2

Glossary of Nail Pathology

Condition	Description	Occurrence
Beau's lines	Transverse lines or ridges marking repeated disturbances of nail growth	Systemic diseases, toxic or nutritional deficiency states of many types, trauma (from manicuring)
Defluvium unguium (onychomadesis)	Complete loss of nails	Certain systemic diseases such as scarlet fever, syphilis, leprosy, alopecia areata, and exfoliative dermatitis
Diffusion of lunula unguis	"Spreading" of lunula	Dystrophies of the extremities
Eggshell nails	Nail plate thin, semitransparent bluish-white, with a tendency to curve upward at the distal edge	Syphilis
Fragilitas unguium	Friable or brittle nails	Dietary deficiency, local trauma
Hapalonychia	Nails very soft, split easily	Following contact with strong alkalis; endocrine disturbances, malnutrition, syphilis, chronic arthritis
Hippocratic nails	"Watch-glass nails" associated with "drumstick fingers"	Chronic respiratory and circulatory diseases, especially pulmonary tuberculosis; hepatic cirrhosis
Koilonychia	"Spoon nails"; nails are concave on the outer surface	Dysendocrinisms (acromegaly), trauma, dermatoses, syphilis, nutritional deficiencies, hypothyroidism
Leukonychia	White spots or striations or rarely the whole nail may turn white (congenital type)	Local trauma, hepatic cirrhosis, nutritional deficiencies, and many systemic diseases
Mees' lines	Transverse white bands	Hodgkin's granuloma, arsenic and thallium toxicity, high fevers, local nutritional derangement
Moniliasis of nails	Infections (usually paronychial) caused by yeast forms (*Candida albicans*)	Occupational (common in food-handlers, dentists, dishwashers, and gardeners)
Onychatrophia	Atrophy or failure of development of nails	Trauma, infection, dysendocrinism, gonadal aplasia, and many systemic disorders
Onychauxis	Nail plate is greatly thickened	Mild persistent trauma, systemic diseases such as peripheral stasis, peripheral neuritis, syphilis, leprosy, hemiplegia, or at times may be congenital
Onychia	Inflammation of the nail matrix causing deformity of the nail plate	Trauma, infection, many systemic diseases
Onychodystrophy	Any deformity of the nail plate, nail bed, or nail matrix	Many diseases, trauma, or chemical agents (poisoning, allergy)
Onychogryposis	"Claw nails"—extreme degree of hypertrophy, sometimes with horny projections arising from the nail surface	May be congenital or related to many chronic systemic diseases (see onychauxis)
Onycholysis	Loosening of the nail plate beginning at the distal or free edge	Trauma, injury by chemical agents, many systemic diseases
Onychomadesis	Shedding of all the nails (defluvium unguium)	Dermatoses such as exfoliative dermatitis, alopecia areata, psoriasis, eczema, nail infection, severe systemic diseases, arsenic poisoning
Onychophagia	Nail biting	Neurosis
Onychorrhexis	Longitudinal ridging and splitting of the nails	Dermatoses, nail infections, many systemic diseases, senility, injury by chemical agents, hyperthyroidism
Onychoschizia	Lamination and scaling away of nails in thin layers	Dermatoses, syphilis, injury by chemical agents

Table 7-2—Cont'd

Condition	Description	Occurrence
Onychotillomania	Alteration of the nail structures caused by persistent neurotic picking of the nails	Neurosis
Pachyonychia	Extreme thickening of all the nails; the nails are more solid and more regular than in onychogryposis	Usually congenital and associated with hyperkeratosis of the palms and soles
Pterygium unguis	Thinning of the nail fold and spreading of the cuticle over the nail plate	Associated with vasospastic conditions such as Raynaud's phenomenon and occasionally with hypothyroidism

From Berry TJ: *The hand as mirror of systemic disease*, Philadelphia, 1963, F.A. Davis.

Figure 7-12
Swan-neck deformity. Note the hyperextension at the proximal interphalangeal joint.

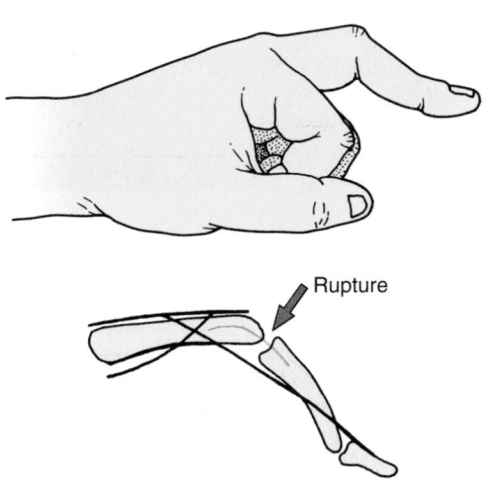

Figure 7-13
Boutonnière deformity. Note the flexion deformity at the proximal interphalangeal joint.

Figure 7-14
Claw fingers (intrinsic minus hand). Fingers are hyperextended at the metacarpophalangeal joints and flexed at the interphalangeal joints.

Figure 7-15
Longitudinal and transverse arches of the hand (lateral view).

Figure 7-16
Ape hand deformity.

Figure 7-17
Bishop's hand or benediction hand deformity.

occurs because of ulnar nerve palsy (Figure 7-17). Flexion of the fourth and fifth fingers is the most obvious resulting change.

Drop-Wrist Deformity. The extensor muscles of the wrist are paralyzed as a result of a radial nerve palsy, and the wrist and fingers cannot be actively extended by the patient (Figure 7-18).

Figure 7-18
Drop-wrist deformity.

Myelopathy Hand. This deformity is a dysfunction of the hand caused by cervical spinal cord pathology in conjunction with cervical spondylosis. The patient shows an inability to extend and adduct the ring and little finger and sometimes the middle finger, especially rapidly, despite good function of the wrist, thumb, and index finger. In addition, the patient shows an exaggerated triceps reflex and positive pathological reflexes (e.g., Hoffman's reflex).[20]

Zigzag Deformity of the Thumb. The thumb is flexed at the carpometacarpal joint and hyperextended at the metacarpophalangeal joint (Fig. 7-19). The deformity is associated with rheumatoid arthritis. A "Z" deformity is due to hypermobility and may be familial Figure 7-20).

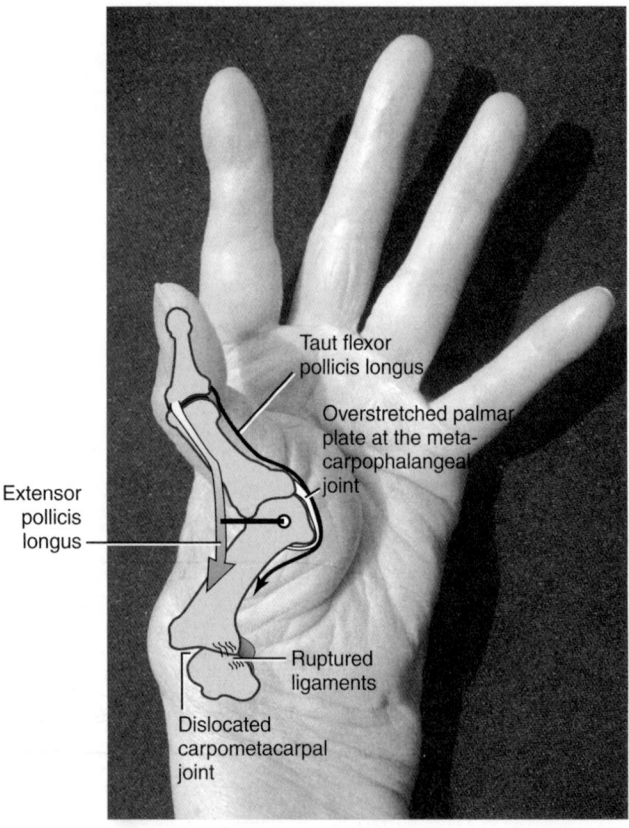

Figure 7-19
Palmar view showing the pathomechanics of a common "zigzag" deformity of the thumb caused by rheumatoid arthritis. The thumb metacarpal dislocates laterally at the carpometacarpal joint, causing hyperextension at the metacarpophalangeal joint. The interphalangeal joint remains partially flexed owing to the passive tension in the stretched and taut flexor pollicis longus. Note that the "bowstringing" of the tendon of the extensor pollicis longus across the metacarpophalangeal joint creates a large extensor moment arm, thereby magnifying the mechanics of the deformity. (From Neumann DA: *Kinesiology of the musculoskeletal system—foundations for physical rehabilitation*, p. 237, St Louis, 2002, C.V. Mosby.)

Figure 7-20
"Z" deformity of the thumb.

A

B

Figure 7-22
Mallet finger. **A,** Patient actively attempting to extend finger.
B, Mechanism of injury. Tendon is ruptured or avulsed from bone.

Force

Dupuytren's Contracture. This condition is the result of contracture of the palmar fascia. There is a fixed flexion deformity of the metacarpophalangeal and proximal interphalangeal joints (Figure 7-21). Dupuytren's contracture is usually seen in the ring or little finger, and the skin is often adherent to the fascia. It affects men more often than women and is usually seen in the 50- to 70-year-old age group.

Mallet Finger [21] A mallet finger deformity is the result of a rupture or avulsion of the extensor tendon where it inserts into the distal phalanx of the finger. The distal phalanx rests in a flexed position (Figure 7-22).

Polydactyly and Triphalangism. Polydactyly is a congenital anomaly characterized by the presence of more than the normal number of fingers or, in the case of the foot, toes. Triphalangism implies there are three phalanges instead of the normal two as would be seen in the thumb.[22]

Figure 7-21
Dupuytren's contracture in both hands, showing flexion contractures of the fourth and fifth digits of the left hand and less severe contractures in the third, fourth, and fifth digits of the right hand. Note the puckering of palmar skin and the presence of bands extending from the concavity of the palm to the proximal interphalangeal joints of the third and fourth digits of the right hand. (From Polley HF, Hunder GG: *Rheumatologic interviewing and physical examination of the joints,* p. 98, Philadelphia, 1978, W.B. Saunders.)

Other Physical Findings

The hand is the terminal part of the upper limb. Many pathological conditions manifest themselves in this structure and may lead the examiner to suspect pathological conditions elsewhere in the body. It is important for the examiner to take the time to view the hands when assessing any joint, especially if an abnormal pattern is presented or the history gives an indication that more than one joint may be involved. For example, if a patient presents with insidious neck pain and demonstrates nail changes that indicate psoriasis, the examiner should consider the possibility of psoriatic arthritis affecting the cervical spine as well as the hand. Some conditions involving the hand include the following:

1. Generalized or continued body exposure to radiation produces brittle nails, longitudinal nail ridges, skin keratosis (thickening), and ulceration.
2. The Plummer-Vinson syndrome produces spoon-shaped nails (see Figure 7-10). This condition is a dysphagia with atrophy in the mouth, pharynx, and upper esophagus.
3. Psoriasis may cause scaling, deformity, and fragmentation and detachment of the nails. Psoriasis may lead to psoriatic arthritis affecting spinal and peripheral joints.
4. Hyperthyroidism produces nail atrophy and ridging with warm, moist hands.
5. Vasospastic conditions produce a thin nail fold and pterygium (abnormal extension) of the cuticle.
6. Trauma to the nail bed, toxic radiation, acute illness, prolonged fever, avitaminosis, and chronic alcoholism produce transverse, or Beau's lines in the nails (Figure 7-23).
7. Many arterial diseases produce a lack of linear growth with thick, dark nails.
8. Lues (syphilis) produces a hypertrophic overgrowth of the nail plate. The nails break and crumple easily.

9. Chronic respiratory disorders produce clubbing of the nails (see Figure 7-11).
10. Subacute bacterial endocarditis may produce Osler's nodes, which are small, tender nodes in the finger pads.
11. Congenital heart disease may produce cyanosis and nail clubbing.
12. Neurocirculatory aesthesia (loss of strength and energy) produces cold, damp hands.
13. Parkinson's disease produces a typical hand tremor known as "pill rolling hand" (Figure 7-24).
14. Causalgic states produce a painful, swollen, hot hand.
15. "Opera glove" anesthesia is seen in hysteria, leprosy, and diabetes. It is a condition in which there is numbness from the elbow to the fingers (Figure 7-25).
16. Raynaud's disease produces a cold, mottled, painful hand. It is an idiopathic vascular disorder characterized by intermittent attacks of pallor and cyanosis of the extremities brought on by cold or emotion.
17. Rheumatoid arthritis produces a warm, wet hand as well as joint swelling, dislocations or subluxations, and ulnar deviation or drift of the wrist (see Figure 7-9).
18. The deformed hand of Volkmann's ischemic contracture is one that is very typical for a compartment syndrome after a fracture or dislocation of the elbow (Figure 7-26).

Box 7-1 gives further examples of physical findings of the hand.

Examination

The examination of the forearm, wrist, and hand may be very extensive, or it may be limited to one or two joints, depending on the area and degree of injury. Regardless, because of its functional importance, the examiner must take extra care when examining this area. Not only must clinical limitations be determined, but functional limitations brought on by trauma, nerve injuries, or other factors must be carefully considered to

Figure 7-24
"Pill rolling hand", seen in Parkinson's disease.

Depression

Figure 7-23
Beau's lines.

Figure 7-25

"Opera glove anesthesia," showing area of abnormal sensation.

Figure 7-26

Deformity seen with Volkmann's ischemic contracture. Note clawed fingers.

have an appropriate outcome functionally, cosmetically, and clinically.

Because there are so many joints, bones, muscles, and ligaments involved, the examiner must develop a working knowledge of all of these tissues and how they interact with one another. The examiner should remember that adduction of the hand (ulnar deviation) is greater than abduction (radial deviation) because of shortness of the ulnar styloid process. Supination of the forearm is stronger than pronation, whereas abduction has a greater ROM in supination than pronation. Adduction and abduction ROM is minimal when the wrist is fully extended or flexed. Both flexion and extension at the fingers are maximal when the wrist is in a neutral position (not abducted or adducted); flexion and extension of the wrist are minimal when the wrist is in pronation.

The wrist and hand have both a fixed (stable) and a mobile segment. The fixed segment consists of the distal row of carpal bones (trapezium, trapezoid, capitate, and hamate) and the second and third metacarpals. This is the **stable segment** of the wrist and hand (Figure 7-27), and movement between these bones is less than that between the bones of the mobile segment. This arrangement allows stability without rigidity, enables the hand to

move more discretely and with suppleness, and enhances the function of the thumb and fingers when they are used for power and/or precision grip. The **mobile segment** is made up of the five phalanges and the first, fourth, and fifth metacarpal bones.

The **functional position** of the wrist is extension to between 20° and 35° with ulnar deviation of 10° to 15°.[14] This position, sometimes called the **position of rest**, minimizes the restraining action of the long extensor tendons and allows complete flexion of the finger; thus, the greatest power of grip occurs when the wrist is in this position (Figure 7-28). In this position, the pulps of the index finger and thumb come into contact to facilitate thumb-finger action. The position of **wrist immobilization** (Figure 7-29) is further extension than is seen in the position of rest, with the metacarpophalangeal joints more flexed and the interphalangeal joints extended. In this way, when the joints are immobilized, the potential for contracture is kept to a minimum.

During extension at the wrist (Figure 7-30), most of the movement occurs in the radiocarpal joint (approximately 40°) and less occurs in the midcarpal joint (approximately 20°).[13] The motion of extension is accompanied by slight radial deviation and pronation of the forearm. During wrist flexion (see Figure 7-30), most of the movement occurs in the midcarpal joint (approximately 40°) and less occurs in the radiocarpal joint (approximately 30°).[13] This movement is accompanied by slight ulnar deviation and supination of the forearm. Radial deviation occurs primarily between the proximal and distal rows of carpal bones (0°–20°), with the proximal row moving toward the ulna and the distal row moving radially. Ulnar deviation occurs primarily at the radiocarpal joint (0°–37°).[14]

Active Movements

Active movements are sometimes referred to as physiological movements. If there is pathology to only one area of the hand or wrist, only that area needs to be assessed, provided the examiner is satisfied that the pathology is not affecting or has not affected the function of the

Box 7-1
Outline of Physical Findings of the Hand

I. **Variations in size and shape of hand**
  A. *Large, blunt fingers (spade hand)*
    1. Acromegaly
    2. Hurler's disease (gargoylism)
  B. *Gross irregularity of shape and size*
    1. Paget's disease of bone
    2. Maffucci's syndrome
    3. Neurofibromatosis
  C. *Spider fingers, slender palm (arachnodactyly)*
    1. Hypopituitarism
    2. Eunuchism
    3. Ehlers-Danlos syndrome, pseudoxanthoma elasticum
    4. Tuberculosis
    5. Asthenic habitus
    6. Osteogenesis imperfecta
  D. *Sausage-shaped phalanges*
    1. Rickets (beading of joints)
    2. Granulomatous dactylitis (tuberculosis, syphilis)
  E. *Spindliform joints (fingers)*
    1. Early rheumatoid arthritis
    2. Systemic lupus erythematosus
    3. Psoriasis
    4. Rubella
    5. Boeck's sarcoidosis
    6. Osteoarthritis
  F. *Cone-shaped fingers*
    1. Pituitary obesity
    2. Fröhlich's dystrophy
  G. *Unilateral enlargement of hand*
    1. Arteriovenous aneurysm
    2. Maffucci's syndrome
  H. *Square, dry hands*
    1. Cretinism
    2. Myxedema
  I. *Single, widened, flattened distal phalanx*
    1. Sarcoidosis
  J. *Shortened fourth and fifth metacarpals (bradymetacarpalism)*
    1. Pseudohypoparathyroidism
    2. Pseudopseudohypoparathyroidism
  K. *Shortened, incurved fifth finger (symptom of Du Bois)*
    1. Mongolism
    2. "Behavioral problem"
    3. Gargoylism (broad, short, thick-skinned hand)
  L. *Malposition and abduction, fifth finger*
    1. Turner's syndrome (gonadal dysgenesis, webbed neck, etc.)
  M. *Syndactylism*
    1. Congenital malformations of the heart, great vessels
    2. Multiple congenital deformities
    3. Laurence-Moon-Biedl syndrome
    4. In normal individuals as an inherited trait
  N. *Clubbed fingers*
    1. Subacute bacterial endocarditis
    2. Pulmonary causes
      a. Tuberculosis
      b. Pulmonary arteriovenous fistula
      c. Pulmonic abscess
      d. Pulmonic cysts
      e. Bullous emphysema

      f. Pulmonary hypertrophic osteoarthropathy
      g. Bronchogenic carcinoma
    3. Alveolocapillary block
      a. Interstitial pulmonary fibrosis
      b. Sarcoidosis
      c. Beryllium poisoning
      d. Sclerodermatous lung
      e. Asbestosis
      f. Miliary tuberculosis
      g. Alveolar cell carcinoma
    4. Cardiovascular causes
      a. Patent ductus arteriosus
      b. Tetralogy of Fallot
      c. Taussig-Bing complex
      d. Pulmonic stenosis
      e. Ventricular septal defect
    5. Diarrheal states
      a. Ulcerative colitis
      b. Tuberculous enteritis
      c. Sprue
      d. Amebic dysentery
      e. Bacillary dysentery
      f. Parasitic infestation (gastrointestinal tract)
    6. Hepatic cirrhosis
    7. Myxedema
    8. Polycythemia
    9. Chronic urinary tract infections (upper and lower)
      a. Chronic nephritis
    10. Hyperparathyroidism (telescopy of distal phalanx)
    11. Pachydermoperiostosis (syndrome of Touraine, Solente, and Golé)
  O. *Joint disturbances*
    1. Arthritides
      a. Osteoarthritis
      b. Rheumatoid arthritis
      c. Systemic lupus erythematosus
      d. Gout
      e. Psoriasis
      f. Sarcoidosis
      g. Endocrinopathy (acromegaly)
      h. Rheumatic fever
      i. Reiter's syndrome
      j. Dermatomyositis
    2. Anaphylactic reaction-serum sickness
    3. Scleroderma

II. **Edema of the hand**
  A. *Cardiac disease (congestive heart failure)*
  B. *Hepatic disease*
  C. *Renal disease*
    1. Nephritis
    2. Nephrosis
  D. *Hemiplegic hand*
  E. *Syringomyelia*
  F. *Superior vena caval syndrome*
    1. Superior thoracic outlet tumor
    2. Mediastinal tumor or inflammation
    3. Pulmonary apex tumor
    4. Aneurysm

G. *Generalized anasarca, hypoproteinemia*
H. *Postoperative lymphedema (radical breast amputation)*
I. *Ischemic paralysis (cold, blue, swollen, numb)*
J. *Lymphatic obstruction*
    1. Lymphomatous masses in axilla
K. *Axillary mass*
    1. Metastatic tumor, abscess, leukemia, Hodgkin's disease
L. *Aneurysm of ascending or transverse aorta, or of axillary artery*
M. *Pressure on innominate or subclavian vessels*
N. *Raynaud's disease*
O. *Myositis*
P. *Cervical rib*
Q. *Trichiniasis*
R. *Scalenus anticus syndrome*

III. **Neuromuscular effects**
    A. *Atrophy*
        1. Painless
            a. Amyotrophic lateral sclerosis
            b. Charcot-Marie-Tooth peroneal atrophy
            c. Syringomyelia (loss of heat, cold, and pain sensation)
            d. Neural leprosy
        2. Painful
            a. Peripheral nerve disease
                1. Radial nerve (wrist drop)
                    a. Lead poisoning, alcoholism, polyneuritis, trauma
                    b. Diphtheria, polyarteritis, neurosyphilis, anterior poliomyelitis
                2. Ulnar nerve (benediction palsy)
                    a. Polyneuritis, trauma
                3. Median nerve (claw hand)
                    a. Carpal tunnel syndrome
                        1. Rheumatoid arthritis
                        2. Tenosynovitis at wrist
                        3. Amyloidosis
                        4. Gout
                        5. Plasmacytoma
                        6. Anaphylactic reaction
                        7. Menopause syndrome
                        8. Myxedema
    B. *Extrinsic pressure on the nerve (cervical, axillary, supraclavicular, or brachial)*
        1. Pancoast tumor (pulmonary apex)
        2. Aneurysms of subclavian arteries, axillary vessels, or thoracic aorta
        3. Costoclavicular syndrome
        4. Superior thoracic outlet syndrome
        5. Cervical rib
        6. Degenerative arthritis of cervical spine
        7. Herniation of cervical intervertebral disc
    C. *Shoulder-hand syndrome*
        1. Myocardial infarction
        2. Pancoast tumor
        3. Brain tumor
        4. Intrathoracic neoplasms
        5. Discogenetic disease
        6. Cervical spondylosis

        7. Febrile panniculitis
        8. Senility
        9. Vascular occlusion
        10. Hemiplegia
        11. Osteoarthritis
        12. Herpes zoster
    D. *Ischemic contractures (sensory loss in fingers)*
        1. Tight plaster cast applications
    E. *Polyarteritis nodosa*
    F. *Polyneuritis*
        1. Carcinoma of lung
        2. Hodgkin's disease
        3. Pregnancy
        4. Gastric carcinoma
        5. Reticuloses
        6. Diabetes mellitus
        7. Chemical neuritis
            a. Antimony, benzene, bismuth, carbon tetrachloride, heavy metals, alcohol, arsenic, lead, gold, emetine
        8. Ischemic neuropathy
        9. Vitamin B deficiency
        10. Atheromata
        11. Arteriosclerosis
        12. Embolic
    G. *Carpodigital (carpopedal spasm) tetany*
        1. Hypoparathyroidism
        2. Hyperventilation
        3. Uremia
        4. Nephritis
        5. Nephrosis
        6. Rickets
        7. Sprue
        8. Malabsorption syndrome
        9. Pregnancy
        10. Lactation
        11. Osteomalacia
        12. Protracted vomiting
        13. Pyloric obstruction
        14. Alkali poisoning
        15. Chemical toxicity
            a. Morphine, lead, alcohol
    H. *Tremor*
        1. Parkinsonism
        2. Familial disorder
        3. Hypoglycemia
        4. Hyperthyroidism
        5. Wilson's disease (hepatolenticular degeneration)
        6. Anxiety
        7. Ataxia
        8. Athetosis
        9. Alcoholism, narcotic addiction
        10. Multiple sclerosis
        11. Chorea (Sydenham's, Huntington's)

Modified from Berry TJ: *The hand as a mirror of systemic disease,* Philadelphia, 1963, F.A. Davis.

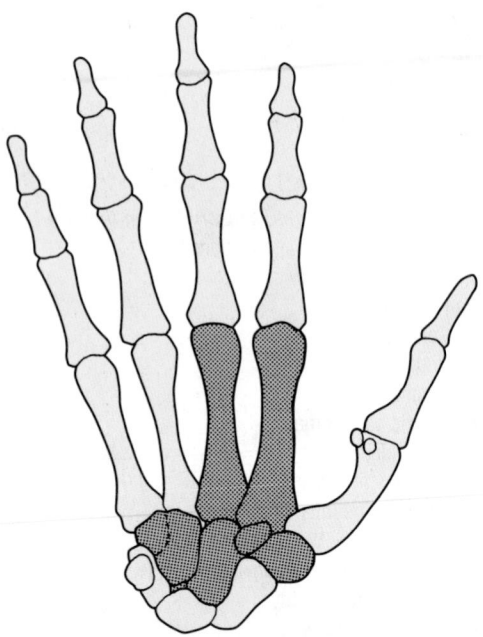

Figure 7-27
Palmar view of hand, showing stable segment (stippled areas).

Figure 7-29
Position of immobilization.

injury to these other areas. Also, if the injury is chronic, adaptive changes may have occurred in adjacent joints.

Examination is accomplished with the patient in the sitting position. As always, the most painful movements are done last. When the examiner is determining the movements of the hand, the middle finger is considered to be midline (Figure 7-31). Wrist flexion decreases as the fingers are flexed just as finger flexion decreases as the wrist flexes, and movements of flexion and extension are limited, usually by the antagonistic muscles and ligaments. In addition, pathology to structures other than the joint may restrict ROM (e.g., muscle spasm, tight ligaments/capsules). If the examiner suspects these structures, passive movement end feels will help differentiate the problem. The patient should actively perform

other areas of the forearm, wrist, and hand. For example, if the patient has suffered a FOOSH injury to the wrist, the examiner spends most of the examination looking at the wrist. However, because positioning of the wrist can affect the function of the rest of the hand and forearm, the examiner must determine the functional effect of the

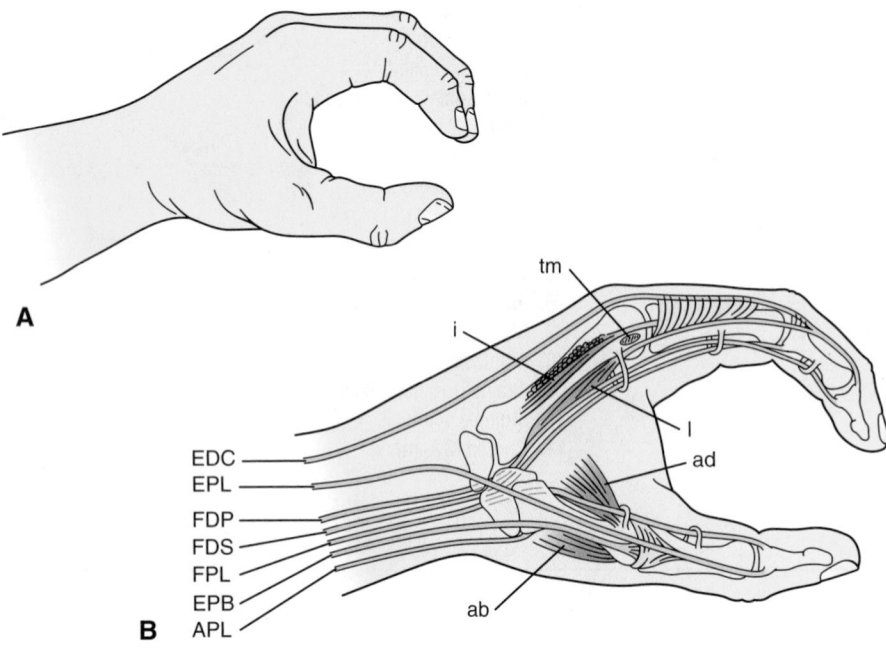

A

B

EDC
EPL
FDP
FDS
FPL
EPB
APL

tm
i
l
ad
ab

Figure 7-28
Position of function of the hand. **A,** Normal view. **B,** The hand is in the position of function. Notice in particular that a very small amount of motion in the thumb and fingers is useful motion in that it can be used in pinch and grasp. Notice the close relation of the tendons to bone. The flexor tendons are held close to bone by a pulley-like thickening of the flexor sheath as represented schematically. With the hand in this position, intrinsic and extrinsic musculature is in balance, and all muscles are acting within their physiological resting length. *EDC,* Extensor digitorum communis; *EPL,* extensor pollicis longus; *FDP,* flexor digitorum profundus; *FDS,* flexor digitorum sublimis; *FPL,* flexor pollicis longus; *EPB,* extensor pollicis brevis; *APL,* abductor pollicis longus; *i,* interossei; *tm,* transverse metacarpal ligament; *l,* lumbrical; *ad,* adductor pollicis brevis; *ab,* abductor pollicis brevis. (**B,** Redrawn from O'Donoghue DH: *Treatment of injuries to athletes,* Philadelphia, p. 287, 1984, W.B. Saunders.)

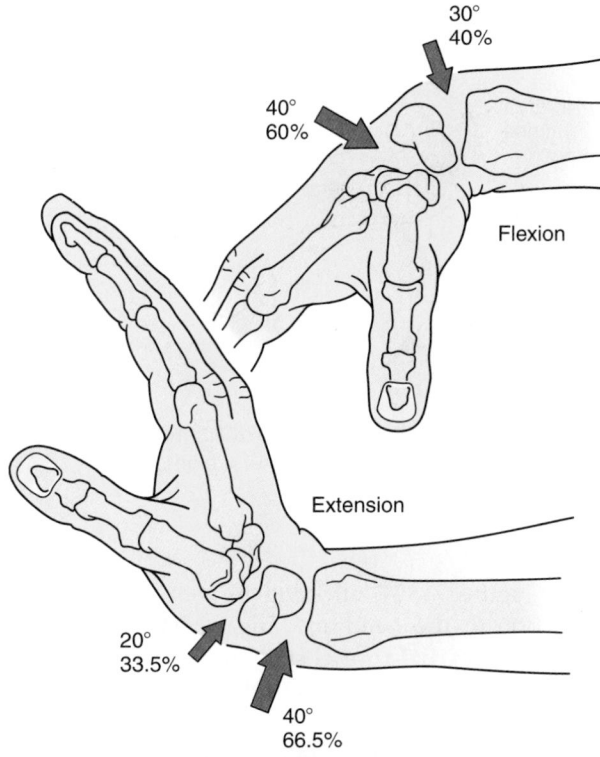

Figure 7-30
During flexion of the wrist, the motion is more midcarpal and less radiocarpal. During extension of the wrist, the motion is more radiocarpal and less midcarpal. (Modified from Sarrafian SK, Melamed JL, Goshgarian GM: Study of wrist motion in flexion and extension, *Clin Orthop* 126:156, 1977.)

the various movements. Initially, the active movements of the forearm, wrist, and hand may be performed in a "scanning" fashion by having the patient make a fist and then open the hand wide. As the patient does these two movements, the examiner notes any restrictions, deviations, or pain. Depending on the results, the examiner can then do a detailed examination of the affected joints. This detailed examination is initiated by selection of the appropriate active movements to be performed, keeping in mind the effect one joint can have on others.

Active pronation and supination of the forearm and wrist are approximately 85° to 90°, although there is variability between individuals and it is more important to compare the movement with that of the normal side. Approximately 75° of supination or pronation occurs in the forearm articulations. The remaining 15° is the result of wrist action. If the patient complains of pain on supination, the examiner can differentiate between the distal radioulnar joint and the radiocarpal joints by passively supinating the ulna on the radius with no stress on the radiocarpal joint. If this passive movement is painful, the problem is in the distal radioulnar joint, not the radiocarpal joints. The normal end feel of both movements is tissue stretch, although in thin patients, the end feel of pronation may be bone-to-bone.

Radial and ulnar deviations of the wrist are 15° and 30° to 45°, respectively. The normal end feel of these movements is bone-to-bone.

Active Movements of the Forearm, Wrist, and Hand

- Pronation of the forearm (85°–90°)
- Supination of the forearm (85°–90°)
- Wrist abduction or radial deviation (15°)
- Wrist adduction or ulnar deviation (30°–45°)
- Wrist flexion (80°–90°)
- Wrist extension (70°–90°)
- Finger flexion (MCP, 85°–90°; PIP, 100°–115°; DIP, 80°–90°)
- Finger extension (MCP, 30°–45°; PIP, 0°; DIP, 20°)
- Finger abduction (20°–30°)
- Finger adduction (0°)
- Thumb flexion (CMC, 45°–50°; MCP, 50°–55°; IP, 85°–90°)
- Thumb extension (MCP, 0°; IP, 0°–5°)
- Thumb abduction (60°–70°)
- Thumb adduction (30°)
- Opposition of little finger and thumb (tip-to-tip)
- Combined movements (if necessary)
- Repetitive movements (if necessary)
- Sustained positions (if necessary)

CMC, Carpometacarpal; *DIP*, distal interphalangeal; *IP*, interphalangeal; *MCP*, metacarpophalangeal; *PIP*, proximal interphalangeal.

Figure 7-31
Axis or reference position of the hand. The middle finger provides a central reference from which the other fingers abduct and adduct.

Wrist flexion is 80° to 90°; **wrist extension** is 70° to 90°. The end feel of each movement is tissue stretch. Midcarpal instability may be evident on ulnar deviation. If there is midcarpal instability as the wrist is taken into ulnar deviation, the proximal row of carpals stays flexed longer and then audibly snaps or clunks into dorsiflexion (known as a "catch up clunk").[9,23,24]

Flexion of the fingers occurs at the metacarpophalangeal joints (85°–90°), followed by the proximal interphalangeal joints (100°–115°) and the distal interphalangeal joints (80°–90°). This sequence enables the hand to grasp large and small objects. **Extension** occurs at the metacarpophalangeal joints (30°–45°), the proximal interphalangeal joints (0°), and the distal interphalangeal joints (20°). Hyperextension at the proximal interphalangeal joints can lead to a swan-neck deformity. This hyperextension is usually prevented by the volar plates.[3] The end feel of finger flexion and extension is tissue stretch. **Finger abduction** occurs at the metacarpophalangeal joints (20°–30°); the end feel is tissue stretch. **Finger adduction** (0°) occurs at the same joint.

The digits are medially deviated slightly in relation to the metacarpal bones (see Figure 7-5). When the fingers are flexed, they should point toward the scaphoid tubercle. In addition, the metacarpals are at an angle to each other. These positions increase the dexterity of the hand and oblique flexion of the medial four digits but contribute to deformities (e.g., ulnar drift) in conditions such as rheumatoid arthritis.

Thumb flexion occurs at the carpometacarpal joint (45°–50°), the metacarpophalangeal joint (50°–55°), and the interphalangeal joint (80°–90°). It is associated with medial rotation of the thumb as a result of the saddle shape of the carpometacarpal joint. **Extension of the thumb** occurs at the interphalangeal joint (0°–5°); it is associated with lateral rotation. Flexion and extension take place in a plane parallel to the palm of the hand. **Thumb abduction** is 60° to 70°; **thumb adduction** is 30°. These movements occur in a plane at right angles to the flexion-extension plane.[14] The thumb is controlled by three nerves, a situation that is unique among the digits. The radial nerve controls extension and opening of the thumb as it does for the other digits. The ulnar nerve controls adduction, produces closure of pinch, and gives power to the grip; the median nerve controls flexion and opposition, producing precision with any grip.[3] The intrinsic muscles are stronger than the extrinsic muscles of the thumb; the opposite is true for the fingers.[3]

If the history has indicated that combined or repetitive movements and/or sustained postures have resulted in symptoms, these movements should also be tested.

The examiner must be aware that active movements may be affected because of neurological as well as contractile tissue problems. For example, the median nerve is sometimes compressed as it passes through the carpal

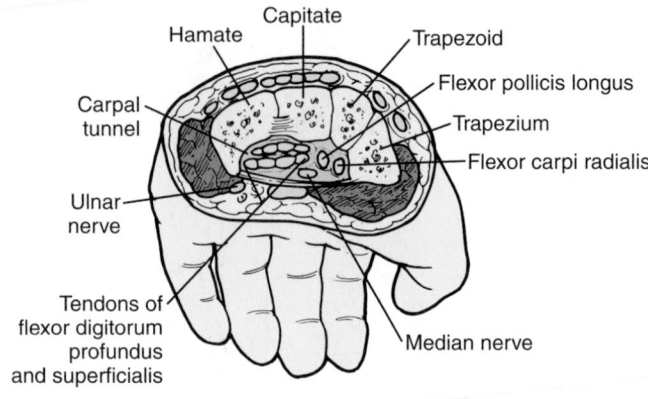

Figure 7-32

Cross section of the wrist showing the carpal tunnel.

tunnel (Figure 7-32), affecting its motor and sensory distribution in the hand and fingers. The condition is referred to as **carpal tunnel syndrome.**

If the patient does not have full active ROM and it is difficult to measure ROM because of swelling, pain, or contracture, the examiner can use a ruler or tape measure to record the distance from the fingertip to one of the palmar creases (Figure 7-33).[25] This measurement provides baseline data for any effect of treatment. It is important to note on the chart which crease was used in the measurement. The majority of functional activities of the hand require the fingers and thumb to open at least 5 cm (2 inches), and the fingers should be able to flex within 1 to 2 cm (0.4–0.8 inch) of the distal palmar crease.[26]

Passive Movements

If, when watching the patient perform the active movements, the examiner believes the ROM is full, overpressure can be gently applied to test the end feel of the joint in each direction. If the movement is not full, passive movements must be carefully performed by the examiner to test the end feel. At the same time, the examiner must watch for the presence of a capsular pattern. The passive movements are the same as the active movements, and the examiner must remember to test each individual joint.

The capsular pattern of the distal radioulnar joint is full ROM with pain at the extremes of supination and pronation. At the wrist, the capsular pattern is equal limitation of flexion and extension. At the metacarpophalangeal and interphalangeal joints, the capsular pattern is flexion more limited than extension. At the trapeziometacarpal joint of the thumb, the capsular pattern is abduction more limited than extension.

In some cases, the examiner may want to test the length of the long extensor and flexor muscles of the wrist (Figure 7-34). If the length of the muscles is normal, the passive

Passive Movements of the Forearm, Wrist, and Hand and Normal End Feel

- Pronation (tissue stretch)
- Supination (tissue stretch)
- Radial deviation (bone-to-bone)
- Ulnar deviation (bone-to-bone)
- Wrist flexion (tissue stretch)
- Wrist extension (tissue stretch)
- Finger flexion (tissue stretch)
- Finger extension (tissue stretch)
- Finger abduction (tissue stretch)
- Thumb flexion (tissue stretch)
- Thumb extension (tissue stretch)
- Thumb abduction (tissue stretch)
- Thumb adduction (tissue approximation)
- Opposition (tissue stretch)

Figure 7-33

A, Gross flexion is measured as the distance between fingertips and proximal palmar crease. **B,** Gross extension is measured as the distance between fingertips and dorsal plane. (From Wadsworth CT: Wrist and hand examination and interpretation, *J Orthop Sports Phys Ther* 5:115, 1983.)

Figure 7-34

Testing the length of the long extensor (**A**) and flexor (**B**) muscles of the wrist.

range on testing will be full and the end feel will be the normal joint tissue stretch end feel. If the muscles are tight, the end feel will be muscle stretch, which is not as "stretchy" as tissue or capsular stretch, and the ROM will be restricted.

To test the length of the long wrist extensors, the patient is placed in supine lying with the elbow extended. The examiner passively flexes the fingers and then flexes the wrist.[27] If the muscles are tight, wrist flexion will be restricted.

To test the length of the long wrist flexors, the patient is placed in supine lying with the elbow extended. The examiner passively extends the fingers and then extends the wrist.[27] If the muscles are tight, wrist extension will be limited.

Conjunct rotation can be tested by folding and fanning the hand (Figure 7-35). To do this, the examiner holds the scaphoid and trapezium with the index and middle finger of one hand and the pisiform and hamate of the other hand while the capitate is held with the thumbs on the dorsum of the hand. The examiner then folds and fans the hand feeling the movement.[28]

Resisted Isometric Movements

As with the active movements, the resisted isometric movements to the forearm, wrist, and hand are done with the patient in the sitting position. Not all resisted isometric movements need to be tested, but the examiner must keep in mind that the actions of the fingers and thumb and the wrist are controlled by extrinsic muscles (wrist, fingers, thumb) and intrinsic muscles (fingers, thumb), so injury affecting these structures requires testing of the appropriate muscles. The movements must be isometric and must be performed in the neutral position (Figures 7-36 and 7-37). If the history has indicated that concentric,

A   **B**

Figure 7-35
A, Fanning and. **B,** folding of the hand.

A   **B**

Figure 7-36
Resisted isometric movements of the wrist. **A,** Flexion. **B,** Extension.

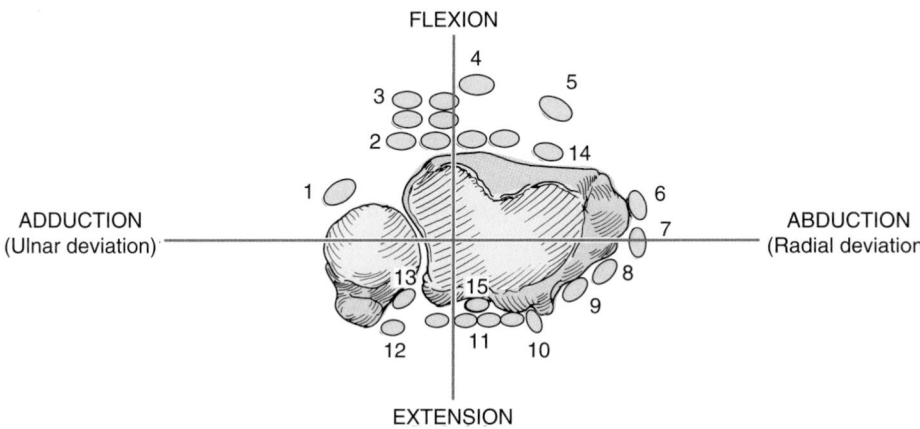

FLEXION

ADDUCTION
(Ulnar deviation)

ABDUCTION
(Radial deviation)

EXTENSION

Figure 7-37
Muscles and their actions at the wrist.
1, Flexor carpi ulnaris. *2*, Flexor
digitorum profundus. *3*, Flexor
digitorum superficialis. *4*, Palmaris
longus. *5*, Flexor carpi radialis.
6, Abductor pollicis longus. *7*,
Extensor pollicis brevis. *8*, Extensor
carpi radialis longus. *9*, Extensor carpi
radialis brevis. *10*, Extensor pollicis
longus. *11*, Extensor digitorum.
12, Extensor digiti minimi. *13*,
Extensor carpi ulnaris. *14*, Flexor
pollicis longus. *15*, Extensor indices.

eccentric, or econcentric movements have caused symptoms, these different types of resisted movement should be tested, but only after the movements have been tested isometrically.

Resisted Isometric Movements of the Forearm, Wrist, and Hand

- Pronation of the forearm
- Supination of the forearm
- Wrist abduction (radial deviation)
- Wrist adduction (ulnar deviation)
- Wrist flexion
- Wrist extension
- Finger flexion
- Finger extension
- Finger abduction
- Finger adduction
- Thumb flexion
- Thumb extension
- Thumb abduction
- Thumb adduction
- Opposition of the little finger and thumb

Table 7-3 shows the muscles and their actions for differentiation during resisted isometric testing. If measured by test instruments, the strength ratio of wrist extensors to wrist flexors is approximately 50%, whereas the strength ratio of ulnar deviators to radial deviators is approximately 80%. The greatest torque is produced by the wrist flexors, followed by the radial deviators, ulnar deviators, and finally the wrist extensors.[29]

Functional Assessment (Grip)

Having completed the basic movement testing of active, passive, and resisted isometric movements, the examiner then assesses the patient's functional active movements. Functionally, the thumb is the most important digit. Because of its relation with the other digits, its mobility, and the force it can bring to bear, its loss can affect hand function greatly. The index finger is the second most important digit because of its musculature, its strength, and its interaction with the thumb. Its loss greatly affects lateral and pulp-to-pulp pinch and power grip. In flexion, the middle finger is strongest, and it is important for both precision and power grips. The ring finger has the least functional role in the hand. The little finger, because of its peripheral position, greatly enhances power grip, affects the capacity of the hand, and holds objects against the hypothenar eminence.[3] In terms of **functional impairment**, the loss of thumb function affects about 40% to 50% of hand function. The loss of index finger function accounts for about 20% of hand function; the middle finger, about 20%; the ring finger, about 10%; and the little finger, about 10%. Loss of the hand accounts for about 90% loss of upper limb function.[30]

Functional Wrist and Hand Scan

- Wrist flexion and extension
- Wrist ulnar and radial deviation
- Making a standard fist
- Making a hook grasp
- Making a straight fist
- Pulp-to-pulp thumb to all fingers pinch
- Tip-to-tip thumb to all fingers pinch

Hand function can be quickly assessed by performing a number of movements to test overall function of the wrist and hand (Functional Hand and Wrist Scan) (Figure 7-38).

Table 7-3

Muscles of the Forearm, Wrist, and Hand: Their Actions, Nerve Supply, and Nerve Root Derivation

Action	Muscles Acting	Nerve Supply	Nerve Root Deviation
Supination of forearm	1. Supinator	Posterior interosseous (radial)	C5–C6
	2. Biceps brachii	Musculocutaneous	C5–C6
Pronation of forearm	1. Pronator quadratus	Anterior interosseous (median)	C8, T1
	2. Pronator teres	Median	C6–C7
	3. Flexor carpi radialis	Median	C6–C7
Extension of wrist	1. Extensor carpi radialis longus	Radial	C6–C7
	2. Extensor carpi radialis brevis	Posterior interosseous (radial)	C7–C8
	3. Extensor carpi ulnaris	Posterior interosseous (radial)	C7–C8
Flexion of wrist	1. Flexor carpi radialis	Median	C6–C7
	2. Flexor carpi ulnaris	Ulnar	C7–C8
Ulnar deviation of wrist	1. Flexor carpi ulnaris	Ulnar	C7–C8
	2. Extensor carpi ulnaris	Posterior interosseous (radial)	C7–C8
Radial deviation of wrist	1. Flexor carpi radialis	Median	C6–C7
	2. Extensor carpi radialis longus	Radial	C6–C7
	3. Abductor pollicis longus	Posterior interosseous (radial)	C7–C8
	4. Extensor pollicis brevis	Posterior interosseous (radial)	C7–C8
Extension of fingers	1. Extensor digitorum communis	Posterior interosseous (radial)	C7–C8
	2. Extensor indices (second finger)	Posterior interosseous (radial)	C7–C8
	3. Extensor digiti minimi (little finger)	Posterior interosseous (radial)	C7–C8
Flexion of fingers	1. Flexor digitorum profundus	Anterior interosseous (median)	C8, T1
		Anterior interosseous (median): lateral two digits	C8, T1
		Ulnar: medial two digits	C8, T1
	2. Flexor digitorum superficialis	Median	C7–C8, T1
			C8, T1
	3. Lumbricals	First and second: median; third and fourth: ulnar (deep terminal branch)	C8, T1
	4. Interossei	Ulnar (deep terminal branch)	C8, T1
	5. Flexor digiti minimi (little finger)	Ulnar (deep terminal branch)	C8, T1
Abduction of fingers (with fingers extended)	1. Dorsal interossei	Ulnar (deep terminal branch)	C8, T1
	2. Abductor digiti minimi (little finger)	Ulnar (deep terminal branch)	C8, T1
Adduction of fingers (with fingers extended)	1. Palmar interossei	Ulnar (deep terminal branch)	C8, T1
Extension of thumb	1. Extensor pollicis longus	Posterior interosseous (radial)	C7–C8
	2. Extensor pollicis brevis	Posterior interosseous (radial)	C7–C8
	3. Abductor pollicis longus	Posterior interosseous (radial)	C7–C8
Flexion of thumb	1. Flexor pollicis brevis	Superficial head: median (lateral terminal branch)	C8, T1
		Deep head: ulnar	C8, T1
	2. Flexor pollicis longus	Anterior interosseous (median)	C8, T1
	3. Opponens pollicis	Median (lateral terminal branch)	C8, T1

Table 7-3—Cont'd

Action	Muscles Acting	Nerve Supply	Nerve Root Deviation
Abduction of thumb	1. Abductor pollicis longus	Posterior interosseous (radial)	C7–C8
	2. Abductor pollicis brevis	Median (lateral terminal branch)	C8, T1
Adduction of thumb	1. Adductor pollicis	Ulnar (deep terminal branch)	C8, T1
Opposition of thumb and little finger	1. Opponens pollicis	Median (lateral terminal branch)	C8, T1
	2. Flexor pollicis brevis	Superficial head: median (lateral terminal branch)	C8, T1
	3. Abductor pollicis brevis	Median (lateral terminal branch)	C8, T1
	4. Opponens digiti minimi	Ulnar (deep terminal branch)	C8, T1

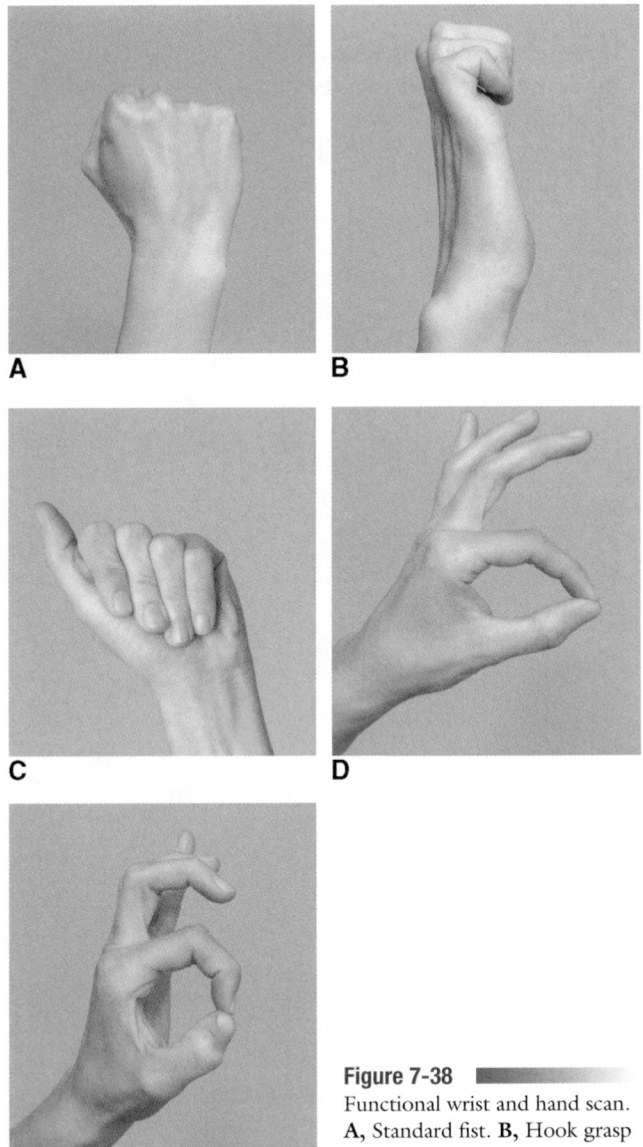

Figure 7-38

Functional wrist and hand scan. **A,** Standard fist. **B,** Hook grasp fist. **C,** Straight fist. **D,** Pulp-to-pulp pinch. **E,** Tip-to-tip pinch.

Although the wrist, hand, and finger joints have the ability to move through a relatively large ROM, most functional daily tasks do not require full ROM. The optimum functional ROM at the wrist is approximately 10° flexion to 35° extension along with 10° of radial deviation and 15° of ulnar deviation.[31-34] Normally, the wrist is held in slight extension (10°–15°) and slight ulnar deviation and is stabilized in this position to provide maximum function for the fingers and thumb. Excessive radial deviation, like ulnar drift of the fingers, can affect grip strength adversely.[35] Functional flexion at the metacarpophalangeal and proximal interphalangeal joints is approximately 60°. Functional flexion at the distal interphalangeal joint is approximately 40°. For the thumb, functional flexion at the metacarpophalangeal and interphalangeal joints is approximately 20°.[26] Within these ROMs, the hand is able to perform most of its grip[14,36] and other functional activities.

The thumb, although not always used in gripping, adds another important dimension when it is used. It gives stability and helps control the direction in which the object moves. Both of these factors are necessary for precision movements. The thumb also increases the power of a grip by acting as a buttress, resisting the pressure of an object held between it and the fingers.

The nerve distribution and the functions of the digits also present interesting patterns. Flexion and sensation of the ulnar digits are controlled by the ulnar nerve and are more related to power grip. Flexion and sensation of the radial digits are controlled by the median nerve and are more related to precision grip. The muscles of the thumb, often used in both types of grip, are supplied by both nerves. In all cases of gripping, opening of the hand or release of grip depends on the radial nerve.

Stages of Grip

1. Opening of the hand, which requires the simultaneous action of the intrinsic muscles of the hand and the long extensor muscles
2. Positioning and closing of the fingers and thumb to grasp the object and adapt to the object's shape, which involves intrinsic and extrinsic flexor and opposition muscles
3. Exerted force, which varies depending on the weight, surface characteristics, fragility, and use of the object, again involving the extrinsic and intrinsic flexor and opposition muscles
4. Release, in which the hand opens to let go of the object, involving the same muscles as for opening of the hand

Power Grip. A power grip requires firm control and gives greater flexor asymmetry to the hand (Figure 7-39). During power grip, the ulnar side of the hand works with the radial side to give stronger stability. The ulnar digits tend to work together to provide support and static control.[3,14,36,37] This grip is used whenever strength or force is the primary consideration. With this grip, the digits maintain the object against the palm; the thumb may or may not be involved, and the extrinsic (forearm) muscles are more important. The combined effect of joint position brings the hand into line with the forearm. For a power grip to be formed, the fingers are flexed and the wrist is in ulnar deviation and slightly extended. Examples of power grips include the **hook grasp,** in which all or the second and third fingers are used as a hook controlled by the forearm flexors and extensors. The hook grasp may involve the interphalangeal joints only or the interphalangeal and metacarpophalangeal joints (the thumb is not involved). In the **cylinder grasp,** a type of **palmar prehension,** the thumb is used, and the entire hand wraps around an object. With the **fist grasp,** or **digital palmar prehension,** the hand moves around a narrow object. Another type of power grip is the **spherical grasp,** another type of palmar prehension, in which there is more opposition and the hand moves around the sphere.

Precision or Prehension Grip. The precision grip is an activity limited mainly to the metacarpophalangeal joints and involves primarily the radial side of the hand (Figure 7-40).[14,36,37] This grip is used whenever accuracy and precision are required. The radial digits

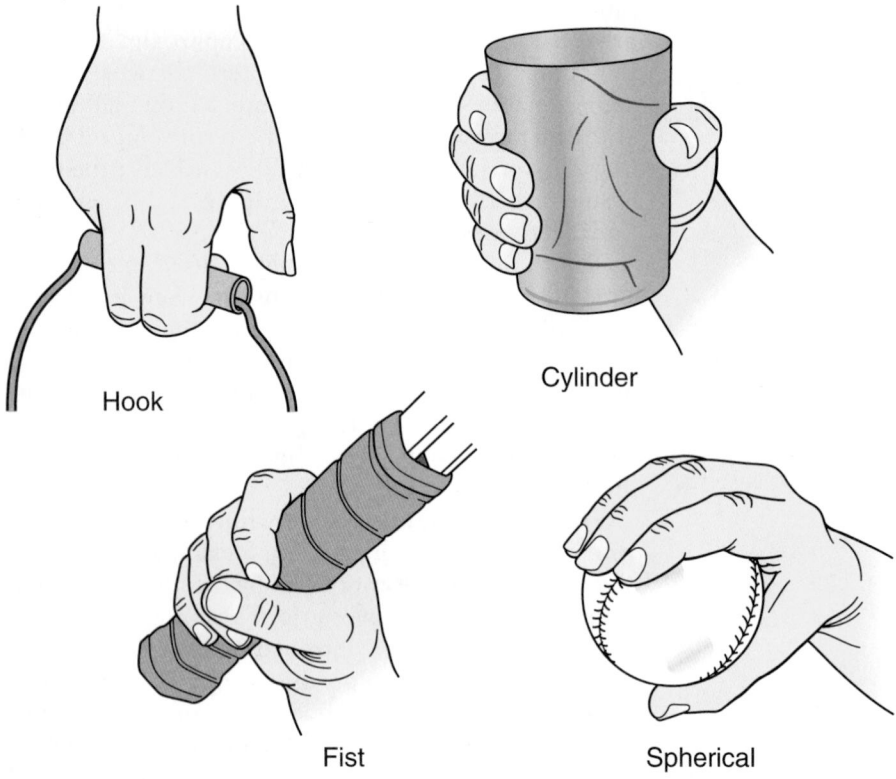

Hook

Cylinder

Fist

Spherical

Figure 7-39
Types of power grips.

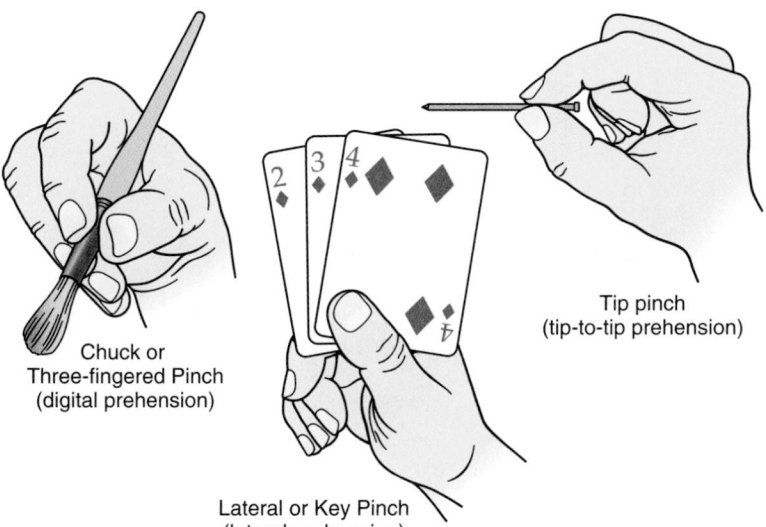

Chuck or
Three-fingered Pinch
(digital prehension)

Lateral or Key Pinch
(lateral prehension)

Tip pinch
(tip-to-tip prehension)

Figure 7-40
Types of precision grips or pinches.

(index and long fingers) provide control by working in concert with the thumb to form a "dynamic tripod" for precision handling.[3] With precision grips, the thumb and fingers are used and the palm may or may not be involved; there is pulp-to-pulp contact between the thumb and fingers, and the thumb opposes the fingers. The intrinsic muscles are more important in precision than in power grips. The thumb is essential for precision grips because it provides stability and control of direction and can act as a buttress, providing power to the grip.[3] There are three types of **pinch grip**. The first is called a **three-point chuck,** three-fingered, or **digital prehension,** in which palmar pinch, or subterminal opposition, is achieved. With this grip, there is pulp-to-pulp pinch, and opposition of the thumb and fingers is necessary (e.g., holding a pencil). This grip is sometimes called a **precision grip with power**. The second pinch grip is termed **lateral key, pulp-to-side pinch, lateral prehension,** or **subterminolateral opposition**. The thumb and lateral side of the index finger come into contact. No opposition is needed. An example of this movement is holding keys or a card. The third pinch grip is called the **tip pinch, tip-to-tip prehension,** or **terminal opposition**. With this positioning, the tip of the thumb is brought into opposition with the tip of another finger. This pinch is used for activities requiring fine coordination rather than power.

Testing Grip Strength

When testing grip strength using the grip dynamometer, the examiner should use the five adjustable hand spacings in consecutive order with the patient grasping the dynamometer with maximum force (Figure 7-41). Both hands are tested alternately, and each force is recorded.[38,39] Care must be taken to ensure that the patient does not fatigue. The results normally form a bell curve (Figure 7-42), with the greatest strength readings at the middle (second and third) spacings and the weakest at the beginning and at the end. There should be a 5% to 10% difference between the dominant and nondominant hands.[40] With injury, the bell curve should still be present, but the force exerted is less. If the patient does not exert maximum force for each test, the typical bell curve will not be produced, nor will the values obtained be consistent. Discrepancies of more than 20% in a test-retest situation indicate that the patient is not exerting maximal force.[39,41] Usually, the mean value of three trials is recorded, and both hands are compared.[26] Table 7-4 gives normal values by age group and gender.

Testing Pinch Strength

The strength of the pinch may be tested with the use of a pinch meter (Figure 7-43). Average values are given for pulp-to-pulp pinch of each finger with the thumb (Table 7-5), lateral prehension (Table 7-6), and pulp-to-pulp pinch (Table 7-7) for different occupational levels. Normally, the mean value of three trials is recorded, and both hands are compared.

Other Functional Testing Methods

In addition to testing grip and pinch strength, the examiner may want to perform a full functional assessment

Figure 7-41
Jamar dynamometer. Arm should be held at the patient's side with elbow flexed at approximately 90° when grip is measured.

Figure 7-42

A, The grip strengths of a patient's uninjured hand *(a)* and injured hand *(b)* are plotted. Despite the patient's decrease in grip strength because of injury, curve b maintains a bell-shaped pattern and parallels that of the normal hand. These curves are reproducible in repeated examinations, with minimal change in values. A great fluctuation in the size of the curve or absence of a bell-shaped pattern casts doubt on the patient's compliance with the examination and may indicate malingering. **B,** If the patient has an exceptionally large hand, the curve shifts to the right *(d)*; with a very small hand, the curve shifts to the left *(c)*. In both cases, the bell-shaped pattern is maintained. (Redrawn from Aulicino PL, DuPuy TE: Clinical examination of the hand. *In* Hunter J et al, editors: *Rehabilitation of the hand: surgery and therapy*, p. 45, St Louis, 1990, C.V. Mosby.)

of the patient. Figures 7-44 and 7-45 give examples of functional assessment forms for the hand. These forms are not numerical scoring charts, but they do include some functional aspects. Levine et al.[42] have developed a severity questionnaire including a functional component to measure severity of symptoms and functional disability for a nerve—in this case, the median nerve in the carpal tunnel (Figure 7-46). Chung et al.[43] have developed

a very comprehensive hand outcomes questionnaire—the Michigan Hand Outcomes Questionnaire, which gives the patient's evaluation of his or her outcome based on overall hand function, activities of daily living,

Text continued on page 428

Table 7-4

Normal Values by Age Group (Years) and Gender for Combined Right and Left Hand Grip Strength (kg)

	Ages 15–19		Ages 20–29		Ages 30–39		Ages 40–49		Ages 50–59		Ages 60–69	
	Male	Female	Male	Female	Male	Female	Male	Female	Male	Female	Male	Female
Excellent	≥113	≥71	≥124	≥71	≥123	≥73	≥119	≥73	≥110	≥65	≥102	≥60
Above average	103–112	64–70	113–123	65–70	113–122	66–72	110–118	65–72	102–109	59–64	93–101	54–59
Average	95–102	59–63	106–112	61–64	105–112	61–65	102–109	59–64	96–101	55–58	86–92	51–53
Below average	84–94	54–58	97–105	55–60	97–104	56–60	94–101	55–58	87–95	51–54	79–85	48–50
Poor	≤83	≤53	≤96	≤54	≤96	≤55	≤93	≤54	≤86	≤50	≤78	≤47

Modified from Canadian Standardized Test of Fitness: *Operations manual,* p. 36, Ottawa, 1986, Fitness and Amateur Sport Canada.

Figure 7-43
Commercial pinch meter to test pinch strength.

Table 7-6

Average Strength of Lateral Prehension Pinch by Occupation (100 Subjects)

	Lateral Prehension Pinch (kg)			
	Male Hand		Female Hand	
Occupation	Major	Minor	Major	Minor
Skilled	6.6	6.4	4.4	4.3
Sedentary	6.3	6.1	4.1	3.9
Manual	8.5	7.7	6.0	5.5
Average	7.5	7.1	4.9	4.7

From Hunter J et al, editors: *Rehabilitation of the hand: surgery and therapy,* p. 114, St Louis, 1990, C.V. Mosby.

Table 7-5

Average Strength of Chuck (Pulp-to-Pulp) Pinch with Separate Digits (100 Subjects)

	Pulp-to-Pulp Pinch (kg)			
	Male Hand		Female Hand	
Digit	Major	Minor	Major	Minor
II	5.3	4.8	3.6	3.3
III	5.6	5.7	3.8	3.4
IV	3.8	3.6	2.5	2.4
V	2.3	2.2	1.7	1.6

From Hunter J et al, editors: *Rehabilitation of the hand: surgery and therapy,* St Louis, p. 115, 1990, C.V. Mosby.

Table 7-7

Average Strength of Chuck (Pulp-to-Pulp) Pinch by Occupation (100 Subjects)

	Pulp-to-Pulp Pinch (kg)			
	Male Hand		Female Hand	
Occupation	Major	Minor	Major	Minor
Skilled	7.3	7.2	5.4	4.6
Sedentary	8.4	7.3	4.2	4.0
Manual	8.5	7.6	6.1	5.6
Average	7.9	7.5	5.2	4.9

From Hunter J et al, editors: *Rehabilitation of the hand: surgery and therapy,* p. 114, St Louis, 1990, C.V. Mosby.

Rheumatoid Arthritis Evaluation Record
Preoperative Silastic Implants

Name _____ Sex: [ ] Male [ ] Female Date _____ Birth date _____

Address _____

Occupation _____ Dominant hand: [ ] R [ ] L Hospital _____ Examiner _____

Diagnosis: [ ] Juvenile rheumatoid [ ] Adult rheumatoid [ ] Erosive arthritis [ ] Osteoarthritis [ ] Psoriatic arthritis
[ ] Ankylosing spondylitis [ ] Sjögren's syndrome [ ] Systemic lupus erythematosus [ ] Trauma

Onset date: _____ Sedimentation rate: [ ] Wintrobe [ ] Westergren [ ] Rourke

Rheumatoid test [ ] (+) [ ] (−) Family Hx [ ] (+) [ ] (−)

Onset distribution: [ ] Peripheral [ ] Central [ ] Both: Remission [ ] Yes [ ] No: Anemia [ ] Yes [ ] No:

Check if the following has been completed: [ ] X-rays [ ] Photographs [ ] Movies [ ] Cineradiography

Range of motion (ROM): use neutral zero method of American Academy of Orthopedic Surgeons, 1965.
Codes 1–25 represent observed and measured abnormalities. Use as indicated in appropriate sections.
Severity indices mild, moderate, and severe are represented by a, b, and c and further categorize codes 1–25.
This evaluation record has been designed for computer analysis. Responses must be complete.

THUMB: Codes: 1, 2, 3, 9–14, 19, 22	Code R	Code L	Abd (degrees) Add (cm) Opp (cm) Joints	ROM R	ROM L
			MC Abd		
			Add		
			Opp		
			MP		
			IP		

FINGER: Codes: 3–15, 19, 22–25

Index			MP		
			PIP		
			DIP		
Flex DIP crease to palmar crease (cm)					
Middle			MP		
			PIP		
			DIP		
Flex DIP crease to palmar crease (cm)					
Ring			MP		
			PIP		
			DIP		
Flex DIP crease to palmar crease (cm)					
Little			MP		
			PIP		
			DIP		
Flex DIP crease to palmar crease (cm)					
WRIST: Codes: 3, 7–14, 19, 20, 22, 23			Flex		
			Ext		
			U. Dev		
			R. Dev		

Prehensile patterns: Check if able to perform

		R	L
GRASP: Cylinders	2.5 cm		
	5 cm		
	7.5 cm		
	10 cm		
Spheres	5 cm		
	7.5 cm		
	10 cm		
	12.5 cm		

STRENGTH: [ ] Lb [ ] Kg [ ] mm Hg

		R	L
Pulp pinch	Index		
	Middle		
	Ring		
	Little		
Lateral or key pinch			
Grip			

ADL: I: Independent A: Assisted U: Unable

Dress	I	A	U	Hygiene	I	A	U
Upper ext				Teeth			
Trunk				Hair			
Lower ext				Shave			
Bathe				Pick up coin			
Shower				Turn key			
Eat				Doorknob			
Toilet				Car door			
Telephone				Screw-top jar			
Typewrite				Aerosol can			
Write				Fasteners			

Ambulatory status:
[ ] Independent [ ] Wheelchair with partial walking
[ ] Assisted walk [ ] Bedfast

Code for clinical abnormality:
1— Swan-neck, thumb
2—Thumb boutonnière
3—Subluxation–dislocation
4—Swan-neck, finger
5—Boutonnière, finger
6—Intrinsic tightness
7—Ulnar drift
8—Radial drift
9—Ankylosis
10—Instability
11—Tendon rupture
12—Constrictive tenosynovitis
13—Synovial hypertrophy
14—Crepitation with motion
15—Extensor tendon subluxation
16—Varus angle
17—Valgus angle
18—Rotational deformity
19—Erosions
20—Joint narrowing
21—Subchondral sclerosis
22—Painful joint with motion
23—Nerve compression—M, U, R
24—Vasculitis
25—Nodules

Severity index:
a—Mild
b—Moderate
c—Severe

Sketch implant into appropriate site

Palm R   Palm L

Figure 7-44

Functional assessment form for the hand, designed for evaluation of rheumatoid and arthritic hands. (Modified from Swanson AB: *Flexible implant resection arthroplasty in the hand and extremities*, St Louis, 1973, C.V. Mosby.)

HAND EVALUATION RECORD

Name _____ Age _____ Date _____ Major hand _____
Occupation _____ X-rays _____ Photographs _____
History:

Shoulder:	L	R	Wrist:			Circ:		
For	____	____	DF	____	____	Biceps	____	____
Back	____	____	PF	____	____	Forearm	____	____
Abd	____	____	RD	____	____	Grip: L	____	____
Add	____	____	UD	____	____	R	____	____
Rotation Int	____	____	Elbow: Ext	____	____	Forearm: Pro	____	____
Ext	____	____	Flex	____	____	Sup	____	____

		MP	IP			% Impairment
Thumb	Ext			Abd		
	Flex			Add		
	Ankylosis			Opp		

		MP	PIP	DIP	Flex pulp to midpalmar crease	
Index	Ext					
	Flex					
	Ankylosis					
Middle	Ext					
	Flex					
	Ankylosis					
Ring	Ext					
	Flex					
	Ankylosis					
Little	Ext					
	Flex					
	Ankylosis					

Total %

Chart:
1. Amputations
2. Scars
3. Skin—subcutaneous loss
4. Nail bed injury
5. Major nerve loss: R, M, U
6. Digital bundle loss
7. Neuroma
8. Pain and tenderness
9. Bone damage
10. Joint damage
11. Flexor tendon loss
12. Extensor tendon loss
13. Ligament injury
14. Sensibility—pickup
        two-point
        Ninhydrin
15. Prehension:
    Grasp—small
          large
    Pinch—pulp
          tip
          lateral
    Hook—distal
          proximal
    Scoop
16. Maximum improvement
17. Rehabilitation needed
18. Further treatment
19. Classification
NOTE: Degrees of motion
      recorded as left/right

Dorsum R hand
or
Palmar L hand

Dorsum L hand
or
Palmar R hand

Figure 7-45
This form is designed for posttraumatic conditions and other disorders of the hand. (Modified from Swanson AB: *Flexible implant resection arthroplasty in the hand and extremities*, St Louis, 1973, C.V. Mosby.)

pain, work performance, esthetics, and patient satisfaction (Figure 7-47). Likewise, Dias et al.[44] have developed the Patient Evaluation Measure (PEM) Questionnaire (Figure 7-48). Table 7-8 provides a functional testing method. These strength values would be considered normal for an average population. They would be considered low for an athletic population or for persons in occupations subjecting the forearm, wrist, and hand to high repetitive loads.

Functional coordinated movements may be tested by asking the patient to perform simple activities, such as

Estimated Use of Grips for Activities of Daily Living[43]	
20% Pulp-to-pulp pinch:	20%
Three lateral pinch:	20%
Five-finger pinch:	15%
Fist grip:	15%
Cylinder grip:	14%
Three-fingered (thumb, index finger, middle finger) pinch:	10%
Spherical grip:	4%
Hook grip:	2%

Carpal Tunnel (Median Nerve) Function Disability Form

Symptom Severity Scale

The following questions refer to your symptoms for a typical twenty-four-hour period during the past two weeks (circle one answer to each question)

How severe is the hand or wrist pain that you have at night?
1   I do not have hand or wrist pain at night
2   Mild pain
3   Moderate pain
4   Severe pain
5   Very severe pain

How often did hand or wrist pain wake you up during a typical night in the past two weeks?
1   Never
2   Once
3   Two or three times
4   Four or five times
5   More than five times

Do you typically have pain in your hand or wrist during the daytime?
1   I never have pain during the day
2   I have mild pain during the day
3   I have moderate pain during the day
4   I have severe pain during the day
5   I have very severe pain during the day

How often do you have hand or wrist pain during the daytime?
1   Never
2   Once or twice a day
3   Three to five times a day
4   More than five times a day
5   The pain is constant

How long, on average, does an episode of pain last during the daytime?
1   I never get pain during the day
2   Less than 10 minutes
3   10 to 60 minutes
4   Greater than 60 minutes
5   The pain is constant throughout the day

Do you have numbness (loss of sensation) in your hand?
1   No
2   I have mild numbness
3   I have moderate numbness
4   I have severe numbness
5   I have very severe numbness

Do you have weakness in your hand or wrist?
1   No weakness
2   Mild weakness
3   Moderate weakness
4   Severe weakness
5   Very severe weakness

Do you have tingling sensations in your hand?
1   No tingling
2   Mild tingling
3   Moderate tingling
4   Severe tingling
5   Very severe tingling

Figure 7-46

Carpal tunnel (median nerve) function disability form. (Modified from Levine DW et al: A self-administered questionnaire for the assessment of severity of symptoms and functional status in carpal tunnel syndrome, *J Bone Joint Surg Am* 75:1586–1587, 1993.)

Symptom Severity Scale *Continued*

How severe is numbness (loss of sensation) or tingling at night?
1   I have no numbness or tingling at night
2   Mild
3   Moderate
4   Severe
5   Very severe

How often did hand numbness or tingling wake you up during a typical night during the past two weeks?
1   Never
2   Once
3   Two or three times
4   Four or five times
5   More than five times

Do you have difficulty with the grasping and use of small objects such as keys or pens?
1   No difficulty
2   Mild difficulty
3   Moderate difficulty
4   Severe difficulty
5   Very severe difficulty

Functional Status Scale

On a typical day during the past two weeks have hand and wrist symptoms caused you to have any difficulty doing the activities listed below? Please circle one number that best describes your ability to do the activity.

Activity	No Difficulty	Mild Difficulty	Moderate Difficulty	Severe Difficulty	Cannot Do at All Due to Hand or Wrist Symptoms
Writing	1	2	3	4	5
Buttoning of clothes	1	2	3	4	5
Holding a book while reading	1	2	3	4	5
Gripping of a telephone handle	1	2	3	4	5
Opening of jars	1	2	3	4	5
Household chores	1	2	3	4	5
Carrying of grocery bags	1	2	3	4	5
Bathing and dressing	1	2	3	4	5

Figure 7-46 cont'd

---

fastening a button, tying a shoelace, or tracing a diagram. Different prehension patterns are used regularly during daily activities.[45]

These tests may also be graded on a four-point scale.[45] This scale is particularly suitable if the patient has difficulty with one of the subtests, and the subtests can be scale-graded:

Unable to perform task: 0
Completes task partially: 1
Completes task but is slow and clumsy: 2
Performs task normally: 3

As part of the functional assessment, manual dexterity tests may be performed. Many standardized tests have been developed to assess manual dexterity and coordination. If comparison with other subjects is desired, the examiner must ensure that the patient is compared with a similar group of patients in terms of age, disability, and occupation. Each of these tests has its supporters and detractors. Some of the more common tests include the ones on pages 429 and 435.

Jebson-Taylor Hand Function Test. This easily administered test involves seven functional areas: (1) writing; (2) card turning; (3) picking up small objects; (4) simulated feeding; (5) stacking; (6) picking up large, light objects; and (7) picking up large, heavy objects. The subtests are timed for each limb. This test primarily measures

Text continued on page 435

Michigan Hand Outcomes Questionnaire

Instructions: This survey asks for your views about your hands and your health. This information will help keep track of how you feel and how well you are able to do your usual activities. Answer *every* question by marking the answer as indicated. If you are unsure about how to answer a question, please give the best answer you can.

I. The following questions refer to the function of your hand(s)/wrist(s) *during the past week*. (Please circle one answer for each question.)

A. The following questions refer to your *right* hand/wrist.

	Very Good	Good	Fair	Poor	Very Poor
1. Overall, how well did your *right* hand work?	1	2	3	4	5
2. How well did your *right* fingers move?	1	2	3	4	5
3. How well did your *right* wrist move?	1	2	3	4	5
4. How was the strength in your *right* hand?	1	2	3	4	5
5. How was the sensation (feeling) in your *right* hand?	1	2	3	4	5

B. The following questions refer to your *left* hand/wrist.

	Very Good	Good	Fair	Poor	Very Poor
1. Overall, how well did your *left* hand work?	1	2	3	4	5
2. How well did your *left* fingers move?	1	2	3	4	5
3. How well did your *left* wrist move?	1	2	3	4	5
4. How was the strength in your *left* hand?	1	2	3	4	5
5. How was the sensation (feeling) in your *left* hand?	1	2	3	4	5

II. The following questions refer to the ability of your hand(s) to do certain tasks *during the past week*. (Please circle one answer for each question.)

A. How difficult was it for you to perform the following activities using your *right* hand?

	Not at All Difficult	A Little Difficult	Somewhat Difficult	Moderately Difficult	Very Difficult
1. Turn a door knob	1	2	3	4	5
2. Pick up a coin	1	2	3	4	5
3. Hold a glass of water	1	2	3	4	5
4. Turn a key in a lock	1	2	3	4	5
5. Hold a frying pan	1	2	3	4	5

B. How difficult was it for you to perform the following activities using your *left* hand?

	Not at All Difficult	A Little Difficult	Somewhat Difficult	Moderately Difficult	Very Difficult
1. Turn a door knob	1	2	3	4	5
2. Pick up a coin	1	2	3	4	5
3. Hold a glass of water	1	2	3	4	5
4. Turn a key in a lock	1	2	3	4	5
5. Hold a frying pan	1	2	3	4	5

C. How difficult was it for you to perform the following activities using *both of your* hands?

	Not at All Difficult	A Little Difficult	Somewhat Difficult	Moderately Difficult	Very Difficult
1. Open a jar	1	2	3	4	5
2. Button a shirt/blouse	1	2	3	4	5
3. Eat with a knife/fork	1	2	3	4	5
4. Carry a grocery bag	1	2	3	4	5
5. Wash dishes	1	2	3	4	5
6. Wash your hair	1	2	3	4	5
7. Tie shoelaces/knots	1	2	3	4	5

Figure 7-47

Michigan Hand Outcomes Questionnaire. (From Chung KC, Pillsbury MS, Walter MR, Hayward RA: Reliability and validity testing of the Michigan hand outcomes questionnaire, *J Hand Surg Am* 23:584–587, 1998.)

III. The following questions refer to how you did in your *normal work* (including both housework and school work) during the *past 4 weeks*. (Please circle one answer for each question.)

	Always	Often	Sometimes	Rarely	Never
1. How often were you unable to do your work because of problems with your hand(s)/wrist(s)?	1	2	3	4	5
2. How often did you have to shorten your work day because of problems with your hand(s)/wrist(s)?	1	2	3	4	5
3. How often did you have to take it easy at your work because of problems with your hand(s)/wrist(s)?	1	2	3	4	5
4. How often did you accomplish less in your work because of problems with your hand(s)/wrist(s)?	1	2	3	4	5
5. How often did you take longer to do the tasks in your work because of problems with your hand(s)/wrist(s)?	1	2	3	4	5

IV. The following questions refer to how much *pain* you had in your hand(s)/wrist(s) *during the past week*. (Please circle one answer for each question.)

1. How often did you have pain in your hand(s)/wrist(s)?
   1. Always
   2. Often
   3. Sometimes
   4. Rarely
   5. Never

If you answered *never* to question IV-1 above, please skip the following questions and go to the next page.

2. Please describe the pain you have in your hand(s)/wrist(s)?
   1. Very mild
   2. Mild
   3. Moderate
   4. Severe
   5. Very severe

	Always	Often	Sometimes	Rarely	Never
3. How often did the pain in your hand(s)/wrist(s) interfere with your sleep?	1	2	3	4	5
4. How often did the pain in your hand(s)/wrist(s) interfere with your daily activities (such as eating or bathing)?	1	2	3	4	5
5. How often did the pain in your hand(s)/wrist(s) make you unhappy?	1	2	3	4	5

V. A. The following questions refer to the appearance (look) of your *right* hand *during the past week*. (Please circle one answer for each question.)

	Strongly Agree	Agree	Neither Agree Nor Disagree	Disagree	Strongly Disagree
1. I was satisfied with the appearance (look) of my *right* hand.	1	2	3	4	5
2. The appearance (look) of my *right* hand sometimes made me uncomfortable in public.	1	2	3	4	5
3. The appearance (look) of my *right* hand made me depressed.	1	2	3	4	5
4. The appearance (look) of my *right* hand interfered with my normal social activities.	1	2	3	4	5

Figure 7-47 cont'd ▬▬▬▬▬▬▬▬

Continued

B. The following questions refer to the appearance (look) of your *left* hand *during the past week.* (Please circle one answer for each question.)

	Strongly Agree	Agree	Neither Agree Nor Disagree	Disagree	Strongly Disagree
1. I was satisfied with the appearance (look) of my *left* hand.	1	2	3	4	5
2. The appearance (look) of my *left* hand sometimes made me uncomfortable in public.	1	2	3	4	5
3. The appearance (look) of my *left* hand made me depressed.	1	2	3	4	5
4. The appearance (look) of my *left* hand interfered with my normal social activities.	1	2	3	4	5

VI. A. The following questions refer to your satisfaction with your *right* hand/wrist *during the past week.* (Please circle one answer for each question.)

	Very Satisfied	Somewhat Satisfied	Neither Satisfied Nor Dissatisfied	Somewhat Dissatisfied	Very Dissatisfied
1. Overall function of your *right* hand	1	2	3	4	5
2. Motion of the fingers in your *right* hand	1	2	3	4	5
3. Motion of your *right* wrist	1	2	3	4	5
4. Strength of your *right* hand	1	2	3	4	5
5. Pain level of your *right* hand	1	2	3	4	5
6. Sensation (feeling) of your *right* hand	1	2	3	4	5

B. The following questions refer to your satisfaction with your *left* hand/wrist *during the past week.* (Please circle one answer for each question.)

	Very Satisfied	Somewhat Satisfied	Neither Satisfied Nor Dissatisfied	Somewhat Dissatisfied	Very Dissatisfied
1. Overall function of your *left* hand	1	2	3	4	5
2. Motion of the fingers in your *left* hand	1	2	3	4	5
3. Motion of your *left* wrist	1	2	3	4	5
4. Strength of your *left* hand	1	2	3	4	5
5. Pain level of your *left* hand	1	2	3	4	5
6. Sensation (feeling) of your *left* hand	1	2	3	4	5

VII. Please provide the following information about yourself. (Please circle one answer for each question.)

1. Are you right-handed or left-handed?
   a. Right-handed
   b. Left-handed
   c. Both

2. Which hand gives you the most problem?
   a. Right hand
   b. Left hand
   c. Both

3. Have you changed your job since you had problems with your hand(s)?
   a. Yes
   b. No

   Please describe the type of job you did *before* you had problems with your hand(s) _____

   _____

   Please describe the type of job you are doing *now* _____

   _____

Figure 7-47 cont'd ▬▬▬▬

Part one – treatment

Please put a circle around the number that is closest to the way you feel about how things have been for you. There are no right or wrong answers.

1. Throughout my treatment I have seen the same doctor:

   1   2   3   4   5   6   7
   Every time   Not at all

2. When the doctor saw me, he or she knew about my case:

   1   2   3   4   5   6   7
   Very well   Not at all

3. When I was with the doctor, he or she gave me the chance to talk:

   1   2   3   4   5   6   7
   As much as I wanted   Not at all

4. When I did talk to the doctor, he or she listened and understood me:

   1   2   3   4   5   6   7
   Very much   Not at all

5. I was given information about my treatment and progress:

   1   2   3   4   5   6   7
   All that I wanted   Not at all

Part two – how is your hand now

Hand health profile

1. The feeling in my hand is now:

   1   2   3   4   5   6   7
   Normal   Absent

2. When my hand is cold and/or damp, the pain is now:

   1   2   3   4   5   6   7
   Non-existent   Unbearable

3. Most of the time, the pain in my hand is now:

   1   2   3   4   5   6   7
   Non-existent   Unbearable

4. The duration my pain is present is:

   1   2   3   4   5   6   7
   Never   All the time

(Part two cont'd)

5. When I try to use my hand for fiddly things, it is now:

   1   2   3   4   5   6   7
   Skillful   Clumsy

6. Generally, when I move my hand it is:

   1   2   3   4   5   6   7
   Flexible   Stiff

7. The grip in my hand is now:

   1   2   3   4   5   6   7
   Strong   Weak

8. For everyday activities, my hand is now:

   1   2   3   4   5   6   7
   No problem   Useless

9. For my work, my hand is now:

   1   2   3   4   5   6   7
   No problem   Useless

10. When I look at the appearance of my hand now, I feel:

    1   2   3   4   5   6   7
    Unconcerned   Embarrassed & self-conscious

11. Generally, when I think about my hand I feel:

    1   2   3   4   5   6   7
    Unconcerned   Very upset

Part three – overall assessment

1. Generally, my treatment at the hospital has been:

   1   2   3   4   5   6   7
   Very satisfactory   Very unsatisfactory

2. Generally, my hand is now:

   1   2   3   4   5   6   7
   Very satisfactory   Very unsatisfactory

3. Bearing in mind my original injury or condition, I feel my hand is now:

   1   2   3   4   5   6   7
   Better than I expected   Worse than I expected

Figure 7-48

The PEM Questionnaire. (From Dias JJ et al: Assessing the outcome of disorders of the hands—is the patient evaluation measure reliable, responsive, and without bias? *J Bone Joint Surg Br* 83:236, 2001.)

Table 7-8

Functional Testing of the Wrist and Hand

Starting Position	Action	Functional Test
1. Forearm supinated, resting on table	Wrist flexion	Lift 0 lb: Nonfunctional Lift 1 to 2 lb: Functionally poor Life 3 to 4 lb: Functionally fair Lift 5+ lb: Functional
2. Forearm pronated, resting on table	Wrist extension lifting 1 to 2 lb	0 Repetitions: Nonfunctional 1 to 2 Repetitions: Functionally poor 3 to 4 Repetitions: Functionally fair 5+ Repetitions: Functional
3. Forearm between supination and pronation, resting on table	Radial deviation lifting 1 to 2 lb	0 Repetitions: Nonfunctional 1 to 2 Repetitions: Functionally poor 3 to 4 Repetitions: Functionally fair 5+ Repetitions: Functional
4. Forearm between supination and pronation, resting on table	Thumb flexion with resistance from rubber band* around thumb	0 Repetitions: Nonfunctional 1 to 2 Repetitions: Functionally poor 3 to 4 Repetitions: Functionally fair 5+ Repetitions: Functional
5. Forearm resting on table, rubber band around thumb and index finger	Thumb extension against resistance of rubber band*	0 Repetitions: Nonfunctional 1 to 2 Repetitions: Functionally poor 3 to 4 Repetitions: Functionally fair 5+ Repetitions: Functional
6. Forearm resting on table, rubber band around thumb and index finger	Thumb abduction against resistance of rubber band*	0 Repetitions: Nonfunctional 1 to 2 Repetitions: Functionally poor 3 to 4 Repetitions: Functionally fair 5+ Repetitions: Functional
7. Forearm resting on table	Thumb adduction, lateral pinch of piece of paper	Hold 0 sec: Nonfunctional Hold 1 to 2 sec: Functionally poor Hold 3 to 4 sec: Functionally fair Hold 5+ sec: Functional
8. Forearm resting on table	Thumb opposition, pulp-to-pulp pinch of piece of paper	Hold 0 sec: Nonfunctional Hold 1 to 2 sec: Functionally poor Hold 3 to 4 sec: Functionally fair Hold 5+ sec: Functional
9. Forearm resting on table	Finger flexion, patient grasps mug or glass using cylindrical grasp and lifts off table	0 Repetitions: Nonfunctional 1 to 2 Repetitions: Functionally poor 3 to 4 Repetitions: Functionally fair 5+ Repetitions: Functional
10. Forearm resting on table	Patient attempts to put on rubber glove keeping fingers straight	21+ sec: Nonfunctional 10 to 20 sec: Functionally poor 4 to 8 sec: Functionally poor 2 to 4 sec: Functional
11. Forearm resting on table	Patient attempts to pull fingers apart (finger abduction) against resistance of rubber band* and holds	Hold 0 sec: Nonfunctional Hold 1 to 2 sec: Functionally poor Hold 3 to 4 sec: Functionally fair Hold 5+ sec: Functional
12. Forearm resting on table	Patient holds piece of paper between fingers while examiner pulls on paper	Hold 0 sec: Nonfunctional Hold 1 to 2 sec: Functionally poor Hold 3 to 4 sec: Functionally fair Hold 5+ sec: Functional

Data from Palmer ML, Epler M: *Clinical assessment procedures in physical therapy,* pp. 140–144, Philadelphia, 1990, J.B. Lippincott.
*Rubber band should be at least 1 cm wide.

gross coordination, assessing prehension and manipulative skills with functional tests. It does not test bilateral integration.[26,46-48] Anyone wishing to perform the test should consult the original article[49] for details of administration.

Minnesota Rate of Manipulation Test. This test involves five activities: (1) placing, (2) turning, (3) displacing, (4) one-hand turning and placing, and (5) two-hand turning and placing. The activities are timed for both limbs and compared with normal values. The test primarily measures gross coordination and dexterity.[26,46,47]

Purdue Pegboard Test. This test measures fine coordination with the use of small pins, washers, and collars. The assessment categories of the test are (1) right hand, (2) left hand, (3) both hands, (4) right, left, and both, and (5) assembly. The subtests are timed and compared with normal values based on gender and occupation.[26,46,47]

Crawford Small Parts Dexterity Test. This test measures fine coordination, including the use of tools such as tweezers and screwdrivers to assemble things, to adjust equipment, and to do engraving.[26,46]

Simulated Activities of Daily Living Examination. This test consists of 19 subtests, including standing, walking, putting on a shirt, buttoning, zipping, putting on gloves, dialing a telephone, tying a bow, manipulating safety pins, manipulating coins, threading a needle, unwrapping a Band-Aid, squeezing toothpaste, and using a knife and fork. Each subtask is timed.[45]

Moberg's Pickup Test. An assortment of 9 or 10 objects (e.g., bolts, nuts, screws, buttons, coins, pens, paper clips, keys) is used. The patient is timed for the following tests:
1. Putting objects in a box with the affected hand
2. Putting objects in a box with the unaffected hand
3. Putting objects in a box with the affected hand with eyes closed

The examiner notes which digits are used for prehension. Digits with altered sensation are less likely to be used. The test is used for median or combined median and ulnar nerve lesions.[50]

Box and Block Test. This is a test for gross manual dexterity in which 150 blocks, each measuring 2.5 cm (1 inch) on a side, are used. The patient has 1 minute in which to individually transfer the blocks from one side of a divided box to the other. The number of blocks transferred is given as the score. Patients are given a 15-second practice trial before the test.[48]

Nine-Hole Peg Test. This test is used to assess finger dexterity. The patient places nine 3.2-cm (1.3-inch) pegs in a 12.7 × 12.7 cm (5 × 5 inch) board and then removes them. The score is the time taken to do this task. Each hand is tested separately.[48]

Special Tests

For the forearm, wrist, and hand, no special tests exist that are commonly done with each assessment.

Depending on the history, observation, and examination to this point, certain special tests may be performed. The examiner picks the appropriate test or tests to help confirm the diagnosis. As with all special tests, however, the examiner must keep in mind that they are confirming tests. When they are positive, they are highly suggestive that the problem exists, but if they are negative, they do not rule out the problem. This is especially true for the tests of neurological dysfunction. The reliability, validity, specificity and sensitivity of some special/diagnostic tests used in the forearm, wrist, and hand are outlined in Appendix 7-1.

Tests for Ligament, Capsule, and Joint Instability

Ligamentous Instability Test for the Fingers. The examiner stabilizes the finger with one hand proximal to the joint to be tested. With the other hand, the examiner grasps the finger distal to the joint to be tested. The examiner's distal hand is then used to apply a varus or valgus stress to the joint (proximal or distal interphalangeal) to test the integrity of the collateral ligaments. The results are compared for laxity with those of the uninvolved hand, which is tested first.

Thumb Ulnar Collateral Ligament Laxity or Instability Test. The patient sits while the examiner stabilizes the patient's hand with one hand and takes the patient's thumb into extension with the other hand. While holding the thumb in extension, the examiner applies a valgus stress to the metacarpophalangeal joint of the thumb, stressing the ulnar collateral ligament and accessory collateral ligament. If the valgus movement is greater than 30° to 35°, it indicates a complete tear of the ulnar collateral and accessory collateral ligaments.[51] If the ligament is only partially torn, the laxity would be less than 30° to 35°. In this case, laxity would still be greater than the unaffected side (normal laxity in extension is about 15°) but not as much as with a complete tear. To test the collateral ligament in isolation, the carpometacarpal joint is flexed to 30° and a valgus stress is applied.[52] This is a test for gamekeeper's or skier's thumb (Figure 7-49).

Test for Tight Retinacular (Collateral) Ligaments (Haines-Zancolli Test).[53] This test tests the structures around the proximal interphalangeal joint. The proximal interphalangeal joint is held in a neutral position while the distal interphalangeal joint is flexed by the examiner (Figure 7-50). If the distal interphalangeal joint does not flex, the retinacular (collateral) ligaments or proximal interphalangeal capsule are tight. If the proximal interphalangeal joint is flexed and the distal interphalangeal joint flexes easily, the retinacular ligaments are tight and the capsule is normal. During the test, the patient remains passive and does no active movements.

Lunotriquetral Ballottement (Reagan's) Test. This test is used to determine the integrity of the lunotriquetral

Figure 7-49

A and **B,** Testing stability of the ulnar collateral ligament in the thumb of a normal individual. In extension, the thumb was stable, but in flexion, it appeared to be unstable. This was caused by the laxity of the dorsal capsule at the metacarpophalangeal joint. (From Nicholas JA, Hershman EB [eds]: *Upper extremity in sports medicine,* p. 580. St Louis, 1989, C.V. Mosby.)

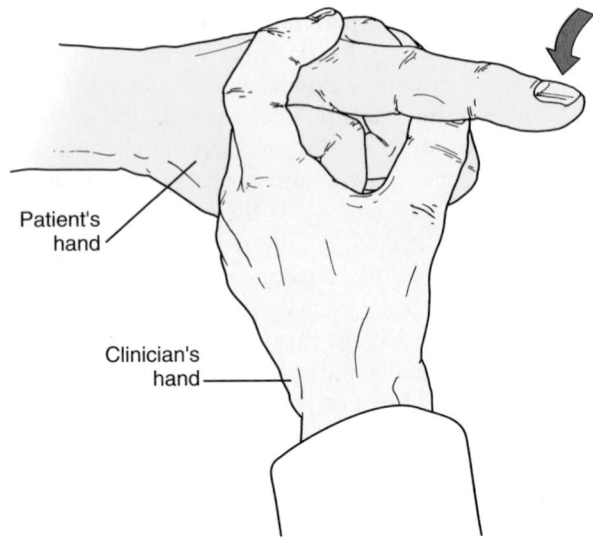

Figure 7-50
Test for retinacular ligaments.

Figure 7-51
Lunatotriquetral ballottement test for lunatotriquetral interosseous membrane dissociations.

ligament.[54] The examiner grasps the triquetrum between the thumb and second finger of one hand and the lunate with the thumb and second finger of the other hand (Figure 7-51). The examiner then moves the lunate up and down (anteriorly and posteriorly), noting any laxity, crepitus, or pain, which indicates a positive test for lunotriquetral instability.[55,56]

Lunotriquetral Shear Test.[54,57] This test also tests the integrity of the lunotriquetral ligament. The patient is seated with the elbow flexed in neutral rotation and resting on the examining table. With one hand, the examiner grasps the patient's wrist so that the thumb rests in the patient's palm and the fingers are placed over the dorsum of the proximal row of carpals to support the

Figure 7-52
Lunotriquetral shear test.

lunate. The thumb of the examiner's opposite hand loads the pisotriquetral joint on the palmar aspect, applying a shearing force to the lunotriquetral joint (Figure 7-52). Pain, crepitus, or abnormal movement are considered positive tests.

Finger Extension or "Shuck" Test.[58] The patient is placed in sitting. The examiner holds the patient's wrist flexed and asks the patient to actively extend the fingers against resistance-loading the radiocarpal joints. Pain would indicate a positive test for radiocarpal or midcarpal instability, scaphoid instability, inflammation, or Kienböck's disease (Figure 7-53).

Murphy's Sign. The patient is asked to make a fist. If the head of the third metacarpal is level with the second and fourth metacarpals, the sign is positive and indicative of a lunate dislocation.[59] Normally, the third metacarpal would project beyond (or further distally) the second and fourth metacarpals.

Watson (Scaphoid Shift) Test.[60] The patient sits with the elbow resting on the table and forearm pronated. The examiner faces the patient. With one hand, the examiner takes the patient's wrist into full ulnar deviation and slight extension while holding the metacarpals. The examiner presses the thumb of the other hand against the distal pole of the scaphoid on the palmar side to prevent it from moving toward the palm while the fingers provide a counter pressure on the dorsum of the forearm. With the first hand, the examiner radially deviates and slightly flexes the patient's hand while maintaining pressure on the scaphoid. This creates a subluxation stress if the scaphoid is unstable. If the scaphoid (and lunate) are unstable, the dorsal pole of the scaphoid subluxes or "shifts" over the dorsal rim of the radius and the patient complains of pain, indicating a positive test (Figure 7-54).[17,56,61,62] If the scaphoid subluxes with the thumb pressure when the thumb is removed, the scaphoid commonly returns to its normal position with a "thunk." If the ligamentous tissue is intact, the scaphoid will normally move forward, pushing the thumb forward with it.

Figure 7-53
Finger extension or "shuck" test.

Figure 7-54
Watson (scaphoid shift) test.

Scaphoid Stress Test. This test is a modification of the Watson test, done actively by the patient. The patient sits and the examiner holds the patient's wrist with one hand so that the thumb applies pressure over the distal pole of the scaphoid. The patient then attempts to radially deviate the wrist. Normally, the patient is unable to deviate the wrist. If excessive laxity is present, the scaphoid is forced dorsally out of the scaphoid fossa of the radius with a resulting "clunk" and pain, indicating a positive test for scaphoid instability.[62,63]

Dorsal Capitate Displacement Apprehension Test. This test is used to determine the stability of the capitate bone.[64] The patient sits facing the examiner. The examiner holds the forearm (radius and ulna) with one hand. The thumb of the examiner's other hand is placed over the palmar aspect of the capitate while the fingers of that hand hold the patient's hand in neutral (no flexion or extension, no radial or ulnar deviation) and apply a counter pressure when the examiner pushes the capitate posteriorly with the thumb (Figure 7-55). Reproduction of the patient's symptoms, apprehension, or pain indicates a positive test. A click or snap may also be heard when pressure is applied.

"Piano Keys" Test. The patient sits with both arms in pronation. The examiner stabilizes the patient's arm with one hand so that the examiner's index finger can push down on the distal ulna. The examiner's other hand supports the patient's hand. The examiner pushes down on the distal ulna as one would push down on a piano key. The results are compared with the nonsymptomatic side. A positive test is indicated by a difference in mobility and the production of pain and/or tenderness.

A positive test indicates instability of the distal radioulnar joint.[16]

Supination Lift Test.[65] This test is used to determine pathology in the triangular fibrocartilage complex-TFCC (also called the triangular cartilaginous disc). The patient is seated with elbows flexed to 90° and forearms supinated. The patient is asked to place the palms flat on the underside of a heavy table (or flat against the examiner's hands). The patient is then asked to lift the table (or push up against the resisting examiner's hands). Localized pain on the ulnar side of the wrist and difficulty applying the force are positive indications for a dorsal TFCC tear. Pain on forced ulnar deviation causing ulnar impaction is a symptom of TFCC tears (Figure 7-56).

Triangular Fibrocartilage Complex (TFCC) Load Test.[66] The examiner holds the patient's forearm with one hand and the patient's hand with the other hand. The examiner then axially loads and ulnarly deviates the wrist while moving it dorsally and palmarly or by rotating the forearm. A positive test is indicated by pain, clicking, or crepitus in the area of the TFCC.

Figure 7-55
Dorsal capitate displacement apprehension test. Note the position of the examiner's thumb over the capitate to push it posteriorly.

Figure 7-56
Supination lift test.

Figure 7-57
Ulnar impaction test.

Figure 7-58
Linscheid test.

Ulnar Impaction Test.[28] The patient is seated with the elbow flexed to 90° and the wrist in ulnar deviation. The examiner holds the patient's forearm with one hand and then applies an axial compression force through the 4th and 5th metacarpals (Figure 7-57). A positive test is indicated by pain and may be related to a TFCC injury or ulnar impaction syndrome.

Axial Load Test. The patient sits while the examiner stabilizes the patient's wrist with one hand. With the other hand, the examiner carefully grasps the patient's thumb and applies axial compression. Pain and/or crepitation indicate a positive test for a fracture of metacarpal or adjacent carpal bones or joint arthrosis. A similar test may be performed for the fingers.

Pivot Shift Test of the Midcarpal Joint. The patient is seated with the elbow flexed to 90° and resting on a firm surface and the hand fully supinated. The examiner stabilizes the forearm with one hand and with the other hand takes the patient's hand into full radial deviation with the wrist in neutral. While the examiner maintains the patient's hand position, the patient's hand is taken into full ulnar deviation. A positive test results if the capitate "shifts" away from the lunate, indicating injury to the anterior capsule and interosseous ligaments.[3]

Thumb Grind Test. The examiner holds the patient's hand with one hand and grasps the patient's thumb below the metacarpophalangeal joint with the other hand. The examiner then applies axial compression and rotation to the metacarpophalangeal joint. If pain is elicited, the test is positive and indicative of degenerative joint disease in the metacarpophalangeal or metacarpotrapezial joint.[41,67] Axial compression with rotation to any of the wrist and hand joints may also indicate positive tests to those joints for the same condition.

Linscheid Test.[66,68] This test is used to detect ligamentous instability of the second and third carpometacarpal joints. The examiner supports the metacarpal shafts with one hand. With the other hand, the examiner pushes the metacarpal heads dorsally, then palmarly (Figure 7-58). Pain localized to the carpometacarpal joints is a positive test.

Lichtman Test.[28] The test is used to detect midcarpal instability. The patient's forearm is pronated with the hand held in support by the examiner. The examiner moves the patient's hand from radial to ulnar deviation while axially compressing the carpus into the radius. If the distal carpal row jumps or snaps dorsally (from its subluxed position palmarly), the test is considered positive.

Sitting Hands Test.[66] The patient places both hands on the arms of a stable chair and pushes off, suspending the body while using only the hands for support (Figure 7-59). This test places a great deal of stress in the wrist (and elbow; see elbow instability tests) and is too difficult to do in the presence of significant wrist synovitis or wrist pathology.

Tests for Tendons and Muscles

Finkelstein Test. The Finkelstein test[69] is used to determine the presence of de Quervain's or Hoffmann's disease, a paratenonitis in the thumb.[19] The patient

Figure 7-59
Sitting hands test.

makes a fist with the thumb inside the fingers (Figure 7-60). The examiner stabilizes the forearm and deviates the wrist toward the ulnar side. A positive test is indicated by pain over the abductor pollicis longus and extensor pollicis brevis tendons at the wrist and is indicative of a paratenonitis of these two tendons. Because the test can cause some discomfort in normal individuals, the examiner should compare the pain caused on the affected side with that of the normal side. Only if the patient's symptoms are produced is the test considered positive.

Sweater Finger Sign. The patient is asked to make a fist. If the distal phalanx of one of the fingers does not flex, the sign is positive for a ruptured flexor digitorum profundus tendon (Figure 7-61). It occurs most often to the ring finger.

Test for Extensor Hood Rupture.[70] The finger to be examined is flexed to 90° at the proximal interphalangeal joint over the edge of a table. The finger is held in position by the examiner. The patient is asked to carefully extend the proximal interphalangeal joint while the examiner palpates the middle phalanx. A positive test for a torn central extensor hood is the examiner's feeling little pressure from the middle phalanx while the distal interphalangeal joint is extending.

Boyes Test.[70,71] This test also tests the central slip of the extensor hood. The examiner holds the finger to be examined in slight extension at the proximal interphalangeal joint. The patient is then asked to flex the distal interphalangeal joint. If the patient is unable or has difficulty flexing the distal interphalangeal joint, it is considered a positive test.

Bunnel-Littler (Finochietto-Bunnel) Test. This test tests the structures around the metacarpophalangeal joint. The metacarpophalangeal joint is held slightly extended while the examiner moves the

Figure 7-60
Finkelstein test.

Figure 7-61

Sweater finger sign. Rupture of the flexor profundus tendon in the ring finger of a football player.

Figure 7-62

Positioning for the Bunnel-Littler test.

proximal interphalangeal joint into flexion, if possible (Figure 7-62).[72] If the test is positive, which is indicated by inability to flex the proximal interphalangeal joint, there is a tight intrinsic muscle or contracture of the joint capsule. If the metacarpophalangeal joints are slightly flexed, the proximal interphalangeal joint flexes fully if the intrinsic muscles are tight, but it does not flex fully

if the capsule is tight. The patient remains passive during the test. This test is also called the **intrinsic-plus test**.[3]

Linburg's Sign. The patient flexes the thumb maximally onto the hypothenar eminence and actively extends the index finger as far as possible. If limited index finger extension and pain are noted, the sign is positive for paratenonitis at the interconnection between flexor pollicis longus and flexor indices (an anomalous tendon condition seen in 10% to 15% of hands).[55,73]

Tests for Neurological Dysfunction

Tests for neurological dysfunction are highly suggestive of a particular nerve lesion if they are positive, but they do not rule out the problem if they are negative. In fact, they may be negative 50% of the time, or more, when the condition actually exists. Electrodiagnostic tests are more conclusive.[74,75]

Tinel's Sign (at the Wrist).[69] The examiner taps over the carpal tunnel at the wrist (Figure 7-63). A positive test causes tingling or paresthesia into the thumb, index finger (forefinger), and middle and lateral half of the ring finger (median nerve distribution). Tinel's sign at the wrist is indicative of a carpal tunnel syndrome. The tingling or paresthesia must be felt distal to the point of pressure for a positive test. The test gives an indication of the rate of regeneration of sensory fibers of the median nerve. The most distal point at which the abnormal sensation is felt represents the limit of nerve regeneration.

Figure 7-63

Tinel's sign at the wrist. Light percussion is applied along nerve starting at "A" and progressing proximally. The point at which paresthesia is elicited is the level of axonal regrowth.

Figure 7-64
Phalen's test.

Figure 7-65
Carpal compression test.

Phalen's (Wrist Flexion) Test. The examiner flexes the patient's wrists maximally and holds this position for 1 minute by pushing the patient's wrists together (Figure 7-64). A positive test is indicated by tingling in the thumb, index finger, and middle and lateral half of the ring finger and is indicative of carpal tunnel syndrome caused by pressure on the median nerve.[76]

Reverse Phalen's (Prayer) Test. The examiner extends the patient's wrist while asking the patient to grip the examiner's hand. The examiner then applies direct pressure over the carpal tunnel for 1 minute. The test is also described by having the patient put both hands together and bringing the hands down towards the waist while keeping the palms in full contact, causing extension of the wrist. Doing the test this way does not put as much pressure on the carpal tunnel. A positive test produces the same symptoms as those seen in Phalen's test and is indicative of pathology of the median nerve.[55]

Carpal Compression Test.[77] The examiner holds the supinated wrist in both hands and applies direct, even pressure over the median nerve in the carpal tunnel for up to 30 seconds (Figure 7-65). Production of the patient's symptoms is considered to be a positive test for carpal tunnel syndrome. This test is a modification of the reverse Phalen's test.

Froment's Sign. The patient attempts to grasp a piece of paper between the thumb and index finger (Figure 7-66).[78] When the examiner attempts to pull away the paper, the terminal phalanx of the thumb flexes because of paralysis of the adductor pollicis muscle, indicating

a positive test. If, at the same time, the metacarpophalangeal joint of the thumb hyperextends, the hyperextension is noted as a positive **Jeanne's sign**.[41] Both tests, if positive, are indicative of ulnar nerve paralysis.

Egawa's Sign. The patient flexes the middle digit and then alternately deviates the finger radially and ulnarly. If the patient is unable to do this, the interossei are affected. A positive sign is indicative of ulnar nerve palsy.

Wrinkle (Shrivel) Test. The patient's fingers are placed in warm water for approximately 5 to 20 minutes. The examiner then removes the patient's fingers from the water and observes whether the skin over the pulp is wrinkled (Figure 7-67). Normal fingers show wrinkling, but denervated ones do not. The test is valid only within the first few months after injury.[79]

Ninhydrin Sweat Test. The patient's hand is cleaned thoroughly and wiped with alcohol. The patient then waits 5 to 30 minutes with the fingertips not in contact with any surface. This allows time for the sweating process to ensue. After the waiting period, the fingertips are pressed with moderate pressure against good-quality bond paper that has not been touched. The fingertips are held in place for 15 seconds and traced with a pencil. The paper is then sprayed with triketohydrindene (Ninhydrin) spray reagent and allowed to dry (24 hours). The sweat areas stain purple. If the change in color (from white to purple) does not occur, it is considered a positive test for a nerve lesion.[50,80] The reagent must be fixed if a permanent record is required.

Figure 7-66
Froment's sign. **A,** Start position. **B,** Thumb flexes when paper is pulled away (positive test).

Figure 7-67
The wrinkle test may be reliable for digital nerve sympathetic function if the fingers (in this case, the radial digital nerve of the fourth and fifth digits) are completely denervated. (From Waylett-Rendall J: Sensibility evaluation and rehabilitation, *Orthop Clin North Am* 19:48, 1988.)

Figure 7-68
Devices used to test two-point discrimination. **A,** The Disk-Criminator is a set of two plastic discs, each containing a series of metal rods at varying intervals from 1 to 25 mm apart. This device evaluates both moving and static two-point discrimination. **B,** Two-point esthesiometer.

Weber's (Moberg's) Two-Point Discrimination Test.
The examiner uses a paper clip, two-point discriminator, or calipers (Figure 7-68) to simultaneously apply pressure on two adjacent points in a longitudinal direction or perpendicular to the long axis of the finger; the examiner

Figure 7-69

Two-point discrimination. **A,** Technique of performing the two-point discrimination test of Weber (after Moberg). **B,** Values of discrimination in the Weber test in millimeters in the different zones of the palm. The largest figure indicates the average values, the other two figures the minimum and maximum values (after Moberg). (From Tubiana R: *The hand*, pp. 645–646, Philadelphia, 1981, W.B. Saunders.)

moves proximal to distal in an attempt to find the minimal distance at which the patient can distinguish between the two stimuli.[36] This distance is called the threshold for discrimination. Coverage values are shown in Figure 7-69. The patient must concentrate on feeling the points and must not be able to see the area being tested. Only the fingertips need to be tested. The patient's hand should be immobile on a hard surface. For accurate results, the examiner must ensure that the two points touch the skin simultaneously. There should be no blanching of the skin indicating too much pressure when the points are applied. The distance between the points is decreased or increased depending on the response of the patient. The starting distance between the points is one that the patient can easily distinguish (e.g., 15 mm). If the patient is hesitant to respond or becomes inaccurate, the patient is required to respond accurately on 7 or 8 of 10 trials before the distance is narrowed and the test repeated.[26,50,81,82] Normal discrimination distance recognition is less than 6 mm, but this varies from person to person. This test is best for hand sensation involving static holding of an object between the fingers and thumb and requiring pinch strength. Table 7-9 demonstrates some two-point discrimination normal values and distances required for certain tasks.

Dellon's Moving Two-Point Discrimination Test. This test is used to predict functional recovery; it measures the quickly adapting mechanoreceptor system.[36] The test is similar to Weber's two-point discrimination test except

Table 7-9

Two-Point Discrimination Normal Values and Discrimination Distances Required for Certain Tasks

Normal	<6 mm
Fair	6–10 mm
Poor	11–15 mm
Protective	1 point perceived
Anesthetic	0 points perceived
Winding a watch	6 mm
Sewing	6–8 mm
Handling precision tools	12 mm
Gross tool handling	>15 mm

Adapted from Callahan AD: Sensibility assessment for nerve lesions-in-continuity and nerve lacerations. *In* Mackin EJ et al (eds): *Hunter-Mackin-Callahan rehabilitation of the hand and upper extremity*, p. 233, St Louis, 2002, Mosby.

that the two points are moved during the test. This test is best for hand sensation related to activity and movement. The examiner moves two blunt points from proximal to distal along the long axis of the limb or digit, starting with a distance of 8 mm between the points. The distance between the points is increased or decreased, depending on the response of the patient, until the two points can no longer be distinguished. During the test, the patient's eyes are closed and the hand is cradled in the examiner's hand. The two smooth points, whether paper clip, two-point discriminator, or calipers, are gently placed longitudinally. There should be no blanching of the skin indicating too much pressure when the points are applied. The patient is asked whether one or two points are felt. If the patient is hesitant to respond or becomes inaccurate, the patient is required to respond accurately 7 or 8 of 10 times before the distance is narrowed and the test repeated.[26,50,81,83]

Normal discrimination distance recognition is 2 to 5 mm.[82] The values obtained for this test are slightly lower than those obtained for Weber's static two-point discrimination test.[81] Although the entire hand may be tested, it is more common to test only the anterior digital pulp.

Tests for Circulation and Swelling

Allen Test. The patient is asked to open and close the hand several times as quickly as possible and then squeeze the hand tightly (Figure 7-70).[76,84] The examiner's thumb

Clinician's hand

Figure 7-70

Allen test. **A,** The patient opens and closes the hand. **B,** While the patient holds the hand closed, the examiner compresses the radial and ulnar arteries. **C,** One artery (in this case, the radial artery) is then released and the examiner notes the filling pattern of the hand until the circulation is normal. **D,** The process is then repeated with the other artery. **E,** Alternative hand hold.

and index finger are placed over the radial and ulnar arteries, compressing them. As an alternative technique, the examiner may use both hands, placing one thumb over each artery to compress the artery and placing the fingers on the posterior aspect of the arm for stability. The patient then opens the hand while pressure is maintained over the arteries. One artery is tested by releasing the pressure over that artery to see if the hand flushes. The other artery is then tested in a similar fashion. Both hands should be tested for comparison. This test determines the patency of the radial and ulnar arteries and determines which artery provides the major blood supply to the hand.

Digit Blood Flow. To test distal blood flow, the examiner compresses the nail bed and notes the time taken for color to return to the nail. Normally, when the pressure is released, color should return to the nail bed within 3 seconds. If return takes longer, arterial insufficiency to the fingers should be suspected. Comparison with the normal side gives some indication of restricted flow.

Hand Volume Test. If the examiner is concerned about changes in hand size, a volumeter (Figure 7-71) may be used. This device can be used to assess change in hand size resulting from localized swelling, generalized edema, or atrophy.[46] Comparisons with the normal limb give the examiner an idea of changes occurring in the affected hand. Care must be taken when doing this test to ensure accurate readings. There is often a 10-mL difference between right and left hands and between dominant and nondominant hands. If swelling is the problem, differences of 30 to 50 mL can be noted.[26,85]

Figure 7-71
Volumeter used to measure hand volume.

Measurement for Swelling. Swelling may also be measured with a tape measure, as long as the examiner is consistent with the measuring points. When assessing swelling, the examiner commonly measures around the proximal interphalangeal joints individually, around the metacarpophalangeal joints as a group, and around the palm and wrist. The values for both sides are compared.

Reflexes and Cutaneous Distribution

Although it is possible to obtain reflexes from the tendons crossing the wrist, this is not commonly done. In fact, no deep tendon reflexes are routinely tested in the forearm, wrist, and hand. The only reflex that may be tested in the hand is Hoffman's reflex, which is a pathological reflex. This reflex may be tested if an upper motor neuron lesion is suspected. To test the reflex, the examiner "flicks" the terminal phalanx of the index, middle, or ring finger. A positive test is indicated by reflex flexion of the distal phalanx of the thumb or a finger that was not "flicked."

The examiner must be aware of the sensory distribution of the ulnar, median, and radial nerves in the hand (Figure 7-72) and must be prepared to compare peripheral nerve sensory distribution with nerve root sensory (dermatome) distributions. As previously mentioned, there is variability in both distributions. It has been reported, however, that each peripheral nerve of the upper limb has a "constant" area in the hand that is always affected if the nerve is injured. For the radial nerve, it is on the dorsum of the thumb near the apex of the anatomical snuff box; for the median nerve, it is the tip of the index finger; and for the ulnar nerve, it is the tip of the little finger.[86]

The median nerve gives off a sensory branch above the wrist before it passes through the carpal tunnel. This sensory branch supplies the skin of the palm (Figure 7-73). Thus, most commonly, carpal tunnel syndrome does not affect the median sensory distribution in the palm but results in altered sensation in the fingers.

Several sensation tests may be carried out in the hand. Table 7-10 illustrates the tests used and the sensation and nerve fibers tested. Pinprick is used to test for pain. Constant light touch, which is a component of fine discrimination, may be tested in the hand using a Semmes-Weinstein pressure esthesiometer (Von Frey test). This kit has 20 probes, each with different thicknesses of nylon monofilament (Figure 7-74). The patient is blindfolded or otherwise unable to see the hand, and each filament is applied perpendicularly to the finger, with the smallest filament being used first. The filament is pushed against the finger until the filament bends. The next filament is then used, and so on until the patient feels one before or just as it bends.[27,51] The test is repeated three times to ensure a positive result.[82] Normal values vary between probes 2.44 and 2.83 (Table 7-11). When doing the

Dorsal surface   Palmar surface

— Radial nerve

— Median nerve

— Ulnar nerve

Figure 7-72
Peripheral nerve distribution in the hand.

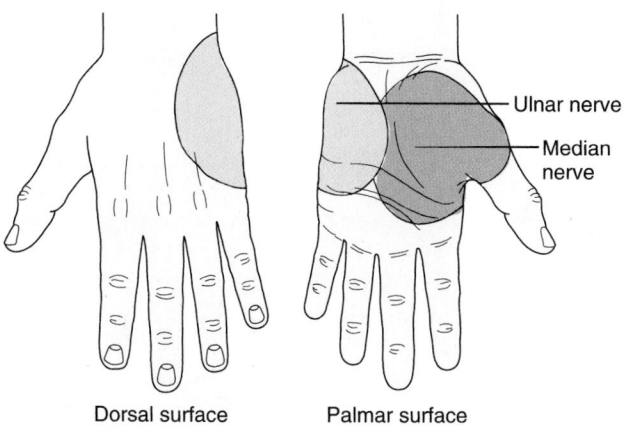

Dorsal surface   Palmar surface

— Ulnar nerve

— Median nerve

Figure 7-73
Sensory distribution of branches of the ulnar and median nerves given off above the wrist.

Figure 7-74
The Semmes-Weinstein monofilament is applied perpendicular to the skin for 1 to 1.5 seconds, held in place for 1 to 1.5 seconds, and lifted for 1 to 1.5 seconds.

Table 7-10

Tests for Cutaneous Sensibility

Test	Sensation	Fiber/Receptor Type
Pin	Pain	Free nerve endings
Warm/cold	Temperature	Free nerve endings
Cotton wool	Moving touch	Quick adapting
Finger stroking	Moving touch	Quick adapting
Dellon's test	Moving touch	Quick adapting
Tuning fork	Vibration	Quick adapting
Von Frey	Constant touch	Slow adapting
Weber's test	Constant touch	Slow adapting
Pick-up test	Constant touch	Slow adapting
Precision sensory grip	Constant touch	Slow adapting
Gross grip	Constant touch	Slow adapting

Modified from Dellon AL: The paper clip: Light hardware to evaluate sensibility in the hand, *Contemp Orthop* 1:40, 1979.

Semmes-Weinstein test, the hand and fingers are commonly divided into a grid (Figure 7-75), and only one point (usually in the center) is tested in each square. It is primarily the palmar aspect of the hand that is tested.

Stereognosis or tactile gnosis, which is the ability to identify common objects by touch, should also be tested. Objects are placed in the patient's hand while the patient is blindfolded or otherwise unable to see the object. The time taken to recognize the object is noted. Normal subjects can usually name the object within 3 seconds of contact.[81]

Vibratory sense is tested using a 256-cps (high frequency) or 30-cps (low-frequency) tuning fork. The patient, who cannot see the test site, indicates when

Table 7-11

Light Touch Testing Using Semmes-Weinstein Pressure Esthesiometer

Esthesiometer Probe No.	Calculated Pressure (g/mm²)	Interpretation
2.44–2.83	3.25–4.86	Normal light touch
3.22–4.56	11.1–47.3	Diminished light touch, point localization* intact
4.74–6.10	68.0–243.0	Minimal light touch, area localization† intact
6.10–6.65	243.0–439.0	Sensation but no localization sensibility

From Omer GE: Report of the Committee for Evaluation of the Clinical Result in Peripheral Nerve Injury, *J Hand Surg Am* 8:755, 1983.
*Point localization: the dowel is in contact with the skin point stimulated.
†Area localization: the dowel is in contact with any point inside the zone of the area being tested (in the hand or foot).

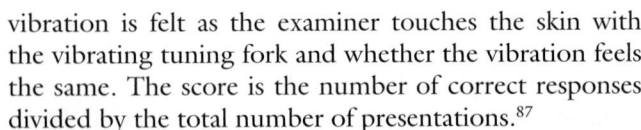

Palmar aspect

Figure 7-75
Grid pattern used for recording results of light touch sensation testing.

Figure 7-76
Symptoms can be referred to the wrist and hand from the elbow, shoulder, and cervical spine.

vibration is felt as the examiner touches the skin with the vibrating tuning fork and whether the vibration feels the same. The score is the number of correct responses divided by the total number of presentations.[87]

To test moving touch, the examiner's fingers stroke the patient's finger. The patient notes whether the stroking was felt and what it felt like.

It must be remembered that pain may be referred to the wrist and hand from the cervical or upper thoracic spine, shoulder, and elbow. Seldom is wrist or hand pain referred up the limb (Figure 7-76). Table 7-12 shows the muscles acting on the forearm, wrist, and hand and their pain referral patterns when injured.

The examiner can attempt a differential diagnosis of paresthesia in the hand if altered sensation is present. A comparison with a normal dermatome chart should be made, and the examiner should remember that there is a fair amount of variability and overlap with dermatomes (Figure 7-77). In addition, there are areas of the hand where sensation is more important (Figure 7-78). Abnormal sensation may mean the following:

Table 7-12

Forearm, Wrist, and Hand Muscles and Referral of Pain

Muscles	Referral Pattern
Brachioradialis	Lateral epicondyle, lateral forearm, and web space between thumb and index finger
Extensor carpi ulnaris	Medial side of dorsum of wrist
Extensor carpi radialis brevis	Middle of dorsum of wrist
Extensor carpi radialis longus	Lateral epicondyle, forearm, and lateral dorsum of hand
Extensor digitorum	Forearm, wrist to appropriate digit
Extensor indices	Dorsum of wrist to index finger
Palmaris longus	Anterior aspect of forearm to palm
Flexor carpi ulnaris	Anteromedial wrist into lateral palm
Flexor carpi radialis	Forearm to anterolateral wrist
Flexor digitorum superficialis	Palm into appropriate digit
Flexor pollicis longus	Thumb
Adductor pollicis	Anterolateral and posterolateral palm into thumb
Opponens pollicis	Anterolateral wrist into anterior thumb
Abductor digiti minimi	Dorsomedial surface of hand into little finger
Interossei	Into adjacent digit, and for first interossei, dorsum of hand

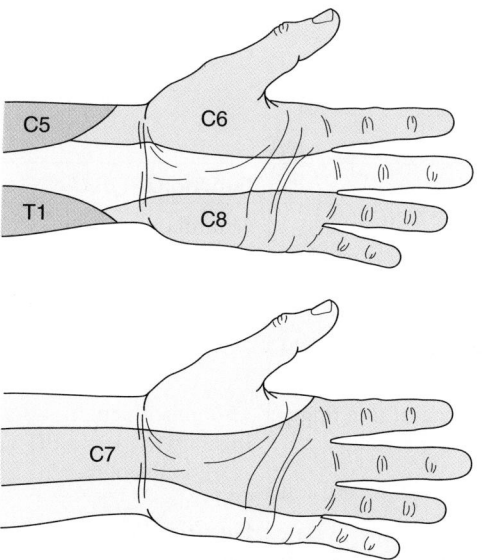

Figure 7-77

Dermatomes of the hand. Note overlap at dermatomes. Both views are palmar.

Figure 7-78

Importance of hand sensation. Darker areas indicate where sensation is most important; lighter areas, where sensation is a little less important; and white areas, where sensation is least important. (Redrawn from Tubiana R: *The hand*, p. 74, Philadelphia, 1981, W.B. Saunders.)

1. Numbness in the thumb only may be caused by pressure on the digital nerve on the outer aspect of the thumb.

2. A "pins and needles" feeling in the thumb may be caused by a contusion of the thenar branch of the median nerve.

3. Paresthesia in the thumb and index finger may be caused by a C5 disc lesion or C6 nerve root palsy.

4. Paresthesia in the thumb, index finger, and middle finger may be caused by a C5 disc lesion, C6 nerve root palsy, or thoracic outlet syndrome.

5. Paresthesia of the thumb, index finger, middle finger, and half of the ring finger on the palmar aspect may be caused by an injury to the median nerve, possibly through the carpal tunnel; on the dorsal aspect, it could be caused by injury to the radial nerve.

6. Numbness of the thumb and middle finger may be caused by a tumor of the humerus.

7. Paresthesia on all five digits in one or both hands may be caused by a thoracic outlet syndrome. If it is in both hands, it may be caused by a central cervical disc protrusion. The level of protrusion would be indicated by the distribution of the paresthesia.

8. Paresthesia of the index and middle fingers may be caused by a trigger finger or "stick" palsy, if it is on the palmar aspect, or by a C6 disc lesion or C7 nerve root palsy. On the dorsal aspect of the hand, it may be caused by a carpal exostosis or subluxation. Stick palsy is the result of an inordinate amount of pressure from a cane or crutches on the ulnar nerve as it passes through the palm.

9. Paresthesia of the index, middle, and ring fingers may be caused by a C6 disc lesion, C7 nerve root injury, or carpal tunnel syndrome.

10. Paresthesia of all four fingers may be caused by a C6 disc lesion or injury to the C7 nerve root.

11. Paresthesia of the middle finger only may be caused by a C6 disc lesion or C7 nerve root lesion.

12. Paresthesia of the middle and ring fingers may be caused by a C6 disc lesion, C7 nerve root lesion, or stick palsy.

13. Paresthesia of the middle, ring, and little fingers may be caused by a C7 disc lesion or C8 nerve root palsy. The same would be true if there were paralysis of the ring and little fingers. This paresthesia may also be the result of a thoracic outlet syndrome.

14. Paresthesia on the ulnar side of the ring finger and the entire little finger may be caused by pressure of the ulnar nerve at the elbow or in the palm.

Peripheral Nerve Injuries of the Forearm, Wrist, and Hand

Carpal Tunnel Syndrome. The most common "tunnel" syndrome in the body is the carpal tunnel syndrome, in which the median nerve is compressed under the flexor retinaculum at the wrist (see Figure 7-32). This compression may follow trauma (for example, a Colles fracture or lunate dislocation), flexor tendon paratenonitis, a ganglion, arthritis (osteoarthritis or rheumatoid arthritis), or collagen disease. As many as 20% of pregnant women may experience median nerve symptoms because compression of the nerve as a result of fluid retention causes swelling in the carpal tunnel. With carpal tunnel syndrome, the symptoms, which are primarily distal to the wrist, are usually worse at night and include burning, tingling, pins and needles, and numbness into the median nerve sensory distribution (Table 7-13). In severe cases, pain may be referred to the forearm.

Symptoms are often aggravated by wrist movements, and long-standing cases show atrophy and weakness of the thenar muscles (flexor and abductor pollicis brevis, opponens pollicis) and the lateral two lumbricals. The condition is most common in women between 40 and 60 years of age, and, although it may occur bilaterally, it is seen most commonly in the dominant hand. It is also commonly seen in younger patients who use their wrists a great deal in repetitive manual labor or are exposed to vibration.[88] Because of the apparent connection between carpal tunnel syndrome and cervical lesions resulting in double crush syndromes, the examiner should take care to include cervical assessment if the history appears to warrant such inclusion.[89-91]

Guyon's (Pisohamate) Canal. The ulnar nerve is sometimes compressed as it passes through the pisohamate, or Guyon's canal (Figure 7-79). The nerve may be compressed from trauma (e.g., fractured hook of hamate), use of crutches, or chronic pressure, as in people who cycle long distances while leaning on the handlebars or who use pneumatic jackhammers. The ulnar nerve gives off two sensory branches above the wrist. These branches supply the palmar and dorsal aspects of the hand, as illustrated in Figure 7-73, and do not pass through Guyon's canal. Therefore, if the ulnar nerve is compressed in the canal, only the fingers show an altered sensation (see Table 7-13). Motor loss includes the muscles of the hypothenar eminence (flexor digiti minimi, abductor digiti minimi, opponens digiti minimi), adductor pollicis, the interossei, medial two lumbricals, and palmaris brevis.

Table 7-13

Nerve Injuries (Neuropathy) About the Wrist and Hand

Nerve	Motor Loss	Sensory Loss	Functional Loss
Median nerve (C6–C8, T1; carpal tunnel)	Flexor pollicis brevis Abductor pollicis brevis Opponens pollicis Lateral two lumbricals	Palmar and dorsal thumb, index, middle, and lateral half of ring finger If lesion above carpal tunnel, palmar sensation also affected	Thumb opposition Thumb flexion Weak or no pinch Weak grip
Ulnar nerve (C7, C8, T1; pisohamate canal)	Flexor digiti minimi Abductor digiti minimi Opponens digiti minimi Adductor pollicis Interossei Medial two lumbricals Palmaris brevis	Little finger, half of ring finger Palm often not affected	Thumb adduction Inability to extend PIP and DIP joints of fourth and fifth fingers Finger abduction Finger adduction Flexion of little finger

DIP, Distal interphalangeal; *PIP,* proximal interphalangeal.

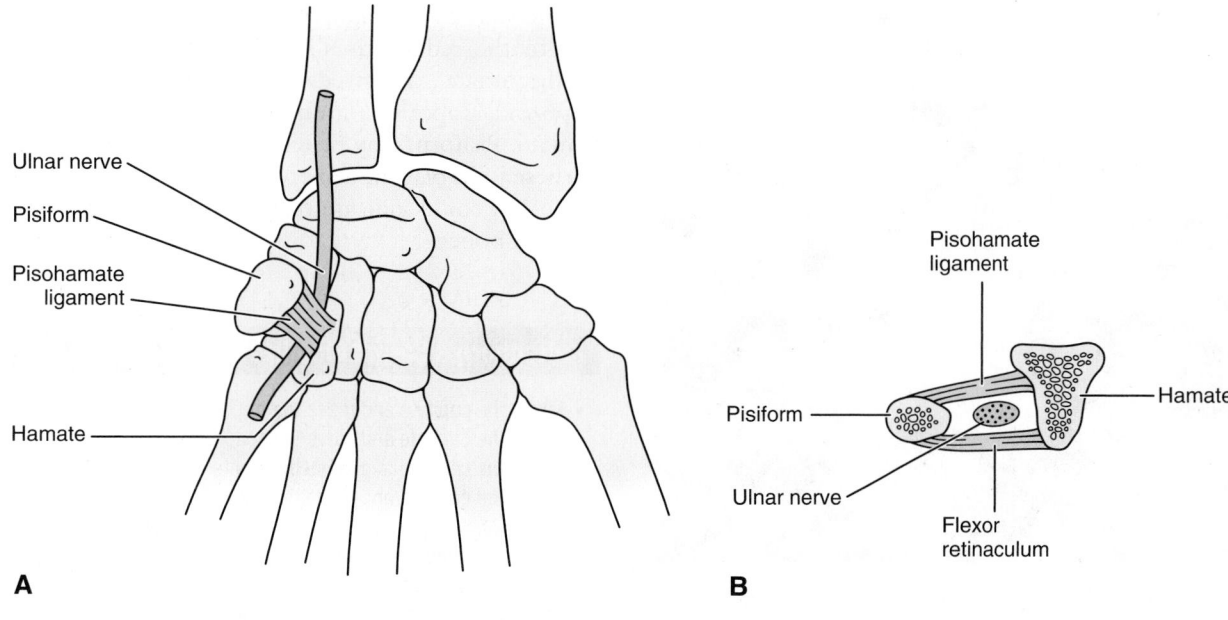

Figure 7-79
Guyon's canal. **A,** Palmar view. **B,** Section view showing position of nerve relative to pisohamate ligament and flexor retinaculum.

Joint Play Movements

When assessing joint play movements, the examiner should remember that if the patient complains of inability or pain on wrist flexion, the lesion is probably in the midcarpal joints. If the patient complains of inability or pain on wrist extension, the lesion is probably in the radiocarpal joints, because it is in these joints that most of the movement occurs during these actions. If the patient complains of pain or inability on supination and pronation, the lesion is probably in the ulnameniscocarpal joint or inferior radioulnar joint.

Joint Play Movements of the Hand

Wrist
• Long-axis extension (traction or distraction)
• Anteroposterior glide
• Side glide
• Side tilt

Intermetacarpal Joints
• Anteroposterior glide

Fingers
• Long-axis extension (traction or distraction)
• Anteroposterior glide
• Rotation
• Side glide

The amount of movement obtained by the joint play should be compared with that of the normal side and considered significant only if there is a difference between the two sides. Reproduction of the patient's symptoms would also give an indication of the joints at fault.

Wrist

To perform **long-axis extension** at the wrist, the examiner stabilizes the radius and ulna with one hand (the patient's elbow may be flexed to 90°, and stabilization may be applied at the elbow if there is no pathology at the elbow) and places the other hand just distal to the wrist. The examiner then applies a longitudinal traction movement with the distal hand.

Anteroposterior glide is applied at the wrist in two positions. The examiner first places the stabilizing hand around the distal end of the radius and ulna just proximal to the radiocarpal joint and then places the other hand around the proximal row of carpal bones. If the examiner's hands are positioned properly, they should touch each other (Figure 7-80). The examiner applies an anteroposterior gliding movement of the proximal row of carpal bones on the radius and ulna, testing the amount of movement and end feel. Then, the stabilizing hand is moved slightly distally (<1 cm) so that it is around the proximal row of carpal bones. The examiner places the mobilizing hand around the distal row of carpal bones. An anteroposterior gliding movement is applied to the

Figure 7-80
Position for testing joint play movements of the wrist. Note that there is no gap between the web spaces of the two hands.

people start by testing the movement of the lunate relative to the radius, then move to the capitate (relative to the lunate), followed by scaphoid-radius, scaphoid-trapezoid/trapezium, triquetrum-radius, and triquetrum-hamate. Pisiform may be tested individually. Pain on any of these joint play movements done in neutral, flexion, or extension could indicate pathology in the joint between the two bones.[28]

Kaltenborn's Carpal Mobilization

- Fixate the capitate and move the trapezoid
- Fixate the capitate and move the scaphoid
- Fixate the capitate and move the lunate
- Fixate the capitate and move the hamate
- Fixate the scaphoid and move the trapezoid and trapezium
- Fixate the radius and move the scaphoid
- Fixate the radius and move the lunate
- Fixate the ulna and move the triquetrum
- Fixate the triquetrum and move the hamate
- Fixate the triquetrum and move the pisiform

---

distal row of carpal bones on the proximal row to test the amount of movement and end feel. These movements are sometimes called the **anteroposterior drawer tests** of the wrist.[3] If the examiner then moves the stabilizing hand slightly distally (<1 cm) again, the hand will be around the distal carpal bones. The mobilizing hand is then placed around the metacarpals, and an anteroposterior gliding movement is applied to the base of the metacarpals to test the amount of joint play and end feel.

Side glide is performed in a similar fashion, except that a side-to-side movement is performed instead of an anteroposterior movement. To perform **side tilting** of the carpals on the radius and ulna, the examiner stabilizes the radius and ulna by placing the stabilizing hand around the distal radius and ulna just proximal to the radiocarpal joint and the mobilizing hand around the patient's hand and then radially and ulnarly deviating the hand on the radius and ulna.

The joint play movements just described are general ones involving different "rows" of carpal bones. To check the joint play movements of the individual carpal bones, a technique such as **Kaltenborn's technique** should be used. Kaltenborn[92] suggested 10 tests to determine the mobility of each of the carpal bones. The movement of each of the bones is determined in a sequential manner, and both sides are tested for comparison. These tests are sometimes referred to as **ballottement tests** or **shear tests**.[3] The examiner may use Kaltenborn's order or any other order as long as each bone and its relationship to adjacent bones is tested individually. For example, some

Intermetacarpal Joints

To accomplish **anteroposterior glide** at the intermetacarpal joints, the examiner stabilizes one metacarpal bone and moves the adjacent metacarpal anteriorly and posteriorly in relation to the fixed bone to determine the amount of joint play and the end feel. The process is repeated for each joint.

Fingers

The joint play movements for the fingers are the same for the metacarpophalangeal, proximal interphalangeal, and distal interphalangeal joints; the hand position of the examiner simply moves farther distally.

To perform **long-axis extension,** the examiner stabilizes the proximal segment or bone using one hand while placing the second hand around the distal segment or bone of the particular joint to be tested. With the mobilizing hand, the examiner applies a longitudinal traction to the joint.

Anteroposterior glide is accomplished by stabilizing the proximal bone with one hand. The mobilizing hand is placed around the distal segment of the joint, and the examiner applies an anterior and/or posterior movement to the distal segment, being sure to maintain the joint surfaces parallel to one another while determining the amount of movement and end feel (Figure 7-81). A minimal amount of traction may be applied to bring about slight separation of the joint surfaces.

Rotation of the joints of the fingers is accomplished by stabilizing the proximal segment with one hand. With

Figure 7-81
Position for testing joint play movements of the fingers.

Figure 7-82
Palpation of the wrist.

the other hand, the examiner applies slight traction to the joint to distract the joint surfaces and then rotates the distal segment on the proximal segment to determine the end feel and joint play.

To perform **side glide** joint play to the joints of the fingers, the proximal segment is stabilized with one hand. The examiner then applies slight traction to the joint with the mobilizing hand to distract the joint surfaces and then moves the distal segment sideways, keeping the joint surfaces parallel to one another to determine joint play and end feel.

Palpation

To palpate the forearm, wrist, and hand, the examiner starts proximally and works distally, first on the dorsal surface and then on the anterior surface (Figure 7-82). The muscles of the forearm are palpated first for any signs of tenderness or pathology.

Dorsal Surface

On the dorsal aspect, the examiner begins on the thumb side of the hand and palpates the "snuff box," the carpal bones, and the metacarpal bones and phalanges.

Anatomic Snuff Box. The snuff box is located between the tendons of extensor pollicis longus and extensor pollicis brevis and can best be seen by having the patient actively extend the thumb (Figure 7-83). The scaphoid bone may be palpated inside the snuff box. Tenderness of the scaphoid bone is often treated as a fracture until proven otherwise because of the possibility of avascular necrosis of the bone, especially the anterior fragment or pole.[93] With the wrist in anatomic position, proximal palpation is used to find the radial styloid on

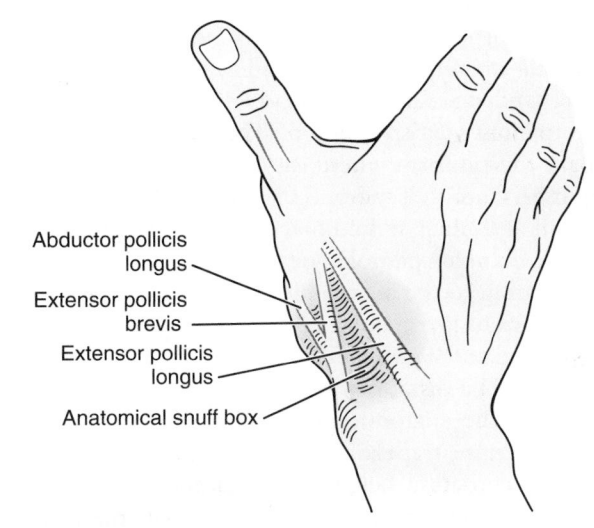

Figure 7-83
The anatomic snuff box. Note how the tendons of the abductor pollicis longus and extensor pollicis brevis diverge in proceeding distally. (Redrawn from Gardner E et al: *Anatomy: a regional study of human structure,* p. 135, London, 1975, W.B. Saunders.)

the lateral aspect. Moving medially over the radius, the examiner comes to the radial (Lister's) tubercle. The extensor pollicis longus tendon moves around the tubercle to enter the thumb, which gives it a different angle of pull from that of the extensor pollicis brevis. With the wrist in anatomic position, the ulnar styloid is palpated on the medial aspect. The radial styloid extends farther distally than the ulnar styloid. By palpating over the dorsum of the wrist, crossing the radius and ulna, the examiner should attempt to palpate the six extensor tendon tunnels (noting any crepitus or restriction to movement), moving lateral to medial (see Figure 7-37):

Tunnel 1: abductor pollicis longus and extensor pollicis brevis

Tunnel 2: extensor carpi radialis longus and brevis

Tunnel 3: extensor pollicis longus

Tunnel 4: extensor digitorum and extensor indices

Tunnel 5: extensor digiti minimi

Tunnel 6: extensor carpi ulnaris

Carpal Bones. In the anatomic snuff box, the examiner can begin palpating the proximal row of carpal bones, starting with the scaphoid bone. When palpating the carpal bones, the examiner usually palpates them on the anterior and dorsal surfaces at the same time by applying anteroposterior joint play-like movements. The proximal row of carpal bones from lateral to medial (in the anatomic position) are the scaphoid, lunate, triquetrum (just below the ulnar styloid), and pisiform.

On the anterior aspect, the examiner should take care to ensure proper positioning of the lunate bone. If it dislocates or subluxes, it tends to move anteriorly into the carpal tunnel, which may lead to symptoms of carpal tunnel syndrome. The pisiform is often easier to palpate if the patient's wrist is flexed. The examiner may then palpate the pisiform where the flexor carpi ulnaris tendon inserts into it. Tenderness in the hollow between the pisiform and ulnar styloid may indicate triangular fibrocartilage complex pathology.[11]

Returning to the anatomic snuff box and moving distally, the examiner palpates the trapezium bone. As this is done, the radial pulse is often palpated in the anatomic snuff box. The distal row of carpal bones from lateral to medial (in the anatomic position) is palpated individually: trapezium, trapezoid, capitate (distal to lunate and a slight indentation before the metacarpal), and hamate (distal to triquetrum; the hook of the hamate on the anterior surface is the easiest part to palpate). The hamate is most commonly injured by direct trauma.[53,94]

On the dorsal aspect, the examiner could begin palpation at the distal row of carpals. If the examiner places a finger over the middle metacarpal and slides along it until the finger drops into a "hole" or depression, this depression is the capitate bone. Moving medially (hamate) and laterally (trapezoid, trapezium), the other bones of the distal row may be palpated again by making anteroposterior joint play-like movements. If the examiner then moves proximally from the capitate, the finger will rest on the lunate. Moving medially (triquetrum) and laterally (scaphoid), these carpals may be palpated.

Metacarpal Bones and Phalanges. The examiner returns to the trapezium bone and moves farther distally

Figure 7-84
Palpation of the proximal interphalangeal joint of the second finger.

to palpate the first metacarpal joint and the first metacarpal bone. Moving medially, the examiner palpates each metacarpal bone on the anterior and dorsal surface in turn. A similar procedure is carried out for the metacarpophalangeal and interphalangeal joints and the phalanges. These structures are also palpated on their medial and lateral aspects for tenderness, swelling, altered temperature, or other signs of pathology (Figure 7-84).

Anterior Surface

Pulses. Proximally, the radial and ulnar pulses are palpated first. The radial pulse on the anterolateral aspect of the wrist on top of the radius is easiest to palpate and is the one most frequently used when taking a pulse. It runs between the tendons of flexor carpi radialis and abductor pollicis longus. The ulnar pulse may be palpated lateral to the tendon of flexor carpi ulnaris. It is more difficult to palpate because it runs deeper and lies under the pisiform and the palmar fascia.

Tendons. Moving across the anterior aspect, the examiner may be able to palpate the long flexor tendons (see Figure 7-37) in a lateral-to-medial direction: flexor carpi radialis, flexor pollicis longus, flexor digitorum superficialis, flexor digitorum profundus, palmaris longus, and flexor carpi ulnaris (inserts into pisiform). The examiner should also palpate the hollow between the flexor carpi ulnaris, the pisiform, and the ulnar styloid. In this hollow lies the triangular cartilaginous disc or complex (TFCC).[65] The palmaris longus (if present) lies over the tendons of the flexor digitorum superficialis, which lie over the tendons of the flexor digitorum profundus. The palmaris longus tendon may sometimes be used for tendon repairs or transfers.

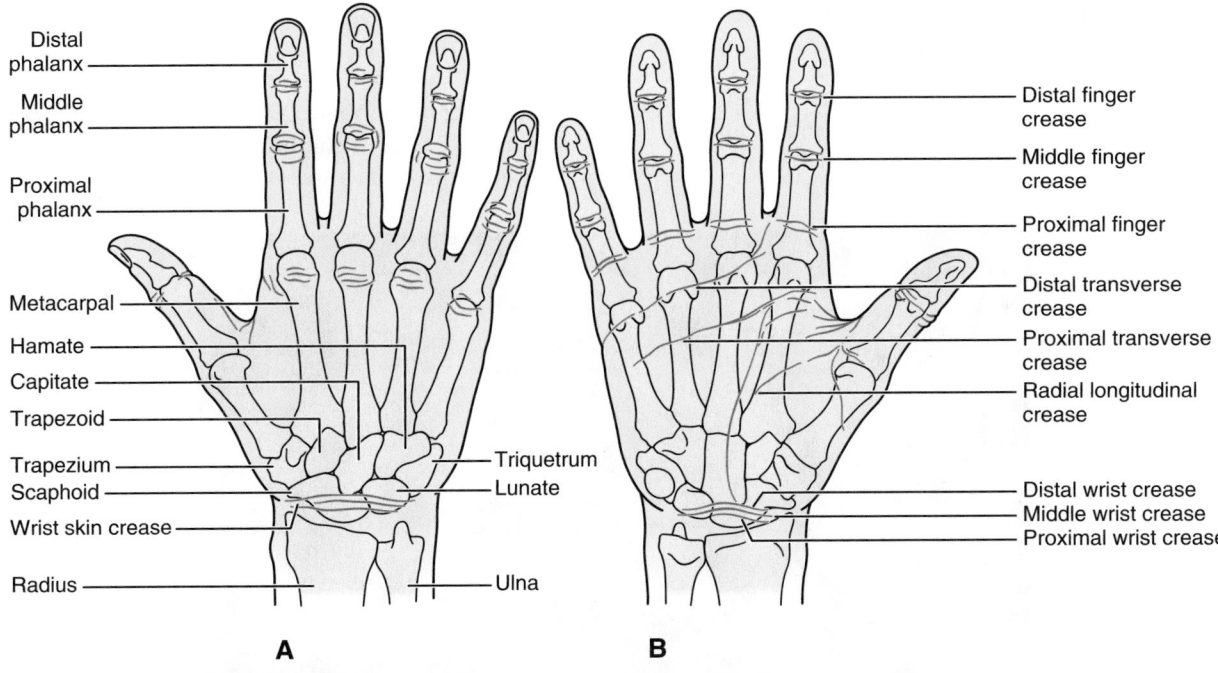

Figure 7-85
Bony landmarks and skin creases of the hand and wrist. **A,** Dorsal view. **B,** Palmar view. (Adapted from Tubiana R: *The hand,* p. 619, Philadelphia, 1981, W.B. Saunders.)

Palmar Fascia and Intrinsic Muscles. The examiner should then move distally to palpate the palmar fascia and intrinsic muscles of the thenar and hypothenar eminences for indications of pathology.

Skin Flexion Creases. From an anatomic point of view, the examiner should note the various skin flexion creases of the wrist, hand, and fingers (Figure 7-85). The flexion creases indicate lines of adherence between the skin and fascia with no intervening adipose tissue. The following creases should be noted:

1. The proximal skin crease of the wrist indicates the upper limit of the synovial sheaths of the flexor tendons.
2. The middle skin crease of the wrist indicates the wrist (radiocarpal) joint.
3. The distal skin crease of the wrist indicates the upper margin of the flexor retinaculum.
4. The radial longitudinal skin crease of the palm encircles the thenar eminence. (Palm readers refer to this line as the "life line.")
5. The proximal transverse line of the palm runs across the shafts of the metacarpal bones, indicating the superficial palmar arterial arch. (Palm readers refer to this line as the "head line.")
6. The distal transverse line of the palm lies over the heads of the second to fourth metacarpals. (Palm readers refer to this line as the "love line.")

7. The proximal skin crease of the fingers is 2 cm (0.8 inch) distal to the metacarpophalangeal joints.
8. The middle skin crease of the fingers is made up of two lines and lies over the proximal interphalangeal joints.
9. The distal skin crease of the fingers lies over the distal interphalangeal joints.
10. On the flexor and extensor aspects, the skin creases over the proximal and distal interphalangeal joints lie proximal to the joint. On the extensor aspect, the metacarpophalangeal creases lie proximal to the joint; on the flexor aspect, they lie distal to the joint.

Arches. In addition, the examiner should ensure the viability of the arches of the hand (see Figure 7-15). The carpal transverse arch is the result of the shape of the carpal bones, which in part forms the carpal tunnel. The flexor retinaculum forms the roof for the tunnel. The metacarpal transverse arch is formed by the metacarpal bones, and its shape can have great variability because of the mobility of these bones. This arch is most evident when the palm is cupped. The longitudinal arch is made of the carpal bones, metacarpal bones, and phalanges. The keystone of this arch is the metacarpophalangeal joints, which provide stability and support for the arch. Weakness or atrophy of the intrinsic muscles of the hand leads to a loss of these arches. The deformity is most obvious with paralysis of the median and ulnar nerve, which results in an "ape hand" deformity.

Diagnostic Imaging

Plain Film Radiography

A routine wrist series of x-rays involves the following views; anteroposterior (AP), lateral, and scaphoid.[95] Other possible views include the carpal tunnel view, clenched-fist (AP) view, and radial and ulnar deviation views. Motion views are sometimes taken, especially if instability is suspected.

Anteroposterior View.[96] The examiner should note the shape and position of the bones (Figure 7-86), watching for any evidence of fractures (Figure 7-87) or displacement,

Figure 7-86

Radiograph showing the bones of both hands. The thumb metacarpal is the shortest, and the index metacarpal is by far the longest. The first and second phalanges of the middle and ring fingers are longer than those of the index finger. Note the interlocking design of the carpometacarpal articulations and the saddle shape in opposing planes of the articular surfaces of the trapezium and the base of the first metacarpal. (From Tubiana R: *The hand*, p. 21, Philadelphia, 1981, W.B. Saunders.)

A

B

Figure 7-87

Wrist fracture: Colles' fracture. **A,** Observe the transverse fracture of the distal portion of the radius (*open arrows*), with extension into the radiocarpal joint (*arrowhead*). **B,** In the lateral projection, dorsal angulation of the articular surface of the radius (*solid arrows*) is apparent and caused by compaction of bone dorsally. This injury is a three-part fracture. The ulnar styloid process is intact, and no evidence of subluxation of the distal portion of the ulna can be seen. (From Resnick D, Kransdorf MJ: *Bone and joint imaging,* p. 851, Philadelphia, 2005, W.B. Saunders.)

Figure 7-88

Wrist arcs. Three arcuate lines can normally be constructed along the carpal articular surfaces: *(1)* along the proximal margins of the scaphoid, lunate, and triquetrum; *(2)* along the distal aspects of these bones; and *(3)* along the proximal margins of the capitate and hamate. (From Weissman BNW, Sledge CB: *Orthopedic radiology,* p. 117, Philadelphia, 1986, W.B. Saunders.)

in Kienböck's disease (Figure 7-90, *B*).[48] In some cases, the triangular fibrocartilage complex may be visualized (Figure 7-91). The AP view may also be used to show dislocations of the lunate (Figure 7-92, *A*), the distal ulna (Figure 7-92, *B*), the lunatotriquetral relation (Figure 7-92, *C*), and ulnar variance (length of ulna in relation to radius).[97]

The AP view of the wrist and hand is also used to determine the skeletal age of a patient.[40] The left hand and wrist are used for study because they are thought to be less influenced by environmental factors. The method used in this technique is based on the fact that after an **ossification center** appears (Figure 7-93), it changes its shape and size in a systematic manner as the ossification gradually spreads throughout the cartilaginous parts of the skeleton. The wrist and hand are studied because several bones are available for overall comparison, including the carpal bones, the metacarpal growth plates (seen at distal end of bone), and the phalangeal growth plates (seen at proximal end of bone). The patient's hand is compared with standard plates[53] until one plate is found that best approximates that of the patient. There is one standard for males and another for females. In two thirds of the population, skeletal age is no more than 1 year above or below chronologic age. Acceleration or retardation of 3 years or more is considered abnormal. At birth, none of the carpal bones is visible (see Figure 1-23). This method may be used up to age 20, when the bones of the hand and wrist have fused.

decrease in the joint spaces, or change in bone density, which may be caused by avascular necrosis. The arcs of the wrist (Figure 7-88) show the normal relation of the carpal bones in the AP view. If avascular necrosis is present, there is rarefaction and increased density of the bone (increased whiteness) and possibly sclerosis (patchy appearance) of the bone. Avascular necrosis is often seen in the scaphoid bone (Figures 7-89 and 7-90, *A*) after a fracture or in the lunate

Lateral View. The examiner should note the shape and position of bones for any evidence of fracture and/or displacement (Figure 7-94, *A*). The lateral view is also useful in detecting swelling around the carpal bones and for measuring the relation of the scaphoid and lunate to the radius and metacarpals (Figure 7-95).[97]

A   **B**

Figure 7-89

Radiographs of the normal scaphoid. **A,** Posteroanterior view. **B,** Lateral view. (From Tubiana R: *The hand,* p. 659, Philadelphia, 1981, W.B. Saunders.)

A

RADIAL
DEVIATION

NEUTRAL

ULNAR
DEVIATION

B ANTEROPOSTERIOR
VIEW

LATERAL
VIEW

Figure 7-90

Avascular necrosis of the carpal bones. **A,** Scaphoid fracture shown in three positions. **B,** Lunate fracture and sclerosis in Kienböck's disease. (**A,** from Cooney WP, Dobyns JH, Linscheid RL: Fractures of the scaphoid: A rational approach to management, *Clin Orthop* 149:92, 1980. **B,** from Beckenbaugh RD, Shives TC, Dobyns JH, Linscheid RL: Kienböck's disease, the natural history of Kienböck's disease and consideration of lunate fractures, *Clin Orthop* 149:99, 1980.)

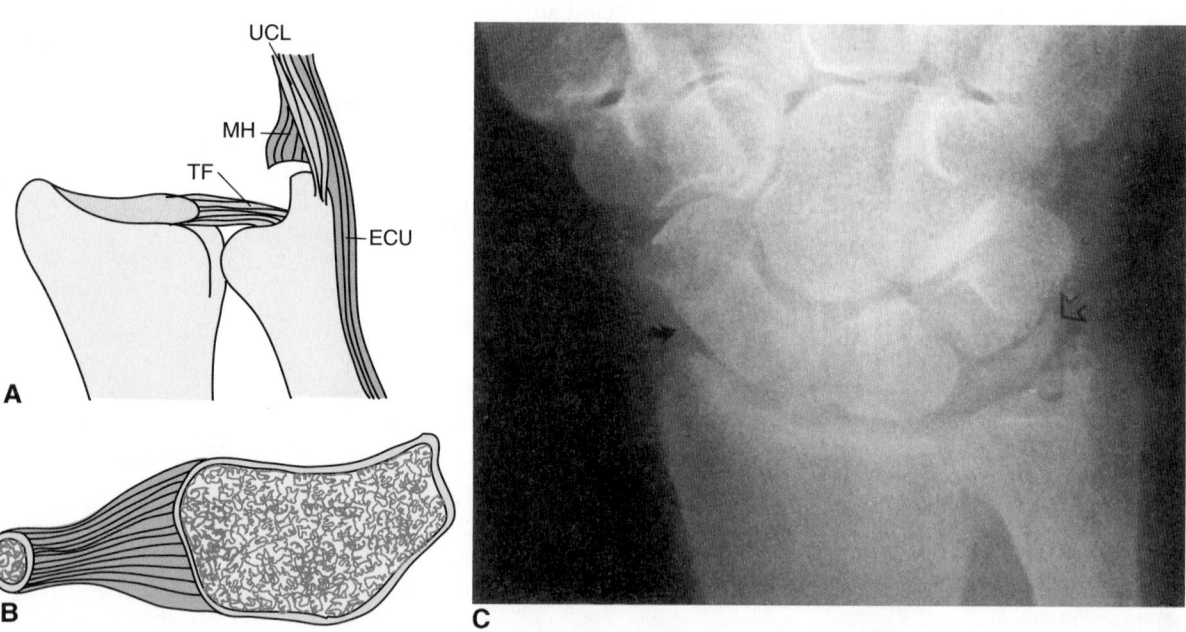

Figure 7-91

Triangular fibrocartilage complex. **A,** This complex includes the triangular fibrocartilage (articular disc, *TF*), the meniscus homolog *(MH)*, the ulnar collateral ligament *(UCL)*, and the dorsal and volar radioulnar ligaments (not shown). The extensor carpi ulnaris tendon (ECU) is shown. **B,** The triangular fibrocartilage *(dotted area)* attaches to the ulnar border of the radius and the distal ulna. The triangular shape is evident on this transverse section through the radius and ulnar styloid. The volar aspect of the wrist is at the top. **C,** Chondrocalcinosis. There is heavy calcification of the articular cartilage *(curved arrow)* and the area of the triangular fibrocartilage complex *(open arrow)*. (From Weissman BNW, Sledge CB: *Orthopedic radiology,* p. 115, Philadelphia, 1986, W.B. Saunders.)

Figure 7-92

A, Scapholunate dissociation. The scaphoid is palmar flexed, producing a cortical ring sign. A gap is present between the scaphoid and the lunate. The lunate appears trapezoidal. **B,** Ulnar translocation can be identified radiographically from the ratio of the distance between the center of the capitate and a line along the longitudinal axis of the ulna *(L2)* divided by the length of the third metacarpal *(L1)*. In normal wrists, this ratio is 0.30 ± 0.03; it is decreased in wrists with ulnar translocation. **C,** Lunatotriquetral instability. Shortened scaphoid and cortical ring sign are present without scapholunate widening. Lunate appears triangular. Lunatotriquetral widening is not present. (© 1993 American Academy of Orthopaedic Surgeons. Reprinted from the *Journal of the American Academy of Orthopaedic Surgeons: A Comprehensive Review*, 1[1], pp. 14–15 with permission.)

Scaphoid View. This view isolates the scaphoid to show a possible fracture (see Figure 7-89).

Carpal Tunnel (Axial) View. This view is used to show the margins of the carpal tunnel and is useful for determining fractures of the hook of hamate and trapezium (Figure 7-96).

Clenched-Fist (AP) View. This view is sometimes useful to show increased gapping between the carpal bones, indicating instability.[98]

Arthrography

If the history and clinical assessment suggest a ligament or fibrocartilage problem of the wrist, arthrography can help to confirm the diagnosis (Figure 7-97). Arthrograms, especially of the wrist, can demonstrate compartment communication, tendon sheaths, synovial irregularity, loose bodies, and cartilage abnormalities.

Computed Tomography

Computed tomography can be used to visualize bones and soft tissue; by making computer-assisted "slices," it allows tissues to be better visualized (Figure 7-98).

Magnetic Resonance Imaging

Magnetic resonance imaging is a noninvasive technique that is useful for visualizing the soft tissues of the wrist and hand and provides the best means of delineating the soft tissues (primarily ligaments and the triangular fibrocartilage complex) as well as showing instability problems and bone.[99-101] For example, it can show swelling of the median nerve in carpal tunnel syndrome, tears in the triangular fibrocartilage (Figure 7-99), and thickening of tendon sheaths (Figure 7-100).

Figure 7-93

Ossification centers of the hand. **A,** Dates of appearance of ossification centers are shown, with dates of fusion in parentheses. Note the different proximal and distal locations of growth plates. **B,** Radiographs of the hand and wrist of a 4- to 5-year-old boy or 3- to 4-year-old girl *(left)* and of an adult *(right). C,* Capitate; *H,* hamate; *L,* lunate; *M,* metacarpal; *P,* phalanx; *Pi,* pisiform; *R,* radius; *S,* scaphoid; *Td,* trapezoid; *Tm,* trapezium; *Tq,* triquetrum; *U,* ulna. (**A,** Redrawn from Tubiana R: *The hand,* p. 11, Philadelphia, 1981, W.B. Saunders, **B,** From Liebgott B: *The anatomical basis of dentistry,* St Louis, 1986, C.V. Mosby.)

Figure 7-94

A, Lateral radiographs showing wrist flexion *(left)* and extension *(right)*. **B,** Posteroanterior views of wrist in radial *(left)* and ulnar *(right)* deviation. Note the change in the form of the lunate, indicating a slipping toward the front in the radial slant and toward the rear in the ulnar slant. (From Tubiana R: *The hand,* p. 655, Philadelphia, 1981, W.B. Saunders.)

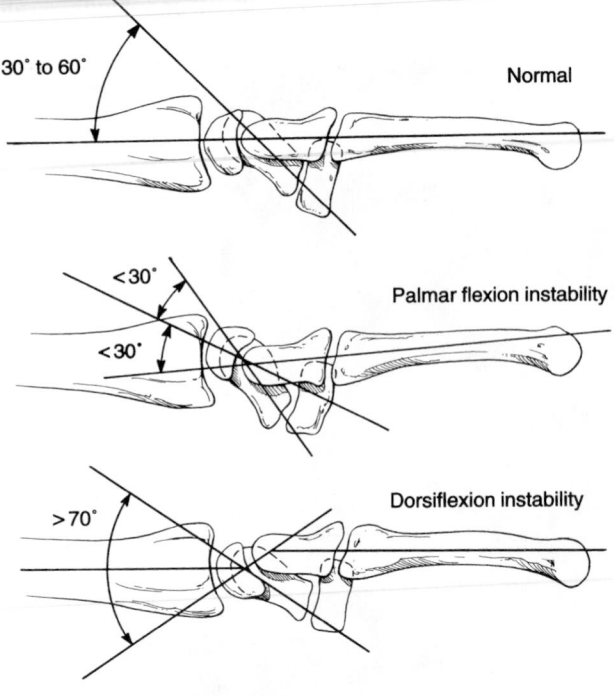

Normal

30° to 60°

<30°

<30°

Palmar flexion instability

>70°

Dorsiflexion instability

Figure 7-95

Scapholunate angle measurement in normal wrist and in carpal instability. (© 1993 American Academy of Orthopaedic Surgeons. Reprinted from the *Journal of the American Academy of Orthopaedic Surgeons: A Comprehensive Review,* 1 [1], p. 14 with permission.)

Figure 7-96

Carpal tunnel or axial radiographic view. (From Tubiana R: *The hand,* p. 662, Philadelphia, 1981, W.B. Saunders.)

A

B

C

Figure 7-97

A, Posteroanterior view of the wrist after a normal radiocarpal joint arthrogram. Contrast remains confined to the radiocarpal space. **B,** After a radiocarpal joint space injection, contrast tracks *(arrowheads)* through a disrupted scapholunate ligament to fill the midcarpal and carpometacarpal joint spaces. **C,** After a radiocarpal joint space arthrogram, the scapholunate ligament is intact because contrast has not yet filled the scapholunate space *(arrowhead)*; however, contrast tracks through the lunatotriquetral joint space *(arrow)* as a result of lunatotriquetral ligament disruption. (From Lightman DM: *The wrist and its disorders,* p. 89, Philadelphia, 1988, W.B. Saunders.)

Figure 7-98

A fracture of the left hamate hook *(arrow)* as shown by a computed tomographic (CT) scan. In this instance, fracture was suspected on the carpal tunnel view but was not demonstrated as well as it was by CT scan. (From Zemel NP, Stark HH: Fractures and dislocations of the carpal bones, *Clin Sports Med* 5:720, 1986.)

Figure 7-100

Tendon rupture. Coronal T1-weighted (TR/TE, 500/14) spin echo from MR image of the hand shows rupture of the flexor tendon of the little finger. The free edge of the thickened, retracted, ruptured tendon *(arrow)* is well seen. (From Resnick D, Kransdor MJf: *Bone and joint imaging,* p. 913, Philadelphia, 2005, W.B. Saunders.)

Figure 7-99

Triangular fibrocartilage complex: normal appearance. On a coronal intermediate-weighted (TR/TE, 2000/20) spin echo MR image, observe the low-signal intensity of the triangular fibrocartilage *(arrow)*, with bifurcated bands of low-signal intensity *(arrowheads)* attaching to or near the styloid process of the ulna. The scapholunate and lunotriquetral interosseous ligaments are not well seen on this image. Note the two bone islands, which appear as foci of low-signal intensity, in the lunate and capitate. (From Resnick D, Kransdorf MJ: *Bone and joint imaging,* p. 907, Philadelphia, 2005, W.B. Saunders Courtesy of AG Bergman, MD, Stanford, CA.)

Précis of the Forearm, Wrist, and Hand Assessment*

History (sitting)
Observation (sitting)
Examination (sitting)
  Active movements
    Pronation of the forearm
    Supination of the forearm
    Wrist flexion
    Wrist extension
    Radial deviation of wrist
    Ulnar deviation of wrist
    Finger flexion (at MCP, PIP, and DIP joints)
    Flexion extension (at MCP, PIP, and DIP joints)
    Finger abduction
    Finger adduction
    Thumb flexion
    Thumb extension
    Thumb abduction
    Thumb adduction
    Opposition of the thumb and little finger
  Passive movements (as in active movements)
  Resisted isometric movements (as in active movements, in
    the neutral position)
  Functional testing
    Functional grip tests
    Pinch tests
    Coordination tests

Special tests (sitting)
Reflexes and cutaneous distribution (sitting)
  Reflexes
  Sensory scan
  Nerve injuries
  Median nerve
  Ulnar nerve
  Radial nerve
Joint play movements (sitting)
  Long-axis extension at the wrist and fingers (MCP, PIP, and DIP joints)
  Anteroposterior glide at the wrist and fingers (MCP, PIP, and DIP joints)
  Side glide at the wrist and fingers (MCP, PIP, and DIP joints)
  Side tilt at the wrist
  Anteroposterior glide at the intermetacarpal joints
  Rotation at the MCP, PIP, and DIP joints
  Individual carpal bone mobility
Palpation (sitting)
Diagnostic imaging
After any examination, the patient should be warned of the possibility of exacerbation of symptoms as a result of the assessment.

---

*DIP, Distal interphalangeal; *MCP*, metacarpophalangeal; *PIP*, proximal interphalangeal.

Case Studies

When doing these case studies, the examiner should list the appropriate questions to be asked and why they are being asked, what to look for and why, and what things should be tested and why. Depending on the answers of the patient (and the examiner should consider different responses), several possible causes of the patient's problem may become evident (examples are given in parentheses). A differential diagnosis chart should be made up. The examiner can then decide how different diagnoses may affect the treatment plan. For example, a 26-year-old man comes to you complaining of pain and clicking in his wrist. He is a carpenter, and it especially bothers him when he uses a screwdriver. See Table 7-14 for an example of a differential diagnosis chart for this patient.

1. A 31-year-old pregnant woman complains of pain in the right hand of 3 months' duration. The pain awakens her at night and is relieved only by vigorous rubbing of her hand and motion of the fingers and wrist. There is some tingling in the index and middle fingers. Describe your assessment for this patient (carpal tunnel syndrome versus lunate subluxation).

2. An 18-year-old man comes to you after suffering a right scaphoid fracture. He has been in a cast for 12 weeks, and clinical union has been achieved. Describe your assessment for this patient.

3. A 16-year-old girl comes to you complaining of thumb pain. She was skiing during the weekend and fell, landing on her ski pole. She hurt her thumb when she fell. Describe your assessment for this patient (ulnar collateral ligament sprain versus Bennett's fracture).

4. A 48-year-old man comes to you complaining of a painful hand. He happened to hit it against a metal door jam as he was going outside. During the next few days, the hand became swollen and painful, and he has become very protective of it. Describe your assessment of this patient (Sudeck's atrophy versus hand aneurysm).

5. A 52-year-old woman who has rheumatoid arthritis comes to you because her hands hurt and she has difficulty doing things functionally. Describe your assessment of this patient.

6. A 14-year-old boy comes to you complaining of wrist pain with swelling on the dorsum of the hand. He says he tripped and fell on the outstretched hand. He states the wrist hurt, the pain decreased, and then the swelling came on over 2 or 3 days. Describe your assessment of this patient (scaphoid fracture versus ganglion).

Case Studies—cont'd

7. A 28-year-old man was in an industrial accident and lacerated the flexor tendons in the palm of his hand. Describe your assessment of this patient.
8. A 37-year-old woman comes to you complaining of pain and grating on the radial side of the wrist.

Describe your assessment of this patient (cartilaginous disc versus scaphoid fracture).
9. A 72-year-old woman comes to you with a left Colles fracture. Describe your assessment of this patient.

Table 7-14

Differential Diagosis of Wrist Cartilaginous Disc and Degenerative Osteoarthritis

	Wrist Cartilaginous Disc	Degenerative Osteoarthritis
Mechanism of injury	Compression and pronation	Vibration, repetitive compression
Age affected	25 years and older	35 years and older
Active movement	Pain on compression and pronation Limited wrist extension more than flexion	Limited wrist flexion and extension
Passive movement	Pain on extension overpressure Pain on compression and pronation Tissue stretch end feel	Capsular pattern of wrist End feel is soft early, hard later
Resisted isometric movement	Pain on pronation	Possibly weak on wrist movements
Special tests	None	None
Reflexes and sensory distribution	Normal	Normal
Joint play	Pain on anteroposterior glide of radiocarpal joint	Pain on anteroposterior glide of radiocarpal and midcarpal joints
Palpation	Pain over lunate	Pain over affected carpal bones

References

To enhance this text and add value for the reader, all references have been incorporated into a CD-ROM that is provided with this text. The reader can view the reference source and access it online whenever possible. There are a total of 127 cited and other general references for this chapter.

APPENDIX 7-1

RELIABILITY, VALIDITY, SPECIFICITY, AND SENSITIVITY OF SPECIAL/DIAGNOSTIC TESTS USED IN THE FOREARM, WRIST, AND HAND

BOX AND BLOCK TEST

Reliability	Validity
• Test retest for able-bodied subjects ICC = 0.79, impaired subjects ICC = 0.91[102]	• Correlation with the autonomy measurement system for activities of daily living r = 0.42, the autonomy measurement system of institutionalized people r = 0.47, the action research arm test r = 0.89[102]

CARPAL COMPRESSION TEST

Reliability	Validity
• Interrater k = 0.63[103]	• No association between severity of carpal tunnel syndrome and test result $p > .51$[103]

COMMERCIAL VOLUMETER (IDYLLWILD, CA)

Reliability

• Interrater ICC = 0.99, intrarater ICC = 0.99[104]

COMMERCIAL VOLUMETER (KIMAX USA)

Reliability

• Test retest ICC = 0.99[105]

DURKAN'S TEST

Specificity	Sensitivity	Odds Ratio
• Carpal tunnel syndrome normal subjects 91%, carpal tunnel syndromes × normal × other hand problem 66%[106]	• Carpal tunnel syndrome normal subjects 89%, carpal tunnel syndrome × normal × other hand problem 89%[106]	• Positive likelihood ratio for carpal tunnel syndrome × normal subjects 9.89, carpal tunnel syndrome × normal × other hand problems 2.62; negative likelihood ratio for carpal tunnel syndrome × normal subjects 0.12, carpal tunnel syndrome × normal × other hand problems 0.17

FIGURE-OF-EIGHT METHOD (HAND SIZE)

Reliability	Validity
• Intrarater ICC = 0.98, interrater ICC = 0.99[107]	• Concurrent validity comparing with volumetric measurement r = 0.93[107]

GRIP STRENGTH

Reliability

• Test retest dominant r = 0.70–0.86, nondominant r = 0.84–0.94[108]

HAND DIAGRAM

Specificity	Sensitivity	Odds Ratio
• Carpal tunnel syndrome normal subjects 98%, carpal tunnel syndromes × normal × other hand problem 84%[106]	• Carpal tunnel syndrome normal subjects 76%, carpal tunnel syndrome × normal × other hand problem 76%[106]	• Positive likelihood ratio for carpal tunnel syndrome × normal subjects 38, carpal tunnel syndrome × normal × other hand problems 4.75; negative likelihood ratio for carpal tunnel syndrome × normal subjects 0.24, carpal tunnel syndrome × normal × other hand problems 0.28

MEDIAN NERVE COMPRESSION TEST

Specificity	Sensitivity	Odds Ratio
• 100%[109]	• 79%[109]	• Positive likelihood ratio 79, negative likelihood ratio 0.79

MICHIGAN HAND OUTCOMES QUESTIONNAIRE

Reliability	Validity
• Test retest overall hand function ICC=0.89, activities of daily living ICC=0.94, work performance ICC=0.93, pain ICC=0.91, aesthetics ICC=0.81, satisfaction with hand function ICC=0.96[110]	• Correlation between self assessment and score change in the questionnaire r<0.43[111] • Internal consistency Cronbach's alpha overall hand function 0.93, activities of daily living 0.95, work performance 0.94, pain 0.86, aesthetics 0.87, satisfaction with hand function 0.93[105] • Concurrent validity with SF-12 activities of daily living r=0.64, work performance 0.54, pain 0.79[110]

MIDCARPAL SHIFT TEST

Validity
• There was a significant association of maximum slope in an instrument to measure instability and the clinical grade of midcarpal laxity $p=.007$[112]

MINNESOTA RATE OF MANIPULATION TEST

Reliability	Validity
• Test retest placing test ICC=0.83, turning test ICC=0.79[113]	• Correlation with box and block test with the placing test r=−0.63, Purdue pegboard test with placing test r=−0.64, turning test r=−0.63[113]

MODIFIED ALLEN TEST

Validity	Specificity	Sensitivity	Odds Ratio
• The test was significantly different between patients with no flow and increased, decreased and reversed flow groups according to Doppler ultrasonography dynamic test $p<.02$, but not between the decreased, increased and reversed flow groups $p>.4$[114]	• Ulnar artery 97.1%, superficial palmar branch of RA 96.6%, dorsal digital thumb artery 97.1%[114]	• Ulnar artery 66.7%, superficial palmar branch of RA 28.6%, dorsal digital thumb artery 100%[114]	• Positive likelihood ratio for ulnar artery 23, superficial palmar branch of RA 8.41, dorsal digital thumb artery 34.48; negative likelihood ratio for ulnar artery 0.34, superficial palmar branch of RA 0.74, dorsal digital thumb artery 0

Continued

APPENDIX 7-1—cont'd

MODIFIED JEBSEN TEST OF HAND FUNCTION

Reliability	Validity
• Test retest r = 0.95[115]	• Construct validity (grip strength r = 0.44, nine hole peg test r = 0.86, University of Maryland arm questionnaire r = 0.10)[115]

MURPHY'S SIGN

Specificity	Sensitivity	Odds Ratio
• 54%[116]	• 49%[116]	• Positive likelihood ratio 1.06, negative likelihood ratio 0.94

NINE HOLD PEG TEST

Reliability	Validity
• Interrater r = 0.99, test retest r = 0.79[117]	• Concurrent validity with Purdue pegboard test r = 0.74[117]

PATIENT-RATED WRIST EVALUATION

Reliability	Validity
• Test retest acute fracture ICC = 0.90, treated fracture ICC = 0.97, 1 year scaphoid ICC = 0.91[118]	• PRWE × SF-36 bodily pain r = −0.64, SF-36 physical function r = −0.48, SF-36 physical summary score r = −0.57, SF-36 mental summary score r = 0.41[118]

PHALEN'S (WRIST FLEXION) TEST

Reliability	Validity	Specificity	Sensitivity	Odds Ratio
• Intrarater k = 0.53, interrater k = 0.65[119] • Interrater k = 0.88[120] • Interrater k = 0.58[103]	• More severe carpal tunnel syndrome more likely to have test positive $p < .05$[103]	• Carpal tunnel syndrome normal subjects 95%, carpal tunnel syndrome × normal × other hand problem 71%[106] • 76%[121] • 54%[116] • 100%[109] • Tester 1 90%, tester 2 86%[120]	• Carpal tunnel syndrome normal subjects 75%, carpal tunnel syndromes × normal × other hand problem 75%[106] • 51%[121] • 58%[116] • 71%[109] • Tester 1 87%, tester 2 86%[120]	• Positive likelihood ratio for carpal tunnel syndrome × normal subjects 15, carpal tunnel syndrome × normal × other hand problems 2.59; negative likelihood ratio for carpal tunnel syndrome × normal subjects 0.26, carpal tunnel syndrome × normal × other hand problems 0.35 • Positive likelihood ratio 2.12, negative likelihood ratio 0.64 • Positive likelihood ratio 1.03, negative likelihood ratio 0.77 • Positive likelihood ratio 71, negative likelihood ratio 0.29 • Positive likelihood ratio tester 1 8.7, tester 2 6.14; negative likelihood ratio tester 1 0.14, tester 2 0.16

PINCH STRENGTH

Reliability	Specificity	Sensitivity	Odds Ratio
• k = 0.76[120]	• Tester 1 88%, tester 2 78%[120]	• Tester 1 72%, tester 2 70%[120]	• Positive likelihood ratio tester 1 6, tester 2 3.18; negative likelihood ratio tester 1 0.31, tester 2 1.36

POWER GRIP

Reliability	Validity
• Test retest ICC = 0.90–0.96[122]	• Stronger results with wrist 15 or 30 degrees of extension with neutral radioulnar deviation than wrist 15 degrees of ulnar deviation with or without extension $p = .021–.004$[122]

PURDUE PEGBOARD TEST

Reliability	Validity
• Test retest female right r = 0.76, left r = 0.79, both r = 0.81; male right r = 0.63, left r = 0.64, both r = 0.66[123] • Test retest ICC = 0.66–0.90[124] • Test retest one trial ICC = 0.85–0.90, sum of three trials ICC = 0.92–0.96[125] • Test retest one trial right hand ICC = 0.37, left hand ICC = 0.61, both hands ICC = 0.58, right+left+both ICC = 0.70, assembly ICC = 0.51; sum of three trials right hand ICC = 0.82, left hand ICC = 0.89, both hands ICC = 0.85, right+left+both ICC = 0.89, assembly ICC = 0.81[126] • Test retest dominant r = 0.59–0.88, nondominant r = 0.35–0.77[108]	• There was no significant difference between groups of patients with or without sensation decrease $p = .22$[127]

SEMMES WEINSTEIN MONOFILAMENT

Reliability	Specificity	Sensitivity	Odds Ratio
• Interrater ICC = 0.15, intrarater ICC = 0.71[119]	• 59%[116]	• 59%[116]	• Positive likelihood ratio 1.44, negative likelihood ratio 0.69

SQUARE-SHAPED WRIST

Specificity	Sensitivity	Odds Ratio
• 73%[121]	• 69%[121]	• Positive likelihood ratio 2.55, negative likelihood ratio 0.42

Continued

APPENDIX 7-1—cont'd

TINEL'S SIGN

Reliability	Validity	Specificity	Sensitivity	Odds Ratio
• Intrarater k = 0.80, interrater k = 0.77[119] • k = 0.81[120] • Interrater k = 0.51[103]	• No association with the severity of carpal tunnel syndrome and test results $p > .11$[103]	• Carpal tunnel syndrome normal subjects 99%, carpal tunnel syndromes × normal × other hand problem 83%[106] • 87%[121] • 63%[116] • 100%[109] • Tester 1 92%, tester 2 94%[120]	• Carpal tunnel syndrome normal subjects 64%, carpal tunnel syndromes × normal × other hand problem 64%[106] • 23%[121] • 42%[116] • 71%[109] • Tester 1 59%, tester 2 41%[120]	• Positive likelihood ratio for carpal tunnel syndrome x normal subjects 64, carpal tunnel syndrome × normal × other hand problems 3.76; negative likelihood ratio for carpal tunnel syndrome × normal subjects 0.36, carpal tunnel syndrome × normal × other hand problems 0.43 • Positive likelihood ratio 1, negative likelihood ratio 1 • Positive likelihood ratio 1.13, negative likelihood ratio 0.92 • Positive likelihood ratio 71, negative likelihood ratio 0.29 • Positive likelihood ratio tester 1 7.35 tester 2 6.83; negative likelihood ratio tester 1 0.44, tester 2 0.63

THORACIC (DORSAL) SPINE

Assessment of the thoracic spine involves examination of the part of the spine that is most rigid because of the associated rib cage. The rib cage in turn provides protection for the heart and lungs. Normally, the thoracic spine, being one of the primary curves, exhibits a mild **kyphosis** (posterior curvature); the cervical and lumbar sections, being secondary curves, exhibit a mild **lordosis** (anterior curvature). When the examiner assesses the thoracic spine, it is essential that the cervical and/or lumbar spines be evaluated at the same time (Figure 8-1, see Figure 3-7).

Applied Anatomy

The **costovertebral joints** are synovial plane joints located between the ribs and the vertebral bodies (Figure 8-2). There are 24 of these joints, and they are divided into two parts. Ribs 1, 10, 11, and 12 articulate with a single vertebra. The other articulations have no intra-articular ligament that divides the joint into two parts, so each of ribs 2 through 9 articulates with two adjacent vertebrae and the intervening intervertebral disc. The main ligament of the costovertebral joint is the radiate ligament, which joins the anterior aspect of the head of the rib radiating to the sides of the vertebral bodies and disc in between. For ribs 10, 11, and 12, it attaches only to the adjacent vertebral body. The intra-articular ligament divides the joint and attaches to the disc.

The **costotransverse joints** are synovial joints found between the ribs and the transverse processes of the vertebra of the same level for ribs 1 through 10 (see Figure 8-2). Because ribs 11 and 12 do not articulate with the transverse processes, this joint does not exist for these two

levels. The costotransverse joints are supported by three ligaments. The superior costotransverse ligament runs from the lower border of the transverse process above to the upper border of the rib and its neck. The costotransverse ligament runs between the neck of the rib and the transverse process at the same level. The lateral costotransverse ligament runs from the tip of the transverse process to the adjacent rib.

The **costochondral joints** lie between the ribs and the costal cartilage (Figure 8-3). The **sternocostal joints** are found between the costal cartilage and the sternum. Joints 2 through 6 are synovial, whereas the first costal cartilage is united with the sternum by a synchondrosis. Where a rib articulates with an adjacent rib or costal cartilage (ribs 5 through 9), a synovial interchondral joint exists.

As in the cervical and lumbar spines, the two **apophyseal or facet joints** make up the main tri-joint complex along with the disc between the vertebrae. The superior facet of the T1 vertebra is similar to a facet of the cervical spine. Because of this, T1 is classified as a **transitional vertebra.** The superior facet faces up and back; the inferior facet faces down and forward. The T2–T11 superior facets face up, back, and slightly laterally; the inferior facets face down, forward, and slightly medially (Figure 8-4). This shape enables slight rotation in the thoracic spine. Thoracic vertebrae T11 and T12 are classified as transitional, and the facets of these vertebrae become positioned in a way similar to those of the lumbar facets. The superior facets of these two vertebrae face up, back, and more medially; the inferior facets face forward and slightly laterally. The ligaments between the vertebral bodies include the ligamentum flavum, the anterior

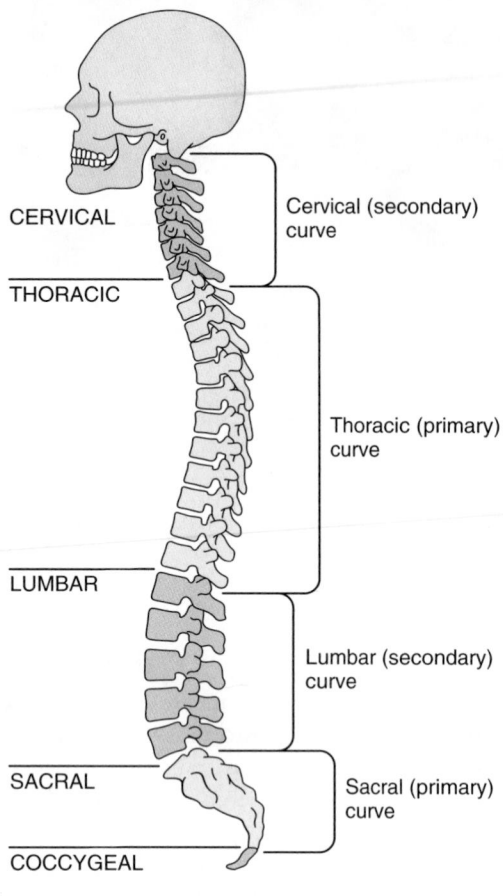

CERVICAL

Cervical (secondary) curve

THORACIC

Thoracic (primary) curve

LUMBAR

Lumbar (secondary) curve

SACRAL

Sacral (primary) curve

COCCYGEAL

Figure 8-1

The articulated spine.

and posterior longitudinal ligaments, the interspinous and supraspinous ligaments and the intertransverse ligament. These ligaments are found in the cervical, thoracic, and lumbar spine. The close packed position of the facet joints in the thoracic spine is extension.

Facet Joints of the Thoracic Spine	
Resting position:	Midway between flexion and extension
Close packed position:	Extension
Capsular pattern:	Side flexion and rotation equally limited, then extension

Within the thoracic spine, there are 12 vertebrae, which diminish in size from T1 to T3 and then increase progressively in size to T12. These vertebrae are distinctive in having facets on the body and transverse processes for articulation with the ribs. The spinous processes of these vertebrae face obliquely downward (Figure 8-5). T7 has the greatest spinous process angulation, whereas the upper three thoracic vertebrae have spinous processes that project directly posteriorly. In other words, the spinous process of these vertebra is on the same plane as the transverse processes of the same vertebrae.

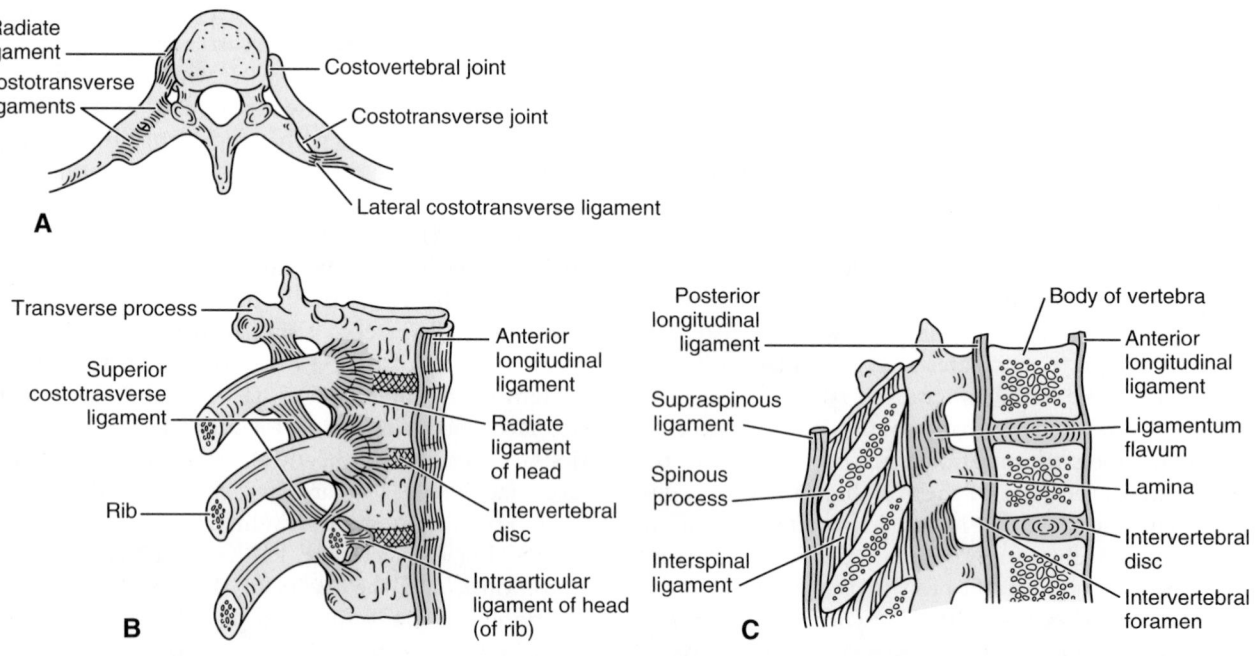

A

Radiate ligament

Costotransverse ligaments

Costovertebral joint

Costotransverse joint

Lateral costotransverse ligament

B

Transverse process

Superior costotrasverse ligament

Rib

Anterior longitudinal ligament

Radiate ligament of head

Intervertebral disc

Intraarticular ligament of head (of rib)

C

Posterior longitudinal ligament

Supraspinous ligament

Spinous process

Interspinal ligament

Body of vertebra

Anterior longitudinal ligament

Ligamentum flavum

Lamina

Intervertebral disc

Intervertebral foramen

Figure 8-2

Joints and ligaments of the thoracic vertebrae and ribs. **A,** Superior view. **B,** Anterolateral aspect. **C,** Median section through vertebra.

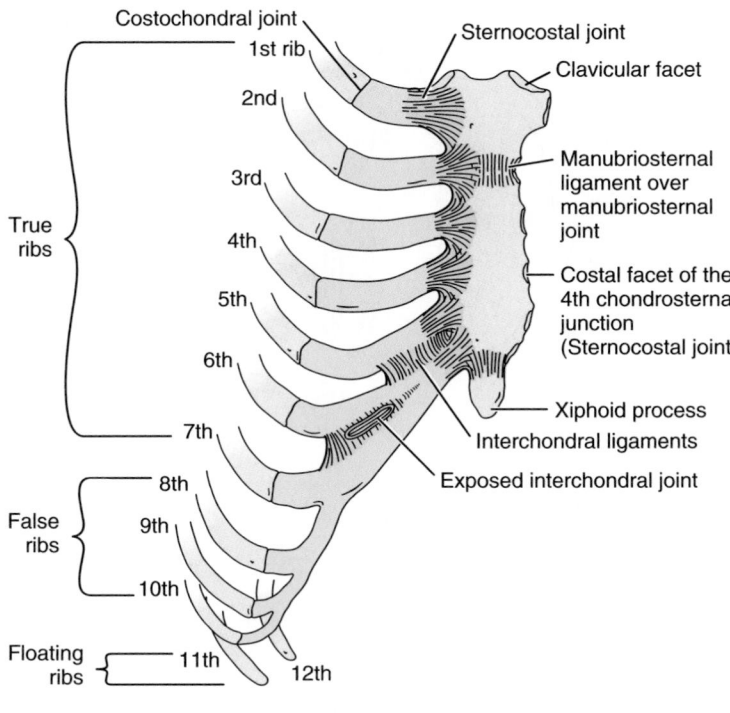

Figure 8-3
Anterior view of the part of the thoracic wall highlights the manubriosternal joint, sternocostal joints with costochondral and chondrosternal joints, and interchondral joints. The ribs are removed on the left side to expose the costal facets. (Modified from Neumann DA: *Kinesiology of the musculoskeletal system—foundations for physical rehabilitation*, p. 370, St Louis, 2002, C.V. Mosby.)

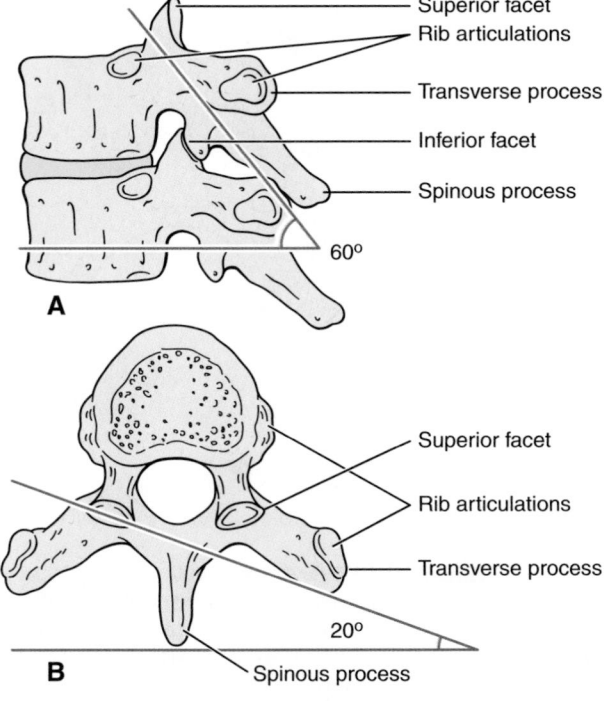

Figure 8-4
Thoracic vertebra. **A,** Side view. **B,** Superior view.

Figure 8-5
Spinous process of one thoracic vertebra at level of body of vertebra below (T7-T9).

T4-T6 vertebrae have spinous processes that project downward slightly. In this case, the tips of the spinous processes are on a plane halfway between their own transverse processes and the transverse processes of the vertebrae below. For T7, T8, and T9 vertebrae, the spinous processes project downward, the tip of the spinous processes being on a plane of the transverse processes of the vertebrae below. For the T10 spinous process, the arrangement is similar to that of the T9 spinous process (i.e., the spinous process is level with the transverse process of the vertebra below). For T11, the arrangement is similar to that of T6 (i.e., the spinous process is halfway between the two transverse processes of the vertebra), and T12 is similar to T3 (i.e., the spinous process is level with the transverse process of the same vertebra). The location of the spinous processes becomes important if the examiner wishes to perform posteroanterior central vertebral pressures. For example, if the examiner pushes on the spinous process of T8, the body of T9 will also move. In fact, the vertebral body of T8 will probably arc backwards slightly, whereas T9 will move in an anterior direction. T7 is sometimes classified as a transitional vertebra because it is the point at which the lower limb axial rotation alternates with the upper limb axial rotation (Figure 8-6).

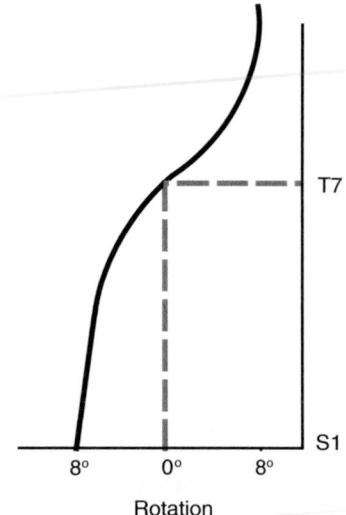

Figure 8-6

Axial rotation of the spine going from left to right on heel strike.

The ribs, which help to stiffen the thoracic spine, articulate with the demifacets on vertebrae T2-T9. For T1 and T10, there is a whole facet for ribs 1 and 10, respectively. The first rib articulates with T1 only, the second rib articulates with T1 and T2, the third rib articulates with T2 and T3, and so on. Ribs 1 through 7 articulate with the sternum directly and are classified as **true ribs** (see Figure 8-3). Ribs 8 through 10 join directly with the costocartilage of the rib above and are classified as **false ribs.** Ribs 11 and 12 are classified as **floating ribs** because they do not attach to either the sternum or the costal cartilage at their distal ends. Ribs 11 and 12 articulate only with the bodies of the T11 and T12 vertebrae, not with the transverse processes of the vertebrae nor with the costocartilage of the rib above. The ribs are held by ligaments to the body of the vertebra and to the transverse processes of the same vertebrae. Some of these ligaments also bind the rib to the vertebra above.

At the top of the rib cage, the ribs are relatively horizontal. As the rib cage descends, they run more and more obliquely downward. By the 12th rib, the ribs are more vertical than horizontal. With inspiration, the ribs are pulled up and forward; this increases the anteroposterior diameter of the ribs. The first six ribs increase the anteroposterior dimension of the chest, mainly by rotating around their long axes. Rotation downward of the rib neck is associated with depression, whereas rotation upward of the same portion is associated with elevation. These movements are known as a **pump handle action** and are accompanied by elevation of the manubrium sternum upward and forward (Figure 8-7, *A*).[1-3] Ribs 7 through 10 mainly increase in lateral, or transverse, dimension. To accomplish this, the ribs move upward, backward,

Figure 8-7

Actions of the ribs. **A,** Pump handle action (T1-T6). **B,** Bucket handle action (T7-T10). **C,** Caliper action (T11-T12). (**A** and **B,** Modified from Williams P, Warwick R [eds]: *Gray's anatomy,* 37th British ed, p. 498, Edinburgh, 1989, Churchill Livingstone.)

and medially to increase the infrasternal angle or downward, forward, and laterally to decrease the angle. These movements are known as a **bucket handle action.** This action is also performed by ribs 2 through 6 but to a much lesser degree (Figure 8-7, *B*). The lower ribs (ribs 8 through 12) move laterally, in what is known as a **caliper action,** to increase lateral diameter (Figure 8-7, *C*).[2]

The ribs are quite elastic in children, but they become increasingly brittle with age. In the anterior half of the chest, the ribs are subcutaneous; in the posterior half, they are covered by muscles.

Patient History

A thorough and complete history should include past and present problems. By listening carefully, the examiner is often able to identify the patient's problem, develop a working diagnosis, and then use the observation and examination to confirm or refute the impressions established from the history. All information concerning the present pain and its site, nature, and behavior is important. If any part of the history implicates the cervical or lumbar spine, the examiner must include these areas in the assessment as well.

In addition to the questions listed under Patient History in Chapter 1, the examiner should obtain the following information from the patient.

1. *What are the patient's age and occupation?* For example, conditions such as Scheuermann's disease occur in young people between 13 and 16 years of age. Idiopathic scoliosis is most commonly seen in adolescent females.

2. *What was the mechanism of injury?* Most commonly, rib injuries are caused by trauma. Thoracic spine problems may result from disease processes (e.g., scoliosis) and may have an insidious onset. Pain from true thoracic trauma tends to be localized to the area of injury. Facet syndromes present as stiffness and local pain, which can be referred.[4,5]

3. *What are the details of the present pain and other symptoms? What are the sites and boundaries of the pain? Have the patient point to the location or locations. Is there any radiation of pain?* The examiner should remember that many of the abdominal structures, such as the stomach, liver, and pancreas, may refer pain to the thoracic region. With thoracic disc lesions, because of the rigidity of the thoracic spine, active movements do not often show the characteristic pain pattern, and sensory and strength deficits are difficult if not impossible to detect.[6] Thoracic root involvement or spondylosis usually causes pain that follows the path of the ribs or a deep, "through-the-chest" pain.

4. *Does the pain occur on inspiration, expiration, or both?* Pain related to breathing may signal pulmonary problems or may be related to movement of the ribs. Pain referred around the chest wall tends to be costovertebral in origin. Does the patient have any difficulty in breathing? If a breathing problem exists, it may be caused by a structural deformity (e.g., scoliosis); thoracic trauma such as disc lesions, fractures, or contusions; or thoracic pathology such as pneumothorax, pleurisy, tumors, or pericarditis.

5. *Is the pain deep, superficial, shooting, burning, or aching?* Thoracic nerve root pain is often severe and is referred in a sloping band along an intercostal space. Pain between the scapulae may be the result of a cervical lesion. It has been reported that any symptoms above a line joining the inferior angles of the scapula should be considered of cervical origin until proven otherwise, especially if there is no history of trauma.[7]

6. *Is the pain affected by coughing, sneezing, or straining?* Dural pain is often accentuated by these maneuvers.

7. *Which activities aggravate the problem?* Active use of the arms sometimes irritates a thoracic lesion. Pulling and pushing activities can be especially bothersome to a patient with thoracic problems. Costal pain is often elicited by breathing and/or overhand arm motion.

8. *Which activities ease the problem?* For example, bracing the arms often makes breathing easier because this facilitates the action of the accessory muscles of respiration.

9. *Is the condition improving, becoming worse, or staying the same?*

10. *Does any particular posture bother the patient?*

11. *Is there any paresthesia or other abnormal sensation that may indicate a disc lesion or radiculopathy?*

12. *Are the patient's symptoms referred to the legs, arms, or head and neck?* If so, it is imperative that the examiner assess these areas as well. For example, shoulder movements may be restricted with thoracic spine problems.

13. *Does the patient have any problems with digestion?* Pain may be referred to the thoracic spine or ribs from pathological conditions within the thorax or abdomen. Visceral pain tends to be vague, dull, and indiscrete and may be accompanied by nausea and sweating. It tends to follow dermatome patterns in its referral. For example, cardiac pain is referred to the shoulder (C4) and posteriorly to T2. Stomach pain is referred to T6-T8 posteriorly. Ulcers may be referred to T4-T6 posteriorly.[4]

14. *Is the skin in the thorax area normal?* Conditions such as herpes zoster can cause unilateral, spontaneous pain. In the observation, the examiner should watch for erythema and grouped vesicles.[6]

Observation

The patient must be suitably undressed so that the body is exposed as much as possible. In the case of a female, the bra is often removed to provide a better view of the spine and rib cage. The patient is usually observed first standing and then sitting.

As with any observation, the examiner should note any alteration in the overall spinal posture (see Chapter 15) because it may lead to problems in the thoracic spine. It is important to observe the total body posture from the head to the toes and look for any deviation from normal (Figure 8-8). Posteriorly, the medial edge of the spine of the scapula should be level with the T3 spinous

A **B** **C**

Figure 8-8
Normal posture. **A,** Front view. **B,** Posterior view. **C,** Side view.

process, whereas the inferior angle of the scapula is level with the T7-T9 spinous process, depending on the size of the scapula. The medial border of the scapula is parallel to the spine and approximately 5 cm lateral to the spinous processes.

Kyphosis

Kyphosis is a condition that is most prevalent in the thoracic spine (Figure 8-9). The examiner must ensure that a kyphosis is actually present, remembering that a slight kyphosis, or posterior curvature, is normal and is found in every individual. In addition, some people have "flat" scapulae, which give the appearance of an excessive kyphosis, as does winging of the scapulae. The examiner must ensure that it is actually the spine that has the excessive curvature. Types of kyphotic deformities are shown in Figure 8-10 and listed below[8]:

1. **Round back** is decreased pelvic inclination (20°) with a thoracolumbar or thoracic kyphosis (Figure 8-11). Most forms of kyphosis seen show a decreased pelvic inclination. To compensate and maintain the body's center of gravity, a structural kyphosis, usually caused by tight soft tissues from prolonged postural change or by a growth disturbance (e.g., Scheuermann's disease), results, causing a round back deformity.

2. **Hump back** is a localized, sharp, posterior angulation called a **gibbus.** This kyphotic deformity is usually structural and often results from an anterior wedging of the body of one or two thoracic vertebrae. The wedging may be caused by a fracture, tumor, or bone disease. The pelvic inclination is usually normal (30°).

3. **Flat back** is decreased pelvic inclination (20°) with a mobile spine. This kyphotic deformity is similar to round back, except that the thoracic spine remains mobile and is able to compensate throughout its length for the altered center of gravity caused by the decreased pelvic inclination. Therefore, although a kyphosis is or should be present, it does not have the appearance of an excessive kyphotic curve.

4. **Dowager's hump** results from postmenopausal osteoporosis. Because of the osteoporosis, anterior wedge

Figure 8-9
Congenital thoracic kyphosis. (From Bradford DS et al: *Moe's textbook of scoliosis and other spinal deformities,* p. 263, Philadelphia, 1987, W.B. Saunders.)

Figure 8-11
Lateral view of patient with ankylosing (rheumatoid) spondylitis showing forward protrusion of head, flattening of anterior chest wall, thoracic kyphosis, protrusion of abdomen, and flattening of lumbar lordosis. This patient also has slight flexion of the hips on the pelvis. (From Polley HF, Hunder GG: *Rheumatologic interviewing and physical examination of the joints,* p. 161, Philadelphia, 1978, W.B. Saunders.)

KYPHOSIS   GIBBUS   DOWAGER'S HUMP

Figure 8-10 Kyphotic deformities.

fractures occur to several vertebrae, usually in the upper to middle thoracic spine, causing a structural scoliosis that also contributes to a decrease in height.

Scoliosis

Scoliosis is a deformity in which there are one or more lateral curvatures of the lumbar or thoracic spine; it is this spinal deformity that was suffered by the "Hunchback of Notre Dame." (In the cervical spine, the condition is called **torticollis.**) The curvature may occur in the thoracic spine alone, in the thoracolumbar area, or in the lumbar spine alone (Figure 8-12). Scoliosis may be

nonstructural (i.e., relatively easily correctable once the cause is determined) or structural. Poor posture, hysteria, nerve root irritation, inflammation in the spine area, leg length discrepancy, or hip contracture can cause nonstructural scoliosis. Structural changes may be genetic, idiopathic, or caused by some congenital problem such as a wedge vertebra, hemivertebra, or failure of vertebral segmentation. In other words, there is a structural change in the bone, and normal flexibility of the spine is lost.[9]

A number of curve patterns may be present with scoliosis (Figure 8-13).[9] The curve patterns are designated according to the level of the apex of the curve (Table 8-1). A right thoracic curve has a convexity toward the right, and the apex of the curve is in the thoracic spine. With a cervical scoliosis, or torticollis, the apex is between C1 and C6. For a cervicothoracic curve, the apex is at C7 or T1. For a thoracic curve, the apex is between T2 and T11. The thoracolumbar curve has its apex at T12 or L1. The lumbar curve has an apex between L2 and L4, and a lumbosacral scoliosis has an apex at L5 or S1. The involvement of the thoracic spine results in a very poor cosmetic appearance or greater visual defect as a result of deformation of the ribs along with the spine. The deformity can vary from a mild rib hump to a severe rotation of the vertebrae, causing a rib deformity called a **razorback spine.**

With a structural scoliosis, the vertebral bodies rotate to the convexity of the curve and become distorted.[10] If

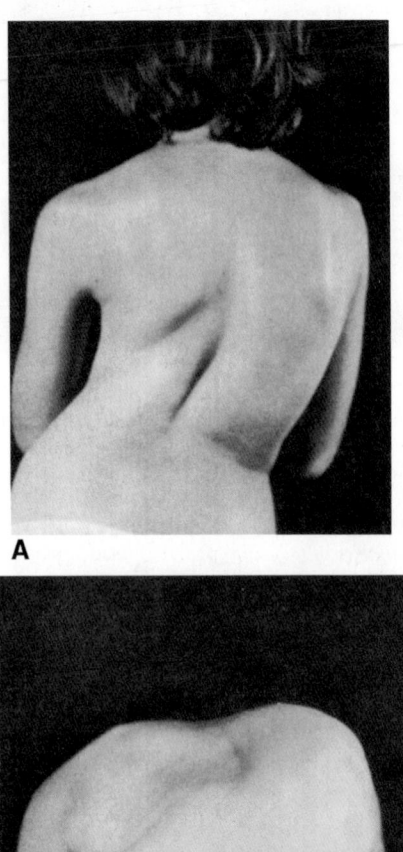

A

B

Figure 8-12
Idiopathic scoliosis. **A,** Postural deformity caused by idiopathic thoracolumbar scoliosis. **B,** Asymmetry of posterior thorax accentuated with patient flexed. Note "hump" on the right and "hollow" on the left. (From Gartland JJ: *Fundamentals of orthopedics*, p. 341, Philadelphia, 1979, W.B. Saunders.)

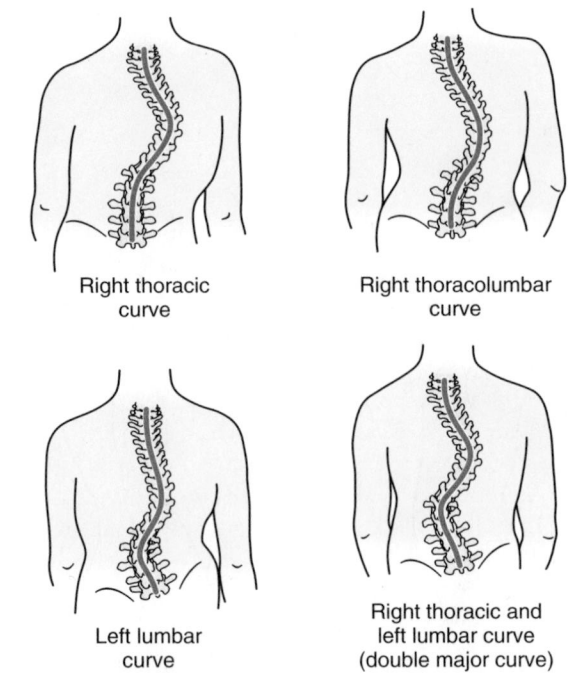

Right thoracic curve

Right thoracolumbar curve

Left lumbar curve

Right thoracic and left lumbar curve (double major curve)

Figure 8-13
Examples of scoliosis curve patterns.

Table 8-1

Curve Patterns and Prognosis in Idiopathic Scoliosis

| | Curve Pattern | | | | |
	Primary Lumbar	Thoracolumbar	Combined Thoracic and Lumbar	Primary Thoracic	Cervicothoracic
Incidence (%)	23.6	16	37	22.1	31.3
Average age curve noted (yr)	13.25	14	12.3	11.1	15.3
Average age curve stabilized (yr)	14.5	16	15.5	16.1	16.3
Extent of curve	T11–L3	T6 or T7–L1 or L1, L2	Thoracic, T6–T10 Lumbar, T11–L4	T6–T11	C7 or T1–T4 or T5
Apex of curve	L1 or L2	T11 or L2	Thoracic, T7 or T8 Lumbar, L2	T8 or T9 (rotation extreme, convexity usually to right)	T3
Average angular value at maturity (degrees)					
Standing	36.8	42.7	Thoracic, 51.9; lumbar, 41.4	81.4	34.6
Supine	29.1	35	Thoracic, 41.4; lumbar, 37.7	73.8	32.2
Prognosis	Most benign and least deforming of all idiopathic curves	Not severely deforming Intermediate between thoracic and lumbar curves	Good Body usually well aligned, curves even if severe tend to compensate each other High percentage of very severe scoliosis if onset before age of 10 yr	Worst Progresses more rapidly, becomes more severe, and produces greater clinical deformity than any other pattern Five years of active growth during which curve could increase	Deformity unsightly Poorly disguised because of high shoulder, elevated scapula, and deformed thoracic cage

Adapted from Ponseti IV Friedman B: Prognosis in idiopathic scoliosis, *J Bone Joint Surg Am* 32:382, 1950.

the thoracic spine is involved, this rotation causes the ribs on the convex side of the curve to push posteriorly, causing a rib "hump" and narrowing the thoracic cage on the convex side. As the vertebral body rotates to the convex side of the curve, the spinous process deviates toward the concave side. The ribs on the concave side move anteriorly, causing a "hollow" and a widening of the thoracic cage on the concave side (Figure 8-14). Lateral deviation may be more evident if the examiner uses a plumb bob (plumbline) from the C7 spinous process or external occipital protuberance (Figure 8-15).

The examiner should note whether the ribs are symmetric and whether the rib contours are normal and equal on the two sides. In idiopathic scoliosis, the rib contours are not normal and there is asymmetry of the ribs. Muscle spasm resulting from injury may also be evident. The bony and soft-tissue contours should be observed for equality on both sides or for any noticeable difference.

The examiner should note whether the patient sits up properly with the normal spinal curves present (Figure 8-16, *A*); whether the tip of the ear, tip of the acromion process, and high point of the iliac crest are in a straight line as they should be; and whether the patient sits in a slumped position (i.e., sag sitting, as in Figure 8-16, *B*).

The skin should be observed for any abnormality or scars (Figure 8-17). If there are scars, are they a result of surgery or trauma? Are they new or old scars? If from surgery, what was the purpose of the surgery?

Breathing

As part of the observation, the examiner should note the patient's breathing pattern. Children tend to breathe abdominally, whereas women tend to do upper thoracic breathing. Men tend to be upper and lower thoracic

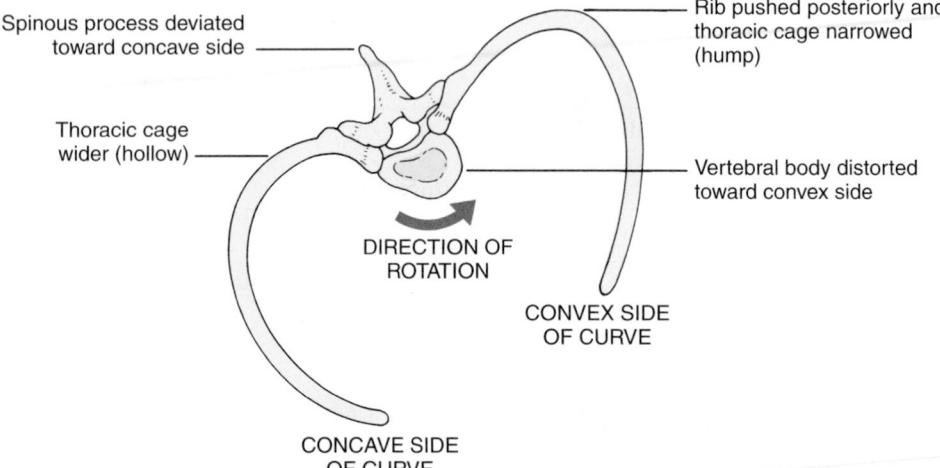

Spinous process deviated toward concave side

Rib pushed posteriorly and thoracic cage narrowed (hump)

Thoracic cage wider (hollow)

Vertebral body distorted toward convex side

DIRECTION OF ROTATION

CONVEX SIDE OF CURVE

CONCAVE SIDE OF CURVE

Figure 8-14
Pathological changes in the ribs and vertebra with idiopathic scoliosis in the thoracic spine.

A   B

Figure 8-15

Right thoracic idiopathic scoliosis (posterior view). **A,** The left shoulder is lower, and the right scapula is more prominent. Note the decreased distance between the right arm and the thorax, with the shift of the thorax to the right. The left iliac crest appears higher, but this results from the shift of the thorax, with fullness on the right and elimination of the waistline; the "high" hip is only apparent, not real. **B,** Plumbline dropped from the prominent vertebra of C7 (vertebra prominens) measures the decompensation of the thorax over the pelvis. The distance from the vertical plumbline to the gluteal cleft is measured in centimeters and is recorded along with the direction of deviation. If there is a cervical or cervicothoracic curve, the plumb should fall from the occipital protuberance (inion). (From Moe JH et al: *Scoliosis and other spinal deformities*, p. 14, Philadelphia, 1978, W.B. Saunders.)

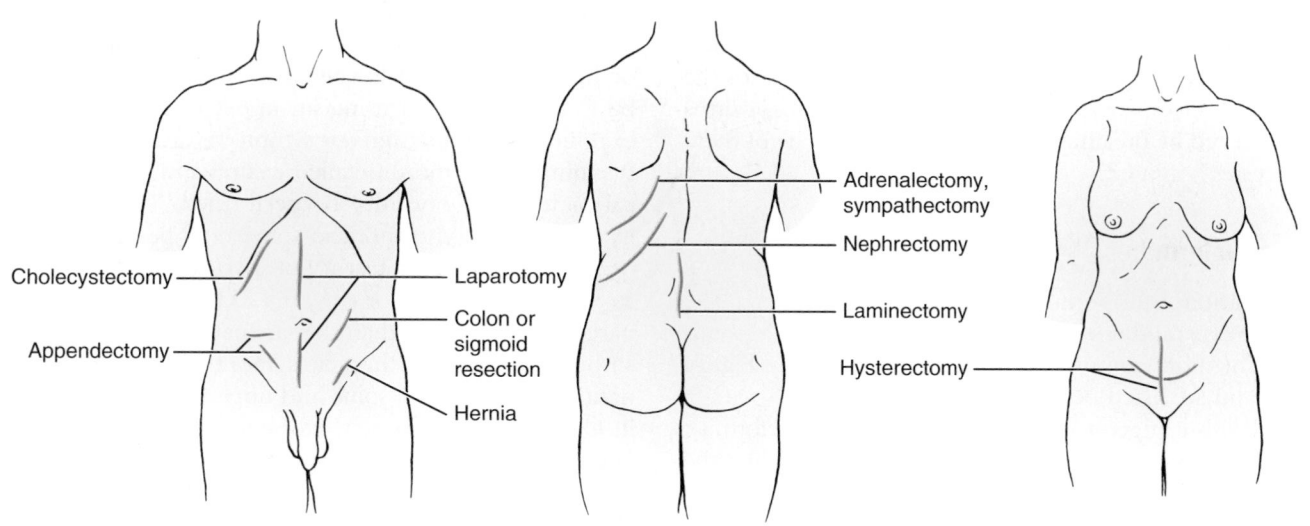

Figure 8-16

Sitting posture. **A,** Normal position. **B,** Sag sitting.

Cholecystectomy
Appendectomy

Laparotomy
Colon or sigmoid resection
Hernia

Adrenalectomy, sympathectomy
Nephrectomy
Laminectomy
Hysterectomy

Figure 8-17

Common surgical scars of the abdomen and thorax. (Redrawn from Judge RD et al: *Clinical diagnosis: a physiologic approach*, p. 295, Boston, 1982, Little, Brown.)

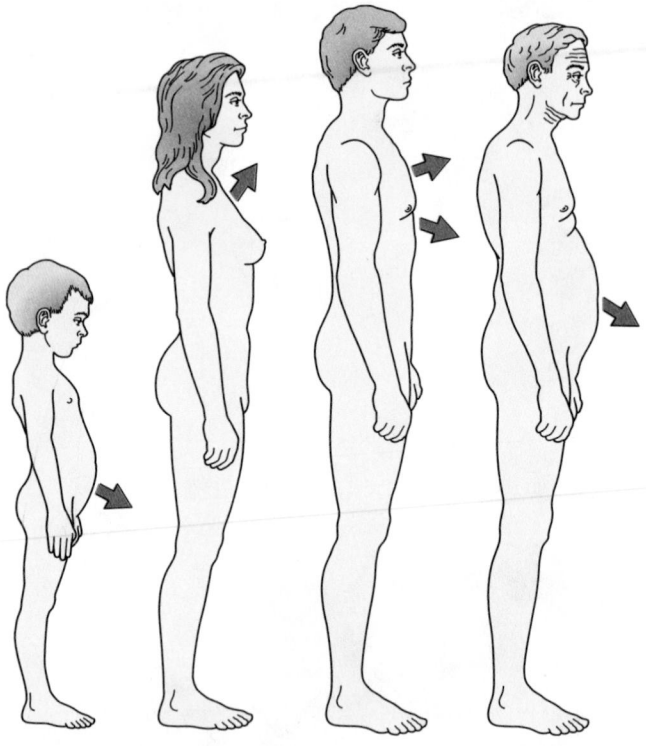

Figure 8-18
Normal breathing patterns for child, adult female, adult male, and elderly person.

Table 8-2
Muscles of Respiration

	Primary	Secondary
Inspiration	Diaphragm	Scaleni
	Levator costorum	Sternocleidomastoid
	External intercostals	Trapezius
	Internal intercostals (anterior)	Serratus anterior and posterior
		Pectoralis major
		Pectoralis minor
		Subclavius
Both		Latissimus dorsi
Expiration	Internal obliques	Serratus posterior inferior
	External obliques	
	Rectus abdominus	Quadratus lumborum
	Transverse abdominus	Iliocostalis lumborum
	Transversus thoracis	
	Transverse intercostals	
	Internal intercostals (posterior)	

breathers. In the aged, breathing tends to be in the lower thoracic and abdominal regions (Figure 8-18). The examiner should note the quality of the respiratory movements as well as the rate, rhythm, and effort required to inhale and exhale. The examiner should also note whether the patient is using the primary muscles of respiration and/or the accessory muscles of respiration, since this will help indicate the ease of the patient's breathing (Table 8-2). In addition, the presence of any coughing or noisy or abnormal breathing patterns should be noted. Because the chest wall movement that occurs during breathing displaces the pleural surfaces, thoracic muscles, nerve, and ribs, pain is accentuated by breathing and coughing if any one of these structures is injured.

Chest Deformities

In addition to rib movements during breathing, the examiner should note the presence of any chest deformities. The more common deformities are shown in Figure 8-19 and are listed below:

1. With a **pigeon chest** (pectus carinatum) deformity, the sternum projects forward and downward like the heel of a boot, increasing the anteroposterior dimension of the chest. This congenital deformity impairs the effectiveness of breathing by restricting ventilation volume.

2. The **funnel chest** (pectus excavatum) is a congenital deformity that results from the sternum's being pushed posteriorly by an overgrowth of the ribs.[11] The anteroposterior dimension of the chest is decreased, and the heart may be displaced. On inspiration, this deformity causes a depression of the sternum that affects respiration and may result in kyphosis.

3. With the **barrel chest** deformity, the sternum projects forward and upward so that the anteroposterior diameter is increased. It is seen in pathological conditions such as emphysema.

Examination

Although the assessment is primarily of the thorax and thoracic spine, if the history, observation, or examination indicates symptoms into or from the neck, upper limb, or lumbar spine and lower limb, these structures must be examined as well using an upper or lower scanning examination. If any signs or symptoms are elicited in the scanning exam, more detailed examination of the cervical or lumbar spine may be performed. Therefore, the examination of the thoracic spine may be an extensive one. Unless there is a history of specific trauma or injury to the thoracic spine or ribs, the examiner must be prepared to assess more than that area alone. If a problem is suspected above the thoracic spine, the scanning examination of the cervical spine and upper limb (as described in Chapter 3) should be performed. If a problem is suspected below the thoracic spine, the scanning examination of the lumbar spine and lower limb (as described in Chapter 9) should be performed. Only examination of the thoracic spine is described here.

PECTUS CARINATUM

PECTUS EXCAVATUM

BARREL CHEST

Figure 8-19
Chest deformities. Lower vertical views show change in chest wall contours with deformity.

Active Movements

The active movements of the thoracic spine are usually done with the patient standing. Movement in the thoracic spine is limited by the rib cage and the long spinous processes of the thoracic spine. When assessing the thoracic spine, the examiner should be sure to note whether the movement occurs in the spine or in the hips. A patient can touch the toes with a completely rigid spine if there is sufficient range of motion (ROM) in the hip joints. Likewise, tight hamstrings may alter the results. The movements may be done with the patient sitting, in which case the effect of hip movement is eliminated or decreased. Similarly, shoulder motion may be restricted if the upper thoracic segments or ribs are hypomobile.[12] As with any examination, the most painful movements are done last. The active movements to be carried out in the thoracic spine are shown in Figure 8-20.

Forward Flexion

The normal ROM of forward flexion (forward bending) in the thoracic spine is 20° to 45° (Figure 8-21). Because the ROM at each vertebra is difficult to measure, the examiner can use a tape measure to derive an indication of overall movement (Figure 8-22). The examiner first measures the length of the spine from the C7 spinous process to the T12 spinous process with the patient in the normal standing posture. The patient is then asked to bend forward

> **Active Movements of the Thoracic Spine**
>
> - Forward flexion (20°–45°)
> - Extension (25°–45°)
> - Side flexion, left and right (20°–40°)
> - Rotation, left and right (35°–50°)
> - Costovertebral expansion (3–7.5 cm)
> - Rib motion (pump handle, bucket handle, and caliper)
> - Combined movements (if necessary)
> - Repetitive movements (if necessary)
> - Sustained postures (if necessary)

and the spine is again measured. A 2.7-cm (1.1-inch) difference in tape measure length is considered normal.

If the examiner wishes, the spine may be measured from the C7 to S1 spinous process with the patient in the normal standing position. The patient is then asked to bend forward, and the spine is again measured. A 10-cm (4-inch) difference in tape measure length is considered normal. In this case, the examiner is measuring movement in the lumbar spine as well as in the thoracic spine; most movement, approximately 7.5 cm (3 inches), occurs between T12 and S1.

A third method of measuring spinal flexion is to ask the patient to bend forward and try to touch the toes

Figure 8-20

Active movement. **A,** Forward flexion. **B,** Extension.
C, Rotation (standing). **D,** Rotation (sitting).

Figure 8-21

Average range of motion in the thoracic spine. (Adapted from Grieve GP: *Common vertebral joint problems*, pp. 41–42, Edinburgh, 1981, Churchill Livingstone.)

A

B

Figure 8-22

Tape measurements for thoracic spine movement. **A,** Positioning of tape measure for determining flexion and extension in the thoracic spine. **B,** Positioning of tape measure for determining flexion or extension in the thoracic and lumbar spines combined.

Continued

Figure 8-22 cont'd

C, Forward flexion measurement of thoracic and lumbar spines. **D,** Forward flexion measurement of thoracic and lumbar spines and hips (fingertips to floor).

while keeping the knees straight. The examiner then measures from the fingertips to the floor and records the distance. The examiner must keep in mind that with this method, in addition to the thoracic spine movement, the movement may also occur in the lumbar spine and hips; in fact, movement could occur totally in the hips.

Each of these methods is indirect. To measure the ROM at each vertebral segment, a series of radiographs would be necessary. The examiner can decide which method to use. It is of primary importance, however, to note on the patient's chart how the measuring was done and which reference points were used.

While the patient is flexed forward, the examiner can observe the spine from the "skyline" view (Figure 8-23). With nonstructural scoliosis, the scoliotic curve disappears on forward flexion; with structural scoliosis, it

remains. With the skyline view, the examiner is looking for a hump on one side (convex side of curve) and a hollow (concave side of curve) on the other. This "hump and hollow" sequence is caused by vertebral rotation in idiopathic scoliosis, which pushes the ribs and muscles out on one side and causes the paravertebral valley on the opposite side. The vertebral rotation is most evident in the flexed position.

When the patient flexes forward, the thoracic spine should curve forward in a smooth, even manner with no rotation or side flexion (Figure 8-24). The examiner should look for any apparent tightness or sharp angulation such as a gibbus when the movement is performed. If the patient has an excessive kyphosis to begin with, very little forward flexion movement occurs in the thoracic spine. McKenzie[7] advocates doing flexion while sitting

E

Figure 8-22 cont'd
E, Side flexion measurement (fingertips to floor).

Figure 8-23
Examiner performing skyline view of spine for assessment of scoliosis.

A

B

Figure 8-24
Side view in forward bending position for assessment of kyphosis.
A, Normal thoracic roundness is demonstrated with a gentle curve
to the whole spine. **B,** An area of increased bending is seen in the
thoracic spine, indicating structural changes-Scheuermann's disease,
in this example. (From Moe JH et al: *Scoliosis and other spinal
deformities,* p. 18, Philadelphia, 1978, W.B. Saunders.)

to decrease pelvic and hip movements. The patient then
slouches forward flexing the thoracic spine. The patient
can put the hands around the neck to apply overpressure
at the end of flexion. If symptoms arise from forward
flexion on the spine with the neck flexed by the hands,
the examiner should repeat the movement with the neck
slightly extended and the hands removed. This will help
differentiate between cervical and thoracic pain.

Extension

Extension (backward bending) in the thoracic spine is
normally 25° to 45°. Because this movement occurs
over 12 vertebrae, the movement between the individual

vertebrae is difficult to detect visually. As with flexion, the examiner can use a tape measure and obtain the distance between the same two points (the C7 and T12 spinous processes). Again, a 2.5-cm (1-inch) difference in tape measure length between standing and extension is considered normal. McKenzie[7] advocates having the patient place the hands in the small of the back to add stability while performing the backward movement or to do extension while sitting or prone lying (sphinx position).

As the patient extends, the thoracic curve should curve backward or at least straighten in a smooth, even manner with no rotation or side flexion. Lee[13] advocates asking the patient to fully forward flex the arms during extension to facilitate extension. The examiner should look for any apparent tightness or angulation when the movement is performed. If the patient shows excessive kyphosis (Figure 8-25), the kyphotic curvature remains on extension; that is, the thoracic spine remains flexed, whether the movement is tested while the patient is standing or lying prone (see Figure 8-25).

If extension is tested in prone lying, the normal thoracic kyphosis should, for the most part, disappear. McKenzie[7] advocates doing prone extension by using a modified push up straightening the arms and allowing the spine to "sag down" toward the bed (Figure 8-26).

Figure 8-25
Kyphosis and lordosis. **A,** On physical examination, definite increases in thoracic kyphosis and lumbar lordosis are visualized. **B,** Thoracic kyphosis does not fully correct on thoracic extension. **C,** Lumbar lordosis, on the other hand, usually corrects on forward bending; in this case, some lordosis remains. (From Moe JH et al: *Scoliosis and other spinal deformities,* p. 339, Philadelphia, 1978, W.B. Saunders.)

Figure 8-26

Thoracic extension in prone lying. **A,** Prone extension. **B,** McKenzie's prone extension.

Side Flexion

Side (lateral) flexion is approximately 20° to 40° to the right and left in the thoracic spine. The patient is asked to run the hand down the side of the leg as far as possible without bending forward or backward. The examiner can then estimate the angle of side flexion or use a tape measure to determine the length from the fingertips to the floor and compare it with that of the other side (see Figure 8-22, *E*). Normally, the distances should be equal. In either case, the examiner must remember that movement in the lumbar spine as well as in the thoracic spine is being measured. As the patient bends sideways, the spine should curve sideways in a smooth, even, sequential manner. The examiner should look for any tightness or abnormal angulation, which may indicate hypomobility or hypermobility at a specific segment when the movement is performed. If, on side flexion, the ipsilateral paraspinal muscles tighten or their contracture is evident **(Forestier's bowstring sign)**, ankylosing spondylitis or pathology causing muscle spasm should be considered.[14]

Rotation

Rotation in the thoracic spine is approximately 35° to 50°. The patient is asked to cross the arms in front or place the hands on opposite shoulders and then rotate to the right and left while the examiner looks at the amount of rotation, comparing both ways. Again, the examiner must remember that movement in the lumbar spine and hips as well as in the thoracic spine is occurring. To eliminate or decrease the amount of the hip movement, rotation may be done in sitting.

If the history indicated that repetitive motion, sustained postures, or combined movements caused aggravation of symptoms, then these movements should also be tested, but only after the original movements of flexion, extension, side flexion, and rotation have been completed. Combined movements that may be tested in the thoracic spine include forward flexion and side bending, backward bending and side flexion, and lateral bending with flexion and lateral bending with extension. Any restriction of motion, excessive movement (hypermobility) or curve abnormality should be noted. These movements would be similar to the H and I test described in the lumbar spine (see Chapter 9).

Costovertebral Expansion

Costovertebral joint movement is usually determined by measuring chest expansion (Figure 8-27). The examiner places the tape measure around the chest at the level of the fourth intercostal space. The patient is asked to exhale as much as possible, and the examiner takes a measurement. The patient is then asked to inhale as much as possible and hold the breath while the second measurement is taken. The normal difference between inspiration and expiration is 3 to 7.5 cm (1 to 3 inches).

A second method of measuring chest expansion is to measure at three different levels. If this method is used, the examiner must take care to ensure that the levels of measurement are noted for consistency. The levels are (1) under the axillae for apical expansion, (2) at the nipple line or xiphisternal junction for midthoracic expansion, and (3) at the T10 rib level for lower thoracic expansion. As before, the measurements are taken after expiration and inspiration.

After the measurement of chest expansion, it is worthwhile for the patient to take a deep breath and cough so that the examiner can determine whether this action causes or alters any pain. If it does, the examiner may suspect a respiratory-related problem or a problem increasing intrathecal pressure in the spine.

Evjenth and Gloeck[15] have noted a way to differentiate thoracic spine and rib pain during movement. If the

Figure 8-27

Measuring chest expansion. **A,** Fourth lateral intercostal space. **B,** Axilla. **C,** Nipple line. **D,** Tenth rib.

patient has pain on flexion, the patient is returned to neutral and is asked to take a deep breath and hold it. While holding the breath, the patient flexes until pain is felt. At this point, the patient stops flexing and exhales. If further flexion can be accomplished after exhaling, the problem is more likely to be the ribs than the thoracic spine. Extension can be tested in a similar fashion.

Rib Motion

The patient is asked to lie supine. The examiner's hands are placed in a relaxed fashion over the upper chest. In this position, the examiner is feeling anteroposterior movement of the ribs (Figure 8-28). As the patient inhales and exhales, the examiner should compare both sides to see whether the movement is equal. Any restriction or difference in motion should be noted. If a rib stops moving relative to the other ribs on inhalation, it is classified as a **depressed rib.** If a rib stops moving relative to the other ribs on exhalation, it is classified as an **elevated rib.** It must be remembered that restriction of one rib affects the adjacent ribs. If a depressed rib is implicated, it is usually the highest restricted rib that causes the greatest problem. If an elevated rib is present, it is usually the lowest restricted rib that causes the greatest problem.[3,16] The examiner then moves his or her hands down the patient's chest, testing the movement in the middle and lower ribs in a similar fashion.

To test lateral movement of the ribs, the examiner's hands are placed around the sides of the rib cage approximately 45° to the vertical axis of the patient's body. The examiner begins at the level of the axilla and works down the lateral aspect of the ribs, feeling the movement of the ribs during inspiration and expiration and noting any restriction.

Rib dysfunctions may be divided into structural, torsional, and respiratory (Table 8-3).[17] Structural rib dysfunctions are due to joint subluxation or dislocation. Torsional rib dysfunctions are due to thoracic vertebra dysfunction as a result of hypomobility or hypermobility. Respiratory rib dysfunctions are due to either hypomobility between the ribs (e.g., intercostal shortening) or hypomobility at the costotransverse or costovertebral joints.[17]

To test the movement of the ribs relative to the thoracic spine, the patient is placed in a sitting position. The examiner places one thumb or finger on the transverse process and the thumb of the other hand just lateral to the tubercle of the rib. The patient is asked to forward flex the head (for the upper thoracic spine) and thorax (for lower thoracic spine) while the examiner feels the movement of the rib (Figure 8-29). Normally, the rib will rotate anteriorly and the rib tubercle will stay at the same level as the transverse process on the forward movement. If the rib is hypermobile, the rib will elevate relative to the transverse process.

A

B

C

Figure 8-28
Feeling rib movement. **A,** Upper ribs. **B,** Middle ribs. **C,** Lower ribs.

Table 8-3
Rib Dysfunction

Structural Rib Dysfunction

Dysfunction	Rib Angle	Midaxillary Line	Intercostal Space	Anterior Rib
Anterior subluxation	Less prominent	Symmetric	Tender, often with intercostal neuralgia	More prominent
Posterior subluxation	More prominent	Symmetric	Tender, often with intercostal neuralgia	Less prominent
Superior first rib subluxation	Superior aspect of first rib elevated (5 mm)	Hypertonicity of the scalene muscles on the same side	—	Marked tenderness of the superior aspect
Anterior-posterior rib compression	Less prominent	Prominent	Tender, often with intercostal neuralgia	Less prominent
Lateral compression	More prominent	Less prominent	Tender	More prominent
Laterally elevated	Tender	Prominent	Narrow above, wide below	Exquisitely tender at pectoral minor

Torsional Rib Dysfunction

Dysfunction	Rib Angle	Midaxillary Line	Intercostal Space
External rib torsion	Superior border prominent and tender	Symmetric	Wide above, narrow below
Internal rib torsion	Inferior border prominent and tender	Symmetric	Narrow above, wide below

Respiratory Rib Function

Dysfunction	Rib Angle	Key Rib
Inhalation restriction	During inspiration the rib or group of ribs that cease rising	Top or superior rib
Exhalation restriction	During exhalation the rib or group of ribs that stop falling	Bottom or inferior rib

Modified from Bookhout MR: Evaluation of the thoracic spine and rib cage. *In* Flynn TW (ed): *The thoracic spine and rib cage*, pp. 163, 165, 166, Boston, 1996, Butterworth-Heinemann.

If the rib is hypomobile, its motion will stop before the thoracic spine.[13] Extension may also be tested in a similar fashion, but the rib will rotate posteriorly.

Passive Movements

Because passive movements in the thoracic spine are difficult to perform in a gross fashion, the movement between each pair of vertebrae may be assessed. With the patient sitting, the examiner places one hand on the patient's forehead or on top of the head (Figure 8-30). With the other hand, the examiner palpates over and between the spinous processes of the lower cervical and upper thoracic spines (C5-T3) and feels for movement between the spinous processes while flexing (move apart) and extending (move together) the patient's head. Rotation (one side moves forward, the other moves back) and side flexion (one side moves apart, one side moves together) may be tested by rotating and side flexing the patient's head. To test the movement properly, the examiner places the middle finger over the spinous process of the vertebra being tested and the index and ring fingers on each side of it, between the spinous processes of the two adjacent vertebrae. The examiner should feel the movement occurring, assess its quality, and note whether the movement is hypomobile or hypermobile relative to the adjacent vertebra. The hypomobility or hypermobility may be indicative of pathology.[16]

Figure 8-29
Testing mobility of rib relative to thoracic vertebra. Note one thumb is on the transverse process of the vertebra and one thumb is on the rib. **A,** Upper ribs. **B,** Lower ribs.

Figure 8-30
Passive flexion/extension movement of the thoracic spine. **A,** Upper thoracic spine. **B,** Middle and lower thoracic spine.

Passive Movements of the Thoracic Spine and Normal End Feel

- Forward flexion (tissue stretch)
- Extension (tissue stretch)
- Side flexion, left and right (tissue stretch)
- Rotation, left and right (tissue stretch)

If, when the spinous processes are palpated, one process appears to be out of alignment, the examiner can then palpate the transverse processes on each side and compare them with the levels above and below to determine whether the vertebrae is truly rotated or side flexed. For example, if the spinous process of T5 is shifted to the right and if rotation has occurred at that level, the left transverse process would be more superficial posteriorly whereas the right one would appear deeper. If the spinous process rotation was an anomaly, the transverse processes would be equal as would the ribs. Passive or active movement of the spine while palpating the transverse processes will also help to indicate abnormal movement when comparing both sides or when comparing one level to another. If the alignment is normal to begin with and becomes abnormal with movement or if it is abnormal

to begin with and becomes normal with movement, it indicates a functional asymmetry rather than a structural one. Generally, a structural asymmetry would be evident if it remains through all movements.[17]

To test the movement of the vertebrae between T3 and T11, the patient sits with the fingers clasped behind the neck and the elbows together in front. The examiner places one hand and arm around the patient's elbows while palpating over and between the spinous processes, as previously described. The examiner then flexes and extends the spine by lifting and lowering the patient's elbows.

Side flexion and rotation of the trunk may be performed in a similar fashion to test these movements. The patient sits with the hands clasped behind the head. The examiner uses the thumb on one side of the spinous process and/or the index finger and/or the middle finger on the other side to palpate just lateral to the interspinous space. For side flexion, the examiner moves the patient into right side flexion and then left side flexion and by palpation compares the amount and quality of right and left movement including adjacent segments (Figure 8-31, *A*). For rotation, the examiner rotates the patient's shoulders to the right or left, comparing by palpation the amount and quality of movement of each segment as well as that of adjacent segments (Figure 8-31, *B*).[16]

A

B

Figure 8-31

A, Passive side flexion of the thoracic spine. **B,** Passive rotation of the thoracic spine.

Resisted Isometric Movements

Resisted isometric movements are performed with the patient in the sitting position. The examiner places one leg behind the patient's buttocks and the upper limbs around the patient's chest and back (Figure 8-32). The examiner then instructs the patient, "Don't let me move you," and isometrically tests the movements, noting any alteration in strength and occurrence of pain.

Resisted Isometric Movements of the Thoracic Spine

- Forward flexion
- Extension
- Side flexion, left and right
- Rotation, left and right

The thoracic spine should be tested in a neutral position, and the most painful movements are done last. Table 8-4 lists the muscles of the thoracic spine, their actions, and their innervations. It must be remembered that the resisted isometric testing of the spine is in reality a very gross test, and subtle alterations in strength are almost impossible to detect. However, if the muscles being tested have been strained (1° or 2°), contraction of the muscle commonly produces pain. In some cases, however, the spine and thorax may have to be repositioned to isolate a particular muscle.

Functional Assessment

When doing specific activities, the thoracic spine primarily plays a stabilization role. Therefore, activities involving the cervical spine, lumbar spine, and shoulder may be impaired as a result of thoracic lesions. Functional activities involving these three areas should be reviewed or considered if functional impairment appears to be related to the thoracic spine or ribs. Activities such as lifting, rotating the thorax, doing heavy work; any activity requiring stabilization of the thorax; or any activity increasing cardiopulmonary output are most likely to provoke thoracic symptoms.

Functional disability scales such as the Roland-Morris Disability Questionnaire[18] (Figure 8-33) and the Oswestry Disability Questionnaire (see Chapter 9), although designed for the lumbar spine, could be used to test functional capacity in the thoracic spine as well.[18–21] The Roland-Morris Disability Questionnaire is better suited for mild to moderate disability, whereas the Oswestry Disability Questionnaire is better suited for persistent severe disability.[19] The Functional Rating Index (Figure 8-34) has been designed to show clinical change in conditions affecting the spine, whether cervical, thoracic, or lumbar.[22]

Figure 8-32
Positioning for resisted isometric movements.

Special Tests

Tests for Neurological Involvement

If the examiner suspects a problem with movement of the spinal cord, any of the neurodynamic tests that stretch the cord may be performed. These include the straight leg raising test and the Kernig sign (see Chapter 9). Either neck flexion from above or straight leg raising from below stretches the spinal cord within the thoracic spine. The following tests should be performed only if the examiner believes they are relevant.

The reliability and validity of some special/diagnostic tests used in the thoracic spine are outlined in Appendix 8-1.

Table 8-4

Muscles of the Thorax and Abdomen: Their Actions and Nerve Root Derivation/Nerve Supply in the Thoracic Spine

Action	Muscles Acting	Nerve Root Derivation
Flexion of thoracic spine	1. Rectus abdominis	T6–T12
	2. External abdominal oblique (both sides acting together)	T7–T12
	3. Internal abdominal oblique (both sides acting together)	T7–T12, L1
Extension of thoracic spine	1. Spinalis thoracis	T1–T12
	2. Iliocostalis thoracis (both sides acting together)	T1–T12
	3. Longissimus thoracis (both sides acting together)	T1–T12
	4. Semispinalis thoracis (both sides acting together)	T1–T12
	5. Multifidus (both sides acting together)	T1–T12
	6. Rotatores (both sides acting together)	T1–T12
	7. Interspinalis	T1–T12
Rotation and side flexion of thoracic spine	1. Iliocostalis thoracis (to same side)	T1–T12
	2. Longissimus thoracis (to same side)	T1–T12
	3. Intertransverse (to same side)	T1–T12
	4. Internal abdominal oblique (to same side)	T7–T12, L1
	5. Semispinalis thoracis (to opposite side)	T1–T12
	6. Multifidus (to opposite side)	T1–T12
	7. Rotatores (to opposite side)	T1–T12
	8. External abdominal oblique (to opposite side)	T7–T12
	9. Transverse abdominis (to opposite side)	T7–T12, L1
Elevation of ribs	1. Scalenus anterior (1st rib)	C4–C6
	2. Scalenus medius (1st rib)	C3–C8
	3. Scalenus posterior (2nd rib)	C6–C8
	4. Serratus posterior superior (2nd to 5th ribs)	2–5 intercostal
	5. Iliocostalis cervicis (1st to 6th rib)	C6–C8
	6. Levatores costarum (all ribs)	T1–T12
	7. Pectoralis major (if arm fixed)	Lateral pectoral (C6–C7) Medial pectoral (C7–C8, T1)
	8. Serratus anterior (lower ribs if scapula fixed)	Long thoracic (C5–C7)
	9. Pectoralis minor (2nd to 5th ribs if scapula fixed)	Lateral pectoral (C6–C7) Medial pectoral (C7–C8)
	10. Sternocleidomastoid (if head fixed)	Accessory C2–C3
Depression of ribs	1. Serratus posterior inferior (lower 4 ribs)	T9–T12
	2. Iliocostalis lumborum (lower 6 ribs)	L1–L3
	3. Longissimus thoracis	T1–T12
	4. Rectus abdominis	T6–T12
	5. External abdominal oblique (lower 5 to 6 ribs)	T7–T12
	6. Internal abdominal oblique (lower 5 to 6 ribs)	T7–T12, L1
	7. Transverse abdominal (all acting to depress lower ribs)	T7–T12, L1
	8. Quadratus lumborum (12th rib)	T12, L1–L4
	9. Transverse thoracis	T1–T12
Approximation of ribs	1. Iliocostalis thoracis	T1–T12
	2. Intercostals (internal and external)	1–11 intercostal
	3. Diaphragm	Phrenic
Inspiration	1. External intercostals	1–11 intercostal
	2. Transverse thoracis (sternocostalis)	1–11 intercostal
	3. Diaphragm	Phrenic
	4. Sternocleidomastoid	Accessory C2–C3
	5. Scalenus anterior	C4–C6
	6. Scalenus medius	C3–C8
	7. Scalenus posterior	C6–C8

Table 8-4—cont'd

Muscles of the Thorax and Abdomen: Their Actions and Nerve Root Derivation/Nerve Supply in the Thoracic Spine

Action	Muscles Acting	Nerve Root Derivation
	8. Pectoralis major	Lateral pectoral (C5–C6)
		Medial pectoral (C7–C8, T1)
	9. Pectoralis minor	Lateral pectoral (C6–C7)
		Medial pectoral (C7–C8)
	10. Serratus anterior	Long thoracic (C5–C7)
	11. Latissimus dorsi	Thoracodorsal (C6–C8)
	12. Serratus posterior superior	2–5 intercostal
	13. Iliocostalis thoracis	T1–T12
Expiration	1. Internal intercostals	1–11 intercostal
	2. Rectus abdominis	T6–T12
	3. External abdominal oblique	T7–T12
	4. Internal abdominal oblique	T7–T12, L1
	5. Iliocostalis lumborum	L1–L3
	6. Longissimus	T1–L3
	7. Serratus posterior inferior	T9–T12
	8. Quadratus lumborum	T12, L1–L4

Special Tests Commonly Performed on the Thoracic Spine

• Slump test

Slump Test (Sitting Dural Stretch Test). The patient sits on the examining table and is asked to "slump" so that the spine flexes and the shoulders sag forward while the examiner holds the chin and head erect. The patient is asked if any symptoms are produced. If no symptoms are produced, the examiner flexes the patient's neck and holds the head down and shoulders slumped to see if symptoms are produced. If no symptoms are produced, the examiner passively extends one of the patient's knees to see if symptoms are produced. If no symptoms are produced, the examiner then passively dorsiflexes the foot of the same leg to see if symptoms are produced (Figure 8-35). The process is repeated with the other leg. Symptoms of sciatic pain or reproduction of the patient's symptoms indicates a positive test, implicating impingement of the dura and spinal cord or nerve roots.[23] Butler[24] suggested that when testing the thoracic spine while the patient is in the slump position that trunk rotation left and right should be added. He felt this maneuver increased the stress on the intercostal nerves. The pain is usually produced at the site of the lesion in a positive test.

Passive Scapular Approximation. The patient lies prone while the examiner passively approximates the scapulae by lifting the shoulders up and back. Pain in the scapular area may be indicative of a T1 or T2 nerve root problem on the side on which the pain is being experienced.[25]

First Thoracic Nerve Root Stretch. The patient abducts the arm to 90° and flexes the pronated forearm to 90°. No symptoms should appear in this position. The patient then fully flexes the elbow, putting the hand behind the neck. This action stretches the ulnar nerve and T1 nerve root. Pain into the scapular area or arm is indicative of a positive test for T1 nerve root.[25]

If the patient has upper limb symptoms that have become evident at the same time as thoracic symptoms, upper limb tension tests should also be considered to rule out referral of neurological symptoms from the thoracic spine.[26]

Upper Limb Tension Test (ULTT4). See the cervical spine chapter (Chapter 3) for a description of the test.

Tests for Failed Load Transfer (Loss of Movement Control)

These tests have been designed to demonstrate the transfer of load through the thoracic spine as part of the kinetic chain. The tests identify the site within the thorax where there are load transfer problems and where in the thoracic area stabilization does not occur during movement.

The Sitting Arm Lift (SAL) Test.[27] The patient sits on the bed with the hands resting on the thighs. The examiner asks the patient to lift one arm (the unaffected side first) into elevation through shoulder flexion with the arm straight and the thumb up. The patient then does the same movement with the opposite side. The examiner asks the patient whether one arm feels heavier to lift than the other. The examiner notes whether any symptoms are produced and which arm requires more effort to lift. If one arm is heavier and requires more effort to lift, the first part of the test is considered positive. The patient is

Text continued on page 501

Roland and Morris Disability Questionnaire (with instructions)

When your back hurts, you may find it difficult to do some of the things you normally do.

This list contains some sentences that people have used to describe themselves when they have back pain. When you read them, you may find that some stand out because they describe you *today*. As you read the list, think of yourself today. When you read a sentence that describes you today, put a tick against it. If the sentence does not describe you, then leave the space blank and go on to the next one. Remember, only tick the sentence if you are sure that it describes you *today*.

Because of my back or leg pain (sciatica) today:

YES	NO	
		1. I stay at home most of the time because of my back.
		2. I change position frequently to try to get my back comfortable.
		3. I walk more slowly than usual because of my back.
		4. Because of my back, I am not doing any of the jobs that I usually do around the house.
		5. Because of my back, I use a handrail to get upstairs.
		6. Because of my back, I lie down to rest more often.
		7. Because of my back, I have to hold on to something to get out of an easy chair.
		8. Because of my back, I try to get other people to do things for me.
		9. I get dressed more slowly than usual because of my back.
		10. I only stand up for short periods of time because of my back.
		11. Because of my back, I try not to bend or kneel down.
		12. I find it difficult to get out of a chair because of my back.
		13. My back is painful almost all the time.
		14. I find it difficult to turn over in bed because of my back.
		15. My appetite is not very good because of my back pain.
		16. I have trouble putting on my socks (or stockings) because of the pain in my back.
		17. I only walk short distances because of my back pain.
		18. I sleep less well because of my back.
		19. Because of my back pain, I get dressed with help from someone else.
		20. I sit down for most of the day because of my back.
		21. I avoid heavy jobs around the house because of my back.
		22. Because of my back pain, I am more irritable and bad tempered with people than usual.
		23. Because of my back, I go upstairs more slowly than usual.
		24. I stay in bed most of the time because of my back.

Figure 8-33

Roland-Morris Disability Questionnaire (with instructions). The higher the number of "yes" responses, the greater the disability. (From Roland M, Morris R: A study of the natural history of back pain. Part I: Development of a reliable and sensitive measure of disability in low back pain, *Spine* 8:144, 1983.)

Functional Rating Index (for use with neck and/or back problems only)

In order to properly assess your condition, we must understand how much your <u>neck and/or back problems</u> have affected your ability to manage everyday activities. For each item below, please circle the number which most closely describes your condition *right now*.

1. Pain Intensity

0	1	2	3	4
No pain	Mild pain	Moderate pain	Severe pain	Worst possible pain

2. Sleeping

0	1	2	3	4
Perfect sleep	Mildly disturbed sleep	Moderately disturbed sleep	Greatly disturbed sleep	Totally disturbed sleep

3. Personal Care (washing, dressing, etc.)

0	1	2	3	4
No pain; no restrictions	Mild pain; no restrictions	Moderate pain; need to go slowly	Moderate pain; need some assistance	Severe pain; need 100% assistance

4. Travel (driving, etc.)

0	1	2	3	4
No pain on long trips	Mild pain on long trips	Moderate pain on long trips	Moderate pain on short trips	Severe pain on short trips

5. Work

0	1	2	3	4
Can do usual work plus unlimited extra work	Can do usual work; no extra work	Can do 50% of usual work	Can do 25% of usual work	Cannot work

Figure 8-34

Functional Rating Index. (Modified from Feise RJ, Menke JM: Functional rating index—A new valid and reliable instrument to measure the magnitude of clinical change in spinal conditions. *Spine* 26:85–86, 2001. © 1999 Institute of Evidence-Based Chiropractic; www.chiroevidence.com.)

Continued

6. Recreation

| 0 | 1 | 2 | 3 | 4 |
| Can do all activities | Can do most activities | Can do some activities | Can do a few activities | Cannot do any activities |

7. Frequency of pain

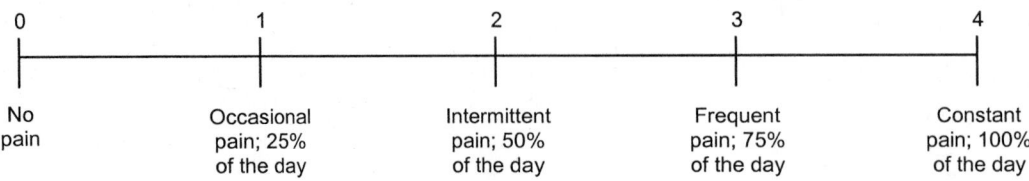

| 0 | 1 | 2 | 3 | 4 |
| No pain | Occasional pain; 25% of the day | Intermittent pain; 50% of the day | Frequent pain; 75% of the day | Constant pain; 100% of the day |

8. Lifting

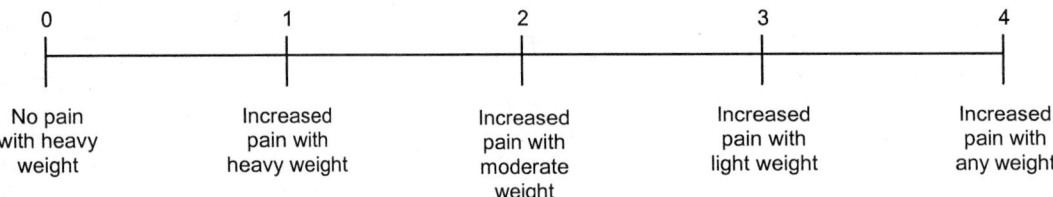

| 0 | 1 | 2 | 3 | 4 |
| No pain with heavy weight | Increased pain with heavy weight | Increased pain with moderate weight | Increased pain with light weight | Increased pain with any weight |

9. Walking

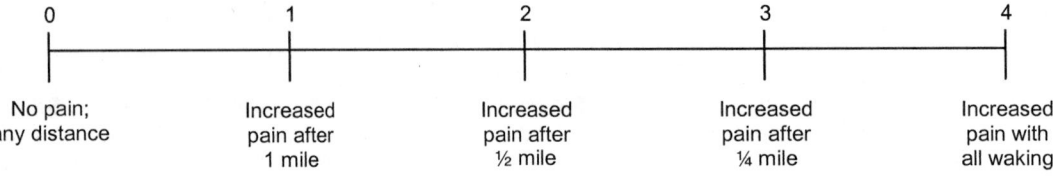

| 0 | 1 | 2 | 3 | 4 |
| No pain; any distance | Increased pain after 1 mile | Increased pain after ½ mile | Increased pain after ¼ mile | Increased pain with all waking |

10. Standing

| 0 | 1 | 2 | 3 | 4 |
| No pain after several hours | Increased pain after several hours | Increased pain after 1 hour | Increased pain after ½ hour | Increased pain with any standing |

To calculate score: $\dfrac{\text{Total Score of 10 Items}}{40}$ x 100%

_____   _____
Patient's Signature   Date

Figure 8-34 cont'd ▬▬▬▬▬

A   B

Figure 8-35
Slump test. **A,** Classic test. **B,** Trunk rotation added to classic test.

then asked to repeat the movement several times while the examiner palpates the ribs individually by placing the thumb on the spinous process and index finger along the rib, noting whether there is any translation of the rib, especially in the first 90° of movement. Normally, when the patient lifts the arm, the muscles of the thorax are activated, stabilizing the thoracic spine so there is no translation. A positive test for the second part of the test would be indicated by one or more of the thoracic rings (i.e., ribs or vertebrae) translating along any axis or rotating in any plane during the test. The examiner should note the level and direction of the loss of control. Normally what is seen is loss of rotational control with concurrent lateral translation either to the same side as the arm lift or to the contralateral side. This loss of control is usually seen between 0° and 90° of forward flexion.

The SAL test may also be used to demonstrate stability in the scapula, glenohumeral joint, and cervical spine. For the scapula, the examiner should watch the movement of the scapula to determine if there is any scapular dyskinesia indicating a loss of control. For the glenohumeral joint, the head of the humerus should remain centered in the glenoid fossa throughout the full forward flexion into elevation movement. To test the cervical spine, the examiner palpates the lateral aspect of the articular pillars of the cervical spine vertebra bilaterally while the patient does the movement. If there is translation of one vertebra relative to another when the patient does the SAL test, it indicates a lack of control of that individual segment.

The Prone Arm Lift (PAL) Test.[27] This test is a modification of the SAL test. It assesses the ability of the arm to take a load in a higher angle of shoulder flexion. This test is especially useful in people who do overhead activities or who complain of problems when they try to lift heavy loads or try to move the arm too quickly. The patient lies prone with the arms overhead at approximately 140° of flexion and fully supported on the bed. The patient is then asked to lift one arm 2 cm and then lower it. This is repeated with the other side. If one arm is heavier than the other, it is considered the positive side. The examiner can then proceed to do an assessment like the second part of the SAL test, palpating the ribs for abnormal translation, watching the movement of the scapula for scapular dyskinesia, ensuring that the head of the humerus remains centralized in the glenoid, and palpating the cervical spine for abnormal translation.

Reflexes and Cutaneous Distribution

Within the thoracic spine, there is a great deal of overlap of the dermatomes (Figure 8-36). The dermatomes tend to follow the ribs, and the absence of only one dermatome may lead to no loss of sensation. Pain may be referred to the thoracic spine from various abdominal organs (Figure 8-37; Table 8-5). Although there are no reflexes to test in conjunction with the thoracic spine, the examiner would be wise to test the lumbar reflexes—the patellar reflex (L3-L4), the medial hamstrings reflex (L5-S1), and the

Figure 8-36

The cutaneous areas (dermatomes) supplied by the thoracic nerve roots (after Foerster). By comparing both sides, the degree of overlapping and the area of exclusive supply of any individual nerve root may be estimated. (Adapted from Williams P, Warwick R [eds]: *Gray's anatomy,* p. 1150, 37th British ed. Edinburgh, 1989, Churchill Livingstone.)

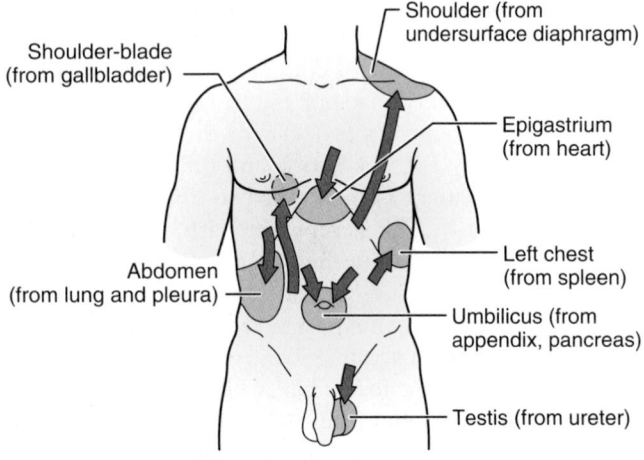

Figure 8-37

Referred pain in the thorax and chest. (Modified from Judge RD et al: *Clinical diagnosis: a physiologic approach,* p. 285, Boston, 1982, Little, Brown.)

Achilles reflex (S1–S2)—because pathology in the thoracic spine can affect these reflexes.

Thoracic nerve root symptoms tend to follow the course of the ribs and may be referred as follows[28]:

T10–T11: Pain in epigastric area
T5: Pain around nipple
T7–T8: Pain in epigastric area

Table 8-5

Differences in Pain Perception

Structure	Effective Stimulus*	Conscious Pain Perception
Skin	Discrete touch, prick, heat, cold	Precisely localized, superficial, burning, sharp
Chest wall (muscles, ribs, ligaments, parietal pleura)	Movement, deep pressure	Intermediate in localization and depth; aching, sharp, or dull
Thoracic viscera	Ischemia, distension, muscle spasm	Vague, diffuse, deep, aching, usually dull

From Levene DL: *Chest pain: an integrated diagnostic approach,* Philadelphia, 1977, Lea & Febiger.
*The effectiveness of a stimulus is heightened by the presence of inflammation.

T10–T11: Pain in umbilical area
T12: Pain in the groin
Muscles of the thoracic spine may also refer pain into adjacent areas (Table 8-6).

Joint Play Movements

The joint play movements performed on the thoracic spine are specific ones that were developed by Maitland.[28] They are sometimes called passive accessory intervertebral movements (PAIVMs). When testing joint play movements, the examiner should note any decreased ROM, muscle spasm, pain, or difference in end feel. The normal end feel is tissue stretch.

Joint Play Movements of the Thoracic Spine

- Posteroanterior central vertebral pressure (PACVP)
- Posteroanterior unilateral vertebral pressure (PAUVP)
- Transverse vertebral pressure (TVP)
- Rib springing

For the vertebral movements, the patient lies prone. The examiner palpates the thoracic spinous processes, starting at C6 and working down to L1 or L2. The occurrence of muscle spasm and/or pain on application of the vertebral pressure gives the examiner an indication of where the pathology may lie. The examiner must take care, however, because the pain and/or muscle spasm at one level may be the result of compensation for a lesion at another level. For example, if one level

Table 8-6

Thoracic Muscles and Referral of Pain

Muscles	Referral Pattern
Levator scapulae	Neck shoulder angle to posterior shoulder and along medial edge of scapula
Latissimus dorsi	Inferior angle of scapula to posterior shoulder; iliac crest
Rhomboids	Medial border of scapula
Trapezius	Upper thoracic spine to medial border of scapula
Serratus anterior	Lateral chest wall to lower medial border of scapula
Serratus posterior	Medial border of arm to medial two fingers
Serratus superior	Scapular area to posterior and anterior arm down to little finger
Multifidus	Adjacent to spinal column
Iliocostalis	Spinal column to line along medial border of scapula

is hypomobile as a result of trauma, another level may become hypermobile to compensate for the decreased movement at the traumatized level. It is probable that both the hypomobile and the hypermobile segments will cause pain and/or muscle spasm. It is then important to determine which joint complex is hypomobile and which is hypermobile, because the treatment for each is different.

Posteroanterior Central Vertebral Pressure (PACVP)

The examiner's hands, fingers, and thumbs are positioned as in Figure 8-38, *A*. The examiner then applies pressure to the spinous process through the thumbs, pushing the vertebra forward. Care must be taken to apply pressure slowly and with careful control, so that the movement, which is minimal, can be felt. This springing test may be repeated several times to determine the quality of the movement. The load applied to the spinous process is primarily taken up by the thoracic spine, although part of it is taken up by the rib cage.[29] Each spinous process is done in turn, starting at C6 and working down to L1 or L2. When doing this test, the examiner must keep in mind that the thoracic spinous processes are not always at the level of the same vertebral body. For example, the spinous processes of T1, T2, T3, and T12 are at the same levels as the T1, T2, T3, and T12 vertebral bodies, but the spinous processes of T7, T8, T9, and T10 are at the same levels as the T8, T9, T10, and T11 vertebral bodies, respectively.

Posteroanterior Unilateral Vertebral Pressure (PAUVP)

The examiner's fingers are moved laterally away from the tip of the spinous process so that the thumbs rest on the appropriate lamina or transverse process of the thoracic vertebra (Figures 8-38, *B* and 8-39). The same anterior springing pressure is applied as in the posteroanterior central vertebral pressure technique. Again, each vertebra

A

B

Figure 8-38

Hand, finger, and thumb positions for joint play movements. **A,** Posteroanterior central vertebral pressure. **B,** Posteroanterior unilateral vertebral pressure.

Continued

C

D

Figure 8-38 cont'd

C, Transverse vertebral pressure. **D**, Rib springing (prone).

Figure 8-39

Direction of pressure during joint play movements. *PACVP*, Posteroanterior central vertebral pressure; *PAUVP*, posteroanterior unilateral vertebral pressure; *TVP*, transverse vertebral pressure.

is done in turn. The two sides should be examined and compared. It must be remembered that in the thoracic area, the spinous process is not necessarily at the same level as the transverse process on the same vertebra. For example, the T9 spinous process is at the level of the T10 transverse process. Therefore, it is necessary to move the fingers up and out from the tip of the T9 spinous process to the T9 transverse process, which is at the level of the T8 spinous process. This difference does not hold true

for the entire thoracic spine. It is also important to realize that a PAUVP applies a rotary force to the vertebra; it therefore places a greater stress at the costotransverse joints, because the ribs are also stressed where they attach to the vertebrae. A PAUVP applied to the right transverse process will cause the vertebral body to rotate to the left.

Transverse Vertebral Pressure (TVP)

The examiner's fingers are placed along the side of the spinous process, as shown in Figures 8-38, *C* and 8-39. The examiner then applies a transverse springing pressure to the side of the spinous process, feeling for the quality of movement. As before, each vertebra is assessed in turn, starting at C6 and working down to L1 or L2. Pressure should be applied to both sides of the spinous process to compare the movement. This technique also applies a rotary force to the vertebra, but in the opposite direction to that caused by the PAUVP. A TVP applied to the right side of the spinous process will cause the spinous process to rotate to the left and the vertebral body to rotate to the right.

The **individual apophyseal** joints may also be tested (Figure 8-40). The patient is placed in a prone lying position with the thoracic spine in neutral. To test the superior glide at the apophyseal joint (i.e., to test the ability of the inferior articular process of the superior vertebra [e.g., T6] to glide superiorly on the superior articular process of the inferior vertebra [e.g., T7]), the examiner stabilizes the transverse process of the inferior vertebra (e.g., T7) with one thumb while the other thumb glides the inferior articular process of the superior vertebra (e.g., T6) superoanteriorly, noting the end feel and quality of the motion (see Figure 8-40, *A*).[13]

Figure 8-40
A, Superior glide of inferior facet of superior vertebra on inferior vertebra. **B,** Inferior glide of inferior facet of superior vertebra on inferior vertebra.

To test the inferior glide at the apophyseal joint (i.e., to test the ability of the inferior articular process of the superior vertebra [e.g., T6] to glide inferiorly on the superior articular process of the inferior vertebra [e.g., T7]), the examiner stabilizes the transverse process of the inferior vertebra (e.g., T7) with one thumb while the other thumb glides the inferior articular process of the superior vertebra (e.g., T6) inferiorly, noting the end feel and quality of the movement (see Figure 8-40, *B*).[13]

To test the costotransverse joints, the patient is placed in a prone lying position with the spine in neutral. The examiner stabilizes the thoracic vertebra by placing one thumb along or against the side of the transverse process. The other thumb is placed over the posterior and/ or superior aspect of the rib just lateral to the tubercle. Some examiners may find it easier to cross thumbs. An anterior or inferior glide is applied to the rib, causing an anterior or inferior movement (Figure 8-41).

Figure 8-41
Testing costotransverse joints. **A,** Anterior glide with crossed thumbs. **B,** Inferior glide.

Rib Springing

The patient lies prone or on the side while the examiner's hands are placed around the posterolateral aspect of the rib cage (see Figure 8-38, *D*). The examiner's hands are approximately 45° to the vertical axis of the patient's body. The examination begins at the top of the rib cage and extends inferiorly, springing the ribs by pushing in with the hands on each side in turn and then quickly releasing. The amount and quality of movement occurring on both sides should be noted. If one rib appears hypomobile or hypermobile in relation to the others being tested, it or all the ribs can be tested individually by compressing them individually anteriorly and/or posteriorly.

Palpation

As with any palpation technique, the examiner is looking for tenderness, muscle spasm, temperature alteration, swelling, or other signs that may indicate disease. Palpation should begin on the anterior chest wall, move around the lateral chest wall, and finish with the posterior structures (Figure 8-42). Palpation is usually done with the patient sitting, although it may be done by combining the supine and prone lying positions. At the same time, the thorax may be divided into sections (Figure 8-43) to give some idea, in charting, where the pathology may lie.

Anterior Aspect

Sternum. In the midline of the chest, the manubrium sternum, body of the sternum, and xiphoid process should be palpated for any abnormality or tenderness.

Ribs and Costal Cartilage. Adjacent to the sternum, the examiner should palpate the sternocostal and costochondral articulations, noting any swelling, tenderness, or abnormality. These "articulations" are sometimes sprained or subluxed, or a costochondritis (e.g., Tietze's syndrome) may be evident. The ribs should be palpated as they extend around the chest wall, with any potential pathology or crepitations (e.g., subcutaneous emphysema) noted.

Clavicle. The clavicle should be palpated along its length for abnormal bumps (e.g., fracture, callus) or tenderness.

Abdomen. The abdomen should be palpated for tenderness or other signs indicating pathology. The palpation is done in a systematic fashion, using the fingers of one hand to feel the tissues while the other hand is used to apply pressure. Palpation is carried out to a depth of 1 to 3 cm (0.5–1.5 inches) to reveal areas of tenderness and abnormal masses. Palpation is usually carried out using the four quadrant or the nine-region system (Figure 8-44).

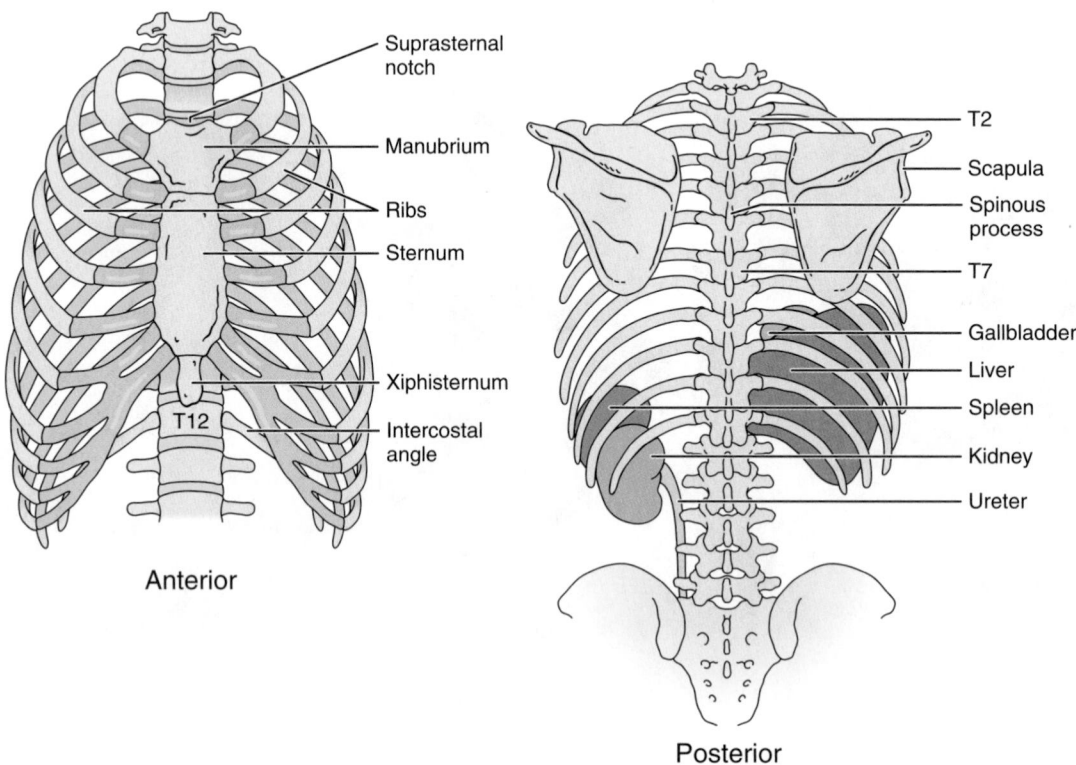

Anterior

Posterior

Figure 8-42

Landmarks of the thoracic spine.

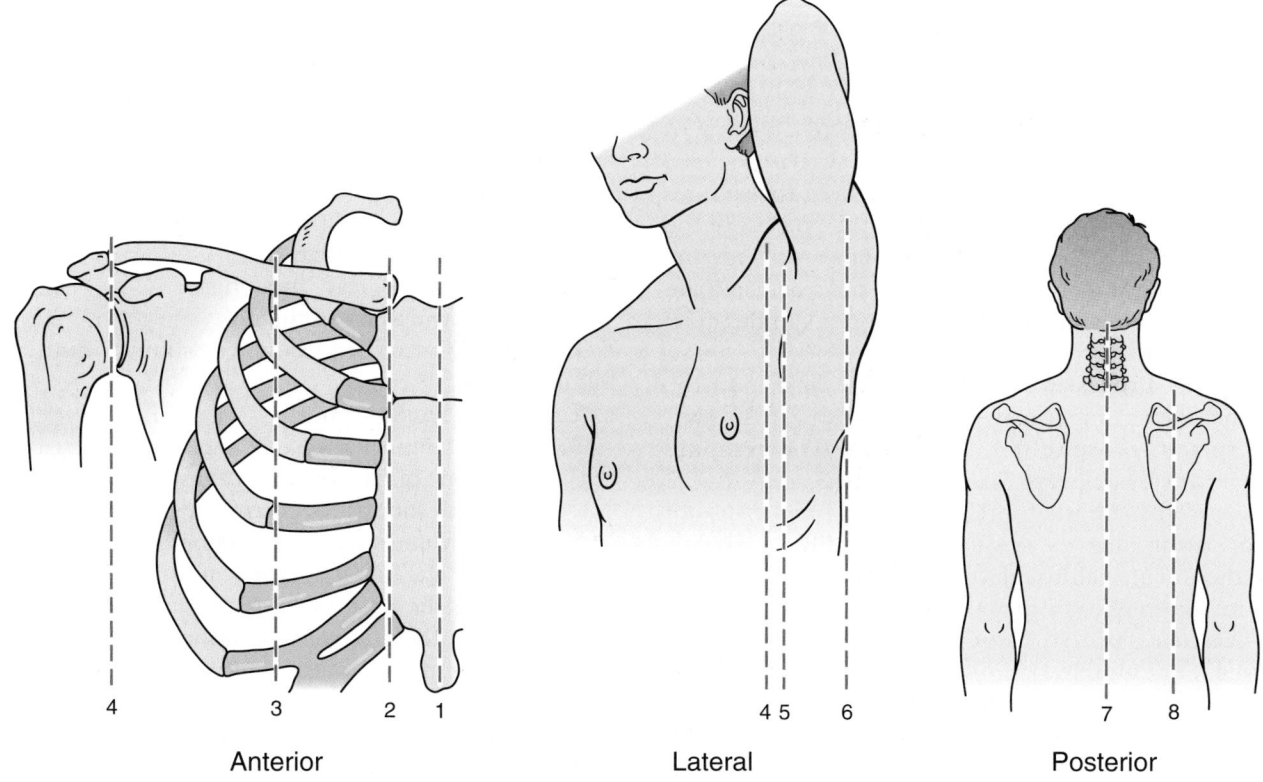

Figure 8-43

Lines of reference in the thoracic area: *(1)* midtarsal line; *(2)* parasternal line; *(3)* midclavicular line; *(4)* anterior axillary line; *(5)* midaxillary line; *(6)* posterior axillary line; *(7)* midspinal (vertebral) line; *(8)* midscapular line.

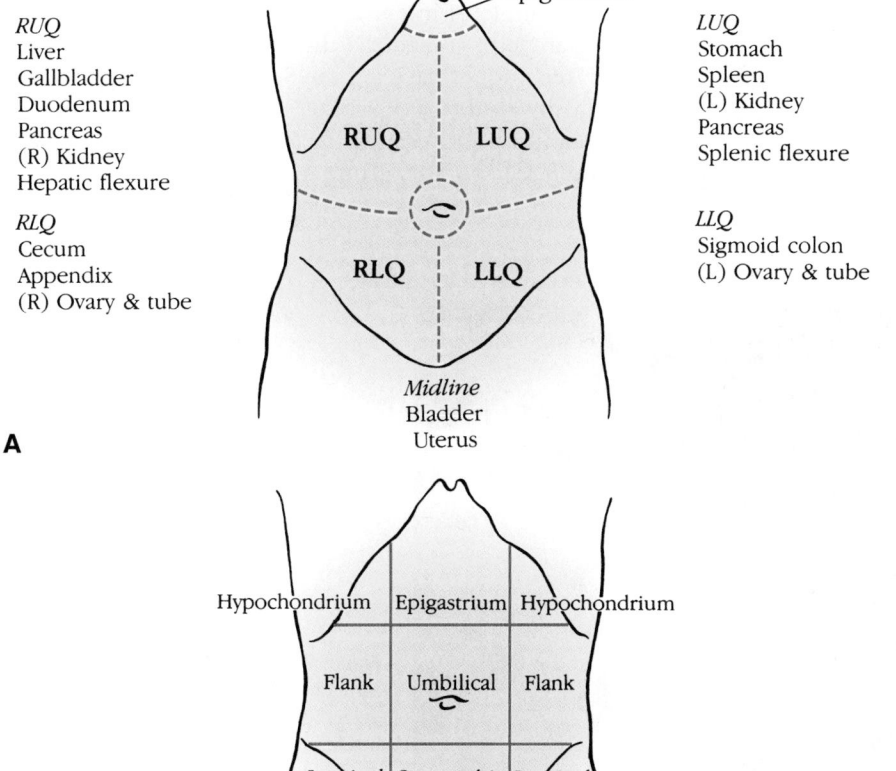

RUQ
Liver
Gallbladder
Duodenum
Pancreas
(R) Kidney
Hepatic flexure

RLQ
Cecum
Appendix
(R) Ovary & tube

LUQ
Stomach
Spleen
(L) Kidney
Pancreas
Splenic flexure

LLQ
Sigmoid colon
(L) Ovary & tube

Midline
Bladder
Uterus

A

B

Figure 8-44

Superficial topography of the abdomen. **A,** Four-quadrant system. *RUQ,* Right upper quadrant; *RLQ,* right lower quadrant; *LUQ,* left upper quadrant; *LLQ,* left lower quadrant. **B,** Nine-regions system. (From Judge RD et al: *Clinical diagnosis: a physiologic approach,* p. 284, Boston, 1982, Little, Brown.)

Posterior Aspect

Scapula. The medial, lateral, and superior borders of the scapula should be palpated for any swelling or tenderness. The scapula normally extends from the spinous process of T2 to that of T7–T9. After the borders of the scapula have been palpated, the examiner palpates the posterior surface of the scapula. Structures palpated are the supraspinatus and infraspinatus muscles and the spine of the scapula.

Spinous Processes of the Thoracic Spine. In the midline, the examiner may posteriorly palpate the thoracic spinous processes for abnormality. The examiner then moves laterally approximately 2 to 3 cm (0.8–1.2 inches) to palpate the thoracic facet joints. Because of the overlying muscles, it is usually very difficult to palpate these joints, although the examiner may be able to palpate for muscle spasm and tenderness. Muscle spasm may also be elicited if some internal structures are injured. For example, pathology affecting the following structures can cause muscle spasm in the surrounding area: gallbladder (spasm on the right side in the area of the eighth and ninth costal cartilages), spleen (spasm at the level of ribs 9 through 11 on the left side), and kidneys (spasm at the level of ribs 11 and 12 on both sides at the level of the L3 vertebra). Evidence of positive findings with no comparable history of musculoskeletal origin could lead the examiner to believe the problem was not of a musculoskeletal origin.

Diagnostic Imaging

Plain Film Radiography

Anteroposterior View. With this view (Figure 8-45), the examiner should note the following:

1. Any wedging of the vertebrae
2. Whether the disc spaces appear normal
3. Whether the ring epiphysis, if present, is normal
4. Whether there is a "bamboo" spine, indicative of ankylosing spondylitis (Figure 8-46)
5. Any scoliosis (Figure 8-47)
6. Malposition of heart and lungs
7. Normal symmetry of the ribs

Lateral View. The examiner should note the following:

1. A normal mild kyphosis
2. Any wedging of the vertebrae, which may be an indication of structural kyphosis resulting from conditions such as Scheuermann's disease or wedge fracture from trauma or osteoporosis (Figure 8-48)
3. Whether the disc spaces appear normal
4. Whether the ring epiphysis, if present, is normal
5. Whether there are any **Schmorl's nodules,** indicating herniation of the intervertebral disc into the vertebral body
6. Angle of the ribs
7. Any osteophytes

Measurement of Spinal Curvature for Scoliosis. With the Cobb method (Figure 8-49), an anteroposterior view is used.[9,30,31] A line is drawn parallel to the superior cortical plate of the proximal end vertebra and to the inferior cortical plate of the distal end vertebra. A perpendicular line is erected to each of these lines, and the angle of intersection of the perpendicular lines is the angle of spinal curvature resulting from scoliosis. Such techniques have led the Scoliosis Research Society to classify all forms of scoliosis according to the degree of curvature: group 1, 0° to 20°; group 2, 21° to 30°; group 3, 31° to 50°; group 4, 51° to 75°; group 5, 76°

Figure 8-45

Structural scoliosis caused by congenital defect. **A,** Left midlumbar and right lumbosacral hemivertebrae in a 3-year-old child (example of hemimetameric shift). **B,** A first cousin also demonstrates a midlumbar hemivertebra as well as asymmetric development of the upper sacrum.

Figure 8-45 cont'd

C, This girl has a semisegmented hemivertebra *(arrow)* in the midlumbar spine with a mild 12° curve. **D,** Her identical twin sister showed no congenital anomalies of the spine. (From Moe JH et al: *Scoliosis and other spinal deformities,* p. 134, Philadelphia, 1978, W.B. Saunders.)

to 100°; group 6, 101° to 125°; and group 7, 126° or greater.[10] Other noninvasive methods of measuring the curve have been advocated. However, the examiner should use the same method each time for consistency and reliability.[32,33]

The rotation of the vertebrae may also be estimated from an anteroposterior view (Figure 8-50). This estimation is best done by the **pedicle method,** in which the examiner determines the relation of the pedicles to the lateral margins of the vertebral bodies. The ver-

tebra is in neutral position when the pedicles appear to be at equal distance from the lateral margin of the peripheral bodies on the film. If rotation is evident, the pedicles appear to move laterally toward the concavity of the curve.

Computed Tomography

Computed tomography is of primary use in evaluating the bony spine, the spinal contents, and the surrounding soft tissues in cross-sectional views.

Figure 8-46

Ankylosing spondylitis of spine. Note the bony encasement of vertebral bodies on the lateral view **(A)** and the bamboo effect on the anteroposterior view **(B).** (From Gartland JJ: *Fundamentals of orthopedics,* p. 147, Philadelphia, 1979, W.B. Saunders.)

Figure 8-47

The natural history of idiopathic scoliosis. **A,** Note the mild degree of vertebral rotation and curvature and the imbalance of the upper torso. **B,** Note the rather dramatic increase in curvature and the increased rotation of the apical vertebrae 1 year later. **C,** Further progression of the curvature has occurred, and the opportunity for brace treatment has been missed. (From Bunnel WP: Treatment of idiopathic scoliosis, *Orthop Clin North Am* 10:817, 1979.)

Figure 8-48

Classic radiographic appearance of the spine in a patient with Scheuermann's disease. Note the wedged vertebra, Schmorl's nodules, and marked irregularity of the vertebral end plates. (From Moe JH et al: *Scoliosis and other spinal deformities,* p. 32, Philadelphia, 1978, W.B. Saunders.)

A

B

Figure 8-49

A, Cobb method of measuring scoliotic curve. **B,** Measurement of idiopathic scoliosis (Cobb's method). This 10-year-old girl has a T4–T11 right spinal curvature of 20° and a T11–L4 left spinal curvature of 27°. Note that T11 is included in both curve measurements. Minimal rotation occurs in the thoracic region, and essentially none in the lumbar segment. (**B,** From Ozonoff MB: *Pediatric orthopedic radiology,* 2nd ed. Philadelphia, 1992, W.B. Saunders.)

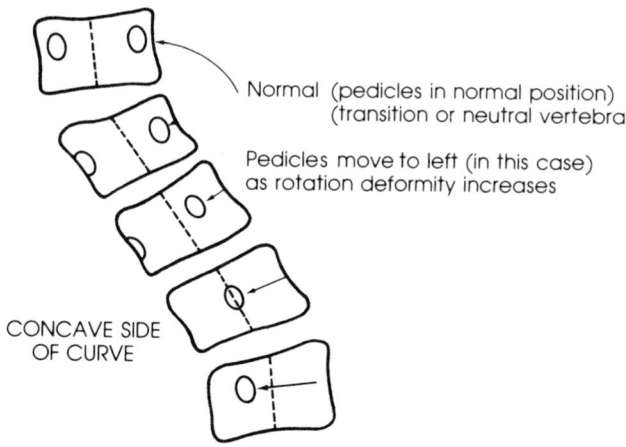

Normal (pedicles in normal position)
(transition or neutral vertebra)

Pedicles move to left (in this case)
as rotation deformity increases

CONCAVE SIDE
OF CURVE

Figure 8-50

Rotation of vertebra in scoliosis. On radiography, the pedicles appear to be off center as the curve progresses.

Magnetic Resonance Imaging

Magnetic resonance imaging (MRI) is a noninvasive technique that is useful for delineating soft tissue, including herniated discs and intrinsic spinal cord lesions, as well as bony tissue (Figure 8-51). However, MRI should be used only to confirm a clinical diagnosis, because conditions such as disc herniation have been demonstrated on MRI in the absence of clinical symptoms.[34,35]

Figure 8-51

Osteoporotic compression fracture of thoracic spine. Midline sagittal T1-weighted magnetic resonance image (SE 500/30) shows compression fracture of upper thoracic vertebral body (*arrowhead*), indicated by anterior wedging. Marrow signal intensity is maintained (*arrowhead*). Schmorl's nodule is incidentally noted at a lower level (*arrow*). (From Bassett LW et al: *MRI atlas of the musculoskeletal system,* p. 49, London, 1989, Martin Dunitz.)

Précis of the Thoracic Spine Assessment*

History
Observation (standing)
Examination
  Active movements (standing or sitting)
    Forward flexion
    Extension
    Side flexion (left and right)
    Rotation (left and right)
    Combined movements (if necessary)
    Repetitive movements (if necessary)
    Sustained postures (if necessary)
  Passive movements (sitting)
    Forward flexion
    Extension
    Side flexion (left and right)
    Rotation (left and right)
  Resisted isometric movements (sitting)
    Forward flexion
    Extension
    Side flexion (left and right)

    Rotation (left and right)
  Special tests (sitting)
  Reflexes and cutaneous distribution (sitting)
    Reflex testing (?)
    Sensation scan
  Special tests (prone lying)
  Joint play movements (prone lying)
    Posteroanterior central vertebral pressure
    Posteroanterior unilateral vertebral pressure
    Transverse vertebral pressure
    Rib springing
  Palpation (prone lying)
  Palpation (supine lying)
  Diagnostic imaging
After any assessment, the patient should be warned of the possibility of exacerbation of symptoms as a result of assessment.

_____

*The précis is shown in an order that limits the amount of movement that the patient has to do but ensures that all necessary structures are tested.

Case Studies

When doing these case studies, the examiner should list the appropriate questions to be asked and why they are being asked, what to look for and why, and what things should be tested and why. Depending on the answers of the patient (and the examiner should consider different responses), several possible causes of the patient's problems may be evident (examples are given in parentheses). If so, a differential diagnosis chart (see Table 8-7 as an example) should be made up. The examiner can then decide how different diagnoses may affect the treatment plan.

1. A 33-year-old patient comes to you complaining of stiffness in the lower spine that is extending into the thoracic spine. Describe your assessment plan for this patient (ankylosing spondylitis versus thoracic spinal stenosis).

2. A 14-year-old boy presents complaining of a severe aching pain in the middorsal spine of several weeks' duration. He is neurologically normal. X-rays reveal a narrowing and anterior wedging at T5 with a Schmorl's nodule into T4. Describe your assessment plan for this patient (kyphosis versus Scheuermann's disease).

3. A 23-year-old woman has a structural scoliosis with a single C curve having its apex at T7. Describe your assessment plan before beginning treatment. How would you measure the curve and the amount of rotation?

4. A 38-year-old woman comes to your clinic complaining of chest pain with tenderness at the costochondral junction of two ribs on the left side. Describe your assessment plan for this patient (Tietze's syndrome versus rib hypomobility).

5. A 26-year-old male ice hockey player comes to you complaining of back pain that is referred around the chest. He explains that he was "boarded" (hit between another player and the boards). He did not notice the pain and stiffness until the next day. He has had the problem for 2 weeks. Describe your assessment plan for this patient (rib hypomobility versus ligament sprain).

6. A 21-year-old female synchronized swimmer comes to you complaining of pain in her side. She says she was kicked when she helped boost another athlete out of the water 5 days ago. Describe your assessment plan for this patient (rib fracture versus rib hypomobility).

Table 8-7

Differential Diagnosis of Ankylosing Spondylitis and Thoracic Spinal Stenosis

	Ankylosing Spondylitis	Thoracic Spinal Stenosis
History	Morning stiffness Intermittent aching pain Male predominance Sharp pain→ache Bilateral sacroiliac pain may refer to posterior thigh	Intermittent aching pain Pain may refer to both legs with walking (neurogenic intermittent claudication)
Active movements	Restricted	May be normal
Passive movements	Restricted	May be normal
Resisted isometric movements	Normal	Normal
Special tests	None	Bicycle test of van Gelderen may be positive Stoop test may be positive
Reflexes	Normal	May be affected in long-standing cases
Sensory deficit	None	Usually temporary
Diagnostic imaging	Plain films are diagnostic	Computed tomography scans are diagnostic

References

To enhance this text and add value for the reader, all references have been incorporated into a CD-ROM that is provided with this text. The reader can view the reference source and access it online whenever possible. There are a total of 37 cited and other general references for this chapter.

APPENDIX 8-1

RELIABILITY, VALIDITY, SPECIFICITY, AND SENSITIVITY OF SPECIAL/DIAGNOSTIC TESTS USED IN THE THORACIC SPINE

SLUMP TEST (SITTING DURAL STRETCH TEST)

Reliability

- Interrater for reproduction of symptoms and subsequent reduction with cervical extension k=0.89, increase with knee extension k=0.83[36]

SRS-22

Reliability	Validity
• Internal consistency, Cronbach's alpha for subscales: pain 0.67, self image 0.76, function 0.79, mental health 0.83[37] • Reliability of the subscales: function r=0.95, self image r=0.95, mental health r=0.92, pain r=0.90, satisfaction r=0.84[37]	• Correlation with SF-12 subscales: r=0.79, mental health r=0.87, pain r=0.73[37] • Correlation with Oswestry subscale for function r=0.87[37]

LUMBAR SPINE

Back pain is one of the great human afflictions. Almost anyone born today in Europe or North America has a great chance of suffering a disabling back injury regardless of occupation.[1] The lumbar spine supports the upper body and transmits the weight of the upper body to the pelvis and lower limbs. Because of the strategic location of the lumbar spine, this structure should be included in any examination of the spine as a whole (i.e., posture) or in any examination of the hip or sacroiliac joints. Unless there is a definite history of trauma, it is often difficult to determine whether an injury originates in the lumbar spine, sacroiliac joints, or hip joints; therefore, all three should be examined in a sequential fashion.

Applied Anatomy

There are 10 (five pairs) facet joints (also called apophyseal or zygoapophyseal joints) in the lumbar spine (Figure 9-1).[2] These diarthrodial joints consist of superior and inferior facets and a capsule. The facets are located on the vertebral arches. With a normal intact disc, the facet joints carry about 20% to 25% of the axial load, but this may reach 70% with degeneration of the disc. The facet joints also provide 40% of the torsional and shear strength.[3] Injury, degeneration, or trauma to the **motion segment** (the facet joints and disc) may lead to **spondylosis** (degeneration of the intervertebral disc), **spondylolysis** (a defect in the pars interarticularis or the arch of the vertebra), **spondylolisthesis** (a forward displacement of one vertebra over another), or **retrolisthesis** (backward displacement of one vertebra on another). The superior facets, or articular processes, face medially and

backward and in general, are concave; the inferior facets face laterally and forward and are convex (Figure 9-2). There are, however, abnormalities, or **tropisms,** that can occur in the shape of the facets, especially at the L5-S1 level (Figures 9-3 and 9-4).[4] In the lumbar spine, the transverse processes are virtually at the same level as the spinous processes.

These posterior facet joints direct the movement that occurs in the lumbar spine. Because of the shape of the facets, rotation in the lumbar spine is minimal and is accomplished only by a shearing force. Side flexion, extension, and flexion can occur in the lumbar spine, but the facet joints control the direction of movement. The close packed position of the facet joints in the lumbar spine is extension. Normally, the facet joints carry only a small amount of weight; with increased extension, however, they begin to have a greater weight-bearing function. The resting position is midway between flexion and extension. The capsular pattern is side flexion and rotation equally limited, followed by extension. However, if only one facet joint in the lumbar spine has a capsular restriction, the amount of observable restriction is minimal. The first sacral segment is usually included in discussions of the lumbar spine, and it is at this joint that the fixed segment of the sacrum joins with the mobile segments of the lumbar spine. In some cases, the S1 segment may be mobile. This occurrence is called **lumbarization** of S1, and it results in a sixth "lumbar" vertebra. At other times, the fifth lumbar segment may be fused to the sacrum or ilium, resulting in a **sacralization** of that vertebra. Sacralization results in four mobile lumbar vertebrae. These abnormalities are sometimes called transitional vertebra.[5]

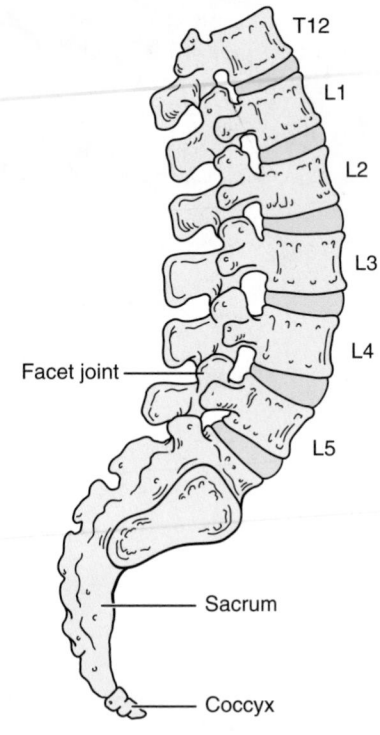

Figure 9-1
Lateral view of the lumbar spine.

The main ligaments of the lumbar spine are the same as those in the lower cervical and thoracic spine (excluding the ribs). These ligaments include the anterior and posterior longitudinal ligaments, the ligamentum flavum, the supraspinous and interspinous ligaments, and the intertransverse ligaments (Figure 9-5). In addition, there is an important ligament unique to the lumbar spine and pelvis—the iliolumbar ligament (Figure 9-6), which connects the transverse process of L5 to the posterior ilium.[6] This ligament helps stabilize L5 with the ilium and helps prevent anterior displacement of L5.[7]

The intervertebral discs make up approximately 20% to 25% of the total length of the vertebral column.

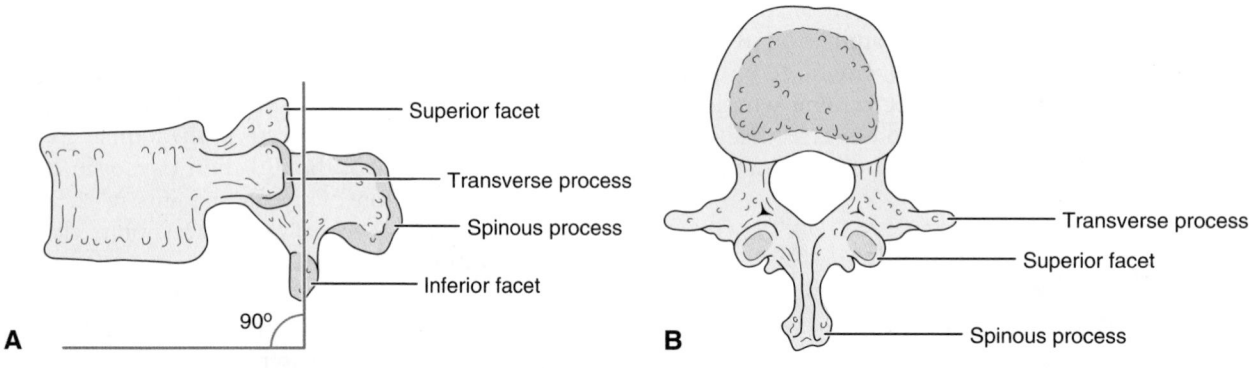

Figure 9-2
Lumbar vertebra. **A,** Side view. **B,** Superior view.

Figure 9-3
Facet anomalies (tropisms) at L5-S1.

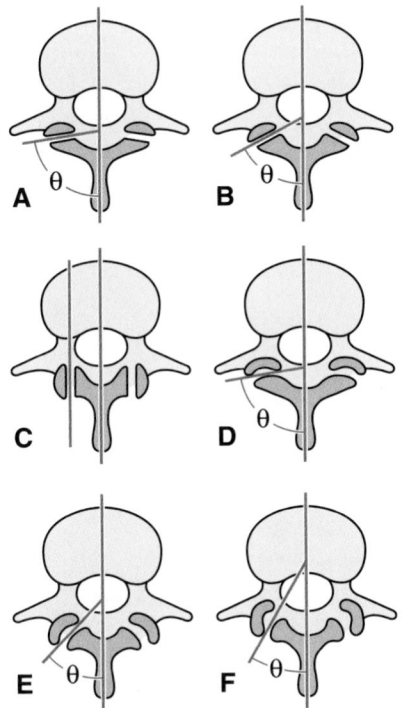

Figure 9-4

The varieties of orientation and curvature of the lumbar zygapophyseal joints. **A,** Flat joints oriented close to 90° to the sagittal plane. **B,** Flat joints orientated at 60° to the sagittal plane. **C,** Flat joints orientated parallel (0°) to the sagittal plane. **D,** Slightly curved joints with an average orientation close to 90° to the sagittal plane. **E,** "C"-shaped joints orientated at 45° to the sagittal plane. **F,** "J"-shaped joints orientated at 30° to the sagittal plane. (Redrawn from Bogduk N, Twomey LT: *Clinical anatomy of the lumbar spine,* p. 26, New York, 1987, Churchill Livingstone.)

The function of the intervertebral disc is to act as a shock absorber distributing and absorbing some of the load applied to the spine, to hold the vertebrae together and allow movement between the bones, to separate the vertebra as part of a **functional segmental** unit acting in concert with the facet joints (Figure 9-7), and, by separating the vertebrae, to allow the free passage of the nerve roots out from the spinal cord through the intervertebral foramina. With age, the percentage of spinal length attributable to the discs decreases as a result of disc degeneration and loss of hydrophilic action in the disc.

The **annulus fibrosus,** the outer laminated portion of the disc, consists of three zones: (1) an outer zone made up of fibrocartilage (classified as **Sharpey's fibers**) that attaches to the outer or peripheral aspect of the vertebral body and contains increasing numbers of cartilage cells in the fibrous strands with increasing depth, (2) an intermediate zone made up of another layer of fibrocartilage, and (3) an inner zone primarily made up of fibrocartilage and containing the largest number of cartilage cells.[8] The annulus fibrosus contains 20 concentric, collar-like rings of collagenous fibers that criss-cross each other to increase their strength and accommodate torsion movements.[9]

The **nucleus pulposus** is well developed in both the cervical and the lumbar spines. At birth, it is made up of a hydrophilic mucoid tissue, which is gradually replaced by fibrocartilage. With increasing age, the nucleus pulposus increasingly resembles the annulus fibrosus. The water-binding capacity of the disc decreases with age, and degenerative changes (spondylosis) begin to occur after the second decade of life. Initially, the disc contains approximately 85% to 90% water, but the amount decreases to 65% with age.[10] In addition, the disc contains a high proportion of mucopolysaccharides, which cause the disc to act as an incompressible fluid. However, these mucopolysaccharides decrease with age and are replaced with collagen. The nucleus pulposus lies slightly posterior to the center of rotation of the disc in the lumbar spine.

The shape of the disc corresponds to that of the body to which it is attached. The disc adheres to the vertebral body by means of the cartilaginous end plate. The end plates consist of thin layers of cartilage covering the majority of the inferior and superior surfaces of the

Anterior longitudinal ligament

Posterior longitudinal ligament

Nerve root

Ligamentum flavum

Interspinal ligament

Intervertebral foramen

Supraspinous ligament

Figure 9-5

Ligaments of the lumbar spine.

Anterior longitudinal ligament

Iliolumbar ligament

Lumbosacral ligament

Anterior sacroiliac ligament

Sacrotuberous ligament

Sacrospinous ligament

A

Anterior

Iliolumbar ligament

Supraspinous ligament

Short posterior sacroiliac ligament

Long posterior sacroiliac ligament

Sacrospinous ligament

Sacrotuberous ligament

B

Posterior

Figure 9-6
Ligaments of the sacrum, coccyx, and some in the lumbar spine.

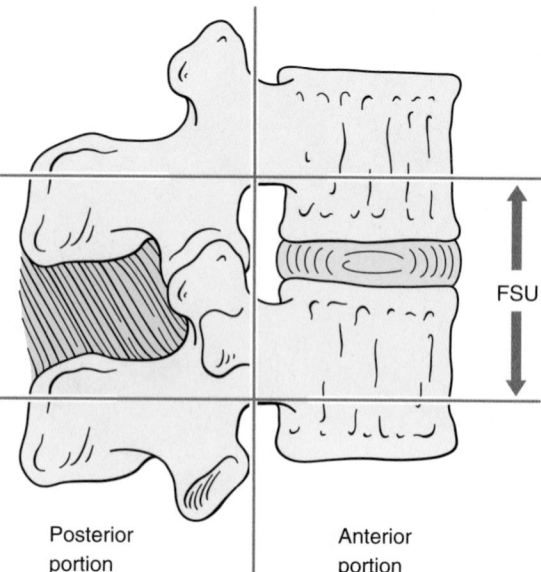

Posterior portion

Anterior portion

FSU

Figure 9-7
Functional segmental unit (three-joint complex) in the lumbar spine. Such a complex may also be seen in the cervical and thoracic spines.

vertebral body. The cartilaginous end plates are approximately 1 mm thick and allow fluid to move between the disc and the vertebral body. The discs are primarily avascular, with only the periphery receiving a blood supply. The remainder of the disc receives nutrition by diffusion, primarily through the cartilaginous end plate. Until the age of 8 years, the intervertebral discs have some vascularity; however, with age this vascularity decreases.

Usually, the intervertebral disc has no nerve supply, although the peripheral posterior aspect of the annulus fibrosus may be innervated by a few nerve fibers from the sinuvertebral nerve.[11,12] The lateral aspects of the disc are innervated peripherally by the branches of the anterior rami and gray rami communicants. The pain-sensitive structures around the intervertebral disc are the anterior longitudinal ligament, posterior longitudinal ligament, vertebral body, nerve root, and cartilage of the facet joint.

With the movement of fluid vertically through the cartilaginous end plate, the pressure on the disc decreases as the patient assumes the natural lordotic posture in the lumbar spine. Direct vertical pressure on the disc can cause the disc to push fluid into the vertebral body. If the pressure is great enough, defects may occur in the cartilaginous end plate, resulting in **Schmorl's nodules,** which are herniations of the nucleus pulposus into the vertebral body. Normally, an adult is 1 to 2 cm (0.4 to 0.8 inch) taller in the morning than in the evening (20% diurnal variation).[3,13] This change results from fluid movement in and out of the disc during the day through the cartilaginous end plate. This fluid shift acts as a pressure safety valve to protect the disc.

If there is an injury to the disc, four problems can result, all of which can cause symptoms.[14] There may be a **protrusion** of the disc, in which the disc bulges posteriorly without rupture of the annulus fibrosus. In the case of a disc **prolapse,** only the outermost fibers of the annulus fibrosus contain the nucleus. With a disc **extrusion,** the annulus fibrosus is perforated, and discal material (part of the nucleus pulposus) moves into the epidural space. The fourth problem is a **se**questrated disc, or a formation of discal fragments from the annulus fibrosus and nucleus pulposus outside the disc proper (Figure 9-8).[15] These injuries can result in pressure on the spinal cord itself (upper lumbar spine) leading to a myelopathy, pressure on the cauda equina leading to **cauda equina syndrome,** or pressure on the nerve roots (most common). The amount of pressure on the neurological tissues determines the severity of the neurological deficit.[16] The pressure may be the result of the disc injury itself or in combination with the inflammatory response

Activity and Percentage Increase in Disc Pressure at L3	
Coughing or straining:	5% to 35%
Laughing:	40% to 50%
Walking:	15%
Side bending:	25%
Small jumps:	40%
Bending forward:	150%
Rotation:	20%
Lifting a 20-kg weight with the back straight and knees bent:	73%
Lifting a 20-kg weight with the back bent and knees straight:	169%

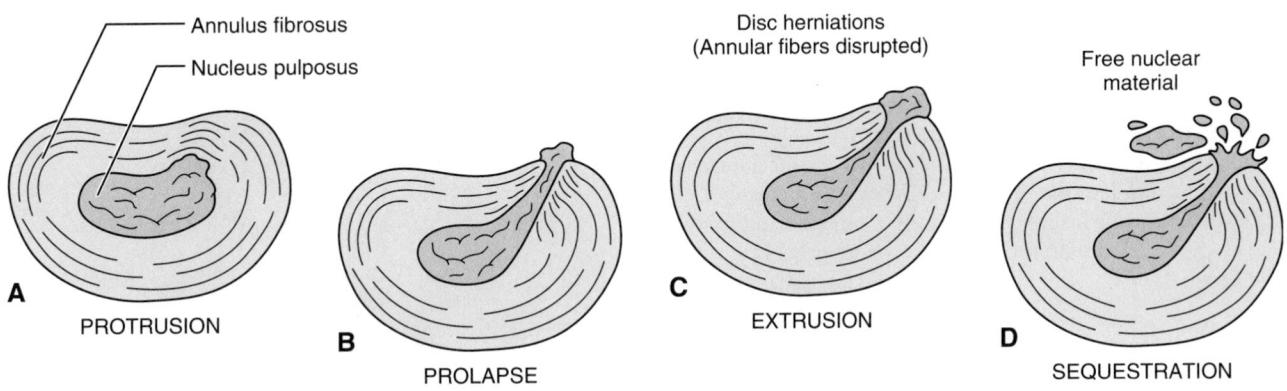

Figure 9-8
Types of disc herniations.

of the injury. Saal has outlined favorable, unfavorable, and neutral factors for positive-outcome prognostic factors for nonoperative lumbar disc herniation (Table 9-1).[14]

Within the lumbar spine, different postures can increase the pressure on the intervertebral disc (Figure 9-9). This information is based on the work of Nachemson and coworkers,[17,18] who performed studies of intradiscal pressure changes in the L3 disc with changes in posture. The pressure in the standing position is classified as the norm, and the values given are increases or decreases above or below this norm that occur with the change in posture.

In the lumbar spine, the nerve roots exit through relatively large intervertebral foramina, and as in the thoracic spine, each one is named for the vertebra above it (in the cervical spine, the nerve roots are named for the vertebra below). For example, the L4 nerve root exits between the L4 and L5 vertebrae. Because of the course of the nerve root as it exits, the L4 disc (between L4 and L5) only rarely compresses the L4 nerve root; it is more likely to compress the L5 nerve root (Figure 9-10).

In general, the L5-S1 segment is the most common site of problems in the vertebral column because this level bears more weight than any other vertebral level. The center of gravity passes directly through this vertebra, which is of benefit because it may decrease the shearing stresses to this segment. There is a transition from the mobile segment, L5, to the stable or fixed segment of the sacrum (S1), which can increase the stress on this area. Because the angle between L5 and S1 is greater than those between the other vertebrae, this joint has a greater chance of having stress applied to it. Another factor that increases the amount of stress on this area is the relatively greater amount of movement that occurs at this level compared with other levels of the lumbar spine.

Patient History

Problems of the lumbar spine are difficult to diagnose. Most of the examination commonly revolves around differentiating symptoms of a herniated disc (or space occupying lesion), which refers radicular symptoms into the leg from other conditions (e.g., inflammatory reaction, sprains, strains, facet syndrome) more likely to cause localized pain.[19] If there are no radicular

Table 9-1

Prognostic Factors for Positive Outcome with Nonoperative Care for Lumbar Disc Herniation

Favorable Factors	Unfavorable Factors	Neutral Factors	Questionable Factors
Absence of crossed SLR	Positive crossed SLR	Degree of SLR	Actual size of LDH
Spinal motion in extension that does not reproduce leg pain	Leg pain produced in spinal extension	Response to bed rest	Canal position of LDH
Large extrusion or sequestration	Subligamentous contained LDH	Response to passive care	Spinal level of LDH
Relief of >50% reduction in leg pain within the first 6 weeks of onset	Lack of >50% reduction in leg pain within the first six weeks of onset	Gender	Multilevel disc abnormalities
Positive response to corticosteroid treatment	Negative response to corticosteroid treatment	Age	LDH material
Limited psychosocial issues	Overbearing psychosocial issues	Degree of neurological deficit (except progressive deficit and cauda equina syndrome)	
Self-employed	Worker's compensation		
Motivated to recover and return to function	Unmotivated to return to function		
Educational level >12 years	Educational level <12 years		
Good fitness level	Illiteracy		
Motivated to exercise and participate in recovery	Unreasonable expectation of recovery time frames		
Absence of spinal stenosis	Poorly motivated and passive in recovery process		
Progressive return from neurological deficit within the first 12 weeks	Concomitant spinal stenosis		
	Progressive neurological deficit		
	Cauda equina syndrome		

Modified from Saal JA: Natural history and nonoperative treatment of lumbar disc herniation, *Spine* 21(24S):7S, 1996.
SLR, Straight leg raise; *LDH,* lumbar disc herniation.

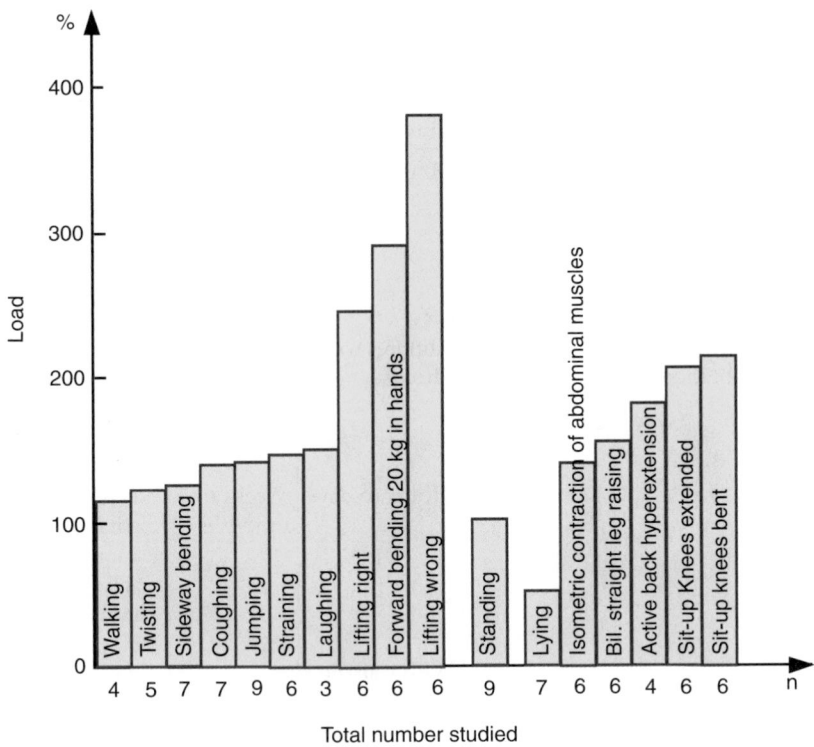

Figure 9-9

Mean change in load on L3 disc with various activities, compared with upright standing. (From Nachemson A, Elfstrom C: Intravital dynamic pressure measurements in lumbar discs, *Scand J Rehabil Med* [suppl. 1]:31, 1970.)

symptoms below the knee, it often becomes difficult for the examiner to determine where in the spine the problem is, or for that matter, whether the problem is truly in the lumbar spine or coming from problems in the pelvic joints, primarily the sacroiliac joints, or the hips. Waddell

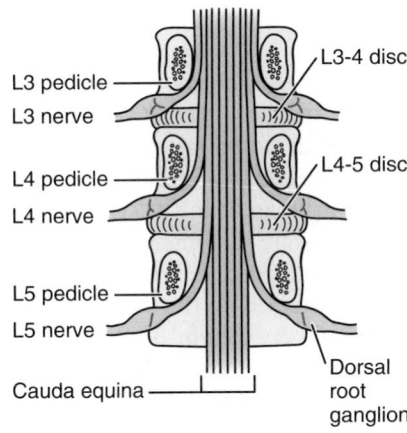

Figure 9-10

A coronal schematic view of the exiting lumbar spinal nerve roots. Note that the exiting root takes the name of the vertebral body under which it travels into the neural foramen. Because of the way the nerve roots exit, L4-L5 disc pathology usually affects the L5 root rather than the L4 root. (Redrawn from Borenstein DG et al. *Low back pain: medical diagnosis and comprehensive management*, p. 5, Philadelphia, 1995, WB Saunders.)

pointed out that in only about 15% of cases can a definitive diagnosis as to the pathology of back pain be made.[3] Hall broke low back pain into four categories—two of which are **back pain dominant** and two of which are **leg pain dominant** (Table 9-2).[20] Pattern 1 suggests disc involvement, whereas pattern 2 suggests facet joint involvement. Pattern 3 suggests nerve root involvement (primarily by a disc or some other space occupying lesion or an injury accompanied by inflammatory swelling), and pattern 4 suggests neurogenic intermittent claudication (pressure on the cauda equina). Thus, only by taking a careful history, followed by a detailed examination, is the examiner able to determine the cause of the problem.[21-23] Even then, some doubt may remain.

In addition to the questions listed under Patient History in Chapter 1, the examiner should obtain the following information from the patient:

1. *What is the patient's age?*[24] Different conditions affect patients at different ages. For example, disc problems usually occur between the ages of 15 and 40 years, and ankylosing spondylitis is evident between 18 and 45 years. Osteoarthritis and spondylosis are more evident in people older than 45 years of age, and malignancy of the spine is most common in people older than 50 years of age.

2. *What is the patient's occupation?*[3,25] Back pain tends to be more prevalent in people with strenuous occupations,[26] although it has been reported that familial

Table 9-2

Patterns of Back Pain

	Pattern	Where Pain Worst	Aggravating Movement	Relieving Movement	Onset	Duration	Probable Cause
Back Dominant Pain/Mechanical Cause	1	Back/buttocks (>90% back pain) Myotomes seldom affected Dermatomes not affected	Flexion Stiff in morning	Extension	Hours to days	Days to months (sudden or slow)	Disc involvement (minor herniation, spondylosis), sprain, strain
	2	Back/buttocks Myotomes seldom affected Dermatomes not affected	Extension/ Rotation	Flexion	Minutes to hours	Days to weeks (sudden)	Facet joint involvement, strain
Leg Pain Dominant/ Nonmechanical Cause	3	Leg (usually below knee) Myotomes commonly affected (especially in chronic cases) Pain in dermatomes	Flexion	Extension	Hours to days	Weeks to months	Nerve root irritation (most likely cause—disc herniation)
	4	Leg (usually below knee) (May be bilateral) Myotomes commonly affected (especially in chronic cases) Pain in dermatomes	Walking (extension)	Rest (sitting) or postural change	With walking	?	Neurogenic intermittent claudication (stenosis)

Modified from Hall H: A simple approach to back pain management, *Patient Care* 15:77–91, 1992.

influences have an effect as well as occupation.[27,28] For example, truck drivers (vibration) and warehouse workers have a high incidence of back injury.[29] Patients who have chronic low back pain develop a **deconditioning syndrome,** which compounds the problem as it leads to decreased muscle strength, impaired motor control, and decreased coordination and postural control.[30] How active is the patient at work (usual job, light duties, full time, frequent days off because of back pain, unemployed because of back, retired)?

3. *What is the patient's sex?* Lower back pain has a higher incidence in women. Female patients should be asked about any changes that occur with menstruation, such as altered pain patterns, irregular menses, and swelling of the abdomen or breasts. Knowledge of the date of the most recent pelvic examination is also useful. Ankylosing spondylitis is more common in men.

4. *What was the mechanism of injury?* Lifting commonly causes low back pain (Tables 9-3 and 9-4). This is not surprising when one considers the forces exerted on the lumbar spine and disc. For example, a 77-kg (170-lb) man lifting a 91-kg (200-lb) weight approximately 36 cm (14 inches) from the intervertebral disc exerts a force of 940 kg (2072 lb) on that disc. The force exerted on the disc can be calculated as roughly 10 times the weight being lifted. Pressure on the intervertebral discs varies depending on the position of the spine. Nachemson and colleagues showed that pressure on the disc can be decreased by increasing the supported inclination of the back rest (e.g., an angle of 130° decreases the pressure on the disc by 50%).[17,18] Using the arms for support can also decrease the pressure on the disc. When one is standing, the disc pressure is approximately 35% of the pressure that occurs in the relaxed sitting position. The examiner

Text continued on page 524

Table 9-3

Some Implications of Painful Reactions

Activity	Reaction of Pain	Possible Structural and Pathological Implications
Lying sleeping	↓	Decreased compressive forces—low intradiscal pressures
		Absence of forces produced by muscle activity
	↑	Change of position—noxious mechanical stress
		Decreased mechanoreceptor input
		Motor segment "relaxed" into a position compromising affected structure
		Poor external support (bed)
		Nonmusculoskeletal cause
First rising (stiffness)	↑	Nocturnal imbibition of fluid, disc volume greatest
		Mechanical inflammatory component (apophyseal joints)
		Prolonged stiffness, active inflammatory disease (e.g., ankylosing spondylitis)
Sitting	↑	Compressive forces
		High intradiscal pressure
With extension	↓	Intradiscal pressure reduced
		Decreased paraspinal muscle activity
	↑	Greater compromise of structures of lateral and central canals
		Compressive forces on lower apophyseal joints
With flexion	↓	Little compressive load on lower apophyseal joints
		Greater volume lateral and central canals
		Reduced disc bulge posteriorly
	↑	Very high intradiscal pressures
		Increased compressive loads upper and mid apophyseal joints
		Mechanical deformation of spine
Prolonged sitting	↑	Gradual creep of tissues
Sitting to standing	↑	Creep, time for reversal, difficulty in straightening up
		Extension of spine, increase disc bulge posteriorly
Walking	↑	Shock loads greater than body weight
		Compressive loads (vertical creep)
		Leg pain
		Neurological claudication
		Vascular claudication
Driving	↑	Sitting: compressive forces
		Vibration: vibro creep repetitive loading, decreased hysteresis loading, decreased hysteresis
		Increased dural tension sitting with legs extended
		Short hamstrings: pull lumbar spine into greater flexion
Coughing, sneezing, straining	↑	Increased pressure subarachnoid space (increased blood flow, Batson's plexus, compromises space in lateral and central canal)
		Increased intradiscal pressure
		Mechanical "jarring" of sudden uncontrolled movement

From Jull GA: Examination of the lumbar spine. In Grieve GP, editor: *Modern manual therapy of the vertebral column,* p. 553, Edinburgh, 1986, Churchill Livingstone.

Table 9-4

Some Mechanisms of Musculoskeletal Pain

Behavior of Pain	Possible Mechanisms
Constant ache	Inflammatory process, venous hypertension
Pain on movement	Noxious mechanical stimulus (stretch, pressure, crush)
Pain accumulates with activity	Repeated mechanical stress
	Inflammatory process
	Degenerative disc—hysteresis decreased, less protection from repetitive loading
Pain increases with sustained postures	Fatigue of supporting muscles
	Gradual creep of tissues may stress affected part of motor unit
Latent nerve root pain	Movement has produced an acute and temporary neurapraxia

From Jull GA: Examination of the lumbar spine. In Grieve, GP, editor: *Modern manual therapy of the vertebral column,* p. 553, Edinburgh, 1986, Churchill Livingstone.

should also keep in mind that stress on the lower back tends to be 15% to 20% higher in men than in women because men are taller and their weight is distributed higher in the body.

5. *How long has the problem bothered the patient?* Acute back pain lasts 3 to 4 weeks. Subacute back pain lasts up to 12 weeks. Chronic pain is anything longer than 3 months. Waddell has outlined predictors (yellow flags) of chronicity with back pain patients.[3]

Predictors of Chronicity Within the First 6 to 8 Weeks ("Yellow Flags")[3]

- Nerve root pain or specific spinal pathology
- Reported severity of pain at the acute stage
- Beliefs about pain being work related
- Psychological distress
- Psychosocial aspects of work
- Compensation
- Time off work
- The longer someone is off work with back pain, the lower the probability that they will return to work

---

6. *Where are the sites and boundaries of pain?* Have the patient point to the location or locations. Note whether the patient indicates a specific joint or whether the pain is more general. The more specific the pain, the easier it is to localize the area of pathology. Unilateral pain with no referral below the knee may be caused by injury to muscles (strain) or ligaments (sprain), the facet joint, or, in some cases, the sacroiliac joints. This is called **mechanical low back pain** (in older books it is called "lumbago"). With each of these injuries, there is seldom if ever peripheralization of the symptoms. The symptoms tend to stay centralized in the back. If the muscles and ligaments are affected, movement will decrease and pain will increase with repeated movements. If the pain extends to the hip, the hip must be cleared by examination. With facet joint problems, the range of motion remains the same (it may be restricted from the beginning), as does the pain with repeated movements. Pain on standing that improves with walking and pain on forward flexion with no substantial muscle tenderness suggests disc involvement.[31] The sacroiliac joints will show pain when pain-provoking (stress) tests are used. A minor disc injury (protrusion) may show the same symptoms, but the pain is more likely to be bilateral if it is a central protrusion.[32]

"Mechanical" Low Back Pain[3]

- Pain is usually cyclic.
- Low back pain is often referred to the buttocks and thighs.
- Morning stiffness or pain is common.
- Start pain (i.e., when starting movement) is common.
- There is pain on forward flexion and often also on returning to the erect position.
- Pain is often produced or aggravated by extension, side flexion, rotation, standing, walking, sitting, and exercise in general.
- Pain usually becomes worse over the course of the day.
- Pain is relieved by a change of position.
- Pain is relieved by lying down, especially in the fetal position.

---

7. *Is there any radiation of pain? Is the pain centralizing or peripheralizing* (Figure 9-11)?[33,34] **Centralization** implies the pain is moving toward or is centered in the lumbar spine.[35-37] **Peripheralization** implies the pain is being referred or is moving into the limb. If so, it is helpful for the examiner to remember and correlate this information with dermatome findings when evaluating sensation. The examiner must be careful when looking at the lumbar spine that he or she does not consider every back problem a disc problem. It has been reported that disc problems account for only about 5% of low back pain cases.[38] Some authors feel the only definitive clinical diagnosis of a disc problem is neurological pain extending below the knee.[20] This means that although there may be pain in the back and in the leg, the leg pain is dominant.[3] Pain on the anterolateral aspect of the leg is highly suggestive of L4 disc problems, whereas pain radiating to the posterior aspect of the foot suggests L5 disc problems if the history indicates a disc may be injured.[39] Pain radiating into the leg below the knee is highly suggestive of a disc lesion, but isolated back or buttock pain does not rule out the disc. Minor injuries such as protrusion of the disc may result only in back or buttock pain.[39] Such an injury makes diagnoses more difficult because such pain may also result from muscle or ligament injury or from injury or degeneration to the adjacent facet joints.

Lumbar and sacroiliac pain tend to be referred to the buttock and posterior leg (and sometimes to the lateral aspect of the leg). Hip pain tends to be in the groin and anterior thigh although it may be referred to the knee (usually medial side). The hip can be ruled out later in the examination by the absence of a hip capsular pattern and a negative sign of the buttock.[40] The examiner must also determine whether the musculoskeletal system is involved or whether the pain is being referred from another structure or system (e.g., abdominal organs). Abnormal signs and symptoms or red flags (see Table 1-1)

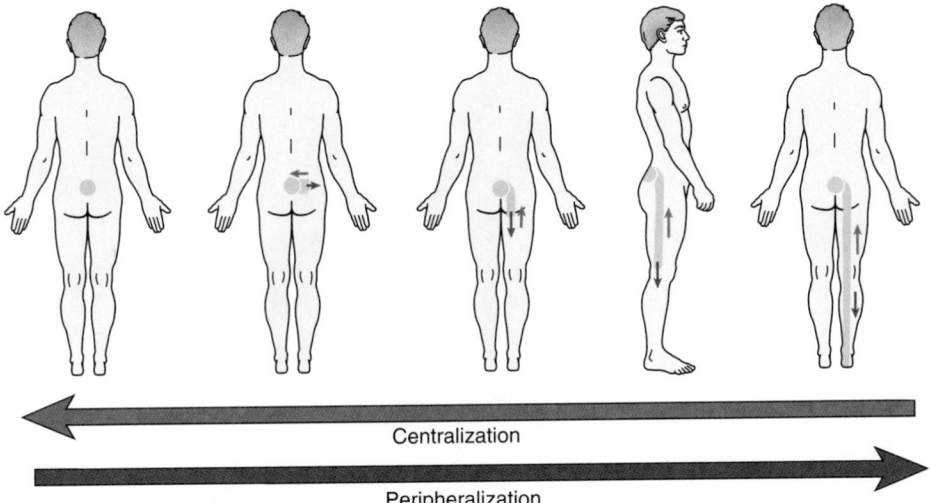

Centralization

Peripheralization

Figure 9-11
Centralization of pain is the progressive retreat of the most distal extent of referred or radicular pain toward the lumbar midline. Peripheralization of pain moves in the opposite direction.

would lead the examiner to consider causes other than the musculoskeletal system.

8. *Is the pain deep? Superficial? Shooting? Burning? Aching?* Questions related to the depth and type of pain often help to locate the structure injured and the source of pain.

9. *Is the pain improving? Worsening? Staying the same?* The answers to these questions will indicate whether the condition is settling down and improving, or they may indicate that the condition is in the inflammation phase (acute) or in the healing phase. Does the patient complain of more pain than the injury would suggest should occur? If so, psychosocial testing may be appropriate.

10. *Is there any increase in pain with coughing? Sneezing? Deep breathing? Laughing?* All of these actions increase the **intrathecal pressure** (the pressure inside the covering of the spinal cord) and would indicate the problem is in the lumbar spine and affecting the neurological tissue.

11. *Are there any postures or actions that specifically increase or decrease the pain or cause difficulty?*[33,41] For example, if sitting increases the pain and other symptoms, the examiner may suspect that sustained flexion is causing mechanical deformation of the spine or increasing the intradiscal pressure.[42] Classically, disc pathology causes increased pain on sitting, lifting, twisting, and bending.[43] It is the most common space-occupying lesion in the lumbar spine and therefore is the most common cause of radiating pain below the knee. If standing increases the pain and other symptoms, the examiner may suspect that extension, especially relaxed standing, is the cause. If walking increases the pain and other symptoms, extension is probably causing the mechanical deformation, because walk-

ing accentuates extension. If lying (especially prone lying) increases the pain and other symptoms, extension may be the cause. Persistent pain or progressive increases in pain while the patient is in the supine position may lead the examiner to suspect neurogenic or space-occupying lesions, such as an infection, swelling, or tumor. Remember that pain may radiate to the lumbar spine from pathological conditions in other areas as well as from direct mechanical problems. For example, tumors of the pancreas refer pain to the low back. Stiffness or pain after rest may indicate ankylosing spondylitis or Scheuermann's disease. Pain from mechanical breakdown tends to increase with activity and decrease with rest. Discogenic pain increases if the patient maintains a single posture (especially flexion) for a long period. Pain arising from the spine almost always is influenced by posture and movement.

The normal lumbosacral angle in the standing position is 140°, the normal lumbar lordotic curve is about 50°, the normal sacral angle is 30° (some call this the lumbosacral angle[44]) (Figure 9-12), and the normal pelvic angle is 30°. In this position, the pelvis would be said to be in neutral (**neutral pelvis**). The pelvis is the key to proper back posture. For the pelvis to "sit" properly on the femora, the abdominal, hip flexor, hip extensor, and back extensor muscles must be strong, supple, and balanced (Figure 9-13). Any deviation in the normal alignment should be noted and recorded. What types of shoes does the patient wear? Heel heights can modify the pelvic angle and lumbar curve, altering the stress on the spine.[45]

12. *Is the pain worse in the morning or evening? Does the pain get better or worse as the day progresses?* For example, osteoarthritis of the facet joints leads to morning stiffness, which in turn is relieved by activity.

Figure 9-12

Normal angles of the spine and sacrum. *a,* Lumbosacral angle (140°); *b,* Lumbar lordotic curve (50°); *c,* sacral angle (30°); *d,* pelvic angle (30°).

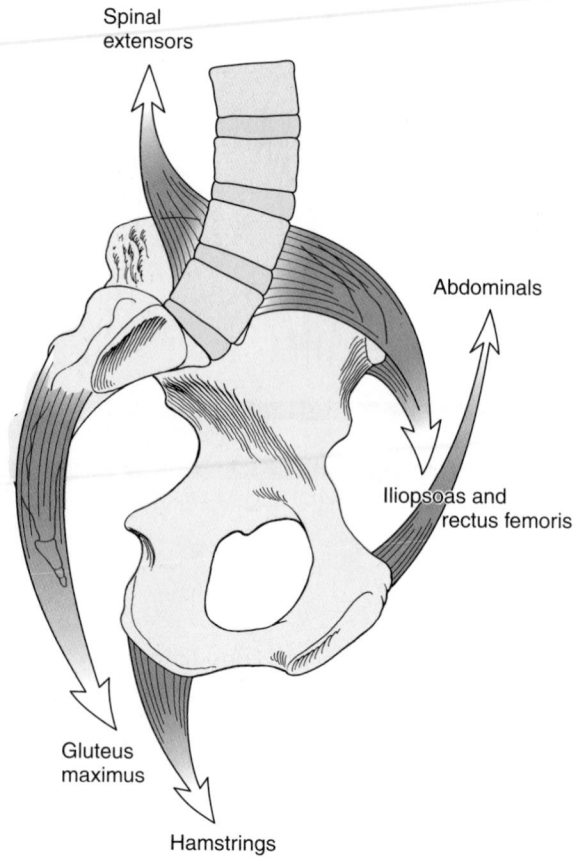

Figure 9-13

Muscles "balancing" the pelvis. (Modified from Dyrek DA, Micheli LJ, Magee DJ: Injuries to the thoracolumbar spine and pelvis. In Zachazewski JE, Magee DJ, WS Quillen, editors: *Athletic injuries and rehabilitation,* p. 470, Philadelphia, 1996, WB Saunders.)

13. *Which movements hurt? Which movements are stiff?* Table 9-5 demonstrates some of the causes of mechanical low back pain and their symptoms. The examiner must help the patient differentiate between true pain and discomfort that is caused by stretching. **Postural,** or **static, muscles** (e.g., iliopsoas) tend to respond to pathology with tightness in the form of spasm or adaptive shortening; **dynamic,** or **phasic,** muscles (e.g., abdominals) tend to respond with atrophy. Pathology affecting both types of muscles can lead to a **"pelvic crossed syndrome"** (discussed later). Does the patient describe a painful arc of movement on forward or side flexion? If so, it may indicate a disc protrusion with a nerve root riding over the bulge or instability in part of the range of motion.[41] Patients with lumbar instability or lumbar muscle spasm have trouble moving to the seated position, whereas patients with discogenic pain usually have pain in flexion (e.g., sitting) and the pain may increase the longer they are seated.

14. *Is paresthesia (a "pins and needles" feeling) or anesthesia present?* A patient may experience a sensation or a lack of sensation if there is pressure on a nerve root. Paresthesia occurs if pressure is relieved from a nerve trunk, whereas if the pressure is on the nerve trunk, the patient experiences a numb sensation. Does the patient experience any paresthesia or tingling and numbness in the extremities, perineal (saddle) area, or pelvic area? Abnormal sensations in the perineal area often have associated micturition (urination) problems. These symptoms may indicate a myelopathy and are considered by many to be an emergency surgical situation because of potential long-term bowel and bladder problems if the pressure on the spinal cord is not relieved as soon as possible.[46,47] The examiner must remember that the adult spinal cord ends at the bottom of the L1 vertebra and becomes the cauda equina within the spinal column. The nerve roots extend in such a way that it is rare for the disc to pinch on the nerve root of the same level. For example, the L5 nerve root is more likely to be compressed by the L4 intervertebral disc than by the L5 intervertebral disc (Figure 9-14). Seldom is the nerve root compressed by the disc at the same level, except when the protrusion is more lateral.

15. *Has the patient noticed any weakness or decrease in strength?* This may be the result of an injury to the muscles themselves, their nerve supply, or reflex inhibition caused by pain.[23,48]

Table 9-5

Differential Diagnosis of Mechanical Low Back Pain

	Muscle Strain	Herniated Nucleus Pulposus	Osteoarthritis	Spinal Stenosis	Spondylolisthesis	Scoliosis
Age (yr)	20–40	30–50	>50	>60	20	30
Pain pattern						
Location	Back (unilateral)	Back, leg (unilateral)	Back (unilateral)	Leg (bilateral)	Back	Back
Onset	Acute	Acute (prior episodes)	Insidious	Insidious	Insidious	Insidious
Standing	↑	↓	↑	↑	↑	↑
Sitting	↓	↑	↓	↓	↓	↓
Bending	↑	↑	↓	↓	↑	↑
Straight leg raise	–	+	–	+ (Stress)	–	–
Plain x-ray	–	–	+	+	+	+

From Borenstein DG et al: *Low back pain: medical diagnosis and comprehensive management,* p. 189, Philadelphia, 1995, WB Saunders.

16. *What is the patient's usual activity or pastime? Before the injury, did the patient modify or perform any unusual repetitive or high-stress activity?* Such questions help the examiner determine whether the cause of injury was macrotrauma, microtrauma, or a combination of both.

17. *Which activities aggravate the pain? Is there anything in the patient's lifestyle that increases the pain?* Many common positions assumed by patients are similar to those in some of the provocative special tests. For example, getting into and sitting in a car is similar to the slump test and straight leg raise test. Long sitting

Figure 9-14

Possible effects of disc herniation. **A,** Herniation of the disc between L4 and L5 compresses the fifth lumbar root. **B,** Large herniation of the L5-S1 disc compromises not only the nerve root crossing it (first sacral nerve root) but also the nerve root emerging through the same foramen (fifth lumbar nerve root). **C,** Massive central sequestration of the disc at the L4-L5 level involves all of the nerve roots in the cauda equina and may result in bowel and bladder paralysis. (Redrawn from MacNab I: *Backache,* pp. 96–97, Baltimore, 1977, Williams & Wilkins.)

in bed is a form of straight leg raise. Reaching up into a cupboard can be similar to an upper limb tension test. A word of caution: There can be a 10° to 20° difference in straight leg raise in lying and sitting because of the change in lordosis and position of the pelvis.[3]

18. *Which activities ease the pain?* If there are positions that relieve the pain, the examiner should use an understanding of anatomy to determine which tissues would have stress taken off them in the pain-relieving postures, and these postures may later be used as resting postures during the treatment.

19. *What is the patient's sleeping position? Does the patient have any problems sleeping? What type of mattress does the patient use (hard, soft)?* The best sleeping position is in side lying with the legs bent in a semifetal position. If the patient lies prone, the lumbar spine often falls into extension increasing the stress on the posterior elements of the vertebrae. In supine lying, the spine tends to flatten out, decreasing the stress on the posterior elements.

20. *Does the patient have any difficulty with micturition?* If so, the examiner should proceed with caution, because the condition may involve more than the lumbar spine (e.g., a myelopathy, cauda equina syndrome, tabes dorsalis, tumor, multiple sclerosis). Conversely, these symptoms may result from a disc protrusion or spinal stenosis with minimal or no back pain or sciatica. A disc derangement can cause total urinary retention; chronic, longstanding partial retention; vesicular irritability; or the loss of desire or awareness of the necessity to void.

21. *Is the patient receiving any medication?* For example, the long-term use of steroid therapy can lead to osteoporosis. Also, if the patient has taken medication just before the assessment, the examiner may not get a true reading of the pain.

22. *Is the patient able to cope during daily activities?* Psychosocial issues often play a role in low back pain, especially if it is chronic.[49-52] Haggman et al. felt that two questions were particularly significant to ask the patient to screen for depressive symptoms[53]: "During the past month, have you often been bothered by feeling down, depressed, or hopeless?" and "During the past month, have you been bothered by little interest or pleasure in doing things?"[31,54] If the answers to these questions are positive, the patient should be monitored closely and if progress does not occur, then further psychological follow-ups should be considered.[55] Does the patient have trouble with work, leisure activities, washing, or dressing? How far can the patient walk before the pain begins?[56] What is the patient's level of disability? Disability implies the effect of the pathology on activity, not pain. Thus, disability testing commonly revolves around activities of daily living and functional activities. Thus, this question may be tied in with the use of the questions in the functional assessment discussed later.

Finally, the examiner must be aware that although in most cases, people who have low back pain have simple mechanical back problems or have nerve root problems involving the disc, there is always the possibility of non-musculoskeletal causes (e.g., kidney stones, abdominal aortic aneurysm) or serious spinal pathology.[31] Waddell outlined signs and symptoms that would lead the examiner to conclude that more serious pathology is present in the lumbar spine (Table 9-6).[3]

Observation

The patient must be suitably undressed. Males must wear only shorts, and females must wear only a bra and shorts.

Table 9-6

Indications of Serious Spinal Pathology

Red Flags	Cauda Equina Syndrome/ Widespread Neurological Disorder	Inflammatory Disorders (Ankylosing Spondylitis and Related Disorders)
Presentation age <20 years or onset >55 years	Difficulty with micturition	Gradual onset before age 40 years
Violent trauma, such as a fall from a height, car accident	Loss of anal sphincter tone or fecal incontinence	Marked morning stiffness
Constant, progressive, nonmechanical pain	Saddle anesthesia about the anus, perineum or genitals	Persisting limitation of spinal movements in all directions
Thoracic pain	Widespread (> one nerve root) or progressive motor weakness in the legs or gait disturbance	Peripheral joint involvement
Previous history carcinoma, systemic steroids, drug abuse, HIV	Sensory level	Iritis, skin rashes (psoriasis), colitis, urethral discharge
Systematically unwell weight loss		Family history
Persisting severe restriction of lumbar flexion		
Widespread neurology		
Structural deformity		
Investigations when required sedimentation rate (ESR) >25 plain x-ray: vertebral collapse or bone destruction		

From Waddell G: *The back pain revolution*, p. 12, New York, 1998, Churchill Livingstone.

When doing the observation, the examiner should note the patient's willingness to move and the pattern of movement. The patient should be observed for the following traits, first in the standing and then in the sitting position.

Body Type

There are three general body types (see Figure 15-24): **ectomorphic**—thin body build, characterized by relative prominence of structures developed from the embryonic ectoderm; **mesomorphic**—muscular or sturdy body build, characterized by relative prominence of structures developed from the embryonic mesoderm; and **endomorphic**—heavy (fat) body build, characterized by relative prominence of structures developed from the embryonic endoderm.

Gait

Does the gait appear to be normal when the patient walks into the examination area, or is it altered in some way? If it is altered, the examiner must take time to find out whether the problem is in the limb or whether the gait is altered to relieve symptoms elsewhere.

Attitude

What is the patient's appearance? Is the patient tense, bored, lethargic, healthy looking, emaciated, overweight?

Total Spinal Posture

The patient should be examined in the habitual relaxed posture (see Chapter 15) that he or she would usually adopt. With acute back pain, the patient presents with some degree of antalgic (painful) posturing. Usually, a loss of lumbar lordosis is present, and there may be a lateral shift or scoliosis. This posturing is involuntary and often cannot be reduced because of the muscle spasm.[57,58]

The patient should be observed anteriorly, laterally, and posteriorly (Figure 9-15). During the observation, the examiner should pay particular attention to whether the patient holds the pelvis "in neutral" naturally; if not, is he or she able to achieve the **neutral pelvis** position (normal lordotic curve with the anterior superior iliac spines [ASISs] being slightly lower than the posterior superior iliac spines [PSISs]). Many people with back pain are unable to maintain

Figure 9-15

Views of the patient in the standing position. **A,** Anterior view. **B,** Posterior view. **C,** Lateral view.

a neutral pelvis position. Anteriorly, the head should be straight on the shoulders, and the nose should be in line with the manubrium, sternum, and xiphisternum or umbilicus. The shoulders and clavicle should be level and equal, although the dominant side may be slightly lower. The waist angles should be equal. Does the patient show a lateral shift or list (Figure 9-16)? Such a shift may be straight lateral movement or it may be a scoliosis (rotation involved). The straight shift is more likely to be caused by mechanical dysfunction and muscle spasm and is likely to disappear on lying down or hanging.[3,59] True scoliosis commonly has compensating curves and does not change with hanging or lying down. The arbitrary "high" points on both iliac crests should be the same height. If they are not, the possibility of unequal leg length should be considered. The difference in height would indicate a functional limb length discrepancy. This discrepancy could be caused by altered bone length, altered mechanics (e.g., pronated foot on one side), or joint dysfunction (Table 9-7). The ASISs should be level. The patellae should point straight ahead. The lower limbs should be straight and not in genu varum or genu valgum. The heads of the fibulae should be level. The medial malleoli should be level, as should be the lateral malleoli. The medial longitudinal arches of the feet should be evident, and the feet should angle out equally. The arms should be an equal distance from the trunk and equally medially or laterally rotated. Any protrusion or depression of the

sternum, ribs, or costicartilage, as well as any bowing of bones, should be noted. The bony or soft-tissue contours should be equal on both sides.

From the side, the examiner should look at the head to ensure that the ear lobe is in line with the tip of the shoulder (acromion process) and the arbitrary highpoint of the iliac crest. Each segment of the spine should have a normal curve. Are any of the curves exaggerated or decreased? Is lordosis present? Kyphosis? Do the shoulders droop forward? Normally with a neutral pelvis, the ASISs are slightly lower than the PSISs. Are the knees straight, flexed, or in recurvatum (hyperextended)?

From behind, the examiner should note the level of the shoulders, spines and inferior angles of the scapula, and any deformities (e.g., a Sprengel's deformity). Any lateral spinal curve (scoliosis) should be noted (Figure 9-17). If the scoliotic curve is because of a disc herniation, the herniation usually occurs on the convex side of the curve.[60] The waist angles should be equal from the posterior aspect, as they were from the anterior aspect. The PSISs should be level. The examiner should note whether the PSISs are higher or lower than the ASISs and the patient's ability to maintain a neutral pelvis. The gluteal folds and knee joints should be level. The Achilles tendons and heels should appear to be straight. The examiner should note whether there is any protrusion of the ribs or bowing of bones. Any deviation in the normal spinal postural alignment should be noted and recorded. The various possible sources of pathology related to posture are discussed in Chapter 15.

Janda and Jull described a lumbar or **pelvic crossed syndrome** (Figure 9-18) to show the effect of muscle imbalance on the ability of a patient to hold and maintain a neutral pelvis.[61] With this syndrome, they hypothesized that there was a combination of weak, long

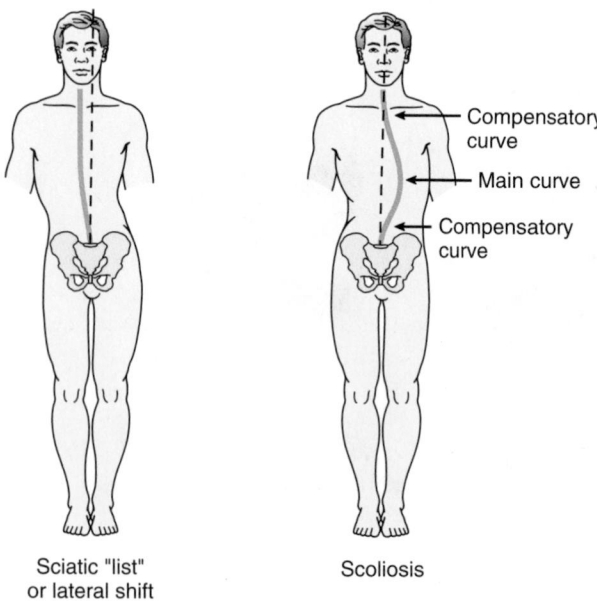

Sciatic "list" or lateral shift

Scoliosis

Figure 9-16 ▬
Lateral shift or list.

Table 9-7

Functional Limb Length Difference

Joint	Functional Lengthening	Functional Shortening
Foot	Supination	Pronation
Knee	Extension	Flexion
Hip	Lowering	Lifting
	Extension	Flexion
	Lateral rotation	Medial rotation
Sacroiliac	Anterior rotation	Posterior rotation

From Wallace LA: Lower quarter pain: mechanical evaluation and treatment. In Grieve GP, editor: *Modern manual therapy of the vertebral column*, p. 467, Edinburgh, 1986, Churchill Livingstone.

Figure 9-17
Congenital scoliosis and a diastematomyelia in a 9-year-old girl. This type of hairy patch strongly indicates a congenital maldevelopment of the neural axis. (From Rothman RH, Simeone FA: *The spine*, p. 371, Philadelphia, 1982, WB Saunders.)

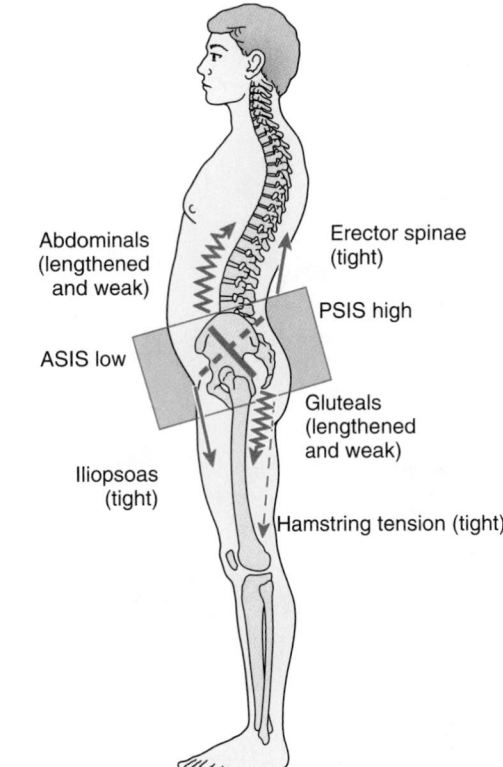

Figure 9-18
The pelvic crossed syndrome as described by Janda and Jull.

muscles and short, strong muscles, which resulted in an imbalance pattern leading to low back pain.[62] They felt that only by treating the different groups appropriately could the back pain be relieved. The weak, long inhibited muscles were the abdominals and gluteus maximus, whereas the strong tight (shortened) muscles were the hip flexors (primarily iliopsoas) and the back extensors. The imbalance pattern promotes increased lumbar lordosis because of the forward pelvic tilt and hip flexion contracture and overactivity of the hip flexors compensating for the weak abdominals. The weak gluteals result in increased activity in the hamstrings and erector spinae as compensation to assist hip extension. Interestingly, although the long spinal extensors show increased activity, the short lumbar muscles (e.g., multifidus, rotatores) show weakness. Also, the hamstrings show tightness as they attempt to pull the pelvis backward to compensate for the anterior rotation caused by the tight hip flexors. Weakness of gluteus medius results in increased activity of the quadratus lumborum and tensor fasciae latae on the same side. This syndrome is often seen in con-

junction with **upper crossed syndrome** (see Chapter 3, Cervical Spine). The two syndromes together are called the layer syndrome.[61]

Markings

A "faun's beard" (tuft of hair) may indicate a spina bifida occulta or diastematomyelia (see Figure 9-17).[63] Café au lait spots may indicate neurofibromatosis or collagen disease (Figure 9-19). Unusual skin markings or the presence of skin lesions in the midline may lead the examiner to consider the possibility of underlying neural and mesodermal anomalies. Musculoskeletal anomalies tend to form at the same time embryologically. Thus, if the examiner finds one anomaly, he or she must consider the possibility of other anomalies.

Step Deformity

A step deformity in the lumbar spine may indicate a spondylolisthesis. The "step" occurs because the spinous process of one vertebra becomes prominent when either the vertebra above (for example, spondylitic spondylolisthesis)

Figure 9-19
Neurofibromatosis with scoliosis. Note the café au lait spots on the right side of the trunk. (From Tachdjian MO: *Pediatric orthopedics,* p. 1290, Philadelphia, 1990, WB Saunders.)

or the affected vertebra (for example, spondylolytic spondylolisthesis) slips forward on the one below (Figure 9-20).

Examination

When assessing the lumbar spine, the examiner must remember that referral of symptoms or the presence of neurological symptoms often makes it necessary to "clear" or rule the lower limb pathology. Many of the symptoms that occur in the lower limb may originate in the lumbar spine. Unless there is a history of definitive trauma to a peripheral joint, a screening or scanning examination must accompany assessment of that joint to rule out problems within the lumbar spine referring symptoms to that joint. It is often helpful at this stage to ask the patient to demonstrate the movements that produce or have produced the pain. When asking the patient

to do this, the examiner must allow time for symptoms to disappear before completing the examination.

Active Movements

Active movements are performed with the patient standing (Figure 9-21). The examiner is looking for differences in range of motion (ROM) and the patient's willingness to do the movement. The ROM taking place during the active movement is normally the summation of the movements of the entire lumbar spine, not just movement at one level, along with hip movement. The most painful movements are done last. If the problem is mechanical, at least one or more of the movements will be painful.[22]

While the patient is doing the active movements, the examiner looks for limitation of movement and its possible causes, such as pain, spasm, stiffness, or blocking.

A

B

Figure 9-20
Step deformity in the lumbar spine. **A,** Caused by spondylosis. **B,** Caused by spondylolisthesis.

Figure 9-20 cont'd
C, Spinous process protrusion caused by step deformity.

As the patient reaches the full range of active movement, passive overpressure may be applied, but only if the active movements appear to be full and pain free. The overpressure must be applied with extreme care, because the upper body weight is already being applied to the lumbar joints by virtue of their position and gravity. If the patient reports that a sustained position increases the symptoms, then the examiner should consider having the patient maintain the position (e.g., flexion) at the end of the ROM for 10 to 20 seconds to see whether symptoms increase. Likewise, if repetitive motion or combined movements have been reported in the history as causing symptoms, these movements should be performed as well, but only after the patient has completed the basic movements.

The greatest motion in the lumbar spine occurs between the L4 and L5 vertebrae and between L5 and S1. There is considerable individual variability in the ROM of the lumbar spine (Figure 9-22).[64–68] In reality,

little obvious movement occurs in the lumbar spine especially in the individual segments because of the shape of the facet joints, tightness of the ligaments, presence of the intervertebral discs, and size of the vertebral bodies.

For flexion (forward bending), the maximum ROM in the lumbar spine is normally 40° to 60°. The examiner must differentiate the movement occurring in the lumbar spine from that occurring in the hips or thoracic spine. Some patients can touch their toes by flexing the hips, even if no movement occurs in the spine. On forward flexion, the lumbar spine should move from its normal lordotic curvature to at least a straight or slightly flexed curve (Figure 9-23).[69] If this change in the spine does not occur, there is probably some hypomobility in the lumbar spine resulting from either tight structures or muscle spasm. The degree of injury also has an effect. For example, the more severely a disc is injured (for example, if sequestration has occurred rather than a protrusion), the greater the limitation of movement.[70] With disc degeneration, intersegmental motion may increase as disc degeneration increases up to a certain point and follows Kirkaldy-Willis's description of degenerative changes in the disc.[71] He divided the changes into three stages: dysfunctional, unstable, and stable. During the first two phases, intersegmental motion increases in flexion, rotation, and side flexion[72] and then decreases in the final stabilization phase. During the unstable phase, it is often possible to see an **instability jog** during one or more movements, especially flexion, returning to neutral from flexion, or side flexion.[73,74] An instability "jog" is a sudden movement shift or "rippling" of the muscles during active movement, indicating an unstable segment.[69,75] Similarly, muscle twitching during movement or complaints of something "slipping out" during lumbar spine movement may indicate instability.[76] If the patient bends one or both knees on forward flexion, the examiner should watch for nerve root symptoms or tight hamstrings, especially if spinal flexion is decreased when the knees are straight. If tight hamstrings or nerve root symptoms are suspected, the examiner should perform suitable tests (see "Special Tests" section) to determine if the hamstrings or nerve root restriction (see the discussion of knee flexion test) are the cause of the problem. When returning to the upright

Figure 9-21

Active movements of the lumbar spine. **A** and **B,** Measuring forward flexion using tape measure. **C,** Extension. **D,** Side flexion (anterior view). **E,** Side flexion (posterior view). **F,** Rotation (standing). **G,** Rotation (sitting).

posture from forward flexion, the patient with no back pain first rotates the hips and pelvis to about 45° of flexion; during the last 45° of extension, the low back resumes its lordosis. In patients with back pain, commonly, most movement occurs in the hips, accompanied by knee flexion, and sometimes with hand support working up the thighs.[77] As with the thoracic spine, the examiner may use a tape measure to determine the increase in spacing of the spinous processes on forward flexion. Normally, the measurement should increase 7 to 8 cm (2.8 to 3.1 inches) if it is taken between the T12 spinous process and S1 (see Figures 9-21, *A* and *B*). The examiner should note how far forward the patient is able to bend (i.e., to midthigh, knees, midtibia, or floor) and compare this finding with the results of straight leg raising tests (see "Special Tests" section). Straight leg raising, especially if bilateral, is

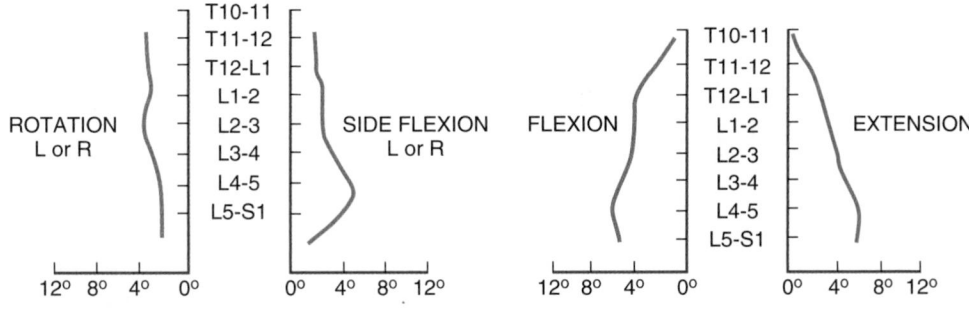

Figure 9-22

Average range of motion in the lumbar spine. (Adapted from Grieve GP: *Common vertebral joint problems,* Edinburgh, 1981, Churchill Livingstone.)

Figure 9-23

On forward flexion, the lumbar curve should normally flatten or go into slight flexion, as shown.

essentially the same movement done passively, except that it is a movement occurring from below upward instead of from above downward.

During the active movements, especially during flexion or extension, the examiner should watch for a **painful arc.** The pain seen in a lumbar painful arc tends to be neurologically based (i.e., it is lancinating or lightening-like), but it may also be caused by instability. If it does occur on movement in the lumbar spine, it is likely that a space-occupying lesion (most likely a small herniation of the disc) is pinching the nerve root in part of the range as the nerve root moves with the motion.[59]

Maigne described an active movement flexion maneuver to help confirm lumbar movement and control.[57] In this **"happy round maneuver,"** the patient bends forward and places the hands on a bed or on the back of a chair. The patient then attempts to arch or hunch the back. Most patients with lumbar pathology are unable to sustain the hunched position.

Extension (backward bending) is normally limited to 20° to 35° in the lumbar spine. While performing the movement, the patient is asked to place the hands in the small of the back to help stabilize the back. Bourdillon and Day have advocated doing this movement in the prone lying position to hyperextend the spine.[78] They called the resulting position the **sphinx position.** The

patient hyperextends the spine by resting on the elbows with the hands holding the chin (Figure 9-24) and allows the abdominal wall to relax. The position is held for 10 to 20 seconds to see if symptoms occur or, if present, become worse.

Side (lateral) flexion or side bending is approximately 15° to 20° in the lumbar spine. The patient is asked to run the hand down the side of the leg and not to bend forward or backward while performing the movement. The examiner can then eyeball the movement and compare it with that of the other side. The distance from the fingertips to the floor on both sides may also be measured, noting any difference. In the spine, the movement of side flexion is a **coupled movement** with rotation. Because of the position of the facet joints, both side flexion and rotation occur together although the amount of movement and direction of movement may not be the same. Table 9-8 shows how different authors interpret the coupled movement in the spine. As the patient side flexes, the examiner should watch the lumbar curve. Normally, the lumbar curve forms a smooth curve on side flexion, and there should be no obvious sharp angulation at only one level. If angulation does occur, it may indicate hypomobility below the level or hypermobility above the level in the lumbar spine (Figure 9-25). Mulvein and Jull advocated having the patient do a lateral shift (Figure 9-26) in addition to side flexion.[79] Their viewpoint is that lateral shift in the lumbar spine focuses the movement more in the lower spine (L4-S1) and helps eliminate the compensating movements in the rest of the spine.

Rotation in the lumbar spine is normally 3° to 18° to the left or right, and it is accomplished by a shearing movement of the lumbar vertebrae on each other. Although the patient is usually in the standing position, rotation may be performed while sitting to eliminate pelvic and hip movement. If the patient stands, the examiner must take care to watch for this accessory movement and try to eliminate it by stabilizing the pelvis.

If a movement such as side flexion toward the painful side increases the symptoms, the lesion is probably

Figure 9-24
The sphinx position.

intra-articular, because the muscles and ligaments on that side are relaxed. If a disc protrusion is present and lateral to the nerve root, side flexion to the painful side increases the pain and radicular symptoms on that side. If a movement such as side flexion away from the painful side alters the symptoms, the lesion may be articular or muscular in origin, or it may be a disc protrusion medial to the nerve root (Figure 9-27).

McKenzie advocated repeating the active movements, especially flexion and extension, 10 times to see whether the movement increases or decreases the symptoms.[33] He also advocated, like Mulvein and Jull,[79] a side gliding movement in which the head and feet remain in position and the patient shifts the pelvis to the left and to the right.

If the examiner finds that side flexion and rotation have been equally limited and extension has been limited

to a lesser extent, a capsular pattern may be suspected. A capsular pattern in one lumbar segment, however, is difficult to detect.

Because back injuries rarely occur during a "pure" movement such as flexion, extension, side flexion, or rotation, it has been advocated that **combined movements** of the spine should be included in the examination.[80,81] The examiner may want to test the following more habitual combined movements: lateral flexion in flexion, lateral flexion in extension, flexion and rotation, and extension and rotation. These combined movements (Figure 9-28) may cause signs and symptoms different from those produced by single plane movements and are definitely indicated if the patient has shown that a combined movement is what causes the symptoms. For example, if the patient is suffering from a facet syndrome, combined extension and rotation is the movement most likely to exacerbate symptoms.[82] Other symptoms that would indicate facet involvement include absence of radicular signs or neurological deficit, hip and buttock pain, and sometimes leg pain above the knee, no paresthesia, and low back stiffness.[83,84]

While the patient is standing, the examiner may perform a **quick test** of the lower peripheral joints (Figure 9-29), provided the examiner feels the patient has the ability to do the test. The patient squats down as far as possible, bounces two or three times, and returns to the standing position. This action quickly tests the ankles, knees, and hips as well as the sacrum for any pathological condition. If the patient can fully squat and bounce without any signs and symptoms, these joints are probably free of pathology related to the complaint. However, this test should be used only with caution and should not be done with patients suspected of having arthritis or pathology in the lower limb joints, pregnant patients, or older patients who exhibit weakness and hypomobility. If this test is negative, there is no need to test the peripheral

Table 9-8

Coupled Movements (Side Flexion and Rotation) Believed to Occur in the Spine in Different Positions (Note the Differences)

Author	In Neutral	In Flexion	In Extension
MacConnaill		Ipsilateral	Contralateral
Farfan		Contralateral	Contralateral
Kaltenborn		Ipsilateral	Ipsilateral
Grieve		Ipsilateral	Contralateral
Fryette	Contralateral	Ipsilateral	Ipsilateral
Pearcy		Ipsilateral (L5-S1) Contralateral (L4, 5)	
Oxland		Ipsilateral (L5-S1)* Contralateral (L5-S1)†	

Ipsilateral implies both movements occur in the same direction, contralateral implies they occur in opposite directions.
*If side flexion induced first.
†If rotation induced first.

Figure 9-25
Lateral (side) flexion. Note that lower lumbar spine stays straight and upper lumbar and lower thoracic spine side flexes. This finding would indicate hypomobility in the lower lumbar spine.

joints (peripheral joint scan) with the patient in the lying position.

The patient is then asked to balance on one leg and to go up and down on the toes four or five times. This is, in effect, a **modified Trendelenberg test.** While the patient does this, the examiner watches for **Trendelenburg's sign** (Figure 9-30). A positive Trendelenburg sign is shown by the nonstance side ilium dropping down instead of elevating as it normally would when standing on the leg. A weak gluteus medius muscle or a coxa vara (abnormal shaft-neck angle of the femur) on the stance leg side may produce a positive sign. If the patient is unable to complete the movement by going up and down on the toes, the examiner should suspect an S1 nerve root lesion. Both legs are tested.

McKenzie advocated doing flexion movements with the patient in the supine lying position as well.[33] In the standing position, flexion in the spine takes place from above downward, so pain at the end of the ROM indicates that L5-S1 is affected. When the patient is in the supine lying position, with the knees being lifted to the chest, flexion takes place from below upward so that pain at the beginning of movement indicates that L5-S1 is affected. Remember that greater stretch is placed on L5-S1 when the patient is in the lying position.

During the observation stage of the assessment, the examiner will have noted any changes in functional limb length (see Table 9-7). Wallace developed a method for measuring **functional leg length.**[85] The patient is first assessed in a

Figure 9-26
Lumbar lateral shift.

relaxed stance. In this position, the examiner palpates the ASISs and the PSISs, noting any asymmetry. The examiner then places the patient in a symmetric stance, ensuring that the subtalar joint is in the neutral position (see Chapter 13), the toes are straight ahead, and the knees are extended. The ASISs and PSISs are again assessed for asymmetry. If differences are still noted, the examiner should check for structural leg length differences (see Chapters 10 and 11), sacroiliac joint dysfunction, or weak gluteus medius or quadratus lumborum (Figure 9-31). The pelvis may also be leveled with the use of calibrated blocks or cards so that the functional length difference can be recorded.

Passive Movements

In the lumbar spine, passive movements are difficult to perform because of the weight of the body. If active movements are full and pain free, overpressure can be attempted with care. However, it is safer to check the end feel of the individual vertebrae in the lumbar spine during the assessment of joint play movements. The end feel is the same, but the examiner has better control of the patient and is less likely to overstress the joints.

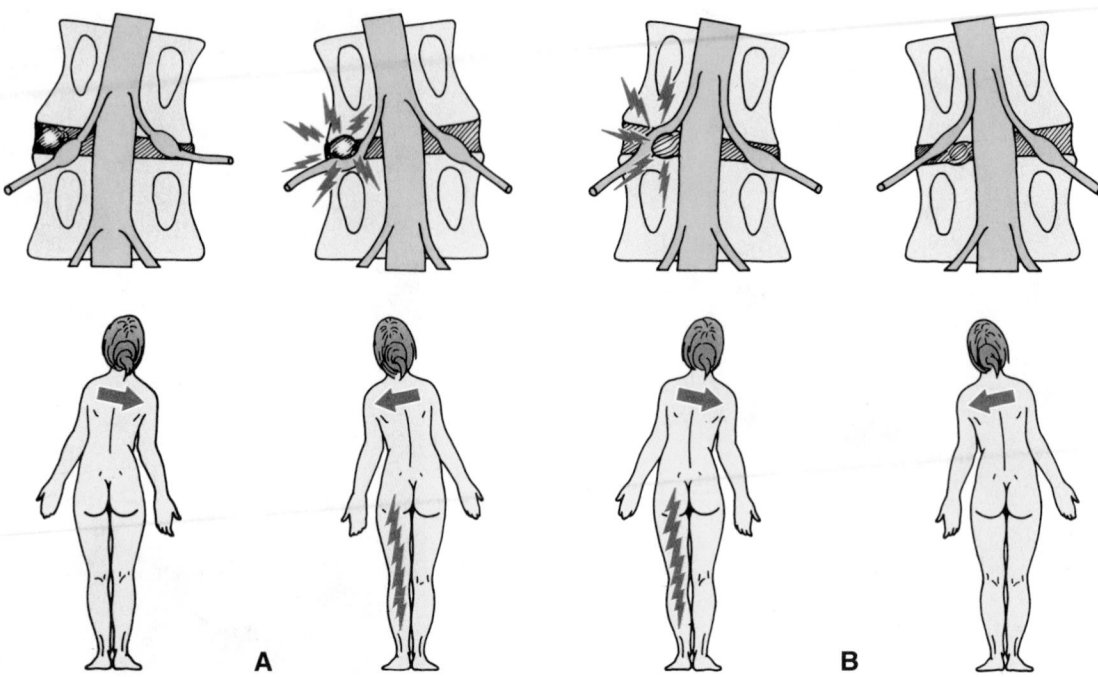

Figure 9-27

Patients with herniated disc problems may sometimes list to one side. This is a voluntary or involuntary mechanism to alleviate nerve root irritation. The list in some patients is toward the side of the sciatica; in others, it is toward the opposite side. A reasonable hypothesis suggests that when the herniation is lateral to the nerve root **(A)**, the list is to the side opposite the sciatica because a list to the same side would elicit pain. Conversely, when the herniation is medial to the nerve root **(B)**, the list is toward the side of the sciatica because tilting away would irritate the root and cause pain. (Redrawn from White AA, Panjabi MM: Clinical biomechanics of the spine, ed 2, p. 415, Philadelphia, 1990, JB Lippincott.) (© Augustus A White III and MM Panjabi.)

Figure 9-28

Combined active movements. **A,** Lateral flexion in flexion. **B,** Lateral flexion in extension. **C,** Rotation and flexion. **D,** Rotation and extension.

Figure 9-29
Quick test.

Passive Movements of the Lumbar Spine and Normal End Feel

- Flexion (tissue stretch)
- Extension (tissue stretch)
- Side flexion (tissue stretch)
- Rotation (tissue stretch)

Resisted Isometric Movements

Resisted isometric muscle strength of the lumbar spine is first tested in the neutral position. The patient is seated. The contraction must be resisted and isometric so that no movement occurs (Figure 9-32). Because of the strength of the trunk muscles, the examiner should say, "Don't let me move you," so that movement is minimized. The examiner tests flexion, extension, side flexion, and rotation. Figure 9-33 shows the axes of movement of the lumbar spine. The lumbar spine should be in a neutral position, and the painful movements should be done last. The examiner should keep in mind that strong abdominal muscles help to reduce the load on the lumbar spine by approximately 30%, and on the thoracic spine by approximately 50%, as a result of the increased intrathoracic and intra-abdominal pressures caused by the contraction of these muscles. Table 9-9 lists the muscles acting on the lumbar vertebrae.

Provided neutral isometric testing is normal or only causes a small amount of pain, the examiner can go on to other tests, which will place greater stress on the muscles. These tests are often dynamic and provide both

A   B   C

Figure 9-30
Trendelenburg and S1 nerve root test. **A,** Anterior view, negative test. **B,** Side view, negative test. **C,** Posterior view, positive test for a weak right gluteus medius.

Figure 9-31

Effect of different leg lengths and posture. Note the presence of scoliosis on the side with the "short" limb.
A, Normal. **B,** Short left femur. **C,** Short left tibia. **D,** Pronation of left foot.

concentric and eccentric work for the muscles supporting the spine. With all of the following tests, the examiner should ensure that the patient can hold a neutral pelvis. If there is excessive movement of the ASIS (supine) or PSIS (prone) when doing the test, the patient should not be allowed to do them. In normal individuals, the ASIS or PSIS should not move when doing the tests. Motivation may also affect the results.[86]

Resisted Isometric Movements of the Lumbar Spine

- Forward flexion
- Extension
- Side flexion (left and right)
- Rotation (left and right)
- Dynamic abdominal endurance
- Double straight leg lowering
- Dynamic extensor endurance
- Isotonic horizontal side support
- Internal/external abdominal oblique test

Dynamic Abdominal Endurance Test [87,88] This test checks the endurance of the abdominals. The patient is in supine with the hips at 45° and knees at 90° and hands at sides. A line is drawn 8 cm (for patients over 40 years of age) or 12 cm (for patients under 40 years of age) distal to the fingers. The patient tucks in the chin and curls the trunk to touch the line with the fingers (Figure 9-34) and repeats as many curls as possible using a cadence of 25 repetitions per minute. The number of repetitions possible before cheating (holding breath, altered mechanics) or fatigue occurs is recorded as the score. The test may also be done as an isometric test (Figure 9-35) by assuming the end position and holding it. The grading for this **isometric abdominal test** would be as follows:[89–91]

Normal (5) = Arms crossed over chest, until scapulae

Normal (5) = Hands behind neck, until scapulae clear table (20 to 30 second hold)

Good (4) = Arms crossed over chest, until scapulae clear table (15 to 20 second hold)

Fair (3) = Arms straight, until scapulae clear table (10 to 15 second hold)

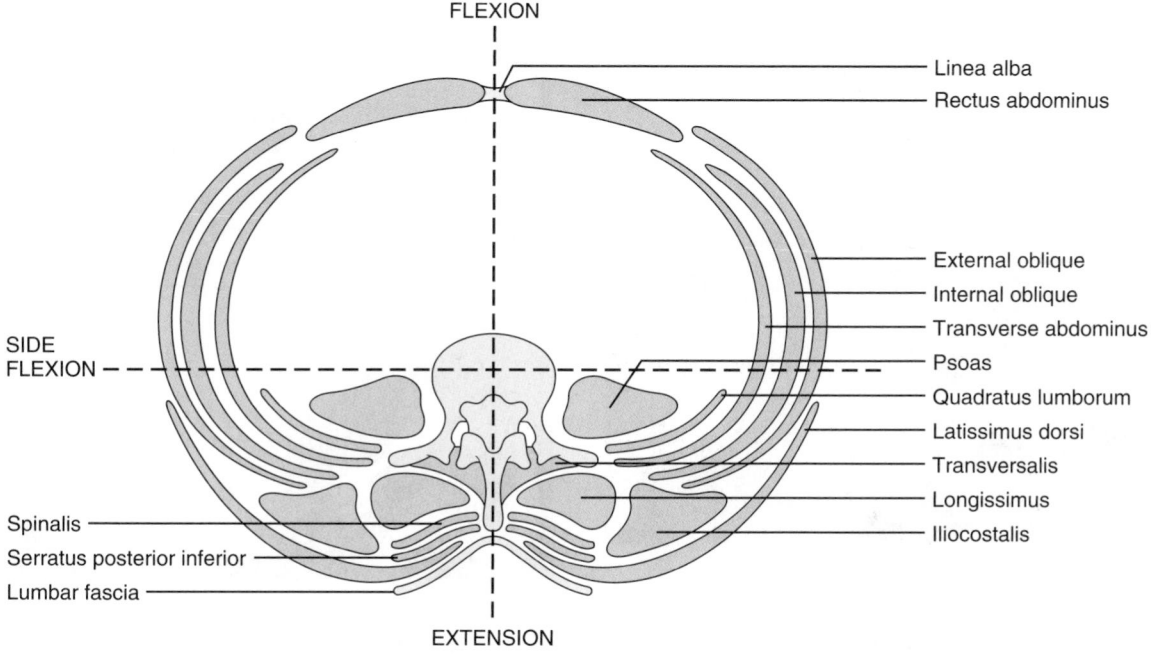

Figure 9-32

Positioning for resisted isometric movements of the lumbar spine. **A,** Flexion, extension, and side flexion.
B, Rotation to right.

FLEXION

Linea alba
Rectus abdominus

External oblique
Internal oblique
Transverse abdominus
Psoas
Quadratus lumborum
Latissimus dorsi
Transversalis
Longissimus
Iliocostalis

SIDE FLEXION

Spinalis
Serratus posterior inferior
Lumbar fascia

EXTENSION

Figure 9-33

Diagram of relations of the lumbar spine showing movement.

Table 9-9

Muscles of the Lumbar Spine: Their Actions and Nerve Root Derivations

Action	Muscles Acting	Nerve Root Derivation
Forward flexion	1. Psoas major	L1-L3
	2. Rectus abdominis	T6-T12
	3. External abdominal oblique	T7-T12
	4. Internal abdominal oblique	T7-T12, L1
	5. Transversus abdominis	T7-T12, L1
	6. Intertransversarii	L1-L5
Extension	1. Latissimus dorsi	Thoracodorsal (C6-C8)
	2. Erector spinae	L1-L3
	iliocostalis lumborum	L1-L3
	longissimus thoracis	L1-L5
	3. Transversospinalis	L1-L5
	4. Interspinales	L1-L5
	5. Quadratus lumborum	T12, L1-L4
	6. Multifidus	L1-L5
	7. Rotatores	L1-L5
	8. Gluteus maximus	L1-L5
Side flexion	1. Latissimus dorsi	Thoracodorsal (C6-C8)
	2. Erector spinae	L1-L3
	iliocostalis lumborum	L1-L3
	longissimus thoracis	L1-L5
	3. Transversalis	L1-L5
	4. Intertransversarii	L1-L5
	5. Quadratus lumborum	T12, L1-L4
	6. Psoas major	L1-L3
	7. External abdominal oblique	T7-T12
Rotation*	1. Transversalis	L1-L5
	2. Rotatores	L1-L5
	3. Multifidus	L1-L5

*Little rotation occurs in the lumbar spine because of the shape of the facet joints. Any rotation would be a result of shearing movement.

Figure 9-34
Dynamic abdominal endurance test. The patient tucks in the chin and curls up the trunk lifting the trunk off the bed. Ideally, the scapula should clear the bed.

A

Figure 9-35
Isometric abdominal test. **A,** Hands behind neck.

Figure 9-35 cont'd
B, Arms crossed over chest, scapulae off table. **C,** Arms straight, scapulae off table. **D,** Hands behind head, top of scapulae off table. **E,** Arms straight, only head off table.

Poor (2) = Arms extended, toward knees, until top of scapulae lift from table (1 to 10 second hold)

Trace (1) = Unable to raise more than head off table

Dynamic Extensor Endurance Test [87,92,93] This test is designed to test the strength of iliocostalis lumborum (erector spinae) and multifidus. The patient is placed in prone lying with the hips and iliac crests resting on the end of the examining table and the hips and pelvis stabilized with straps (Figure 9-36). Initially, the patient's hands support the upper body in 30° flexion on a chair or bench (see Figure 9-36, *A*). Keeping the spine straight, the examiner instructs the patient to extend the trunk to neutral and then lower the head to the start position. During the exercise, the patient's arms are crossed at the chest. The cadence is 25 repetitions per minute. The number of repetitions possible before cheating (holding breath, altered mechanics) or fatigue occurs is recorded as the score. The test may also be done isometrically, and the examiner times how long the patient can hold the contraction without pelvic or spinal movement. This test may also be done with the patient beginning in prone lying and extending the spine if

the preceding test is too hard.[94,95] In this case, the patient can start with the hands by the side, moving the hands in the small of the back, and finally moving the hands behind the head for increasing difficulty. The test, if done isometrically **(isometric extensor test)** (Figure 9-37), would be graded as follows:[89-91]

Normal (5) = Arms crossed over chest, until scapulae

Normal (5) = With hands clasped behind the head, extends the lumbar spine, lifting the head, chest, and ribs from the floor (20 to 30 second hold)

Good (4) = With hands at the side, extends the lumbar spine, lifting the head, chest, and ribs from the floor (15 to 20 second hold)

Fair (3) = With hands at the side, extends the lumbar spine, lifting the sternum off the floor (10 to 15 second hold)

Poor (2) = With hands at the side, extends the lumbar spine, lifting the head off the floor (1 to 10 second hold)

Trace (1) = Only slight contraction of the muscle with no movement

Figure 9-36
Dynamic extensor endurance test. **A,** Starting position. **B,** End position.

Biering and Sorensen described a similar test (**Biering-Sorensen fatigue test**) in which the subject had arms by the side, and the time the patient was able to hold the straight position before fatigue was recorded (i.e., the patient could not hold the position).[96,97] The start position is the same as for the dynamic test.

Double Straight Leg Lowering Test [94,95,98] (NOTE: This test checks the abdominals. It should only be per-

formed if the patient receives a "normal" grade in the dynamic abdominal endurance test or the abdominal isometric test.) This is an abdominal eccentric test that can place a great deal of stress on the spine so the examiner must ensure the patient is able to hold a neutral pelvis before doing the exercise. It also causes greater abdominal activation than curlups.[99] The patient lies supine and flexes the hips to 90° (Figure 9-38, *A*) and then straightens

Figure 9-37
Isometric extensor test. **A,** Hands behind head, lift head, chest and ribs off bed. **B,** Hands at side, lift head, chest and ribs off bed. **C,** Hands at side, lift sternum off bed. **D,** Hands at side, lift head off bed.

the knees (Figure 9-38, *B*). The patient then positions the pelvis in neutral (i.e., the PSISs are slightly superior to the ASISs) by doing a posterior pelvic tilt and holding the spinous processes tightly against the examining table. The straight legs are eccentrically lowered (Figure 9-38, *C*). As soon as the ASISs start to rotate forward, the test is stopped, the angle measured (plinth to thigh angle), and the knees bent. The test must be done slowly, and the patient must not hold his or her breath. The grading of the test is as follows:[90]

Normal (5) = Arms crossed over chest, until scapulae
Normal (5) = Able to reach 0° to 15° from table before pelvis tilts
Good (4) = Able to reach 16° to 45° from table before pelvis tilts
Fair (3) = Able to reach 46° to 75° from table before pelvis tilts

Poor (2) = Able to reach 75° to 90° from table before pelvis tilts
Trace (1) = Unable to hold pelvis in neutral at all

Internal/External Abdominal Obliques Test [94,95]

This test checks the combined action of the internal oblique muscle of one side and the external oblique muscle on the opposite side. The patient is in supine lying with hands by the side. The patient is asked to lift the head and shoulder on one side and reach over and touch the fingernails of the other hand (Figure 9-39, *A*). The examiner counts the number of repetitions the patient performs. The patient's feet should not be supported and the patient should breathe normally. The test can be made more difficult by asking the patient to put the hands on the opposite shoulders across the chest (Figure 9-39, *B*) and do the test by taking the elbow toward where the fingers would have rested beside the body or, more difficult still, by putting

Figure 9-38
Double straight leg lowering test. **A,** Flexing hips to 90°. **B,** Start position with knees straight. **C,** Example of leg lowering. Note how the examiner is watching for anterior pelvic rotation, indicating an inability to hold a neutral pelvis.

the hands behind the head and taking the elbows toward the position where the fingernails would have rested beside the body (Figure 9-39, *C*). The grading of the test, if done isometrically **(isometric internal/external abdominal oblique test)**, would be as follows:[90]

Normal (5) = Arms crossed over chest, until scapulae

Normal (5) = Flexes and rotates the lumbar spine fully with hands behind head (20 to 30-second hold)

Good (4) = Flexes and rotates the lumbar spine fully with hands across chest (15 to 20-second hold)

Fair (3) = Flexes and rotates the lumbar spine fully with arms reaching forward (10- to 15-second hold)

Poor (2) = Unable to flex and rotate fully

Trace (1) = Only slight contraction of the muscle with no movement

(0) = No contraction of the muscle

Dynamic Horizontal Side Support (Side Bridge) Test [100] This movement tests the quadratus lumborum muscle. The patient is in a side lying position resting the upper body on his or her elbow (Figure 9-40). To begin, the patient side lies with the knees flexed to 90°. The examiner asks the patient to lift the pelvis off the examining table (see Figure 9-40, *B*) and straighten the spine. The patient should not roll forward or backward when doing the test. The patient repeats the movement as many times as possible in a dynamic test or holds for as long as possible in an isometric test. In younger, more fit patients, the test can be made more difficult by having the legs straight and asking the patient to lift the knees

and pelvis off the examining table with the feet as the base so the whole body is straight (see Figure 9-40, *C*). As an isometric test, the test would be graded as follows:

Normal (5) = Arms crossed over chest, until scapulae

Normal (5) = Able to lift pelvis off examining table and hold spine straight (10 to 20-second hold)

Good (4) = Able to lift pelvis off examining table but has difficulty holding spine straight (5- to 10-second hold)

Fair (3) = Able to lift pelvis off examining table and cannot hold spine straight (<5-second hold)

Poor (2) = Unable to lift pelvis off examining table

McGill reported that the side bridge should be able to be held 65% of the extensor time for men and 39% for women and 99% of the flexor time for men and 79% for women.[101]

Back Rotators/Multifidus Test This test checks the ability of the lumbar rotators and multifidus to stabilize the trunk during dynamic extremity movement. The patient assumes the quadriped position (Figure 9-41, *A*) and is asked to hold the neutral pelvis position and breathe normally. The patient is then asked to do the following movements (Figure 9-41, *B-D*):

1. Single straight arm lift and hold
2. Single straight leg lift and hold
3. Contralateral straight arm and straight leg lift and hold

The scoring for the test would be as follows:

Normal (5) = Arms crossed over chest, until scapulae

Figure 9-39

Internal/external abdominal oblique test. **A,** Test position with hands at side. **B,** Test position with hands on shoulders. **C,** Test position with hands behind head.

Figure 9-40
Dynamic horizontal side support. **A,** Start position. **B,** Lifting pelvis off bed using knees as support. **C,** Lifting pelvis off bed using feet and ankles as support.

Normal (5) = Able to do contralateral arm and leg, both sides while maintaining neutral pelvis (20- to 30-second hold)

Good (4) = Able to maintain neutral pelvis while doing single leg lift but not able to hold neutral pelvis when doing contralateral arm and leg (20-second hold)

Fair (3) = Able to do single arm lift and maintain neutral pelvis (20-second hold)

Poor (2) = Unable to maintain neutral pelvis while doing single arm lift

If tested isokinetically, the back extensors are stronger than the flexors. Men produce a force equal to approximately 65% of body weight in flexion, whereas women produce approximately 65% to 70% of their body weight in flexion. In extension, men produce approximately 90% to 95% of their body weight, and women produce 80% to 95% of their body weight, depending on the speed tested. In rotation, men produce approximately 55% to 65% of their body weight, whereas women produce approximately 40% to 55% of their body weight, depending on the speed tested.[102]

Peripheral Joint Scanning Examination

After the resisted isometric movements of the lumbar spine have been completed, if the examiner did not use the quick test to test the peripheral joints or is unsure of the findings or whether the peripheral joints are involved, the peripheral joints should be quickly scanned to rule out obvious pathology in the extremities. Any deviation from normal should lead the examiner to do a detailed examination of that joint. The following joints are scanned.[103]

Lower Limb Scanning Examination

- Sacroiliac joints
- Hip joints
- Knee joints
- Ankle joints
- Foot joints

Figure 9-41
Back rotators/multifidus test. **A,** Start position. **B,** Single straight arm lift. **C,** Single straight leg lift.
D, Contralateral straight arm and leg lift.

Sacroiliac Joints

With the patient standing, the examiner palpates the PSIS on one side with one thumb and one of the sacral spines with the other thumb. The patient then fully flexes the hip on that side, and the examiner notes whether the PSIS drops as it normally should or whether it elevates, indicating fixation of the sacroiliac joint on that side (Figure 9-42). The examiner then compares the other side. The examiner next places one thumb on one of the patient's ischial tuberosities and one thumb on the sacral apex. The patient is then asked to flex the hip on that side again. If the movement is normal, the thumb on the ischial tuberosity moves laterally. If the sacroiliac joint on that side is fixed, the thumb moves up. The other side is then tested for comparison. This test has also been called **Gillet's** or the **sacral fixation** test (see Chapter 10).

Hip Joints

These joints are actively moved through flexion, extension, abduction, adduction, and medial and lateral rotation in as full a ROM as possible. Any pattern of restriction or pain should be noted. As the patient flexes the hip, the examiner may palpate the ilium, sacrum, and lumbar spine to determine when movement begins at the sacroiliac joint on that side and at the lumbar spine during the hip movement. The two sides should be compared.

Knee Joints

The patient actively moves the knee joints through as full a range of flexion and extension as possible. Any restric-

tion of movement or abnormal signs and symptoms should be noted.

Foot and Ankle Joints

Plantar flexion, dorsiflexion, supination, and pronation of the foot and ankle as well as flexion and extension of the toes are actively performed through a full ROM. Again, any alteration in signs and symptoms should be noted.

Myotomes

Having completed the scanning examination of the peripheral joints, the examiner next tests the patient's muscle power for possible neurological weakness (Table 9-10).[103] With the patient lying supine, the myotomes are assessed individually (Figure 9-43). When testing myotomes (Table 9-11), the examiner should place the test joint or joints in a neutral or resting position and then apply a resisted isometric pressure. The contraction should be held for *at least 5 seconds* to show any weakness. If feasible, the examiner should test the two sides simultaneously to provide a comparison. The simultaneous bilateral comparison is not possible for movements involving the hip and knee joints because of the weight of the limbs and stress to the low back, so both sides must be done individually. The examiner should not apply pressure over the joints, because this action may mask symptoms.

Remember that the examiner has previously tested the S1 myotome with the patient standing and has tested for a positive Trendelenburg's sign (modified

Figure 9-42

Tests to demonstrate left sacroiliac fixation. **A,** Examiner places the left thumb on the posterior superior iliac spine and the right thumb over one of the sacral spinous processes. **B,** With normal movement, the examiner's left thumb moves downward as the patient raises the left leg with full hip flexion. **C,** If the joint is fixed, the examiner's left thumb moves upward as the patient raises the left leg. **D,** The examiner places the left thumb over the ischial tuberosity and the right thumb over the apex of the sacrum. **E,** With normal movement, the examiner's left thumb moves laterally as the patient raises the left leg with full hip flexion. **F,** If the joint is fixed, the examiner's left thumb moves slightly upward as the patient raises the left leg. (Modified from Kirkaldy-Willis WH: *Managing low back pain,* p. 94, New York, 1983, Churchill Livingstone.)

Myotomes of the Lumbar and Sacral Spines

- L2: Hip flexion
- L3: Knee extension
- L4: Ankle dorsiflexion
- L5: Great toe extension
- S1: Ankle plantar flexion, ankle eversion, hip extension
- S2: Knee flexion

Trendelenburg test); these movements are repeated here only if the examiner is unsure of the result and wants to test again. The ankle movements should be tested with the knee flexed approximately 30°, especially if the patient complains of sciatic pain, because full dorsiflexion is considered a provocative maneuver for stretching of neurological tissue. Likewise, the extended knee increases the stretch on the sciatic nerve and may result in false signs, such as weakness that results from pain rather than from pressure on the nerve root. Rainville et al. have recommended testing the L3 and L4 nerve roots at the same time by doing a **single leg sit-to-stand test** to check for unilateral quadriceps weakness

(Figure 9-44).[104] Note that the patient can hold the examiner's hands for balance.

If the patient is in extreme pain, all tests with the patient in the supine position should be completed before the patient is tested in prone. This reduces the amount of movement the patient must do, decreasing the patient's discomfort. Ideally, all tests in the standing position should be performed first, followed by tests in the sitting, supine, side lying, and prone positions. This procedure is shown in the précis at the end of the chapter.

To test hip flexion (L2 myotome), the examiner flexes the patient's hip to 30° to 40°. The examiner then applies a resisted force into extension proximal to the knee while ensuring that the heel of the patient's foot is not resting on the examining table (see Figure 9-43, *A*). The other side is then tested for comparison. To prevent excessive stress on the lumbar spine, the examiner must ensure that the patient does not increase the lumbar lordosis while doing the test and that only one leg at a time is tested.

To test knee extension or the L3 myotome, the examiner flexes the patient's knee to 25° to 35° and then applies a resisted flexion force at the midshaft of the tibia ensuring the heel is not resting on the examining table (see Figure 9-43, *B*). The other side is tested for comparison.

Table 9-10

Lumbar Root Syndromes

Root	Dermatome	Muscle Weakness	Reflexes/Special Tests Affected	Paresthesias
L1	Back, over trochanter, groin	None	None	Groin, after holding posture, which causes pain
L2	Back, front of thigh to knee	Psoas, hip adductors	None	Occasionally front of thigh
L3	Back, upper buttock, front of thigh and knee, medial lower leg	Psoas, quadriceps—thigh wasting	Knee jerk sluggish, PKB positive, pain on full SLR	Inner knee, anterior lower leg
L4	Inner buttock, outer thigh, inside of leg, dorsum of foot, big toe	Tibialis anterior, extensor hallucis	SLR limited, neck-flexion pain, weak knee jerk; side flexion limited	Medial aspect of calf and ankle
L5	Buttock, back and side of thigh, lateral aspect of leg, dorsum of foot, inner half of sole and first, second, and third toes	Extensor hallucis, peroneals, gluteus medius, ankle dorsiflexors, hamstrings—calf wasting	SLR limited to one side, neck-flexion pain, ankle jerk decreased, crossed-leg raising—pain	Lateral aspect of leg, medial three toes
S1	Buttock, back of thigh, and lower leg	Calf and hamstrings, wasting of gluteals, peroneals, plantar flexors	SLR limited	Lateral two toes, lateral foot, lateral leg to knee, plantar aspect of foot
S2	Same as S1	Same as S1 except peroneals	Same as S1	Lateral leg, knee, heel
S3	Groin, inner thigh to knee	None	None	None
S4	Perineum, genitals, lower sacrum	Bladder, rectum	None	Saddle area, genitals, anus, impotence

Manipulation and traction are contraindicated if S4 or massive posterior displacement causes bilateral sciatica and S3 pain.

PKB, prone knee bendings; *SLR,* straight leg raising.

To test ankle dorsiflexion (L4 myotome), the examiner asks the patient to place the feet at 90° relative to the leg (plantigrade position). The examiner applies a resisted force to the dorsum of each foot and compares the two sides (see Figure 9-43, *C*). Ankle plantar flexion (S1 myotome) is compared in a similar fashion, but the resistance is applied to the sole of the foot. Because of the strength of the plantar flexor muscles, it is better to test this myotome with the patient standing. The patient slowly moves up and down on the toes of each foot (for at least 5 seconds) in turn (**modified Trendelenburg test**), and the examiner compares the differences as previously described. Ankle eversion (S1 myotome) is tested with the patient in the supine lying position, and the examiner applies a force to move the foot into inversion (see Figure 9-43, *D*).

Toe extension (L5 myotome) is tested with the patient holding both big toes in a neutral position. The examiner applies resistance to the nails of both toes and compares the two sides (see Figure 9-43, *E*). It is imperative that the resistance be isometric, so the amount of force in this case is less than that applied during knee extension, for example.

Hip extension (S1 myotome) is tested with the patient lying prone. This test needs to be done only if the patient is unable to do plantar flexion testing in standing or ankle eversion. The knee is flexed to 90°. The examiner then lifts the patient's thigh slightly off the examining table while stabilizing the leg. A downward force is applied to the patient's posterior thigh with one hand while the other hand ensures that the patient's thigh is not resting on the table (see Figure 9-43, *F*).

Knee flexion (S1–S2 myotomes) is tested in the same position (prone) with the knee flexed to 90°. An extension isometric force is applied just above the ankle (see Figure 9-43, *G*). Although it is possible to test both knee flexors at the same time, it is not advisable to do this because the stress on the lumbar spine is too great.

Functional Assessment

Injury to the lumbar spine can greatly affect the patient's ability to function. Activities such as standing, walking, bending, lifting, traveling, socializing, dressing, and sexual intercourse can be affected. Numerical scoring tables may be used to determine the degree of pain caused by lumbar spine pathology or disability. Care must be taken when selecting one of these scales to ensure that it measures the disability from the patient's perspective.[105–108] Examples are the Oswestry Disability Index (Figure 9-45), the Roland-Morris Disability Questionnaire[109] (see Figure 8-33), and the Hendler 10-Minute Screening Test for Chronic Back Pain Patients (Figure 9-46).[107,110,111] It has been reported that the Hendler test helps to differentiate

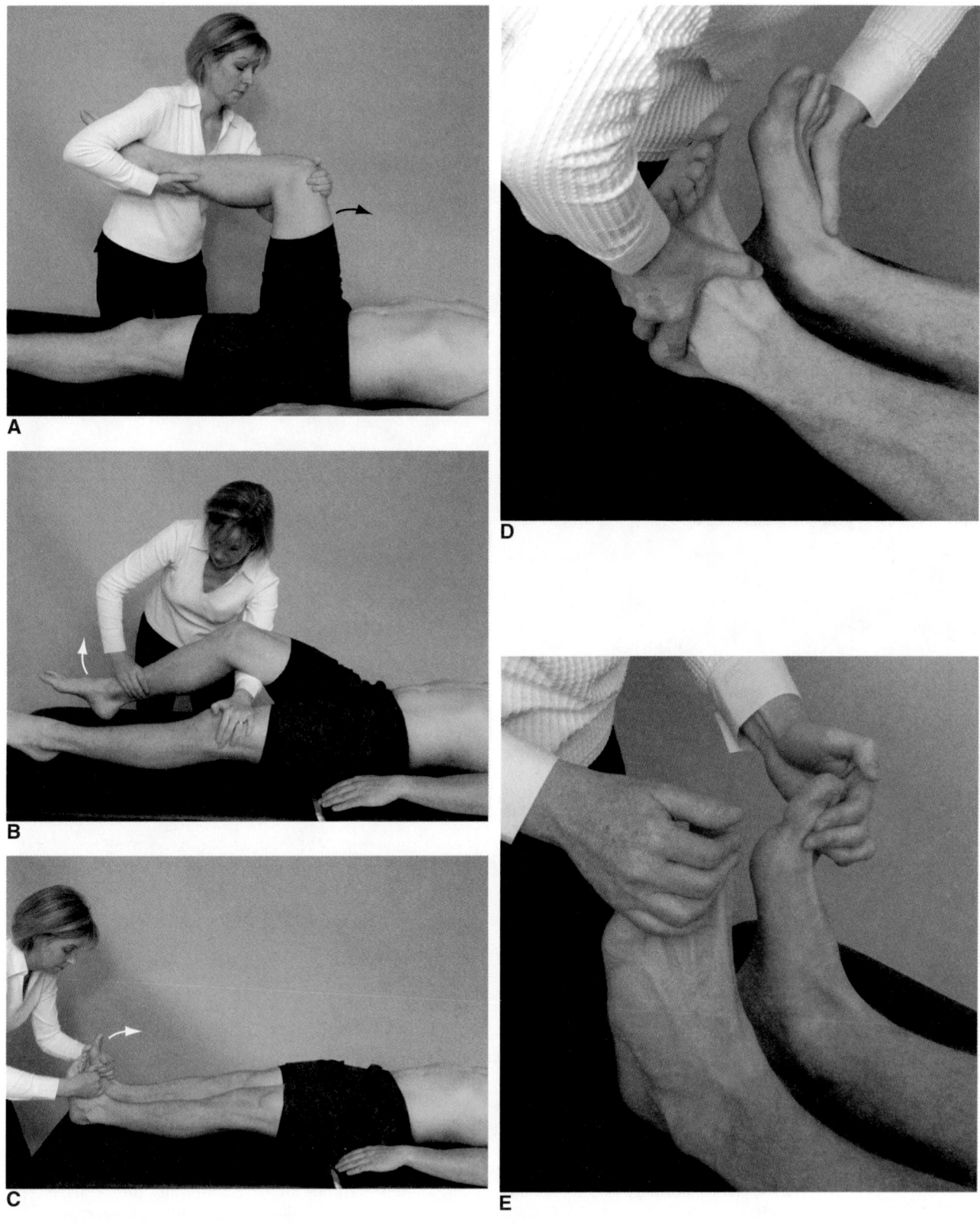

Figure 9-43

Positioning to test myotomes. **A,** Hip flexion (L2). **B,** Knee extension (L3). **C,** Foot dorsiflexion (L4).
D, Ankle eversion (S1). **E,** Extension of the big toe (L5).

Continued

Figure 9-43 cont'd
F, Hip extension (S1). **G,** Knee flexion (S1-S2).

Table 9-11
Myotomes of the Lower Limb

Nerve Root	Test Action	Muscles
L1-L2	Hip flexion	Psoas, iliacus, sartorius, gracilis, pectineus, adductor longus, adductor brevis
L3	Knee extension	Quadriceps, adductor longus, magnus, and brevis
L4	Ankle dorsiflexion	Tibialis anterior, quadriceps, tensor fasciae latae, adductor magnus, obturator externus, tibialis posterior
L5	Toe extension	Extensor hallucis longus, extensor digitorum longus, gluteus medius and minimus, obturator internus, semimembranosus, semitendinosus, peroneus tertius, popliteus
S1	Ankle plantar flexion Ankle eversion Hip extension Knee flexion	Gastrocnemius, soleus, gluteus maximus, obturator internus, piriformis, biceps femoris, semitendinosus, popliteus, peroneus longus and brevis, extensor digitorum brevis
S2	Knee flexion	Biceps femoris, piriformis, soleus, gastrocnemius, flexor digitorum longus, flexor hallucis longus, intrinsic foot muscles
S3		Intrinsic foot muscles (except abductor hallucis), flexor hallucis brevis, flexor digitorum brevis, extensor digitorum brevis

A **B**

Figure 9-44
Single leg sit-to-stand test.

organic from functional low back pain.[112] The Oswestry Disability Index is a good functional scale because it deals with activities of daily living and therefore is based on the patient's response and concerns affecting daily life. It is the most commonly used functional back scale. The disability index is calculated by dividing the total score (each section is worth from 1 to 6 points) by the number of sections answered and multiplying by 100. The Roland-Morris Disability Questionnaire is short and simple, and it is suitable for following up on progress in clinical settings and for combining with other measures of function (e.g., work disability).[109,113] Other numerical back pain scales include the Functional Rating Index,[114,115] the Dallas Pain Questionnaire,[116] the Million Index,[117] the Japanese Orthopedic Association Scale,[118] the Iowa Low Back Rating Scale,[119] the Bournemouth Questionnaire,[120,121] the Quebec Back Pain Disability Scale,[122] the Scoliosis Research Society form (SRS-22 for those with spinal deformity),[123–125] the Lumbar Spinal Stenosis Questionnaire,[126] and the Aberdeen Back Pain Scale.[127] Thomas provide a good review of these and other scales.[107] Lehman and colleagues developed a rating scale for lumbar dysfunction (Figure 9-47) that includes assessment criteria, physician criteria, and, perhaps more

importantly, patient criteria for determining the degree of dysfunction.[119] These criteria can be evaluated during the normal assessment for the patient.

Waddell and colleagues developed a series of tests to differentiate between organic and nonorganic back pain.[128] Each test counts +1 if positive or 0 if negative:
1. Superficial skin tenderness to light pinch over wide area of lumbar spine
2. Deep tenderness over wide area, often extending to thoracic spine, sacrum, or pelvis
3. Low back pain on axial loading of spine in standing
4. Straight leg raising test positive when specifically tested, but not when patient is seated with knee extended to test Babinski reflex
5. Abnormal neurological (motor or sensory) patterns
6. Overreaction

Positive findings of +3 or more should be investigated for nonorganic cause; these patients may also have social and psychological components to their complaint.[3,129,130]

Waddell also described a simple clinical functional capacity evaluation (Figure 9-48),[3] which examiners may find useful for testing patients.[131]

Simmonds et al. came up with several functional tests or physical performance measures which they felt would

Text continued on page 558

Oswestry Disability Index

Section 1 - Pain intensity
- [ ] I have no pain at the moment.
- [ ] The pain is very mild at the moment.
- [ ] The pain is moderate at the moment.
- [ ] The pain is fairly severe at the moment.
- [ ] The pain is very severe at the moment.
- [ ] The pain is the worst imaginable at the moment.

Section 2 - Personal care (washing, dressing, etc.)
- [ ] I can look after myself normally without causing extra pain.
- [ ] I can look after myself normally but it is very painful.
- [ ] It is painful to look after myself and I am slow and careful.
- [ ] I need some help but manage most of my personal care.
- [ ] I need help every day in most aspects of self care.
- [ ] I do not get dressed, wash with difficulty, and stay in bed.

Section 3 - Lifting
- [ ] I can lift heavy weights without extra pain.
- [ ] I can lift heavy weights but it gives extra pain.
- [ ] Pain prevents me from lifting heavy weights off the floor but I can manage if they are conveniently positioned, e.g., on a table.
- [ ] Pain prevents me from lifting heavy weights but I can manage light to medium weights if they are conveniently positioned.
- [ ] I can lift only very light weights.
- [ ] I cannot lift or carry anything at all.

Section 4 - Walking
- [ ] Pain does not prevent me walking any distance.
- [ ] Pain prevents me walking more than 1 mile.
- [ ] Pain prevents me walking more than ¼ of a mile.
- [ ] Pain prevents me walking more than 100 yards.
- [ ] I can only walk using a stick or crutches.
- [ ] I am in bed most of the time and have to crawl to the toilet.

Section 5 - Sitting
- [ ] I can sit in any chair as long as I like.
- [ ] I can sit in my favorite chair as long as I like.
- [ ] Pain prevents me from sitting for more than 1 hour.
- [ ] Pain prevents me from sitting for more than ½ an hour.
- [ ] Pain prevents me from sitting for more than 10 minutes.
- [ ] Pain prevents me from sitting at all.

Section 6 - Standing
- [ ] I can stand as long as I want without extra pain.
- [ ] I can stand as long as I want but it gives me extra pain.
- [ ] Pain prevents me from standing for more than 1 hour.
- [ ] Pain prevents me from standing for more than ½ an hour.
- [ ] Pain prevents me from standing for more than 10 minutes.
- [ ] Pain prevents me from standing at all.

Section 7 - Sleeping
- [ ] My sleep is never disturbed by pain.
- [ ] My sleep is occasionally disturbed by pain.
- [ ] Because of pain I have less than 6 hours sleep.
- [ ] Because of pain I have less than 4 hours sleep.
- [ ] Because of pain I have less than 2 hours sleep.
- [ ] Pain prevents me from sleeping at all.

Section 8 - Sex life (if applicable)
- [ ] My sex life is normal and causes no extra pain.
- [ ] My sex life is normal but causes some extra pain.
- [ ] My sex life is nearly normal but is very painful.
- [ ] My sex life is severely restricted by pain.
- [ ] My sex life is nearly absent because of pain.
- [ ] Pain prevents any sex life at all.

Section 9 - Social life
- [ ] My social life is normal and causes me no extra pain.
- [ ] My social life is normal but increases the degree of pain.
- [ ] Pain has no significant effect on my social life apart from limiting my more energetic interests, e.g., sport.
- [ ] Pain has restricted my social life and I do not go out as often.
- [ ] Pain has restricted social life to my home.
- [ ] I have no social life because of pain.

Section 10 - Traveling
- [ ] I can travel anywhere without pain.
- [ ] I can travel anywhere but it gives extra pain.
- [ ] Pain is bad but I manage journeys of over two hours.
- [ ] Pain restricts me to journeys of less than one hour.
- [ ] Pain restricts me to short necessary journeys under 30 minutes.
- [ ] Pain prevents me from traveling except to receive treatment.

Section 11 - Previous treatment
Over the past three months have you received treatment, tablets, or medicines of any kind for your back or leg pain? Please tick the appropriate box.
- [ ] No
- [ ] Yes (if yes, please state the type of treatment you have received)

Figure 9-45 ▬▬▬▬▬▬

Oswestry Disability Index. (Redrawn from Fairbank JC, Couper J, Davies JB et al: The Oswestry low back pain disability questionnaire, *Physiotherapy* 66:271–273, 1980.)

Hendler 10-Minute Screening Test for Chronic Back Pain Patients

Instructions: Each question is asked by an examiner, and the patient is given points according to the response that he makes. The number of points to be awarded for the various responses is shown in the column at the right. At the end of the test, the examiner calculates the total number of points. The results are interpreted as explained in the Key.

		Points
I	**How did the pain that you now experience occur?**	
	(a) Sudden onset with accident or definable event	0
	(b) Slow, progressive onset without acute exacerbation	1
	(c) Slow, progressive onset with acute exacerbation without accident or event	2
	(d) Sudden onset without an accident or definable event	3
II	**Where do you experience the pain?**	
	(a) One site, specific, well-defined, consistent with anatomical distribution	0
	(b) More than one site, each well-defined and consistent with anatomical distribution	1
	(c) One site, inconsistent with anatomical considerations, or not well-defined	2
	(d) Vague description, more than one site, of which one is inconsistent with anatomical considerations, or not well-defined or anatomically explainable	3
III	**Do you ever have trouble falling asleep at night, or are you ever awakened from sleep?**	

If the answer is "no," score 3 points and go to question IV. If the answer is "yes," proceed:

What keeps you from falling asleep, or what awakens you from sleep?

		Points
IIIA	(a) Trouble falling asleep every night due to pain	0
	(b) Trouble falling asleep due to pain more than three times a week	1
	(c) Trouble falling asleep due to pain less than three times a week	2
	(d) No trouble falling asleep due to pain	3
	(e) Trouble falling asleep which is not related to pain	4
IIIB	(a) Awakened by pain every night	0
	(b) Awakened from sleep by pain more than three times a week	1
	(c) Not awakened from sleep by pain more than twice a week	2
	(d) Not awakened from sleep by pain	3
	(e) Restless sleep, or early morning awakening with or without being able to return to sleep, both unrelated to pain	4
IV	**Does weather have any effect on your pain?**	
	(a) The pain is always worse in both cold and damp weather.	0
	(b) The pain is always worse with damp weather or with cold weather.	1
	(c) The pain is occasionally worse with cold or damp weather.	2
	(d) The weather has no effect on the pain.	3
V	**How would you describe the type of pain that you have?**	
	(a) Burning; or sharp, shooting pain; or pins and needles; or coldness; or numbness	0

		Points
	(b) Dull, aching pain, with occasional sharp, shooting pains not helped by heat; or, the patient is experiencing hyperesthesia	1
	(c) Spasm-type pain, tension-type pain, or numbness over the area, relieved by massage or heat	2
	(d) Nagging or bothersome pain	3
	(e) Excruciating, overwhelming, or unbearable pain, relieved by massage or heat	4
VI	**How frequently do you have your pain?**	
	(a) The pain is constant.	0
	(b) The pain is nearly constant, occurring 50–80% of the time.	1
	(c) The pain is intermittent, occurring 25–50% of the time.	2
	(d) The pain is only occasionally present, occurring less than 25% of the time.	3
VII	**Does movement or position have any effect on the pain?**	
	(a) The pain is unrelieved by position change or rest, and there have been previous operations for the pain.	0
	(b) The pain is worsened by use, standing, or walking; and is relieved by lying down or resting the part.	1
	(c) Position change and use have variable effects on the pain.	2
	(d) The pain is not altered by use or position change, and there have been no previous operations for the pain.	3
VIII	**What medications have you used in the past month?**	
	(a) No medications at all	0
	(b) Use of non-narcotic pain relievers; non-benzodiazepine tranquilizers; or use of antidepressants	1
	(c) Less than three-times-a-week use of a narcotic, hypnotic, or benzodiazepine	2
	(d) Greater than four-times-a-week use of a narcotic, hypnotic, or benzodiazepine	3
IX	**What hobbies do you have, and can you still participate in them?**	
	(a) Unable to participate in any hobbies that were formerly enjoyed	0
	(b) Reduced number of hobbies or activities relating to a hobby	1
	(c) Still able to participate in hobbies but with some discomfort	2
	(d) Participate in hobbies as before	3
X	**How frequently did you have sex and orgasms before the pain, and how frequently do you have sex and orgasms now?**	
	(a^1) Sexual contact, prior to pain, three to four times a week, with no difficulty with orgasm; now sexual contact is 50% or less than previously, and coitus is interrupted by pain	0

Figure 9-46

Hendler 10-Minute Screening Test for Chronic Back Pain Patients. (Redrawn from Hendler N, Vierstein M, Gucer P et al: A preoperative screening test for chronic back pain patients, *Psychosomatics* 20:806–808, 1979. Copyright © Nelson Hendler, M.D., 1979.)

Continued

Points

(a²) (For people over 45) Sexual contact twice a week, with a 50% reduction in frequency since the pain — 0

(a³) (For people over 60) Sexual contact once a week, with a 50% reduction in frequency of coitus since the onset of pain — 0

(b) Pre-pain adjustment as defined above (a¹–a³), with no difficulty with orgasm; now loss of interest in sex and/or difficulty with orgasm or erection — 1

(c) No change in sexual activity now as opposed to before the onset of pain — 2

(d) Unable to have sexual contact since the onset of pain, and difficulty with orgasm or erection prior to the pain — 3

(e) No sexual contact prior to the pain, or absence of orgasm prior to the pain — 4

XI Are you still working or doing your household chores?

(a) Works every day at the same pre-pain job or same level of household duties — 0

(b) Works every day but the job is not the same as pre-pain job, with reduced responsibility or physical activity — 1

(c) Works sporadically or does a reduced amount of household chores — 2

(d) Not at work, or all household chores are now performed by others — 3

XII What is your income now compared with before your injury or the onset of pain, and what are your sources of income?

(a) Any one of the following answers scores — 0
  1. Experiencing financial difficulty with family income 50% or less than previously
  2. Was retired and is still retired
  3. Patient is still working and is not having financial difficulties

(b) Experiencing financial difficulty with family income only 50–75% of the pre-pain income — 1

(c) Patient unable to work, and receives some compensation so that the family income is at least 75% of the pre-pain income — 2

(d) Patient unable to work and receives no compensation, but the spouse works and

Points

family income is still 75% of the pre-pain income — 3

(e) Patient doesn't work, yet the income from disability or other compensation sources is 80% or more of gross pay before the pain; the spouse does not work — 4

XIII Are you suing anyone, or is anyone suing you, or do you have an attorney helping you with compensation or disability payments?

(a) No suit pending, and does not have an attorney — 0

(b) Litigation is pending, but is not related to the pain — 1

(c) The patient is being sued as the result of an accident — 2

(d) Litigation is pending or workmen's compensation case with a lawyer involved — 3

XIV If you had three wishes for anything in the world, what would you wish for?

(a) "Get rid of the pain" is the only wish. — 0

(b) "Get rid of the pain" is one of the three wishes. — 1

(c) Doesn't mention getting rid of the pain, but has specific wishes usually of a personal nature such as for more money, a better relationship with spouse or children, etc. — 2

(d) Does not mention pain, but offers general, nonpersonal wishes such as for world peace — 3

XV Have you ever been depressed or thought of suicide?

(a) Admits to depression; or has a history of depression secondary to pain and associated with crying spells and thoughts of suicide — 0

(b) Admits to depression, guilt, and anger secondary to the pain — 1

(c) Prior history of depression before the pain or a financial or personal loss prior to the pain; now admits to some depression — 2

(d) Denies depression, crying spells, or "feeling blue" — 3

(e) History of a suicide attempt prior to the onset of pain — 4

POINT TOTAL

Key to Hendler Screening Test for Chronic Back Pain

A score of 18 pts or less suggests that the patient is an objective pain patient and is reporting a normal response to chronic pain. One may proceed surgically if indicated, and usually finds the patient quite willing to participate in all modalities of therapy, including exercise and psychotherapy. Occasionally, a person with conversion reaction or posttraumatic neurosis will score less than 18 points; this is because subjective distress is being experienced on an unconscious level. Persons scoring 14 points or less can be considered objective pain patients with more certainty than those at the upper range (14–18) of this group.

A score of 15–20 points suggests that the patient has features of an objective pain patient as well as of an exaggerating pain patient. This implies that a person with a poor premorbid adjustment has an organic lesion that has produced the normal response to pain; however, because of the person's poor pre-pain adjustment, the chronic pain produces a more extreme response than would otherwise occur.

A score of 19–31 points suggests that the patient is an exaggerating pain patient. Surgical or other interventions may be carried out with caution. This type of patient usually has a premorbid (pre-pain) personality that may increase his likelihood of using or benefiting from the complaint of chronic pain. The patient may show improvement after treatment in a chronic pain treatment center, where the main emphasis is placed on an attitude change toward the chronic pain.

A score of 32 points or more suggests that a psychiatric consultation is needed. These patients freely admit to a great many pre-pain problems, and show considerable difficulty in coping with the chronic pain they now experience. Surgical or other interventions should not be carried out without prior approval of a psychiatric consultant. Severe depression, suicide, and psychosis are potential problems in this group of affective pain patients.

Test copyright 1979 by Nelson Hendler, M.D., M.S.

Figure 9-46 cont'd

FUNCTIONAL RATING SCALE FOR THE LUMBAR SPINE

A. Physical criteria   _____
B. Patient's perception   _____
C. Physician's perception   _____
   TOTAL   _____

A. PHYSICAL CRITERIA (Max: 30)
   1. Range of motion—Total flexion and   _____
      extension in degrees
      Points (1 point for every 10 degrees— _____
      15 points maximum)
   2. Trunk strength—Total flexion and extension _____
      in kilograms
      Points (1 point for every 8 kg, male
      patients—15 points maximum)
      Points (1 point for every 4 kg, female
      patients—15 points maximum)

B. PATIENT'S PERCEPTION (Max: 40)
   1. Average pain (visual-analog scale)   (15) _____
   2. How disabled: _____
      No disability, able to work full-time   (10)
      Able to work full-time but at a lower   (8)
      level
      Able to work part-time but at usual   (6)
      level
      Able to work only part-time and at   (4)
      lower level
      Not able to work at all   (0)
   3. Activities you can perform—1 point   _____
      for each **Yes** answer

C. PHYSICIAN'S PERCEPTION (Max: 30)
   1. How much pain would you expect for this   _____
      patient at this time? (visual-analog scale)
   2. At the present time, what is the degree   _____
      of impairment?
      None   (10)
      Mild but should not affect most activities (8)
      Moderate, cannot perform some strenuous
      activities   (6)
      Only light activities, cannot perform any
      strenuous activities   (2)
      Severely limited, cannot perform most light
      activities or some activities of daily living (0)
   3. Current drugs and daily doses (quantity):   _____
      Analgesics (occasional) use = less than 5
      times per week)
      Major narcotic, regular use   (0)
      Major narcotic, occasional use   (2)
      Minor narcotic, regular use   (4)
      Minor narcotic, occasional use   (6)
      Nonnarcotic, regular use   (8)
      Nonnarcotic, occasional use   (10)

TOTAL   _____

Figure 9-47

Functional rating scale for the lumbar spine. (Modified from Lehmann TR, Brand RA, German TW: A low back rating scale, *Spine* 8:309, 1983.)

A Simple Clinical Functional Capacity Evaluation

The test area should be quiet and free of passing people. Put up warning signs for staff and other patients when tests are taking place. The patient should not need to walk a long distance to reach the test area or between the different tests. Ask the patient to wear comfortable shoes and loose clothing.

- *Five minutes of walking.* The distance walked up and down between marks 20 m apart in 5 min. Choose a quiet, empty corridor with a non-slip surface or hard carpet. There should be walls or doors on either side that can be used if necessary for support, but not handrails. Patients should not use walking aids but can use the walls for support or can sit down for a rest. Inform the patient of the time at the end of each lap or every minute if they are slower (mean, 185 m).

- *One minute of stair climbing.* Climbing up and down a straight flight of standard stairs with one handrail and an opposite wall within easy reach. Have a chair available for resting if the patient needs it. Count the number of steps up and down, eg. 20 up and 15 down = 35 steps (mean, 48 steps).

- *One minute of stand-ups.* The number of times the patient can stand up from a chair in 1 min. Use a firm, upright chair with a padded seat and back rest but no arm rests. The seat height should be about 45 cm, or 18 inches. There should not be any wall or other furniture within reach that the patient could use for support (mean, 11 stand-ups).

Standardization of test instructions. The tester should have written instructions. The test should have written instructions. The tester must respond neutrally at all times and maintain a 'test' atmosphere. Do not give the patient any advice or encouragement during the tests as feedback influences their performance. Only give information on the time to help patients to pace themselves if they are able. Tell the patient this is a test of current performance. It is a measure of how much they can manage, bearing in mind the journey home after their assessment. These instructions are designed to prevent anxiety and over-exertion.

Figure 9-48

Simple clinical functional capacity evaluation as described by Waddell. (From Waddell G: *The back Pain Revolution*, p. 41, New York, 1998, Churchill Livingstone.)

be useful and discriminate between individuals with and without low back pain:[132]

Timed 15 meter (50 foot) Walk. Patient walks 7.5 m (25 ft) as fast as he or she can, turns, and returns to the starting position while being timed.

Loaded Reach Test. Patient stands next to a wall, which has a meter ruler at shoulder height. The patient reaches forward with weight at shoulder height as far as he or she can while keeping the heels on the floor. The weight should not exceed a maximum of 5% of body weight or 4.5 kg (9.9 lbs).

Repeated Sit-to-Stand. This timed test involves the patient starting by sitting in a chair. The patient then stands fully and returns to sitting, repeating the sequence as fast as possible. The average value of two trials is used as the time.

Repeated Trunk Flexion.[133] This timed test involves the patient starting in a standing position and then flexing forward as far as possible and returning to the upright posture as fast as tolerable, repeating the motion 10 times. The average value of two trials is used as the time.

Biering-Sorensen Fatigue Test. Described previously under "Resisted Isometric Movements."

Special Tests

Special tests should always be considered as an integral part of a much larger examination process.[134] They should never be used in isolation. Because these are clinical tests and commonly depend on the skill of the examiner, many of them show low reliability and validity.[135–137] The reliability, validity, specificity, and sensitivity of some special/diagnostic tests used in the lumbar spine are outlined in Appendix 9–1.

When the examiner performs special tests in the lumbar assessment, the straight leg raising test, the prone knee bending test, and the slump test should always be done, especially if there are neurological symptoms. The other tests need be done only if the examiner believes they are relevant or to confirm a diagnosis.

Tests for Neurological Dysfunction (Neurodynamic Tests)

Neurodynamic tests check the mechanical movement of the neurological tissues as well as their sensitivity to mechanical stress or compression.[138,139] These neurodynamic tests, along with relevant history and decreased range of motion, are considered by some to be the most important physical signs of disc herniation,[140] regardless of the degree of disc injury. Most of the special tests for neurological involvement are progressive or sequential. The patient is positioned, and one maneuver is tried; if no symptoms result, a second provocative, enhancing, or sensitizing maneuver is carried out, and so on, while the examiner watches to see if the patient's symptoms

are reproduced. The order in which these maneuvers are done also makes a difference. For example, with straight leg raising, the results are different if the hip is flexed with the knee extended than if the hip is flexed with the knee first flexed and then extended after the hip is in position.

> **Neurodynamic Tests Commonly Performed on the Lumbar Spine**
>
> • Slump test
> • Straight leg raising test
> • Prone knee bending test

Because of **tension points,** the neurological tissues move in different directions (Figure 9-49) depending on where the stress is applied,[139,141] and the direction of movement varies depending on where movement is initiated. For example, when doing the straight leg raising test, movement is toward the hip; with dorsiflexion as a sensitizing maneuver, the neurological tissue moves toward the ankle. If knee extension is performed in the slump test, the neurological tissue moves toward the knee.[138] This movement in different directions or in convergence

Figure 9-49
Postulated neurobiomechanics that occur with slump movement. The approximate points C6, T6, L4, and the knee are where the neural tissue does not move in relation to the movements of the spinal canal. It is important to understand, however, that movement of neurological tissue is toward the joint where movement was initiated. (Modified from Butler DS: *Mobilisation of the nervous system,* pp. 41–42, Melbourne, 1991, Churchill Livingstone.)

toward the joint being moved can produce different symptoms depending on where and in what direction the movement occurs. The neurological tissue may move in one direction for one part of the test and in another direction for the next part of the test. Pathology may restrict this normal movement. Tension points are areas where there is minimal movement of the neurological tissue. According to Butler,[139] these areas are C6, the elbow, the shoulder, T6, L4, and the knee. It is important to realize, however, that the amount of tension placed on these points depends on the position of the extremity.

For a neurodynamic test to be positive, it must reproduce the patient's symptoms. Because these are provocative tests designed to put stress on the neurological tissue, they often cause discomfort or pain, which may be bilateral. However, if the patient's symptoms are not reproduced, the test should be considered negative. As a second check for a positive test, the symptoms that have been produced may be increased or decreased by adding or taking away the sensitizing parts of the test.[142]

The examiner has no need to do all or most of the neurodynamic tests listed. Some examiners will find one method more effective, others will find other tests more effective. The examiner should develop the skill to do two or three tests effectively and develop an understanding of how the neurological tissue is being stretched and which neurological tissue in particular is demonstrating signs and symptoms.

Slump Test. The slump test has become the most common neurological test for the lower limb. The patient is seated on the edge of the examining table with the legs supported, the hips in neutral position (i.e., no rotation, abduction, or adduction), and the hands behind the back (Figure 9-50). The examination is performed in sequential steps. First, the patient is asked to "slump" the back into thoracic and lumbar flexion. The examiner maintains the patient's chin in the neutral position to prevent neck and head flexion. The examiner then uses one arm to apply overpressure across the shoulders to maintain flexion of the thoracic and lumbar spines. While this position is held, the patient is asked to actively flex the cervical spine and head as far as possible (i.e., chin to chest). The examiner then applies overpressure to maintain flexion of all three parts of the spine (cervical, thoracic, and lumbar) using the hand of the same arm to maintain overpressure in the cervical spine. With the other hand, the examiner then holds the patient's foot in maximum dorsiflexion. While the examiner holds these positions, the patient is asked to actively straighten the knee as much as possible. The test is repeated with the other leg and then with both legs at the same time. If the patient is unable to fully extend the knee because of pain, the examiner releases the overpressure to the cervical spine and the patient actively extends the neck. If the knee extends further, the symptoms decrease with neck extension, or if the positioning of the patient increases the patient's symptoms, then the test is considered positive for increased tension in the neuromeningeal tract.[143–146] Some clinicians modify the test to make the knee extension of the test passive. Once the patient is positioned with the three parts of the spine in flexion, the examiner first passively extends the knee. If symptoms do not result, then the examiner passively dorsiflexes the foot. A positive test would indicate the same lesion.

Butler advocated doing bilateral knee extension in the slump position.[139] Any asymmetry in the amount of knee extension is easier to note this way. Also, the effect of releasing neck flexion on the patient's symptoms should be noted. Butler has also suggested modifications to the slump test to stress individual nerves[139] (Table 9-12 and Figure 9-51). In hypermobile patients, more hip flexion (more than 90°), as well as hip adduction and medial rotation may be required to elicit a positive response.[139] It is important that if symptoms are produced in any phase of the sequence, the provocative maneuvers are stopped to prevent undue discomfort to the patient.

When doing the slump test, the examiner is looking for reproduction of the patient's pathological symptoms, not just the production of symptoms.[147] The test does place stress on certain tissues, so some discomfort or pain is not necessarily symptomatic for the problem. For example, nonpathological responses include pain or discomfort in the area of T8-T9 (in 50% of normal patients), pain or discomfort behind the extended knee and hamstrings, symmetric restriction of knee extension, symmetric restriction of ankle dorsiflexion, and symmetric increased range of knee extension and ankle dorsiflexion on release of neck flexion.[139]

Sitting Root Test. This test is a modification of the slump test. The patient sits with a flexed neck. The knee is actively extended while the hip remains flexed at 90°. Increased pain indicates tension on the sciatic nerve. This test is sometimes used to catch the patient unaware. In this case, the examiner passively extends the knee while pretending to examine the foot. Patients with true sciatic pain arch backward and complain of pain into the buttock, posterior thigh, and calf when the leg is straightened, indicating a positive test.[148] The **Bechterewis test** follows a similar pattern.[149] The patient is asked to extend one knee at a time. If no symptoms result, the patient is asked to extend both legs simultaneously. Symptoms in the back or leg indicate a positive response.[150]

Straight Leg Raising Test. Also known as Lasègue's test, the straight leg raising test (Figure 9-52) is done with the patient completely relaxed.[151–158] It is one of the most common neurological tests of the lower limb. It is a passive test, and each leg is tested individually with the normal leg being tested first. With the patient in the supine position, the hip medially rotated and adducted and the knee extended, the examiner flexes the hip until the patient complains of pain or tightness in the back or back of the leg.[139] If the pain is primarily back pain,

Figure 9-50

Sequence of subject postures in the slump test. **A,** Patient sits erect with hands behind back. **B,** Patient slumps lumbar and thoracic spine while either patient or examiner keeps the head in neutral. **C,** Examiner pushes down on shoulders while patient holds head in neutral. **D,** Patient flexes head. **E,** Examiner carefully applies overpressure to cervical spine. **F,** Examiner extends patient's knee while holding the cervical spine flexed. **G,** While holding the knee extended and cervical spine flexed, the examiner dorsiflexes the foot. **H,** Patient extends head, which should relieve any symptoms. If symptoms are reproduced at any stage, further sequential movements are not attempted.

Table 9-12

Slump Test and Its Modifications

	Slump Test (ST1)	Slump Test (ST2)	Side Lying Slump Test (ST3)	Long Sitting Slump Test (ST4)
Cervical spine	Flexion	Flexion	Flexion	Flexion, rotation
Thoracic and lumbar spine	Flexion (slump)	Flexion (slump)	Flexion (slump)	Flexion (slump)
Hip	Flexion (90°+)	Flexion (90°+), abduction	Flexion (20°)	Flexion (90°+)
Knee	Extension	Extension	Flexion	Extension
Ankle	Dorsiflexion	Dorsiflexion	Plantar flexion	Dorsiflexion
Foot	—	—	—	—
Toes	—	—	—	—
Nerve bias	Spinal cord, cervical and lumbar nerve roots, sciatic nerve	Obturator nerve	Femoral nerve	Spinal cord, cervical and lumbar nerve roots, sciatic nerve

Data from Butler DA: *Mobilisation of the nervous system,* Melbourne, 1991, Churchill Livingstone.

it is more likely a disc herniation from pressure on the anterior theca of the spinal cord,[159] or the pathology causing the pressure is more central. "Back pain only" patients who have a disc prolapse have smaller, more central prolapses.[159] If pain is primarily in the leg, it is more likely that the pathology causing the pressure on neurological tissues is more lateral. Disc herniations or pathology causing pressure between the two extremes are more likely to cause pain in both areas.[160] The examiner then slowly and carefully drops the leg back (extends it) slightly until the patient feels no pain or tightness. The patient is then asked to flex the neck so the chin is on the chest, or the examiner may dorsiflex the patient's foot, or both actions may be done simultaneously. Most

Text continued on page 564

A **B**

Figure 9-51

Modifications of the slump test (ST) to stress specific nerve. **A,** Basic ST1 test (spinal cord, nerve roots). **B,** ST2 (obturator nerve).

Continued

Figure 9-51 cont'd
C, ST3 (femoral nerve). **D,** ST4 (spinal cord, nerve roots). See Table 9-12 for movements at each joint.

A

B

C

D

Figure 9-52
Straight leg raising. **A,** Radicular symptoms are precipitated on the same side with straight leg raising. **B,** The leg is lowered slowly until pain is relieved. **C,** The foot is then dorsiflexed, causing a return of symptoms; this indicates a positive test. **D,** To make the symptoms more provocative, the neck can be flexed by lifting the head at the same time as the foot is dorsiflexed.

Table 9-13

Straight Leg Raising (SLR) Test and Its Modifications

	SLR (Basic)	SLR2	SLR3	SLR4	Cross (Well Leg) SLR5
Hip	Flexion and adduction	Flexion	Flexion	Flexion and medial rotation	Flexion
Knee	Extension	Extension	Extension	Extension	Extension
Ankle	Dorsiflexion	Dorsiflexion	Dorsiflexion	Plantar flexion	Dorsiflexion
Foot	—	Eversion	Inversion	Inversion	—
Toes	—	Extension	—	—	—
Nerve bias	Sciatic nerve and tibial nerve	Tibial nerve	Sural nerve	Common peroneal nerve	Nerve root (disc prolapse)

Data from Butler DA: *Mobilisation of the nervous system,* Melbourne, 1991, Churchill Livingstone.

Figure 9-53

Modifications to straight leg raising (SLR) to stress specific nerve. **A,** Basic SLR and SLR2 (sciatic and tibial nerves). **B,** SLR3 (sural nerve). **C,** SLR4 (common peroneal nerve). **D,** SLR5 (intervertebral disc and nerve root). See Table 9-13 for movements at each joint.

commonly, foot dorsiflexion is done first. Both of these maneuvers are considered to be provocative or sensitizing tests for neurological tissue. Table 9-13 and Figure 9-53 show modifications of the straight leg raising test that can be used to stress different peripheral nerves to a greater degree; these are referred to as straight leg raising tests with a particular nerve bias.

The neck flexion movement has also been called **Hyndman's sign, Brudzinski's sign, Lidner's sign,** and the **Soto-Hall test.** If the examiner desires, neck flexion may be done by itself as a passive movement (passive neck flexion). Tension in the cervicothoracic junction is normal and should not be considered a production of symptoms. If lumbar, leg, or arm symptoms are produced, the neurological tissue is involved. The ankle dorsiflexion movement has also been called the **Bragard's test.** Pain that increases with neck flexion, ankle dorsiflexion, or both indicates stretching of the dura mater of the spinal cord or a lesion within the spinal cord (e.g., disc herniation, tumor, meningitis). Pain that does not increase with neck flexion may indicate a lesion in the hamstring area (tight hamstrings) or in the lumbosacral or sacroiliac joints. **Sicard's test** involves straight leg raising and then extension of the big toe instead of foot dorsiflexion. **Turyn's test** involves only extension of the big toe.[161]

With unilateral straight leg raising, the nerve roots, primarily the L5, S1, and S2 nerve roots (sciatic nerve), are normally completely stretched at 70°, having an excursion of approximately 2 to 6 cm (0.8 to 2.4 inches).[156] Pain after 70° is probably joint pain from the lumbar area (e.g., facet joints) or sacroiliac joints (Figure 9-54). However, if the examiner suspects hamstring tightness, the hamstrings must also be cleared by examination (see Chapter 11). The examiner should compare the two legs for any differences. Although the sciatic nerve roots are commonly stretched at 70° hip flexion, the ROM for straight leg raising and the stress placed on the neurological tissue vary greatly from person to person. For example, patients who are very hypermobile (e.g., gymnasts, synchronized swimmers) may not show a positive straight leg raising test until 110° to 120° of hip flexion, even in the presence of nerve root pathology. It is more important to compare left and right sides for symptoms before deciding whether a lesion is caused by stretching of the neurological tissue or arises from the joints or other soft tissues.

During the unilateral straight leg raising test, tension develops in a sequential manner. It first develops in the greater sciatic foramen, then over the ala of the sacrum, next in the area where the nerve crosses over the pedicle, and finally in the intervertebral foramen. The test causes traction on the sciatic nerve, lumbosacral nerve roots, and dura mater. Adhesions within these areas may result from herniation of the intervertebral disc or extradural or meningeal irritation. Pain comes from the dura mater, nerve root, adventitial sheath of the epidural veins, or synovial facet joints. The test is positive if pain extends from the back down into the leg in the sciatic nerve distribution.

A central protrusion of an intervertebral disc (L4 or L5 disc affecting nerve roots from L4 down to S3) leads to pain primarily in the back with the possibility of bowel and bladder symptoms; a protrusion in the intermediate area causes pain in the posterior aspect of the lower limb and low back; and a lateral protrusion causes pain primarily in the posterior leg with pain below the knee.

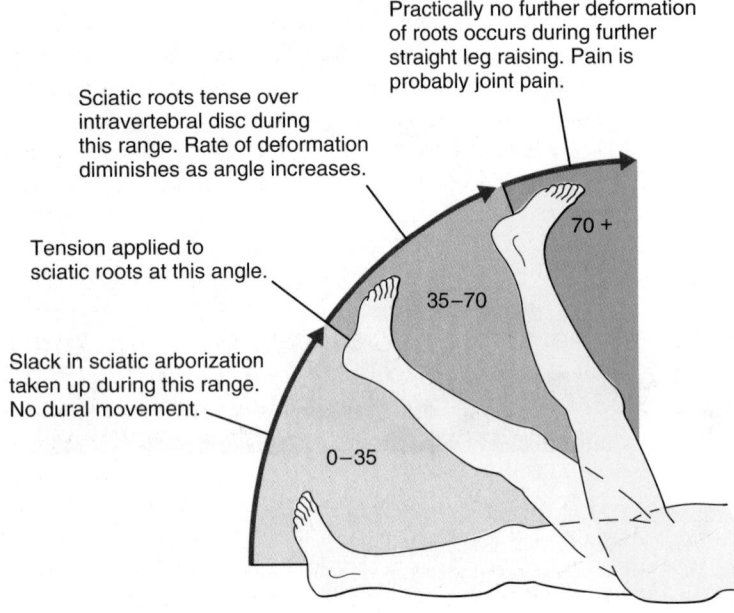

Practically no further deformation of roots occurs during further straight leg raising. Pain is probably joint pain.

Sciatic roots tense over intravertebral disc during this range. Rate of deformation diminishes as angle increases.

Tension applied to sciatic roots at this angle.

Slack in sciatic arborization taken up during this range. No dural movement.

70 +

35–70

0–35

Figure 9-54
Dynamics of single straight leg raising test in most people. (Modified from Fahrni WS: Observations on straight leg raising with special reference to nerve root adhesions, *Can J Surg* 9:44, 1966.)

Figure 9-55

Modified straight leg raising for patients who cannot lie supine. **A,** Starting position with knee flexed to 90°.
B, Knee is extended as far as possible.

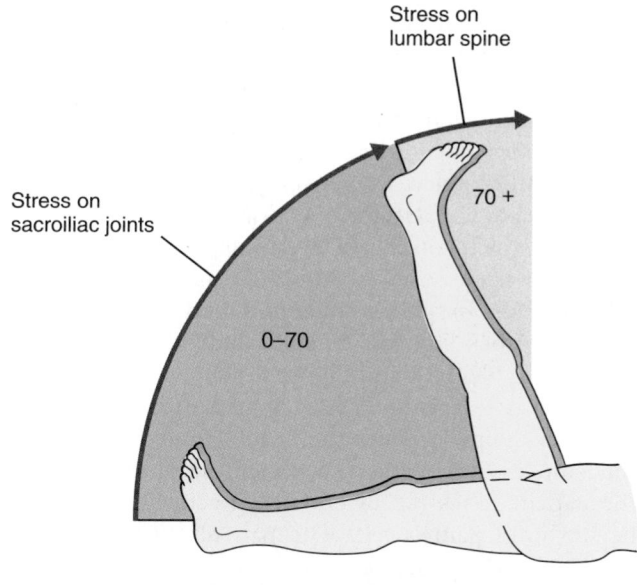

Figure 9-56

Dynamics of the bilateral straight leg raise.

Having said this, however, the examiner must realize that the intervertebral disc is only one cause of back pain.

For patients who have difficulty lying supine, a **modified straight leg raising test** has been suggested.[162] The patient is in a side lying position with the test leg uppermost and the hip and knee at 90°. The lumbosacral spine is in neutral but may be positioned in slight flexion or extension if this is more comfortable for the patient. The examiner then passively extends the patient's knee (Figure 9-55), noting pain, resistance, and reproduction of the patient's symptoms for a positive test. The knee

position (amount of flexion remaining) on the affected side is compared with that on the good side.

The examiner should then test both legs simultaneously (**bilateral straight leg raising,** Figure 9-56). This test must be done with care, because the examiner is lifting the weight of both lower limbs and thereby placing a large stress on the examiner's lumbar spine. With the patient relaxed in the supine position and knees extended, the examiner lifts both of the legs by flexing the patient's hips until the patient complains of pain or tightness. Because both legs are lifted the pelvis is not stabilized (as it would be by one leg in unilateral straight leg raise), so on hip flexion the pelvis is freer to rotate, thereby decreasing the stress on the neurological tissue. If the test causes pain before 70° of hip flexion, the lesion is probably in the sacroiliac joints; if the test causes pain after 70°, the lesion is probably in the lumbar spine area.

With the unilateral straight leg raising test, 80° to 90° of hip flexion is normal. If one leg is lifted and the patient complains of pain on the opposite side, it is an indication of a space-occupying lesion (e.g., a herniated disc, inflammatory swelling). This finding of pain when the examiner is testing the opposite (good) leg may be called the **well leg raising test of Fajersztajn** (Figure 9-57), a **prostrate leg raising test,** a **sciatic phenomenon, Lhermitt's test,** or the **crossover sign.**[148,156,163] It is typically indicates a rather large intervertebral disc protrusion, usually medial to the nerve root (see Figure 9-57), and a poor prognosis for conservative treatment.[156,164] The test causes stretching of the ipsilateral as well as the contralateral nerve root, pulling laterally on the dural sac. A positive Lasègue's and crossover sign can also indicate the degree of disc injury. For example, both are limited to a greater degree if

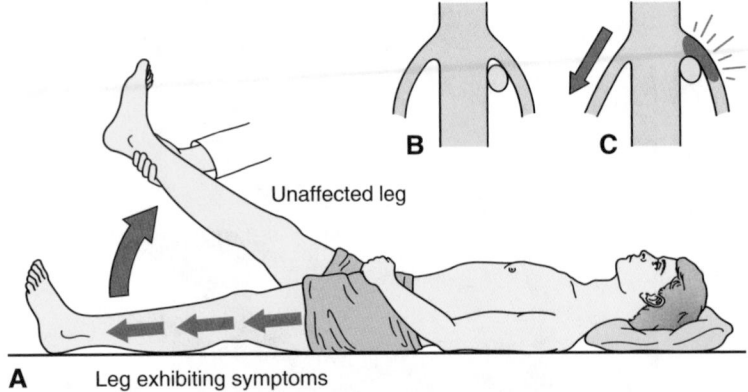

Figure 9-57

Well leg raising test of Fajersztajn. **A,** Movement of nerve roots occurs when the leg on the opposite side is raised. **B,** Position of disc and nerve root before opposite leg is lifted. **C,** When the leg is raised on the unaffected side, the roots on the opposite side slide slightly downward and toward the midline. In the presence of a disc lesion, this movement increases the root tension resulting in radicular signs in the affected leg, which remains on the table. (Modified from DePalma AF, Rothman RH: *The intervertebral disc,* Philadelphia, 1970, WB Saunders.)

Figure 9-58

Prone knee bending test (PKB1), which stresses the femoral nerve and L2-L4 nerve root. The examiner is pointing to where pain may be expected in the lumbar spine with a positive test.

sequestration of the disc occurs.[70] If the examiner finds this test positive, careful questioning about bowel and bladder symptoms is a necessity. Many, but not all, patients with a central protrusion are candidates for surgery, especially if there are bowel and bladder symptoms.

Prone Knee Bending (Nachlas) Test. The patient lies prone while the examiner passively flexes the knee as far as possible so that the patient's heel rests against the buttock.[165,166] At the same time, the examiner should ensure that the patient's hip is not rotated. If the examiner is unable to flex the patient's knee past 90° because of a pathological condition in the hip, the test may be performed by passive extension of the hip while the knee is flexed as much as possible. Unilateral neurological pain in the lumbar area, buttock, or posterior thigh may indicate an L2 or L3 nerve root lesion (Figure 9-58).

This test also stretches the femoral nerve. Pain in the anterior thigh indicates tight quadriceps muscles or stretching of the femoral nerve. A careful history and pain differentiation helps delineate the problem. If the rectus femoris is tight, the examiner should remember that taking the heel to the buttock may cause anterior torsion to the ilium, which could lead to sacroiliac or lumbar pain. The flexed knee position should be maintained for 45 to 60 seconds. Butler has suggested modifications of the prone knee bending test to stress individual peripheral nerves[139] (Table 9-14 and Figure 9-59).

Brudzinski-Kernig Test. The patient is supine with the hands cupped behind the head (Figure 9-60).[167–170] The patient is instructed to flex the head onto the chest. The patient raises the extended leg actively by flexing the hip until pain is felt. The patient then flexes the knee, and if the pain disappears, it is considered a positive test. The mechanics of the Brudzinski-Kernig test are similar to those of the straight leg raising test except that the patient performs the movements actively. Pain is a positive sign and may indicate meningeal irritation, nerve root involvement, or dural irritation. Brudzinski originally described the neck flexion aspect of the test, and Kernig described the hip flexion component. The two parts of the test may be done individually, in which case they are described as the test of the original author.

Naffziger's Test. The patient lies supine while the examiner gently compresses the jugular veins (which lie beside the carotid artery) for approximately 10 seconds (Figure 9-61). The patient's face flushes, and then the patient is asked to cough. If coughing causes pain in the

Table 9-14

Prone Knee Bending (PBK) Test and Its Modification

	Basic Prone Knee Bending (PKB1)	Prone Knee Bending (PKB2)	Prone Knee Extension (PKE)
Cervical spine	Rotation to test side	Rotation to test side	—
Thoracic and lumbar spine	Neutral	Neutral	Neutral
Hip	Neutral	Extension, adduction	Extension, abduction, lateral rotation
Knee	Flexion	Flexion	Extended
Ankle	—	—	Dorsiflexion
Foot	—	—	Eversion
Toes	—	—	—
Nerve bias	Femoral nerve, L2-L4 nerve root	Lateral femoral cutaneous nerve	Saphenous nerve

Data from Butler DA: *Mobilisation of the nervous system,* Melbourne, 1991, Churchill Livingstone.

low back, the spinal theca is being compressed, leading to an increase in intrathecal pressure. The theca is the covering (pia mater, arachnoid mater, and dura mater) around the spinal cord.

Valsalva Maneuver. The seated patient is asked to take a breath, hold it, and then bear down as if evacuating the bowels (Figure 9-62). If pain increases, it indicates increased intrathecal pressure. The symptoms may be accentuated by having the patient first flex the hip to a position just short of that causing pain.[156]

Femoral Nerve Traction Test. The patient lies on the unaffected side with the unaffected limb flexed slightly at the hip and knee (Figure 9-63).[171] The patient's back should be straight, not hyperextended. The patient's head should be slightly flexed. The examiner grasps the patient's affected or painful limb and extends the knee while gently extending the hip approximately 15°. The patient's knee is then flexed on the affected side; this movement further stretches the femoral nerve. Neurological pain radiates down the anterior thigh if the test is positive.

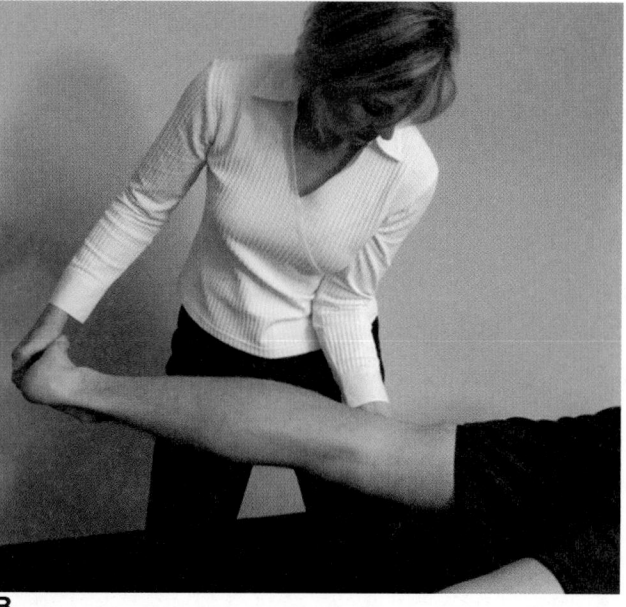

A   **B**

Figure 9-59

Modifications to the prone knee bending (PKB) test to stress specific nerve. **A,** PKB2 (lateral femoral cutaneous nerve). **B,** Prone knee extension, or PKE (saphenous nerve). See Table 9-14 for movements at each joint.

Figure 9-60

Brudzinski-Kernig test. **A,** In Brudzinski's portion of the test, the patient lies supine and elevates the head from the table. When the head is lifted, the patient complains of neck and low back discomfort and attempts to relieve the meningeal irritation by involuntary flexion of the knees and hips. **B,** In the Kernig portion of the test, the patient lies supine with the hip and knee flexed to 90°. The patient then extends the knee. If the patient complains of pain in the lower back, neck, or head on knee extension, it is suggestive of meningeal irritation. Returning to knee flexion will relieve the pain.

Figure 9-62

The Valsalva maneuver. Increased intrathecal pressure leads to symptoms in the sciatic nerve distribution in a positive test.

Figure 9-61

Naffziger's test. This test may be done while the patient is standing or lying down. The examiner applies bilateral compression to the jugular veins, which is hypothesized to increase cerebral spinal fluid pressure. This increased pressure in the subarachnoid space in the root canal may cause back or leg pain by irritating a local mechanical or inflammatory condition.

This is also a traction test for the nerve roots at the midlumbar area (L2-L4). As with the straight leg raising test, there is also a contralateral positive test. That is, when the test is performed, the symptoms occur in the opposite limb. This is called the **crossed femoral** stretching test.[172] Pain in the groin and hip that radiates along the anterior medial thigh indicates an L3 nerve root problem; pain extending to the midtibia indicates an L4 nerve root problem.

This test is similar to Ober's test for a tight iliotibial band, so the examiner must be able to differentiate between the two conditions. If the iliotibial band is tight, the test leg does not adduct but remains elevated away from the table as the tight tendon riding over the greater trochanter keeps the leg abducted. Femoral nerve injury presents with a different history, and the referred pain (anteriorly) tends to be stronger.

"Bowstring" Test (Cram Test or Popliteal Pressure Sign). The examiner carries out a straight leg raising test, and pain results (Figure 9-64).[15,173] While maintaining the thigh in the same position, the examiner flexes the knee slightly (20°), reducing the symptoms. Thumb or finger pressure is then applied to the popliteal area to reestablish the painful radicular symptoms. The test indicates tension or pressure on the sciatic nerve and is a modification of the straight leg raising test.

Figure 9-63
Femoral nerve traction test. **A,** The hip and knee are extended. **B,** Then knee is flexed.

The test may also be done in the sitting position with the examiner passively extending the knee to produce pain. The examiner then slightly flexes the knee so that the pain and symptoms disappear. The examiner holds this slightly flexed position by clasping the patient's leg between the examiner's knees. The examiner then presses the fingers of both hands into the popliteal space. Pain resulting from these maneuvers indicates a positive test and pressure or tension on the sciatic nerve. In this case, the test is called the **sciatic tension test** or **Deyerle's sign.**[58,169,174]

Compression Test.[59] The patient lies supine with the hips and knees flexed. The hips are flexed until the PSISs start to move backward (usually about 100° hip flexion). The examiner then applies direct pressure against the patient's feet or buttocks applying axial compression to the spine. If radicular pain into the posterior leg is produced, the test is thought to be positive for a possible disc herniation.

Flip Sign. While the patient is sitting, the examiner extends the patient's knee and looks for symptoms. The patient is then placed supine, and a unilateral straight leg raising test is performed. For the sign to be positive, both tests must cause pain in the sciatic nerve distribution. If only one test is positive, the examiner should suspect problems in the lower lumbar spine. This is a combination of the classic Lasègue test and the sitting root test.

Knee Flexion Test.[175] The patient, who has complained of sciatica, is in a standing position. The patient is asked to bend forward to touch the toes. If the patient bends the knee on the affected side while forward flexing the spine, the test is positive for sciatic nerve root compression. Likewise, if the patient is not allowed to bend the knee, spinal flexion is decreased.

Babinski Test. The examiner runs a pointed object along the plantar aspect of the patient's foot.[176] A posi-

Figure 9-64
Bowstring sign. **A,** The examiner does a straight leg raise test. If a positive test results, the examiner relieves the pain by flexing the knee slightly. **B,** The examiner then pushes into the popliteal space to increase the stress on the sciatic nerve looking for a return of the same symptoms that present with the straight leg raise test.

tive Babinski test or reflex suggests an upper motor neuron lesion if present on both sides and may be evident in lower motor neuron lesions if seen only on one side. The reflex is demonstrated by extension of the big toe and abduction (splaying) of the other toes. In an infant up to a few weeks old, a positive test is normal. The test is often performed to determine the presence of the Babinski reflex, which is a pathological reflex.

Oppenheim Test. The examiner runs a fingernail along the crest of the patient's tibia.[176] A negative Oppenheim test is indicated by no reaction or no pain. A positive test is indicated by a positive Babinski sign (positive pathological reflex) and suggests an upper motor neuron lesion.

Gluteal Skyline Test. The patient is relaxed in a prone position with the head straight and arms by the sides.[177] The examiner stands at the patient's feet and observes the buttocks from the level of the buttocks. The affected gluteus maximus muscle appears flat as a result of atrophy. The patient is asked to contract the gluteal muscles. The affected side may show less contraction, or it may be atonic and remain flat. If this occurs, the test is positive and may indicate damage to the inferior gluteal nerve or pressure on the L5, S1, or S2 nerve roots.

Tests for Lumbar Instability

Lumbar instability implies that during movement, the patient loses the ability to control the movement for a brief time (milliseconds), or it may mean the segment is structurally unstable. The brief loss of control often results in an **instability jog** or sudden shift of movement in part of the ROM. Pope called this "loss of control in the neutral spine."[178] It commonly occurs with spondylosis owing to degeneration of the disc.[178,179] Structural instability primarily results from spondylolisthesis, and the following tests are designed to test for structural instability.

Common Instability Tests Performed on the Lumbar Spine

- H and I stability test
- Specific torsion test

H and I Stability Tests[59,76]. This set of movements tests for muscle spasm and can be used to detect instability. The H and I monikers relate to the movements that occur (Figure 9-65).

The first part of the test is the "H" movement. The patient stands in the normal resting position, which would be considered the center of the "H". The pain-free side is tested first. The patient is asked, with guidance from the clinician, to side flex as far as possible (the side of

"H"). While in this position, the patient is then asked to flex (the front of the "H") and then move into extension (the back of the "H"). If flexion was more painful than extension, then extension would be done before flexion. The patient then returns to neutral and repeats the movements to the other side. The clinician may stabilize the pelvis with one hand and guide the movement with the other hand on the shoulder.

The second part of the test is the "I" movement. The patient stands in the normal resting position, which would be considered the centre of the "I". Pain-free movement (flexion or extension) is tested first. With guidance from the clinician, the patient is asked to forward flex (or extend) the lumbar spine until the hips start to move (top part of "I"). Once in flexion, the patient is guided into side bending (to the pain free side first "I") followed by return to neutral and then side bending to the opposite side. The patient then returns to neutral standing and does the opposite movement (extension in this case) followed by side bending.

If a hypomobile segment is present, at least two of the movements (the movements into the same quadrant [for example, the top right of the H and I]) would be limited. If instability is present, one quadrant will again be affected, but only by one of the moves (i.e., by the "H" movement or the "I" movement—not both). For example, if the patient had spondylolisthesis instability in anterior shear (a component of forward flexion) and the "I" is attempted, the shear or slip will occur on forward flexion, and there will be little movement during the attempted side bending or flexion. If the "H" is attempted, the side bending will be normal, and the following forward flexion will be full because the shear occurs in the second phase. So, in this case, the "I" movement would be limited but not the "H" movement. This test is primarily for structural instability, but an instability jog may be evident during one of the movements if loss of control occurs. In this case, the end range is commonly normal, but loss of control occurs somewhere in the available ROM.

Specific Lumbar Spine Torsion Test[59,76]. This test stresses specific levels of the lumbar spine. To do this, the specific level must be rotated and stressed. An example would be testing the integrity of left rotation on L5 S1. The patient is placed in a right side lying position with the lumbar spine in slight extension (slight lordosis). To achieve rotation and side bending, the examiner grasps the right arm and pulls it upward and forward at a 45° angle until movement is felt at the L5 spinous process. This "locks" all the vertebrae above L5. The examiner then stabilizes the L5 spinous process by holding the left shoulder back with the examiner's elbow while rotating the pelvis and sacrum forward until S1 starts to move (Figure 9-66) with the opposite hand. Minimal movement should occur, and a normal capsular tissue stretch should be felt when L5 S1 is stressed by carefully

Figure 9-65

H and I stability tests. **A,** H test—side flexion. **B,** H test—side flexion followed by forward flexion. **C,** H test—side flexion followed by extension. **D,** I test—forward flexion. **E,** I test—forward flexion and side flexion. **F,** I test—extension. **G,** I test—extension and side flexion.

A   B

Figure 9-66
Specific lumbar spine torsion test (to L5-S1). **A,** Start position. **B,** Final position.

pushing the shoulder back with the elbow and rotating the pelvis forward with the other arm/hand. This test position is a common position used to manipulate the spine, so the examiner should take care not to overstress the rotation during assessment. In some cases, when doing the test, the examiner may hear a "click" or "pop." This is the same "pop" or "click" that would be heard with a manipulation.

Farfan Torsion Test[9,32]. This nonspecific test stresses the facet joints, joint capsule, supraspinous and interspinous ligaments, neural arch, the longitudinal ligaments, and the disc. The patient lies prone. The examiner stabilizes the ribs and spine (at about T12) with one hand and places the other hand under the anterior aspect of the ilium. The examiner then pulls the ilium backward (Figure 9-67) causing the spine to be rotated on the opposite side producing torque on the opposite side. The test is said

to be positive if it reproduces all or some of the patient's symptoms. The other side is tested for compression.

Lateral Lumbar Spine Stability Test[76]. The patient is placed in side lying with the lumbar spine in neutral. The examiner places the forearm over the side of the thorax at about the L3 level as an example. The examiner then applies a downward pressure to the transverse process of L3, which produces a shear to the side on which the patient is lying for vertebra below L3 and a relative lateral shear in the opposite direction to the segments above L3 (Figure 9-68). The production of the patient's symptoms indicates a positive test.

Test of Anterior Lumbar Spine Instability[76]. The patient is placed in side lying with the hips flexed to 70° and knees flexed. The examiner palpates the desired spinous processes (e.g., L4–5). By pushing the patient's knees posteriorly with the body along the line of the

Figure 9-67
Farfan torsion test.

Figure 9-68
Lateral lumbar spine stability test.

femur, the examiner can feel the relative movement of the L5 spinous process on L4 (Figure 9-69). Normally, there should be little or no movement. Other levels of the spine may be tested in a similar fashion. A problem with the test is that the examiner should ensure that the posterior ligaments of the spine are relatively loose or relaxed. This can be controlled by altering the amount of hip flexion. With greater hip flexion, the posterior ligaments tighten more from the bottom (sacrum) up.

Test of Posterior Lumbar Spine Instability[76]. The patient sits on the edge of the examining table. The examiner stands in front of the patient. The patient places the pronated arms with elbows bent on the anterior aspect of the examiner's shoulders. The examiner puts both hands around the patient so the fingers rest over the lumbar spine and with the heels of the hands gently pull the lumbar spine into full lordosis. To stress L5 on S1, the examiner stabilizes the sacrum with the fingers of both hands and asks the patient to push through the forearm while maintaining the lordotic posture (Figure 9-70). This produces a posterior shear of L5 on S1. Other levels of the spine may be tested in a similar fashion.

Segmental Instability Test. The patient lies prone with the body on the examining table and the legs over the edge resting on the floor (Figure 9-71). The examiner applies pressure to the posterior aspect of the lumbar spine while the patient rests in this position. The patient then lifts the legs off the floor, and the examiner again applies posterior compression to the lumbar spine. If pain is elicited in the resting position only, the test is positive, because the muscle action masks the instability.[180]

Pheasant Test. The patient lies prone. With one hand, the examiner gently applies pressure to the posterior aspect of the lumbar spine. With the other hand,

Figure 9-70
Test of posterior lumbar spine instability.

the examiner passively flexes the patient's knees until the heels touch the buttocks (Figure 9-72). If this hyperextension of the spine causes the patient to feel pain in the leg, the test is considered positive and indicates an unstable spinal segment.[181]

Tests for Joint Dysfunction

One-Leg Standing (Stork Standing) Lumbar Extension Test. The patient stands on one leg and extends the spine while balancing on the leg (Figure 9-73). The test is repeated with the patient standing on the opposite leg. A positive test is indicated by pain in the back and is associated with a pars interarticularis stress

Figure 9-69
Test of anterior lumbar spine stability.

Figure 9-71
Segmental instability test. **A,** Toes on floor. **B,** Feet lifted off floor.

fracture (spondylolisthesis). If the stress fracture is unilateral, standing on the ipsilateral leg causes more pain.[182-184] If rotation is combined with extension and pain results, this indicates possible facet joint pathology on the side to which rotation occurs.

Common Tests for Joint Dysfunction

• One-leg standing lumbar extension test

Quadrant Test. The patient stands with the examiner standing behind. The patient extends the spine while the examiner controls the movement by holding the patient's shoulders. The examiner may use his or her shoulders to hold the occiput and take the weight of the head. Overpressure is applied in extension while the patient side flexes and rotates to the side of pain. The movement is continued until the limit of range is reached or until symptoms are produced (Figure 9-74). The position causes maximum narrowing of the intervertebral foramen and stress on the facet joint to the side on which rotation occurs.[185] The test is positive if symptoms are produced.[186] Cipriano described a similar test as **Kemp's test.**[161]

Schober Test. The Schober test may be used to measure the amount of flexion occurring in the lumbar spine. A point is marked midway between the two PSISs ("dimples of the pelvis"), which is the level of S2; then, points 5 cm (2 inches) below and 10 cm (4 inches) above that level are marked. The distance between the three

Figure 9-72
Pheasant test.

Figure 9-73
One-leg standing lumbar extension test.

Figure 9-74
Quadrant test for the lumbar spine.

points is measured, the patient is asked to flex forward, and the distance is remeasured. The difference between the two measurements indicates the amount of flexion occurring in the lumbar spine. Little reported a modification of the Schober test to measure extension as well.[187] After completion of the flexion movement, the patient extends the spine, and the distance between the marks is noted. Little also advocated using four marking points (one below the dimples and three above) with 10 cm (4 inches) between them.

Yeoman's Test. The patient lies prone while the examiner stabilizes the pelvis and extends each of the patient's hips in turn with the knees extended. The examiner then extends each of the patient's legs in turn with the knee flexed. In both cases, the patient remains passive. A positive test is indicated by pain in the lumbar spine during both parts of the test.

Milgram's Test. The patient lies supine and actively lifts both legs simultaneously off the examining table

5 to 10 cm (2 to 4 inches), holding this position for 30 seconds. The test is positive if the limbs or affected limb cannot be held for 30 seconds or if symptoms are reproduced in the affected limb.[149,150] This test should always be performed with caution because of the high stress load placed on the lumbar spine.

McKenzie's Side Glide Test. The patient stands with the examiner standing to one side. The examiner grasps the patient's pelvis with both hands and places a shoulder against the patient's lower thorax. Using the shoulder as a block, the examiner pulls the pelvis toward the examiner's body (Figure 9-75). The position is held for 10 to 15 seconds, and then the test is

Figure 9-75
McKenzie's side glide test.

repeated on the opposite side.[33,150] If the patient has an evident scoliosis, the side to which the scoliosis curves should be tested first. A positive test is indicated by increased neurological symptoms on the affected side. It also indicates whether the symptoms are actually causing the scoliosis.

Tests for Muscle Tightness

Thomas Test. See Tests for Tight Iliopsoas in Chapter 11.

Ober Test. See Tests for Tight Tensor Fasciae Latae in Chapter 11.

90-90 Straight Leg Raising Test. See Tests for Tight Hamstrings in Chapter 11.

Rectus Femoris Test. See Tests for Tight Rectus Femoris in Chapter 11.

Tests for Muscle Dysfunction

Beevor's Sign. The patient lies supine. The patient flexes the head against resistance, coughs, or attempts to sit up with the hands resting behind the head.[149,188] The sign is positive if the umbilicus does not remain in a straight line when the abdominals contract, indicating pathology in the abdominal muscles (i.e., paralysis).

Tests for Intermittent Claudication

Intermittent claudication implies arterial insufficiency to the tissues. It is most commonly evident when activity occurs because of the increased vascular demand of the tissues. There are two types of intermittent claudication—vascular and neurogenic. The vascular type is most commonly the result of arteriosclerosis, arterial embolism, or thrombo-angiitis obliterans and commonly manifests itself with symptoms in the legs. The neurogenic type is sometimes called **pseudoclaudication** or **cauda equina syndrome** and is commonly associated with spinal stenosis and its effect on circulation to the spinal cord and cauda equina.[189-194] The symptoms in this case may be manifested in the back or sciatic nerve distribution.

Stoop Test. The stoop test is performed to assess neurogenic intermittent claudication to determine whether a relation exists among neurogenic symptoms, posture, and walking.[195] When the patient with neurogenic intermittent claudication walks briskly, pain ensues in the buttock and lower limb within a distance of 50 m (165 feet). To relieve the pain, the patient flexes forward. These symptoms may also be relieved when the patient is sitting and forward flexing. If flexion does not relieve the symptoms, the test is negative. Extension may also be used to bring the symptoms back.

Bicycle Test of van Gelderen[196]. The patient is seated on an exercise bicycle and is asked to pedal against resistance. The patient starts pedaling while leaning backward to accentuate the lumbar lordosis (Figure 9-76). If pain into the buttock and posterior thigh occurs, followed

Figure 9-76

Bicycle test of van Gelderen. **A,** Sitting erect. **B,** Sitting flexed.

by tingling in the affected lower extremity, the first part of the test is positive. The patient is then asked to lean forward while continuing to pedal. If the pain subsides over a short period of time, the second part of the test is positive; if the patient sits upright again, the pain returns. The test determines whether the patient has neurogenic intermittent claudication.

Treadmill Test[197,198]. This test may also be used to determine if the patient has intermittent claudication. Two trials are conducted—one at 1.2 mph and one at the patient's preferred walking speed. The patient walks upright (no leaning forward or holding hand rails is allowed) on the treadmill for 15 minutes or until the onset of severe symptoms (symptoms that would make patient stop walking in usual life situations). Time to first symptoms, total ambulatory time, and precipitating symptoms are recorded.

Tests for Malingering

Hoover Test. The patient lies supine. The examiner places one hand under each calcaneus while the patient's legs remain relaxed on the examining table (Figure 9-77).[199–201] The patient is then asked to lift one leg off the table, keeping the knees straight, as for active straight leg raising. If the patient does not lift the leg or the examiner does not feel pressure under the opposite heel, the patient is probably not really trying or may be a malingerer. If the lifted limb is weaker, however, pressure under the normal heel increases, because of the increased effort to lift the weak leg. The two sides are compared for differences.

Burns Test. The patient is asked to kneel on a chair and then bend forward to touch the floor with the fingers (Figure 9-78). The test is positive for malingering

Figure 9-77

The Hoover test. **A,** Normally, when the patient attempts to elevate one leg, the opposite leg pushes down as a counterbalance. **B,** When the "weak" leg attempts to elevate but the opposite (asymptomatic) leg does not help by pushing down, at least some of the weakness is probably feigned.

Figure 9-78

Burns test.

if the patient is unable to perform the test or the patient overbalances.[150]

Other Tests

Sign of the Buttock. The patient lies supine,[128] and the examiner performs a passive unilateral straight leg raising test. If there is unilateral restriction, the examiner then flexes the knee to see whether hip flexion increases. If the problem is in the lumbar spine or hamstrings, hip flexion increases when the knee is flexed. This finding indicates a negative sign of the buttock test. If hip flexion does not increase when the knee is flexed, it is a positive sign of the buttock test and indicates pathology in the buttock behind the hip joint, such as a bursitis, tumor, or abscess.[202] The patient should also exhibit a noncapsular pattern of the hip.

Reflexes and Cutaneous Distribution

After the special tests, the reflexes should be checked for differences between the two sides (Figure 9-79) if one suspects neurological involvement in the patient's problem.

Reflexes of the Lumbar Spine

- Patellar (L3-L4)
- Medial hamstring (L5-S1)
- Lateral hamstring (S1-S2)
- Posterior tibial (L4-L5)
- Achilles (S1-S2)

The deep tendon reflexes are tested with a reflex hammer, with the patient's muscles and tendons relaxed. The patellar reflex may be performed with the patient sitting or lying, and the hammer strikes the tendon directly. To test the patellar reflex (C3–C4), the knee is flexed to 30° (supine lying) or 90° (sitting). The Achilles reflex (S1–S2) may be tested in prone, sitting, or kneeling position. To test the Achilles reflex, the ankle is at 90° or slightly dorsiflexed. The examiner must ensure that the patient's dorsiflexors are relaxed before doing the test; otherwise, the test will not work. This is done by passively dorsiflexing the foot and feeling for the "springing back" of the foot into plantar flexion. If this does not occur, the dorsiflexors are not relaxed. To test the hamstring reflex (semimembrinosus: L5, S1, and biceps femoris: S1–S2), the examiner places the thumb over the appropriate tendon and taps the thumbnail to elicit the reflex. Again, the knee should be slightly flexed with the hamstrings relaxed to perform the test.

Figure 9-79

Reflexes of the lower limb. **A,** Patellar (L3) in sitting position. **B,** Patellar (L3) in lying position. **C,** Medial hamstrings (L5) in supine lying position. **D,** Lateral hamstrings (S1, S2) in prone lying position.

Continued

Figure 9-79 cont'd

E, Achilles (S1) in sitting position. **F,** Achilles (S1) in kneeling position. **G,** Posterior tibial (L4, L5) in prone lying position.

Neurogenic intermittent claudication may cause the reflexes to be absent soon after exercise (Table 9-15).[203,204] If neurogenic intermittent claudication is suspected, it is necessary to test the reflexes immediately, because reflexes may return within 1 to 3 minutes after stopping the activity.

Another reflex that may be tested is the **superficial cremasteric reflex,** which occurs in males only (Figure 9-80). The patient lies supine while the examiner strokes the inner side of the upper thigh with a pointed object. The test is negative if the scrotal sac on the tested side pulls up. Absence or reduction of the reflex bilaterally suggests an upper motor neuron lesion. A unilateral absence suggests a lower motor neuron lesion between L1 and L2. Absences have increased significance if they are associated with increased deep tendon reflexes.[205]

Two other superficial reflexes are the **superficial abdominal reflex** (Figure 9-81) and the **superficial anal reflex**. To test the superficial abdominal reflex, the examiner uses a pointed object to stroke each quadrant of the abdomen of the supine patient in a triangular fashion around the umbilicus. Absence of the reflex (reflex movement of the skin) indicates an upper motor neuron lesion; unilateral absence indicates a lower motor neuron lesion from T7 to L2, depending on where the absence is noted, as a result of the segmental innervation. The examiner tests the superficial anal reflex by touching the perianal skin. A normal result is shown by contraction of the anal sphincter muscles (S2–S4).

Finally, the examiner should perform one or more of the pathological reflex tests (see Table 1-33) used to determine upper motor lesions or pyramidal tract disease, such as the Babinski or Oppenheim tests (see "Special Tests"). The presence of these reflexes indicates the possible presence of disease or upper motor neuron lesion, whereas their absence reflects the normal situation.

If neurological symptoms are found, the examiner must check the dermatome patterns of the nerve roots as well as the peripheral sensory distribution of

Table 9-15

Differential Diagnosis of Intermittent Claudication

	Vascular	Neurogenic
Pain	Related to exercise; occurs at various sites simultaneously	Related to exercise; sensations spread from area to area
Pulse	Absent after exercise	Present after exercise
Protein content of cerebrospinal fluid	Normal	Raised
Sensory change	Variable	Follows more specific dermatomes
Reflexes	Normal	Decreased but returns quickly

Figure 9-81
Superficial abdominal reflex.

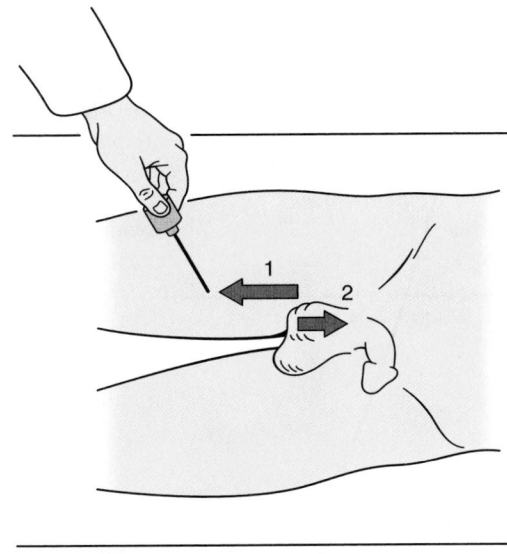

Figure 9-80
Cremasteric reflex. *1,* The examiner runs a sharp object along the inner thigh. *2,* A negative reflex is indicated by the scrotum's rising on that side.

the peripheral nerves (Table 9-16 and Figure 9-82). Remember that dermatomes vary from person to person, and the accompanying representations are estimations only. The examiner tests for sensation by running relaxed hands over the back, abdomen, and lower limbs (front, sides, and back), being sure to cover all aspects of the leg and foot. If any difference between the sides is noted during this **sensation scan,** the examiner may then use a pinwheel, pin, cotton ball, or brush to map out the exact area of sensory

difference and determine the peripheral nerve or nerve root affected.

Pain may be referred from the lumbar spine to the sacroiliac joint and down the leg as far as the foot. Seldom is pain referred up the spine (Figure 9-83). Pain may be referred to the lumbar spine from the abdominal organs, the lower thoracic spine, and the sacroiliac joints. Muscles may also refer pain to the lumbar area (Table 9-17).[206]

Peripheral Nerve Injuries of the Lumbar Spine

Lumbosacral Tunnel Syndrome. This syndrome involves compression of the L5 nerve root as it passes under the iliolumbar ligament in the iliolumbar canal (Figure 9-84). The usual cause of compression is trauma (inflammation), osteophytes, or a tumor. Symptoms are primarily sensory (L5 dermatome) and pain. There is minimal or no effect on the L5 myotome.[207]

Joint Play Movements

The joint play movements have special importance in the lumbar spine because they are used to determine the end feel of joint movement as well as the presence of joint play. They are often used to replace passive movements in the lumbar spine, which are difficult to perform because of the need to move the heavy trunk or lower limbs. As

Table 9-16

Peripheral Nerve Lesions

Nerve (Root Derivation)	Sensory Supply	Sensory Loss	Motor Loss	Reflex Change	Lesion
Lateral cutaneous nerve of thigh (L2–L3)	Lateral thigh	Lateral thigh; often intermittent	None	None	Lateral inguinal entrapment
Posterior cutaneous nerve of thigh (S1–S2)	Posterior thigh	Posterior thigh	None (N.B. sciatic often involved too)	None (N.B. sciatic nerve often involved too)	Local (buttock) trauma Pelvic mass Hip fracture
Obturator nerve (L2–L4)	Medial thigh	Often none ± medial thigh	Thigh adduction	None	Pelvic mass
Femoral nerve (L2–L4)	Anteromedial thigh and leg	Anteromedial thigh and leg	Knee extension ± hip flexion	Diminished knee jerk	Retroperitoneal or pelvic mass Femoral artery aneurysm (or puncture) Diabetic mononeuritis
Saphenous branch of femoral nerve (L2–L4)	Anteromedial knee and medial leg	Medial leg	None (N.B. positive Tinel sign 5 to 10 cm above medial femoral epicondyle of knee)	None (N.B. positive Tinel sign 5 to 10 cm above medial femoral epicondyle of knee)	Local trauma Entrapment above medial femoral condyle
Sciatic nerve (L4–L5, S1)	Anterior and posterior leg Sole and dorsum of foot	Entire foot	Foot dorsiflexion Foot inversion ± plantar flexion ± knee flexion	Diminished ankle jerk	Pelvic mass Hip fracture Piriformis entrapment Misplaced buttock injection
Common peroneal nerve (division of sciatic nerve)	Anterior leg, dorsum of foot	None or dorsal foot	Foot dorsiflexion, inversion, and eversion (N.B. positive Tinel sign at lateral fibular neck)	None (N.B. positive Tinel sign at lateral fibular neck)	Entrapment pressure at neck of fibula Rarely, diabetes, vasculitis, leprosy

From Reilly BM: *Practical strategies in outpatient medicine,* p. 928, Philadelphia, 1991, WB Saunders.

Figure 9-82

Lumbar dermatomes.

Figure 9-83
Referral of pain from and to the lumbar spine.

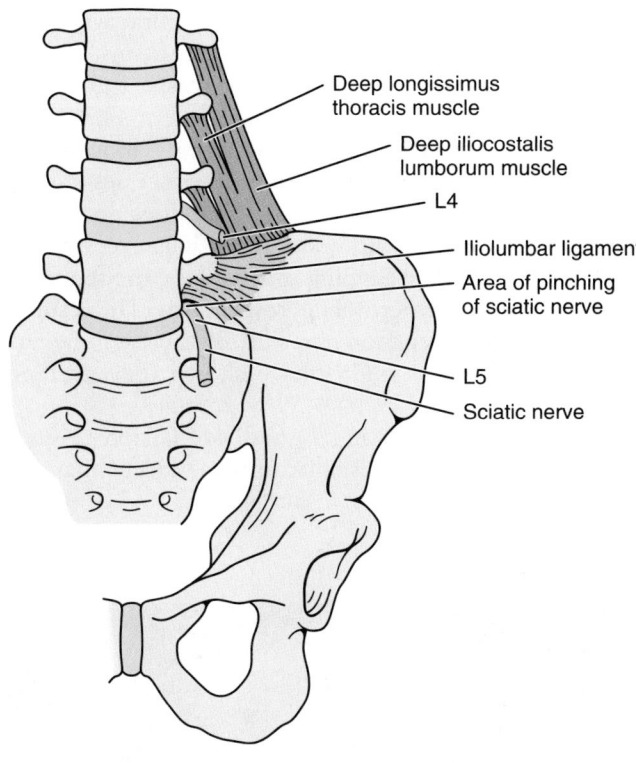

Figure 9-84
Lumbosacral tunnel syndrome. This syndrome involves compression of the L5 nerve root as it passes under the iliolumbar ligament in the iliolumbar canal.

the joint play movements are performed, the examiner should note any decreased ROM, pain, or difference in end feel.

Joint Play Movements of the Lumbar Spine

- Flexion
- Extension
- Side flexion
- Posteroanterior central vertebral pressure
- Posteroanterior unilateral vertebral pressure
- Transverse vertebral pressure

Flexion, Extension, and Side Flexion

The movements tested during these motions are sometimes called **passive intervertebral motions** (PIVMs).[208] Flexion is accomplished with the patient in the side lying position. The examiner flexes both of the patient's bent knees toward the chest by flexing the hips (Figure 9-85, *A*). While palpating between

Table 9-17

Lumbar Muscles and Referral of Pain

Muscle	Referral Pattern
Iliocostalis lumborum	Below T12 ribs lateral to spine down to buttock
Longissimus	Beside spine down to gluteal fold
Multifidus	Lateral to spine, sacrum to gluteal cleft, posterior leg, and lower abdomen
Abdominals	Below xiphisternum and along anterior rib cage down along inguinal ligament to genitals
Serratus posterior inferior	Lateral to spine in T9-T12 posterior rib area

Data from Travell JG, Simons DG: *Myofascial pain and dysfunction: the trigger point manual,* Baltimore, 1983, Williams & Wilkins.

the spinous processes of the lumbar vertebrae with one hand (one finger on the spinous process, one finger above, and one finger below the process), the examiner passively flexes and releases the patient's hips; the examiner's body weight is used to cause the movement. The examiner should feel the spinous processes gap or move apart on flexion. If this gapping does not occur between two spinous processes, or if it is excessive in relation to the other gapping movements, the segment is hypomobile or hypermobile, respectively. The results, however, will depend on the skill of the examiner as interrater reliability studies have shown only average reliability.[208]

Extension (Figure 9-85, *B*) and side flexion (Figure 9-85, *C*) are tested in a similar fashion, except that the movement is passive extension or passive side flexion rather than passive flexion. Side flexion is most easily accomplished by grasping the patient's uppermost leg and rotating the leg upward, which causes side flexion in the lumbar spine by tilting the pelvis. Hip pathology must be ruled out before this is performed.

Central, Unilateral, and Transverse Vertebral Pressure

These movements are sometimes called **passive accessory intervertebral movements** (PAIVMs). To perform the last three joint play movements, the patient lies prone.[209] The lumbar spinous processes are palpated beginning at L5 and working up to L1. If the examiner plans to test end feel over several occasions, the same

Figure 9-85

Joint play movements of the lumbar spine. **A,** Flexion. **B,** Extension. **C,** Side flexion. **D,** Posteroanterior central vertebral pressure.

Figure 9-85 cont'd

E, Posteroanterior unilateral vertebral pressure. **F,** Transverse vertebral pressure.

examining table should be used to improve reliability.[210] Likewise, the patient should be positioned the same way each time. The greatest movement occurs with the spine in neutral.[211] Interrater reliability of these techniques is often low.[212]

The examiner positions the hands, fingers, and thumbs as shown in Figure 9-85, *D,* to perform **posteroanterior central vertebral pressure** (PACVP). Pressure is applied through the thumbs, with the vertebrae being pushed anteriorly (see Figure 8-39). The examiner must apply the pressure slowly and carefully so that the feel of the movement can be recognized. In reality, the movement is minimal. This springing test may be repeated several times to determine the quality of the movement through the range available, and the end feel.

To perform **posteroanterior unilateral vertebral pressure** (PAUVP), the examiner moves the fingers laterally away from the tip of the spinous process about 2.5 to 4.0 cm (1.0 to 1.5 inches) so that the thumbs rest on the muscles overlying the lamina or the transverse process of the lumbar vertebra (Figure 9-85, *E*). The same anterior springing pressure is applied as in the central pressure technique. This springing pressure causes a slight rotation of the vertebra in the opposite direction, which can be confirmed by palpating the spinous process while doing the technique. The two sides should be evaluated and compared.

To perform **transverse vertebral pressure** (TVP), the examiner's fingers are placed along the side of the spinous process of the lumbar spine (Figure 9-85, *F*). The examiner then applies a transverse springing pres-

sure to the side of the spinous process, which causes the vertebra to rotate in the direction of the pressure, feeling for the quality of movement. Pressure should be applied to both sides of the spinous process to compare the quality of movement through the range available and the end feel.

Palpation

If the examiner, having completed the examination of the lumbar spine, decides that the problem is in another joint, palpation should not be done until that joint is completely examined. However, when palpating the lumbar spine, any tenderness, altered temperature, muscle spasm, or other signs and symptoms that may indicate the source of pathology should be noted. If the problem is suspected to be in the lumbar spine area, palpation should be carried out in a systematic fashion, starting on the anterior aspect and working around to the posterior aspect.

Anterior Aspect

With the patient lying supine, the following structures are palpated anteriorly (Figure 9-86).

Umbilicus. The umbilicus lies at the level of the L3–L4 disc space and is the point of intersection of the abdominal quadrants. It is also the point at which the aorta divides into the common iliac arteries. With some patients, the examiner may be able to palpate the anterior aspects of the L4, L5, and S1 vertebrae along with the discs and anterior longitudinal ligament with

T12 vertebra

T12 rib

L2 intravertebral disc

L3 vertebra

Level of L4-5 interspace

Iliac crest

Anterior superior iliac spine

Anterior inferior iliac spine

Acetabulum

Greater trochanter

Anterior view

Figure 9-86
Bony landmarks of the lumbar spine (anterior view).

careful deep palpation. The abdomen may also be carefully palpated for symptoms (e.g., pain, muscle spasm) arising from internal organs. For example, the appendix is palpated in the right lower quadrant and the liver in the right upper quadrant; the kidneys are located in the left and right upper quadrants, and the spleen is found in the left upper quadrant.

Inguinal Area. The inguinal area is located between the ASIS and the symphysis pubis. The examiner should carefully palpate for symptoms of a hernia, abscess, infection (lymph nodes), or other pathological conditions in the area.

Iliac Crest. The examiner palpates the iliac crest from the ASIS, moving posteriorly and looking for any symptoms (e.g., hip pointer or apophysitis).

Symphysis Pubis. The examiner uses both thumbs to palpate the symphysis pubis. Standing at the patient's side, the examiner pushes both thumbs down onto the symphysis pubis so that the thumbs rest on the superior aspect of the pubic bones (see Figure 10-12). In this way, one can ensure that the two pubic bones are level. The symphysis pubis and pubic bones may also be carefully palpated for any tenderness (e.g., osteitis pubis).

Posterior Aspect

The patient is then asked to lie prone, and the following structures are palpated posteriorly (Figure 9-87).

Spinous Processes of the Lumbar Spine. The examiner palpates a point in the midline, which is on a line joining the high point of the two iliac crests. This point is the L4–L5 interspace. After moving down to the first hard mass, the fingers will be resting on the spinous process of L5. Moving toward the head, the interspaces and spinous processes of the remaining lumbar vertebrae can be palpated. In addition to looking for tenderness, muscle spasm, and other signs of pathology, the examiner should watch for signs of a spondylolisthesis, which is most likely to occur at L4–L5 or L5–S1. A visible or palpable dip or protrusion from one spinous process to another may be evident, depending on the type of spondylolisthesis present. In addition, absence of a spinous process may be seen in a spina bifida. If the examiner moves laterally 2 to 3 cm (0.8 to 1.2 inches) from the spinous processes, the fingers will be resting over the lumbar facet joints. These joints should also be palpated for signs of pathology. Because of the depth of these joints, the examiner may have difficulty palpating them. However, pathology in this area results in spasm of the overlying paraspinal muscles, which can be palpated.

Sacrum, Sacral Hiatus, and Coccyx. If the examiner returns to the spinous process of L5 and moves caudally, the fingers will be resting on the sacrum. Like the lumbar spine, the sacrum has spinous processes, but they are much harder to distinguish because there are no interposing soft-tissue spaces between them. The S2 spinous process is at the level of a line joining the two PSISs ("posterior dimples"). Moving distally, the examiner's fingers may palpate the sacral hiatus, which is the caudal portion of the sacral canal. It has an inverted U shape and lies approximately 5 cm (2 inches) above the tip of the

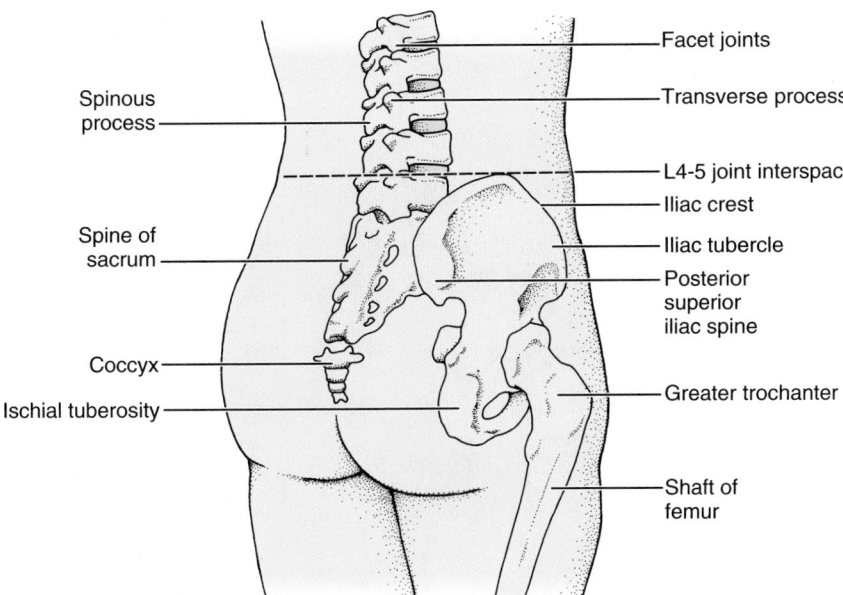

Spinous process

Spine of sacrum

Coccyx

Ischial tuberosity

Facet joints

Transverse process

L4-5 joint interspace

Iliac crest

Iliac tubercle

Posterior superior iliac spine

Greater trochanter

Shaft of femur

Figure 9-87
Bony landmarks of the lumbar spine (posterior view).

coccyx. The two bony prominences on each side of the hiatus are called the **sacral cornua** (see Figure 10-64). As the examiner's fingers move farther distally, they eventually rest on the posterior aspect of the coccyx. Proper palpation of the coccyx requires a rectal examination using a surgical rubber glove (Figure 9-88). The index finger is lubricated and inserted into the anus while the patient's sphincter muscles are relaxed. The finger is inserted as far as possible and then rotated so that the pulpy surface rests against the anterior surface of the coccyx. The examiner then places the thumb of the same hand against the posterior aspect of the sacrum. In this way, the coccyx can be moved back and forth. Any major tenderness (e.g., coccyodynia) should be noted.

Iliac Crest, Ischial Tuberosity, and Sciatic Nerve. Beginning at the PSISs, the examiner moves along the iliac crest, palpating for signs of pathology. Then, moving slightly distally, the examiner palpates the gluteal muscles for spasm, tenderness, or the presence of abnormal nodules. Just under the gluteal folds, the examiner should palpate the ischial tuberosities on both sides for any abnormality. As the examiner moves laterally, the greater trochanter of the femur is palpated. It is often easier to palpate if the hip is flexed to 90°. Midway between the ischial tuberosity and the greater trochanter, the examiner may be able to palpate the path of the sciatic nerve. The nerve itself is not usually palpable. Deep to the gluteal muscles, the piriformis muscle should also be palpated for potential

Ilium

Greater trochanter

Ischial tuberosity

Anus

Sacrum

Coccyx

Figure 9-88
Palpation of the coccyx.

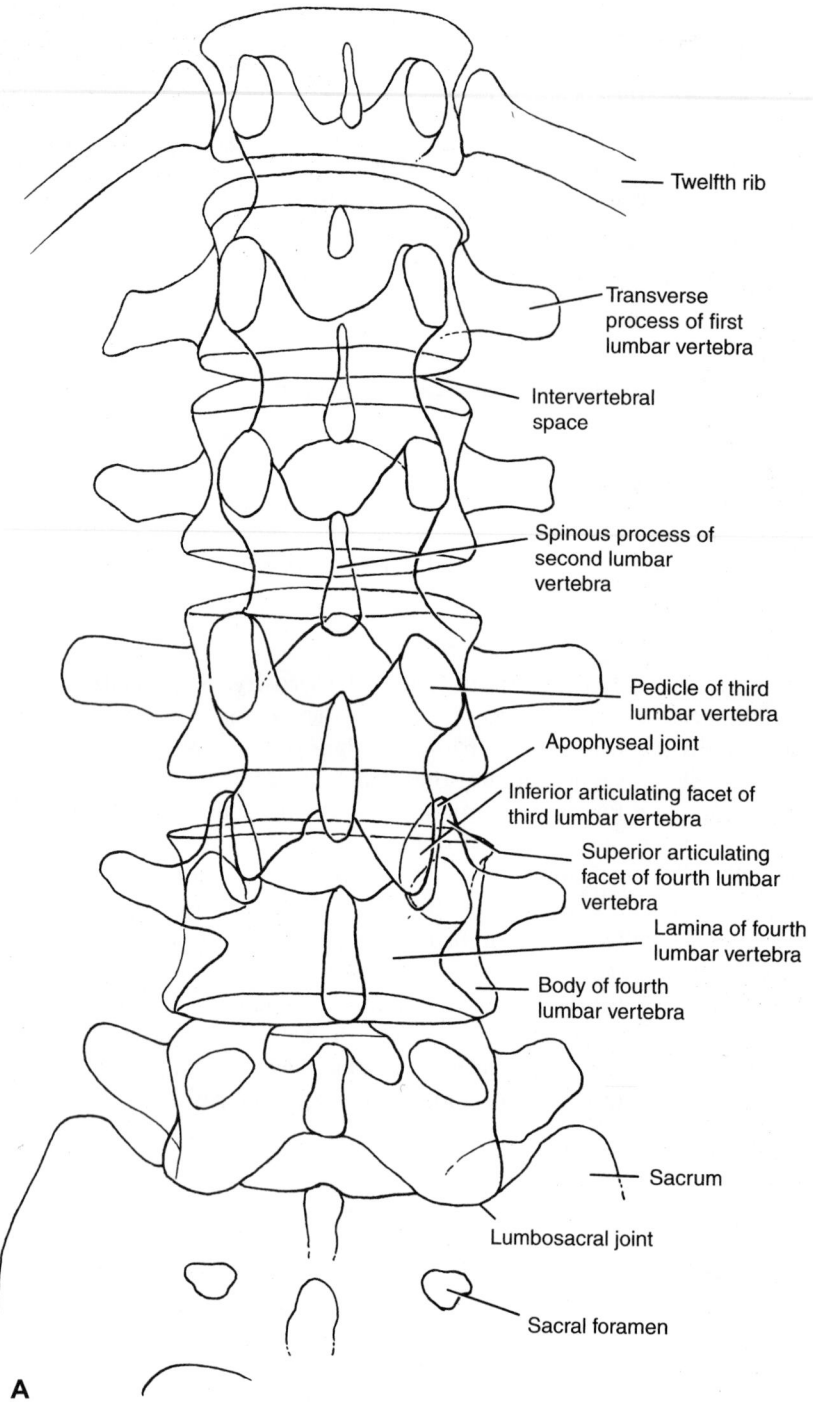

Twelfth rib

Transverse process of first lumbar vertebra

Intervertebral space

Spinous process of second lumbar vertebra

Pedicle of third lumbar vertebra

Apophyseal joint

Inferior articulating facet of third lumbar vertebra

Superior articulating facet of fourth lumbar vertebra

Lamina of fourth lumbar vertebra

Body of fourth lumbar vertebra

Sacrum

Lumbosacral joint

Sacral foramen

A

Figure 9-89 ▬▬▬

Anteroposterior radiograph of the lumbar spine. **A,** Film tracing.

pathology. This muscle is in a line dividing the PSIS of the pelvis and greater trochanter of the femur from the ASIS and ischial tuberosity of the pelvis.

Diagnostic Imaging[213–223]

It is imperative when using diagnostic imaging, to correlate clinical findings with imaging findings, because many anomalies, congenital abnormalities, and aging changes may be present that are not related to the patient's problems.[224]

Plain Film Radiography

Normally, anteroposterior and lateral views are taken. In some cases, two lateral views may be taken, one that shows the whole lumbar spine, and one that focuses on the lower two segments. Oblique views are taken if spondylolysis or spondylolisthesis is suspected.[106]

B

Figure 9-89 cont'd
B, Radiograph. (From Finneson BE: *Low back pain,*
pp. 52–53, Philadelphia, 1973, JB Lippincott.)

Anteroposterior View. With this view (Figure 9-89), the examiner should note the following:

1. Shape of the vertebrae.
2. Any wedging of the vertebrae, possibly resulting from fracture (Figure 9-90).
3. Disc spaces. Do they appear normal, or are there height decreases, as occurs in spondylosis?
4. Any vertebral deformity, such as a hemivertebra or other anomalies (Figures 9-91 through 9-94).
5. The presence of a bamboo spine, as seen in ankylosing spondylitis.
6. Any evidence of lumbarization of S1, making S1–S2 the first mobile segment rather than L5-S1. Lumbarization occurs in 2% to 8% of the population (Figure 9-95).
7. Any evidence of sacralization of L5, making the L4–L5 level the first mobile segment rather than L5-S1. This anomaly occurs in 3% to 6% of the population (Figure 9-96).
8. Any evidence of spina bifida occulta, which occurs in 6% to 10% of the population (see Figure 9-93).

Figure 9-90

Wedging *(arrow)* of a vertebral body. Some wedging may also be seen in the vertebra above.

Lateral View. With this view (Figure 9-97), the examiner should note the following:

1. Any evidence of spondylosis or spondylolisthesis, which occurs in 2% to 4% of the population (Figure 9-98). The degree of slipping can be graded as shown in Figure 9-99.[225]

2. A normal lordosis. Do the intervertebral foramina appear normal?

3. Any wedging of the vertebrae.

4. Normal disc spacing.

5. Alignment of the vertebrae should be noted. Disruption of the curve may indicate spinal instability.

6. Any osteophyte formation or traction spurs (Figure 9-100).[220,226] Traction spurs indicate an unstable lumbar intervertebral segment. A traction spur occurs approximately 1 mm from the disc border; an osteophyte occurs at the disc border with the vertebral body.

Oblique View. With the oblique view (Figure 9-101), the examiner should look for any evidence of spondylolisthesis (sometimes referred to as a "Scottie dog decapitated") or spondylolysis (sometimes referred to as a "Scottie dog with a collar"; Figure 9-102).

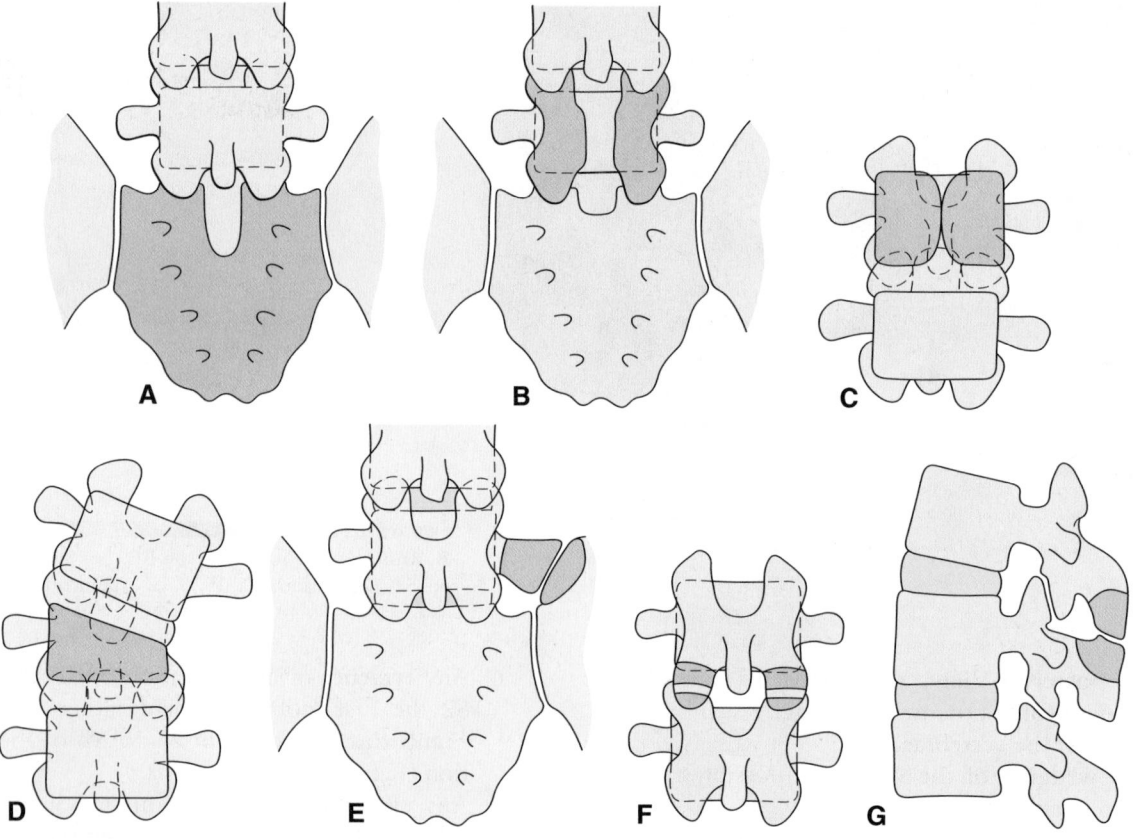

Figure 9-91

Diagrammatic representation of the x-ray appearance of common anatomical anomalies in the lumbosacral spine. **A,** Spina bifida occulta, S1. **B,** Spina bifida, L5. **C,** Anterior spina bifida ("butterfly vertebra"). **D,** Hemivertebra. **E,** Iliotransverse joint (transitional segments). **F,** Ossicles of Oppenheimer. These are free ossicles seen at the tip of the inferior articular facets and are usually found at the level of L3. **G,** "Kissing" spinous processes. (Redrawn from MacNab I: *Backache,* pp. 14–15, Baltimore, 1977, Williams & Wilkins.)

Figure 9-92

Butterfly vertebra. Also note transitional segments *(large arrows)*. (Modified from Jaeger SA: Atlas of radiographic positioning: normal anatomy and developmental variants, p. 333, Norwalk, Conn, 1988, Appleton & Lange.)

Figure 9-93

Spina bifida occulta. (From Jaeger SA: *Atlas of radiographic positioning: normal anatomy and developmental Variants,* p. 317, Norwalk, Conn, 1988, Appleton & Lange.)

Motion Views. In some cases, motion views may be used to demonstrate abnormal spinal motion or structural abnormalities. These are usually lateral views showing flexion and extension to demonstrate instability or spondylolisthesis (Figure 9-103), but they may also include anteroposterior views with side bending.[142,227,228]

Myelography

A myelogram, although seldom used today because of its complications and replacement by computed tomography (CT) scans and magnetic resonance imaging (MRI), can confirm the presence of a protruding intervertebral

Figure 9-94

Hemivertebra shown on an anteroposterior radiograph.

disc, osteophytes, a tumor, or spinal stenosis (Figures 9-104 through 9-106). The examiner must be careful of the side effects of myelograms, which include headache, stiffness, low back pain, cramps, and paresthesia in the lower limbs. Although side effects do occur, no permanent injuries have been noted.

Radionuclide Imaging (Bone Scans)

Bone scans are useful for detecting active bone disease processes and areas of high bone turnover. In children, the epiphyseal and metaphyseal areas of the long bones show increased uptake. In adults, only the metaphyseal area is so affected. Traumatic bone injuries, tumors, metabolic abnormalities (e.g., Paget's disease), infection, and arthritis may be detected on bone scan.[107]

Computed Tomography

A computed tomography (CT) scan may be used to delineate a fracture or to show the presence of spinal stenosis caused by protrusion or a tumor (Figures 9-107 through 9-110). As with plain x-rays, results must be correlated with clinical findings, because the anatomical changes

Text continued on page 597

Figure 9-95
Lumbarization of the S1 vertebra seen on anteroposterior **A,** and lateral **B,** radiographs.

Figure 9-96
Unilateral sacralization of the fifth lumbar vertebra. **A,** Note the massive formation of sacral ala on the left side with a relatively normal transverse process on the right (anteroposterior view). **B,** Lateral view showing the narrow disc space and the massive arches. (From O'Donoghue DH: *Treatment of injuries to athletes,* ed 4, p. 403, Philadelphia, 1984, WB Saunders.)

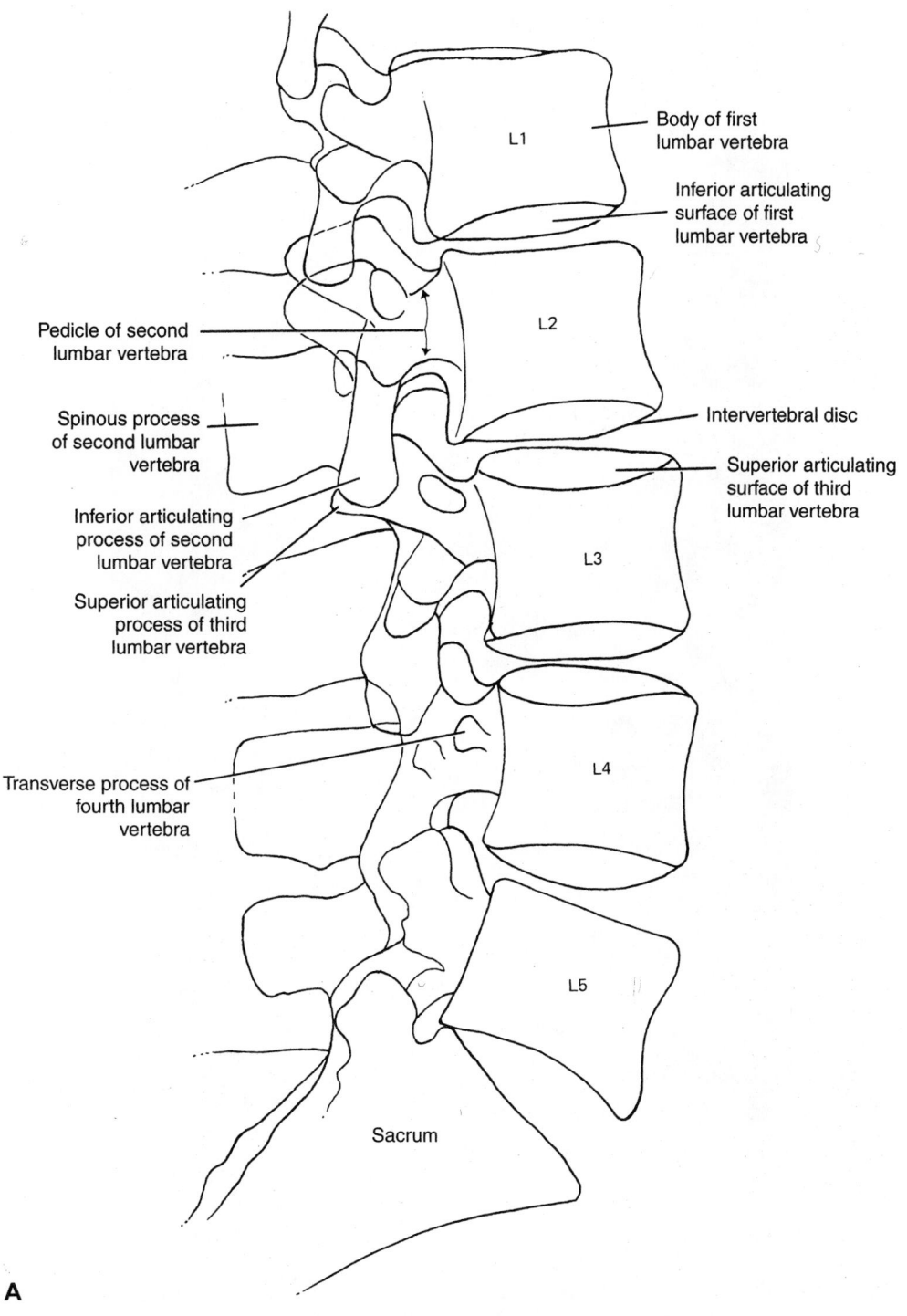

Body of first
lumbar vertebra

Inferior articulating
surface of first
lumbar vertebra

Pedicle of second
lumbar vertebra

Spinous process
of second lumbar
vertebra

Inferior articulating
process of second
lumbar vertebra

Superior articulating
process of third
lumbar vertebra

Intervertebral disc

Superior articulating
surface of third
lumbar vertebra

Transverse process of
fourth lumbar
vertebra

Sacrum

L1

L2

L3

L4

L5

A

Figure 9-97

Lateral radiograph of the lumbar spine. **A,** Film tracing.

Continued

Figure 9-97 cont'd
B, Radiograph. (From Finneson BE: *Low back pain,* pp. 54–55, Philadelphia, 1973, JB Lippincott.)

Figure 9-98

Spondylolisthesis. **A,** Grade 1: Arch defect in L5 with mild forward displacement of L5 on S1; backache but no gross disability. **B,** Grade 2: More forward slipping between L4 and L5 with collapse of the intervertebral disc; definite symptomatic back with restriction of motion, muscle spasm, and curtailment of activities. **C,** Grade 3: More extensive slipping combined with a wide separation at the arch defect and degenerative changes of the disc; grossly symptomatic. **D,** Grade 4: Vertebrae slipped forward more than halfway; severe disability. (From O'Donoghue DH: *Treatment of injuries to athletes,* ed 4, p. 402, Philadelphia, 1984, WB Saunders.)

NORMAL   GRADE 1   GRADE 2

GRADE 3   GRADE 4

Figure 9-99

Meyerding grading system for slipping in spondylolisthesis.

Traction spur

Claw spondylophyte

Figure 9-100

Lateral radiograph of a thin-slice pathological section of lumbar spine. Note traction spur and claw spondylophyte. (From Rothman RH, Simeone FA: *The spine*, p. 512, Philadelphia, 1982, WB Saunders.)

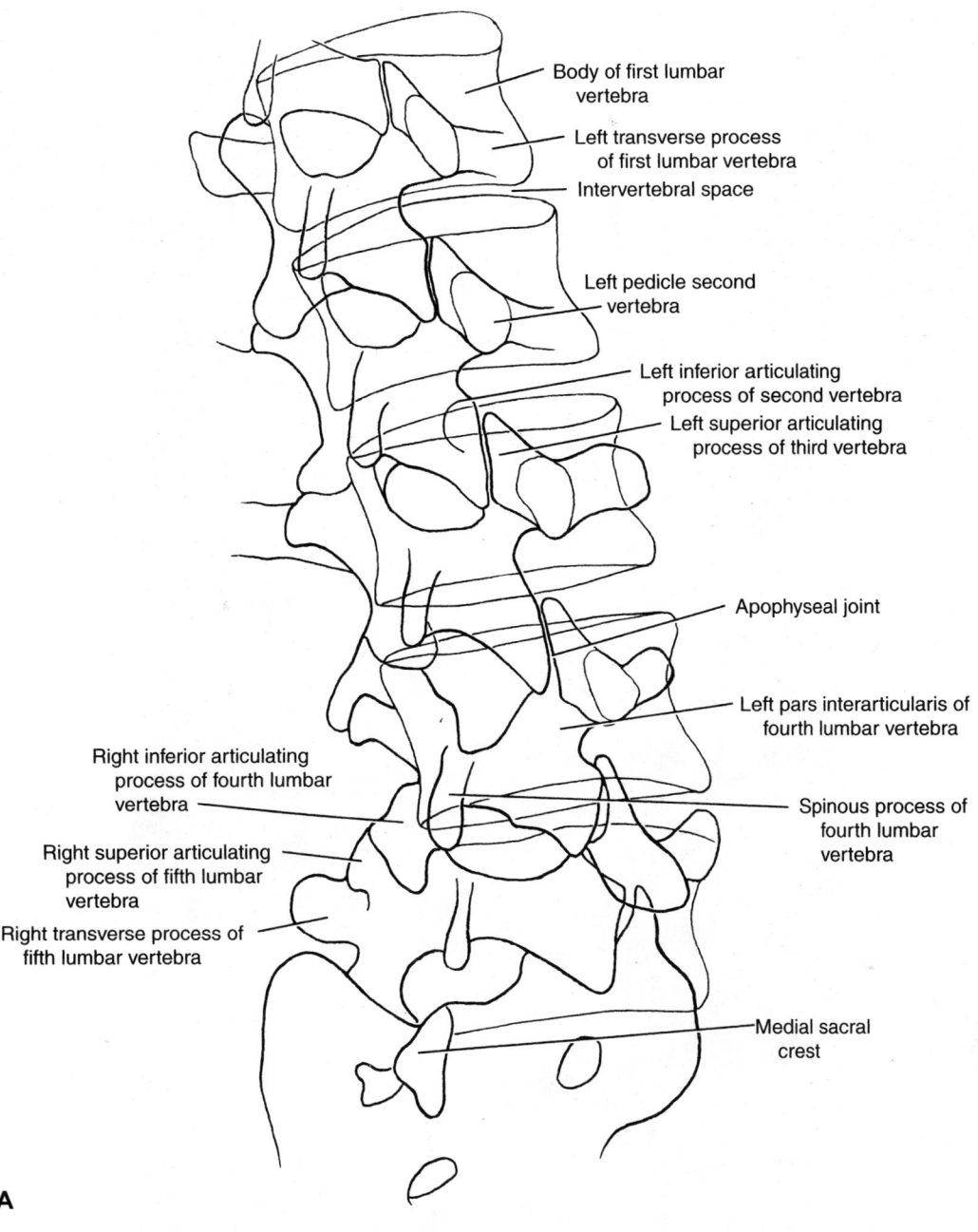

Body of first lumbar
vertebra

Left transverse process
of first lumbar vertebra

Intervertebral space

Left pedicle second
vertebra

Left inferior articulating
process of second vertebra

Left superior articulating
process of third vertebra

Apophyseal joint

Left pars interarticularis of
fourth lumbar vertebra

Right inferior articulating
process of fourth lumbar
vertebra

Spinous process of
fourth lumbar
vertebra

Right superior articulating
process of fifth lumbar
vertebra

Right transverse process of
fifth lumbar vertebra

Medial sacral
crest

A

Figure 9-101

Left posterior oblique radiograph of the lumbar spine. **A,** Film tracing.

Continued

seen are often unassociated with the patient's symptoms.[224,229,230] This technique provides an axial projection of the spine, showing the anatomy of not only the spine but also the paravertebral muscles, vascular structures, and organs of the body cavity. In doing so, it shows more precisely the relation among the intervertebral discs, spinal canal, facet joints, and intervertebral foramina. It may be used to evaluate spinal stenosis, the shape of the spinal canal, epidural scarring (after surgery), facet joint arthritis, tumors, and trauma.[107] It may be used in conjunction with a water-soluble contrast medium (computer-assisted myelography) to further delineate the structures.

Magnetic Resonance Imaging

Magnetic resonance imaging (MRI) is a noninvasive technique that can be used in several planes (transaxial,

B

Figure 9-101 cont'd

B, Radiograph. (From Finneson BE: *Low back pain,* pp. 56–57, Philadelphia, 1973, JB Lippincott.)

coronal, or sagittal) to delineate bony and soft tissues. This technique is commonly used to diagnose tumors, to view the spinal cord within the spinal canal, and to assess for syringomyelia, cord infarction, or traumatic injury.[107] The delineation of soft tissues is much greater with MRI than with CT.[231] For example, with MRI, the nucleus pulposus and the annulus fibrosis are easier to differentiate because of their different water contents, making it the preferred imaging modality for disc disease (Figures 9-111 through 9-114).[232,233] As with other diagnostic imaging techniques, clinical findings must support what is seen before the structural abnormalities can be considered the source of the problem.[224,229,234–236]

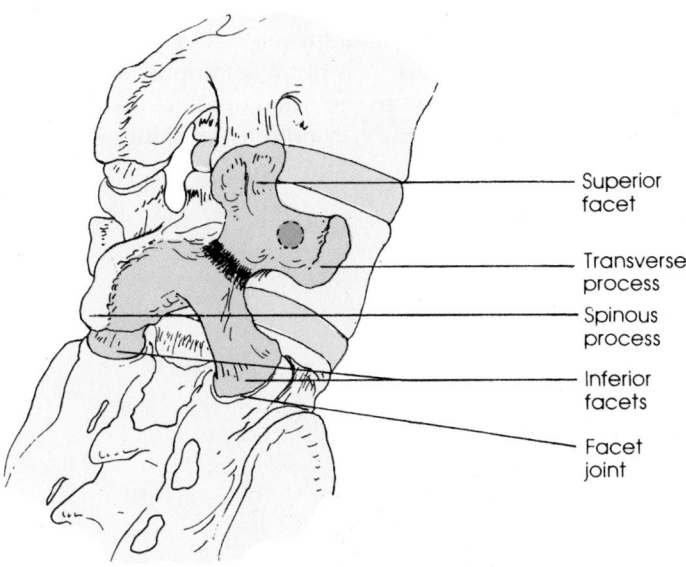

Superior facet

Transverse process

Spinous process

Inferior facets

Facet joint

SPONDYLOLYSIS
"Scottie dog with collar"

A

SPONDYLOLISTHESIS
"Scottie dog decapitated"

B

Figure 9-102

A, Diagrammatic representation (posterior oblique view) of spondylolysis and spondylolisthesis. **B,** Posterior oblique film showing "Scottie dog" at L2. L4 shows Scottie dog with a "collar" *(arrow)*, indicating spondylolysis.

Figure 9-103

Lumbar spine in flexion. Note forward slipping of one vertebra on the one below (*arrow*).

Discography [237]

For discography, radiopaque dye is injected into the nucleus pulposus. It is not a commonly used technique but may be used to see whether injection of dye reproduces the patient's symptoms, making it diagnostic (Figure 9-115).

Figure 9-104

Metrizamide myelograms illustrating a herniated disc at L4-L5 on the right. Note lack of filling of the nerve root sleeve and indentation (*arrow*) of the dural sac. (From Rothman, RH, Simeone FA: *The spine,* p. 550, Philadelphia, 1982, WB Saunders.)

Figure 9-105
Oil myelograms showing the characteristic appearance of chronic disc degeneration and spinal stenosis with diffuse posterior bulging of the annulus and osteophyte formation. **A,** Symmetric wasting of the dye column is shown in the anteroposterior view. Note the hourglass configuration. **B,** Indentation of the dye column of the annulus anteriorly and the buckled ligamentum flavum and facet joints posteriorly (lateral view). (From Rothman RH, Simeone FA: *The spine,* p. 553, Philadelphia, 1982, WB Saunders.)

Figure 9-106
Metrizamide myelograms showing stenotic block at the L4-L5 level as a result of degenerative spondylolisthesis and spinal stenosis at the L4-L5 level. **A,** Note the 4-mm anterior migration of L4 on L5 caused by the degenerative spondylolisthesis. **B** and **C,** The extensive block on the myelogram is caused by spinal stenosis. (From Rothman RH, Simeone FA: *The spine,* p. 553, Philadelphia, 1982, WB Saunders.)

Figure 9-107

Normal disc anatomy on computed tomography (CT). **A,** Scout view. The chosen sections *(dashed lines)* can be planned and angled along the planes of the discs. **B,** CT scan through the L4 vertebral body shows the neural foramina and the L4 nerve root ganglia *(white arrow indicates left ganglion)*. The dural sac (d) and ligamenta flava *(black arrows)* are shown. **C,** CT scan through the L4-L5 disc (labeled *D*) shows very little fat between the posterior margin of the disc *(arrows)* and the dural sac (d). The nerve roots are not clearly shown. **D,** CT scan through the L5 vertebral body and foramina shows the L5 nerve root ganglia *(arrows)*. **E,** CT scan through the L5-S1 disc space (labeled *D*) shows the L5 nerve roots *(straight white arrows)*, the dural sac (d), and the ligamenta flava *(black arrows)*. Small epidural veins are noted *(curved arrows)*. **F,** At the S1 level, the S1 nerve roots *(arrows)* and dural sac (d) are clearly visualized. (From Weissman BNW, Sledge CB: *Orthopedic radiology,* p. 306, Philadelphia, 1986, WB Saunders.)

Figure 9-108

Soft-tissue detail of the L4–L5 intervertebral disc space on computed tomography (CT). **A,** Lateral digital scout view obtained through the lumbosacral spine. The upper and lower scan limits through the L4–L5 region are designated with an electronic cursor. Scan collimation is 5 mm thick; incrementation is 3 mm (2-mm overlap). **B,** Axial CT section of L4. The L4 root ganglia and spinal nerves are seen within the intervertebral foramina *(white arrowheads)* surrounded by abundant epidural fat (e). The thecal sac (t) is bounded anterolaterally by fat in the lateral recess. The posterior arch of L4 consists of inferior facets (if), laminae (l), and spinous process (s). The superior facet of L5 (sf) is just visible. **C,** The next lower axial section demonstrates the L4–L5 facet articulations. The ligamentum flavum (lf) is contiguous with the facet joint capsule. Again, the thecal sac (t) is readily apparent; it is slightly higher in density than the adjacent epidural fat. Note that without subarachnoid contrast media, the intrathecal contents cannot be discerned. **D,** Axial CT section of the L4–L5 disc space. The disc *(multiple black arrowheads)* is a region of central hypodensity surrounded by the cortical margin of L4. The posterior arch of L4 projects below the disc level. The intervertebral foramina (ivf) have begun to close. The cartilaginous articular surfaces *(white arrowhead)* between superior (sf) and inferior (if) facets are poorly demonstrated with these window settings. The ligamentum flavum *(double black arrowheads)* is noted medial to the facet joints. t = Thecal sac; s = spinous process. **E,** The next inferior CT section demonstrates the disc *(multiple arrowheads)* positioned somewhat more anteriorly, marginated posteriorly at this level by the posterosuperior cortical rim of the L5 body. The ligamentum flavum *(double arrowheads)* normally maintains a flat medial surface adjacent to the thecal sac (t). The posterior arch of L4 and its spinous process (s) are still in view. **F,** Axial CT section through the L5 body at the level of the pedicles (p). The canal now completely encloses the thecal sac (t). **G,** Immediately below, only the spinous process (s) of the posterior arch of L4 is visible. The transverse process (tp) of L5 is noted. t = Thecal sac. **H,** At the level of the iliac crest (IC), the posterior arch of L5 *(small arrowheads)* has just begun to form. The transverse processes (tp) are quite large at this level. t = Thecal sac. (From LeMasters DL, Dowart RL: High-resolution, cross-sectional computed tomography of the normal spine, *Orthop Clin North Am* 16:359, 1985.)

Figure 9-109

Computed tomography (CT) anatomy of L4 nerve roots. **A,** Lateral view during metrizamide myelography showing indentations on the anterior aspect of the contrast column *(arrows)* at L3–L4 and L4–L5 resulting from bulging intervertebral discs. The levels for subsequent CT sections *B* and *D* are marked. **B,** CT section through the L4 vertebra and L4–L5 foramina 1 hour after a metrizamide myelogram. Contrast agent fills the left axillary pouch *(white arrow)* and the right nerve root sleeve. Small arrows indicate the filling defects produced by the remaining nerve roots. **C,** CT section slightly more distal than B shows the L4 nerve root ganglia (left ganglion is indicated by arrow). **D,** Section through the L4–L5 disc and the posterior inferior body of L4 shows an abnormally bulging disc without compression of the subarachnoid space. The ligamentum flavum on the left *(arrow),* the superior facet of L5 (sf-5), and the inferior facet of L4 (if-4) are indicated. (From Weissman BNW, Sledge CB: *Orthopedic radiology,* p. 284, Philadelphia, 1986, WB Saunders.)

Figure 9-110

Degenerative spondylolisthesis. Sagittal reformatted image derived from transverse CT scans of the lumbar spine shows degeneration at the L4–L5 level with a vacuum phenomenon. A grade II spondylolisthesis at the L4–L5 level results from osteoarthritis of the facet joints. (From Resnick D, Kransdorf MJ: *Bone and joint imaging,* p. 146, Philadelphia, 2005, WB Saunders.)

Figure 9-111

Magnetic resonance imaging of normal lumbar spine. **A,** Level of neural canal.

Continued

Vertebral body

Pedicle

Nerve roots surrounded
by CSF

Apophyseal joint

Epidural fat

Figure 9-111 cont'd

B, Level of pedicle. CSF = Cerebrospinal fluid. (From Bassett LW, Gold RH, Seeger LL: *MRI atlas of the musculoskeletal system,* p. 40, London, 1989, Martin Dunitz.)

Figure 9-112

Disc degeneration viewed by magnetic resonance imaging. **A,** T1-weighted image. There is little difference in intensity between the intervertebral discs. A grade 1 spondylolisthesis is present at L5–S1. **B,** T2-weighted image. The L4–L5 and L5–S1 discs *(arrowheads)* are darker than the other, normal discs. A degenerating disc dehydrates, which shortens the T2 and consequently decreases the signal intensity on a T2-weighted image. (From Gillespy T, Genant HK, Chafetz NI: Magnetic resonance imaging atlas of the lumbar spine. In Jayson M, editor: *The lumbar spine and back pain,* p. 292, Edinburgh, Churchill Livingstone, 1987.)

Figure 9-113

Type II vertebral endplates. Sagittal T1-weighted (**A**) and T2-weighted (**B**) spin echo MR images of the lumbar spine show signal intensity changes at the L4–L5 level that are typical of a type II end plate. The signal intensity of subchondral bone at this level is identical to that of fat. There is also evidence of degeneration of the intervertebral disc at this level, with a decrease in disc space height and loss of disc signal on the T2-weighted image. (From Resnick D, Kransdorf MJ: *Bone and joint imaging,* p. 144, Philadelphia, 2005, WB Saunders.)

Figure 9-114

Normal and abnormal intervertebral disc: sagittal T2-weighted (TR/TE, 3400/96) spin echo MR imaging technique. In discs that are relatively normal (L1–L2, L3–L4, and L4–L5), a central portion of high signal intensity containing a horizontal line of low signal intensity is evident. In the disc (L2–L3) with mild intervertebral (osteo)chondrosis, minimal loss of signal intensity is shown, particularly in its anterior third. With severe intervertebral (osteo)chondrosis (L5–S1), the disc is of low signal intensity and diminished in height. A large posterior extruded disc *(arrow)* with low signal intensity is also evident. (From Resnick D, Kransdorf MJ: *Bone and joint imaging,* p. 399, Philadelphia, 2005, WB Saunders.)

Figure 9-115

Lumbar discography. **A,** Lateral lumbar spine with discographic needle entry low in the posterior disc margin. Note the normal unilocular appearance of the nucleogram. **B,** Normal bilocular appearance of the nucleogram. The anterior arrows identify anterior vacuum phenomena in the anulus fibrosus, consistent with peripheral annular tears that were asymptomatic at discography. (From Resnick D, Kransdorf MJ: *Bone and joint imaging,* p. 164, Philadelphia, 2005, WB Saunders.)

Précis of the Lumbar Spine Assessment*

History (sitting)
Observation (standing)
Examination
  Active movements (standing)
    Forward flexion
    Extension
    Side flexion (left and right)
    Rotation (left and right)
    Quick test (if possible)
    Trendelenburg's test and S1 nerve root test
      (modified Trendelenburg test)
  Passive movements (only with care and caution)
  Peripheral joint scan (standing)
    Sacroiliac joints
  Special tests (standing)
    One leg standing lumbar extension test
    H and I test
  Resisted isometric movements (sitting)
    Forward flexion
    Extension
    Side flexion (left and right)
    Rotation (left and right)
  Special tests (sitting)
    Slump test
    Sitting root test
  Resisted isometric movements (supine lying)
    Dynamic abdominal endurance

    Double straight leg lowering
    Internal/external abdominal obliques test
  Peripheral joint scan (supine lying)
    Hip joints (flexion, abduction, adduction, and medial
      and lateral rotation)
    Knee joints (flexion and extension)
    Ankle joints (dorsiflexion and plantar flexion)
    Foot joints (supination, pronation)
    Toe joints (flexion, extension)
  Myotomes (supine lying)
    Hip flexion (L2)
    Knee extension (L3)
    Ankle dorsiflexion (L4)
    Toe extension (L5)
    Ankle eversion or plantar flexion (S1)
  Special tests (supine lying)
    Straight leg raise test and its variants
    Sign of the buttock
  Reflexes and cutaneous distribution (anterior and side aspects)
  Palpation (supine lying)
  Resisted isometric movements (side lying)
    Horizontal side support
  Special tests (side lying)
    Femoral nerve traction test
    Specific torsion test
  Joint play movements (side lying)
    Flexion

Précis of the Shoulder Assessment* cont'd

Examination cont'd
Peripheral joint scan (prone lying)
  Hip joints (extension, medial and lateral rotation)
Myotomes (prone lying)
  Hip extension (S1)
  Knee flexion (S1–S2)
Resisted isometric movements
  Dynamic extension test
Special tests (prone lying)
  Prone knee bending test
Reflexes and cutaneous distribution (prone lying) (posterior aspect)

Joint play movements (prone lying)
  Posteroanterior central vertebral pressure (PACVP)
  Posteroanterior unilateral vertebral pressure (PAUVP)
  Transverse vertebral pressure (TVP)
Palpation (prone lying)
Resisted isometric movements (quadriped position)
  Back rotators/multifidus test
Diagnostic imaging

After any examination, the patient should be warned of the possibility that symptoms may exacerbate as a result of the assessment.

_____

*The précis is shown in an order that limits the amount of movement that the patient has to do but ensures that all necessary structures are tested.

Case Studies

When doing these case studies, the examiner should list the appropriate questions to ask and should specify why they are being asked, what to look for and why, and what things should be tested and why. Depending on the patient's answers (and the examiner should consider different responses), several possible causes of the patient's problem may become evident (examples given in parentheses). The examiner should prepare a differential diagnosis chart and then decide how different diagnoses may affect the treatment plan. For example, an 18-year-old female synchronized swimmer was "boosting" another swimmer out of the water and felt a sharp pain in her back. She found that she could no longer swim because of the pain. She demonstrated paresthesia on the dorsum of the foot and lateral aspect of the leg. Describe your assessment plan for this patient (acute disc herniation versus lumbar strain) (Table 9-18).

1. A 23-year-old man comes to you complaining of a low backache. He works as a dishwasher, and although the pain has been present for 5 months, he has not missed any work. The pain gets worse as the day progresses and is relieved by rest. X-rays reveal some sclerosis in the area of the sacroiliac joints. Describe your assessment plan for this patient (ankylosing spondylitis versus lumbar sprain).

2. A 36-year-old woman comes to you complaining of a chronic backache of 6 months' duration. The pain has been gradually increasing in severity and is worse at rest and in the morning on arising from bed. When present, the pain is centered in her low back and radiates into her buttocks and posterior left thigh. Describe your assessment plan for this patient (lumbar stenosis versus lumbar disc lesion).

3. A 13-year-old female gymnast comes to you complaining of low back pain. The pain increases when she extends the spine. Like most gymnasts, she is hypermobile in most of her joints. Describe your assessment plan for this patient (spondylolisthesis versus lumbar sprain).

4. A 56-year-old male steel worker comes to you complaining of low back pain that was brought on when he slipped on ice and twisted his trunk while trying to avoid falling. The injury occurred 2 days earlier, and he has right-sided sciatica. X-rays show some lipping at L4–L5 and L5–S1 with slight narrowing of the L5 disc. He has difficulty bending forward. Describe your assessment plan for this patient (lumbar spondylosis versus acute lumbar disc herniation).

5. A 28-year-old man had a laminectomy for a herniated L5 disc 2 days earlier. He is still an inpatient. Describe your assessment plan for this patient.

6. A 32-year-old man comes to you complaining of back pain and stiffness, especially with activity. He has a desk job and has no history of unusual activity. Describe your assessment plan for this patient (chronic lumbar sprain versus lumbar spina bifida occulta).

7. A 39-year-old male electrician comes to you complaining of back pain after a motor vehicle accident in which he was hit from behind while stopped for a red light. The accident occurred 3 days earlier. Describe your assessment program for this patient (lumbar sprain versus lumbar stenosis).

8. A 26-year-old woman comes to you complaining of low back pain. She appears to have a functional leg length difference. Describe your assessment plan for this patient (lumbar sprain versus congenital anomaly).

Table 9-18

Differential Diagnosis of Lumbar Strain and Posterolateral Lumbar Disc Herniation at L5-S1

	Lumbar Strain	Lumbar Disc (L5-S1)
History	Mechanism of injury: flexion, side flexion, and/or rotation under load or without control	Quick movement into flexion, rotation, side flexion, or extension (may or may not be under load)
Pain	In lumbar spine, may be referred into buttocks	In lumbar spine with referral into posterior leg to foot (radicular pain)
	May increase with extension (muscle contraction) or flexion (stretch)	Increases with extension
Observation	Scoliosis may be present	Scoliosis may be present
	Muscle spasm	Muscle guarding
Active movement	Pain especially on stretch (flexion, side flexion, and rotation)	Pain especially on extension and flexion
	Pain on unguarded movement	Side flexion and rotation may be affected
	Limited range of motion	Limited range of motion
Resisted isometric movement	Pain on muscle contraction (often minimal pain)	Minimal pain unless large protrusion
	Myotomes normal	L5-S1 myotomes may be affected
Special tests	Neurological tests negative	SLR and slump test often positive
Sensation	Normal	L5-S1 dermatomes may be affected
Reflexes	Normal	L5-S1 reflexes may be affected
Joint play	Muscle guarding	Muscle guarding

SLR = straight leg raising.

References

To enhance this text and add value for the reader, all references have been incorporated into a CD-ROM that is provided with this text. The reader can view the reference source and access it online whenever possible. There are a total of 276 cited references and other general references for this chapter.

APPENDIX 9-1

RELIABILITY, VALIDITY, SPECIFICITY, AND SENSITIVITY OF SPECIAL/DIAGNOSTIC TESTS USED IN THE LUMBAR SPINE

BACK PERFORMANCE SCALE

Reliability	Validity
• Intertester ICC = 0.996, test-retest ICC = 0.91[238]	• Roland Morris Disability Questionnaire p = 0.454, fear avoidance beliefs questionnaire p = 0.05[238]

CRAMP FINDING

Sensitivity	Specificity	Responsiveness	Odds Ratio
• 100% (MRI)[239]	• 72% (MRI)[239]	• 72% (MRI)[239]	• Positive likelihood ratios 72, negative likelihood ratios 0.28

CRANIOSACRAL RHYTHM

Reliability

• Intrarater ICC = 0.78, interrater ICC = 0.22[240]

DOUBLE STRAIGHT LEG LOWERING TEST

Validity

• The EMG of abdominal muscles increases according to the increase of level of the test, different muscles act differently at each stage[241]

DYNAMIC ABDOMINAL ENDURANCE TEST

Reliability

• Interrater ICC = 0.59[87]

DYNAMIC EXTENSOR ENDURANCE TEST

Reliability

• Interrater ICC = 0.78[87]

EXTENSION (ATTRACTION METHOD FOR MEANS LUMBAR SPINE BACK BEND)

Reliability

• Interrater ICC = 0.94, intrarater ICC = 0.90[242]

FINGER TO FLOOR

Reliability	Validity	Responsiveness
• Test-retest r = 0.88[243] • Intrarater ICC = 0.99, • Interrater ICC = 0.99[114]	• Criterion validity correlation with radiography r = −0.96[114]	• Effect size = 0.87, SRM = 0.97[114]

FUNCTIONAL LEG LENGTH

Reliability	Validity
• Interrater ICC = 0.84, intrarater ICC = 0.77[244]	• Relationship with radiographic measurements ICC = 0.64[244]

Continued

APPENDIX 9-1—cont'd

FUNCTIONAL RATING INDEX

Reliability	Validity	Responsiveness
• Test-retest ICC = 0.99[114] • ICC = 0.67, SEM = 3.52[245]	• Internal consistency Cronbach's alpha 0.92, correlation with SF-12 PCS r = 0.76, SF-12 MCS r = 0.36[114]	• Overall SRM = 1.24, cervical SRM = 1.26, thoracic SRM = 1.61, lumbar SRM = 1.24[114]

FUNCTIONAL RATING INDEX INTRACLASS

Reliability	Validity
• Test-retest ICC = 0.99[114]	• Internal consistency Cronbach's alpha 0.92, correlation with disability rating index r = 0.76 and SF-12 r = 0.36[114]

GENERAL FUNCTION SCORE

Reliability	Validity	Responsiveness
• Test-retest ICC = 0.87[246] • Test-retest ICC = 0.87[247]	• Criterion validity r > 0.41 for subitems (correlation with the questionnaire with preadmission self-rating score, postperformance test self rating, observer postperformance test rating)[246] • Construct validity correlation with Oswestry disability index r = 0.61, Million scale r = 0.54[246]	• Spondylolisthesis effect size = 0.82, disc herniation effect size = 0.55[246]

ISOMETRIC ABDOMINAL TEST

Reliability
• Interrater ICC = 0.25[87]

ISOMETRIC EXTENSOR TEST

Reliability
• Interrater ICC = 0.24[87]

KRAUS SITUP TEST

Validity
• Female (concentric isokinetic r = 0.42, eccentric isokinetic r = 0.40); male (concentric isokinetic r = −0.18, eccentric isokinetic r = −0.21)[248]

LOW BACK OUTCOME SCORE

Reliability	Validity
• Test-retest r = 0.92 (kappa for all items separately ranged from 0.51 to 0.86)[249]	• Internal consistency Cronbach's alpha 0.79[249]

MCKENZIE EVALUATION

	Reliability
• Syndrome categories	• k = 1[250] • k = 0.6[251] • k = 0.84 (lumbar patients k = 1, cervical patients k = 0.63)[252]
• Type of subsyndromes	• k = 0.7[250] • k = 0.7[251] • k = 0.87 (lumbar patients k = 0.89, cervical patients k = 0.84)[252]
• Lateral shift	• Presence k = 0.52, relevance k = 0.85[250] • Presence of clinical relevance k = 0.16[253] • Presence k = 0.2, direction k = 0.4, relevance k = 0.7[251]
• Lateral component	• Presence k = 0.95[250]
• Centralization	• k = 0.7[251]
• Direction preference	• k = 0.9[251]

NUMERICAL PAIN RATING SCALE FOR LOW BACK PAIN

Responsiveness

• Effect size 1 week 0.95, 4 weeks 1.2[254]

OSWESTRY DISABILITY INDEX

Reliability	Validity	Responsiveness
• Test-retest Cronbach's alpha 0.86[255] • Test-retest ICC = 0.94[247] • Test-retest ICC = 0.83[256] • Test-retest ICC = 0.84, SEM = 9[257]	• Internal consistency Cronbach's alpha 0.86[255]	• Effect size 0.39[255] • SRM = 0.52[257]

PHYSICAL IMPAIRMENT INDEX (FOR ACUTE LOW BACK PAIN)

Reliability	Validity	Responsiveness
• Interrater ICC = 0.89 (for individual components ICC between 0.35 and 0.91)[258]	• Correlation with OSD r = 0.43, SF-36 r = 0, pain rating r = 0.47, depressive symptoms r = –0.05, fear avoidance r = 0.24, nonorganic signs r = 0.36[258]	• Area under the curve 0.88[258]

PRESSURE CHANGE (mmHg) TRANSVERSUS ABDOMINIS

Validity

• EMG latency test, correlation is r = 0.48[259]

QUEBEC BACK PAIN DISABILITY SCALE

Reliability	Responsiveness
• Test-retest ICC = 0.84, SEM = 11[257]	• SRM = 0.49[257]

REPETITIVE ARCHUP

Reliability

• Intrarater r = 0.65[260]

REPETITIVE SITUP

Reliability

• Intrarater r = 0.84[260]

Continued

APPENDIX 9-1—cont'd

REPETITIVE SQUATTING

Reliability

- Intrarater r = 0.47[260]

ROBERTSON CURLUP TEST

Validity

- Female (concentric isokinetic r = −0.07, eccentric isokinetic r = −0.08); male (concentric isokinetic r = −0.41, eccentric isokinetic r = −0.38)[248]

ROLAND MORRIS DISABILITY QUESTIONNAIRE

Reliability	Validity	Specificity	Sensitivity	Responsiveness	Odds Ratio
• Test-retest ICC = 0.53 SEM = 5.2[257] • Test-retest ICC = 0.42, SEM = 5.4[261] • Test-retest ICC = 0.91, limits of agreement/ normal variation over sessions ± 5.4[262] • ICC = 0.68, SEM = 2.72[115] • Test-retest ICC = 0.92[113]	• Internal consistency Cronbach's alpha coefficient 0.87[261]	• Scale interval from (0–24) 62%; (0–8) 88%, (5–12) 81%, (9–16) 77%, (13–29) 80%, (14–17) 78%[263]	• Scale interval from (0–24) 60%; (0–8) 64%, (5–12) 69%, (9–16) 85%, (13–29) 80%, (14–17) 100%[263]	• SRM = 0.55[257]	• Positive likelihood ratios scale from (0–24) 1.58, from (0–8) 5.33, from (5–12) 3.63, from (9–16) 3.69, (13–29) 4, from (14–17) 4.54; negative likelihood ratios scale from (0–24) 0.64, from (0–8) 0.41, from (5–12) 0.38, from (9–16) 0.19, (13–29) 0.25, from (14–17) 2.28

SCHOBER TEST

Reliability	Responsiveness
• Test-retest r = 0.65[264] • Test-retest (flexion ICC = 0.78, extension ICC = 0.69); interrater (flexion ICC = 0.72, extension ICC = 0.76)[265]	• Effect size = 0.75, SRM = 0.69[266]

SF-36

Validity

- 68% of subjects presented worst score possible showing floor effect[257]

SF-36 BODILY PAIN SCALE

Reliability	Validity	Responsiveness
• Test-retest ICC = 0.37, SEM = 25[257]	• Internal consistency Cronbach's alpha 0.79[255]	• Effect size 0.44[255] • SRM = 0.67[257]

SF-36 PHYSICAL FUNCTIONING SCALE

Reliability	Validity	Responsiveness
• Test-retest ICC = 0.83, SEM = 14[257]	• Internal consistency Cronbach's alpha 0.91[255]	• Effect size 0.27[255] • SRM = 0.44[257]

SF-36 ROLE LIMITATIONS-PHYSICAL SCALE

Reliability	Validity	Responsiveness
• Test-retest ICC = 0.39, SEM = 40[257]	• Internal consistency Cronbach's alpha 0.85[255]	• Effect size 0.03[255] • SRM = 0.45[257]

SF-36 SHORT FORM

Validity

• Correlation with modified Harris hip score (r = 0.71)[267]

SHUTTLE WALKING TEST

Reliability	Responsiveness
• Test-retest of distance to walk ICC = 0.99[268] • Claudication distance ICC > 0.68, maximum walking distance ICC > 0.87[269]	• Fitness effect size = 1.42, control effect size = 0.23, orthopaedic clinical effect size = 0.94[268]

SITUP TEST

Validity

• Female (concentric isokinetic r = 0.27, eccentric isokinetic r = 0.32); male (concentric isokinetic r = –0.25, eccentric isokinetic r = –0.28)[248]

SLUMP TEST

Reliability

• Interrater ICC = 0.92 SEM = 3, test-retest ICC = 0.80 SEM = 5[270]

STANDING FLEXION TEST

Reliability

• Interrater k = 0.052, intrarater k = 0.46[271]

STATIC BACK ENDURANCE

Reliability

• Intrarater r = 0.63[260]

STRAIGHT LEG RAISING TEST

Reliability	Validity	Specificity	Sensitivity	Odds Ratio
• Positive agreement 33%, negative agreement 96%, interrater k = 0.33[272] • For patients with radiating pain k = 0.33, positive agreement 40%, negative agreement 94%; for patients without radiating pain, negative agreement 98%[272] • Interrater of passive test ICC = 0.93 SEM = 4, test-retest ICC = 0.91 SEM = 4[270]	• 98% of positive correlation of the test with presence of disc protrusion[160]	• 87%[273]	• 33%[273]	• Positive likelihood ratios 2.53, negative likelihood ratios 0.77

Continued

APPENDIX 9-1—cont'd

THOMAS TEST

Reliability

- Interrater ICC = 0.90 SEM = 3, test-retest ICC = 0.69 SEM = 5[270]

TREADMILL TEST

Reliability	Sensitivity	Specificity	Odds Ratio
• Concordance correlation coefficient (CCC) (1.2 mph time first symptom CCC = 0.9; 1.2 mph total ambulation time CCC = 0.89) (preferred speed TFS CCC = 0.98; TAT CCC = 0.96)[274] • Claudication distance ICC > 0.86, maximum walking distance ICC > 0.87[269]	• Diagnose stenotic and nonstenotic patients (earlier onset of symptoms with level walking 83.3%, longer total walking time during inclined walking 92.3%, prolonged recovery after level walking 68.4%)[275]	• Diagnose stenotic and nonstenotic patients (earlier onset of symptoms with level walking 68%, longer total walking time during inclined walking 50%, prolonged recovery after level walking 81.8%)[275]	• Positive likelihood ratios for diagnose stenotic and nonstenotic patients (earlier onset of symptoms with level walking 4.07, longer total walking time during inclined walking 6.49, prolonged recovery after level walking 2.59); negative likelihood ratios for diagnose stenotic and nonstenotic patients (earlier onset of symptoms with level walking 0.38, longer total walking time during inclined walking 0.54, prolonged recovery after level walking 0.26)

TREATMENT-BASED CLASSIFICATION (TBC) TEST

Reliability

- Intrarater for inexperienced physical therapist k = 0.45[276]

WADDELL DISABILITY INDEX

Reliability	Responsiveness
• Test-retest ICC = 0.74, SEM = 1.7[257]	• SRM = 0.35[257]

CHAPTER 10

PELVIS

The sacroiliac joints form the "key" of the arch between the two pelvic bones; with the symphysis pubis, they help to transfer the weight from the spine to the lower limbs and provide elasticity to the pelvic ring. This triad of joints also acts as a buffer to decrease the force of jars and bumps to the spine and upper body caused by contact of the lower limbs with the ground. Because of this shock-absorbing function, the structure of the sacroiliac and symphysis pubis joints is different from that of most joints that are assessed. Assessment of the sacroiliac joints and symphysis pubis should be included in the examination of the lumbar spine and/or hips if there is no direct trauma to either one of these joints.[1] Normally, a comprehensive examination of the sacroiliac joints is not made until examination of the lumbar spine and/or hip has been completed. If both of these joints are examined and the problem still appears to be present and remains undiagnosed, an examination of the pelvis should be initiated.

Applied Anatomy

The **sacroiliac joints** are part synovial joint and part syndesmosis. A syndesmosis is a type of fibrous joint in which the intervening fibrous connective tissue forms an interosseous membrane or ligament. The synovial portion of the joint is C-shaped, with the convex iliac surface of the C facing anteriorly and inferiorly. Kapandji[2] states that the greater or the more acute the angle of the C, the more stable the joint and the less the likelihood of a lesion to the joint. The sacral surface is slightly concave.

The size, shape, and roughness of the articular surfaces vary greatly among individuals. In the child, these surfaces are smooth. In the adult, they become irregular depressions and elevations that fit into one another; by so doing, they restrict movement at the joint and add strength to the joint for transferring weight from the lower limb to the spine. The articular surface of the ilium is covered with fibrocartilage; the articular surface of the sacrum is covered with hyaline cartilage that is three times thicker than that of the ilium. In older persons, parts of the joint surfaces may be obliterated by adhesions.

Sacroiliac Joint	
Resting position:	Neutral
Capsular pattern:	Pain when joints are stressed
Close pack:	Nutation
Loose pack:	Counternutation

Although the sacroiliac joints are relatively mobile in young people, they become progressively stiffer with age. In some cases, ankylosis results. The movements that occur in the sacroiliac and symphysis pubis joints are slight compared with the movements occurring in the spinal joints.

The sacroiliac joints are supported by several strong ligaments (Figure 10-1)—the long posterior sacroiliac ligaments that limit anterior pelvic rotation[3] or sacral counternutation, the short posterior sacroiliac ligament that limits all pelvic and sacral movement, the posterior interosseous

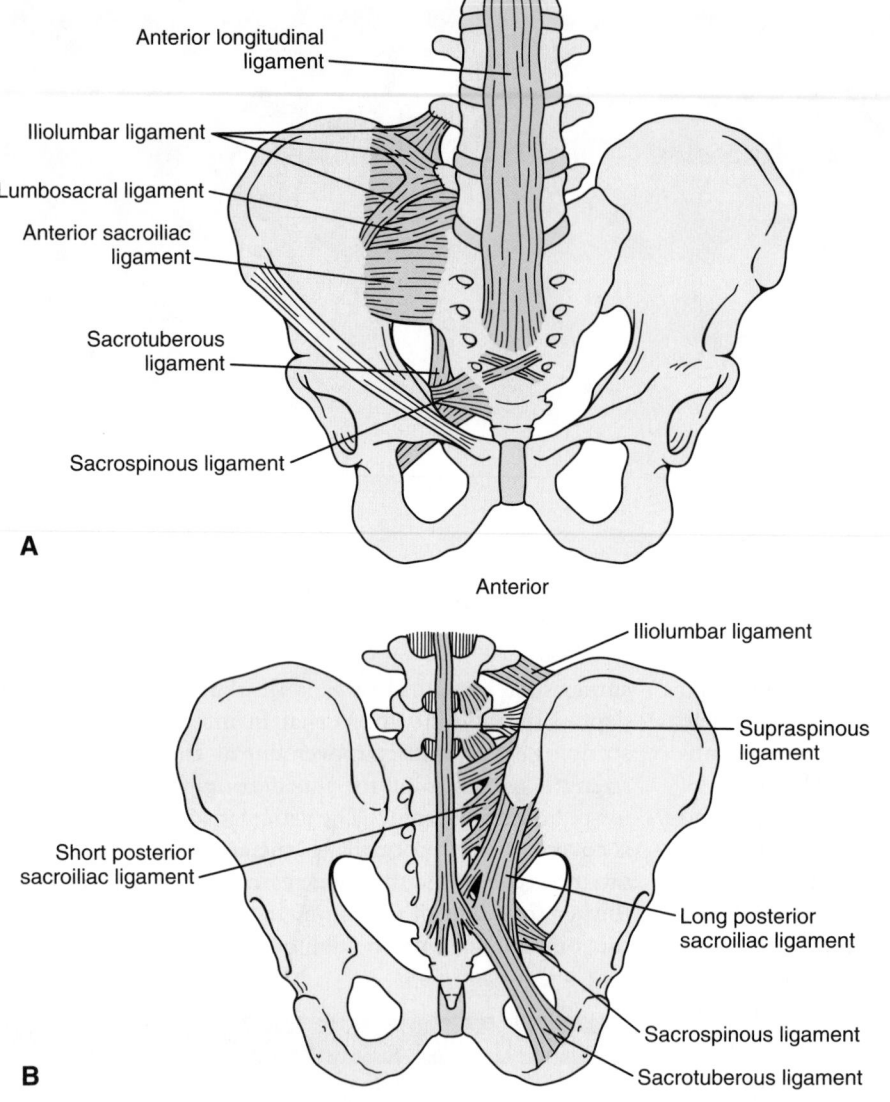

Anterior longitudinal ligament

Iliolumbar ligament

Lumbosacral ligament

Anterior sacroiliac ligament

Sacrotuberous ligament

Sacrospinous ligament

A

Anterior

Iliolumbar ligament

Supraspinous ligament

Short posterior sacroiliac ligament

Long posterior sacroiliac ligament

Sacrospinous ligament

Sacrotuberous ligament

B

Posterior

Figure 10-1
Ligaments of the pelvis. **A,** Anterior view.
B, Posterior view.

ligament that forms part of the sacroiliac articulation (the syndesmosis), and the anterior sacroiliac ligaments.[4] The sacrotuberous ligament and sacrospinous ligament limit nutation and posterior innominate rotation.[4] The iliolumbar ligament stabilizes L5 on the ilium.[4]

The sacroiliac joints and symphysis pubis have no muscles that control their movements directly, although the muscles do provide pelvic stability. However, they are influenced by the action of the muscles moving the lumbar spine and hip, because many of these muscles attach to the sacrum and pelvis (Table 10-1).

The muscles that support the pelvic girdle as well as the lumbar spine and hips can be divided into groups.[5-7] The inner group consists of deep muscles—transverse abdominus, diaphragm, multifidus, and pelvic floor muscles.

The outer group consists of four groupings, which act primarily in crossing or oblique patterns of force couples to stabilize the pelvis. The deep longitudinal system consists of the erector spinae, thoracolumbar fascia, and the hamstring muscles, along with the sacrotuberous ligament (Figure 10-2). The superficial posterior oblique system includes the latissimus dorsi, gluteus maximus, and the intervening thoracolumbar fascia (Figure 10-3, *A*). The anterior oblique system consists of the internal and external obliques, the contralateral adductors, and the abdominal fascia in between (Figure 10-3, *B*). The lateral system consists of gluteus medius and minimus and the contralateral adductors (Figure 10-4). The innermost muscles consist of the multifidus, transverse abdominus, diaphragm, and pelvic floor

Table 10-1

Muscles Attaching to the Pelvis

Muscles	Nerve Root Derivation
Latissimus dorsi	Thoracodorsal (C6–C8)
Erector spinae	L1–L3
Multifidus	L1–L5
External oblique	T7–T12
Internal oblique	T7–T12, L1
Transverse abdominis	T7–T12, L1
Rectus abdominis	T6–T12
Pyramidalis	Subcostal (T12)
Quadratus lumborum	T12, L1–L4
Psoas minor	L1
Iliacus	Femoral (L2–L3)
Levator ani	S4, inferior rectal nerve/pudendal nerve
Sphincter ani externus	S2–S4
Superficial transverse perineal ischiocavernous	S2–S4
Coccygeus	S4–S5
Gluteus maximus	Inferior gluteal (L5, S1–S2)
Gluteus medius	Superior gluteal (L5, S1)
Gluteus minimus	Superior gluteal (L5, S1)
Obturator internus	Nerve to obturator internus (L5, S1)
Obturator externus	Obturator (L3–L4)
Piriformis	L5, S1–S2
Interior gemellus	Nerve to quadratus femoris (L5, S1)
Superior gemellus	Nerve to obturator internus (L5, S1)
Pectineus	Femoral (L2, L3)
Semimembranosus	Sciatic (L5, S1–S2)
Semitendinosus	Sciatic (L5, S1–S2)
Biceps femoris	Sciatic (L5, S1–S2)
Tensor fascia lata	Superior gluteal (L4–L5)
Sartorius	Femoral (L2–L3)
Rectus femoris	Femoral (L2–L4)
Gracilis	Obturator (L2–L3)
Adductor magnus	Obturator/Sciatic (L2–L4)
Adductor longus	Obturator (L2–L4)
Adductor brevis	Obturator (L2–L4)

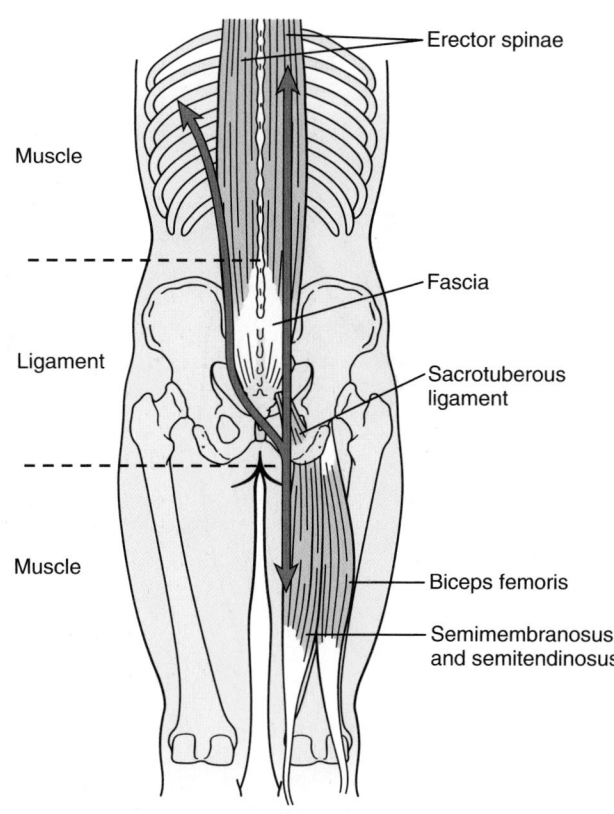

Figure 10-2

The deep longitudinal muscle system of the outer group (includes the erector spinae, deep lamina of the thoracolumbar fascia, sacrotuberous ligament, and biceps femoris muscle).

muscles (Figure 10-5). These muscle systems help to actively stabilize the pelvic joints and contribute significantly to load transfer during gait and pelvic rotational activities.[5]

The **symphysis pubis** is a cartilaginous joint. There is a disc of fibrocartilage between the two joint surfaces called the **interpubic disc.**

The **sacrococcygeal joint** is usually a fused line (symphysis) united by a fibrocartilaginous disc. It is found between the apex of the sacrum and the base of the coccyx. Occasionally, the joint is freely movable and synovial. With advanced age, the joint may fuse and be obliterated.

Patient History

In addition to the questions listed under Patient History in Chapter 1, the examiner should obtain the following information from the patient:

1. *Was there any known mechanism of injury? Has there been more than one episode?* For example, the sacroiliac joints are commonly injured by a sudden jar caused by inadvertently stepping off a curb, an overzealous kick (either missing the object or hitting the ground), a fall on the buttocks, or a lift and twist maneuver.[8] Has the patient experienced any recent falls, twists, or strains? These movements increase the chance of sacroiliac joint sprains.

2. *Where is the pain, and does it radiate?* With a lesion of the sacroiliac joint, deep, dull, undefined pain tends to be unilateral and can be referred to the posterior thigh, iliac fossa, and buttock on the affected side. Sacroiliac pain does not commonly extend below the knee.

3. *When does the pain occur? Does the pain keep the patient awake?* Pain that is caused by sacroiliac joint problems is usually felt when turning in bed, getting out of bed, or stepping up with the affected leg. Often, the pain is constant and unrelated to

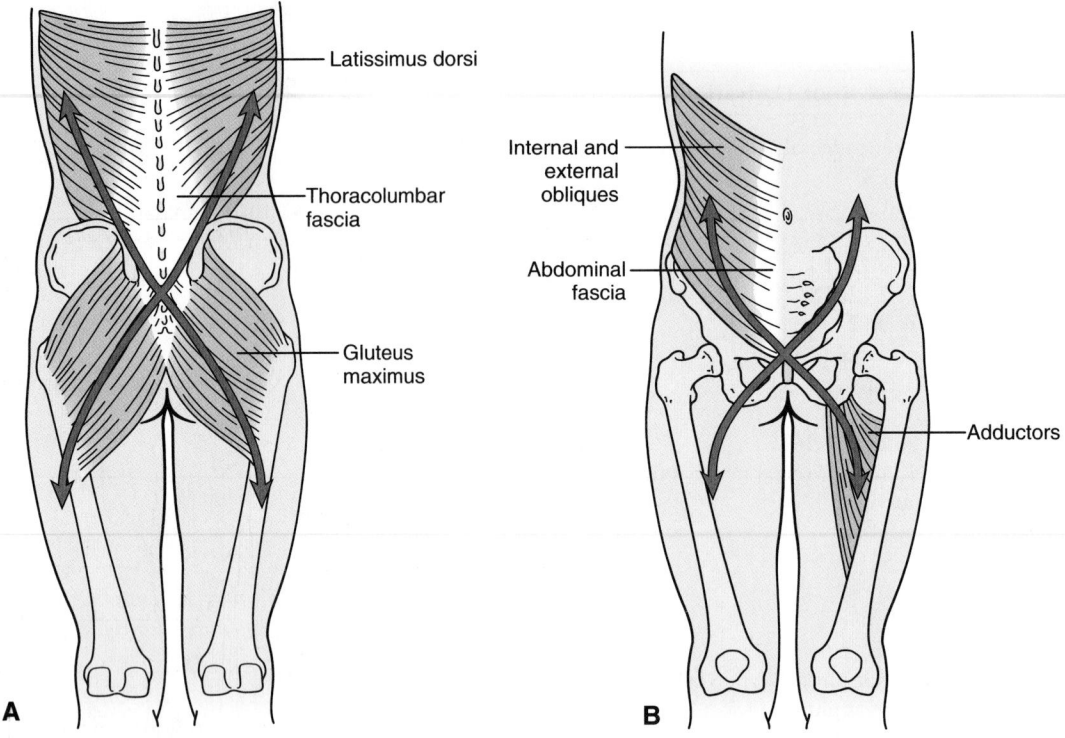

Figure 10-3

A, The posterior oblique muscle system of the outer group (includes the latissimus dorsi, gluteus maximus, and intervening thoracolumbar fascia). **B,** The anterior oblique muscle system of the outer group (includes the external and internal obliques, contralateral adductors of the thigh, and intervening anterior abdominal fascia).

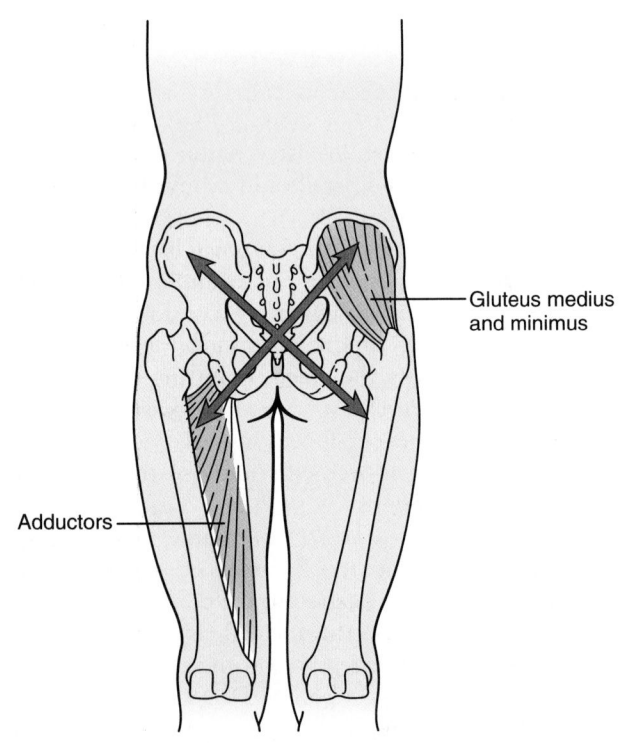

Figure 10-4

The lateral muscle system of the outer group (includes the gluteus medius and minimus and contralateral adductors of the thigh).

position. Symphysis pubis pain tends to be localized and increases with any movement involving the adductor or rectus abdominus muscles.

4. *What is the patient's habitual working stance? Is a great deal of sitting or twisting involved?* The examiner should look for postures that potentially increase the stress on the sacroiliac joints (e.g., standing, especially on one leg).

5. *What is the patient's usual activity or pastime?* Again, would any of these activities stress the sacroiliac joints?

6. *Is there any particular position or activity that aggravates the condition?* Climbing or descending stairs, walking, and standing from a sitting position all stress the sacroiliac joint (Tables 10-2 and 10-3).

7. *What is the patient's age?* Apophyseal injuries and avulsion fractures of the pelvis can occur in young athletes.[9] Ankylosing spondylitis is found primarily in men between the ages of 15 and 35 years. Hypomobility is likely to be seen in men between 40 and 50 and in women after 50 years of age.[10]

8. *Does the patient have or feel any weakness in the lower limbs?* Neurological deficit in the limbs can be present if the sacroiliac joint is affected.

9. *Has the patient had any difficulty with micturition?* It has been reported that sacroiliac joint dysfunction can lead to urinary problems.[11]

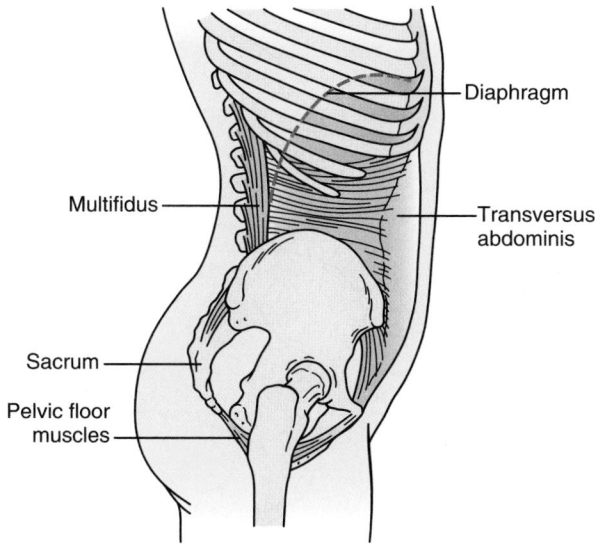

Figure 10-5
The inner muscle unit including multifidus, transverse abdominus, and the pelvis floor muscles.

Table 10-2

Pelvic Motions with Lumbar Spine Movement

Lumbar Spine	Innominate	Sacrum
Flexion	Anterior rotation	Nutation followed by counternutation
Extension	Posterior rotation (slight)	Nutation
Rotation	Same side: posterior rotation Opposite side: anterior rotation	Nutation on same side
Side flexion	Same side: anterior rotation Opposite side: posterior rotation	Side bend

Adapted from Dutton M: *Orthopedic examination, evaluation and intervention*, New York, 2004, McGraw-Hill.

Table 10-3

Pelvic Motions with Hip Movement

Hip	Innominate
Flexion	Posterior rotation
Extension	Anterior rotation
Medial rotation	Inflare (medial rotation)
Lateral rotation	Outflare (lateral rotation)
Abduction	Superior glide
Adduction	Inferior glide

Adapted from Dutton M: *Orthopedic examination, evaluation and intervention*, New York, 2004, McGraw-Hill.

10. *Has there been a recent pregnancy?* In females, sprain of the sacroiliac ligaments can be the result of increased laxity of the ligaments caused by hormonal changes. It may take 3 to 4 months or longer for the ligaments to return to their normal state after a pregnancy.

11. *Does the patient have a past history of rheumatoid arthritis, Reiter's disease, or ankylosing spondylitis?* Each of these conditions can involve the sacroiliac joints.

12. *Are there any psychosocial issues that are relevant in the presence of pathology?* Questions about anxiety, depression, and other psychosocial issues should be addressed if considered important.[12]

Observation

The patient must be suitably undressed. For the sacroiliac joints to be observed properly, the patient is often required to be nude from the midchest to the toes. If he or she wishes to wear shorts, they must be rolled down as far as possible so that the sacroiliac joints are visible. The posterior, superior, and inferior iliac spines must be visible. The patient stands and is viewed from the front, side, and back. The examiner should note the following:

1. Are the posture (see Chapter 15) and gait (see Chapter 14) normal? Nutation[5,13] (sacral locking) is the forward motion of the base of the sacrum into the pelvis; it could also be described as the backward rotation of the ilium on the sacrum (Figure 10-6). When moving from supine lying to standing, the sacrum normally moves bilaterally, just as it does in early movement of trunk flexion. The ilia move closer together and the ischial tuberosities move farther apart.[10] Unilaterally, the sacrum normally moves with hip flexion of the lower limb.[5] Pathologically, if nutation occurs only on one side, where it should occur bilaterally, the examiner will find that the anterior superior iliac spine (ASIS) is higher and the posterior superior iliac spine (PSIS) is lower on that side.[13] The result is an apparent or functional short leg on the same side.[14] Nutation is limited by the anterior sacroiliac ligaments, the sacrospinous ligament, and the sacrotuberous ligament and is more stable than counternutation. Nutation occurs when a person assumes a "pelvic tilt" position. During nutation, the sacrum will slide down its short part and then posteriorly along its long part (Figure 10-7).[5]

Counternutation (sacral unlocking), or contranutation as it is sometimes called, is the opposite movement to nutation. It indicates an anterior rotation of the ilium on the sacrum or backward motion of the base of the sacrum out of the pelvis.[5] The iliac bones move farther apart, and the ischial tuberosities approximate.[10] Pathologically, if counternutation occurs only on one side as it does

Nutation

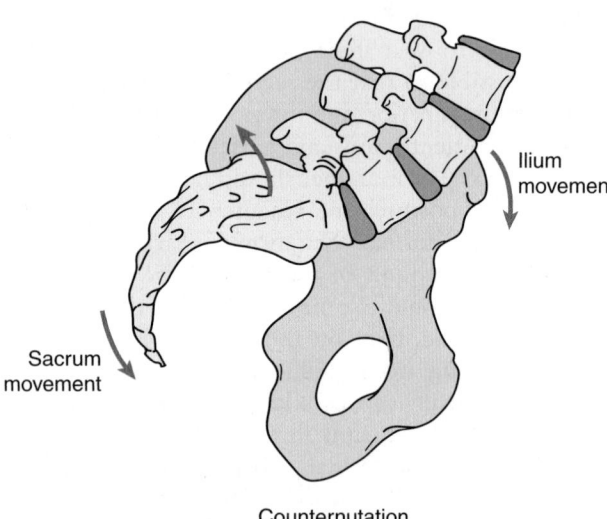

Counternutation

Figure 10-6

Movements of nutation and counternutation occurring at the sacroiliac joint.

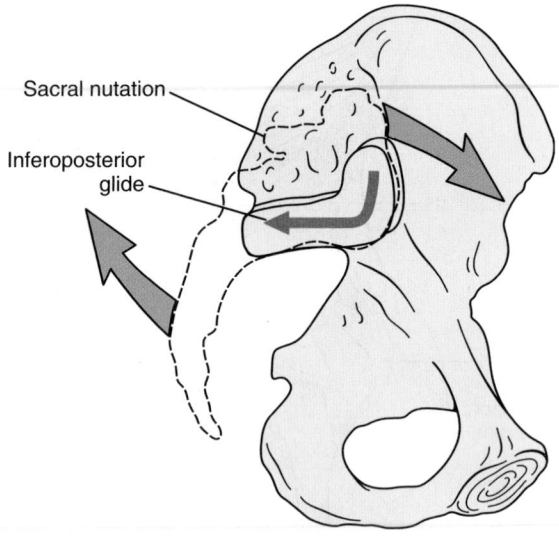

Figure 10-7

When the sacrum nutates, its articular surface glides inferoposteriorly relative to the innominate bones. (Redrawn from Lee D: *The pelvic girdle*, ed. 3, p. 60, Edinburgh, 2004, Churchill Livingstone.)

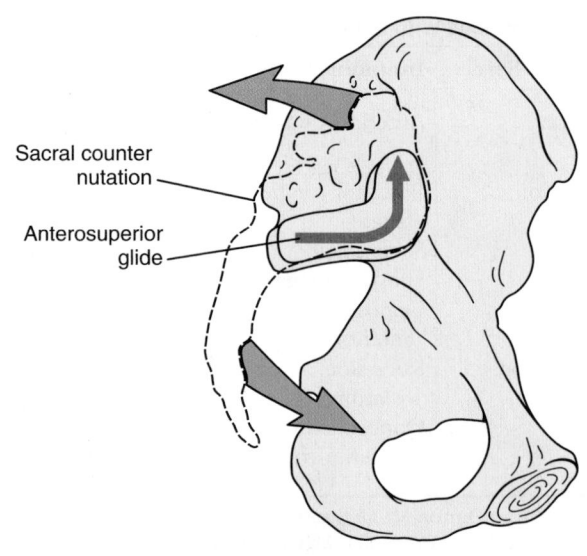

Figure 10-8

When the sacrum counternutates, its articular surface glides anterosuperiorly relative to the innominate bones. (Redrawn from Lee D: *The pelvic girdle*, ed. 3, p. 60, Edinburgh, 2004, Churchill Livingstone.)

during extension of the extremity on that side, the lower limb on that side will probably be medially rotated.[5] Pathological or abnormal counternutation on one side occurs when the ASIS is lower and the PSIS is higher on one side.[13] Counternutation is limited by the posterior sacroiliac ligaments. Counternutation occurs when a person assumes a "lordotic" or "anterior pelvic tilt" position. During counternutation, the sacrum will slide anteriorly along its long arm and then superiorly up its short arm (Figure 10-8).[5] This motion is resisted by the long posterior sacroiliac ligament supported by the multifidus (contraction of multifidus causes nutation of the sacrum).[5]

Levine and Whittle[15] found that anterior and posterior pelvic tilt has an effect on lumbar lordosis with an aver-age change of 20° being possible (9° posteriorly and 11° anteriorly). Thus, looking for the **"neutral** pelvis" position becomes important especially for later rehabilitation. Based on their data, a neutral pelvis would be somewhere between the two extremes. Pelvic tilt is the angle between a line joining the ASIS and PSIS, and a horizontal line (Figure 10-9). Average pelvic tilt is 11° ± 4°.[15,16] Ideal pelvic alignment would see the ASIS on the same vertical plane as the symphysis pubis.[17]

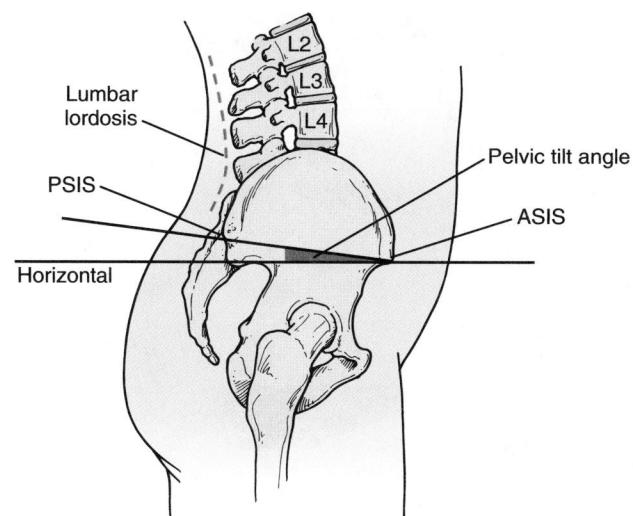

Figure 10-9
Pelvic tilt angle (7°–15°).

Gait is often affected if the pathology involves the pelvis. If the sacroiliac joints are not free to move, the stride length is decreased and a vertical limp may be present.[8] A painful sacroiliac joint may also cause reflex inhibition of the gluteus medius, leading to a Trendelenburg's gait or lurch.

2. Are the ASISs level when viewed anteriorly (Figure 10-10)? On the affected side, the ASIS often tends to be higher and slightly forward. The examiner must remember this difference, if present, when the patient is viewed from behind (Figure 10-11). If the ASIS and PSIS on one side are higher than the ASIS and PSIS on the other side, this indicates an **upslip** of the ilium on the sacrum on the high side, a short leg on the opposite side, or muscle spasm caused by lumbar pathology (e.g., disc lesion).[18-21] If the ASIS is higher on one side and the PSIS is lower at the same time, it indicates an **anterior torsion** of the sacrum (pathological nutation) on that side.[18] This torsion may result in a spinal scoliosis or an altered functional leg length, or both. Anterior rotational dysfunction is seen most frequently following a posterior horizontal thrust of the femur (dashboard injury), golf or baseball swing, or any forced anterior diagonal pattern.[19] The sacrum is lower on the side of the pelvis that has rotated backward. The most common rotation of the innominate bones is left posterior torsion or rotation (pathological counternutation). The posterior rotational dysfunctions are usually the result of falling on an ischial tuberosity, lifting when forward flexed with the knees straight, repeated standing on one leg, vertical thrusting onto an extended leg, or sustaining hyperflexion and abduction of hips.

3. Are both pubic bones level at the symphysis pubis? The examiner tests for level equality by placing one finger or thumb on the superior aspect of each pubic bone and comparing the heights (Figure

A   B

Figure 10-10
Anterior observational view. **A,** Level of anterior superior iliac spines. **B,** Level of iliac crests.

Figure 10-11

Posterior observational view. **A,** Level of iliac crests. **B,** Level of posterior superior iliac spines. **C,** Level of ischial tuberosities. **D,** Level of gluteal folds.

10-12). If the ASIS on one side is higher, the pubic bone on that side is suspected to be higher, and this can be confirmed by this procedure, indicating a backward torsion problem of the ilium on that side. This procedure is usually done with the patient lying supine.

4. Does the patient, when standing, have equal weight on both feet, favor one leg, or have a lateral pelvic tilt? This finding may indicate pathology in the sacroiliac joints, the leg, the spine, or a short leg.

5. Are the ASISs equidistant from the center line of the body?

6. What type of pelvis does the patient have?[22] Gynecoid and android types are the most common (as described in Figure 10-13 and Table 10-4).

7. Is the sacrovertebral or lumbosacral angle normal (140°)?

8. Is the pelvic angle or inclination normal (30°)?

9. Is the sacral angle normal (30°) (some call this the lumbosacral angle[23]) (Figure 10-14)?

Figure 10-12
Determining level of pubic bones.

10. Are the iliac crests level? Altered leg length may alter their height.

11. Are the PSISs level?

12. Are the buttock contours or gluteal folds normal? The painful side is often flatter if there is loss of tone in the gluteus maximus muscle.

13. Is there any unilateral or bilateral spasm of the erector spinae muscles?

14. Are the ischial tuberosities level? If one tuberosity is higher, it may indicate an upslip of the ilium on the sacrum on that side.[18]

15. Is there excessive lumbar lordosis? Forward or backward sacral torsion may increase or decrease the lordosis.

16. Are the PSISs equidistant from the center line of the body?

17. Are the sacral sulci equal? If one is deeper, it may indicate a sacral torsion.

18. Do the feet face forward to the same degree? Often, the affected limb is medially rotated. With spasm of the piriformis muscle, the limb is laterally rotated on the affected side.

Examination

Before assessing the pelvic joints, the examiner should first assess the lumbar spine and hip, unless the history definitely indicates that one of the pelvic joints is at fault. The lumbar spine and hip can, and frequently do, refer pain to the sacroiliac joint area. Because the sacroiliac joints are in part a syndesmosis, movements at these joints are minimal compared with those of the other peripheral joints. It should also be remembered that any condition that alters the position of the sacrum relative to the ilium causes a corresponding change in the position of the symphysis pubis.

A Pelvic inlet

B Sacrosciatic notch — Ischial spine

C Subpubic arch

GYNECOID   ANDROID

Figure 10-13
Gynecoid (predominantly female) and android (primarily male) pelvises. **A,** Anterior view. **B,** Lateral view. **C,** Anterior view of the pubis and ischium.

Table 10-4

A Comparison of the Two Most Common Types of Pelvis

Feature	Gynecoid	Android
Inlet	Round	Triangular
Sacrosciatic notch	Average size	Narrow
Sacrum	Average	Forward
Subpubic arch	Inclination curved	Inclination straight

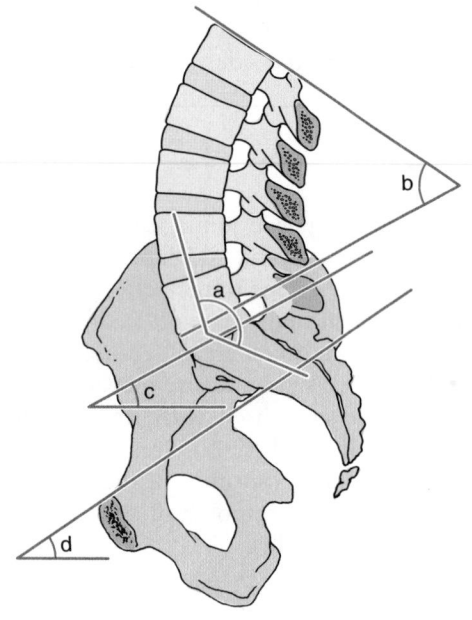

Figure 10-14

Normal angles of the pelvic joints. *a*, Lumbosacral angle (140°). *b*, Lumbar lordotic curve (50°). *c*, Sacral angle (30°). *d*, Pelvic angle (30°).

Although many tests and test movements have been described to help determine if there is sacroiliac dysfunction, many of them are imprecise and their reliability has been questioned.[24-30] At the present time, they are the best tests available. It is important for the examiner to consider all aspects of the assessment, including the history and the patient's symptoms along with the various tests and movements, before diagnosing sacroiliac joint problems.[4,5,24,31-33]

Active Movements

Unlike other peripheral joints, the sacroiliac joints do not have muscles that directly control their movement. However, because contraction of the muscles of the other joints may stress these joints or the symphysis pubis, the examiner must be careful during the active or resisted isometric movements of other joints and must be sure to ask the patient about the exact location of

the pain on each movement. Table 10-1 outlines the muscles that attach to the pelvis. For example, resisted abduction of the hip can cause pain in the sacroiliac joint on the same side if the joint is injured, because the gluteus medius muscle pulls the ilium away from the sacrum when it contracts strongly. In addition, side flexion to the same side increases the shearing stress to the sacroiliac joint on that side. The examiner is attempting to reproduce the patient's symptoms rather than just looking for pain.

The sacroiliac joints move in a "nodding" fashion of anteroposterior rotation. Normally, the PSISs approximate when the patient stands and separate when the patient lies prone. When he or she stands on one leg, the pubic bone on the supported side moves forward in relation to the pubic bone on the opposite side as a result of rotation at the sacroiliac joint.

The stability at the sacroiliac joint is determined by three factors—form closure, force closure, and motor control along with psychological aspects.[12] **Form closure** refers to the close packed position of the joint where no outside forces are necessary to hold the joint stable. Thus, intrinsic factors such as joint shape, coefficient of friction of the joint surfaces, and integrity of the ligaments contribute to form closure.[5,12,34] **Force closure** would be similar to the loose packed position in that extrinsic factors, primarily the **muscles and their neurological control,** along with the capsule are needed to maintain stability of the joint as well as the forces applied to the joint.[5,12,34] These two forms of closure and neurological control enable the sacroiliac joints to self lock as they go into close pack and slightly release, when the joint unlocks.

During the active movements of the pelvic joints, the examiner looks for unequal movement, loss of or increase in movement (hypomobility or hypermobility), tissue contracture, tenderness, or inflammation.

Active Movements That Stress the Sacroiliac Joints

- Forward flexion of the spine (40°–60°)
- Extension of the spine (20°–35°)
- Rotation of the spine, left and right (3°–18°)
- Side flexion of the spine, left and right (15°–20°)
- Flexion of the hip (100°–120°)
- Abduction of the hip (30°–50°)
- Adduction of the hip (30°)
- Extension of the hip (0°–15°)
- Medial rotation of the hip (30°–40°)
- Lateral rotation of the hip (40°–60°)

The movements of the spine put a stress on the sacroiliac joints as well as on the lumbar and lumbosacral

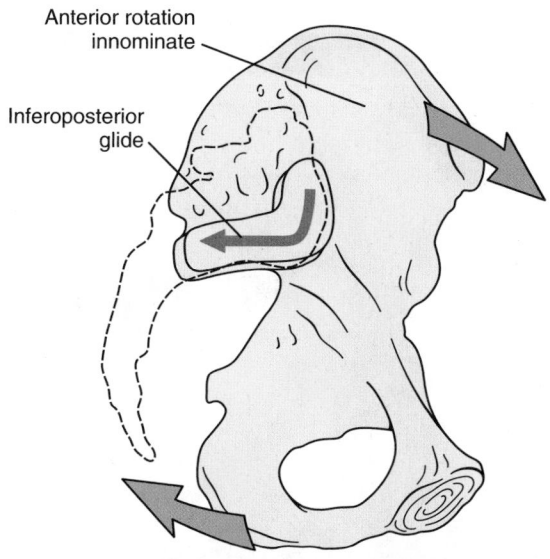

Anterior rotation innominate

Inferoposterior glide

Figure 10-15
When the innominate rotates anteriorly, its articular surface glides inferoposteriorly relative to the sacrum. (Redrawn from Lee D: *The pelvic girdle,* 2nd ed, p. 51, Edinburgh, 1999, Churchill Livingstone.)

Figure 10-16
Examiner palpating PSIS prior to forward flexion.

joints. During forward flexion of the trunk, the innominate bones and pelvic girdle as a whole rotate anteriorly as a unit on the femoral heads bilaterally. The same thing occurs when one rises from supine lying to sitting. If one leg is actively extended at the hip, the innominate on that side will unilaterally rotate anteriorly.[5] During the anterior rotation of the innominate bones (counternutation), the innominate slides posteriorly along its long arm and inferiorly down its short arm (Figure 10-15).[5] Initially, the sacrum nutates up to about 60° of forward flexion, but once the deep posterior structures (deep and posterior oblique muscle systems, thoracolumbar fascia, and the sacrotuberous ligament) become tight, the innominates continue to rotate anteriorly on the femoral heads, but the sacrum begins to counternutate.[5] This counternutation causes the sacroiliac joint to be vulnerable to instability as greater muscle action (force closure) is required to maintain stability with counternutation.[7] Thus, the earlier counternutation occurs during forward flexion, the more vulnerable is the sacroiliac joint to instability problems. Excessive counternutation is more likely to occur in patients who have tight hamstrings.[5]

To test forward flexion, the patient stands with weight equally distributed on both legs. The examiner sits behind the patient and palpates both PSISs (Figure 10-16). The patient is asked to bend forward (see Tables 10-2 and 10-3) and the symmetry of movement of the PSIS superiorly is noted. At the same time, the examiner should note the amount of flexion that has occurred when sacral nutation begins. This can be done by hav-

ing the patient repeat the forward bending motion while the examiner palpates the PSIS (inferior aspect) on one side with one thumb while the other thumb palpates the sacral base so the thumbs are parallel. In the first 45° of forward flexion, the sacrum will move forward (nutate) (Figure 10-17, *A*), but near 60° (normally), the sacrum will begin to counternutate or move backwards (Figure 10-17, *B*).[5] During the sacral counternutation, the two PSISs should move upward equally in relation to the sacrum and toward each other or approximate. At the same time, the ASIS will tend to flare out.

During extension, the opposite movements occur (see Tables 10-2 and 10-3).[5,8] During extension or backward bending of the trunk, the innominate bones (the pelvic girdle) as a whole unit rotate posteriorly (nutation) on the femoral heads bilaterally. If one leg is actively flexed at the hip, the innominate on that side will unilaterally rotate posteriorly.[5] During the posterior rotation of the innominate bones, the innominate slides anteriorly along the long arm and superiorly up the short arm. This movement is the same as sacral nutation (Figure 10-18).

A　　　　　　　　　　　　　　　　　　　**B**

Figure 10-17

Examiner palpating for sacral nutation. One thumb is on the PSIS, other thumb is parallel to it on the sacrum. Examiner is feeling for forward movement (nutation) of the sacrum that occurs early in movement (**A**) and backward movement (counternutation) of the sacrum, which normally occurs around 60° of hip flexion (**B**).

With backward bending, both PSISs move inferiorly an equal amount.

To test backward bending, the patient stands with weight equally distributed on both legs. The examiner sits behind the patient and palpates both PSISs. The patient is asked to bend backwards while the examiner notes any asymmetry (Figure 10-19). Normally, the PSISs move inferiorly. During backward bending, the innominate bones and sacrum remain in the same position so there should be no change in their relationship.[5] The examiner palpates both sides of the sacrum at the level of S1. As the patient extends, the sacrum should normally move forward. This is called the **sacral flexion test**.

Side flexion normally produces a torsion movement between the ilia and the sacrum. As the patient side flexes, the innominate bones bend to the same side and the sacrum rotates slightly in the opposite direction; the thumb of the examiner on the same side (the thumbs are palpating on each side of the sacrum at the level of S1) will move forward. This is called the **sacral rotation test**.[5] If this torsion movement does not occur (e.g., in hypomobility), the patient finds that more effort is required to side flex and it is harder to maintain balance.[8]

During rotation, the pelvic girdle moves in the direction of the rotation causing intrapelvic torsion. The innominate, which is on the side to which rotation is occurring, rotates posteriorly while the opposite innominate rotates anteriorly, pushing the sacrum into rotation in the same direction (i.e., right rotation of the trunk and pelvis causes right rotation of the sacrum).

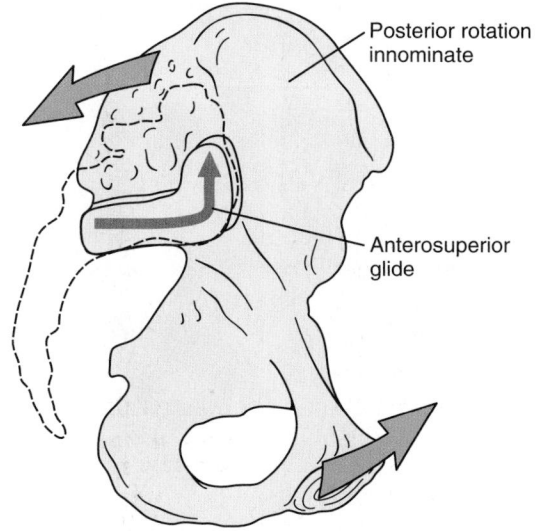

Figure 10-18

When the innominate posteriorly rotates, its articular surface glides anterosuperiorly relative to the sacrum. (Redrawn from Lee D: *The pelvic girdle,* 2nd ed, p. 51, Edinburgh, 1999, Churchill Livingstone.)

Posterior rotation innominate

Anterosuperior glide

Figure 10-19

Examiner palpating PSIS for asymmetric movement on backward bending.

This causes the sacrum to nutate on the side to which rotation occurs and counternutate on the opposite side.[5]

The hip movements performed are also affected by sacroiliac lesions. As the patient flexes each hip maximally, the examiner should observe the range of motion present, the pain produced, and the movement of the PSISs. The examiner first notes whether the PSISs are level before the patient flexes the hip. Normally, flexion of the hip with the knee flexed to 90° or more causes the sacroiliac joint on that side to drop or move caudally in relation to the other sacroiliac joint (**Gillet test**). If this drop does not occur, it may indicate hypomobility on the flexed side. The examiner can observe this movement by placing one thumb over the PSIS and the other thumb over the spinous process of S2 (Figure 10-20, *A*). In the patient with a normal sacroiliac joint, the thumb on the PSIS drops (Figure 10-20, *B*). If it is hypomobile, the thumb moves up on hip flexion. The two sides are compared. Sturesson and colleagues[35] have questioned whether much movement occurs at all because the stress of doing the test on one leg causes "force closure" of the sacroiliac joints, thus limiting movement.

The examiner then leaves the one thumb over the sacral spinous process and moves the other thumb over the ischial tuberosity (Figure 10-20, *C*). The patient is again asked to flex the hip as far as possible. Normally, the thumb over the ischial tuberosity moves laterally (Figure 10-20, *D*). With a fixed or hypomobile joint, the thumb moves superiorly or toward the head. Again, the two sides are compared.

The examiner then sits in front of the standing patient and palpates the ASIS. Testing one leg at a time, the patient pivots the leg on the heel into medial and lateral rotation. When doing these movements, the ASIS should move medially and laterally. Both sides are compared.[5]

The position of the sacrum can then be determined. To do this, the examiner tests the patient in two positions—sitting and prone—doing three movements: flexion, staying in neutral, and extension. Before testing, the examiner palpates the base of the sacrum and the inferior lateral angle (near apex) of the sacrum on both sides (Figure 10-21). Normally, the sacral bone and the inferior lateral angle of the sacrum are level (i.e., one is not more anterior or posterior than the other). The first test involves the patient sitting with the feet supported and the spine fully flexed. The examiner palpates the four points (Figure 10-22) and determines their relationship to one another. The patient is then put in prone lying with the spine in neutral and the relationship of the four points determined. The examiner then asks the patient to fully extend the spine and then determines the relationship of the four points. In any of

Figure 10-20

Active movements demonstrating how to show hypomobility of the sacroiliac joints. **A,** Starting position for sacral spine and posterior superior iliac spine. **B,** Hip flexion; the ilium drops as it normally should *(arrow)*. **C,** Starting position for sacral spine and ischial tuberosity. **D,** Hip flexion. Ischial tuberosity moves laterally *(arrow)*, as expected.

the positions tested, if the examiner found, for example, an anterior left sacral base along with a posterior right inferior lateral angle, it would indicate a left rotated sacrum.[5]

Passive Movements

The passive movements of the pelvic joints involve stressing of the ligaments and the joints themselves. They are not true passive movements, like those done at other joints, but are in reality stress or provocative tests. Lee[12] feels these passive movements or tests should be used to determine symmetry or asymmetry of stiffness rather than normal, hypermobile, or hypomobile. It is her contention that asymmetry at the two sacroiliac joints is the problem, not the amount of movement. Doing the passive movement is more likely to eliminate muscle tension effects that cause compression and increased stiffness.[12] Because of their anatomic makeup, the pelvic joints do not move to the same degree or in the same fashion as other joints of the body. When testing passive movement,

the examiner is looking for the **reproduction of the patient's symptoms**, not just pain or discomfort.[36,37]

Common Stress Tests (Passive Movements) of the Sacroiliac Joints

- Ipsilateral prone kinetic test
- Passive extension and medial rotation of ilium on sacrum
- Passive flexion and lateral rotation of ilium on sacrum
- Gapping test
- Approximation test
- Knee-to-shoulder test

Ipsilateral Prone Kinetic Test.[5,8] This test is designed to assess the ability of the ilium to flex and to rotate laterally or posteriorly. The patient lies prone while the examiner places one thumb on the PSIS and the other thumb parallel to it on the sacrum. The patient is then asked to actively extend the leg on the same side (Figure 10-23).

Figure 10-21
Examiner palpating base of sacrum and inferior lateral angle of the sacrum for anteroposterior symmetry.

Figure 10-22
Examiner palpating position of sacrum in flexed sitting.

Figure 10-23
Ipsilateral prone kinetic test. On extension, the posterior superior iliac spine and sacral crest move superiorly and laterally.

Normally, the PSIS should move superiorly and laterally. If it does not, it indicates hypomobility with a posterior rotated ilium, or **outflare**.

Passive Extension and Medial Rotation of Ilium on Sacrum.[5,8] The patient is in side lying position on the nontest side. The examiner places one hand over the ASIS area of the anterior ilium. The other hand is placed over the PSIS in such a way that the fingers of the hand palpate the posterior ilium and sacrum. The examiner then pulls the ilium forward with the hand over the ASIS and pushes the posterior ilium forward with the other hand while feeling the relative movement of the ilium on the sacrum (Figure 10-24). The unaffected side is then tested for comparison. If the affected side moves less, it indicates hypomobility and a posterior rotated ilium, or **outflare**.

Passive Flexion and Lateral Rotation of Ilium on Sacrum. The patient is positioned as for the previously mentioned test. In this case, the examiner pushes the anterior ilium backward with the anterior hand, and the posterior hand and arm pull the ilium posteriorly while palpating the relative movement (Figure 10-25). The unaffected side is then tested for comparison. If the affected side moves less, it is a sign of hypomobility and an anterior rotated ilium, or **inflare**.

If both this test and the previously mentioned one are positive, it means an **upslip** has occurred to the ilium relative to the sacrum.

Gapping (Transverse Anterior Stress) Test.[5] The patient lies supine while the examiner applies crossed-arm pressure to the ASIS (Figure 10-26, *A*). The examiner pushes down and out with the arms. The test is positive only if unilateral gluteal or posterior leg pain is produced, indicating a sprain of the anterior sacroiliac

Figure 10-24
Passive extension and medial rotation of the ilium on the sacrum. The innominate bone is held in extension and medial rotation. The examiner palpates the sacrum and ilium with the fingers while rotating the ilium forward. With hypomobility, the relative movement is less than on the unaffected side, indicating an outflare.

Figure 10-25
Passive flexion and lateral rotation of the ilium on the sacrum. The innominate bone is held in flexion and lateral rotation. The examiner palpates the sacrum and ilium with the left fingers while rotating the ilium backward. With hypomobility, the relative movement is less than on the unaffected side, indicating an inflare.

A

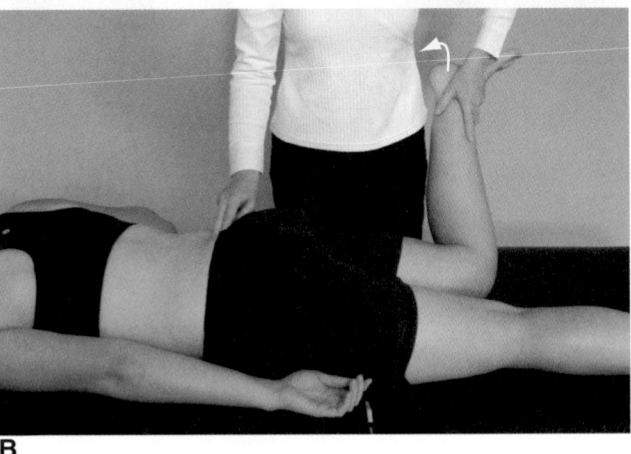

B

Figure 10-26
Gapping test. **A,** Done in supine. **B,** Done in prone.

ligaments. Care must be taken when performing this test. The examiner's hands pushing against the ASIS can elicit pain because the soft tissue is being compressed between the examiner's hands and the patient's pelvis.

Approximation (Transverse Posterior Stress) Test.[5] The patient is in the side lying position and the examiner's hands are placed over the upper part of the iliac crest, pressing toward the floor (Figure 10-27). The movement causes forward pressure on the sacrum. An increased feeling of pressure in the sacroiliac joints indicates a possible sacroiliac lesion and/or a sprain of the posterior sacroiliac ligaments.

Sacroiliac Rocking (Knee-to-Shoulder) Test. This test is also called the **sacrotuberous ligament stress test.** The patient is in a supine position (Figure 10-28). The examiner flexes the patient's knee and hip fully and then adducts the hip. To perform the test properly, both the hip and knee must demonstrate no pathology and have full range of motion. The sacroiliac joint is "rocked" by flexion and adduction of the patient's hip. To do the test properly, the knee is moved toward the patient's opposite shoulder. Some authors[5,38] believe that the hip should be medially rotated as it is flexed and adducted to increase the stress on the sacroiliac joint. Simultaneously, the sacrotuberous ligament may be palpated (see Figure 10-1

Figure 10-27
Approximation test. **A,** Diagram of posterior view. **B,** Anterior view.

for location) for tenderness. Pain in the sacroiliac joints indicates a positive test. Care must be taken, because the test places a great deal of stress on the hip and sacroiliac joints. If a longitudinal force is applied through the hip in a slow, steady manner (for 15 to 20 seconds) in an oblique and lateral direction, further stress is applied to the sacrotuberous ligament.[5] While performing the test, the examiner may palpate the sacroiliac joint on the test side to feel for the slight amount of movement that normally is present.

Prone Gapping (Hibb's) Test. The posterior sacroiliac ligaments may be stressed with the patient in the prone position (Figure 10-26, *B*). To perform the test, the patient's hips must have full range of motion and be pathology free. The patient lies prone, and the examiner stabilizes the pelvis with his or her chest. The patient's knee is flexed to 90° or greater, and the hip is medially rotated as far as possible. While pushing the hip into the very end of medial rotation, the examiner palpates the sacroiliac joint on the same side. The test is repeated on the other side, with the examiner comparing the degree of opening and the quality of the movement at each sacroiliac joint as well as stressing the posterior sacroiliac ligaments.

Passive Lateral Rotation of the Hip. The patient lies supine. The examiner flexes the hip and knee to 90° and then laterally rotates the hip. This movement, provided the hip is normal, stresses the sacroiliac joint on the test side.[10]

"Squish" Test. With the patient in the supine position, the examiner places both hands on the patient's ASISs and iliac crests and pushes down and in at a 45° angle (Figure 10-29). This movement tests the posterior sacroiliac ligaments. A positive test is indicated by pain.

Sacral Apex Pressure (Prone Springing) Test. The patient lies in a prone position on a firm surface while the

Figure 10-28
Sacroiliac rocking (knee-to-shoulder) test.

Figure 10-29
"Squish" test.

examiner places the base of his or her hand at the apex of the patient's sacrum (Figure 10-30). Pressure is then applied to the apex of the sacrum, causing a shear of the sacrum on the ilium. The test may indicate a sacroiliac joint problem if pain is produced over the joint. The test causes a rotational shift of the sacroiliac joints.

Torsion Stress Test.[5] The patient lies prone. The examiner palpates the spinous process of L5, with one thumb holding it stable. The examiner's other hand is placed around the anterior ilium on the opposite side and lifts the contralateral ilium up (Figure 10-31). This rotational movement stresses the lumbosacral junction, the iliolumbar ligament, the anterior sacroiliac ligament, and the sacroiliac joint.

Femoral Shear Test. The patient lies in the supine position. The examiner slightly flexes, abducts, and laterally rotates the patient's thigh at approximately 45° from the midline. The examiner then applies a graded force through the long axis of the femur, which causes an anterior-to-posterior shear stress to the sacroiliac joint on the same side (Figure 10-32).[38]

Figure 10-32
Femoral shear test.

Superoinferior Symphysis Pubis Stress Test.[5,8] The patient lies supine. The examiner places the heel of one hand over the superior pubic ramus of one pubic bone and the heel of the other hand over the inferior pubic ramus of the other pubic bone. The examiner then squeezes the hands together, applying a shearing force to the symphysis pubis (Figure 10-33). Production of pain in the symphysis pubis is considered a positive test.

Resisted Isometric Movements

As previously stated, there are no specific muscles acting directly on the sacroiliac joints and symphysis pubis. However, contraction of adjacent muscles can stress these joints and cause force closure.[34] The examiner performs these movements with the patient supine and attempts to reproduce the patient's symptoms.

Figure 10-30
Sacral apex pressure test. Patient is lying prone.

Figure 10-31
Torsion stress test. Patient is lying prone.

Figure 10-33
Superoinferior symphysis pubis stress test. Patient is lying supine.

Resisted Isometric Movements Stressing the Sacroiliac Joints

- Forward flexion of spine (the abdominals stress the symphysis pubis)
- Flexion of hip (the iliacus stresses the sacroiliac joint)
- Abduction of hip (the gluteus medius stresses the sacroiliac joint)
- Adduction of the hip (the adductors stress the symphysis pubis)
- Extension of hip (the gluteus maximus and erector spinae cause force closure)
- Pelvic floor muscles—transverse abdominus/multifidus force couple causes force closure
- Abdominal obliques cause force closure
- Latissimus dorsi causes force closure

Functional Assessment

Functional assessment of the pelvic joints by themselves is very difficult because these joints do not work in isolation. Functionally, they should be considered part of the lumbar spine or part of the hip joint, depending on the area that the presenting pathology most affects.

Special Tests

The examiner should use only those special tests that are considered necessary to confirm the diagnosis. Few special tests that accurately diagnose sacroiliac joint pathology have been validated.[34] Dreyfuss et al.[31,39] showed that the sacral sulcus (the area of soft tissue just medial to the PSIS) was tender in 89% of sacroiliac joint patients. When performing these tests, especially the stress or provocative tests, the examiner is attempting to reproduce the patient's symptoms. The reliability, validity, specificity, and sensitivity of special/diagnostic tests used in the pelvis are outlined in Appendix 10-1.

If muscle tightness is suspected as part of the problem, muscle should be tested for length.

Special Tests Commonly Performed on the Pelvis

- Straight leg raising test
- Prone knee bending test
- Gillet test
- Ipsilateral anterior rotation test
- Flamingo test
- Leg length tests
- Sign of the buttock
- Trendelenburg's test
- Functional hamstring length
- Thoracolumbar fascia length

Tests for Neurological Involvement

Straight Leg Raising (Lasègue's) Test. Although the Lasègue sign is primarily considered a test of the neurological tissue around the lumbar spine, this test also places a stress on the sacroiliac joints. With the patient in the supine position (Figure 10-34), the examiner passively flexes the patient's hip with the knee extended. Pain occurring after 70° is usually indicative of joint pain. However, in hypermobile persons, joint pain is often not experienced until after 120° of hip flexion. Therefore, it is more important to watch for the production of the patient's symptoms than for the actual range of motion. In addition, the range of motion obtained should be compared with the unaffected side. If the examiner then does a passive bilateral straight leg raising test in a similar fashion, pain occurring before 70° is usually indicative of sacroiliac joint problems. DonTigny[40] has reported that the straight leg raise (SLR) can be affected by sacroiliac

Figure 10-34

Straight leg raising test. **A,** Unilateral (head may be flexed, ankle may be dorsiflexed, or both). **B,** Bilateral.

problems. If, when doing SLR, the pain in the sacroiliac joint is unaltered or decreases, the examiner may suspect an anterior torsion. If the pain increases in the sacroiliac joint, a posterior torsion is possible. If pain increases on the opposite side, an anterior torsion on the opposite side should be suspected.

Lee[5] advocated several modifications to the straight leg test (Figure 10-35, *A*) if sacroiliac joint problems are suspected. These tests are called **active SLR tests** and were originally designed to test for postpartum pelvic problems.[41-43] In the first modification, Lee recommends that the test be done actively by the patient.[12,41-43] As the patient actively lifts the leg, the examiner asks whether the patient notes any "effort differences" between the two sides. The examiner then stabilizes and compresses the pelvis while the patient actively does the SLR providing **form closure** of the joints by squeezing the innominate bones together anteriorly (Figure 10-35, *B*). If the pain decreases or the SLR is easier to do with form closure (with no increased neurological signs), the test is considered positive for possible sacroiliac joint problems.

At the same time, the examiner can check the contraction of the pelvic floor/transverse abdominus/multifidus force couple by palpating medial to the ASIS bilaterally. If the force couple functions properly, tension is felt symmetrically and the abdomen moves inward. If superficial tension is felt, it means the internal obliques are contracting and there is a force-couple imbalance.[12] Multifidus may be palpated close to the spinous process and it should contract when the pelvic floor contracts. Another modification tests **force closure** at the sacroiliac joints.[5] The patient is asked to flex and rotate the trunk toward the side that the SLR is actively being performed. The trunk motion is resisted by the examiner (Figure 10-35, *C*). The two sides are compared for any difference. Force closure tests the ability of the muscles to stabilize the sacroiliac joints during movement.

Lee[5] also advocates doing active hip extension with the leg straight under three conditions. The first condition is hip extension (Figure 10-36, *A*). The second condition includes the same movement as the first with the examiner applying manual compression

A

B

C

Figure 10-35

Functional test of supine-active straight leg raise. **A,** Patient actively does straight leg raise to provide comparison with ease of doing test in other two positions. **B,** With form closure augmented (compression of innominate bones). **C,** With force closure augmented (resisted muscle action).

Figure 10-36

Functional test of prone-active straight leg raise. **A,** Patient actively extends straight leg to provide comparison with ease of doing test in other two positions. **B,** With form closure augmented (compression of innominate bones). **C,** With force closure augmented (resisted muscle action).

to the innominate bones (form closure) (Figure 10-36, *B*). The third condition has the examiner resisting extension of the contralateral medially rotated arm (force closure) as the patient extends the straight leg (Figure 10-36, *C*). If function improves when force closure stabilization is used, exercise will probably benefit the patient.

A more detailed description of the straight leg raising test is given in Chapter 9.

Prone Knee Bending (Nachlas) Test. Normally, this is used to test for a tight rectus femoris, an upper lumbar joint lesion, an upper spine nerve root lesion, or a hypomobile sacroiliac joint. The patient lies prone, and the examiner flexes the knee so that the heel is brought to the buttocks. If pain is felt in the front of the thigh before full range is reached, the problem is in the rectus femoris muscle. If the pain is in the lumbar spine, the problem is in the lumbar spine, usually the L3 nerve root, especially if these are radicular symptoms. If the problem is a hypomobile sacroiliac joint, the ipsilateral pelvic rim (ASIS) rotates forward, usually before the knee reaches 90° flexion.[38,44]

Tests for Sacroiliac Joint Involvement

Lee[12] has reported that active mobility tests should not be used to test the passive mobility of the sacroiliac joints. She felt passive movements used to look for asymmetry were more effective.

Gillet's (Sacral Fixation) Test.[19] This test is also called the ipsilateral posterior rotation test. While the patient stands, the sitting examiner palpates the PSISs with one thumb and the other thumb parallel with the first thumb on the sacrum. The patient is then asked to stand on one leg while pulling the opposite knee up toward the chest. This causes the innominate bone on the same side to rotate posteriorly and the sacrum to rotate to the same side. The test is repeated with the other leg palpating the other PSIS. If the sacroiliac joint on the side on which the knee is flexed (i.e., the ipsilateral side) moves minimally or up, the joint is said to be hypomobile, or "blocked," indicating a positive test.[30] On the normal side, the test PSIS moves down or inferiorly (Figure 10-37). This test is similar to the test performed during hip flexion in active movement; the only difference is the points of palpation during the movement.

Figure 10-37
Gillet's (sacral fixation) test.

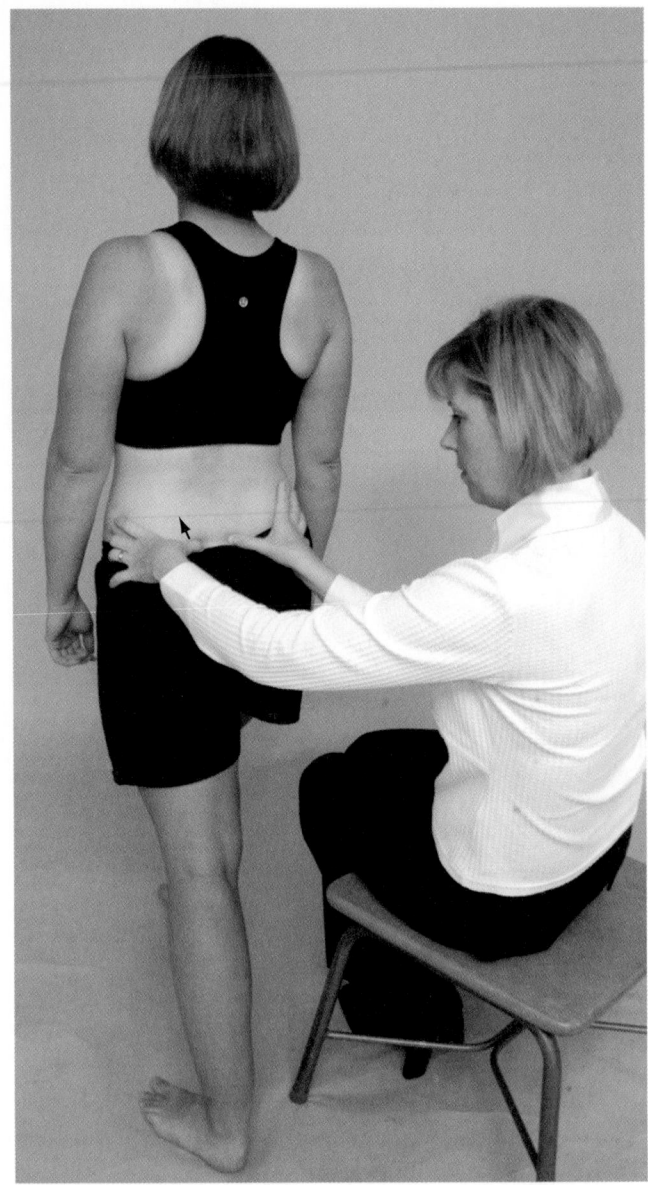

Figure 10-38
Ipsilateral anterior rotation test.

Jackson[4] has suggested a modification to the test. After completing the Gillet's test, he suggests that the examiner palpate the same PSIS and sacrum and ask the patient to do a repeat of the Gillet test using the other leg, which causes the opposite innominate bone to rotate posteriorly. As the patient flexes the hip and knee, the lumbar spine will begin to flex, causing the sacrum to move inferiorly and resulting in the test innominate (side opposite to the leg being flexed) to rotate anteriorly.

Ipsilateral Anterior Rotation Test.[5] The patient stands with weight equally distributed on both feet. The examiner sits behind the patient and palpates one PSIS with one thumb and the sacrum on a parallel line with the other thumb. The patient is asked to extend the ipsilateral leg. Normally, the PSIS should move superiorly and laterally (Figure 10-38). The other side is tested for comparison. This test determines the ability of the innominate on the test side to rotate anteriorly while the sacrum rotates to the opposite side.[5]

Flamingo Test or Maneuver. The patient is asked to stand on one leg (Figure 10-39). When the patient is standing on one leg, the weight of the trunk causes the sacrum to shift forward and distally (caudally) with forward rotation. The ilium moves in the opposite direction. On the nonweight-bearing side, the opposite occurs, but the stress is greatest on the stance side.[10] Pain in the symphysis

pubis or sacroiliac joint indicates a positive test for lesions in whichever structure is painful. The stress may be increased by having the patient hop on one leg. This position is also used to take a stress x-ray of the symphysis pubis.

Piedallu's Sign. The patient is asked to sit on a hard, flat surface (Figure 10-40). This position keeps the muscles (e.g., hamstrings) from affecting the pelvic flexion symmetry and increases the stability of the ilia. In effect, it is a test of the sacrum on the ilia. The examiner palpates the PSISs and compares their heights. If one PSIS, usually the painful one, is lower than the other, the patient is asked to forward flex while remaining seated. If the lower PSIS becomes the higher one on forward flexion, the test is positive; it is that

Figure 10-39
Flamingo test.

Figure 10-40
Piedallu's sign. **A,** Starting position. **B,** Test position.

side that is affected. Because the affected joint does not move properly and is hypomobile, it goes from a low to a high position. This is believed to indicate an abnormality in the torsion movement at the sacroiliac joint.

Gaenslen's Test. The patient lies on the side with the upper leg (test leg) hyperextended at the hip (Figure 10-41, *A*). The patient holds the lower leg flexed against the chest. The examiner stabilizes the pelvis while extending the

hip of the uppermost leg. Pain indicates a positive test. The pain may be caused by an ipsilateral sacroiliac joint lesion, hip pathology, or an L4 nerve root lesion.

Gaenslen's test is sometimes done with the patient supine (Figure 10-41, *B*), but this position may limit the amount of hyperextension available. The patient is positioned so that the test hip extends beyond the edge of the table. The patient draws both legs up onto the chest and then slowly lowers the test leg into extension. The other leg is tested in a similar fashion for comparison. Pain in the sacroiliac joints is indicative of a positive test.

Mazion's Pelvic Maneuver.[45] The patient stands in a straddle position with the limb on the unaffected side forward so that the feet are 0.5 to 1 m (2–3 feet) apart. The patient bends forward, trying to touch the floor, until the heel of the back leg lifts off the floor. If pain is produced in the lower trunk on the affected side, it is considered a positive test for unilateral forward displacement of the ilium relative to the sacrum.

Laguere's Sign. The patient lies supine (Figure 10-42). To test the left sacroiliac joint, the examiner flexes, abducts, and laterally rotates the patient's left hip, applying an overpressure at the end of the range of motion. The examiner must stabilize the pelvis on the opposite side by holding the opposite ASIS down. Pain in the left sacroiliac joint constitutes a positive test. The other side is tested for comparison. This test should be performed with caution for patients with hip pathology, because hip pain may ensue.

Figure 10-41

Gaenslen's test. **A,** With patient in side lying position, examiner extends test leg. **B,** With patient supine, test leg is extended over edge of table.

Figure 10-42

Laguere's sign.

Supine-to-Sit (Long Sitting) Test. The patient lies supine with the legs straight. The examiner ensures that the medial malleoli are level. The patient is asked to sit up, and the examiner observes whether one leg moves up (proximally) farther than the other (Figures 10-43 and 10-44). If so, it is believed that there is a functional leg length difference resulting from a pelvic dysfunction caused by pelvic torsion or rotation.[38,46,47] It may also be caused by spasm of the lumbar muscles in the presence of lumbar pathology.

Goldthwait's Test. The patient lies supine. The examiner places one hand under the lumbar spine so that each finger is in an interspinous space (i.e., L5-S1, L4–L5, L3–L4, and L2–L3 interspaces). The examiner uses the other hand to perform straight leg raising. If pain is elicited before movement occurs at the interspaces, the problem is in the sacroiliac joint. Pain during interspace movement indicates a lumbar spine dysfunction. As with the straight leg raising test, pain may be referred along the course of the sciatic nerve if there is neurological (e.g., nerve root) involvement.[44]

Yeoman's Test. The patient lies prone. The examiner flexes the patient's knee to 90° and extends the hip (Figure 10-45). Pain localized to the sacroiliac joint indicates pathology in the anterior sacroiliac ligaments. Lumbar pain indicates lumbar involvement.[44] Anterior thigh paresthesia may indicate a femoral nerve stretch.

Tests for Limb Length

Leg Length Test. The leg length test, described in detail in Chapter 11, should always be performed if the examiner suspects a sacroiliac joint lesion. Nutation (backward

Text continued on page 642

Figure 10-43
Supine-to-sit test for functional leg length discrepancy. **A,** Initial position. **B,** Final position. **C,** Symmetric leg
lengths. **D,** Asymmetric leg lengths.

Figure 10-44
Supine-to-sit test. Leg length reversal; supine (**A**) versus
sitting (**B**). If the lower limb on the affected side appears
longer when a patient lies supine but shorter when sitting, the
test is positive, implicating anterior innominate rotation of the
affected side. (Redrawn from Wadsworth CT, editor: *Manual
examination and treatment of the spine and extremities,* p. 82,
Baltimore, 1988, Williams & Wilkins.)

Figure 10-45
Yeoman's test.

Figure 10-46
Measuring leg length (anterior superior iliac spine to medial malleolus).

rotation) of the ilium on the sacrum results in a decrease in leg length, as does counternutation (anterior rotation) on the opposite side. If the iliac bone on one side is lower, the leg on that side is usually longer.[40] True leg length is measured by placing the patient in a supine position with the ASISs level and the patient's lower limbs perpendicular to the line joining the ASISs (Figure 10-46). Using a flexible tape measure, the examiner obtains the distance from the ASIS to the medial or lateral malleolus on the same side. The measurement is repeated on the other side, and the results are compared. A difference of 1 to 1.3 cm (0.5–1 inch) is considered normal. It should be remembered, however, that leg length differences within this range may also be pathological if symptoms result.[48]

Functional Limb Length Test.[49] The patient stands relaxed while the examiner palpates the ASISs and PSISs, noting any asymmetry. The patient is then placed in the "correct" stance (subtalar joints neutral, knees fully extended, and toes facing straight ahead), and the ASISs and PSISs are palpated, with the examiner noting whether the asymmetry has been corrected. If the asymmetry has been corrected by "correct" positioning of the limb, the leg is structurally normal (i.e., the bones have proper length) but abnormal joint mechanics (functional deficit) are producing a functional leg length difference. Therefore, if the asymmetry is corrected by proper positioning, the test is positive for a functional leg length difference.

Other Tests

Sign of the Buttock Test. With the patient supine, the examiner performs a passive unilateral straight leg raising test as done previously (Figure 10-47). If restriction or pain is found on one side, the examiner flexes the patient's knee while holding the patient's thigh in the same position. Once the knee is flexed, the examiner tries to flex the hip further. If the problem is in the lumbar spine or hamstrings, hip flexion increases. This finding indicates a negative sign of the buttock test. If hip flexion does not increase when the knee is flexed, it is a positive sign of the buttock test and indicates pathology in the buttock, such as a bursitis, tumor, or abscess. The patient with this pathology would also exhibit a noncapsular pattern of the hip.

Trendelenburg's Test or Sign. The patient is asked to stand or balance first on one leg and then on the other (Figure 10-48). While the patient is balancing on one leg, the examiner watches the movement of the pelvis. If the pelvis on the side of the nonstance leg rises, the test is considered negative, because the gluteus medius muscle on the opposite (stance) side lifts it up as it normally does in one-legged stance. If the pelvis on the side

Figure 10-47

Sign of the buttock test. **A,** Hip is flexed with knee straight until resistance or pain is felt. **B,** The knee is then flexed to see whether further hip flexion can be achieved. If further hip flexion can be achieved, the test is negative.

of the nonstance leg falls, the test is considered positive and is an indication of weakness or instability of the hip abductor muscles, primarily the gluteus medius on the stance side. Therefore, although the examiner is watching what happens on the nonstance side, it is the stance side that is being tested.

Functional Hamstring Length.[5] The patient sits on the examining table with the knees flexed to 90°, no weight on feet, and spine in neutral. The examiner sits behind the patient and palpates the PSIS with one thumb while the other thumb rests parallel on the sacrum. The patient is asked to actively extend the knee (Figure 10-49).

Normally, full knee extension is possible without posterior rotation of the pelvis or flexion of the lumbar spine. Tight hamstrings would cause the pelvis to rotate posteriorly and/or the spine to flex.

Thoracolumbar Fascia Length.[5] The patient sits on the examining table with the knees bent to 90° and a neutral spine. The examiner stands behind the patient. The patient is asked to rotate left and right fully and the examiner notes the range of motion available (Figure 10-50, *A*). The patient is then asked to forward flex the arms to 90° and laterally rotate and adduct the arms so the little fingers touch each other and palms face up (Figure 10-50,

Figure 10-48
Trendelenburg's sign. **A,** Negative test. **B,** Positive test.

Figure 10-49
Test of functional length of hamstrings and the sacrotuberous ligament.

B). Holding this arm position, the patient is again asked to rotate left and right as far as possible. The motion will be restricted in the second set of rotations if the thoracolumbar fascia or latissimus dorsi are tight.

90-90 SLR Test for Hamstring Tightness. See Hip or Knee chapters (See Chapters 11 and 12).

Reflexes and Cutaneous Distribution

There are no reflexes to test for the pelvic joints. However, the examiner must be aware of the dermatomes from the sacral nerve roots (Figure 10-51). Pain may be referred to the sacroiliac joints from the lumbar spine and the hip (Figure 10-52). In addition, the sacroiliac joint may refer pain to these same structures or along the courses of the superior gluteal and obturator nerves. The muscles of the spine may also refer pain to the sacral area (Table 10-5).

Peripheral Nerve Injuries About the Pelvis

Meralgia Paresthetica.[50] This condition is the result of pressure or entrapment of the lateral femoral cutaneous nerve near the ASIS as the nerve passes under the inguinal ligament. It may result from trauma such as that caused by a seat belt in a car accident, during delivery (in stirrups), by tight clothing, or as a complication of surgery (e.g., hernia). This nerve is sensory only, so the patient experiences sensory alteration and/or burning pain on the lateral aspect of the thigh (Figure 10-53).

Ilioinguinal Nerve.[51] This nerve, which lies within the transverse abdominus muscle, may be compressed by spasm of the muscle (Figure 10-54). The nerve is sensory only, and the sensory alteration and/or pain occurs in the superior aspect of the anterior thigh (in the L1 dermatome area) as well as in the scrotum or labia. There have been reports in the literature[52-55] that this nerve may be entrapped with injury to the external oblique muscle aponeurosis (hockey player's syndrome). The patient feels pain especially on ipsilateral hip extension and contralateral torso rotation. The pain may radiate to the groin, scrotum, hip, and back.

Joint Play Movements

The joint play movements (Figure 10-55) are minimal for the sacroiliac joints and are similar to the passive movements in that they are stress or provocative tests.

To test each of these movements, the patient is in the prone position. For the first joint play movement, the examiner places the heel of one hand over the iliac crest and the heel of the other hand over the apex of the sacrum. The ilium is pushed down or caudally with one hand while the sacrum is pushed up or cephalad with the other hand. The test is repeated for the other ilium (see Figure 10-55, *A*). The examiner should feel only minimal movement, and there should be no pain in the

Figure 10-50
Test of functional length of the thoracolumbar fascia and the latissimus dorsi muscle. **A,** Test without stretch. **B,** Test with muscle and fascia under stretch.

joint if the joint is normal. In an affected sacroiliac joint, there is usually pain over the joint and little or no movement. This positioning tests for cephalad movement of the sacrum and caudal movement of the ilium.

To test caudal movement of the sacrum and cephalad movement of the ilium, the examiner places the heel of one hand over the base of the sacrum and the heel of the other hand over the ischial tuberosity (see Figure 10-55, *B*). The examiner then pushes the pelvis cephalad and the sacrum caudally. The test is repeated with the other half of the pelvis being moved. The movement and amount of pain are compared.

Joint Play Movements of the Sacroiliac Joints

- Cephalad movement of the sacrum with caudal movement of the ilium (left and right)
- Cephalad movement of the ilium with caudal movement of the sacrum (left and right)
- Anterior movement of the sacrum on the ilium
- Anteroposterior translation of ilium on sacrum
- Superoinferior translation of ilium on sacrum
- Inferoposterior translation of ilium on sacrum
- Superoanterior translation of ilium on sacrum

Figure 10-51
Posterior sacral dermatomes. Representation in the lower left is an anterior view.

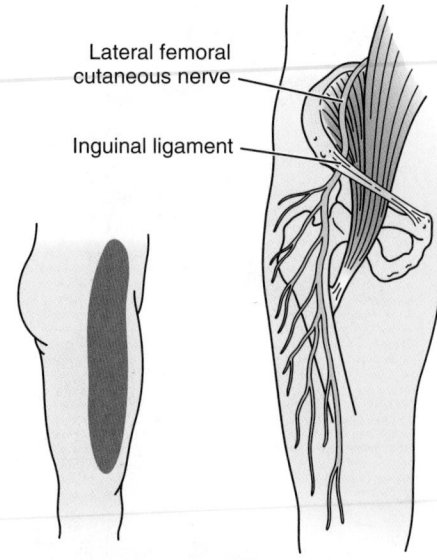

Figure 10-53
Meralgia paresthetica. The lateral femoral cutaneous nerve supplies the skin of the lateral thigh. An area from the inguinal ligament to the knee may be affected.

Figure 10-52
Referred pain from sacroiliac joint (**A**) and to sacroiliac joint (**B**).

Figure 10-54
Ilioinguinal syndrome. The ilioinguinal nerve lies within the transversus abdominis and emerges below the inguinal ligament. An area of skin on the medial thigh near the genitalia is affected.

Table 10-5

Muscles and Referral of Pain to Pelvic Area

Muscle	Referral Pattern
Longissimus thoracis	From lower thoracic spine to posterior iliac crest and gluteal area
Iliocostalis lumborum	From area lateral to lumbar spine to sacral and gluteal area
Multifidus	Sacral area

The anterior movement of the sacrum on the ilium is tested with the patient lying prone (see Figure 10-55, *C*). The examiner places the heel of one hand over the sacrum and places the other hand under the iliac crest in the area of the ASIS on one side. The hand is then pushed down on the sacrum while the other hand lifts up. The process is repeated on the other side, and the results are compared. Similarly, with the patient supine, a wedge may be

Figure 10-55
Joint play movements of the sacroiliac joints. **A,** Cephalad movement of sacrum with caudal movement of ilium. **B,** Cephalad movement of ilium with caudal movement of sacrum. **C,** Anterior movement of sacrum on ilium (left side demonstrated).

used against the sacrum with the patient's body weight acting to push the sacrum forward.

Lee[5,56] has advocated a way to test other translations at the sacroiliac joint. The patient lies supine with the hips and knees in the resting position. The examiner palpates the sacral sulcus just medial to the PSIS with the middle and ring fingers of one hand, and the lumbosacral junction with the index finger of the same hand (Figure 10-56). The middle and ring fingers monitor movement between the sacrum and innominate (ilium) bone while the index finger notes movement between the sacrum and L5.

To test anteroposterior translation of the ilium on the sacrum, the examiner, using the other hand, applies pressure through the iliac crest and ASIS. Posterior movement of the ilium should be noted and end range is achieved at the sacroiliac joint when the pelvis is felt to rotate or move at L5-S1 (Figure 10-57). The motion is compared with the other side.

Figure 10-56
Position of the posterior hand for palpation during mobility and stability testing of the sacroiliac joint.

Figure 10-57

Anteroposterior translation of the ilium on the sacrum.

To test superoinferior translation of the innominate (ilium) bone on the sacrum, the examiner applies a superior force through the ischial tuberosity (Figure 10-58). The end of motion is reached when the pelvic girdle is felt to laterally bend beneath L5-S1. The motion is compared with the opposite side.

Figure 10-58

Superoinferior translation of the ilium on the sacrum.

To test inferoposterior translation of the innominate on the sacrum, the examiner, using the heel of the other hand, applies an anterior rotation force to the ipsilateral ASIS and iliac crest (Figure 10-59). This produces an inferoposterior glide at the sacroiliac joint and is associated with counternutation of the sacrum.

To test superoanterior translation of the innominate on the sacrum, the examiner, using the heel of the other hand, applies a posteriorly rotating force to the ipsilateral ASISs and iliac crest (Figure 10-60). This produces a superoanterior glide at the sacroiliac joint and is associated with nutation of the sacrum.

An unstable sacroiliac joint will have a softer end feel, increased translation, and possible production of symptoms.[56]

Superoinferior Translation of Symphysis Pubis.[5] The patient lies supine. The examiner places the heel of one hand on the superior aspect of the superior ramus of one pubic bone and the heel of the other hand on the inferior aspect of the superior ramus of the opposite pelvic bone. A slow steady inferior force is applied with the uppermost hand while a superior force is applied with the lower hand (Figure 10-61). The examiner is testing the end feel and looking for the production of symptoms.

Figure 10-59

Anterior rotation of the innominate requires an inferoposterior glide at the sacroiliac joint.

Figure 10-60
Posterior rotation of the innominate requires a superoanterior glide at the sacroiliac joint.

Figure 10-61
Superoinferior translation of one pubic bone on the other.

Palpation[57]

Because many structures are included in the assessment of the pelvic joints, palpation of this area may be extensive, beginning on the anterior aspect and concluding posteriorly. While palpating, the examiner should note any tenderness, muscle spasm, or other signs that may indicate the source of pathology.

Anterior Aspect

The following structures should be carefully and thoroughly palpated (Figure 10-62).

Iliac Crest and ASIS. The palpating fingers are placed on the iliac crests on both sides and gently moved anteriorly until each ASIS is reached. "Hip pointers" (crushing or contusion of abdominal muscles that insert into iliac crest) may result in tenderness or pain on palpation of the iliac crest as may undisplaced fractures. The inguinal ligament attaches to the ASIS and runs downward and medially to the symphysis pubis.

McBurney's Point and Baer's Point. The examiner may then draw an imaginary line from the right ASIS to the umbilicus. **McBurney's point** lies along this line approximately one third of the distance from the ASIS and is especially tender in the presence of acute appendicitis. **Baer's point** is located in the right iliac fossa anterior to the right sacroiliac joint and slightly medial to McBurney's point. It is tender in the presence of infection or when there are sprains of the right sacroiliac ligament and indicates spasm and tenderness of the iliacus muscle.

Lymph Nodes, Symphysis Pubis (Pubic Tubercles), Greater Trochanter of the Femur, Trochanteric Bursa, Femoral Triangle, and Surrounding Musculature. The examiner returns to the ASIS and gently palpates the length of the inguinal ligament, feeling for any tenderness or swelling of the lymph nodes or possible inguinal hernia. At the distal end of the inguinal ligament, the examiner comes to the pubic tubercles and symphysis pubis,[58] which should be palpated for tenderness or signs of pathology.

The examiner then places the thumbs over the pubic tubercles and moves the fingers laterally until the bony greater trochanter of the femur is felt. The trochanters are usually level. The trochanteric bursa lies over the greater trochanter and is palpable only if it is swollen.

Returning to the ASIS, the examiner can move on to palpate the **femoral triangle,** which has as its boundaries the inguinal ligament superiorly, the adductor longus muscle medially, and the sartorius muscle laterally. It is in the superior aspect of the triangle that the examiner palpates for swollen lymph nodes. The **femoral pulse** can be palpated deeper in the triangle. Although almost impossible to palpate, the femoral nerve lies lateral to the artery, whereas the femoral vein lies medial to it. The

A

- T 12 vertebra
- 12th rib
- L2 intervertebral disc
- L3 vertebra
- Level of L4–L5 interspace
- Iliac crest
- Lumbosacral joint
- Anterior superior iliac spine
- Sacroiliac joint
- Anterior inferior iliac spine
- Sacrococcygeal joint
- Symphysis pubis
- Ischial tuberosity

B

- Iliac crest
- Posterior superior iliac spine
- Sacroiliac joint
- Posterior inferior iliac spine
- Coccyx
- Ischial tuberosity

Figure 10-62
Landmarks of the sacroiliac joints and symphysis pubis.
A, Anterior view. **B,** Posterior view.

psoas bursa may also be palpated within the femoral triangle, but only if it is swollen. Before moving on to the posterior structures, the examiner should determine whether the adjacent musculature—the abductor, flexor, and adductor muscles—shows any indication of pathology (e.g., muscle spasm, pain).

Posterior Aspect

To complete the posterior palpation, the patient lies in the prone position, and the following structures are palpated.

Iliac Crest and PSIS. Again, the examiner places the fingers on the iliac crest and moves posteriorly until they rest on the PSIS, which is at the level of the S2 spinous process. On many patients, dimples indicate the position of the PSIS.

Ischial Tuberosity. If the examiner then moves distally from the PSIS and down to the level of the gluteal folds, the ischial tuberosities may be palpated. It is important that they be palpated, because the hamstring muscles attach here and the bony prominences are what one "sits on."

Sacral Sulcus and Sacroiliac Joints. Returning to the PSIS as a starting point, the examiner should palpate slightly below it on the sacrum adjacent to the ilium. (This area is sometimes referred to as the sacral sulcus.)

The depth on the right side should be compared with that on the left side. If one side is deeper than the other, sacral torsion or rotation on the ilium around the horizontal plane may be indicated.

If the examiner then moves slightly medially and distal to the PSIS, the fingers will rest adjacent to the sacroiliac joints. To palpate these joints, the patient's knee is flexed to 90° or greater and the hip is passively medially rotated while the examiner palpates the sacroiliac joint on the same side (Figure 10-63). This procedure is identical to the prone gapping test previously described under Passive Movements. The procedure is repeated on the other side, and the two results are compared.

Sacrum, Lumbosacral Joint, Coccyx, Sacral Hiatus, Sacral Cornua, and Sacrotuberous and Sacrospinous Ligaments. The examiner again returns to the PSIS and moves to the midline of the sacrum, where the S2 spinous process can be palpated.

Moving superiorly over two spinous processes, the fingers now rest on the spinous process of L5. As a check, the examiner may look to see if the fingers rest just below a horizontal line drawn from the high point of the iliac crests. This horizontal line normally passes through the interspace between L4 and L5. Having found the L5

Figure 10-63
Palpation of the right sacroiliac joint.

Sacral articular facet
Sacral canal
Sacral spinous process
Sacral foramen
Sacral hiatus
Sacral cornu
Coccyx

Figure 10-64
Posterior view of the sacrum and coccyx.

spinous process, the examiner then palpates between the spinous processes of L5 and S1, feeling for signs of pathology at the lumbosacral joint. Moving laterally approximately 2 to 3 cm (0.8–1.2 inches), the fingers lie over the lumbosacral facet joints, which are not palpable. However, the overlying structures may be palpated for tenderness or spasm, which may indicate pathology of these joints or related structures. In a similar fashion, the spinous processes and facet joints of the other lumbar spines and intervening structures can be palpated.

The examiner then returns to the S2 spinous process or tubercle. Carefully palpating farther distally, just before the coccyx, the examiner may be able to palpate the sacral hiatus lying in the midline. If the fingers are moved slightly laterally, the sacral cornua, which constitute the distal aspect of the sacrum, may be palpated (Figure 10-64).

To palpate the coccyx properly, the examiner performs a rectal examination (Figure 10-65). A rubber glove is put on, and the index finger is lubricated. The index finger is then carefully pushed into the rectum as the patient relaxes the sphincter muscles. The index finger then palpates the anterior surface of the coccyx while the thumb of the same hand palpates its posterior aspect. While holding the coccyx between the finger and thumb, the examiner is able to move it back and forth, rocking it at the sacrococcygeal joint. Normally, this action should not cause pain.

The examiner then returns to the PSIS. Moving straight down or distally from the PSIS, the fingers follow the path of the **sacrotuberous ligament,** which should be palpated for tenderness. Slightly more than halfway between the PSIS and ischial tuberosity and slightly medially, the fingers pass over the **sacrospinous**

Ilium
Greater trochanter
Ischial tuberosity
Anus
Sacrum
Coccyx

Figure 10-65
Palpation of the coccyx.

ligament, which is deep to the sacrotuberous ligament. Tenderness in this area may indicate pathology of this ligament.

Diagnostic Imaging[59]

Plain Film Radiography

On plain film radiography, anteroposterior view (Figures 10-66 and 10-67), the examiner should look for or note the following:

1. Ankylosis of sacroiliac joints (e.g., ankylosing spondylitis; Figure 10-68).
2. Displacement of one sacroiliac joint and/or the symphysis pubis (Figure 10-69).[60]
3. Demineralization, sclerosis, or periosteal reaction of one or both pubic bones at the symphysis pubis (e.g., osteitis pubis; Figure 10-70).
4. Any fracture.
5. Relation of the sacrum to the ilium.

Text continued on page 654

Figure 10-66

Anteroposterior radiograph of the sacroiliac joint.

Figure 10-67

Normal sacroiliac joints. Angled (**A**) and oblique (**B**) anteroposterior views show normally maintained cortices and cartilage spaces. (From Weissman BNW, Sledge CB: *Orthopedic radiology,* p. 347, Philadelphia, 1986, W.B. Saunders.)

Figure 10-68
Fusion of sacroiliac joint spaces in the late stage of sacroiliitis of ankylosing spondylitis (anteroposterior view). The sclerosis has resorbed, and there is slight narrowing of the left hip joint. (From Rothman RH, Simeone FA: *The spine,* p. 921, Philadelphia, 1982, W.B. Saunders.)

Figure 10-69
Anteroposterior radiograph of the pelvis. Note higher left pubic bone.

Figure 10-70
Osteitis pubis. **A,** Anteroposterior view of pelvis showing well-concealed bony lesion at inferior corner of left pubis at the symphysis *(arrowhead).* **B,** Posterior view of same pelvis; bony fragment is well delineated in this view. (From Wiley JJ: Traumatic osteitis pubis: The gracilis syndrome, *Am J Sports Med* 11:361, 1983.)

Précis of the Pelvis Assessment*

History (sitting)
Observation (standing)
Examination
  Active movements (standing)
    Flexion of the spine
    Extension of the spine
    Rotation of the spine (left and right)
    Side flexion of the spine (left and right)
    Flexion of the hip
    Abduction of the hip
    Adduction of the hip
    Extension of the hip
    Medial rotation of the hip
    Lateral rotation of the hip
  Special tests (standing)
  Special tests (sitting)
  Passive movements (supine)
    Gapping test
    Rocking (knee-to-shoulder) test
    Sacral apex pressure test
  Resisted isometric movements (supine)†
    Forward flexion of the spine
    Flexion of the hip
    Abduction of the hip
    Adduction of the hip
    Extension of the hip
  Special tests (supine)
  Passive movements (side lying)
    Approximation test
    Passive extension and medial rotation of ilium
      on sacrum

  Passive flexion and lateral rotation of ilium on sacrum
  Reflexes and cutaneous distribution (supine, then prone)
  Passive movements (prone)
    Ipsilateral prone kinetic test
    Sacral apex pressure test
  Special tests (prone)
  Joint play movements (prone)
    Cephalad movement of the sacrum with caudal
      movement of the ilium
    Cephalad movement of the ilium with caudal move-
      ment of the sacrum
  Palpation (prone, then supine)
  Diagnostic imaging
  As previously stated, assessment of the sacroiliac joints and symphysis pubis is done only after an
assessment of the lumbar spine and hips, unless there has
been specific trauma to the sacroiliac joints or symphysis
pubis. Completion of the examination of the sacroiliac
joints and symphysis pubis therefore may involve only
passive movements, special tests, joint play movements,
and palpation, because the other tests would have been
completed when assessing the other joints.
  After any examination, the patient should be warned of
the possibility of exacerbation of symptoms as a result of
the assessment.

---

*The précis is shown in an order that will limit the amount of
moving or changing position that the patient has to do and yet
ensure that all necessary structures are tested.
†If not done in standing.

Case Studies

When doing these case studies, the examiner should list the appropriate questions to be asked and why they are being asked, what to look for and why, and what things should be tested and why. Depending on the answers of the patient (and the examiner should consider different responses), several possible causes of the patient's problem may become evident (examples are given in parentheses). A differential diagnosis chart (Table 10-6) should be made up. The examiner can then decide how different diagnoses may affect the treatment plan.

1. A 26-year-old male soccer player complains of lower abdominal pain that is referred into the right groin. Sit-ups are painful, and he experiences pain when he kicks the ball. Describe your assessment plan for this patient (abdominal strain versus osteitis pubis).

2. A 35-year-old man complains of "back pain." He complains that his back is stiff and sore when he gets up in the morning and that the stiffness remains for most of the day. Sclerosis of the sacroiliac is evident on x-ray. Describe your assessment plan for this patient (ankylosing spondylitis versus osteoarthritis of the sacroiliac joints).

3. An 18-year-old female figure skater complains of back pain that increases when she is skating; the pain is prominent on one leg. The ASIS and PSIS are higher on the right side. Describe your assessment plan for this patient (sacroiliac dysfunction versus short leg syndrome).

Table 10-6

Differential Diagnosis Between Ankylosing Spondylitis and Sacroiliac Arthritis

	Ankylosing Spondylitis	Sacroiliac Arthritis
History	Bilateral sacroiliac pain that may refer to posterior thigh Morning stiffness Male predominance	Bilateral sacroiliac pain referring to gluteal area (S1–S2 dermatomes) Morning stiffness (prolonged) Coughing painful
Observation	Stiff, controlled movement of pelvis	Controlled movement of pelvis
Active Movement	Decreased	Side flexion and extension full Slight limitation of flexion
Passive Movement	Decreased	Normal
Resisted Isometric Movement	Pain and weakness, especially if sacroiliac joints are stressed	Pain, especially if sacroiliac joints are stressed
Special Tests	Sacral stress tests probably positive	Sacral stress tests probably positive
Sensation and Reflexes	Normal	Normal
Palpation	Tender over sacroiliac joints	Tender over sacroiliac joints
Diagnostic Imaging	X-rays diagnostic	X-rays diagnostic
Lab Tests	Erythrocyte sedimentation rate increased HLA-B27 human leukocyte antigen present in 80%	Normal

References

To enhance this text and add value for the reader, all references have been incorporated into a CD-ROM that is provided with this text. The reader can view the reference source and access it online whenever possible. There are a total of 68 cited references and other general references for this chapter.

APPENDIX 10-1

RELIABILITY, VALIDITY, SPECIFICITY AND SENSITIVITY OF SPECIAL/DIAGNOSTIC TESTS USED IN THE PELVIS

ARM FOSSA

Specificity	Sensitivity	Odds Ratio
• 69%[6]	• 54%[61]	• Positive likelihood ratios 1.74, negative likelihood 0.66

COMPRESSION TEST

Reliability	Specificity	Sensitivity	Odds Ratio
• Test retest k = 0.58[62]	• 69%[63]	• 60%[63]	• Positive likelihood ratios 2.20, negative likelihood ratios 0.46

DISTRACTION TEST

Reliability	Specificity	Sensitivity	Odds Ratio
• Test retest k = 0.46[62]	• 81%[63] • 100%[64]	• 60%[63] • 55%[64]	• Positive likelihood ratio 3.20, negative likelihood ratio 0.49

EXTEND PUSH

Specificity	Sensitivity	Odds Ratio
• 59%[61]	• 56%[61]	• Positive likelihood ratios 1.36, negative likelihood 0.74

EXTEND SUPPORT

Specificity	Sensitivity	Odds Ratio
• 72%[61]	• 46%[61]	• Positive likelihood ratios 1.64, negative likelihood 0.75

FABERE

Specificity	Sensitivity	Odds Ratio
• 86%[61]	• 10%[61]	• Positive likelihood ratios 0.41, negative likelihood 1.05

GAESLEN TEST

Reliability	Specificity	Sensitivity	Odds Ratio
• Test retest k = 0.58[62]	• Right 71%, left 77%[63]	• Right 53%, left 50%[63]	• Positive likelihood ratios right 1.84, left 2.21; negative likelihood ratios right 0.66, left 0.65

GILLET'S TEST (SACRAL FIXATION OR IPSILATERAL POSTERIOR ROTATION TEST)

Reliability
• Intrarater Kappa = 0.08, interrater Kappa = −0.00[65] • Intrarater k = 0.18, interrater k = 0.02[66]

Reliability, Validity, Specificity and Sensitivity of Special/Diagnostic Tests Used in the Pelvis

HELL BUTTOCK

Specificity	Sensitivity	Odds Ratio
• 83%[61]	• 44%[61]	• Positive likelihood ratios 2.59, negative likelihood 0.67

KNEE FLEXION

Specificity	Sensitivity	Odds Ratio
• 79%[61]	• 33%[61]	• Positive likelihood ratios 1.57, negative likelihood 0.85

PALPATION

Reliability

- Intrarater posterior superior iliac spine k=0.33, sacral sulcus k=0.24, sacral inferior lateral angle k=0.21[67]
- Interrater posterior superior iliac spine k=0.04, sacral sulcus k=0.07, sacral inferior lateral angle k=0.08[67]

PATRICK SIGN

Reliability

- Test retest k=0.62[62]

PRONE KNEE FLEXION TEST

Reliability

- Interrater k=0.26[68]

SACRAL BASE SPRING TEST (SBST)

Specificity	Sensitivity	Odds Ratio
• 59%[61]	• 33%[61]	• Positive likelihood ratios 0.80, negative likelihood 1.13

SACRAL THRUST

Specificity	Sensitivity	Odds Ratio
• 75%[63]	• 63%[63]	• Positive likelihood ratios 2.50, negative likelihood 0.50

SI AGGRAVATION

Specificity	Sensitivity	Odds Ratio
• 59%[61]	• 20%[61]	• Positive likelihood ratios 0.49, negative likelihood 1.35

SITTING POSTERIOR SUPERIOR ILIAC SPINE TEST

Reliability

- Interrater k=0.37[68]

STANDING FLEXION TEST

Reliability

- Interrater k=0.32[68]

Continued

SUPINE LONG SITTING TEST

Reliability

• Interrater k = 0.19[68]

THIGH THRUST

Reliability	Specificity	Sensitivity	Odds Ratio
• Test retest k = 0.69[62]	• 71%[63]	• 88%[63]	• Positive likelihood ratios 2.80, negative likelihood ratios 0.66

CHAPTER 11

H~IP~

The hip joint is one of the largest and most stable joints in the body. If it is injured or exhibits pathology, the lesion is usually immediately perceptible during walking. Because pain from the hip can be referred to the sacroiliac joints or the lumbar spine, it is imperative—unless there is evidence of direct trauma to the hip—that these joints be examined along with the hip.

Applied Anatomy

The hip joint is a multiaxial ball-and-socket joint that has maximum stability because of the deep insertion of the head of the femur into the acetabulum (Figure 11-1). In addition, the hip, like the shoulder, has a labrum, which helps to deepen and stabilize the joint.[1,2] It has a strong capsule and very strong muscles that control its actions (Figure 11-2). The acetabulum is formed by fusion of part of the ilium, ischium, and pubis, which taken as a group are sometimes called the innominate bone or pelvis. The acetabulum opens outward, forward, and downward. It is half of a sphere, and the femoral head is two thirds of a sphere. The hip, already a stable joint because of its bony configuration, is supported by three strong ligaments: the iliofemoral, the ischiofemoral, and the pubofemoral ligaments (Figure 11-3). The iliofemoral ligament (Y ligament of Bigelow) is considered to be the strongest ligament in the body. It is positioned to prevent excessive extension and plays a significant role in maintaining upright posture at the hip. The ischiofemoral ligament, the weakest of these three strong ligaments, winds tightly on extension, helping to stabilize the hip in extension. The pubofemoral ligament prevents excessive abduction of the femur and limits extension. All three ligaments also limit medial rotation of the femur.

Hip Joint	
Resting position:	30° flexion, 30° abduction, slight lateral rotation
Close packed position:	Extension, medial rotation, and abduction
Capsular pattern:	Flexion, abduction, medial rotation (order may vary)

Under low loads, the joint surfaces are incongruous; under heavy loads, they become congruous, providing maximum surface contact. The maximum contact brings the load per unit area down to a tolerable level. Depending on the activity, the forces exerted on the hip will vary.[3]

Forces on the Hip	
Standing:	0.3 times the body weight
Standing on one limb:	2.4–2.6 times the body weight
Walking:	1.3–5.8 times the body weight
Walking up stairs:	3 times the body weight
Running:	4.5+ times the body weight

Patient History

In addition to the questions listed under Patient History in Chapter 1, the examiner should obtain the following information from the patient.

659

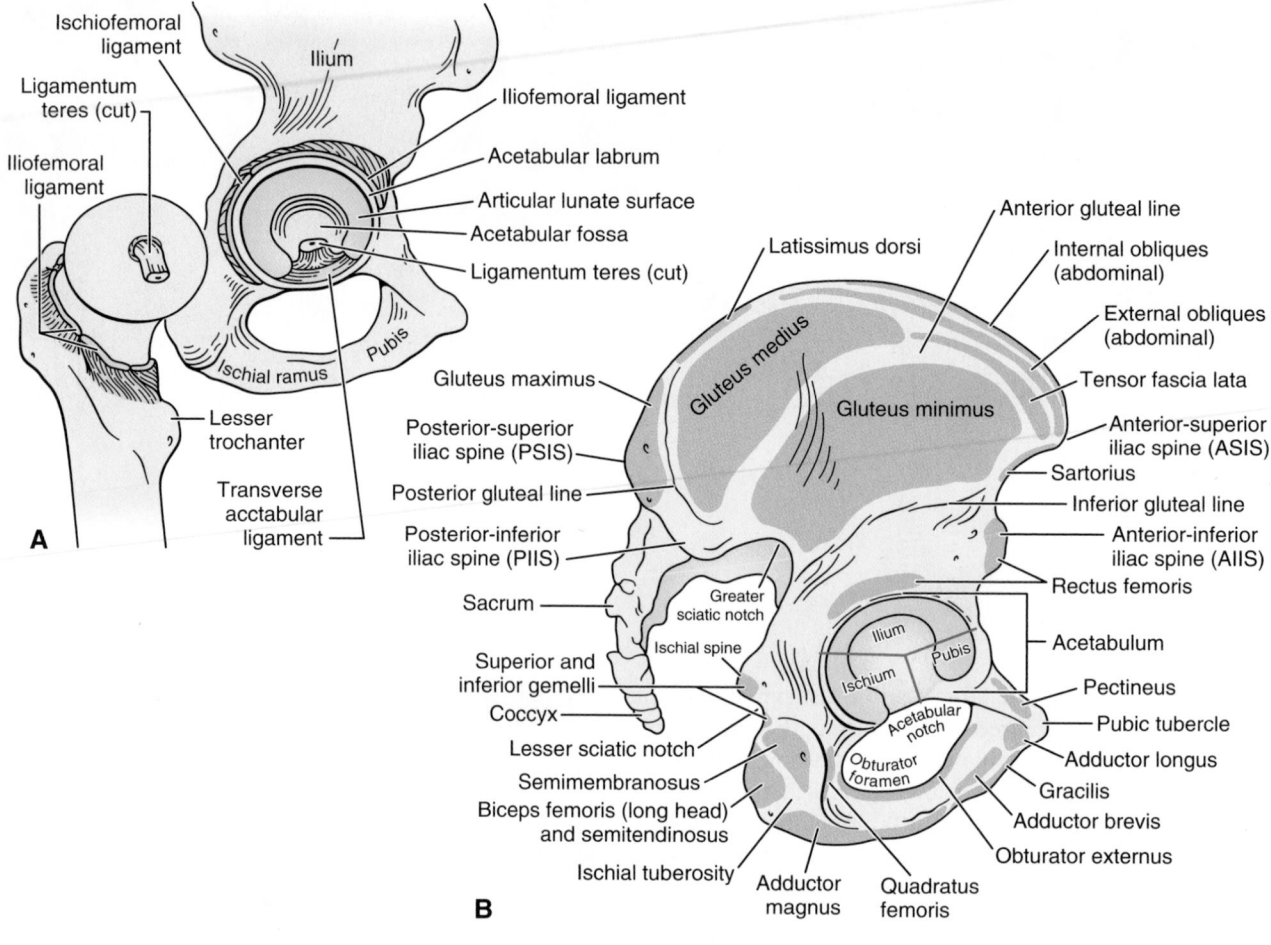

Figure 11-1

Anatomy of the hip. **A,** The right hip opened to show its internal components. **B,** Side view of right innominate bone (pelvis) showing muscle attachments. (Modified from Neumann DA: *Kinesiology of the musculoskeletal system—foundations for physical rehabilitation,* pp. 388, 397, St Louis, 2002, C.V. Mosby.)

1. *What is the age of the patient?* Different conditions occur in different age groups, and range of motion (ROM) decreases with age. For example, congenital hip dysplasia is seen in infancy, primarily in girls; Legg-Calvé-Perthes disease is more common in boys 3 to 12 years old; and elderly women are more prone to osteoporotic femoral neck fractures.

2. *If trauma was involved, what was the mechanism of injury?* Did the patient land on the outside of the hip (e.g., trochanteric bursitis) or land on or hit the knee, thus jarring the hip (e.g., subluxation, acetabular labral tear)? Was the patient involved in repetitive loading activity (e.g., femoral stress fracture) or osteoporotic (insufficiency injury)?[4] A careful determination of the mechanism of injury often leads to a diagnosis of the problem.

3. *What are the details of the present pain and other symptoms (Table 11-1)?*[5] Hip pain, including labral tears and anterior impingement, is felt mainly in the groin and along the front or medial side of the thigh,[1] whereas buttock pain is associated with posterior labral tears and lumbar spine problems.[1,6] Adductor pain may be the result of overactive adductors caused by pelvic instability.[7] Pain may also be referred to the hip area from several structures (Figure 11-4). Pain from the lumbar spine may commonly be referred to the back or lateral aspect of the hip.

Lateral hip pain may be due to a trochanteric bursitis or tear of the gluteus medius tendon, most commonly in older patients.[8] Lateral hip pain may also simulate L4 nerve root pain; therefore, assessment of the back should also be considered for lateral or posterior symptoms. Hip pain may also be referred to the knee or back and may increase on walking. **Clicking** is common with labral tears.[9] **Snapping** in and around the hip (coxa saltans) has many causes (Table 11-2). First and most commonly, it may be caused by slipping of the iliopsoas tendon over the osseous ridge of the lesser trochanter or anterior acetabulum, or the iliofemoral ligament may be riding over the femoral head.[10-12] Some call this **internal snapping**. If due to the iliopsoas tendon or iliofemoral ligament, the snapping often occurs at approximately 45° of flexion when the hip is moving from flexion to extension, especially with the hip abducted and laterally rotated (**snapping hip sign** or **extension test**).[13] The snap, which may be accompanied by pain or a jerk, is palpated anteriorly in the inguinal region.[13,14] Second, the snapping may be caused by a tight iliotibial band or gluteus maximus tendon riding over the greater trochanter of the femur.[10,11] This is sometimes called **external snapping**. This snapping or popping, which

tends to be felt more lateral, occurs during hip flexion and extension, especially if the hip is held in medial rotation, and may be made worse if the trochanteric bursa is inflamed.[14] The third cause of a snapping hip is acetabular labral tears or loose bodies, which may be the result of trauma or degeneration.[11,15-17] This is sometimes referred to as **intra-articular snapping**. In this case, the patient (commonly between 20 to 40 years) complains of a sharp pain into the groin and anterior thigh, especially on pivoting movements. Passively, clicking may be felt and heard when the extended hip is adducted and laterally rotated.[11,14] Each of these conditions may be referred to as **snapping hip syndrome**.

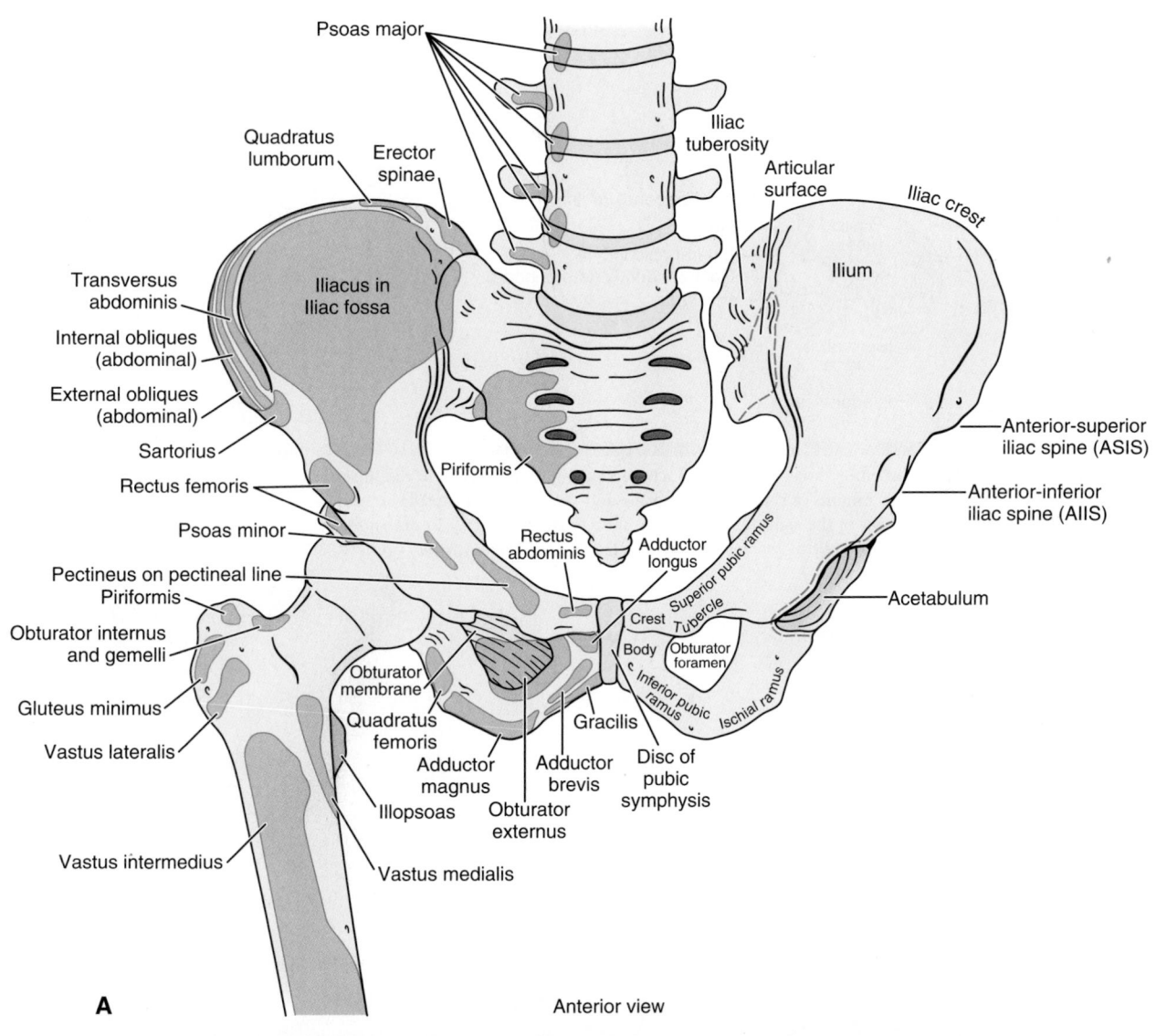

Figure 11-2

A, The anterior aspect of the pelvis, sacrum, and right proximal femur showing muscle attachments (origins are shown in red, insertions are shown in blue). A section of the left side of the sacrum is removed to expose the articular surface of the sacroiliac joint. The pelvic attachments of the capsule around the sacroiliac joint are indicated by dashed lines.

Continued

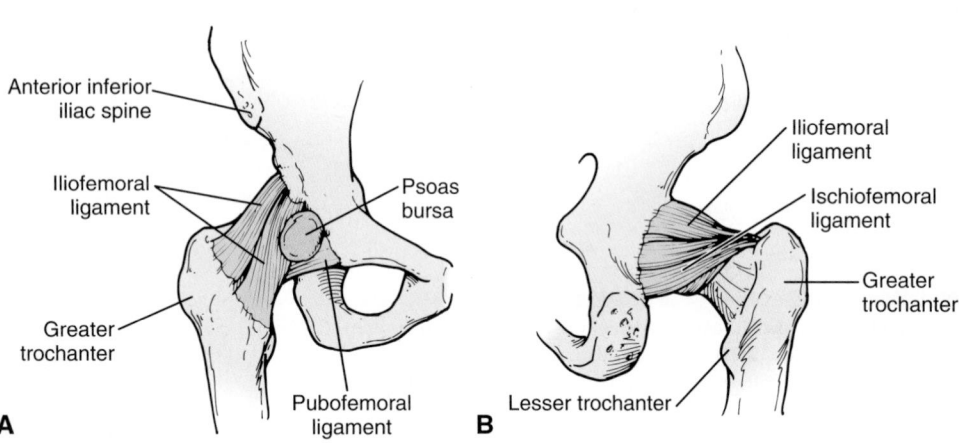

Figure 11-2 cont'd

B, The posterior aspect of the right femur showing muscle attachments (origins are shown in red, insertions are shown in blue). The femoral attachments of the hip joint capsule and the knee joint capsule are indicated by dashed lines. **C,** The superior aspect of the right femur showing muscle attachments. (Redrawn from Neumann DA: *Kinesiology of the musculoskeletal system—foundations for physical rehabilitation*, pp. 389, 393, St Louis, 2002, C.V. Mosby.)

Figure 11-3

Ligaments of the hip. **A,** Anterior view. **B,** Posterior view.

Table 11-1

Diagnostic Clues in Hip Pain

Type of Pain	Possible Causes
Dull, deep, aching	Arthritis, Paget's disease
Sharp, intense, sudden, associated with weight bearing	Fracture
Tingling that radiates	Radiculopathy, spinal stenosis, meralgia paresthetica
Increased pain while sitting with the affected leg crossed	Trochanteric bursitis
Pain at sitting, legs not crossed	Ischiogluteal bursitis
Pain after standing, walking	Hip arthrosis
Pain on attempted weight bearing	Occult fracture, severe arthrosis
Unremitting, long duration	Paget's disease, metastatic carcinoma, severe arthrosis (occasionally)

From Schon L, Zuckerman JD: Hip pain in the elderly: evaluation and diagnosis, *Geriatrics* 43:58, 1988.

Figure 11-4

Pain in the region of the hip can represent different musculoskeletal and non-musculoskeletal problems. (Redrawn from Schon L, and Zuckerman JD: Hip pain in the elderly: evaluation and diagnosis, *Geriatrics* 43:52, 1988.)

Table 11-2

Causes of Snapping Hip (Coxa Saltans) Symptoms

Coxa Saltans		
External	**Internal**	**Intra-articular**
Posterior iliotibial band	Iliopsoas tendon snapping	Labral or ligamentum tears
Anterior gluteus maximus	Iliofemoral ligament snapping	Loose bodies
Trochanteric bursitis	Hamstring syndrome	Synovial chondromatosis
	Iliopsoas bursal/capsular thickening	Displaced fractures
		Capsular instability

From Wahl CJ, et al: Internal coxa saltans (snapping hip) as a result of overtraining, *Am J Sports Med* 32:1303, 2004.

4. *Is the condition improving? Worsening? Staying the same?* Such a question gives the examiner some idea of the present state of the joint and pathology. Table 11-3 outlines criteria for osteoarthritis in patients with hip pain.[18]

5. *Does any type of activity ease the pain or make it worse?* For example, trochanteric bursitis often results from abnormal running mechanics with the feet crossing midline (increased adduction), wide pelvis and genu valgum, or running on tracks with no banking.[14]

6. *Are there any movements that the patient feels are weak or abnormal?* For example, in **piriformis syndrome**, the sciatic nerve may be compressed, the piriformis muscle is tender, and hip abduction and lateral rotation are weak.

7. *What is the patient's usual activity or pastime?* By listening to the patient, the examiner should be able to tell whether repetitive or sustained positions have contributed to the problem. Also, the examiner can develop some idea of the functional impairment felt by the patient.

Observation

As the patient comes into the assessment area, the gait should be observed. If the hip is affected, the weight is lowered carefully on the affected side and the knee bends slightly to absorb the shock. The length of the step on the affected side is shorter so that weight can be taken off the leg quickly. If the hip is stiff, the entire trunk and affected leg swing forward together. It is also important to watch for "balance" of the pelvis on the hip. Pathology in the hip region can lead to tight adductors, iliopsoas, piriformis, tensor fasciae latae, rectus femoris, and hamstrings while, at the same time, the gluteus maximus, medius, and minimus become weak.[19,20] Weak abductors can lead to a Trendelenburg gait or an "abductor lurch." Internal hip pathology or a flexion contracture may lead

Table 11-3

Classification Criteria for Osteoarthritis of the Hip

Clinical (history, physical examination, laboratory) classification criteria for osteoarthritis of the hip, classification tree format*	1. Hip pain, and 2a. Hip internal rotation <15°, and 2b. ESR ≤45 mm/hour (if ESR not available, substitute hip flexion ≤115°), or 3a. Hip internal rotation ≥15°, and 3b. Pain on hip internal rotation, and 3c. Morning stiffness of the hip ≥60 minutes, and 3d. Age >50 years
Combined clinical (history, physical examination, laboratory) and radiographic classification criteria for osteoarthritis of the hip, traditional format†	Hip pain, and At least 2 of the following 3 features: - ESR <20 mm/hr - Radiographic femoral or acetabular osteophytes - Radiographic joint space narrowing (superior, axial, and/or medial)

Modified from Altman R et al.: The American College of Rheumatology criteria for the classification and reporting of osteoarthritis of the hip, *Arth Rheum* 34:51, 1991.

ESR, Erythrocyte sedimentation rate (Westergren).

*This classification method yields a sensitivity of 86% and a specificity of 75%.

†This classification method yields a sensitivity of 89% and a specificity of 91%.

to a "pelvic wink." This is excessive rotation in the axial plane (>40°) toward the affected hip in an attempt by the patient to obtain terminal hip extension.[21] If there is an imbalance of the flexors or extensors in the sagittal plane, the forward–backward motion of the trunk is altered to help maintain balance. For example, a bilateral hip flexion contracture causes the lumbar spine to extend to a greater degree (increased lordosis) as a compensating mechanism. Weak extensors cause the patient to move the trunk backward to maintain balance and avoid falling as a result of the unopposed action of the flexors. If the lateral rotators are significantly stronger than the medial rotators, as is normally the case, excessive toe-out can result. In addition, the patellae may have a "frog eyes" appearance (turn-out). Contracture of either of the rotators may lead to a pivoting at the hip during gait.[22] The different types of gait are discussed in greater detail in Chapter 14.

If the patient uses a cane, it should be held in the hand opposite the affected side to negate some of the force of gravity on the affected hip.[23] The use of a cane can decrease the load on the hip by as much as 40%.[23,24]

The patient should be standing and suitably undressed for the examiner to perform a proper observation. The following aspects are noted from the front, side, and behind:

1. Posture. The examiner should watch for pelvic obliquity caused by, for example, unequal leg length, muscle contractures, or scoliosis (see Chapter 15 for more details). It must be remembered that injury to iliopsoas may also affect the spine. Therefore, when asking patients to do movements involving these muscles, the examiner must watch the effect on the spine and spinal movement (see Thomas test later in this chapter). Tightness of the iliopsoas can cause deviation of the spine to the same side.[25]

2. Whether the patient can or will stand on both legs. Two bathroom scales may be used to check symmetry of weight bearing.

3. Balance. It is important to check the patient's proprioceptive control in the joints being assessed. This control may be evaluated by asking the patient to balance first on one leg (the good one) and then the other leg—first with the eyes open, and then with the eyes closed. Differences should be noted through comparison. Loss of proprioceptive control is especially obvious when the patient's eyes are closed. The use of the **stork standing test**[22] (Figure 11-5) has also been advocated for testing proprioception. This test may also test stability at the sacroiliac joints, the knee, and the ankle and foot. With both methods, the examiner should watch for a positive Trendelenburg's sign, which would negate the proprioceptive tests.

4. Whether the limb positions are equal and symmetric. The position of the limb may indicate the type of injury. With traumatic posterior hip dislocation, the limb is shortened, adducted, and medially rotated, and the greater trochanter is prominent. With an anterior hip dislocation, the limb is abducted and laterally rotated and may appear cyanotic or swollen owing to pressure in the femoral triangle. With intertrochanteric fractures, the limb is shortened and laterally rotated.

5. Any obvious shortening of a leg. Shortening of the leg may be demonstrated by a spinal scoliosis if the shortening is present in only one lower limb. Shortening may be structural or functional. If the hips are unstable (e.g., bilateral unreduced congenital dislocation of the hip [CDH]), an increased lumbar lordosis may be evident because the head of the femur usually rests above and behind the acetabulum, causing the patient to have an increased lordosis to maintain the center of gravity.

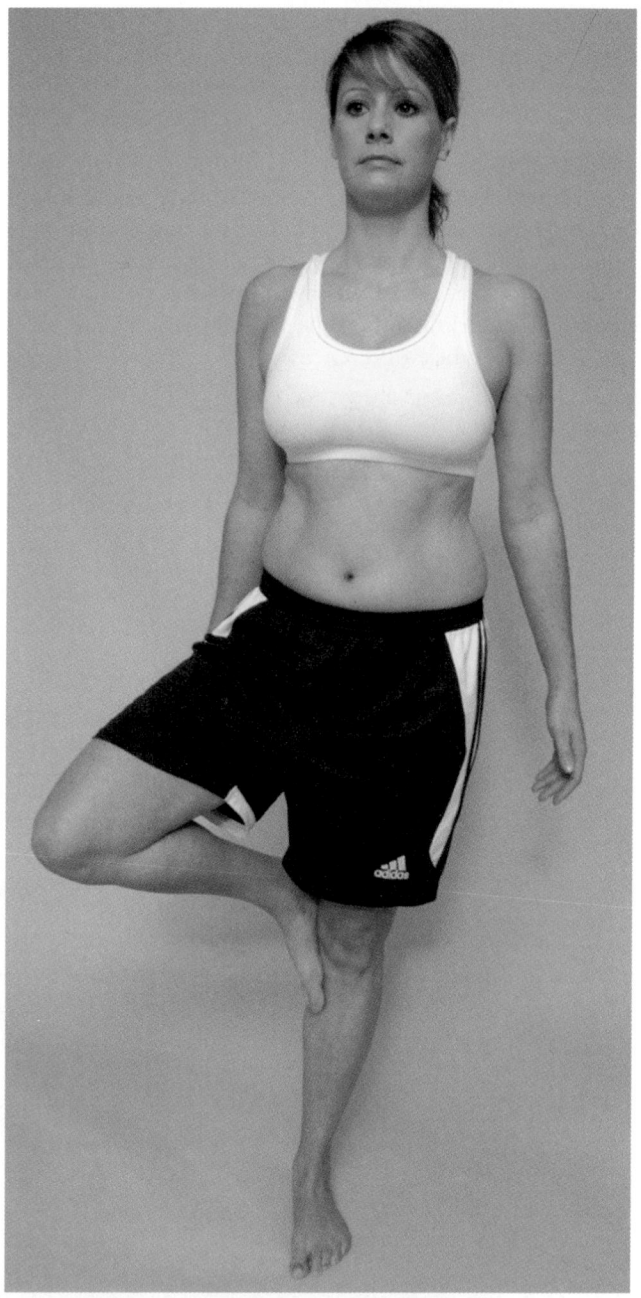

Figure 11-5
Stork standing test.

6. Color and texture of the skin.
7. Any scars or sinuses.
8. The patient's willingness to move. If the hip is painful, the patient has an antalgic gait (see Chapter 14) and does not want to move the hip. If the hip is unstable, the patient has more difficulty controlling its movement.

Anterior View

The examiner should note any abnormality of the bony and soft-tissue contours. With many patients, differences in these contours are difficult to detect because of muscle bulk and other soft-tissue deposition around the hips. The examiner must therefore look closely. The same is true for swelling. Swelling in the hip joint itself is virtually impossible to detect by observation, and swelling resulting from a psoas or trochanteric bursitis can easily be missed if the examiner is not carefully observant.

Lateral View

While the patient is viewed from the side, the contour of the buttock should be observed for any abnormality (gluteus maximus atrophy or atonia). In addition, a hip flexion deformity is best observed from this position. The examiner should take the time to compare the two sides and note any subtle differences.

Posterior View

The position of the hip and the effect, if any, of this position on the spine should be noted. For example, a hip flexion contracture may lead to an increased lumbar lordosis. Any differences in bony and soft-tissue contours should again be noted.

Examination

When doing an examination of the hip, the examiner must keep in mind that pain may be referred to the hip from the sacroiliac joints or the lumbar spine, and vice versa. Therefore, the examination may be an extensive one. If there is any doubt as to the location of the lesion, an assessment of the lumbar spine and sacroiliac joints should be performed along with the hip. It is only through a careful examination of the three areas, especially if there has been no history of trauma, that the examiner can discern the location of the lesion.

As with any examination, the examiner should compare one side of the body with the other, noting any differences. This comparison is necessary because of the individual differences among normal people.

Active Movements

The active movements (Figure 11-6) are done in such a way that the most painful ones are done last. To keep

Figure 11-6
Active movements of the hip. **A,** Flexion. **B,** Extension. **C,** Abduction. **D,** Adduction.

Continued

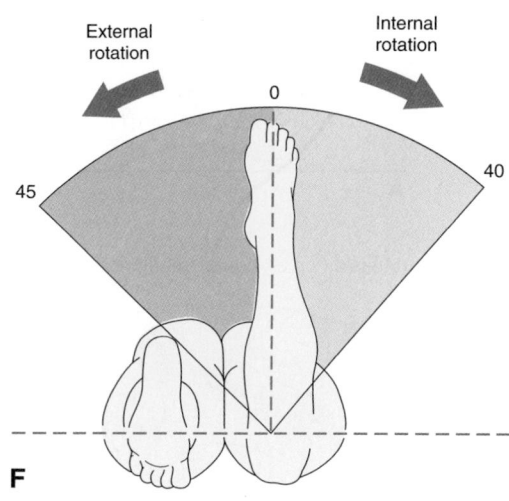

Figure 11-6 cont'd
E, Rotation in the supine position. **F,** Rotation in the prone position. (**A, E,** and **F,** Redrawn from Beetham WP, Polley HF, Slocumb CH, Weaver WF: *Physical examination of the joints*. Philadelphia, 1965, W.B. Saunders, pp. 134, 137, and 138, respectively.)

movement of the patient to a minimum, some movements are tested with the patient in the supine position and others are tested in the prone position. For ease of description, the movements are described together. The examiner should follow the order as stated in the précis at the end of the chapter when examining the patient. If the history has indicated that repetitive movements, sustained postures, or combined movements have caused symptoms, the examiner should ensure that these movements are tested as well. For example, sustained extension of the hip may provoke gluteal pain in the presence of claudication in the common or internal iliac artery.[26] During the active movements, the examiner should always watch for the possibility of muscle or force-couple imbalances that lead to abnormal muscle recruitment patterns. For example, during extension, the normal pattern is contraction of the gluteus maximus followed by the erector spinae on the opposite side and the hamstrings (depending on the load being extended). If the erector spinae contract first, the pelvis will rotate anteriorly and hyperextension of the lumbar spine will occur. When doing the active movements, the examiner should watch the pelvis and the anterior superior (supine) and posterior superior (prone) iliac spines. During hip movement, if the pelvic force-couples are normal, the pelvis and ASIS/PSIS will not move. If they do, it may be an indication of muscle imbalance (Figure 11-7).

Flexion of the hip is tested in the supine position and normally ranges from 110° to 120° with the knee flexed. If the anterior superior iliac spine (ASIS) begins to move, the movement is stopped because pelvic rotation is occurring rather than hip flexion. The patient's knee is flexed during the test to prevent limitation of movement caused by hamstring tightness. If sharp groin pain is elicited on flexion and medial rotation, the pain may be the result of **anterior impingement** of the femoral neck against the acetabular rim.[27-31] During the movement, if the abdominals are weak, the pelvis will rotate anteriorly (see Figure 11-6). If the hip flexors are weak, the pelvis will posteriorly rotate.

Active Movements of the Hip

- Flexion (110°–120°)
- Extension (10°–15°)
- Abduction (30°–50°)
- Adduction (30°)
- Lateral rotation (40°–60°)
- Medial rotation (30°–40°)
- Sustained postures (if necessary)
- Repetitive movements (if necessary)
- Combined movements (if necessary)

Normal activation of muscles during hip flexion

Rectus femoris

Rectus abdominis

Psoas

Iliacus

Flexion

A

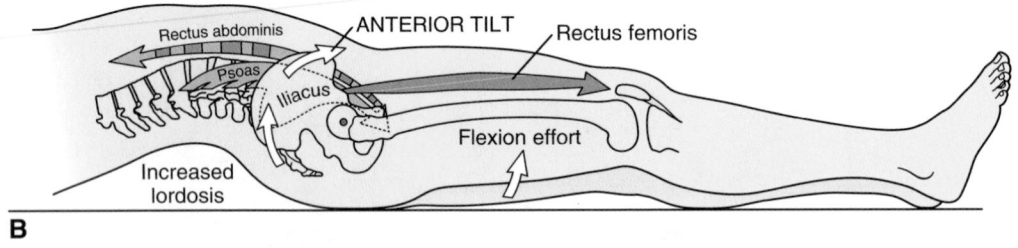

Muscle (force-couple) imbalance pattern (weak rectus abdominus)

Rectus abdominis

Psoas

Iliacus

ANTERIOR TILT

Rectus femoris

Flexion effort

Increased lordosis

B

Figure 11-7

Force-couple action during a unilateral straight leg raise. **A,** With normal activation of the rectus abdominis and the hip flexors (psoas and rectus femoris), the pelvis is stabilized and prevented from anterior tilting by the pull of the hip flexor muscles. **B,** With reduced activation of the rectus abdominis, contraction of the hip flexor muscles causes a marked anterior tilt of the pelvis. Note the increase in lumbar lordosis that accompanies the anterior tilt of the pelvis. (Modified from Neumann DA: *Kinesiology of the musculoskeletal system—foundations for physical rehabilitation*, p. 413, St Louis, 2002, C.V. Mosby.)

Extension of the hip normally ranges from 0° to 15°. The patient is in the prone position, and the examiner must differentiate between hip extension and spinal extension. Patients often have a tendency to extend the lumbar spine at the same time that they are extending the hip, giving the appearance of increased hip extension. Elevation of the pelvis or superior movement of the posterior superior iliac spine indicates the patient has passed the end of hip extension.

Hip abduction normally ranges from 30° to 50° and is tested with the patient in the supine position. Before asking the patient to do the abduction or adduction movement, the examiner should ensure that the patient's pelvis is "balanced" or level, with the anterior superior iliac spines (ASISs) being level and the legs being perpendicular to a line joining the two ASISs. The patient is then asked to abduct one leg at a time. Abduction is stopped when the pelvis begins to move. Pelvic motion is detected by palpation of the ASIS and by telling the patient to stop the movement as soon as the ASIS on either side starts to move. Normally, the ASIS on the movement side will elevate while the opposite ASIS may drop or elevate. When the patient abducts the leg, the opposite ASIS tends to move first; with an **adduction contracture,** this occurs earlier in the range of movement.

If, during abduction, lateral rotation and slight flexion occurs early in the movement, the tensor fascia lata may be stronger and gluteus medius/minimus weak. If lateral rotation occurs later in the ROM, the iliopsoas or piriformis may be overactive. If the pelvis tilts up at the beginning of movement, the quadratus lumborum is overactive. All of these movements demonstrate imbalance patterns.

Hip adduction is normally 30° and is measured from the same starting position as abduction. The patient is asked to adduct one leg over the other while the examiner ensures that the pelvis does not move. An alternative method is for the patient to flex the opposite hip and knee and hold the limb in flexion with the arms; the patient then adducts the test leg under the other leg.

This method is useful only for thin patients. When the patient adducts the leg, the ASIS on the same side moves first. This movement occurs earlier in the ROM if there is an **abduction contracture**. Adduction may also be measured by asking the patient to abduct one leg and leave it abducted; the other leg is then tested for the amount of adduction present. The advantage of this method is that the test leg does not have to be flexed to clear the other leg before doing the adduction movement.

Rotation movements may be performed with the patient supine, prone, or sitting. Medial rotation normally ranges from 30° to 40°, and lateral rotation from 40° to 60°. In the supine position, the patient simply rotates the straight leg on a balanced pelvis. Turning the foot or leg outward tests lateral rotation; turning the foot or leg inward tests medial rotation. In another supine test (see Figure 11-6, E), the patient is asked to flex both the hip and knee to 90° as the patient would do when being tested in sitting.[32] When using this method, it must be recognized that having the patient rotate the leg outward tests medial rotation, whereas having the patient rotate the leg inward tests lateral rotation. With the patient prone, the pelvis is balanced by aligning the legs at right angles to a line joining the posterior superior iliac spines (PSISs). The patient then flexes the knee to 90°. Again, medial rotation is being tested when the leg is rotated outward, and lateral rotation is being tested when the leg is rotated inward (see Figure 11-6, F). Usually, one of these last two methods (sitting or prone) is used to measure hip rotation, because it is easier to measure the angle when performing the test. However, in prone, the measurement is done on a straight leg, whereas in sitting or supine, rotation is measured with the hip flexed to 90°. It has been found that there is a difference in the amount of lateral rotation between the flexed (less) and straight position, whereas medial rotation shows little difference when measured in the two positions.[32]

Passive Movements

If the range of movement was not full and the examiner was unable to test end feel during the active movements, passive movements should be performed to determine the end feel and passive ROM. The passive movements performed are the same as the active movements. All the movements except extension can be tested with the patient in the supine lying position.

The capsular pattern of the hip is flexion, abduction, and medial rotation. These movements are always the ones most limited in a capsular pattern, although the order of restriction may vary. For example, medial rotation may be most limited, followed by flexion and abduction. The hip joint is the only joint to exhibit this altered pattern of the same movements.

Passive Movements of the Hip and Normal End Feel

- Flexion (tissue approximation or tissue stretch)
- Extension (tissue stretch)
- Abduction (tissue stretch)
- Adduction (tissue approximation or tissue stretch)
- Medial rotation (tissue stretch)
- Lateral rotation (tissue stretch)

The pelvis should not move during hip movements. Groin discomfort and a limited ROM on medial rotation are good indications of hip problems. Passive hip flexion, adduction, and medial rotation, if painful, may indicate acetabular rim problems or labral tears, especially if clicking and pain into the groin is elicited.[33]

Intra-abdominal inflammation in the lower pelvis, as in the case of an abscess, may cause pain on passive medial and lateral rotation of the hip when the patient is supine with the hip and knee at 90°.

Resisted Isometric Movements

The resisted isometric movements are performed with the patient in the supine position (Figure 11-8). Because the hip muscles are very strong and there are many of them (Figure 11-9; Table 11-4), the examiner should position the patient's hip properly and say to the patient, "Don't let me move your hip," to ensure that the movement is isometric. By carefully noting which movements cause pain or show weakness when the tests are done isometrically, the examiner should be able to determine which muscle, if any, is at fault (see Table 11-4). For example, the gluteus maximus is the only muscle that is involved in all of the following movements: extension, adduction, and lateral rotation. Therefore, if pain resulted from only these three movements, the examiner would suspect the gluteus maximus muscle. As with active movements, the most painful movements are performed last.

Text continued on page 672

Resisted Isometric Movements of the Hip

- Flexion of the hip
- Extension of the hip
- Abduction of the hip
- Adduction of the hip
- Medial rotation of the hip
- Lateral rotation of the hip
- Flexion of the knee
- Extension of the knee

Figure 11-8

Resisted isometric movements around the hip. **A,** Flexion. **B,** Extension. **C** Adduction. **D,** Abduction. **E,** Medial rotation. **F,** Lateral rotation. **G,** Knee flexion. **H,** Knee extension.

Psoas minor

Psoas major

Iliacus

Piriformis

Tensor
fascia lata

Pectineus

Gracilis

Adductor longus

Sartorius

Iliotibial band

Vastus lateralis

Rectus femoris

Vastus medialis

Psoas major

Iliacus

Sartorius (cut)

Iliofemoral
ligament

Pectineus (cut)

Obturator externus

Adductor longus
(cut)

Gracilis (cut)

Adductor brevis

Adductor magnus

Vastus lateralis (cut)

Iliotibial band (cut)

Rectus femoris (cut)

Vastus medialis (cut)

Sartorius (cut)

A   Anterior

Gluteus
medius

Gluteus
maximus

Adductor
magnus

Iliotibial band

Biceps femoris
(long head)

Semitendinosus

Semimembranosus

Gracilis

Gluteus medius

Gluteus maximus (cut)

Piriformis

Gemellus superior

Obturator internus

Gemellus inferior

Quadratus femoris

Gluteus maximus (cut)

Biceps femoris
Semitendinosus   }(cut)
Semimembranosus

Adductor magnus

Biceps femoris
(short head)

Biceps femoris
(long head) (cut)

Gracilis (cut)

Semitendinosus (cut)

Semimembranosus (cut)

B   Posterior

Figure 11-9
Muscles of the hip region. **A,** Anterior view.
The right side shows the primary flexors
and adductor muscles of the hip. Many
muscles on the left side are cut to expose
the adductor brevis and adductor magnus.
B, Posterior view. The left side highlights
the gluteus maximus and hamstring muscles
(long head of biceps femoris, semitendinosis,
and semimembranosus). The right side
shows the hamstring muscles cut to expose
the adductor magnus and short head of
the biceps femoris. The right side shows
the gluteus medius and five of the six
short external rotators (i.e., piriformis,
gemellus superior and inferior, obturator
internus, and quadratus femoris). (Redrawn
from Neumann DA: *Kinesiology of the
musculoskeletal system—foundations for
physical rehabilitation*, pp. 411, 419,
St Louis, 2002, C.V. Mosby.)

Table 11-4

Muscles of the Hip: Their Actions, Innervation, and Nerve Root Derivation

Action	Muscles Acting	Innervation	Nerve Root Deviation
Flexion of hip	1. Psoas	L1–L3	L1–L3
	2. Iliacus	Femoral	L2–L3
	3. Rectus femoris	Femoral	L2–L4
	4. Sartorius	Femoral	L2–L3
	5. Pectineus	Femoral	L2–L3
	6. Adductor longus	Obturator	L2–L4
	7. Adductor brevis	Obturator	L2–L3, L5
	8. Gracilis	Obturator	L2–L3
Extension of hip	1. Biceps femoris	Sciatic	L5, S1–S2
	2. Semimembranosus	Sciatic	L5, S1–S2
	3. Semitendinosus	Sciatic	L5, S1–S2
	4. Gluteus maximus	Inferior gluteal	L5, S1–S2
	5. Gluteus medius (posterior part)	Superior gluteal	L5, S1
	6. Adductor magnus (ischiocondylar part)	Sciatic	L2–L4
Abduction of hip	1. Tensor fasciae latae	Superior gluteal	L4–L5
	2. Gluteus minimus	Superior gluteal	L5, S1
	3. Gluteus medius	Superior gluteal	L5, S1
	4. Gluteus maximus	Inferior gluteal	L5, S1–S2
	5. Sartorius	Femoral	L2–L3
Adduction of hip	1. Adductor longus	Obturator	L2–L4
	2. Adductor brevis	Obturator	L2–L4
	3. Adductor magnus (ischiofemoral part)	Obturator	L2–L4
	4. Gracilis	Obturator	L2–L3
	5. Pectineus	Femoral	L2–L3
Medial rotation of hip	1. Adductor longus	Obturator	L2–L4
	2. Adductor brevis	Obturator	L2–L4
	3. Adductor magnus	Obturator and sciatic	L2–L4
	4. Gluteus medius (anterior part)	Superior gluteal	L5, S1
	5. Gluteus minimus (anterior part)	Superior gluteal	L5, S1
	6. Tensor fasciae latae	Superior gluteal	L4–L5
	7. Pectineus	Femoral	L2–L3
	8. Gracilis	Obturator	L2–L3
Lateral rotation of hip	1. Gluteus maximus	Inferior gluteal	L5, S1–S2
	2. Obturator internus	N. to obturator internus	L5, S1
	3. Obturator externus	Obturator	L3–L4
	4. Quadratus femoris	N. to quadratus femoris	L5, S1
	5. Piriformis	L5, S1–S2	L5, S1–S2
	6. Gemellus superior	N. to obturator internus	L5, S1
	7. Gemellus inferior	N. to quadratus femoris	L5, S1
	8. Sartorius	Femoral	L2–L3
	9. Gluteus medius (posterior part)	Superior gluteal	L5, S1

Resisted isometric flexion and extension of the knee must also be performed, because there are two joint muscles (hamstrings and rectus femoris) that act over the knee as well as the hip. If the history has indicated that concentric, eccentric, or econcentric movement causes symptoms, these movements should also be tested, but only after the isometric tests have been completed. For example, strength of the hamstrings may be determined by doing a **supine plank test** in which the patient is in crook lying, resting on his or her elbows (Figure 11-10).[34] The patient then lifts the buttocks off the table while maintaining the body weight on the elbows and heels. The patient then alternately lifts the injured leg and then the good leg. If pain occurs at the ischial origin or in

Figure 11-10

The supine plank test is used to assess hamstring strength. The patient elevates the pelvis while keeping the body weight on the elbows and heels. The legs are alternately lifted, starting with lifting the injured leg (this tests the good leg first). Pelvic collapse or rotation or pain at the hamstring origin as the contralateral leg is lifted indicates hamstring weakness.

Table 11-5

Range of Motion Necessary at the Hip for Selected Activities

Activity	Average Range of Motion Necessary
Shoe tying	120° of flexion
Sitting (average seat height)	112° of flexion
Stooping	125° of flexion
Squatting	115° of flexion/20° of abduction/20° of medial rotation
Ascending stairs (average stair height)	67° of flexion
Descending stairs (average stair height)	36° of flexion
Putting foot on opposite thigh	120° of flexion/20° of abduction/20° of lateral rotation
Putting on trousers	90° of flexion

the hamstrings musculature, or if pelvic "collapse" or rotation occurs, the test is positive for a weak hamstrings.

The examiner must be aware that intra-abdominal inflammation in the area of the psoas muscle may cause pain on resisted hip flexion. Intra-abdominal inflammation may also result in a rigid abdominal wall. It has been reported that hip flexors and hip extensors are almost equal in strength[35] and that the adductors are 2.5 times as strong as the abductors.[36] These ratios may vary depending on whether the movement is tested isometrically or isokinetically.

Functional Assessment

Hip motion is necessary for more activities than just ambulation. In fact, more hip ROM is required for daily living activities than is required for gait; activities such as shoe tying, sitting, getting up from a chair, and picking up things from the floor all require a greater ROM. Table 11-5 illustrates the ranges of motion necessary for various activities. Ideally, the patient should have functional ranges of 120° of flexion, 20° of abduction, and 20° of lateral rotation.

There are several numerical rating scales with which to rate hip function.[37-43] These rating methods are based primarily on pain, mobility, and gait. Tables 11-6 through 11-8 and Figures 11-11 and 11-12 illustrate three different rating scales. D'Aubigné and Postel[37] (see Tables 11-6 through 11-8) developed one of the first hip rating scales based on pain, mobility, and ability to walk.[38] The Harris hip function scale[39] (see Figure 11-11) is useful for rating hips before and after surgery. This scale is most often used because it emphasizes pain and function. The Western Ontario and McMaster Universities Osteoarthritis Index (WOMAC)[44-48] and the Lower

Table 11-6

Method of Grading Functional Value of Hip*

Grade	Pain	Mobility	Ability to Walk
0	Pain is intense and permanent	Ankylosis with bad position of the hip	None
1	Pain is severe, even at night	No movement; pain or slight deformity	Only with crutches
2	Pain is severe when walking; prevents any activity	Flexion less than 40°	Only with canes
3	Pain is tolerable with limited activity	Flexion between 40° and 60°	With one cane, for less than 1 hour; very difficult without a cane
4	Pain is mild when walking; it disappears with rest	Flexion between 60° and 80°; patient can reach own foot	A long time with a cane; a short time without cane and with limp
5	Pain is mild and inconstant; normal activity	Flexion between 80° and 90°; abduction at least 15°	Without cane but with slight limp
6	No pain	Flexion more than 90°; abduction to 30°	Normal

* Values used in conjunction with Table 11-7.

From D'Aubigné RM, Postel M: Functional results of hip arthroplasty with acrylic prosthesis, *J Bone Joint Surg Am* 36:459, 1954.

Table 11-7

D'Aubigné and Postel Scale for Functional Grading of the Hip

Pain (P)	Ability to Walk (W)	Mobility Normal or Nearly Normal	Grade
		Very Good	P+W = 11 or 12
6	6	Walk without cane, with no pain and no limp	
6	5	Walk without cane, with no pain but slight limp	
5	6	Walk without cane, with no limp but slight pain when starting	
		Good	P+W = 10
5	5	Walk without cane, with slight pain and slight limp	
4	6	Walk without cane, with pain but no limp	
6	4*	Walk without cane, without pain; a cane used to go outdoors	
		Medium	P+W = 9
5	4	Slight pain; a cane is used outdoors	
4	5	Pain after walking some minutes; no cane is used, but there is a slight limp	
6	3†	No pain; a cane used all the time	
		Fair	P+W = 8
5	3	Slight pain; a cane is used all the time	
4	4	Pain after walking; a cane is used outdoors	
≤3	≤3	*Poor*	P+W = 7 or less

* If the mobility is reduced to 4, the result is classified one grade lower.
† If the mobility is reduced to 3 or less, the result is classified two grades lower.
Adapted from D'Aubigné RM, Postel M: Functional results of hip arthroplasty with acrylic prosthesis, *J Bone Joint Surg Am* 36:460, 1954.

Table 11-8

Method of Evaluating Improvement Brought About by Operation in Problems of the Hip (Relative Result)

	Preoperative Grading	Postoperative Grading	Difference	Improvement
Pain	3	5	$2 \times 2 = 4$	
Mobility	2	5	$3 = 3$	= 9
Ability to walk	3	4	$1 \times 2 = 2$	

Very great improvement = 12 or more, great improvement = 7 to 11, fair improvement = 3 to 7, failure = less than 3.
From D'Aubigné RM, Postel M: Functional results of hip arthroplasty with acrylic prosthesis, *J Bone Joint Surg Am* 36:461, 1954.

Extremity Function Scale (LEFS) (Figure 11-13)[49] were developed to evaluate clinically important and patient-relevant changes in health status primarily with arthroplasties of the hip and knee. The WOMAC scale is made up of three sections with scores ranging from one (none) to five (extreme). The sum of three scores is called the index or global score. The higher the score, the greater the disability. The SF-36 questionnaire is also sometimes used as a functional assessment tool in arthroplasty cases.[48,50] The Iowa scale (see Figure 11-12) provides a single rating value. The Mayo hip score[40] for hip arthroplasty makes use of greater patient (functional) input and

radiographic input (to predict long-term results). This score correlates well with the Harris scale.[38,40] Johanson and colleagues[41] developed a numerical scale that is related to what patients are able to do functionally after total hip replacement. Its value comes from its focus on the outcome from the patient's perspective (Figure 11-14). As Burton and co-workers[42] pointed out, the notion of expectations is more important than the notion of success. Table 11-9 gives a functional strength and endurance testing scheme for the hip.

Several **walking tests** have been developed, especially for the elderly, to give an indication of musculoskeletal

Harris Hip Function Scale

(Circle one in each group)

Pain (44 points maximum)

None/ignores	44
Slight, occasional, no compromise in activity	40
Mild, no effect on ordinary activity, pain after unusual activity, uses aspirin	30
Moderate, tolerable, makes concessions, occasional codeine	20
Marked, serious limitations	10
Totally disabled	0

Function (47 points maximum)

Gait (walking maximum distance) (33 points maximum)

1. Limp:
   - None — 11
   - Slight — 8
   - Moderate — 5
   - Unable to walk — 0
2. Support:
   - None — 11
   - Cane, long walks — 7
   - Cane, full time — 5
   - Crutch — 4
   - Two canes — 2
   - Two crutches — 0
   - Unable to walk — 0
3. Distance walked:
   - Unlimited — 11
   - Six blocks — 8
   - Two to three blocks — 5
   - Indoors only — 2
   - Bed and chair — 0

Functional Activities (14 points maximum)

1. Stairs:
   - Normally — 4
   - Normally with banister — 2
   - Any method — 1
   - Not able — 0
2. Socks and tie shoes:
   - With ease — 4
   - With difficulty — 2
   - Unable — 0
3. Sitting:
   - Any chair, 1 hour — 5
   - High chair, ½ hour — 3
   - Unable to sit ½ hour any chair — 0
4. Enter public transport
   - Able to use public transportation — 1
   - Not able to use public transportation — 0

Absence of Deformity (requires all four) (4 points maximum)

1. Fixed adduction <10° — 4
2. Fixed internal rotation in extension <10° — 0
3. Leg length discrepancy less than 1¼″
4. Pelvic flexion contracture <30°

Range of Motion (5 points maximum)

Instructions

Record 10° of fixed adduction as "—10° abduction, adduction to 10°"

Similarly, 10° of fixed external rotation as "—10° internal rotation, external rotation to 10°"

Similarly, 10° of fixed external rotation with 10° further external rotation as "—10° internal rotation, external rotation to 20°"

	Range	Index Factor	Index Value*
Permanent flexion (1) _____°	_____°		
A. Flexion to			
(0–45°)		1.0	
(45–90°)		0.6	
(90–120°)		0.3	
(120–140°)	_____°	0.0	
B. Abduction to			
(0–15°)		0.8	
(15–30°)		0.3	
(30–60°)		0.0	
C. Adduction to			
(0–15°)	_____°	0.2	
(15–60°)		0.0	
D. External rotation in extension to	_____°		
(0–30°)		0.4	
(30–60°)		0.0	
E. Internal rotation in extension to	_____°		
(0–60°)		0.0	

*Index Value = Range × Index Factor

Total index value (A + B + C + D + E) _____

Total range of motion points (multiply total index value × 0.05) _____

Pain points: _____
Function points: _____
Absence of Deformity points: _____
Range of Motion points: _____
Total points _____
(100 points maximum)
Comments:

Figure 11-11

Harris hip function scale. (Modified from Harris WH: Traumatic arthritis of the hip after dislocation and acetabular fractures: Treatment by mold arthroplasty. An end result study using a new method of result evaluation, *J Bone Joint Surg Am* 51:737–755, 1969.)

impairment.[51] These include the timed up and go test (TUG test),[51,52] 13-metre walk test,[51] 6-minute walk test (6MWT),[51,53–56] self paced walk test,[57–59] 2-minute walk test,[53] 10-metre walk test, and 12-minute walk test.[53]

If the patient is able to perform normal active movements with little difficulty, the examiner may use a series of functional tests to determine whether increased intensity of activity produces pain or other symptoms. These tests must be geared to the individual patient.[60] Older persons should not be expected to perform the last six activities unless they have been doing these movements or similar ones in the recent past.

Text continued on page 679

Iowa Functional Hip Evaluation

Chart 1	Chart 2

Chart 1

Date _____

Name _____ Age _____

100-Point Scale for Hip Evaluation

Total points _____

Function (35 points)
Does most of housework or job that
   requires moving about 5
Dresses unaided (includes tying shoes and
   putting on socks)..................................... 5
Walks enough to be independent 5
Sits with difficulty at table or toilet 4
Picks up objects from floor by squatting 3
Bathes without help 3
Negotiates stairs foot over foot........................... 3
Carries objects comparable to suitcase.................... 2
Gets into car or public conveyance unaided and rides
   comfortably 2
Drives a car 1

_____

Freedom From Pain (35 points) (circle 1 only)
No pain.. 35
Pain only with fatigue 30
Pain only with weight-bearing............................ 20
Pain at rest but not with weight-bearing.............. 15
Pain sitting or in bed 10
Continuous pain.. 0

_____

Gait (10 points) (circle 1 only)
No limp; no support... 10
No limp using cane.. 8
Abductor limp 8
Short leg limp.. 8
Needs two canes 6
Needs two crutches... 4
Cannot walk 0

_____

Absence of Deformity (10 points)
No fixed flexion over 30°..................................... 3
No fixed adduction over 10°................................ 3
No fixed rotation over 10°................................... 2
Not over 1″ shortening (ASIS-MM)*...................... 2

_____

Range of Motion (10 points)
Flexion-extension (normal 140°) .... _____°
Abduction-adduction (normal 80°) .... _____°
External-internal rotation (normal 80°) .... _____°
      Total degrees.................................... _____°
      Points (1 point/30°) .... _____°

_____

Muscle Strength (no points)
Straight leg raising:
  Less than gravity _____Gravity _____
  Gravity + resistance _____
Abduction:
  Less than gravity _____Gravity _____
  Gravity + resistance _____
Extension:
  Less than gravity _____Gravity _____
  Gravity + resistance _____
      TOTAL (100 points maximum) _____

Chart 2

Name _____ Diagnosis _____
Age _____ Sex _____ Date of operation _____
Date of follow-up _____
Previous surgery: Date _____ Type _____
Subsequent surgery: Date _____ Type _____

Pain   40%
  None 40
  Pain with fatigue 35
  Pain with weight-bearing:
    Mild.. 30
    Moderate.................................. 20
    Severe...................................... 10
  Persistence with non–weight-bearing....... 10 (less than above)
  Continuous pain.......................... 0

Ability to Function   30%
  Work and household duties:
    Full day, usual occupation 10
    Modified work or duties 6
    Severe restriction of work or duties 2
  Walking tolerances:
    Long distances 10
    Short distances........................... 6
    Two blocks or less....................... 1
  Self-reliance:
    Dresses self unaided 3
    Help with shoes and socks 2
    Sit at table and toilet 3
  Stairs:
    Normal 2
    One at a time 1
    Gets into car or public conveyance without
      difficulty.................................. 2

Gait   15%
  No limp, no support 15
  No limp, with cane........................ 12
  Limp, mild, without cane 12
  Limp, mild, with cane 9
  Limp, moderate, without cane or crutch 9
  Limp, moderate, with cane or crutch.......... 6
  Limp, severe, without cane or crutch.......... 3
  Limp, severe, with cane or crutch............. 2
  Two canes or crutches 1

Anatomic Assessment   15%
  A. Motion:
    Flexion—up to 80° in range 0–100° × 0.1 ... 8
    Abduction—up to 20° in range 0–30° × 0.1.. 2
  B. Shortening:
    None—½″.................................... 3
    ½″–1″...................................... 2
    1″–2″..................................... 1
  C. Trendelenburg—absent..................... 2

_____
                             100%

Figure 11-12

Iowa functional hip evaluation form. *ASIS-MM*, Anterior superior iliac spine to medial malleolus. (Modified from Larson CB: Rating scale for hip disabilities, *Clin Orthop* 31:86, 1963.)

LOWER EXTREMITY FUNCTION SCALE

We are interested in knowing whether you are having any difficulty at all with the activities listed below *because of your lower limb* problem for which you are currently seeking attention. Please provide an answer for each activity.

Today, *do you or would you* have any difficulty at all with:
(Circle one number on each line)

ACTIVITIES	Extreme Difficulty or Unable to Perform Activity	Quite a Bit of Difficulty	Moderate Difficulty	A Little Bit of Difficulty	No Difficulty
a. Any of your usual work, housework of school activities.	0	1	2	3	4
b. Your usual hobbies, recreational or sporting activities.	0	1	2	3	4
c. Getting into or out of the bath.	0	1	2	3	4
d. Walking between rooms.	0	1	2	3	4
e. Putting on your shoes or socks.	0	1	2	3	4
f. Squatting.	0	1	2	3	4
g. Lifting an object, like a bag of groceries from the floor.	0	1	2	3	4
h. Performing light activities around your home.	0	1	2	3	4
i. Performing heavy activities around your home.	0	1	2	3	4
j. Getting into or out of a car.	0	1	2	3	4
k. Walking 2 blocks.	0	1	2	3	4
l. Walking a mile.	0	1	2	3	4
m. Going up or down 10 stairs (about 1 flight of stairs).	0	1	2	3	4
n. Standing for 1 hour.	0	1	2	3	4
o. Sitting for 1 hour.	0	1	2	3	4
p. Running on even ground.	0	1	2	3	4
q. Running on uneven ground.	0	1	2	3	4
r. Making sharp turns while running fast.	0	1	2	3	4
s. Hopping.	0	1	2	3	4
t. Rolling over in bed.	0	1	2	3	4
Column Totals:					

Score variation ± 6 LEFS points
MDC & MCID = 9 LEFS points

Score: _____ / 80

Figure 11-13 ▬▬▬

Lower Extremity Function Scale. (From Stratford PW et al: Validation of the LEFS on patients with total joint arthroplasty, *Physiother Can* 52:105, 2000.)

A SELF-ADMINISTERED HIP-RATING QUESTIONNAIRE

Which hip is affected by arthritis?
(circle one)

Left   Right   Both

Please answer the following questions about the hip(s) you have just indicated.

1. Considering all of the ways that your hip arthritis affects you, mark (X) on the scale for how well you are doing.

0	25	50	75	100
very well	well	fair	poor	very poor

Circle one response for each question (The score here is determined by subtraction of the number marked from 100, with the number being interpolated, if necessary, if the mark is between printed numbers. The result is divided by 4, and the answer then rounded off to the nearest integer. The maximum is 25 points.)

2. During the past month, how would you describe the usual arthritis pain in your hip? (maximum, 10 points)
   a. Very severe (2 points)
   b. Severe (4 points)
   c. Moderate (6 points)
   d. Mild (8 points)
   e. None (10 points)

3. During the past month, how often have you had to take medication for your arthritis? (maximum, 5 points)
   a. Always (1 point)
   b. Very often (2 points)
   c. Fairly often (3 points)
   d. Sometimes (4 points)
   e. Never (5 points)

4. During the past month, how often have you had severe arthritis pain in your hip? (maximum, 5 points)
   a. Every day (1 point)
   b. Several days per week (2 points)
   c. One day per week (3 points)
   d. One day per month (4 points)
   e. Never (5 points)

5. How often have you had hip arthritis pain at rest, either sitting or lying down? (maximum, 5 points)
   a. Every day (1 point)
   b. Several days per week (2 points)
   c. One day per week (3 points)
   d. One day per month (4 points)
   e. Never (5 points)

6. How far can you walk without resting because of your hip arthritis pain? (maximum, 15 points)
   a. Unable to walk (3 points)
   b. Less than one city block (6 points)
   c. 1 to <10 city blocks (9 points)
   d. 10 to 20 city blocks (12 points)
   e. Unlimited (15 points)

7. How much assistance do you need for walking? (maximum, 10 points)
   a. Unable to walk (1 point)
   b. Walk only with someone's help (2 points)
   c. Two crutches or walker every day (3 points)
   d. Two crutches or walker several days per week (4 points)
   e. Two crutches or walker once per week or less (5 points)
   f. Cane or one crutch every day (6 points)
   g. Cane or one crutch several days per week (7 points)
   h. Cane or one crutch once per week (8 points)
   i. Cane or one crutch once per month (9 points)
   j. No assistance (10 points)

8. How much difficulty do you have going up or down one flight of stairs because of your hip arthritis? (maximum, 5 points)
   a. Unable (1 point)
   b. Require someone's assistance (2 points)
   c. Require crutch or cane (3 points)
   d. Require banister (4 points)
   e. No difficulty (5 points)

9. How much difficulty do you have putting on your shoes and socks because of your hip arthritis? (maximum, 5 points)
   a. Unable (1 point)
   b. Require someone's assistance (2 points)
   c. Require long shoehorn and reacher (3 points)
   d. Some difficulty, but no devices required (4 points)
   e. No difficulty (5 points)

10. Are you able to use public transportation? (maximum, 3 points)
    a. No, because of my hip arthritis (1 point)
    b. No, for some other reason (2 points)
    c. Yes (3 points)

11. When you bathe—either a sponge bath or in a tub or shower—how much help do you need? (maximum, 3 points)
    a. No help at all (3 points)
    b. Help with bathing one part of my body, like back or leg (2 points)
    c. Help with bathing more than one part of my body (1 point)

12. If you had the necessary transportation, under what circumstances could you go shopping for groceries or clothes? (maximum, 3 points)
    a. Without help (taking care of all shopping needs myself) (3 points)
    b. With some help (need someone to go with me to help on all shopping trips) (2 points)
    c. Completely unable to do any shopping (1 point)

13. If you had household tools and appliances (vacuum, mops, and so on) could you do your own housework? (maximum, 3 points)
    a. Without help (can clean floors, windows, refrigerator, and so on) (3 points)
    b. With some help (can do light housework, but need help with some heavy work) (2 points)
    c. Completely unable to do any housework (1 point)

14. How well are you able to move around? (maximum, 3 points)
    a. Able to get in and out of bed or chair without the help of another person (3 points)
    b. Need the help of another person to get in and out of bed or chair (2 points)
    c. Not able to get out of bed (1 point)

This is the end of the Hip-Rating Questionnaire. Thank you for your cooperation

Figure 11-14 ▮▮▮▮

A self-administered hip-rating questionnaire. The maximum score is 100 points and the minimum is 16 points. The point values of the answers are not shown in the questionnaire that is administered to patients. (From Johanson NA, Charlson ME, Szatrowski TP, Ranawat CS: A self-administered hip-rating questionnaire for the assessment of outcome after total hip replacement, *J Bone Joint Surg Am* 74:589, 1992.)

Table 11-9

Functional Testing of the Hip

Starting Position	Action	Functional Test
Standing	Lift foot onto 20-cm step and return (hip flexion–extension)	5 to 6 Repetitions: Functional 3 to 4 Repetitions: Functionally fair 1 to 2 Repetitions: Functionally poor 0 Repetitions: Nonfunctional
Standing	Sit in chair and return to standing (hip extension–flexion)	5 to 6 Repetitions: Functional 3 to 4 Repetitions: Functionally fair 1 to 2 Repetitions: Functionally poor 0 Repetitions: Nonfunctional
Standing	Life leg to balance on one leg keeping pelvis straight (hip abduction)	Hold 1 to 1.5 minutes: Functional Hold 30 to 59 seconds: Functionally fair Hold 1 to 29 seconds: Functionally poor Cannot hold: Nonfunctional
Standing	Walk sideways 6 m (hip adduction/abduction)	6 to 8 m one way: Functional 3 to 6 m one way: Functionally fair 1 to 3 m one way: Functionally poor 0 m: Nonfunctional
Standing	Test leg off floor (patient may hold onto something for balance) medially rotate non–weight-bearing hip	10 to 12 Repetitions: Functional 5 to 9 Repetitions: Functionally fair 1 to 4 Repetitions: Functionally poor 0 Repetitions: Nonfunctional
Standing	Test leg off floor (patient may hold onto something for balance) laterally rotate non–weight-bearing hip	10 to 12 Repetitions: Functional 5 to 9 Repetitions: Functionally fair 1 to 4 Repetitions: Functionally poor 0 Repetitions: Nonfunctional

Data from Palmer ML, Epler M: *Clinical assessment procedures in physical therapy*, pp. 251–254, Philadelphia, 1990, J.B. Lippincott.

Functional Tests of the Hip

- Squatting
- Going up and down stairs one at a time
- Crossing the legs so that the ankle of one foot rests on the knee of the opposite leg
- Going up and down stairs two or more at a time
- Running straight ahead
- Running and decelerating
- Running and twisting
- One-legged hop (time, distance, crossover)
- Jumping

Special Tests

Only those tests that the examiner believes are necessary should be performed when assessing the hip. Most tests are done primarily to confirm a diagnosis or to determine pathology. As with all special tests, if the test is positive, it is highly suggestive that the problem exists, but if it is negative, it does not necessarily rule out the problem. Therefore, special tests should not be taken in isolation but should be used to support the history, observation, and clinical examination. The reliability and validity of some special/diagnostic tests used in the hip are outlined in Appendix 11-1.

Special Tests Commonly Performed on the Hip

- Patrick (Faber) test
- Flexion-adduction test
- Trendelenburg's sign
- Leg length tests
- Thomas test
- Rectus femoris test
- Ober's test
- 90-90 straight leg raise test
- Sign of the buttock (straight leg raising)
- Abduction/adduction tests

ZONES: 3   2   1

Figure 11-15

Patrick's test (Faber or figure-four test) for the detection of limitation of motion in the hip. (Redrawn from Beetham WP et al: *Physical examination of the joints*, p. 139, Philadelphia: 1965, W.B. Saunders.)

Figure 11-16

The normal hip permits the ipsilateral knee to move convincingly across the midline of the body without rolling the pelvis. The knee should enter zone 1 by overlapping the opposite hip and, in the youthful or supple patient, will reach a position lateral to the thigh. Progressive pathologic changes in the hip limit adduction to zones 2 and 3, with the production of pain by this maneuver. (Redrawn from Woods D, Macnicol M: The flexion-adduction test: an early sign of hip disease, *J Pediatr Orthop* 10:181, 2001.)

Tests for Hip Pathology

Patrick's Test (Faber or Figure-Four Test). The patient lies supine, and the examiner places the patient's test leg so that the foot of the test leg is on top of the knee of the opposite leg (Figure 11-15). The examiner then slowly lowers the knee of the test leg toward the examining table. A negative test is indicated by the test leg's knee falling to the table or at least being parallel with the opposite leg. A positive test is indicated by the test leg's knee remaining above the opposite straight leg. If positive, the test indicates that the hip joint may be affected, that there may be iliopsoas spasm, or that the sacroiliac joint may be affected. **Faber** (which stands for flexion, abduction, and external rotation) is the position of the hip at which the patient begins the test. The test is sometimes referred to as **Jansen's test**.[61]

Flexion-Adduction Test.[62] This test is used in older children and young adults as a test for hip disease. The patient lies supine while the examiner flexes the patient's hip to at least 90° with the knee flexed (Figure 11-16). The examiner then adducts the flexed leg. Normally, the knee will pass over the opposite hip without rolling the pelvis. In pathological hips, adduction will be limited and

accompanied by pain or discomfort. Maitland[63] called this test the quadrant or scouring test. He felt the test stressed or compressed the femoral neck against the acetabulum, or pinched adductor longus, pectineus, iliopsoas, sartorius or tensor fascia lata (see joint play movements).

Trendelenburg's Sign.[64] This test assesses the stability of the hip and the ability of the hip abductors to stabilize the pelvis on the femur. The patient is asked to stand on one lower limb. Normally, the pelvis on the opposite side should rise; this finding indicates a negative test (Figure 11-17). If the pelvis on the opposite side (nonstance side) drops when the patient stands on the affected leg, a positive test is indicated. The test should always be performed on the normal side first so that the patient understands what to do. If the pelvis drops on the opposite side, it indicates a weak gluteus medius or an unstable hip (e.g., as a result of hip dislocation) on the affected or stance side.

Stinchfield Resisted Hip Flexion Test.[65-67] The patient lies supine and then actively elevates the straight leg (i.e., flexes the hip) to about 20° to 30° while the examiner applies gentle resistance. In a positive test, pain may be referred into the sensory distribution of the femoral, obturator, or sciatic nerves. A positive test

Figure 11-17

Trendelenburg's sign. **A,** Negative test. **B,** Positive test.

indicates intra-articular pathology, which may include a labral tear, synovitis, arthritis, occult femoral neck fractures, iliopsoas tendinitis/bursitis, and prosthetic failure or loosening.[68]

Anterior Labral Tear Test (FADDIR—Flexion, Adduction, and Internal Rotation Test).[15,21] This test is used to test for anterior–superior impingement syndrome, anterior labial tear, and iliopsoas tendinitis. The patient is placed in supine position. The examiner takes the hip into full flexion, lateral rotation, and full abduction

as a starting position. The examiner then extends the hip combined with medial rotation and adduction (Figure 11-18). A positive test is indicated by the production of pain or the reproduction of the patient's symptoms with or without a click.

Posterior Labral Tear Test.[15] The patient is placed in supine position. The examiner takes the hip into full flexion, adduction, and medial rotation as a starting position. The examiner then takes the hip into extension combined with abduction and lateral rotation (Figure 11-19). A positive test is indicated by the production of groin pain, patient apprehension, or the reproduction of the patient's symptoms, with or without a click. A positive test is an indication of a labral tear, anterior hip instability or posterior–inferior impingement. The test is sometimes called the apprehension test if apprehension occurs toward the end of ROM when doing the test.

McCarthy Hip Extension Sign.[69] The patient lies supine on the bed with both hips flexed. The examiner then takes the good hip and extends it from the flexed position, first in combination with lateral rotation, and then repeats the test in combination with medial rotation. The test is repeated with the affected hip. A positive test would be the reproduction of the patient's pain. McCarthy et al[69] believed there were three positive tests that would help to predict labral pathology: pain with the McCarthy hip extension test, painful impingement with hip flexion abduction and lateral rotation (the anterior labial tear test), and inguinal pain on resisted straight leg raise (Stinchfield resisted in flexion test).

Craig's Test. Craig's test measures femoral **anteversion** or forward torsion of the femoral neck (Figure 11-20).

Figure 11-18

Anterior labral tear test. **A,** Starting position. **B,** End position.

Figure 11-19

Posterior labral tear test. **A,** Starting position. **B,** End position.

Degree of anteversion

Palpate greater trochanter
parallel to table

Figure 11-20

Craig's test to measure femoral anteversion.

Anteversion of the hip is measured by the angle made by the femoral neck with the femoral condyles (Figure 11-21). It is the degree of forward projection of the femoral neck from the coronal plane of the shaft (Figure 11-22), and it decreases during the growing period. At birth, the mean angle is approximately 30°; in the adult, the mean angle is 8° to 15° (Figure 11-23). Increased anteversion leads to squinting patellae and toeing-in (Figure 11-24).[70] Excessive anteversion is twice as common in girls as in boys. A common clinical finding of excessive anteversion is excessive medial hip rotation (more than 60°) and decreased lateral rotation in extension.[70] Gelberman

et al[71] pointed out, however, that rotation should be viewed both in neutral (as in the Craig's test) and with 90° of hip flexion, since rotation will show greater variability in flexion. They felt that greater medial rotation than lateral rotation in both positions was a better indicator of increased femoral anteversion. In retroversion, the plane of the femoral neck rotates backward in relation to the coronal condylar plane (see Figure 11-24) or the acetabulum itself may be retroverted.[72–76]

For Craig's test, which has been found to correlate well with x-rays (within 4°) in children,[77] the patient lies prone with the knee flexed to 90°. The examiner

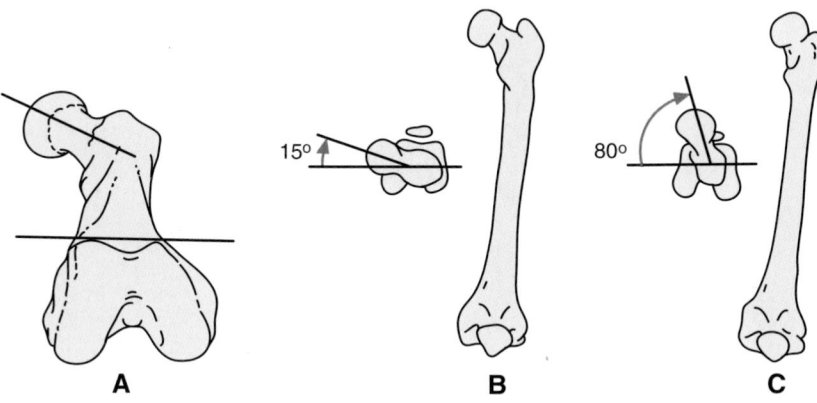

Figure 11-21
Anteversion of the hip. **A,** Femoral anteversion angle. **B,** Normal angle. **C,** Excessive angle. (**A,** Redrawn from the American Orthopaedic Association: *Manual of Orthopaedic Surgery,* p. 45, Chicago, 1979.)

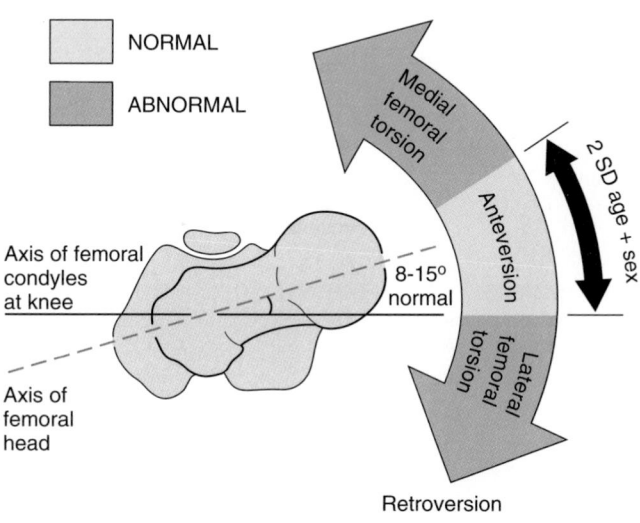

Figure 11-22
Axial view of right femur showing approximately normal angle of anteversion and torsional deformity beyond. (Redrawn from Staheli LT: Medial femoral torsion, *Orthop Clin North Am* 11:40, 1980.)

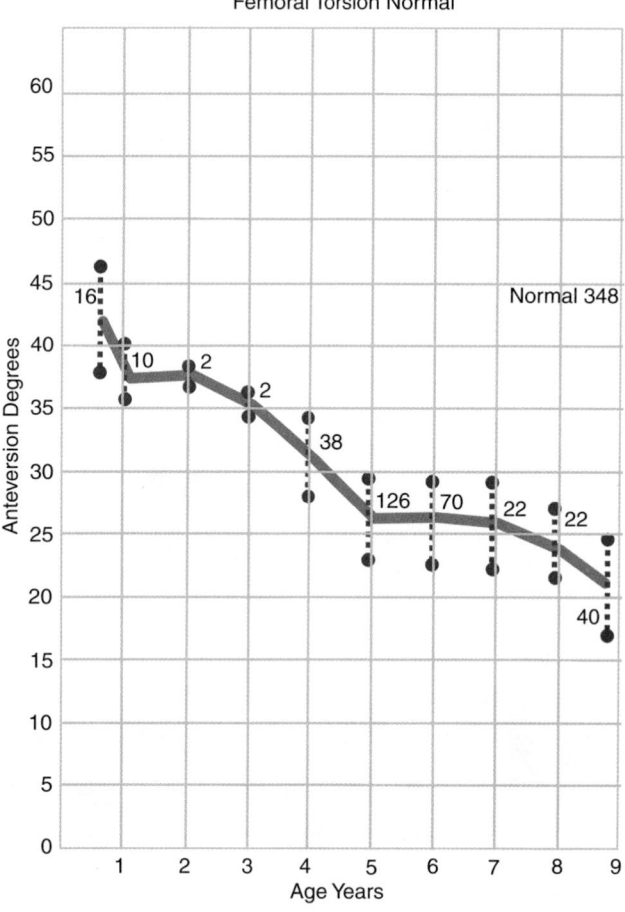

Figure 11-23
The degree of normal femoral torsion in relation to age. Solid lines represent the mean, vertical lines the standard deviation. (Redrawn from Crane L: Femoral torsion and its relation to toeing-in and toeing-out, *J Bone Joint Surg Am* 41:423, 1959.)

palpates the posterior aspect of the greater trochanter of the femur. The hip is then passively rotated medially and laterally until the greater trochanter is parallel with the examining table or reaches its most lateral position. The degree of anteversion can then be estimated, based on the angle of the lower leg with the vertical. The test is also called the **Ryder method** for measuring anteversion or retroversion.

Torque Test. The patient lies supine close to the edge of the examining table with the femur of the test leg extended over the edge of the table (Figure 11-25). The test leg is extended until the pelvis (i.e., the ASIS)

A, Positions of femoral neck.

Anteverted hip

"Toeing in" due to anteverted hip

Retroverted hip

"Toeing out" due to retroverted hip

Figure 11-24
Torsion angles of the hip. **A,** Positions of femoral neck. **B,** Different foot positions with anteversion and retroversion at the hip (coronal views). (Redrawn from Echternach J, editor: *Physical therapy of the hip*, p. 25, New York, 1990, Churchill Livingstone.)

Figure 11-25
Torque test.

begins to move. The examiner uses one hand to medially rotate the femur to the end of range and the other hand to apply a slow posterolateral pressure along the line of the neck of the femur for 20 seconds to stress the capsular ligaments and test the stability of the hip joint.[78]

Nélaton's Line. Nélaton's line is an imaginary line drawn from the ischial tuberosity of the pelvis to the ASIS of the pelvis on the same side (Figure 11-26).[73] If the greater trochanter of the femur is palpated well above the line, it is an indication of a dislocated hip or coxa vara. The two sides should be compared.

Bryant's Triangle. With the patient lying supine, the examiner drops an imaginary perpendicular line from the ASIS of the pelvis to the examining table.[75] A second imaginary line is projected up from the tip of the greater trochanter of the femur to meet the first line at a right angle (Figure 11-27). This line is measured, and the two sides are compared. Differences may indicate conditions such as coxa vara or CDH. This measurement can be done with

Figure 11-26
Nélaton's line.

Figure 11-27
Bryant's triangle.

radiographs, in which case the lines may be drawn on the radiograph.

Rotational Deformities. Rotational deformities can occur anywhere between the hip and the foot (Table 11-10). Many of these deformities are hereditary. The patient lies supine with the lower limbs straight while the examiner looks at the patellae.[74] If the patellae face in (squinting patellae), it is a possible indication of medial rotation of the femur or the tibia. If the patellae face up, out, and away from each other ("frog eyes" or "grasshopper eyes"),

Table 11-10

Hip Malalignment

Malalignment	Related Posture	Possible Compensating Postures
Excessive anteversion	Toeing-in Subtalar pronation Lateral patellar subluxation Medial tibial torsion Medial femoral torsion	Lateral tibial torsion Lateral rotation at knee Lateral rotation of tibia, femur, and/or pelvis Lumbar rotation on same side
Excessive retroversion	Toeing-out Subtalar supination Lateral tibial torsion Lateral femoral torsion	Medial rotation at knee Medial rotation of tibia, femur, and/or pelvis Lumbar rotation on opposite side
Coxa vara	Pronated subtalar joint Medial rotation of leg Short ipsilateral leg Anterior pelvic rotation	Ipsilateral subtalar supination Contralateral subtalar pronation Ipsilateral plantar flexion Contralateral genu recurvatum Contralateral hip and/or knee flexion Ipsilateral posterior pelvic rotation and ipsilateral lumbar rotation
Coxa valga	Supinated subtalar joint Lateral rotation of leg Long ipsilateral leg Posterior pelvic tilt	Ipsilateral subtalar pronation Contralateral subtalar supination Contralateral plantar flexion Ipsilateral genu recurvatum Ipsilateral hip and/or knee flexion Ipsilateral anterior pelvic rotation and contralateral lumbar rotation

Adapted from Reigger-Krugh C, Keysor JJ: Skeletal malalignments of the lower quarter: Correlated and compensatory motions and postures, *J Orthop Sports Phys Ther* 23:166–167, 1996.

Figure 11-28
Clinical appearance of excessive femoral torsion in a girl. **A,** With the knees in full extension and the feet aligned (pointing straight forward), the legs appear bowed and the patellae face inward (squinting patella). **B,** On lateral rotation of the hips so that the patellae are facing to the front, the feet and legs point outward and the bowleg appearance is corrected. (From Tachdjian MO: *Pediatric orthopedics,* p. 2802, Philadelphia, 1990, W.B. Saunders.)

it is a possible indication of lateral rotation of the femur or the tibia. If the tibia is affected, the feet face in ("pigeon toes") for medial rotation and face out more than 10° for excessive lateral rotation of the tibia (Figure 11-28) while the patellae face straight ahead. Normally, the feet angle out 5° to 10° **(Fick angle)** for better balance.

Pediatric Tests for Hip Pathology

Orthopedic tests are commonly performed in newborns to detect problems, especially CDH or developmental dysplasia of the hip (DDH) that covers more than congenital problems, which may be amenable to conservative treatment if caught early.[79,80]

Ortolani's Sign. Ortolani's test can determine whether an infant has a CDH (Figures 11-29, *A* and *B*).[74] With the infant supine, the examiner flexes the hips and grasps the legs so that the examiner's thumbs are against the insides of the knees and thighs and the fingers are placed along the outsides of the thighs to the buttocks. With gentle traction, the thighs are abducted and pressure is applied against the greater trochanters of the femora. Resistance to abduction and lateral rotation begins to be felt at approximately 30° to 40°. The examiner may feel a click, clunk, or jerk, which indicates a positive test and that the hip has reduced; in addition, increased abduction

of the hip is obtained. The femoral head has slipped over the acetabular ridge into the acetabulum, and normal abduction of 70° to 90° can be obtained.

This test is valid only for the first few weeks after birth and only for dislocated and lax hips, not for dislocations that are difficult to reduce. The examiner should take care to feel the quality of the click. Soft clicks may occur without dislocation and are thought to be caused by the iliofemoral ligament's clicking over the anterior surface of the head of the femur as it is laterally rotated. Soft clicking usually occurs without the prior resistance that is seen with dislocations. By repeated rotation of the hip, the exact location of the click can be palpated. However, Ortolani's test should not be repeated too often because it could lead to damage of the articular cartilage of the femoral head. As with all clinical tests, if the test is positive, it is highly suggestive that the problem (i.e., CDH) exists, but if it is negative, it does not necessarily rule out the problem.

Barlow's Test. Barlow's test is a modification of Ortolani's test[74] (see Figure 11-29) used for DDH.[80] The infant lies supine with the legs facing the examiner. The hips are flexed to 90°, and the knees are fully flexed. Each hip is evaluated individually while the examiner's other hand steadies the opposite femur and

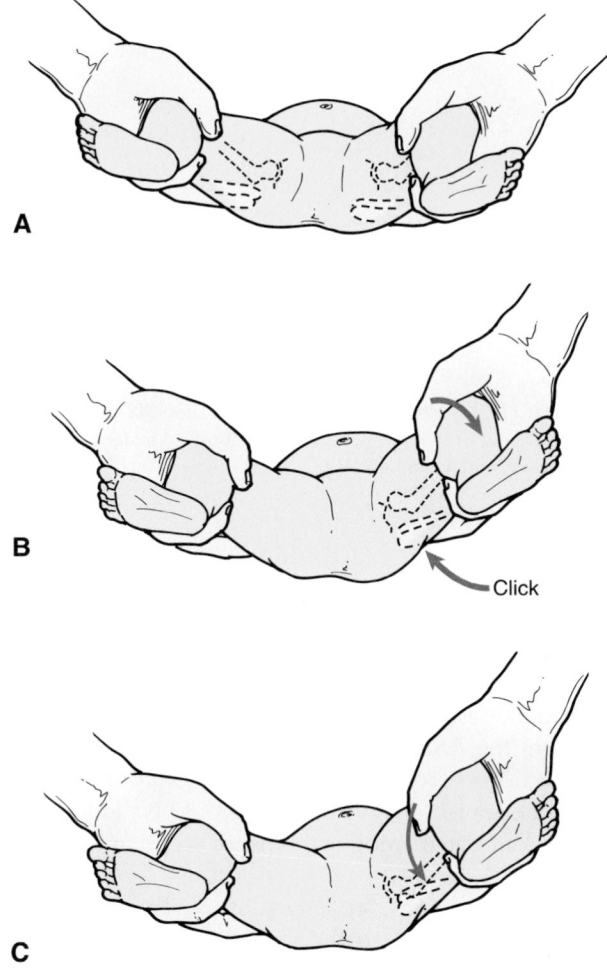

Figure 11-29
Ortolani's sign and Barlow's test. **A,** In the newborn, the two hips can be equally flexed, abducted, and laterally rotated without producing a "click." **B,** Ortolani's sign or first part of Barlow's test. **C,** Second part of Barlow's test.

This test may be used for infants up to 6 months of age. It should not be repeated too often because it may result in a dislocated hip as well as articular damage to the head of the femur.[81]

Galeazzi Sign (Allis or Galeazzi Test). The Galeazzi test is good only for assessing unilateral CDH or unilateral DDH and may be used in children from 3 to 18 months of age.[68] The child lies supine with the knees flexed and the hips flexed to 90°. A positive test is indicated if one knee is higher than the other (Figure 11-30).

Telescoping Sign (Piston or Dupuytren's Test).[82] The telescoping sign is evident in a child with a dislocated hip. The child lies in the supine position. The examiner flexes the knee and hip to 90°. The femur is pushed down onto the examining table. The femur and leg are then lifted up and away from the table (Figure 11-31). With the normal hip, little movement occurs with this action. With the dislocated hip, however, there is a lot of relative movement. This excessive movement is called **telescoping**, or **pistoning**.

Abduction Test (Harts' Sign).[82] If CDH is not diagnosed early or there is DDH, parents often note that when they change the child's diapers, one leg does not abduct as far as the other one.[80] This is the basis for this test. The child lies supine with the hips and knees flexed to 90°. The examiner then passively abducts both legs, noting any asymmetry or limitation of movement. In addition, if one hip is dislocated, the child often demonstrates asymmetry of fat folds in the gluteal and upper leg area because of the "riding up" of the femur on the affected side.

Tests for Leg Length

There are two types of leg length discrepancy. The first, called **true leg length discrepancy** or **true shortening**, is caused by an anatomic or structural change in the lower

the pelvis. The examiner's middle finger of each hand is placed over the greater trochanter, and the thumb is placed adjacent to the inner side of the knee and thigh opposite the lesser trochanter. The hip is taken into abduction while the examiner's middle finger applies forward pressure behind the greater trochanter. If the femoral head slips forward into the acetabulum with a click, clunk, or jerk, the test is positive, indicating that the hip was dislocated. This part of the test is identical to Ortolani's test. The examiner then uses the thumb to apply pressure backward and outward on the inner thigh. If the femoral head slips out over the posterior lip of the acetabulum and then reduces again when pressure is removed, the hip is classified as unstable. The hip is not dislocated but is dislocatable. The procedure is repeated for the other hip.

Figure 11-30
Galeazzi sign (Allis test).

A   **B**

Figure 11-31
Telescoping of the hip. Because hip is not fixed in acetabulum, it moves down (**A**) and up (**B**).

leg resulting from congenital maldevelopment (e.g., adolescent coxa vara, congenital hip dysplasia, bony abnormality) or trauma (e.g., fracture). Because an anatomic short leg results, the spine and pelvis are often affected, leading to lateral pelvic tilt and scoliosis.[83,84]

The second type of leg length discrepancy is called **functional leg length discrepancy** or **functional shortening**, and it is the result of compensation for a change that may have occurred because of positioning rather than structure. For example, a functional leg length discrepancy could occur because of unilateral foot pronation or spinal scoliosis.[83,84]

True Leg Length. Before any measuring is done, the examiner must set the pelvis square, level, or in balance with the lower limbs.[85–87] The legs should be 15 to 20 cm (4–8 inches) apart and parallel to each other (Figure 11-32). If the legs are not placed in proper relation to the pelvis, apparent shortening of the limb may occur.

The lower limbs must be placed in comparable positions relative to the pelvis because abduction of the hip brings the medial malleolus closer to the ASIS on the same side and adduction of the hip takes the medial malleolus farther from the ASIS on the same side. If one hip is fixed in abduction or adduction as a result of contracture or some other cause, the normal hip should be adducted or abducted an equal amount to ensure accurate leg length measurement.

In North America, leg length measurement is usually taken from the ASIS to the medial malleolus; however, these values may be altered by muscle wasting or obesity. Measuring to the lateral malleolus is less likely to be affected by the muscle bulk. To obtain the leg length, the examiner measures from the ASIS to the lateral or medial malleolus. The flat metal end of the tape measure is placed immediately distal to the ASIS and pushed up against it. The thumb then presses the tape end firmly

A   **B**

Figure 11-32
Measuring true leg length. **A,** Measuring to the medial malleolus. **B,** Measuring to the lateral malleolus.

against the bone, rigidly fixing the tape measure against the bone. The index finger of the other hand is placed immediately distal to the lateral or medial malleolus and pushed against it. The thumbnail is brought down against the tip of the index finger so that the tape measure is pinched between them. A slight difference (as much as 1–1.5 cm) in leg length is considered normal; however, this difference can still cause symptoms.

The **Weber-Barstow maneuver** (visual method) may also be used to measure leg length asymmetry. The patient lies supine with the hips and knees flexed (Figure 11-33). The examiner stands at the patient's feet and palpates the distal aspect of the medial malleoli with the thumbs. The patient then lifts the pelvis from the examining table and returns to the starting position. Next, the examiner passively extends the patient's legs and compares the positions of the malleoli using the borders of the thumbs. Different levels indicate asymmetry.[88]

If one leg is shorter than the other (Figure 11-34), the examiner can determine where the difference is by measuring the following:

1. From the iliac crest to the greater trochanter of the femur (for coxa vara or coxa valga). The neck-shaft angle of the femur (Figure 11-35) is normally 150° to 160° at birth and decreases to between 120° and 135° in the adult (Figure 11-36). If this angle is less than 120° in an adult, it is known as **coxa vara;** if it is more than 135° in the adult, it is known as **coxa valga.**
2. From the greater trochanter of the femur to the knee joint line on the lateral aspect (for femoral shaft shortening)
3. From the knee joint line on the medial side to the medial malleolus (for tibial shaft shortening)

The relative length of the tibia may also be examined with the patient lying prone. The examiner places the thumbs transversely across the soles of the feet just in

Figure 11-33

Weber-Barstow maneuver for leg length asymmetry. **A,** Starting position. **B,** Patient lifts hips off bed. **C,** Comparing height of medial malleoli with the legs extended.

Left shortened
tibia

Right shortened
tibia

Figure 11-34
Leg length discrepancy.

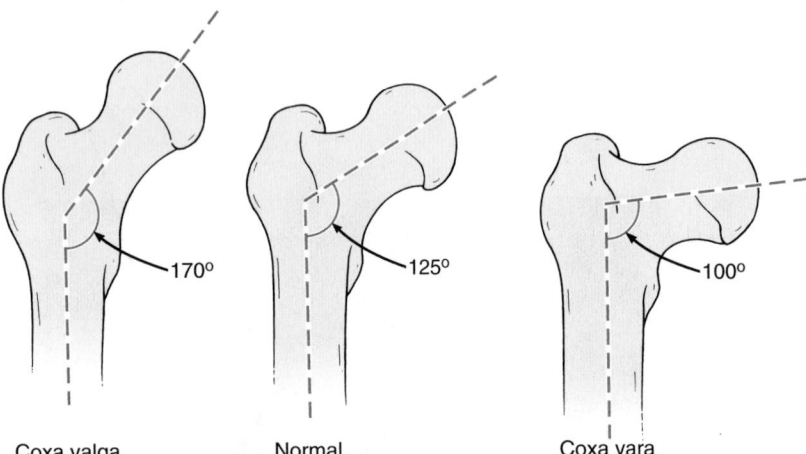

170°

125°

100°

Coxa valga

Normal

Coxa vara

Figure 11-35
Neck-shaft angles of the femur in adults.

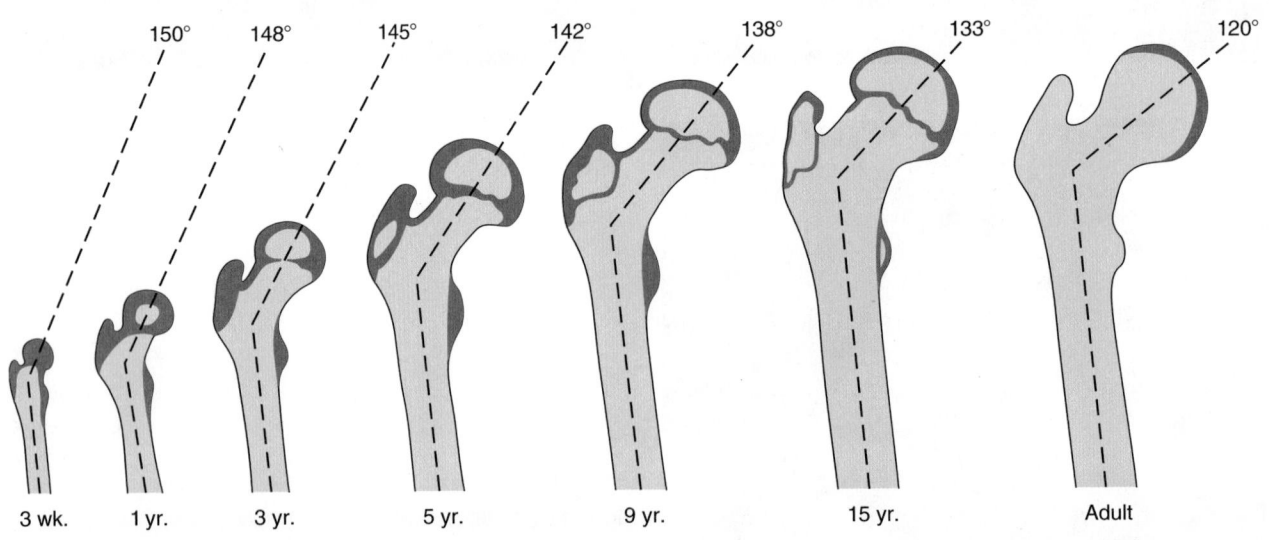

150°   148°   145°   142°   138°   133°   120°

3 wk.   1 yr.   3 yr.   5 yr.   9 yr.   15 yr.   Adult

Figure 11-36
Mean angle of the femoral neck shaft in different age groups. Red area indicates cartilage. (Modified from von
Lanz T, Wachsmuth W: *Praktische anatomie*, p. 143, Berlin, 1938, Julius Springer.)

A **B**

Figure 11-37

Prone knee flexion test for tibial shortening. The prone knee flexion test is completed as the examiner (**A**) passively flexes the patient's knees to 90° and (**B**) sights through the plane of the heel pads to see whether a difference in height is noticeable.

front of the heels. The knees are flexed 90°, and the relative heights of the thumbs are noted. Care must be taken to ensure that the legs are perpendicular to the examining table (Figure 11-37).[88]

Similarly, the femoral lengths can be compared by having the patient lie supine with the hips and knees flexed to 90°. If one femur is longer than the other, its height will be higher (Figure 11-38).[84]

Apparent or functional shortening (Figure 11-39) of the leg is evident if the patient has a lateral pelvic tilt when the measurement is taken. Apparent or functional shortening of the limb is the result of adaptations the patient has made in response to pathology or contracture somewhere in the spine, pelvis, or lower limbs. In reality, there is no structural or anatomic difference in bone lengths. If there were, it would be called true shortening of the limb. When measuring the apparent leg length shortening, the examiner obtains the distance from the tip of the xiphisternum or umbilicus to the medial malleolus (Figure 11-40). If true leg length is normal but the umbilicus-to-malleolus measurements are different, a functional leg length discrepancy is present.[84] Values obtained by these measurements may be affected by muscle wasting, obesity, asymmetric position of the xiphisternum or umbilicus, or asymmetric positioning of the lower limbs.

Standing (Functional) Leg Length. The patient is first assessed while in a relaxed stance. In this position, the examiner palpates the ASIS and the PSIS, noting any asymmetry. The examiner then places the patient

Figure 11-38

Hip flexion test for femoral shortening.

in a symmetric stance, ensuring that the subtalar joint is in neutral position (see Chapter 13), the toes are facing straight ahead, and the knees are extended. The ASIS and PSIS are again assessed for asymmetry. If differences are still noted, the examiner should check for structural leg length differences, sacroiliac joint dysfunction, or weak gluteus medius or quadratus lumborum muscles.

Figure 11-39
Functional shortening due to adduction contracture.
A, Legs crossed. **B,** Legs uncrossed. Note that uncrossing
causes pelvis to elevate on one side, but true leg length
is equal on both sides. (Redrawn from the American
Orthopaedic Association: *Manual of orthopaedic surgery,*
p. 45, Chicago, 1972, AOA.)

Figure 11-40
Measuring functional leg length.

Figure 11-41
Thomas test. **A,** Negative test. **B,** Positive test.

Tests for Muscle Tightness or Pathology

Sign of the Buttock. The patient lies supine and the examiner performs a straight leg raising test. If there is limitation on straight leg raising, the examiner flexes the patient's knee to see whether further hip flexion can be obtained. If hip flexion does not increase, the lesion is in the buttock or the hip, not the sciatic nerve or hamstring muscles. There may also be some limited trunk flexion. Causes of a positive test include ischial bursitis, a neoplasm, an abscess in the buttock, or hip pathology.

Thomas Test. The Thomas test is used to assess a hip flexion contracture, the most common contracture of the hip. The patient lies supine while the examiner checks for excessive lordosis, which is usually present with tight hip flexors. The examiner flexes one of the patient's hips, bringing the knee to the chest to flatten out the lumbar spine and to stabilize the pelvis. The patient holds the flexed hip against the chest. If there is no flexion contracture, the hip being tested (the straight leg) remains on the examining table. If a contracture is present, the patient's straight leg rises off the table and a muscle stretch end feel will be felt (Figure 11-41). The angle of contracture can be measured. If the lower limb is pushed down onto the table, the patient may exhibit an increased lordosis; again, this result indicates a positive test. When doing the test, if measurements are taken, the examiner must be sure the restriction is in the hip and not the pelvis or lumbar spine.[89] If the leg does not lift off the table but abducts as the other leg is flexed to the chest, it is called the **"J" sign** or **stroke** and is indicative of a tight iliotibial band on the extended leg side.

Rectus Femoris Contracture Test (Kendall Test, Method 1). The patient lies supine with the knees bent over the end or edge of the examining table. The patient flexes one knee onto the chest and holds it (Figure 11-42).

Figure 11-42

Rectus femoris contracture. **A,** The movement leg is brought to the chest. The test leg remains bent over the end of the examining table, indicating a negative test. **B,** The test knee extends, indicating a positive test.

The angle of the test knee should remain at 90° when the opposite knee is flexed to the chest. If it does not (i.e., the test knee extends slightly), a contracture is probably present. The examiner may attempt to passively flex the knee to see whether it will remain at 90° of its own volition. The examiner should always palpate for muscle tightness when doing any contracture test. If there is no palpable tightness, the probable cause of restriction is tight joint structures (e.g., the capsule) and the end feel will be different (muscle stretch versus capsular). The two sides should be tested and compared.

Ely's Test (Tight Rectus Femoris, Method 2). The patient lies prone, and the examiner passively flexes the patient's knee (Figure 11-43).[90] On flexion of the knee, the patient's hip on the same side spontaneously flexes, indicating that the rectus femoris muscle is tight on that side and that the test is positive. The two sides should be tested and compared.

Ober's Test. Ober's test assesses the tensor fasciae latae (iliotibial band) for contracture (Figure 11-44).[91] The patient is in the side lying position with the lower leg flexed at the hip and knee for stability. The examiner then passively abducts and extends the patient's upper leg with the knee straight or flexed to 90°. The examiner slowly lowers the upper limb; if a contracture is present, the leg

Figure 11-43

Ely's test for a tight rectus femoris. **A,** Position for the test. **B,** Posture test shown by hip flexion when the knee is flexed.

A

B

C

Figure 11-44
Ober's test. **A,** Knee straight. **B,** The hip is passively extended by the examiner to ensure that the tensor fasciae latae runs over the greater trochanter. A positive test is indicated when the leg remains abducted while the patient's muscles are relaxed. **C,** Test done with the knee flexed.

remains abducted and does not fall to the table. When doing this test, it is important to extend the hip slightly so that the iliotibial band passes over the greater trochanter of the femur. To do this, the examiner stabilizes the pelvis at the same time to stop the pelvis from "falling backward." Ober[91] originally described the test with the knee flexed. However, the iliotibial band has a greater stretch placed on it when the knee is extended. Also, when the knee is flexed during the test, greater stress is placed on the femoral nerve. If neurological signs (i.e., pain, paresthesia) occur during the test, the examiner should consider pathology affecting the femoral nerve. Likewise, tenderness over the greater trochanter should lead the examiner to consider trochanteric bursitis.

Prone Lying Test for Iliotibial Band Contracture.[92] The patient lies prone while the examiner stands on the opposite side to the leg being tested. The examiner holds the ankle of the test leg and maximally abducts it at the hip, while the other hand applies pressure to the buttock on the same side as the test leg to flatten the pelvis and correct any hip flexion deformity (Figure 11-45). While maintaining the hip in neutral rotation and the knee flexed to 90°, the examiner then adducts the hip until there is a firm end feel. The angle is measured relative to the body's vertical axis and compared with the other side.[92] This test is more commonly done in children.

Noble Compression Test. This test is used to determine whether iliotibial band friction syndrome exists near

Figure 11-45
Prone lying test for iliotibial band contracture.

"balancing" implies a line joining the ASIS is perpendicular to the two lines formed by the straight legs (Figure 11-47). If a contracture is present, the affected leg forms an angle of less than 90° with the line joining the two ASISs. If the examiner then attempts to "balance" the lower limb with the pelvis, the pelvis (i.e., ASIS) shifts up on the affected side or down on the unaffected side, and balancing is not possible. Normally, hip abduction should be 30° to 50° before the ASIS moves. If the ASIS moves before this, the adductors are tight if a muscle stretch end feel is felt. This type of contracture can lead to **functional shortening** of the limb rather than true shortening (see Figure 11-39).

the knee (Figure 11-46).[93] This syndrome is a chronic inflammation of the iliotibial band near its insertion, adjacent to the femoral condyle. The patient lies supine and the knee is flexed to 90° accompanied by hip flexion. The examiner then applies pressure with the thumb to the lateral femoral epicondyle or 1 to 2 cm (0.4–0.8 inch) proximal to it. While the pressure is maintained, the patient slowly extends the knee. At approximately 30° of flexion (0° being a straight leg), if the patient complains of severe pain over the lateral femoral condyle, a positive test is indicated. The patient usually says it is the same pain that accompanies the patient's activity (e.g., running).

Adduction Contracture Test. This test is designed to test the length of the adductor muscles (adductor longus, brevis and magnus, and pectineus) of the hip. The patient lies supine with the ASISs level. Normally, the examiner can easily "balance" the pelvis on the legs. This

Figure 11-46
Noble compression test for iliotibial band friction syndrome. The patient extends the knee. The examiner is indicating where pain is felt at about 30° of flexion.

Figure 11-47
Balancing the pelvis on the legs (femora).

Patients, especially children, with adductor spasticity, may also be tested by abduction. The patient is supine. The examiner then quickly abducts the leg. If there is a "grab" or "kicking in" of the stretch reflex at less than 30°, the test for adductor spasticity is considered positive. The test should be repeated with the knee flexed to rule out medial hamstring contracture.[94]

Abduction Contracture Test. This test is used to test the length of the abductor muscles (gluteus medius and minimus) of the hip. The patient lies supine with the ASISs level. If a contracture is present, the affected leg forms an angle of more than 90° with a line joining each ASIS. If the examiner then attempts to balance the lower limb with the pelvis, the pelvis (i.e., the ASIS) shifts down on the affected side or up on the unaffected side, and balancing is not possible. Normally, hip adduction should be about 30° before the ASIS moves. If the ASIS moves before this, the abductors are tight if a muscle stretch end feel is felt. This type of contracture can lead to **functional lengthening** of the limb rather than true lengthening.

Piriformis Test. In about 15% of the population, the sciatic nerve, all or in part, passes through the piriformis muscle rather than below it (Figures 11-48 and 11-49).[14] These people are more likely to suffer from this relatively rare condition, **piriformis syndrome.** The patient is in the side lying position with the test leg uppermost. The patient flexes the test hip to 60° with the knee flexed.

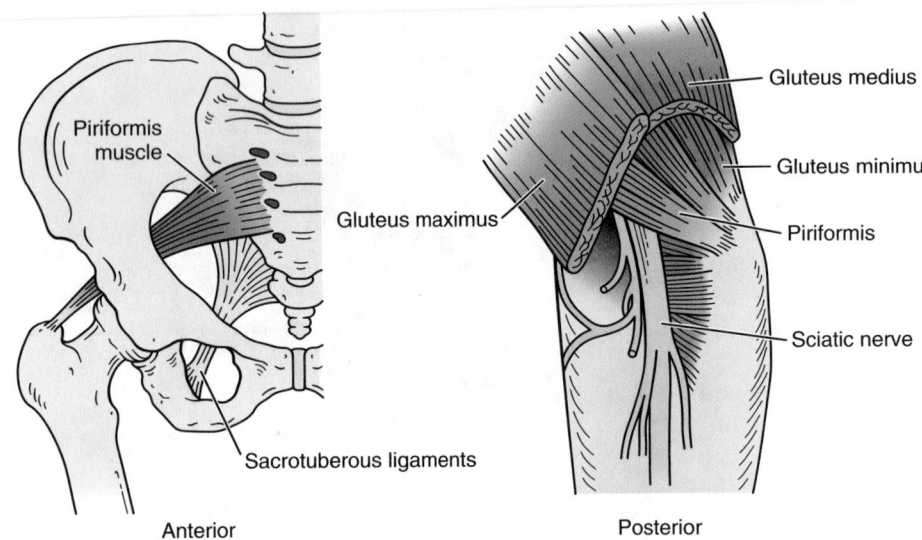

Anterior   Posterior

Figure 11-48
Position of the piriformis muscle. (Redrawn from Norris C: *Sports injuries: diagnosis and management* ed 3, p. 205, London, 2004, Butterworth-Heinemann.)

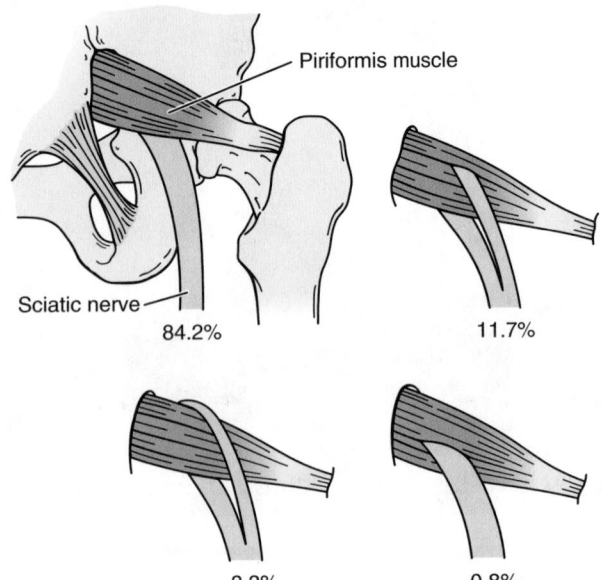

84.2%   11.7%

3.3%   0.8%

Figure 11-49
Sciatic nerve: variations in its relationship with the piriformis muscle. (Redrawn from Levin P: Hip dislocations. In Browner BD, et al. editors: *Skeletal trauma,* p. 1333, Philadelphia, 1992, W.B. Saunders.)

Figure 11-50
Piriformis test.

A

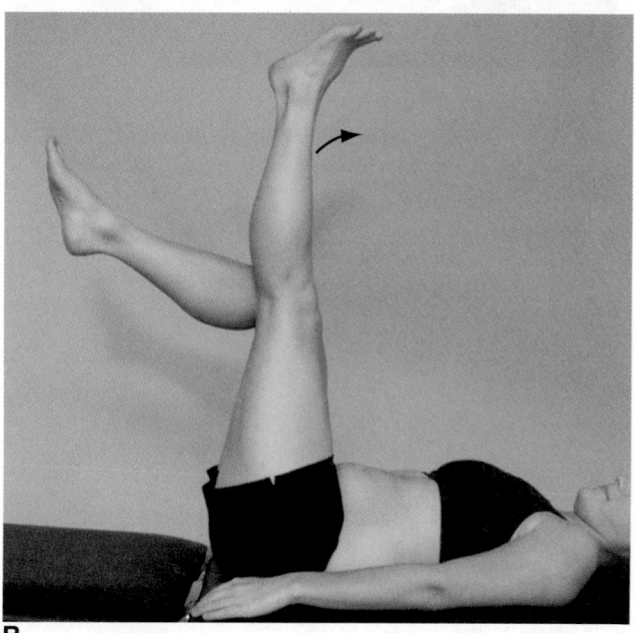

B

Figure 11-51
The 90-90 straight leg raising test.

The examiner stabilizes the hip with one hand and applies a downward pressure to the knee (Figure 11-50). If the piriformis muscle is tight, pain is elicited in the muscle. If the piriformis muscle is pinching the sciatic nerve, pain results in the buttock and sciatica may be experienced by the patient.[22,78] Resisted lateral rotation with the muscle on stretch (hip medially rotated) can cause the same sciatica.[95]

90-90 Straight Leg Raising Test (Hamstrings Contracture, Method 1). The supine patient flexes both hips to 90° while the knees are bent. The patient then grasps behind the knees with both hands to stabilize the hips at 90° of flexion. The patient actively extends each knee in turn as much as possible. For normal flexibility in the hamstrings, knee extension should be within 20° of full extension (Figure 11-51).[22,96] Kuo et al[97] called this angle the popliteal angle (the angle between two lines—one line along the shaft of femur and one line along the line of the tibia). They reported this angle to be 180° from birth to 2 years of age, which then decreased to about 155° by age 6 and remained fairly constant after that. If the angle is less than 125°, the hamstrings were considered to be tight. Normally, or if the hamstrings are tight, the end feel will be muscle stretch. Nerve root symptoms may also result, since this positioning is similar to the slump test done in supine lying instead of sitting.

A modification of this test may also be used to test the length of gluteus maximus. The patient assumes the same starting position. While the examiner palpates the ASIS on the same side, the examiner flexes the hip with the knee flexed (Figure 11-52). If the thigh flexes 110° to 120° before the ASIS moves up, gluteus maximus length is normal. If the ASIS moves up before the thigh reaches the trunk, gluteus maximus is tight. Both sides should be compared.

Janda[19,20] has reported that the gluteus maximus, medius, and minimus are more likely to be weak than tight. To test gluteus maximus strength, the patient is placed in prone with the hip straight and the knee flexed to 90°. The patient is asked to extend the hip, keeping the knee flexed while the examiner applies an anterior force to the posterior thigh. Both legs are tested (good side first) and compared. If the patient attempts to further flex the knee when doing the test, it indicates greater use of hamstrings is occurring. To test the strength of gluteus medius and minimus, the patient is positioned in side lying. The examiner stabilizes the pelvis and asks the patient to abduct the leg against the

Figure 11-52

Testing for length of gluteus maximus. **A,** Negative test. **B,** Positive test.

Figure 11-53

Testing for weakness. **A,** Gluteus maximus. Note examiner is palpating iliac crest *(PSIS)* to ensure no movement. **B,** Gluteus medius and minimus. Note examiner is palpating iliac crest to ensure no movement.

examiner's resistance applied to the lateral aspect of the thigh (Figure 11-53). Both legs are tested (good side first) and compared.

Hamstrings Contracture Test (Method 2). The patient is instructed to sit with one knee flexed against the chest to stabilize the pelvis and the other knee extended (Figure 11-54). The patient then attempts to flex the trunk and touch the toes of the extended lower limb (test leg) with the fingers. The test is repeated on the other side. A comparison is made between the two sides. Normally, the patient should be able to at least touch the toes while keeping the knee extended. If he or she is unable to do so, it is an indication of tight hamstrings on the straight leg.

Tripod Sign (Hamstrings Contracture, Method 3). The patient is seated with both knees flexed to 90° over the edge of the examining table (Figure 11-55).[98] The examiner then passively extends one knee. If the hamstring muscles on that side are tight, the patient extends the trunk to relieve the tension in the hamstring muscles. The leg is returned to its starting position, and the other leg is tested and compared with the first side. Extension of the spine is indicative of a positive test. The examiner must be aware that nerve root problems (stretching of the sciatic nerve) can cause a similar positive sign, although the symptoms will be slightly different.

Bent-Knee Stretch Test for Proximal Hamstrings.[34] The patient lies supine while the examiner flexes the hip and knee of the test leg maximally (Figure 11-56, *A*).

Figure 11-54
Test for hamstring tightness (method 2). **A,** Negative test. **B,** Positive test. **C,** Hypermobility of hamstrings.

Figure 11-55
Tripod sign.

The examiner then slowly extends the knee (Figure 11-56, *B*). Pain in the hamstrings at the ischial origin indicates a positive test. It should be noted that neurological tissues must also be cleared before the test would be considered positive.

"Taking Off the Shoe" (TOST) Test.[99] The patient stands wearing shoes. The patient is asked to remove the shoe on the affected side with the help of the shoe on the opposite side (Figure 11-57) by putting the heel of the affected side into the medial longitudinal arch of the stance (good) leg to pry the shoe off. In this position, the affected hip is laterally rotated about 90° with 20° to 25° flexion at the knee, leading to contraction of the biceps femoris on the affected side. If a sharp pain is felt in the biceps femoris, it indicates a 1° or 2° muscle strain.

Phelps' Test.[61] The patient lies prone with the knees extended. The examiner passively abducts both of the patient's legs as far as possible. The knees are then flexed to 90° (Figure 11-58), and the examiner tries to abduct the hips further. If abduction increases, the

Figure 11-56
The bent-knee stretch test for proximal hamstring tightness is performed with the patient supine. The hip and knee of the test leg are maximally flexed (**A**), and then the examiner slowly straightens the knee (**B**).

Figure 11-57
Patient doing the TOST test while standing. **A,** Anterior view. **B,** Posterior view.

test is considered positive for contracture of the gracilis muscle.

Tightness of Hip Rotators. The medial and lateral hip rotators can be tested by placing the patient in supine lying with the hip and knee flexed to 90°. To test for tightness of the lateral rotators, the patient is asked to medially rotate the hip by rotating the leg outward. If the lateral rotators are tight, medial rotation will be less than 30° to 40° and the end feel will be muscle stretch rather than tissue (capsular) stretch. To test for tightness of the

Figure 11-58
Phelps' test. Hips are abducted and knees are flexed to 90°. If abduction increases with knee flexion, test is positive.

medial rotators, the patient is asked to laterally rotate the hip by rotating the leg inward. If the medial rotators are tight, lateral rotation will be less than 40° to 60° and the end feel will be muscle stretch rather than tissue (capsular) stretch.

Lateral Step Down Maneuver (Pelvis Drop Test).[100] A 20-cm (8-inch) stool or step is placed in front of the patient. The patient is asked to place one foot on the stool and stand up straight on the stool on one foot. The patient then slowly lowers the non-weight-bearing leg to the floor. This should normally be accomplished with the arms by the side and the trunk relatively erect and no hip adduction or medial rotation (Figure 11-59). If, however, on lowering, the arms abduct, and/or the trunk inclines forward, and/or the weight-bearing hip adducts or medially rotates, and/or the pelvis flexes forward or rotates backwards, it is an indication of an unstable hip or weak lateral rotators.

Other Tests

Fulcrum Test of the Hip. The fulcrum test[101] is used to assess for possible stress fracture of the femoral shaft. The patient sits with the knees bent over the end of the bed with feet dangling. The examiner places an arm under the patient's thigh to act as a fulcrum (Figure 11-60). The fulcrum arm is moved from distal to proximal along the thigh as gentle pressure is applied to the dorsum of the knee with the examiner's opposite hand. If a stress fracture is present, the patient complains of a sharp pain and expresses apprehension when the fulcrum arm is under the fracture site. A bone scan confirms the diagnosis.

Reflexes and Cutaneous Distribution

There are no reflexes around the hip that can be evaluated easily. However, the examiner should assess the normal dermatome patterns of the nerve roots (Figure 11-61) as well as the sensory distribution of the peripheral nerves

Figure 11-59

Lateral step down maneuver (pelvic drop test). **A,** Normal (negative test). **B,** Positive test.

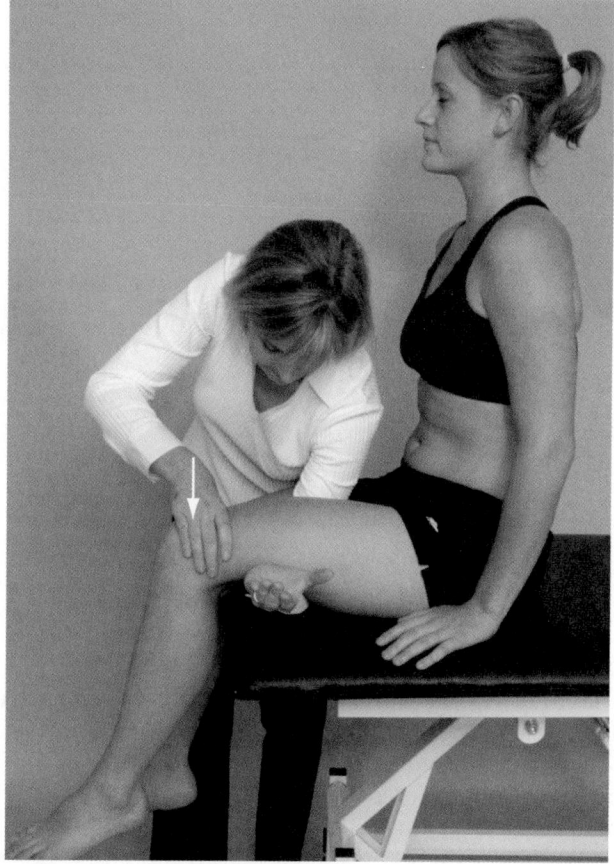

Figure 11-60

Fulcrum test of the hip. Examiner places arm under femur and carefully applies a downward force at the knee.

Figure 11-61
Dermatomes around the hip. Only one side is illustrated.

A

B

Figure 11-62
Sensory distribution of peripheral nerves around the hip.
A, Anterior view. **B**, Posterior view.

(Figure 11-62). Because dermatomes vary from person to person, the accompanying diagrams are estimations only. Testing for altered sensation is performed by running the relaxed hands and fingers of the examiner over the pelvis and legs anteriorly, posteriorly, and laterally in a sensation scanning assessment. Any difference in sensation should be noted and can be mapped out more precisely using a pinwheel, pin, cotton batten, and/or small brush.

True hip pain is usually referred to the groin, but it may also be referred to the ankle, knee, lumbar spine, and sacroiliac joints (Figure 11-63). In children with hip problems (e.g., slipped capital femoral epiphysis,

Legg-Calvé-Perthes disease), sensory symptoms may be manifested only in the knee. Similarly, the knee, sacroiliac joints, and lumbar spine may refer pain to the hip. Table 11-11 illustrates muscles of the hip and their referral pattern if injured.

Peripheral Nerve Injuries About the Hip

Sciatic Nerve (L4 through S3). The sciatic nerve (Figure 11-64 and Table 11-12) may be injured anywhere along its path from the lumbosacral spine down the back of the leg to the knee. It is the most commonly injured nerve in the hip region.[102-104] If it is injured in

Figure 11-63
Referred pain around the hip. Right side demonstrates referral to the hip. Left side shows referral from hip.

sory alteration in the entire foot except the instep and medial malleolus, along with muscle atrophy. Usually, the symptoms are primarily in the common peroneal branch of the sciatic nerve. In the hip region, the sciatic nerve may be compressed by the piriformis muscle (piriformis syndrome) (see Figure 11-49).[105] If piriformis is affected, there will be pain and weakness on abduction and lateral rotation of the hip (**sign of Pace and Nagel**). The pain on passive medial rotation of the extended hip (**Freiberg sign**) will also be elicited because this action stretches the piriformis.[106] Burning pain and hyperesthesia may be felt in the sacral and/or gluteal region as well as in the sciatic nerve distribution. Medial rotation with flexion of the hip accentuates the problem.

Superior Gluteal Nerve (L4 through S1). The superior gluteal nerve may be compressed as it passes between the piriformis and inferior border of the gluteus minimus muscle. It may also be injured during hip surgery.[103] The patient complains of acute gluteal pain that increases with ambulation. The hip is often medially rotated, and there is weakness of the hip abductors, resulting in a Trendelenburg's gait. Tenderness may be palpated just lateral to the greater sciatic notch.

Femoral Nerve (L2 through L4). The femoral nerve (Figure 11-65), although not commonly injured, may be compressed during childbirth or with anterior dislocation of the femur or may be traumatized during hernia surgery, stripping of varicose veins, hip surgery, or fractures.[103] The patient is not able to flex the thigh on the trunk or extend the knee. The deep tendon knee reflex is also lost. Wasting of the quadriceps is most evident. Sensory loss includes the

the pelvis or upper femur area (e.g., posterior hip dislocation), the hamstrings and all muscles below the knee can be affected. The result is a high steppage gait with an inability to stand on the heel or toes. There is sen-

Table 11-11

Hip Muscles and Referral of Pain

Muscle	Referral Pattern
Iliopsoas	Lateral to lumbar spine, anterior thigh
Gluteus maximus	Sacral and gluteal area to lateral aspect of pelvis and posterosuperior thigh
Gluteus medius	Lumbar and sacral gluteal area to lateral aspect of pelvis and upper thigh
Gluteus minimus	Gluteal area to area below iliac crest down lateral aspect of thigh and leg
Piriformis	Sacrum, gluteal area down posterior aspect of thigh
Tensor fasciae latae	Lateral thigh
Sartorius	Anteromedial thigh (along course of muscle)
Pectineus	Groin to upper medial thigh
Rectus femoris	Anterior thigh to knee
Adductor longus and brevis	Anterior thigh to medial thigh to anterior knee to anteromedial leg to ankle
Adductor magnus	Groin along medial thigh to above knee
Gracilis	Anteromedial thigh to knee
Hamstrings	Gluteal area along posterior thigh to knee and posteromedial calf

Figure 11-64
Sciatic nerve.

medial aspect of the distal thigh (**anterior femoral cutaneous nerve**) and the medial aspect of the leg and foot (**saphenous nerve**).

Obturator Nerve (L2 through L4). The obturator nerve (Figure 11-66) may be compressed as it leaves the pelvis and enters the leg in the obturator tunnel. Injury to the nerve may be caused by pelvic or hip surgery, pregnancy (obstetric palsy), fractures, or tumors and has been reported as a cause of groin pain in athletes.[103,105,107] Because the obturator nerve controls primarily the adductors, hip adduction is affected, as are knee flexion (gracilis) and hip lateral rotation (obturator externus). Sensory deficit is small, involving a small area in the middle medial part of the thigh, although the patient may complain of pain from the symphysis pubis to the medial aspect of the knee.

Joint Play Movements of the Hip

- Caudal glide of the femur (long leg traction or long-axis extension)
- Compression
- Lateral distraction
- Quadrant test

Joint Play Movements

The joint play movements (Figure 11-67) are completed with the patient in the supine position. The examiner should attempt to compare the amounts of available movement on the two sides. Small differences may be difficult to detect because of the large muscle bulk in the area.

Table 11-12

Peripheral Nerve Injuries (Neuropathy) About the Hip

	Muscle Weakness	Sensory Alteration	Reflexes Affected
Sciatic nerve (L4 through S3)	Hamstrings Tibialis anterior Extensor digitorum longus Extensor digitorum brevis Extensor hallucis longus Peroneus tertius Peroneus longus Peroneus brevis Gastrocnemius Soleus Plantaris Tibialis posterior Flexor digitorum longus Flexor hallucis longus Flexor accessorius (quadratus plantae) Abductor digiti minimi Flexor digiti minimi Lumbricales Interossei Adductor hallucis Abductor hallucis Flexor digitorum brevis Flexor hallucis brevis	Posterior thigh and leg Whole foot except instep and medial malleolus	Medial hamstrings (L5–S1) Lateral hamstrings (S1–S2) Achilles (S1–S2) Tibialis posterior (L4–L5)
Superior gluteal nerve	Gluteus medius Gluteus minimus Tensor fasciae latae	None	None
Femoral nerve (L2 through L4)	Iliacus Psoas Sartorius Pectineus Quadriceps	Medial side of thigh and leg	Patellar (L3–L4)
Obturator nerve (L2 through L4)	Adductor brevis Adductor magnus Adductor longus Obturator externus Gracilis	Middle thigh on anterior aspect	None

Caudal Glide (Long Leg Traction). The examiner places both hands around the patient's leg, slightly above the ankle. The examiner then leans back, applying a long-axis extension (traction) to the entire lower limb. Part of the movement occurs in the knee. If one suspects some pathology in the knee or the knee is stiff, both hands should be placed around the thigh just proximal to the knee, and traction force should again be applied (see Figure 11-67, *A*). The first method enables the examiner to apply a greater force. During the movement, any telescoping or excessive movement occurring in the hip should be noted, since it may indicate an unstable joint.

Compression. The examiner places the patient's knee in the resting position and then applies a compressive force to the hip through the longitudinal axis of the femur by pushing through the femoral condyles (see Figure 11-67, *B*).

Lateral Distraction. The examiner applies a lateral distraction force to the hip by placing a wide strap around the leg as high up in the groin as possible. The strap is then wrapped around the examiner's

L2
L3
L4

Psoas major

Iliacus

Femoral nerve

Sartorius

Pectineus

Medial cutaneous nerve of the thigh

Vastus lateralis

Rectus femoris

Saphenous nerve

Vastus intermedius

Vastus medialis

Anterior femoral cutaneous nerve

Saphenous nerve

Anterior view

Figure 11-65
Femoral nerve.

the femoral neck against the acetabular rim and pinches the adductor longus, pectineus, iliopsoas, sartorius, and/or tensor fascia lata. Therefore, it should be performed with care.[27–29]

Palpation

During palpation of the hip and associated muscles, the examiner should note any tenderness, temperature, muscle spasm, or other signs and symptoms that may indicate the source of pathology. Intraarticular pain in the hip is rarely palpable.[108]

Anterior Aspect

The following structures should be palpated anteriorly, as shown in Figure 11-68.

Iliac Crest, Greater Trochanter, and Anterior Superior Iliac Spine. The iliac crests are easily palpated and should be level. The crest should be palpated for any tenderness because several muscles insert into this structure. In athletes, a condition called a **"hip pointer"** may be located on the iliac crest. This occurs from a strain or contusion of the muscles that insert into the crest. The iliac tubercle is felt during palpation along the lateral aspect of the crest. The examiner then moves anteriorly to the ASIS. The greater trochanter, located approximately 10 cm (4 inches) distal to the iliac tubercle of the iliac crest, is palpated next. If the examiner's thumbs are placed over each ASIS, the fingers will naturally lie along the lateral aspect of each thigh and the greater trochanter can be felt with the fingers on each side. If the trochanteric bursa is swollen, it may also be palpated over the greater trochanter.

Inguinal Ligament, Femoral Triangle, Hip Joint, and Symphysis Pubis. The examiner's fingers are placed on the ASIS. Palpation gently continues along the inguinal ligament to the pelvic tubercles (symphysis pubis), with the examiner noting any signs of pathology. The psoas bursa, if swollen, is usually palpable under the inguinal ligament at its midpoint. Moving distal to the inguinal ligament, the examiner palpates the femoral triangle, the boundaries of which are the inguinal ligament superiorly, the sartorius muscle laterally, and the adductor longus muscle medially (Figure 11-69). Within the femoral triangle, the examiner may palpate swollen lymph glands (Figure 11-70) and the femoral artery. The femoral nerve lies lateral to the artery and the femoral vein lies medial to it, but neither of these structures is easily palpated. At this stage, the examiner may decide to palpate for an inguinal hernia in the male. The head of the femur is then palpated. Although the hip joint is deep and not easily palpable, the surrounding structures may show signs of pathology. The head of the femur is 1 to

buttocks. The examiner leans back, using the buttocks to apply the distraction force to the hip. The proximal hand is used to palpate the hip or greater trochanter movement, while the distal hand prevents abduction of the leg, and, hence, torque to the hip (see Figure 11-67, C).

Quadrant (Scouring) Test.[63] The examiner flexes and adducts the patient's hip so that the hip faces the patient's opposite shoulder and resistance to the movement is felt. As slight resistance is maintained, the patient's hip is taken into abduction while maintaining flexion in an arc of movement. As the movement is performed, the examiner should look for any irregularity in the movement (e.g., "bumps"), pain, or patient apprehension, which may give an indication of where the pathology is occurring in the hip (see Figure 11-67, D).[63] This motion also causes **impingement** of

Text continued on page 709

Figure 11-66

Obturator nerve. **A,** Anatomy of the obturator nerve. **B,** Cutaneous sensory distribution of the anterior branch of the obturator nerve.

Figure 11-67

Joint play movements of the hip. **A,** Long leg traction (applied above the knee). **B,** Compression.

Continued

Figure 11-67 cont'd
C, Lateral distraction. **D,** Quadrant test.

Iliac tubercle

Greater trochanter

Head of femur

Lesser trochanter

Iliac crest

Anterior superior
Iliac spine

Acetabulum

Symphysis pubis

Ischial tuberosity

Figure 11-68
Landmarks of the hip (anterior view).

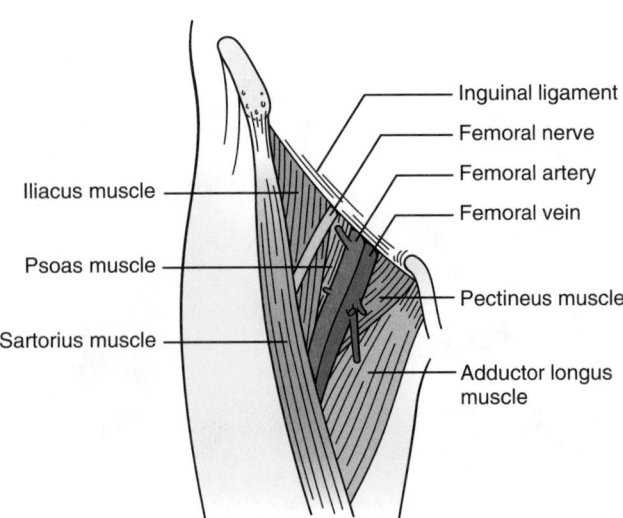

Iliacus muscle

Psoas muscle

Sartorius muscle

Inguinal ligament

Femoral nerve

Femoral artery

Femoral vein

Pectineus muscle

Adductor longus
muscle

Figure 11-69
Femoral triangle containing the femoral artery, vein, and nerve. Note the inguinal ligament above, iliacus and psoas laterally, and adductors medially. The sartorius attaches to the anterosuperior spine, whereas the adductor muscles attach along the pubic ramus. (Modified from Anson BJ: *Atlas of human anatomy*, p. 583, Philadelphia, 1963, W.B. Saunders.)

Figure 11-70
Lymph glands in the groin area.

2 cm (0.4–0.8 inch) below the middle third of the inguinal ligament and is found on a horizontal line running halfway between the pubic tubercle and the greater trochanter.

The examiner concludes the anterior palpation by palpating the hip flexor, adductor, and abductor muscles for signs of pathology.

Posterior Aspect

The patient is then asked to lie in the prone position so that the following structures can be palpated posteriorly.

Iliac Crest, Posterior Superior Iliac Spine, Ischial Tuberosity, and Greater Trochanter. The examiner begins posterior palpation by following the iliac crests, which are easily palpable, posteriorly to the PSIS. On most patients, each PSIS is evident by the presence of overlying skin dimples. As the examiner moves caudally, the ischial tuberosities, which are approximately at the level of the gluteal folds, may be felt. If the ischial bursa is swollen, it is sometimes palpable over the ischial tuberosities. The tuberosities should also be palpated for possible tenderness of the hamstring muscle insertions. Laterally, the posterior aspect of the greater trochanter is felt. If the distance between the ischial tuberosity and greater trochanter is divided in half, the fingers will lie over the sciatic nerve as it enters the lower limb. Normally, the nerve is not palpable. The examiner then palpates upward from the midpoint to determine whether there is any tenderness of the hip lateral rotators, especially the piriformis muscle. In addition, the gluteal

and hamstring muscle bellies should be palpated for signs of pathology.

Sacroiliac, Lumbosacral, and Sacrococcygeal Joints. If the examiner suspects pathology in these joints, they should be palpated. Detailed descriptions of their palpation are given in Chapters 9 and 10.

Diagnostic Imaging

Plain Film Radiography

Normally, the standard views of the hip include anteroposterior views and axial or frog-leg views.

Anteroposterior View. The examiner should compare the two hips, noting the following features:

1. Neck-shaft angle, femoral head uncovering and head-tear drop distance (Figure 11-71). Abnormal head-neck, offset (i.e., flattening of superior femoral head) is called a **pistol grip deformity**.
2. Joint spaces and pelvic lines and other landmarks (Figures 11-72 and 11-73).
3. Presence of any bone disease (i.e., Legg-Calvé-Perthes disease, bony cysts, or tumors; Figure 11-74).
4. Neck-shaft angle.[109] The examiner should note whether the angle is normal or whether the patient exhibits a coxa vara or coxa valga (Figures 11-75 and 11-76).

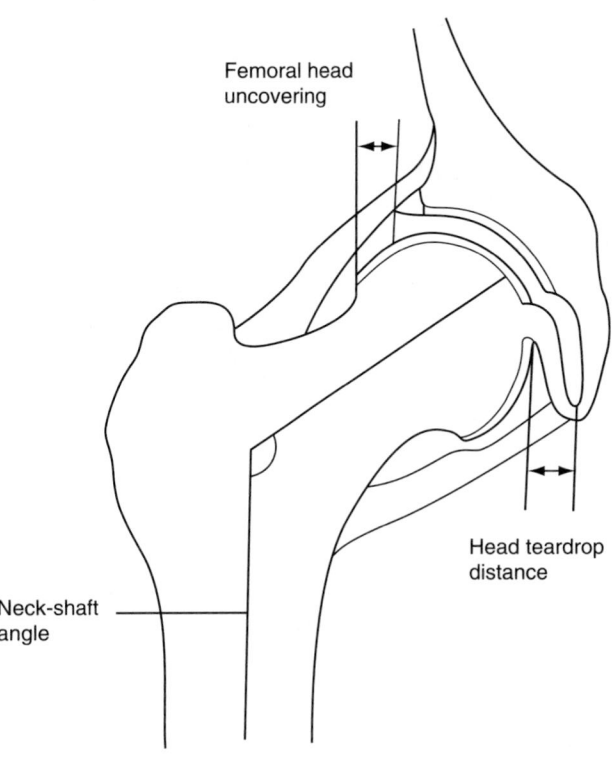

Figure 11-71
Three radiologic measurements of the hip. (From Richardson JK, Iglarsh ZA: *Clinical orthopedic physical therapy*, p. 358, Philadelphia, 1994, W.B. Saunders.)

Figure 11-72 ▰
Pelvic lines. The iliopubic *(ip)* and ilioischial
(ii) lines help in assessing the anterior and
posterior columns. The acetabular dome *(D)*
and anterior *(a)* and posterior *(p)* lips *(rims)*
of the acetabulum are seen. The teardrop
figure *(arrows)* is a composite shadow made up
laterally of the anterior aspect of the acetabular
fossa and medially of the quadrilateral surface
of the ilium. The more posterior aspect of
the quadrilateral surface (represented by the
ilioischial line) is superimposed on the teardrop
in this nonrotated view. (From Weissman
BNW, Sledge CB: *Orthopedic radiology,* p. 343,
Philadelphia, 1986, W.B. Saunders.)

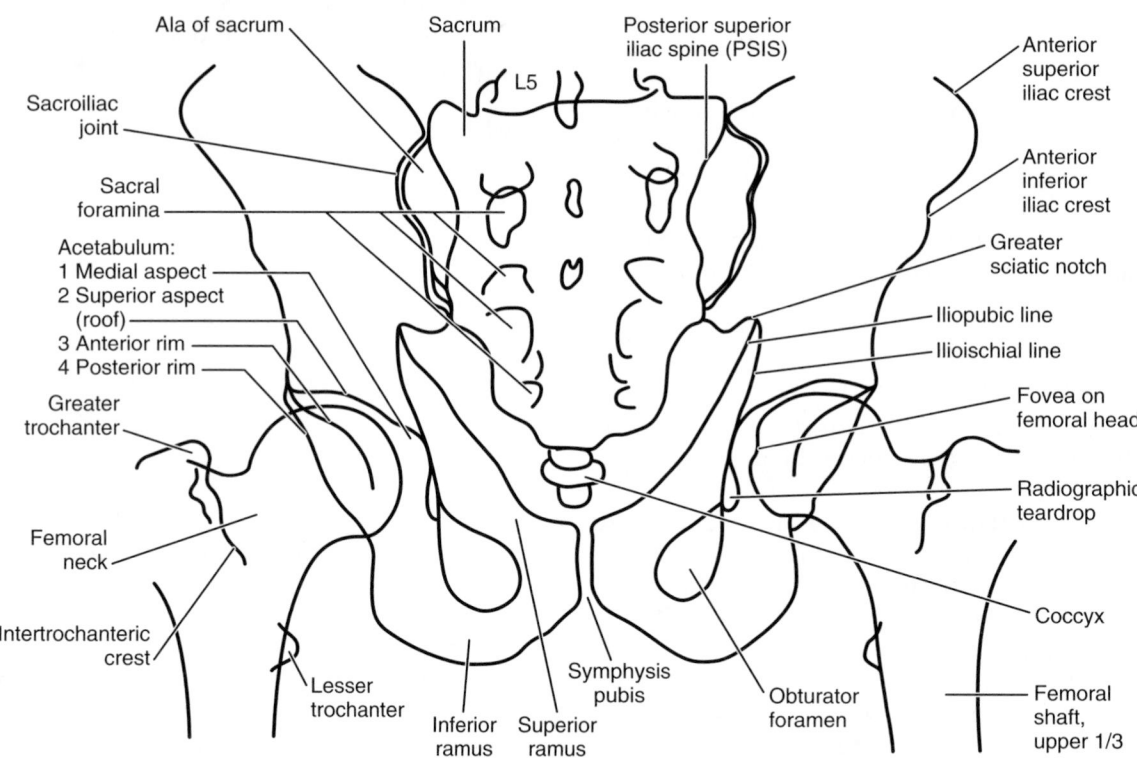

Figure 11-73 ▰
Tracing of anteroposterior radiograph of the pelvis. (Redrawn from McKinnis LN: *Fundamentals of
musculoskeletal imaging,* p. 297, Philadelphia, 2005, F.A. Davis.)

5. Shape of the femoral head.[110]
6. Presence of osteophytes or arthritis (Figure 11-77).
7. Whether **Shenton's line** is normal. Normally,
Shenton's line is curved, drawn along the medial
curved edge of the femur and continuing upward

in a smooth arc along the inferior edge of the pubis
(Figure 11-78). If the head of the femur is dislocated or fractured, two lines form two separate arcs,
indicating a broken line. A broken Shenton's line is
diagnostic of pathology.

Figure 11-74
Legg-Calvé-Perthes disease of the left hip.

Figure 11-75
AP view of the pelvis in an adult patient with coxa vara of the hip joint shows a neck-shaft angle of less than 125° and a decreased trochanteric acetabular distance *(white arrows)*. This configuration contributes to the potential for abnormal joint reaction forces, with an increased risk of a medial osteoarthritis developing at the hip joint. In this patient, the loss of the medial joint space and/or early arthrokatadysis or medial migration of the femoral heads can be seen, as can early development of osteophytes at the acetabulum and femoral head. (From Johnson TR, Steinbach LS: *Essentials of musculoskeletal imaging*, p. 458, Rosemont, Illinois, 2004, American Academy of Orthopedic Surgeons.)

Figure 11-76
AP view of an adult patient with a valgus alignment at the hip joint shows a neck-shaft angle that exceeds 140° *(white dotted arrow)*. Note also the increased portion of the articular aspect of the femoral head that is uncovered *(white arrow)*. This attribute becomes even more important if the superior aspect of the weight-bearing surface of the acetabulum is smaller than normal. In this patient, the trochanteric acetabular distance (the distance from a line drawn parallel to the superior aspect of the weight-bearing surface of the dome to a line parallel to the superior aspect of the tip of the greater trochanter) exceeds 2.5 cm *(arrowheads)*. Normally, the trochanteric acetabular distance in adults averages about 2.2 cm. (From Johnson TR, Steinbach LS: *Essentials of musculoskeletal imaging*, p. 457, Rosemont, Illinois, 2004, American Academy of Orthopedic Surgeons.)

8. Any evidence of fracture or dislocation (Figures 11-79 and 11-80). Is the pelvic ring intact, or has it been disrupted? Disruption of the pelvic ring indicates severe injury.

9. Evidence of pelvic distortion.

10. Whether Hilgenreiner's and Perkins' lines are within normal limits.[111] **Hilgenreiner's line** is horizontal, drawn between the inferior parts of the ilium. **Perkins' line** is vertical, drawn through the upper outer point of the acetabulum (Figure 11-81). Normally, the developing femoral head or ossification center of the femoral head lies in the inner distal quadrant formed by the two lines. If the ossification center lies in the upper outer quadrant, the finding is indicative of a dislocation or DDH.[80] In the newborn, the ossification center is not visible (Figure 11-82).

11. Whether the femoral head and acetabulum are normal on both sides. In development dysplasia of the hip, both structures may show dysplasia, and the **acetabular index** on the affected side may be more than the normal 30°. The acetabular index is determined by first drawing Hilgenreiner's line. An intersecting line is drawn from the lateral to the medial edge of the acetabulum, and the angle formed by the two lines is called the acetabular index, or **Hilgenreiner's angle** (Table 11-13). The greater the slope angle, the less sta-

Figure 11-77
Arthritis of the left hip. **A,** Before surgery. Note decreased joint space and unevenness of femoral head. **B,** After total hip surgery.

Figure 11-79
Trauma to the hip. **A,** Fractured right acetabulum. **B,** Dislocated left femur.

ABNORMAL   NORMAL

Figure 11-78
Shenton's line.

ble the femoral head in the acetabulum. Figure 11-83 shows measurements that may be taken with DDH.

12. **"Sagging rope" sign.** With Legg-Calvé-Perthes disease, only the head of the femur is affected. If avascular necrosis of a developing femoral head occurs, the sagging rope sign may be seen (Figure 11-84). The sign indicates damage to the growth plate with marked metaphyseal reaction. Its presence indicates a severe disease process.

13. **"Teardrop" sign.** Migration of the femoral head upward in relation to the pelvis, caused by degeneration as seen in osteoarthritis, may be detected by the teardrop sign (Figure 11-85). The teardrop is visible at the base of the pubic bone, extending vertically downward to terminate in a round teardrop, or head. The x-ray beam must be centered relative to the pelvis. A line is drawn between the two teardrops and extended to the femoral heads on both sides. The examiner can then measure from the

Figure 11-80
Stress fracture of the femoral neck.

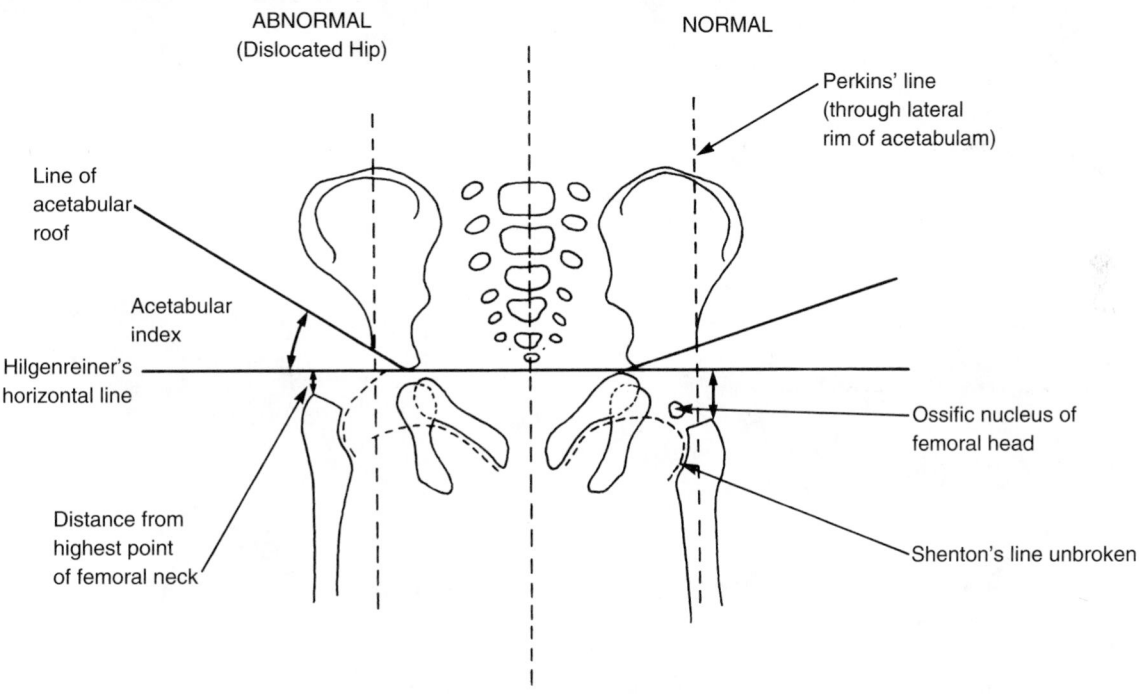

Figure 11-81
Radiological findings in congenital dislocation of the hip compared with normal findings in a 12- to 15-month-old child. Acetabular index: normal = 30°, in newborn = 27.5°. If the ossific nucleus of the femoral head is present, it should sit in the inner lower quadrant.

Figure 11-82
Radiograph of the hip in the newborn. Ossification of the femoral head has not yet developed.

Table 11-13

Average Values of Hilgenreiner's Angle (Acetabular Index)

	Newborn	6 Months Old	1 Year Old
Male	26°	20°	20°
Female	28°	22°	20°

teardrop to the femoral head. A difference of more than 10 mm between the two sides indicates significant migration of the head of the femur. Serial films or films taken over time often show a progression of the migration.

14. **"Head-at-risk" signs.** With Legg-Calvé-Perthes disease, the examiner should note the following radiologic head-at-risk signs on an anteroposterior film:

Figure 11-83

Additional measurements performed on conventional radiographs in patients with developmental dysplasia of the hip. **A,** *1:* Slope of the lateral edge of the acetabulum. The angle formed between a line that is parallel to Hilgenreiner's line and tangent to the roof of the acetabulum and a line that is parallel to the lateral edge of the acetabulum is termed the slope. The normal acetabulum has a slope of the lateral edge that is defined as positive. *2:* Center-edge *(CE)* angle. This angle lies between a line drawn from the center of the femoral head, perpendicular to the line connecting the centers of each femoral head, and a line drawn from the center of the head to the superolateral ossified edge of the acetabulum. The CE angle has a negative value. **B,** *Right hip:* the pelvic midline is drawn vertically through the centers of the sacrum and the symphysis pubis. The lateral displacement of each femoral head is indicated by the length of a line *(A)* drawn horizontally from the pelvic midline to the center of the femoral head. *Left hip:* The *C/B* ratio compared *C,* the distance from the pelvic midline to the medial beak of the femoral metaphysis, and *B,* the distance from the pelvic midline to the lateral acetabular edge. **C,** *1:* The angle that lies between a line connecting the teardrops on the inferior margin of the acetabula and a line drawn from the most superolateral ossified edge of the acetabulum to the teardrop constitutes the adult acetabular index or angle. *2:* The greatest perpendicular distance between the medial articular surface of the acetabulum and a line drawn from the teardrop to the superolateral ossified edge of the acetabulum is the acetabular depth. **D,** Vertical center-edge angle, drawn on a false profile view. It is defined as the angle subtended by a line *(V-C)* drawn from the center of the femoral head extending vertically upward and a line *(C-A)* drawn from the center of the femoral head obliquely to the anterior edge of the acetabulum. The angle lies between the two lines.

Continued

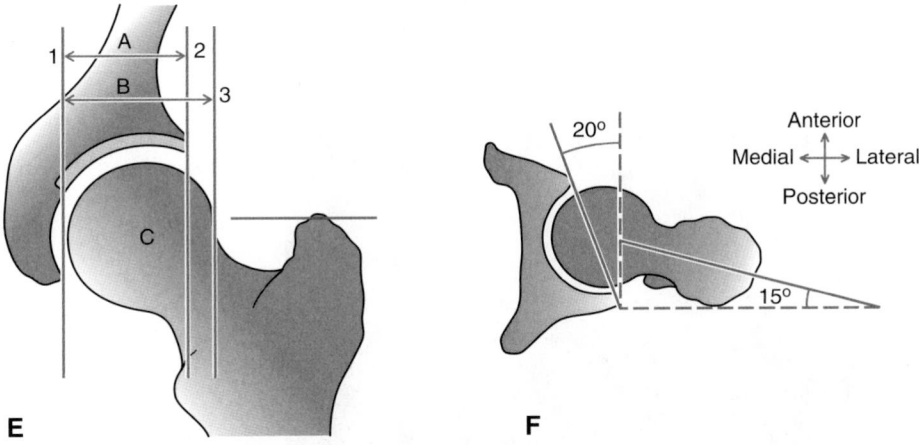

E

F

Figure 11-83 cont'd

E, Percentage of the femoral head covered by the acetabulum. This represents the relative width of the weight-bearing surface of the acetabulum *(A),* represented by line *1-2,* and that of the femoral head, represented by line *1-3.* Normal acetabular coverage is 75% or above when the ratio of *1-2:1-3* is determined. **F,** The acetabular anteversion angle describes the extent to which the acetabulum surrounds the femoral head within the horizontal plane. Measured from above, this angle is normally about 20°. As shown, the angle is formed by the intersection of an anterior-posterior reference line *(stippled)* and a line across the rim of the acetabulum. The 15° of normal anteversion of the proximal femur is also indicated. (**A-D,** Redrawn from Restrick D, Kransdorf MJ: *Bone and joint imaging,* p. 1268. Philadelphia, 2005, Elsevier, Courtesy of N. Lektakul, MD, Bangkok, Thailand. F, Redrawn from Neumann, DA: *Kinesiology of the musculoskeletal System—foundations for physical rehabilitation,* p. 398, St Louis, 2002, C.V. Mosby.)

"SAGGING ROPE"

Figure 11-84

Sagging rope sign.

a. Cage's sign, a small osteoporotic segment on the lateral side of the epiphysis that appears to be translucent (Figure 11-86)

b. Calcification lateral to the epiphysis (if collapse is occurring)

c. Lateral subluxation of the head (an increase in the inferomedial joint space)

d. Angle of the epiphyseal line (horizontal, in this case)

e. Metaphyseal reaction

Patients who exhibit three or more head-at-risk signs have a poor prognosis, and surgery is usually performed.

15. Signs of a **slipped capital femoral epiphysis.**[112] With a slipped capital femoral epiphysis (Figure 11-87), the following x-ray signs may be noted:

a. The epiphyseal line may widen.

b. Lipping or stepping may be seen, as occurs on lateral films.

c. The superior femoral neck line does not transect the overhanging ossified epiphysis as it does in the normal hip.

d. Shenton's line does not describe a continuous arc. (The line is also broken if the hip is dislocated or subluxed.)

In addition to a slipped capital femoral epiphysis causing a coxa vara, fractures or congenital malformations can lead to the same deformity (Figures 11-88 and 11-89).

Lateral (Axial "Frog-Leg") View. For this view, the patient is supine with the hips in flexion, abduction, and lateral rotation. This view provides a true lateral view of the femoral head and neck.[113] The examiner looks for any pelvic distortion or any slipping of the femoral head, as may be seen in slipped capital femoral epiphysis. The lateral view is the first in which slipping may be seen.

Arthrography

Although arthrograms are not routinely done on the hip, they may be done if the hip cannot be reduced following a dislocation (Figure 11-90). The arthrogram may indicate

Text continued on page 719

Figure 11-85

Teardrop sign. **A,** A line has been drawn between the tips of the two "teardrops" and extended into the femoral neck. Osteoarthritis of both hip joints appears to be equal, with equivalent narrowing of the joint space, but the left hip is already at a slightly higher level than the right in relation to the line. **B,** Later, both hips have gradually moved upward as a result of loss of the bone at the apex of each femoral head. The left hip is now at a higher level than the right, confirming the original observation that the process of destruction in the left hip was more advanced. (From Greubel-Lee DM: *Disorders of the hip*, pp. 61, 146, Philadelphia, 1983, J.B. Lippincott.)

Figure 11-86

All of the signs of the "head-at-risk" are present: lateral subluxation, abnormal direction of the growth plates, Cage's sign, lateral calcification, and irregularity of the epiphysis. (From Greubel-Lee DM: *Disorders of the hip*, p. 146, Philadelphia, 1983, J.B. Lippincott.)

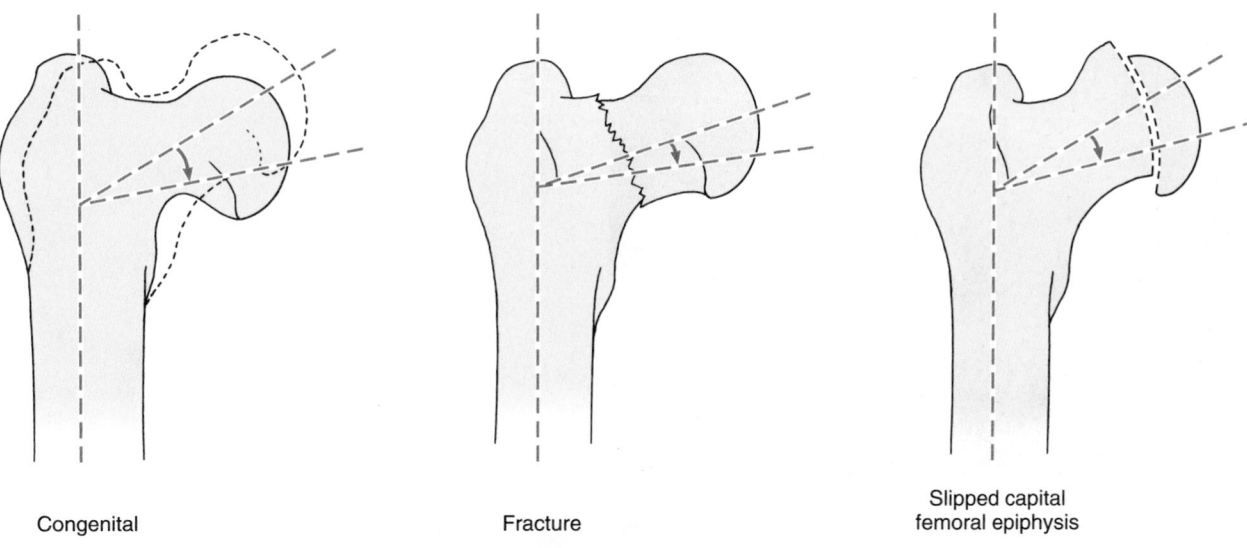

Congenital   Fracture   Slipped capital
                                                          femoral epiphysis

Figure 11-87

Some causes of coxa vara.

Figure 11-88

Acute slipped femoral epiphysis in a 14-year-old boy. After a fall, the patient complained of severe pain in the left groin and anterior thigh and was unable to bear weight on the left lower limb. **A** and **B,** Preoperative radiographs show the severe slip on the left. The patient was placed in bilateral split Russell traction with medial rotation straps on the left thigh and leg. Gradually, within a period of 3 to 4 days, the slip was reduced. **C** and **D,** Postoperative radiographs approximately 6 months later show closure of epiphyseal plate and normal position of femoral head. The hip had full range of motion. (From Tachdjian MO: *Pediatric orthopedics,* p. 470, Philadelphia, 1972, W.B. Saunders.)

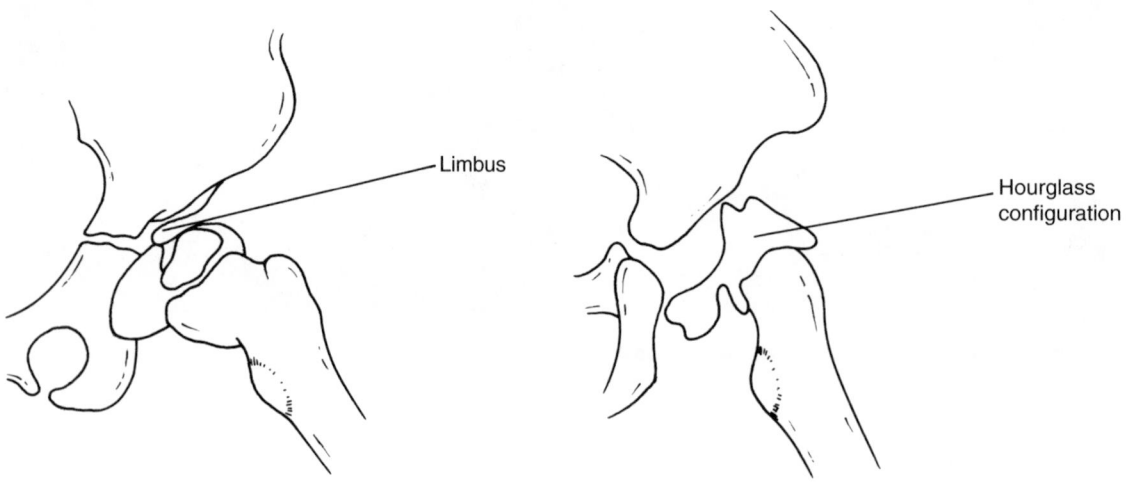

Figure 11-89

Congenital coxa vara of the left hip in an infant. **A,** Anteroposterior radiographs of both hips at 3 months of age, taken because of limited abduction of left hip and suspicion of congenital hip dislocation. It was interpreted to be normal. **B** and **C,** Radiographs of the hips of same patient at 1 year of age when he started walking with a painless gluteus medius lurch on the left. Varus deformity of the left hip is evident. (From Tachdjian MO: *Pediatric orthopedics*, p. 587, Philadelphia, 1972, W.B. Saunders.)

Limbus

Hourglass configuration

Figure 11-90

Drawings of arthrograms in congenital dislocation of the hip.

Figure 11-91

Normal hip arthrogram. Normal examination after intra-articular injection of approximately 6 mL of contrast medium. **A,** Anteroposterior and, **B,** frog lateral views. *c,* Contrast agent outlining articular cartilage (recess capitis); *i,* inferior articular recess; *ir,* recess colli inferior; *l,* acetabular labrum; *lt,* defect on contrast from transverse ligament; *s,* superior articular recess; *sr,* recess colli superior; *z,* zona orbicularis (impression on the intra-articular contrast by the iliofemoral ischiofemoral ligaments of the hip joint capsule). (From Weissman BNW, Sledge CB: *Orthopedic radiology,* p. 396, Philadelphia, 1986, W.B. Saunders.)

a possible inverted limbus (infolding of a meniscus-like structure) or an hourglass configuration from a contracted capsule. It is also useful in CDH to show where the unossified femoral head lies relative to the labrum. A normal hip arthrogram is shown in Figure 11-91.

Computed Tomography

Computed tomography scanning is useful in assessing abnormalities of the hip, especially bony ones.[108] For example, it can be used to measure anteversion and retroversion, and it can show the size and shape of the acetabulum and femoral head as well as the congruity and position of the femoral head relative to the acetabulum (Figures 11-92 and 11-93). In newborns, the lack of ossification limits its use.

Magnetic Resonance Imaging[114]

Magnetic resonance imaging (Figures 11-94 and 11-95) is a useful technique to study the hip because it is able to show soft tissue (e.g., bursitis, tendon lesions) as well as osseous tissue (e.g., osteonecrosis, femoral neck stress fractures, labral tears) (Figure 11-96).[4] This ability makes it an excellent technique to use for congenital abnormalities. It is also the examination of choice for the evaluation of unexplained hip pain.[108] When combined with arthrography (magnetic resonance arthrograph), it is often more sensitive to hip lesions but also produces more false positives.[115]

Scintigraphy (Bone Scan)

Bone scans may be used in the hip to help diagnose stress fractures (especially of femoral neck), necrosis, and tumors (Figures 11-97 and 11-98).

Ultrasonography

Ultrasonography is a nonirradiation technique that may be used to detect hip abnormalities and soft-tissue problems such as swelling.[108,116-118]

Text continued on page 724

Figure 11-92

A, Normal computed tomography (CT) image at the level of the midacetabulum obtained with soft-tissue window settings, showing the homogenous, intermediate signal of musculature. A, Common femoral artery; *gd,* gluteus medius; *gn,* gluteus minimus; *gx,* gluteus maximus; *ip,* iliopsoas; *oi,* obturator internus; *ra,* rectus abdominis; *rf,* rectus femoris; *s,* sartorius; *t,* tensor fasciae latae; *v,* common femoral vein. **B,** Axial CT at bone window settings reveals improved delineation of cortical and medullary osseous details. Note anterior and posterior semilunar acetabular articular surfaces and the central nonarticular acetabular fossa. **C,** Normal midacetabular T1-weighted axial 0.4-T magnetic resonance image (TR, 600 msec; TE, 20 msec) of a different patient shows a normal, high-signal-intensity image of muscle and absence of signal in the cortical bone. The thin articular hyaline cartilage is of intermediate signal intensity *(arrow).* **D,** T2-weighted magnetic resonance image (TR, 2000 msec; TE, 80 msec) shows decreasing high-signal intensity in fatty marrow and subcutaneous tissue with increased signal intensity in the fluid-filled urinary bladder. (From Pitt MJ et al: Imaging of the pelvis and hip, *Orthop Clin North Am* 21:553, 1990.)

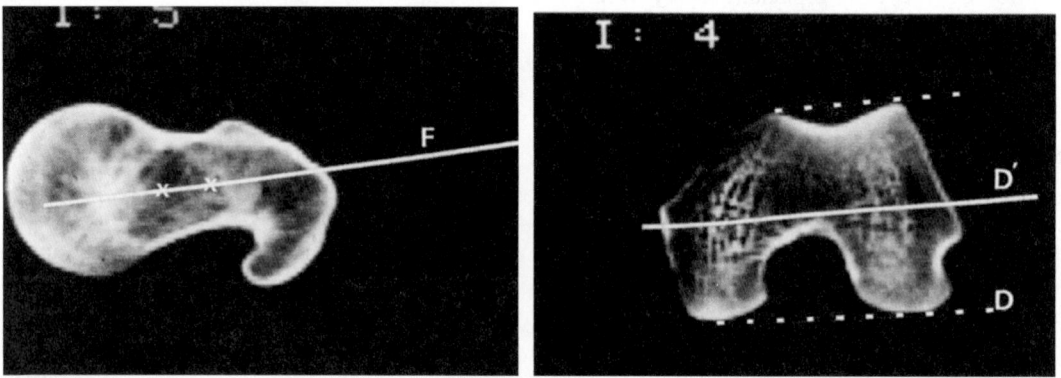

Figure 11-93

Computed tomography for determining femoral anteversion (using a femoral specimen). The diacondylar line *(D)* is drawn along the condyles, although Hernandez and co-workers construct it *(D')* midway between the anterior and posterior femoral surfaces *(dashed lines).* The axis of the femoral neck *(F)* is shown. The angle between the femoral neck axis *(F)* and the diacondylar line is the angle of anteversion. In this case, there is 2° of retroversion. (From Weissman BNW, Sledge CB: *Orthopedic radiology,* p. 399, Philadelphia, 1986, W.B. Saunders.)

Figure 11-94

A, Normal magnetic resonance imaging scan of a young adult. Spin-echo T1-weighted image (600/25). Note the bright signal of fat in the region of the femoral epiphysis and the greater trochanter. The intermediate signal intensity in the femoral neck represents hemopoietic marrow. **B,** Normal elderly woman with same imaging sequence shows replacement of hemopoietic marrow in the femoral neck by fatty marrow. (From Dalinka MK, Neustadter LM: Radiology of the hip. *In* Steinberg ME, editor: *The hip and its disorders*, p. 68, Philadelphia, 1991, W.B. Saunders.)

Figure 11-95

Normal adult bone marrow. **A,** Transaxial T1-weighted (TR/TE, 600/8) spin echo MR image of the pelvis. Yellow marrow within the femoral heads *(F)* is isointense to subcutaneous fat. Red marrow within the acetabula *(A)* has signal intensity between that of muscle and fat. **B,** Transaxial fat-suppressed T2-weighted (TR/TEeff, 4000/60) fast spin echo MR image. The signal intensity of both yellow and red marrow decreases. A small effusion is seen in the left hip *(arrow)*. (From Resnick D, Kransdorf MJ: *Bone and joint imaging*, p. 119, Philadelphia, 2005, Elsevier.)

Figure 11-96

Acetabular labrum: tear and cystic degeneration. **A** and **B,** Partial detachment of the anterosuperior portion of the labrum *(arrows)* is seen on fat-suppressed sagittal **(A)** and coronal **(B)** T1-weighted (TR/TE, 600/16) spin echo MR arthrographic images. **C,** In a different patient, a fat-suppressed coronal T1-weighted (TR/TE, 700/12) spin echo MR arthrographic image demonstrates a massive superior labral tear with a perilabral ganglion cyst. (From Resnick D, Kransdorf MJ: *Bone and joint imaging,* Philadelphia, 2005, Elsevier. **A** and **B,** Courtesy J. Tomanek, MD, Johnson City, Tenn.)

Figure 11-97

Stress fracture. This athletic young woman complained of a persistent hip pain aggravated by activity.
A, Radionuclide examination reveals a focal, sharply marginated area of increased activity in the femoral neck *(arrow)*. **B,** Radiograph of the hip delineates a minimal amount of indistinct new bone formation along the medial aspect of the femoral neck *(arrow)*. (From Resnick D, Kransdorf MJ: *Bone and joint imaging*, p. 797, Philadelphia, 2005, Elsevier.)

Figure 11-98

Femoral neck stress fracture. **A,** In the medial portion of the femoral neck, observe the presence of buttressing and sclerosis *(arrows)*.
B, Coronal intermediate-weighted (TR/TE, 2000/20) spin echo MR image reveals bilateral fatigue fractures *(arrows)* in the medial portion of the femoral neck. The fracture itself and the surrounding marrow edema are of low signal intensity. (From Resnick D, Kransdorf MJ: *Bone and joint imaging*, p. 800, Philadelphia, 2005, Elsevier.)

Précis of the Hip Assessment*

History
Observation
Examination
   Active movements (supine)
      Hip flexion
      Hip abduction
      Hip adduction
      Hip lateral rotation
      Hip medial rotation
   Passive movements (supine) as in active movements (if
     necessary)
   Resisted isometric movements (supine)
      Hip flexion
      Hip extension
      Hip adduction
      Hip abduction
      Hip medial rotation
      Hip lateral rotation
      Knee flexion
      Knee extension
   Special tests (supine)
      Patrick test
      Thomas test
      Leg length tests
      Rectus femoris test
      90-90 straight leg raise test
      Sign of the buttock
      Abduction/Adduction Tests
   Reflexes and cutaneous distribution (supine)
      Reflexes
      Sensory scan
      Peripheral nerves

   Joint play movements (supine)
      Caudal glide
      Compression
      Lateral distraction
      Quadrant test
   Palpation (supine)
   Active movement (prone)
      Hip extension
   Passive movement (prone)
      Hip extension
   Resisted isometric movements (prone)
      Hip medial rotation (if not previously done)
      Hip lateral rotation (if not previously done)
      Knee flexion (if not previously done)
      Knee extension (if not previously done)
      Special tests (prone and side lying)
      Ober's test
   Reflexes and cutaneous distribution (prone)
   Palpation (prone)
   Diagnostic imaging
    After the rest of the examination is completed, the examiner can ask the patient to perform the appropriate functional test.
    After any examination, the patient should be warned of the possibility of exacerbation of symptoms as a result of the assessment.

---

*The précis is shown in an order that limits the amount of moving the patient must do but ensures that all necessary structures are tested.

Case Studies

When doing these case studies, the examiner should list the appropriate questions to be asked and why they are being asked, what to look for and why, and what things should be tested and why. Depending on the answers of the patient (and the examiner should consider different responses), several possible causes of the patient's problem may become evident (examples are given in parentheses). A differential diagnosis chart (Table 11-14) should be made up. The examiner can then decide how different diagnoses may affect the treatment plan.

1. A 14-year-old boy was well until he fell from a chair onto his buttocks. He did not appear hurt, but 1 week later his parents brought him in for assessment because of a limp and pain in his right thigh and knee. The teenager is a tall, thin boy who prefers to walk with the right foot laterally rotated. Design your assessment plan for this patient (slipped capital femoral epiphysis versus ischial bursitis).

2. A 71-year-old woman had an Austin Moore prosthesis inserted into the left hip 1 day ago. The prosthesis has relieved the pain she had in her hip. X-rays reveal that the prosthesis is solid. The surgeon has asked you to get the patient up and moving. Before doing this, however, you must do a bedside assessment. Outline how you would do the assessment.

3. A 7-year-old boy is brought by his parents for assessment. He walks with a limp and has done so during the past 5 weeks at irregular times, the limp becoming more pronounced when the boy becomes tired. The boy also complains of a painful left knee. Describe your assessment plan for this patient (Legg-Calvé-Perthes disease versus slipped capital femoral epiphysis).

Case Studies–cont'd

4. A 3-week-old girl is referred to you to be fitted with a Pavlik harness for CDH. Before you can fit the harness, you must do an assessment. Design your assessment plan for this patient.
5. A 55-year-old man complains of hip and back pain. There is some sciatica with pain into the groin. The pain is especially bad when he walks. He has a desk job but has been very active throughout his life. Describe your assessment plan for this patient (piriformis syndrome versus lumbar spondylosis).
6. A 35-year-old woman complains of lateral hip pain. She states that she was in a motor vehicle accident 2 weeks ago in which she was hit from the passenger side (she was driving) and her car was pushed against a telephone pole. She was wearing a seat belt. Describe your assessment plan for this patient (trochanteric bursitis versus muscle contusion).
7. An 18-year-old man was surfing when he was thrown by a wave and hurt his hip. The hip is medially rotated and shortened. He has some sciatic pain. Describe your assessment plan for this patient (posterior hip dislocation versus trochanteric fracture).
8. A 23-year-old female diver comes to you complaining of hip pain. She says it bothers her when she does any quick flexion of the hip. Describe your assessment plan for this patient (psoas bursitis versus psoas strain).

Table 11-14

Differential Diagnosis of Slipped Capital Femoral Epiphysis and Ischial Bursitis

	Slipped Capital Femoral Epiphysis	Ischial Bursitis
History	Trauma may or may not be a factor	Usually results from trauma (fall)
	Growth spurt may be involved	Usually acute but can become chronic
	More common on boys	Pain over ischial tuberosity and sometimes into hamstrings
	May be acute or chronic	
	Pain into hip, groin, thigh to knee	
Observation	Lurching gait	Gait generally normal although may be antalgic
Active movement	Abduction, medial rotation, and flexion limited	Flexion limited
Passive movement	Capsular pattern	Noncapsular pattern
Resisted isometric movement	Normal but stress may cause pain	Hamstrings contraction sometimes painful
Special tests	True leg length difference	Leg lengths equal
	Trendelenburg's test positive	Trendelenburg's test negative
Sensation	Normal	Normal
Reflexes	Normal	Normal
Joint play movements	May cause pain or relief	Normal
Diagnostic imaging	Diagnostic	Negative

References

To enhance this text and add value for the reader, all references have been incorporated into a CD-ROM that is provided with this text. The reader can view the reference source and access it online whenever possible. There are a total of 124 cited references and other general references for this chapter.

RELIABILITY, VALIDITY, SPECIFICITY, AND SENSITIVITY OF SPECIAL/DIAGNOSTIC TESTS USED IN THE HIP

CRAIG'S TEST

Reliability

- Intrarater ICC = 0.94, interrater ICC = 0.85[119]

DISABILITY RATING INDEX (DRI)

Reliability	**Validity**
• Test-retest r = 0.95, intrarater 0.98, interrater 0.99[120]	• Internal consistency, Cronbach's coefficient 0.84, construct validity correlation with Functional Status Questionnaire 0.46, Oswestry Low Back Pain Disability Questionnaire 0.38, patient score with assessors scores 0.48, perception of ability to perform task of subject and assessor 0.78, self reported and actual performance was 0.69[120]

FUNCTIONAL SQUAT

Reliability

- Intrarater ICC = 0.90 SEM = 0.48[121]

HIP FLEXION

Reliability

- Intrarater ICC = 0.87 SEM = 0.43[121]

HIP SCOUR

Reliability

- Intrarater ICC = 0.87 SEM = 0.57[121]

PATRICK'S TEST (FABER OR FIGURE-FOUR TEST)

Reliability

- Test-retest ICC = 0.93 SEM = 1.33[122]
- Intrarater ICC = 0.87 SEM = 0.58[121]

RADIOGRAPHIC DIAGNOSIS AND CLASSIFICATION OF TROCHLEA DYSPLASIA

Reliability

- Types of trochlea (interrater kappa = 0.17, intrarater kappa = 0.30), trochlear prominence (interrater ICC = 0.62), trochlear depth (interrater ICC = 0.62)[123]

SUPINE LEG LENGTH

Reliability

- Interrater ICC = 0.94, intrarater ICC = 0.7 (intrarater ICC range 0-1)[124]

CHAPTER 12

KNEE

The knee joint is particularly susceptible to traumatic injury because it is located at the ends of two long lever arms, the tibia and the femur. In addition, because the joint connects one long bone "sitting" on another long bone, it depends on the ligaments and muscles that surround it for its strength and stability, not on its bony configuration.[1]

Because the knee joint depends on its ligaments to such a great extent, it is imperative that the ligaments be tested during the examination of the knee. Therefore the ligamentous tests are not included under Special Tests but instead are listed in a separate section to ensure that they are always included in the examination of the knee.

Because of its anatomical arrangement, the knee is a complicated area to assess, and the examiner must take time to ensure that all relevant structures are tested. It must also be remembered that the lumbar spine, hip, and ankle may refer pain to the knee, and these joints must be assessed if it appears that joints other than the knee may be involved. For example, a slipped capital femoral epiphysis at the hip commonly refers pain to the knee, and this knee pain may predominate.

Applied Anatomy

The **tibiofemoral joint** is the largest joint in the body. It is a modified hinge joint having two degrees of freedom. The synovium around the joint is extensive; it communicates with many of the bursae and pouches around the knee joint. Although the synovial membrane "encapsulates" the entire knee joint, its distribution within the knee is such that the cruciate ligaments, which run from the middle of the tibial plateau to the intercondylar area of the femur, are extrasynovial. ("Cruciate" means that the ligaments cross each other.)

The articular surfaces of the tibia and femur are not congruent, which enables the two bones to move different amounts, guided by the muscles and ligaments. The two bones approach congruency in full extension, which is the close packed position. Kaltenborn[2] has stated that the close packed position includes full lateral rotation of the tibia. The lateral femoral condyle projects anteriorly more than the medial femoral condyle to help prevent lateral dislocation of the patella. In females, this enlargement is important because of the female's broader pelvis and increased inward angle of the femur, which allow the femoral condyles to be parallel with the ground (Figure 12-1). The resting position of the joint is approximately 25° of flexion, and the capsular pattern is flexion more limited than extension.

Tibiofemoral Joint	
Resting position:	25° flexion
Close packed position:	full extension, lateral rotation of tibia
Capsular pattern:	flexion, extension

The space between the tibia and femur is partially filled by two menisci that are attached to the tibia to add congruency. The **medial meniscus** is a small part of a large circle (i.e., **C** shaped) and is thicker posteriorly than anteriorly. The **lateral meniscus** is a large part of a small circle (i.e., **O** shaped) and is generally of equal thickness

727

Figure 12-1

Q-angle differences in males and females. Because of the broader pelvis in the female, it is necessary for the femur to come inward at an increased angle to make the distal end of the condyles parallel with the ground. The quadriceps, patella, and patellar tendon form an angle centered at the patella. As the quadriceps contracts, the angle tends to straighten, which forces the patella laterally. (Redrawn from O'Donoghue D.: *Treatment of injuries to athletes*, ed 4, p. 522, Philadelphia, 1984, WB Saunders.)

throughout. Both menisci are thicker along the periphery and thinner along the inner margin.

During the movement from extension to flexion, both menisci move posteriorly, the lateral meniscus being displaced more than the medial meniscus. The lateral meniscus has an excursion of 10 mm, and the medial meniscus has an excursion of 2 mm. The menisci are avascular in their cartilaginous inner two thirds and are partly vascular and fibrous in their outer one third.[3] They are held in place by the coronary ligaments attaching to the tibia.

The menisci serve several functions in the knee. They aid in lubrication and nutrition of the joint and act as shock absorbers (a meniscectomy can reduce shock absorption capacity at the knee by 20%),[4] spreading the stress over the articular cartilage and decreasing cartilage wear. They make the joint surfaces more congruent and improve weight distribution by increasing the area of contact between the condyles. The menisci reduce friction during movement and aid the ligaments and capsule in preventing hyperextension. The menisci prevent the joint capsule from entering the joint and participate in

the "locking" mechanism of the joint into close pack by directing the movement of the femoral articular condyles. Because more recent literature indicates that removal of the entire meniscus can lead to early degeneration of the joint,[5,6] most surgeons today remove only the torn portion of the meniscus, or, if the tear is in the outer one third where there is sufficient circulation to aid healing, the surgeon may attempt to surgically repair (suture) the meniscus.

It is generally believed that the meniscus possesses minimal innervation so there is minimal or no pain when it is damaged unless the coronary ligaments have been damaged as well. Gray[7] has reported, however, that the menisci possess innervation in their outer two thirds with the anterior and posterior horns being well innervated. Because the menisci are primarily avascular, especially in the inner two thirds, there is seldom bloody effusion in injury; however, there may be synovial effusion. Their poor blood supply, especially in the inner two thirds, gives the menisci a low regeneration potential.

The lateral meniscus is not as firmly attached to the tibia as the medial meniscus and therefore is less prone to injury. The coronary ligaments, also referred to as the meniscotibial ligaments, tend to be longer on the lateral aspect, and the horns of the lateral meniscus are closer together.

The **patellofemoral joint** is a modified plane joint, the lateral articular surface of the patella being wider. The patella contains the thickest layer of cartilage in the body and, in reality, is a sesamoid bone found within the patellar tendon. It has five facets, or ridges: superior, inferior, lateral, medial, and odd. It is the odd facet that is most frequently the first part of the patella to be affected in chondromalacia patellae (i.e., premature degeneration of the patellar cartilage) or patellofemoral syndrome.

During the movement from flexion to extension, different parts of the patella articulate with the femoral condyles (Figure 12-2).[8,9] The odd facet does not come into contact with the femoral condyles until at least 135° of flexion is reached. Incorrect alignment or malalignment of the patellar movement over the femoral condyles can lead to patellofemoral arthralgia. The capsule of this joint is continuous with the capsule of the tibiofemoral joint.

The **patella** improves the efficiency of extension during the last 30° of extension (i.e., 30° to 0° of extension, with the straight leg being 0°), because it holds the quadriceps tendon away from the axis of movement. The patella also functions as a guide for the quadriceps or patellar tendon, decreases friction of the quadriceps mechanism, controls capsular tension in the knee, acts as a bony shield for the cartilage of the femoral condyles, and improves the aesthetic appearance of the knee (Figure 12-3).

Figure 12-2

A, Area of contact of the patella during different degrees of flexion. **B,** Articulation between patella and femur. **C,** The circles depicted on the patella indicate the point of maximal contact between the patella and the femur. As the knee is extended, the contact point on the patella migrates from superior to inferior pole. Note the suprapatellar fat pad deep to the quadriceps. **D,** The path and contact areas of the patella on the intercondylar groove of the femur. The degree values 135, 90, 60, and 20 indicate flexed positions of the knee. (**C** and **D** Redrawn from Neumann DA: *Kinesiology of the musculoskeletal system—foundations for physical rehabilitation*, p. 448, St Louis, 2002, Mosby.)

Overall quadriceps force

LATERAL DIRECTED FORCES

Iliotibial band

"Bowstringing" force on the patella

Lateral patellar retinacular fibers

MEDIAL DIRECTED FORCES

Vastus medialis (oblique fibers)

Medial patellar (retinacular fibers)

Patellar ligament force

Figure 12-3

The major guiding forces acting on the patella are shown as it moves through the intercondylar groove of the femur. Each structure has a natural tendency to pull the patella laterally or medially. In most cases, the opposing forces counteract one another so that the patella moves optimally during flexion and extension. (Redrawn from Neumann DA: *Kinesiology of the musculoskeletal system— foundations for physical rehabilitation*, p. 463, St Louis, 2002, Mosby.)

Patellar Loading with Activity

Walking:	0.3 times the body weight
Climbing stairs:	2.5 times the body weight
Descending stairs:	3.5 times the body weight
Squatting:	7 times the body weight

The **superior tibiofibular joint** is a plane synovial joint between the tibia and the head of the fibula. It is supported by anterior and posterior ligaments of the same name. Movement occurs in this joint with any activity involving the ankle. Hypomobility at this joint can lead to pain in the knee area on activity, because the fibula can bear up to one sixth of the body weight. In approximately 10% of the population, the capsule of this joint is continuous with that of the tibiofemoral joint.

Patient History

In addition to the questions listed under Patient History in Chapter 1, the examiner should obtain the following information from the patient:

1. *How did the accident occur, or what was the mechanism of injury?*[10] The primary mechanisms of injury in the knee are a valgus force (with or without rotation), hyperextension, flexion with posterior translation, and a varus force.[11] The first often results in injury to the medial collateral ligament, frequently accompanied by

injury to the posteromedial capsule, medial meniscus, and anterior cruciate ("terrible triad"). The second leads to anterior cruciate injuries, often associated with meniscus tears. The third mechanism of injury often involves the posterior cruciate ligament, and the fourth mechanism involves the lateral collateral ligament, the posterolateral capsule, and the posterior cruciate ligament. Was the injury the result of trauma, such as a direct or an indirect blow? Was the patient bearing weight at the time of injury? From which direction did the injuring force come? For example, meniscal injuries, especially those on the medial side, occur as a result of a torsion injury that combines compression and rotation. Slowly developing forces tend to cause bony avulsions, whereas rapidly developing forces tend to tear ligaments. In young children, injuries to the growth plate or physis may occur instead of injury to the ligaments, especially during a rapid growth spurt when the physis is weaker than the ligaments. Injuries may occur to the distal femoral physis, the proximal tibial physis, and the tibial tubercle apophysis (traction epiphysis).[12,13] Injury to this last structure is called Osgood-Schlatter disease. Table 12-1 lists typical mechanisms of injury to the knee and the structures injured. The lower limb may be viewed as an open (foot off the ground) or a closed (foot on the ground) kinetic chain (Figure 12-4). There is less chance of injury when the lower limb is an open kinetic chain. As a closed kinetic chain, the lower limb is an encapsulated system in which all parts work in concert. Forces applied to one part of the chain must be absorbed by that part as well as by other parts of the closed chain. If the forces are too great, injury results.

Table 12-1

Mechanisms of Injury to the Knee and Structures Possibly Injured

Mechanism of Injury	Structures Possibly Injured
Varus or valgus contact without rotation	1. Collateral ligament 2. Epiphyseal fracture 3. Patellar dislocation or subluxation
Varus or valgus contact with rotation	1. Collateral and cruciate ligaments 2. Collateral ligaments and patellar dislocation or subluxation 3. Meniscus tear
Blow to patellofemoral joint, or fall on flexed knee, foot dorsiflexed	1. Patellar articular injury or osteochondral fracture
Blow to tibial tubercle, or fall on flexed knee, foot plantar flexed	1. Posterior cruciate ligament
Anterior blow to tibia, resulting in knee hyperextension (contact hypertension)	1. Anterior cruciate ligament 2. Anterior and posterior cruciate ligament
Noncontact hyperextension	1. Anterior cruciate ligament 2. Posterior capsule
Noncontact deceleration	1. Anterior cruciate ligament
Noncontact deceleration, with tibial medial rotation or femoral lateral rotation on fixed tibia	1. Anterior cruciate ligament
Noncontact, quickly turning one way with tibia rotated in opposite direction	1. Patellar dislocation or subluxation
Noncontact, rotation with varus or valgus loading	1. Meniscus injury
Noncontact, compressive rotation	1. Meniscus injury 2. Osteochondral fracture
Hyperflexion	1. Meniscus (posterior horn) 2. Anterior cruciate ligament
Forced medial rotation	1. Meniscus injury (lateral meniscus)
Forced lateral rotation	1. Meniscus injury (medial meniscus) 2. Medial collateral ligament and possibly anterior cruciate ligament 3. Patellar dislocation
Flexion-varus-medial rotation	1. Anterolateral instability
Flexion-valgus-lateral rotation	1. Anteromedial instability
Dashboard injury	1. Isolated posterior cruciate ligament 2. Posterior cruciate ligament and posterior capsule 3. Posterolateral instability 4. Posteromedial instability 5. Patellar fracture 6. Tibial fracture (proximal) 7. Tibial plateau fracture 8. Acetabular and pelvic fracture

Adapted from Clancy W.: Evaluation of acute knee injuries. In American Association of Orthopaedic Surgeons, Symposium on Sports Medicine: *The knee*, St Louis, 1985, Mosby; Strobel M, Stedtfeld HW: *Diagnostic evaluation of the knee*, Berlin, 1990, Springer-Verlag.

2. *Has the knee been injured before, or does it have any feeling of weakness?*

3. *What is the patient able or unable to do functionally? Is there disability on running, cutting, pivoting, twisting, climbing, or descending stairs?* Positive responses to these questions should alert the examiner to instability caused by injured ligaments, muscle dysfunction, joint articular problems, or meniscus problems.[14]

4. *Is there any "clicking," or was there a "pop" when the injury occurred?* A distinct pop may indicate an anterior cruciate ligament tear or osteochondral fracture. Popping on the lateral aspect of the knee may be due to the popliteus tendon snapping over the lateral femoral inferoposterior tubercle within 2 cm of the muscle's attachment into the femur.[15]

5. *Did the injury occur during acceleration, during deceleration, or when the patient was moving at a constant speed?* Acceleration and twisting injuries may involve the meniscus. Deceleration injuries often involve the cruciate ligaments. Constant speed with cutting may involve the anterior cruciate ligament.

Figure 12-4

Sagittal plane motion at the knee. **A,** Tibial-on-femoral perspective (open kinetic chain). **B,** Femoral-on-tibial perspective (closed kinetic chain). (Modified from Neumann DA: *Kinesiology of the musculoskeletal system— foundations for physical rehabilitation*, p. 444, St Louis, 2002, Mosby.)

6. *Is there any pain? If so, where? What type is it?* Is it diffuse? Aching? Retropatellar? Aching pain may indicate degenerative changes, whereas sharp, "catching" pain usually indicates a mechanical problem. Arthritic pain is more likely to be associated with stiffness in the morning and eases with activity. Anterior knee pain may be due to patellofemoral problems, bursa (prepatellar, infrapatellar) pathology, fat pad pathology, tendinosis, or Osgood-Schlatter disease.[16,17] Patellofemoral pain tends to be insidious and occurs spontaneously, often from overuse, which makes establishing the source of the problem important.[18,19] Pain at rest is not usually mechanical in origin. Pain during activity is usually seen in structural abnormalities, such as subluxation or patellar tracking disorders. Pain after activity or with overuse is characteristic of inflammatory disorders, such as synovial plica irritation or early tendinosis or paratenonitis-leading to jumper's knee or Sinding-Larsen-Johansson syndrome.[20-25] Generalized pain in the area of the knee is usually characteristic of contusions or partial tears of muscles or ligaments. Instability rather than pain tends to be the major presenting factor in complex ligament disruptions or muscle dysfunction (e.g., quadriceps rupture). Pain in the knee on ankle movements may implicate the superior tibiofibular joint.

7. *Do certain positions or activities have an increased or decreased effect on the pain?* Which activities produce pain? How much activity is needed to produce pain? Which positions or activities ease the pain? Does the pain go away when activity ceases? The examiner must take note of constant pain that is unrelated to activity, time, or posture, because it usually indicates serious pathology, such as a tumor. Does the patient have confidence in the knee? Such a question gives the examiner some idea of the functional impairment from the patient's perspective.[26]

8. *Does the knee "give way"?*[26] This finding usually indicates instability in the knee, meniscus pathology, patellar subluxation (if present when rotation or stopping is involved), undisplaced osteochondritis dissecans, patellofemoral syndrome, plica, or loose body. Giving way when walking uphill or downhill is more likely the result of a retropatellar lesion.[14,27] If the patient complains that the patella "slips out of place," it may be because of patellar subluxation or a pathological plica.[28]

9. *Has the knee ever locked?* True locking of the knee is rare. Loose bodies may cause recurrent locking. Locking must be differentiated from catching, which is momentary locking or giving way as a result of reflex inhibition or pain.[28] **Locking** in the knee usually means that the knee cannot fully extend with flexion often being normal, and it is related to meniscus pathology. Hamstring muscle spasm may also limit extension and is sometimes referred to as **spasm locking**.

10. *On movement, is there any grating or clicking in the knee?* Grating or clicking may be caused by degeneration or by one structure's snapping over another.

11. *Is the joint swollen? Does the swelling occur with activity or several hours after activity, or does the joint*

feel tight at rest? Swelling with activity may be caused by instability, and tightness at rest may be caused by arthritic changes or patellofemoral dysfunction. Is the swelling recurrent? If so, what activity causes it? Swelling with pivoting or twisting may be a result of meniscus problems or instability at the tibiofemoral joint. Recurrent swelling caused by climbing or descending slopes or stairs may be related to patellofemoral dysfunction.[28] Often there is no swelling in the knee after severe injury, because the fluid extravasates into the soft tissues surrounding the joint and because a number of structures around the knee joint are avascular and can be injured without bloody swelling occurring. Synovial swelling may occur 8 to 24 hours after the injury; swelling caused by blood begins to occur almost immediately. Localized swelling may be caused by an inflamed bursa (Figure 12-5).[29] The deep infrapatellar bursa has been noted as a source of anterior knee pain and could be misdiagnosed as patellofemoral arthralgia or Osgood-Schlatter disease.[30,31]

12. *Is the gait normal?* Does the patient put weight on the limb? *Can* the patient extend the knee while walking? Is the stride length altered on the affected limb? All these questions give an indication of the patient's functional disability and how much the knee is bothering the patient.

13. *What type of shoes does the patient wear?* Shoes with negative heels (e.g., "earth shoes") can increase the incidence of patellofemoral syndrome.

Observation

For a proper observation, the patient must be suitably undressed so that the examiner can observe the posture of the spine as well as the hips, knees, and ankles. Initially, the examiner should note whether the patient puts weight on the affected limb or stands with only a slight amount of weight on the affected side. In addition to the common observational items mentioned in Chapter 1, the examiner should look for the following alterations around the knee.

Anterior View, Standing

From the anterior aspect (Figure 12-6), the examiner should note any malalignment, including **genu varum** (bowleg) or **genu valgum** (knock-knee) deformity (Figure 12-7). Any observable malalignment may lead to or be the result of malalignment elsewhere (Table 12-2).[32] These deformities may be unilateral or bilateral. Although in adults the legs should be relatively straight, in the child, the normal development of the knee is from genu varum to straight, to genu valgum, and then to straight. Initially, a child's lower limbs are in genu varum until 18 or 19 months, when they straighten. The knee then goes into genu valgum until about 3 to 4 years of age (Figure 12-8). The limbs should be almost straight by age 6 years and should remain that way. In the adult, the knee is normally in approximately 6° of valgus.

To observe genu varum and genu valgum, the patient is positioned so that the patellae face forward and the medial aspects of the knees and medial malleoli of both limbs are as close together as possible. If the knees touch and the ankles do not, the patient has a genu valgum. A distance of 9 to 10 cm (3.5 to 4 inches) between the ankles is considered excessive. If two or more fingers (4 cm [1.6 inch]) fit between the knees when the ankles

Figure 12-5
The bursae around the knee (medial aspect).

Labels (left): Femur · Semimembranosus muscle · Semimembranosus bursa · Synovial sacs · Medial collateral ligament · Anserine bursa · Gastrocnemius muscle

Labels (right): Quadriceps muscle · Suprapatellar bursa (pouch) · Prepatellar bursa (pouch) · Meniscus · Superficial infrapatellar bursa · Deep infrapatellar bursa and (Hoffa's) fat pad · Tendons of gracilis, sartorius, semitendinosus muscles (pes anserinus)

Figure 12-6
Anterior view of the lower limbs. Note the wider than normal base width.

Figure 12-7
Genu varum and genu valgum. **A,** Tibia vara of proximal third. Genu varum deformity located mainly in proximal tibia. Along with lateral tibial torsion and medial femoral torsion, this gives a "bandy-legged" appearance. **B,** Genu varum of entire lower extremities. **C,** Genu valgum deformity of both lower extremities. (From Hughston JC, Walsh WM, Puddu G: *Patellar subluxation and dislocation,* p. 221, Philadelphia, 1984, WB Saunders.)

are together, the patient has a varus deformity or genu varum.[33] On x-ray studies, the normal **tibiofemoral shaft angle** is approximately 6° (Figure 12-9).

Alignment is often different between males and females.[34] Some of these misalignments, if excessive, can lead to patellofemoral symptoms or instability.[35] These excessive differences are sometimes referred to as **miserable malalignment syndrome** (Figure 12-10).

The patient is asked to extend the knees to see whether the movement can be performed and what effect it has on the knee. Both knees should extend equally. If not, something must be limiting the movement (swelling, loose body, or meniscus). Normally, a person does not stand with the knees fully extended. If, however, the patient has an excessive lordosis, the knees are often hyperextended to maintain the center of gravity. This change can lead to posterior knee pain.

Is there any apparent swelling or ecchymosis in or around the knees (see Figure 1-8)? If there is intracapsular swelling, or at least sufficient swelling, the knee assumes a position of 15° to 25° of flexion, which provides the synovial cavity with the maximum capacity to hold fluid. This position is also called the **resting**

Table 12-2

Malalignment about the Knee and Possible Correlated and Compensatory Motions or Postures

Malalignment	Possible Correlated Motions or Postures	Possible Compensatory Motions or Postures
Genu valgum	Pes planus Excessive subtalar pronation Lateral tibial torsion Lateral patellar subluxation Excessive hip adduction Ipsilateral hip excessive medial rotation Lumbar spine contralateral rotation	Forefoot varus Excessive subtalar supination to allow the lateral heel to contact the ground In-toeing to decrease lateral pelvic sway during gait Ipsilateral pelvic lateral rotation
Genu varum	Excessive lateral angulation of the tibia in the frontal plane; tibial varum Medial tibial torsion Ipsilateral hip lateral rotation Excessive hip abduction	Forefoot valgus Excessive subtalar pronation to allow the medial heel to contact the ground Ipsilateral pelvic medial rotation
Genu recurvatum	Ankle plantar flexion Excessive anterior pelvic tilt	Posterior pelvic tilt Flexed trunk posture Excessive thoracic kyphosis
Lateral tibial torsion	Out-toeing Excessive subtalar supination with related rotation along the lower quarter	Functional forefoot varus Excessive subtalar pronation with relaxed rotation along the lower quarter
Medial tibial torsion	In-toeing Metatarsus adductus Excessive subtalar pronation with related rotation along the lower quarter	Functional forefoot valgus Excessive subtalar supination with relaxed rotation along the lower quarter
Excessive tibial retroversion (posterior slant of tibial plateaus)	Genu recurvatum	
Inadequate tibial retrotorsion (posterior deflection of proximal tibia because of hamstrings pull)	Flexed knee posture	
Inadequate tibial retroflexion (bowing of the tibia)	Altered alignment of Achilles tendon causing altered associated joint motion	
Bowleg deformity of the tibia (tibial varum)	Medial tibial torsion	Forefoot valgus Excessive subtalar pronation

From Riegger-Krugh C, Keysor JJ: Skeletal malalignments of the lower quarter: correlated and compensatory motions and postures, *J Orthop Sports Phys Ther* 23:166–167, 1996.

position of the knee. Is the swelling intracapsular or extracapsular? Intracapsular swelling is evident over the entire joint; extracapsular swelling tends to be more localized. An example of extracapsular swelling is shown in Figure 12-11, which illustrates **prepatellar bursitis**.

The examiner should ask the patient to contract the quadriceps muscles to see whether there is any visible wasting of the muscles, especially of the vastus medialis obliquus. The prominence of the vastus medialis results from the obliquity of the distal fibers, the inferior position of its insertion, and the thinness of the fascial covering compared with the other quadriceps muscles. Muscle defects (third-degree strain or rupture) should also be watched for when the patient contracts the muscles. Third-degree strains may be indicated by muscle "bunch-ing," abnormal mechanics (e.g., unilateral patella alta with patella tendon rupture), or a palpable defect.[28]

The position of the patella should be noted. When viewing the patellae, the examiner should note whether they face straight ahead, tilt outward ("grasshopper eyes" patellae), tilt inward ("squinting" patellae), or are rotated ("spin") in or out[36] (Figure 12-12). Rotation and tilt may be caused by tight structures that alter the position of the patella. These tight structures may include muscles (e.g., rectus femoris, iliotibial band, gastrocnemius) or fascia (e.g., lateral retinaculum). Normally, the patellae should face straight ahead with no lateral tilt or rotation. If these deviations are seen in the observation phase, they are considered static problems, and the examiner should test patellar movement passively and watch the patellae

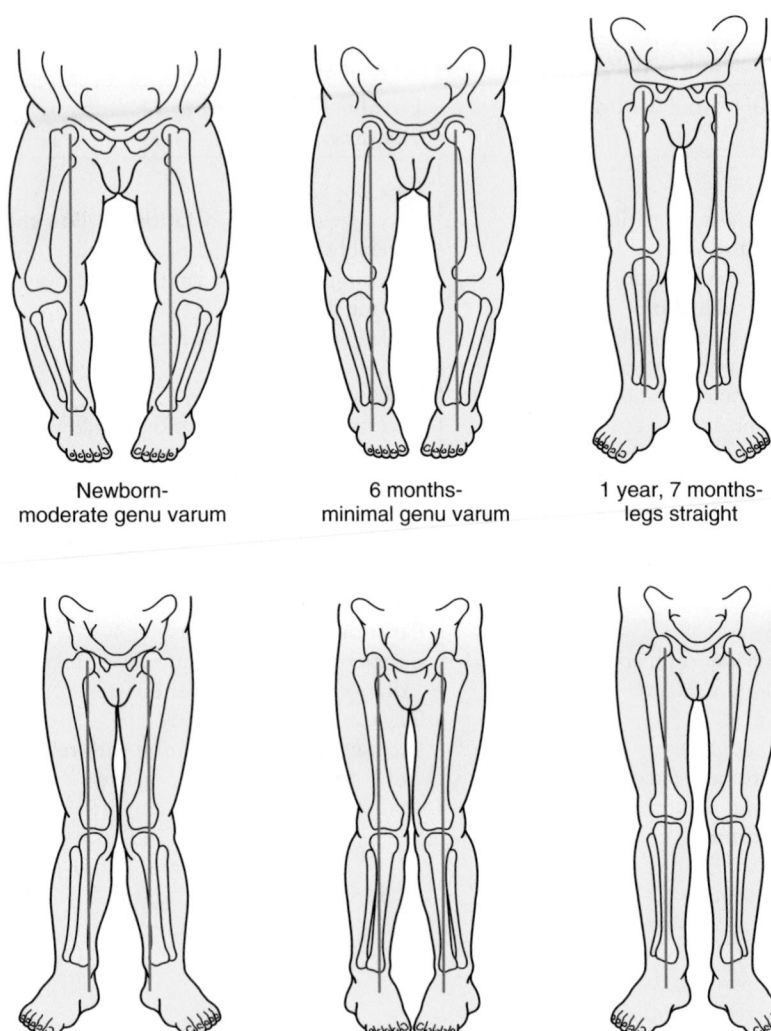

Newborn-
moderate genu varum

6 months-
minimal genu varum

1 year, 7 months-
legs straight

2 years, 6 months-
physiological genu valgum

Protective toeing-in

4 to 6 years-
legs straight with normal
toeing-out

Figure 12-8

Physiological evolution of lower limb alignment at various ages in infancy and childhood. (Redrawn from Tachdjian MO: *Pediatric orthopedics*, p. 1463, Philadelphia, 1972, WB Saunders.)

Lateral

Medial

Genu
valgum

Genu
varum

Normal (6°)

Figure 12-9

Normal tibiofemoral shaft angle.

during active movements to see whether it is a dynamic problem as well.[37] A squinting or rotated patella may indicate medial femoral or lateral tibial torsion (Figure 12-13). Patients with abnormal torsion are prone to patellofemoral instability.

Any bruising or discoloration around the knee should also be noted, as well as any scars or signs indicating recent injury or surgery.

Lateral View, Standing

The examiner then views the patient from both sides for comparison. It should be noted whether **genu recurvatum** (hyperextended knee)[38] is present and whether one or both patellae are higher **(patella alta)** or lower **(patella baja** or **patella infera)**[39] than normal (Figure 12-14). With an abnormally high patella, a **"camel sign"** may be present (Figure 12-15); because of the high patella (one "hump"), the infrapatellar fat pad

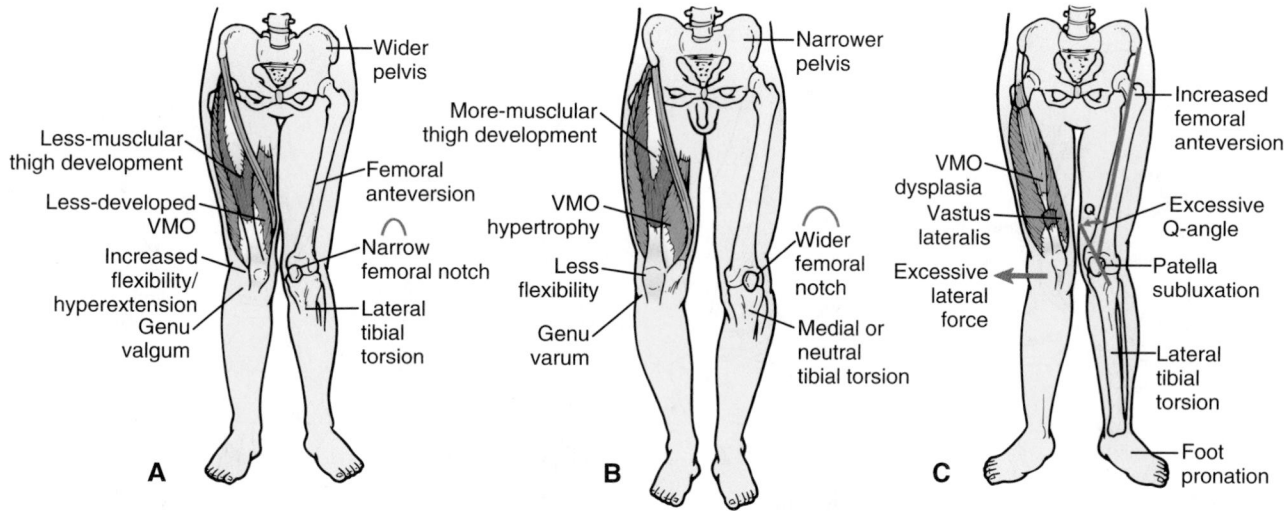

Figure 12-10

A, Normal female alignment with wider pelvis, femoral anteversion, genu valgum, hyperflexibility, lateral tibial torsion, and narrow notch. **B,** Normal male alignment demonstrates a narrower pelvis, more developed musculature, genu varum, medial or neutral tibial torsion, and wider notch. **C,** Miserable malalignment syndrome is a term coined to describe patients who have increased femoral anteversion, genu valgum, vastus medialis obliquus (VMO) dysplasia, lateral tibial torsion, and forefoot pronation. These factors create excessive lateral forces and contribute to patellofemoral dysfunction. (From Griffin LY, editor: *Rehabilitation of the injured knee*, pp 298–299, St Louis, 1995, Mosby.)

(second hump) or an inflamed infrapatellar bursa (just anterior to the fat pad) becomes more prominent. This finding is especially noticeable in females. In this position, the examiner should also note (Figure 12-16) whether the inferior pole of the patella is tilted in (inferior tilt). Ideally, the plane of the patella and that of the femoral condyles should be the same. If the inferior pole tilts in, fat pad irritation may occur.[40] Habitual genu recurvatum may make a patient prone to posterior cruciate tears because of the stretching of the posterior oblique ligament.[28] If one knee (normal) hyperextends and the

other one (injured) does not, it may indicate meniscus pathology that is limiting extension. Osteoarthritic lipping (Figure 12-17) or synovial hypertrophy (rheumatoid arthritis) may also limit movement.

Posterior View, Standing

Next, the examiner views the patient from behind, looking for findings similar to those from the anterior aspect. In addition, the examiner looks for abnormal swellings, such as a popliteal (Baker's) cyst, which is caused by herniation of synovial tissue through a weakening in the posterior capsule wall (Figure 12-18).

Anterior and Lateral Views, Sitting

For the final part of the observation, the patient sits with the knee flexed to 90° and the feet either partially bearing weight (on a stool) or dangling free. The patient is observed from the front and from the side. In this position, the patella should face forward and should rest on the distal end of the femur. With patella alta, the patella becomes more aligned with the anterior surface of the femur (angled upward). If the patella is laterally displaced or laterally displaced with a patella alta, the patellae take on the appearance of "frog eyes" or "grasshopper eyes" (Figure 12-19), meaning that the patellae face upward and outward, away from each other. Patella alta sometimes causes a concavity proximal to the patella in thin patients.[28] Any bony enlargements, such as those seen in Osgood-Schlatter disease (i.e., an enlarged tibial tubercle),

Figure 12-11

Prepatellar bursitis.

Figure 12-12

Assessment of the patellar glide component. Ideally, the patella should be centered on the superior portion of the femoral articular surface at 20° flexion. **A,** Ideal alignment. **B,** Lateral glide of the patella. **C,** Lateral tilt of the patella. **D,** Lateral rotation ("spin") of inferior pole of patella. (From McConnell J, Fulkerson J: The knee: patellofemoral and soft tissue injuries. In Zachazewski JE et al, editors: *Athletic injuries and rehabilitation,* pp. 711–712, Philadelphia, 1996, WB Saunders.)

Figure 12-13

"Squinting" patellae, especially prominent on the patient's left knee. Both patellae point inward in a medial fashion, a sign of excessive femoral anteversion or increased medial femoral torsion. (From Carson WG, James SL, Larsen RL et al: Patellofemoral disorders: physical and radiographic evaluation. I. Physical examination, *Clin Orthop* 185:169, 1984.)

should be noted (Figure 12-20), as should abnormal swelling. Swelling of the pes anserine bursa and a meniscal cyst (Figure 12-21) are best visualized in the seated position.[28,41] Meniscal cysts may also present as isolated medial swelling.[27]

In the same position, any **tibial torsion** should be noted (Figure 12-22).[40,42] If there is tibial torsion, it is medial torsion that is associated with genu varum; genu valgum is associated with lateral tibial torsion. Normally, the patella faces straight ahead while the foot faces slightly laterally (Fick angle). With medial tibial torsion, the feet point toward each other, resulting in a "pigeon-toed" foot deformity. These deformities can be exacerbated by habitual postures. The positions illustrated in Figures 12-23, 12-24, *A* and 12-25 cause problems only if they are used habitually. Excessive tibial torsion can contribute to conditions such as chondromalacia patellae, patellofemoral instability, and fat pad entrapment. When standing, most people exhibit a lateral tibial torsion, the Fick angle (see Figure 13-13), which increases as the child grows. This angle is approximately 5° in babies and as much as 18° in adults. To test for tibial torsion, the examiner aligns the patient's straight legs (knees extended) so that the patellae face straight ahead. The examiner then looks at the feet to determine their angle relative to the shaft of the tibia.

Femoral torsion, or anteversion (discussed in Chapter 11, can also affect the position of the patella relative to the femur and tibia.

Patella baja   Normal   Patella alta

Figure 12-14

The normal patellar posture for exerting deceleration forces in the functional position of 45° of knee flexion places the patellar articular surface squarely against the anterior femur. A lower posture represents patella baja. A higher posture represents patella alta. Patella alta makes the patella less efficient in exerting normal forces. (Redrawn from Hughston JC et al: *Patellar subluxation and dislocation*, p. 8, Philadelphia, 1984, WB Saunders.)

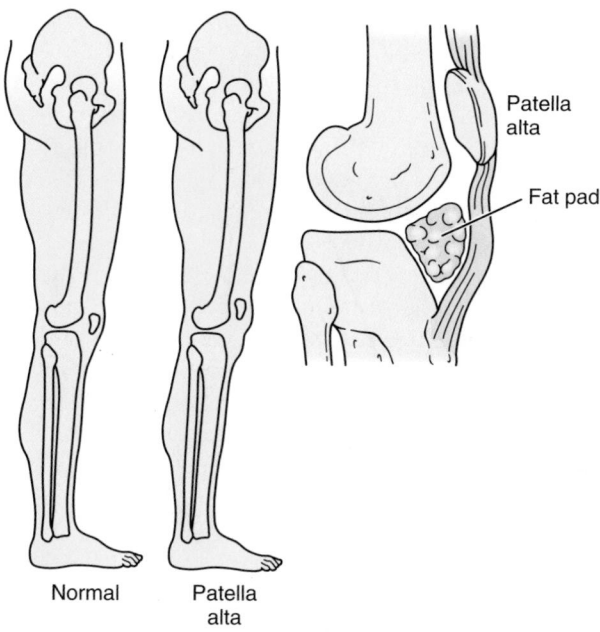

Normal   Patella alta

Patella alta

Fat pad

Figure 12-15

Camel sign. Double hump seen from side caused by high-riding patella and uncovered infrapatellar fat pad. (Modified from Hughston JC et al: *Patellar subluxation and dislocation*, p. 22, Philadelphia, 1984, WB Saunders.)

A   B

Fat pad
Patellar tendon

Figure 12-16

Assessment of the anteroposterior component of the patella. Ideally, the superior and inferior poles of the patella should be parallel in the sagittal plane of the knee, **A.** Commonly, in individuals with patellar malalignment, the inferior patellar pole pushes posteriorly into the infrapatellar fat pad, **B.** This may irritate the fat pad. (Redrawn from McConnell J, Fulkerson J: The knee: patellofemoral and soft tissue injuries. In Zachazewski JE et al, editors: *Athletic injuries and rehabilitation*, p. 712, Philadelphia, 1996, WB Saunders.)

Figure 12-17

Osteophytic lipping in posterior knee limits flexion and produces a bone-to-bone end feel.

Gait

The examiner should also observe the patient's gait (see Chapter 14), noting any differences in stride length, walking speed, cadence, or linear and angular displacement. In addition, the examiner should watch for abnormal patellar movement, indicating possible patellar tracking problems, and abnormal motion of the tibia relative to the femur, indicating possible instability problems.

Movement at the pelvis, hip, and ankle should also be observed. For example, weak hip abductors (positive Trendelenburg's sign) may lead to increased stress on the knee. If this is combined with medial tibial torsion, patellofemoral syndromes may result.[28,43] Tight heel cords may result in gait with the knee flexed, which can put extra pressure on the patellofemoral joint. Similarly, pronation of the foot and lateral tibial torsion may lead to patellofemoral pathology or anteromedial joint pain.[28] Tight hamstrings result in increased knee flexion, which can lead to the need for more ankle dorsiflexion. If no further dorsiflexion is possible, the foot pronates to compensate, thus increasing the **dynamic Q-angle**.[44]

Examination

Although the examination focuses primarily on the knee, the examiner must keep in mind that knee pathology may be the result of biomechanical (e.g., alignment, asymmetry)

A   B

Figure 12-18

Popliteal (Baker's) cysts. **A,** This 74-year-old man presented with the acute onset of calf pain and swelling without knee pain. The initial suspected diagnosis was popliteal thrombosis. A venogram was normal. The arthrogram revealed a collection of dye posterior to the joint space—a popliteal cyst *(arrow)*. **B,** Schematic diagram of Baker's cyst. (**A** from Reilly BM: *Practical strategies in outpatient medicine,* p. 1179, Philadelphia, 1991, WB Saunders.)

Figure 12-19
A, Normal knee seen from side; patella faces straight ahead in line with femur. **B,** Patella alta seen from side; patella points toward ceiling. **C,** Normal patellae seen from front; patellae centered in outline of knees. **D,** High and lateral posturing of patellae seen from front, giving "grasshopper eyes" or "frog eyes" appearance. (From Hughston JC et al: *Patellar subluxation and dislocation*, p. 23, Philadelphia, 1984, WB Saunders.)

Figure 12-20
Osgood-Schlatter disease (enlarged tibial tuberosity).

Figure 12-21
Lateral meniscus cyst. (From Reider B: *The orthopedic physical examination*, p. 209, Philadelphia, 1999, WB Saunders.)

Figure 12-22
Exaggerated lateral tibial torsion. In stance, with the patellae facing straight forward, the feet point outward. (From Tachdjian MO: *Pediatric orthopedics*, p. 2816, Philadelphia, 1990, WB Saunders.)

and pathological (e.g., hypomobility, hypermobility, muscle weakness, instability) issues in other joints in the kinetic chain, including the lumbar spine, pelvis, hips, ankles, and feet. Thus the examination, like the history and observation, may be extensive to rule out other kinetic chain contributors.[45-50] For example, Dutton[51] believed the gracilis and adductor longus and magnus play a significant role along with the iliotibial band in knee stability. Also, several muscles that are two joint muscles acting over the hip and knee (e.g., rectus femoris, hamstrings, sartorius, gracilis) and knee and ankle (gastrocnemius) should be tested for functional mobility, because their action at one joint can affect the other joint (Figure 12-26).

Active Movements

The examination is performed initially with the patient sitting and then with the patient in lying position. During the active movements, the examiner should observe (1) the excursion of the patella, to ensure that it tracks freely and smoothly; (2) the range of motion (ROM) available; (3) whether pain occurs during the movement, and if so, where; and (4) what appears to be limiting the movement. The active movements may be done in the sitting or supine position, and, as always, the most painful movements should be done last (Figure 12-27).

Figure 12-23
"Television" or "W" sitting position may lead to excessive lateral tibial torsion. **A,** Anterior view. **B,** Posterior view.

Figure 12-24
Medial tibial torsion. **A,** Position to be avoided to prevent excessive medial tibial torsion. **B,** Tailor position maintains normal medial tibial torsion.

Active Movements of the Knee Complex

- Flexion (0° to 135°)
- Extension (0° to 15°)
- Medial rotation of the tibia on the femur (20° to 30°)
- Lateral rotation of the tibia on the femur (30° to 40°)
- Repetitive movements (if necessary)
- Sustained postures (if necessary)
- Combined movements (if necessary)

Full knee flexion is 135° (0° being straight knee). As the patient moves the knee through flexion and extension, the examiner should watch the movement of the patella as it "tracks" along the femoral trochlea. The examiner should note whether the movement is smooth from beginning to end or whether there is a lag or abrupt jump of the patella as it attempts to center in the groove.[52] The patella does not follow a straight path as the knee moves from extension to flexion. Normally, it follows a curved pattern moving medially in early flexion and then laterally (Figure 12-28).[53] As in the observation phase, the examiner should note whether dynamic movement causes lateral tilt, anteroposterior tilt, or rotation of the patella during movement.[44,53]

Active knee extension is approximately 0° but may be −15°, especially in women, who are more likely to have hyperextended knees (genu recurvatum). The knee extensor muscles develop the greatest force near 60°, and the knee flexor muscles develop their greatest force at 45° to 10°. To complete the last 15° of knee extension, a 60% increase in force of the quadriceps muscles is required. The examiner should also watch for evidence of **quadriceps lag**, which means the quadriceps muscles are not strong enough to fully extend the knee. The lag results from loss of mechanical advantage, muscle atrophy, decreasing power of the muscle as it shortens, adhesion formation, effusion, or reflex inhibition (Table 12-3). In non–weight bearing, active medial rotation of the tibia on the femur should be 20° to 30°, whereas active lateral rotation should be 30° to 40° at 90° flexion in non-weight-bearing (Figure 12-29A). In weight bearing (closed kinetic chain), the femur will rotate on the tibia (Figure 12-29B).

If, during the history, the patient has complained that repetitive or combined movements or sustained postures have resulted in symptoms, these movements should also be tested.

Passive Movements

If, on active movements, the ROM is full, overpressure may gently be applied to test the end feel of the various movements in the tibiofemoral joint. This action would preclude the need to do passive movements to the tibiofemoral joint. However, the examiner must do movements of the patella passively (Figure 12-30).

Passive Movements of the Knee Complex and Normal End Feel

- Flexion (tissue approximation)
- Extension (tissue stretch)
- Medial rotation of tibia on femur (tissue stretch)
- Lateral rotation of tibia on femur (tissue stretch)
- Patellar movement (tissue stretch—all directions)

Figure 12-25

Traditional Japanese kneeling requires full knee flexion, often accompanied by medial tibial rotation.

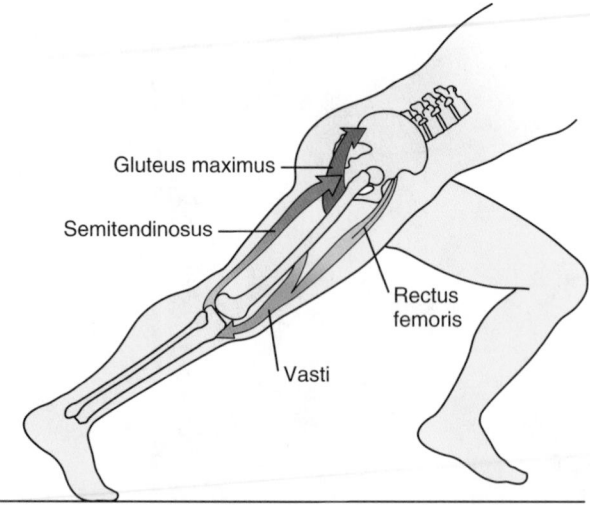

Figure 12-26

The action of several 1 joint and 2 joint muscles is depicted during the hip-and-knee extension phase of running. Observe that the vasti extend the knee, which then stretches the distal end of the semitendinosus. The gluteus maximus extends the hip, which then stretches the proximal end of the rectus femoris. The stretch placed on the active biarticular muscles reduces the rate and amount of their overall contraction. (Redrawn from Neumann D: *Kinesiology of the musculoskeletal system—foundations for physical rehabilitation*, p. 468, St Louis, 2002, Mosby.)

A

B

Figure 12-27

Active movements of the knee. **A,** Extension. **B,** Flexion.

At the tibiofemoral joint, the end feel of flexion is tissue approximation; the end feel of extension and of medial and lateral rotation of the tibia on the femur is tissue stretch. During passive movement, the examiner is also looking for a capsular pattern of the tibiofemoral joint.[54] This pattern is more limitation of flexion than of extension. Passive medial rotation of the tibia on the femur should be approximately 30° when the knee is flexed to 90°. Passive lateral rotation of the tibia on the femur at 90° of knee flexion should be 40°.

Figure 12-28

Multiplanar patellar path during knee flexion. (Redrawn from Stanitski CL et al, editors: *Pediatric and adolescent sports medicine*, p. 307, Philadelphia, 1994, WB Saunders.)

Table 12-3

Selected Factors That Contribute to the Inability to Completely Extend the Knee

Factor	Clinical Examples
Reduced force production from the quadriceps	Disuse atrophy of quadriceps following trauma and/or prolonged immobilization
	Lacerated femoral nerve
	Herniated disc compressing L3 or L4 nerve roots
	Severe pain
	Excessive swelling in the knee
Excessive resistance from connective tissues	Excessive tightness in hamstring or other knee flexor muscles
	Excessive stiffness in the anterior cruciate ligament, posterior capsule, or collateral ligaments
	Scarring of the skin in the popliteal fossa
	Excessive swelling in the knee
Faulty arthrokinematics	Lack of "screw-home" rotation mechanics
	Lack of anterior slide of the tibia*
	Meniscal block or other derangement
	Lack of superior slide of the patella*

From Neumann DA: *Kinesiology of the musculoskeletal system—foundations for physical rehabilitation*, p. 460, St Louis, 2002, Mosby.
*Assume tibial-on-femoral knee extension.

Although full knee extension is usually preferable for everyday activities (e.g., standing, walking), full flexion (135°) is often not necessary except where people kneel back on their heels. However, approximately 117° of flexion is necessary for activities such as squatting to tie a shoelace or to pull on a sock. Sitting in a chair requires approximately 90° of flexion, and climbing stairs (average height) requires approximately 80° of flexion.

Passive medial and lateral movement of the patella is also carried out to determine its mobility and to compare it with the unaffected side. Normally, the patella should move up to half its width medially and laterally in extension (Figure 12-31). When the patella is pushed

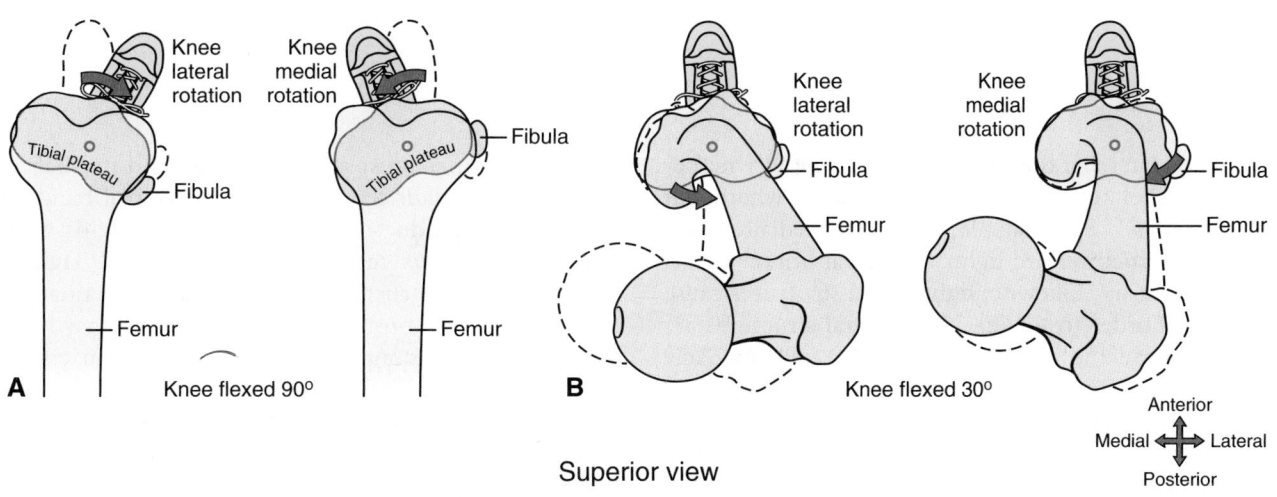

Superior view

Figure 12-29

Horizontal plane (axial) rotation at the knee. **A,** Tibial-on-femoral rotation at 90° flexion (open kinetic chain). **B,** Femoral-on-tibial rotation (closed kinetic chain). (Redrawn from Neumann DA: *Kinesiology of the musculoskeletal system—foundations for physical rehabilitation*, p. 445, St Louis, 2002, Mosby.)

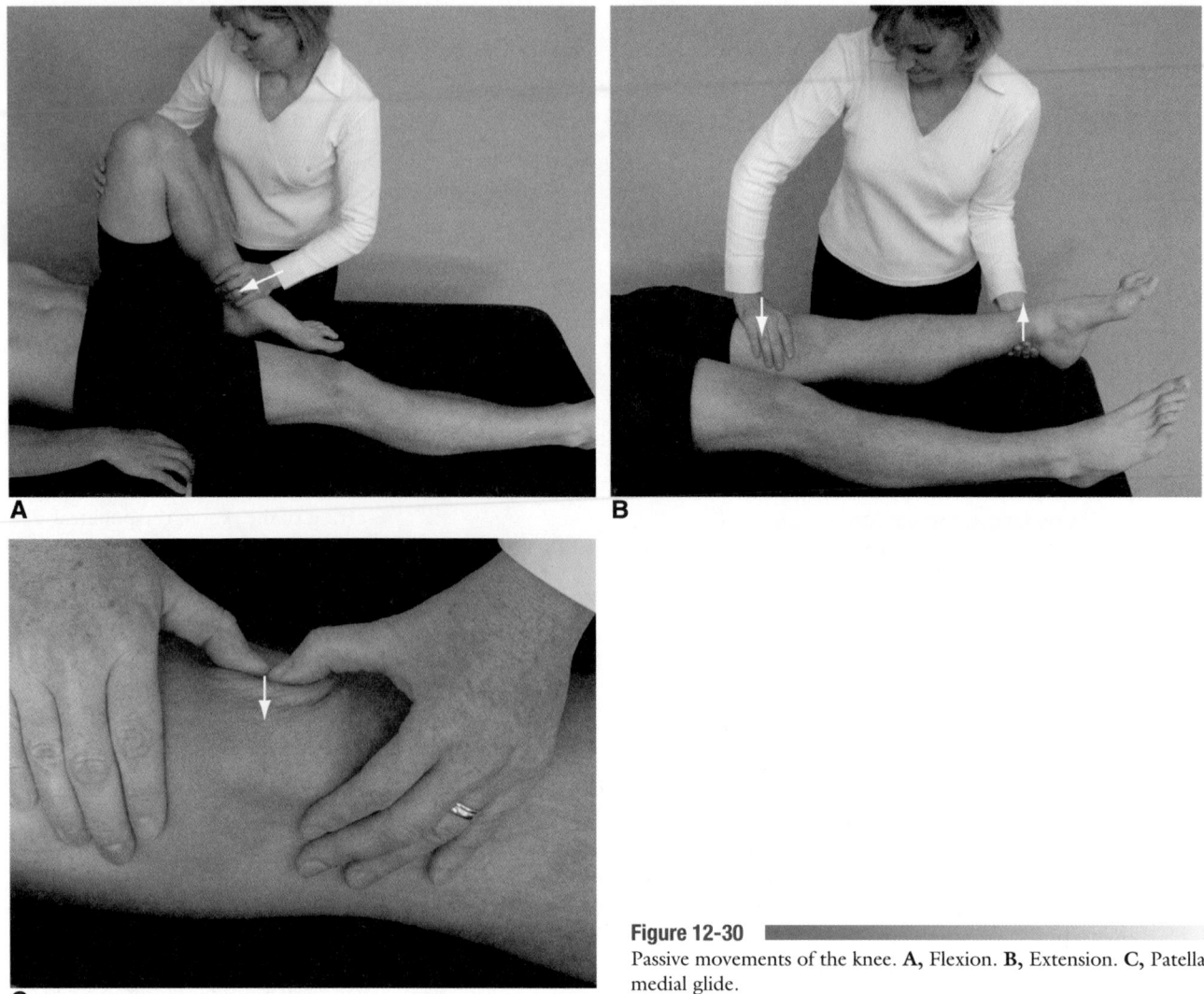

Figure 12-30
Passive movements of the knee. **A,** Flexion. **B,** Extension. **C,** Patella medial glide.

medially or laterally, the examiner should note whether it stays parallel to the femoral condyles or whether it tilts or rotates.[37] For example, if pushed medially when the medial structures are tight, the lateral border of the patella will tilt up. Likewise, tight lateral structures cause the medial border to tilt up. If the lateral structures are tight superiorly, the inferior pole of the patella medially rotates. These are examples of dynamic tilt and rotation problems of the patella. The side-to-side passive motion of the patella should also be tested in 45° of flexion, which is a more functional position and gives a better indication of functional instability of the patella.[55] The end feel of these movements is tissue stretch. Lateral displacement must be performed with care, especially in patients who have experienced a dislocated patella.

The examiner must also ensure full and normal flexibility of the quadriceps, hamstring, iliotibial band, and abductor and adductor muscles of the thigh, as well as the gastrocnemius muscles (Figure 12-32). Tightness of any of these structures or of the lateral retinaculum can alter gait and postural mechanics, which may lead to pathology. For example, tight hamstrings can contribute to patellofemoral pathology because of increased knee flexion at heel strike and during stance phase.[44] Limitation of hip rotation in extension can lead to patellofemoral pathology as well.[28] If the rectus femoris is tight, full excursion of the patella in the trochlea is not possible, especially if the hip is extended. A tight iliotibial band can lead to lateral tracking of the patella.[44,56] Tests for the hamstring, abductor, adductor, and rectus femoris

Figure 12-31

Passive lateral glide test demonstrating a patella being subluxated laterally to its second quadrant. Decreased patellar mobility (hypomobile) is manifested by less than one quadrant of medial and lateral glide; movement of more than two quadrants (one half of patellar width) is considered hypermobile. (Redrawn from Jackson DW, editor: *The anterior cruciate ligament: current and future concepts*, p. 358, New York, 1993, Raven Press.)

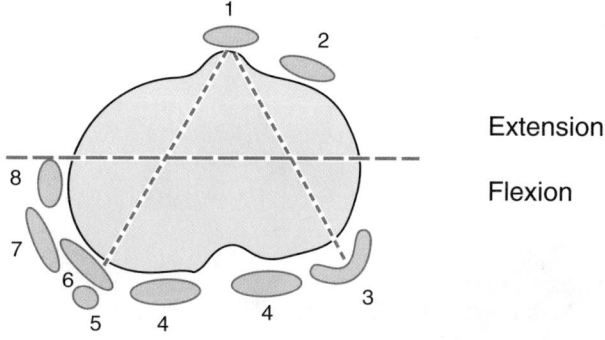

Figure 12-32

Movement diagram of the knee showing quadriceps hamstrings tripod. *1*, Patellar tendon (quadriceps); *2*, iliotibial band; *3*, biceps femoris; *4*, gastrocnemius; *5*, semitendinosus; *6*, semimembranosus; *7*, gracilis; *8*, sartorius.

muscles have been described in Chapter 11. A functional test for the quadriceps (described under Special Tests in this chapter) is also a passive movement test (heel to buttock) for the femoral nerve. To test the gastrocnemius muscle, the examiner extends the patient's knee and, while holding it straight, dorsiflexes the patient's ankle. The examiner should be able to reach at least 90° (plantigrade), although 10° to 15° of dorsiflexion is more common.

Resisted Isometric Movements

For a proper test of the muscles, resisted isometric movements must be performed. The patient should be in the supine position (Figure 12-33).

Resisted Isometric Movements of the Knee Complex

- Flexion of the knee
- Extension of the knee
- Ankle plantar flexion
- Ankle dorsiflexion

Figure 12-33

Resisted isometric movements of the knee. **A,** Knee extension. **B,** Knee flexion.

Continued

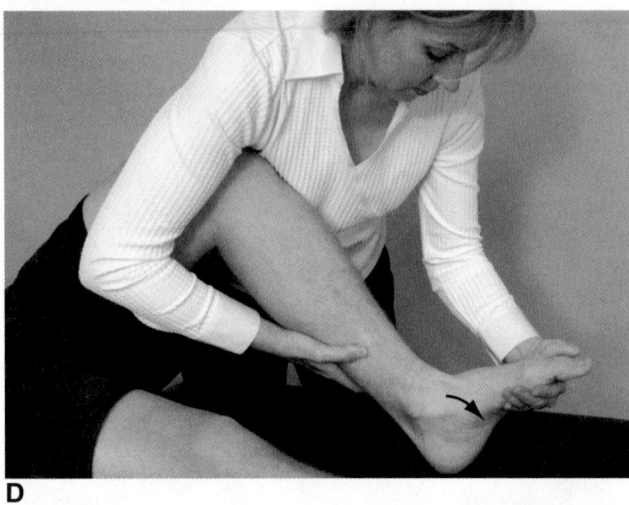

Figure 12-33 cont'd
C, Ankle dorsiflexion. **D,** Ankle plantar flexion.

Figure 12-34

Components of the quadriceps femoris complex. Note the angle of insertion of the various components of the complex. The orientation of the muscle fibers dictates the line of action and pull on the patella. (Redrawn from McConnell J, Fulkerson J: The knee: patellofemoral and soft tissue injuries. In Zachazewski JE et al, editors: *Athletic injuries and rehabilitation*, p. 697, Philadelphia, 1996, WB Saunders.)

Ideally, these resisted isometric movements are performed with the joint in its resting position. Segal and Jacob[57] suggest testing the quadriceps muscle at 0°, 30°, 60°, and 90° while observing any abnormal tibial movement (e.g., ligament instability) or excessive pain from patellar compression (e.g., patellofemoral syndrome). Figure 12-34 shows the quadriceps complex components and their angle of pull. Table 12-4 lists the muscles acting at the knee.

Although these movements are tested with the patient in the supine-lying position, the hamstrings are often tested with the patient prone. If the knee is flexed to 90° and the heel is turned out, the greatest stress is placed on the lateral hamstring muscle (biceps femoris) with resisted knee flexion. If the heel is turned in, the greatest stress is placed on the medial hamstring (semimembranosus and semitendinosus) muscles.

Ankle movements are tested because the gastrocnemius muscle crosses the posterior knee and both plantar and dorsiflexion movements cause movement of the fibula. Dorsiflexion causes the fibula to move up and increases the stress being applied to the ligaments supporting the superior tibiofibular joint. Plantar flexion decreases the stress on these ligaments and also brings the gastrocnemius into play, supporting the posterior knee and assisting knee flexion.

If the history has indicated concentric, eccentric, or econcentric movements have caused symptoms, these types of contractions should be tested as well, but only after isometric testing has been performed.

Kannus and colleagues[58] developed a scoring scale for measuring isokinetic and isometric strength (Figure 12-35). The scale can be used to show improvement in strength over time. When using isokinetic values, different

Table 12-4

Muscles of the Knee: Their Actions, Nerve Supply, and Nerve Root Derivation

Action	Muscles Acting	Nerve Supply	Nerve Root Derivation
Flexion of knee	1. Biceps femoris	Sciatic	L5, S1–S2
	2. Semimembranosus	Sciatic	L5, S1–S2
	3. Semitendinosus	Sciatic	L5, S1–S2
	4. Gracilis	Obturator	L2–L3
	5. Sartorius	Femoral	L2–L3
	6. Popliteus	Tibial	L4–L5, S1
	7. Gastrocnemius	Tibial	S1–S2
	8. Tensor fasciae latae (in 45° to 145° of flexion)	Superior gluteal	L4–L5
	9. Plantaris	Tibial	S1–S2
Extension of knee	1. Rectus femoris	Femoral	L2–L4
	2. Vastus medialis	Femoral	L2–L4
	3. Vastus intermedius	Femoral	L2–L4
	4. Vastus lateralis	Femoral	L2–L4
	5. Tensor fasciae latae (in 0° to 30° of flexion)	Superior gluteal	L4–L5
Medial rotation of flexed leg (non–weight bearing)	1. Popliteus	Tibial	L4–L5
	2. Semimembranosus	Sciatic	L5, S1–S2
	3. Semitendinosus	Sciatic	L5, S1–S2
	4. Sartorius	Femoral	L2–L3
	5. Gracilis	Obturator	L2–L3
Lateral rotation of flexed leg (non–weight bearing)	1. Biceps femoris	Sciatic	L5, S1–S2

Scoring Scale for Isokinetic and Isometric Strength Measurements of the Knee Joint

	Peak Torque		Difference		
	Uninjured	Injured	Absolute	Percent	Score†
Isokinetic					
Extension 60°/sec	_____	_____	_____	_____	_____
Flexion 60°/sec	_____	_____	_____	_____	_____
Extension 180°/sec	_____	_____	_____	_____	_____
Flexion 180°/sec	_____	_____	_____	_____	_____
Isometric					
Extension 60°	_____	_____	_____	_____	_____
Flexion 60°	_____	_____	_____	_____	_____
Total score (maximum 100 points)					_____

†Scoring System
Isometric

Isokinetic
17 points = percent difference (uninjured – injured):	≤2%
15 points = percent difference (uninjured – injured):	3 to 5%
13 points = percent difference (uninjured – injured):	6 to 10%
9 points = percent difference (uninjured – injured):	11 to 25%
5 points = percent difference (uninjured – injured):	26 to 49%
0 points = percent difference (uninjured – injured):	≥50%

Isometric
16 points = percent difference (uninjured – injured):	≤2%
14 points = percent difference (uninjured – injured):	3 to 5%
12 points = percent difference (uninjured – injured):	6 to 10%
8 points = percent difference (uninjured – injured):	11 to 25%
4 points = percent difference (uninjured – injured):	26 to 49%
0 points = percent difference (uninjured – injured):	≥50%

Figure 12-35

Scoring scale for isokinetic and isometric strength measurements of the knee joint. (Modified from Kannus P et al: Knee strength evaluation, *Scand J Sport Sci* 9:9, 1987.)

Isokinetic Test Parameters Commonly Used for the Knee

- Left/right peak torque ratio
- Left/right average (mean) torque ratio
- Ratio of peak torque to body weight
- Torque curve analysis
- Bilateral total work comparison
- Hamstrings/quadriceps ratio (left and right)
- Ratio of average power to body weight
- Time ratio to torque development
- Time to 50% peak torque
- Endurance (fatigue) ratio (first to last repetition)

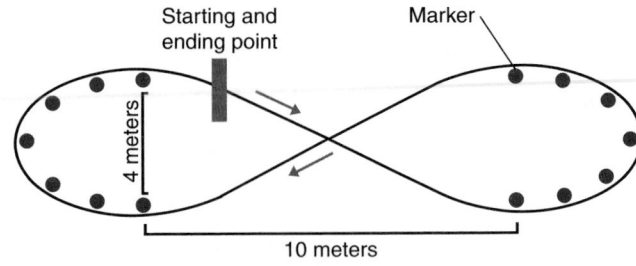

Figure 12-36

Figure-of-eight running track. (Redrawn from Fonseca ST, Magee DJ, Wessel J et al: Validation of a performance test for outcome evaluation of knee function, *Clin J Sport Med* 2:253, 1992.)

test parameters may be used. It is important to realize, however, that most knee isokinetic tests are not done with the knee in a functional position.

Depending on the speed, the hamstring/quadriceps ratio is normally between 50% and 60%.[59] As the speed of isokinetic testing increases, however, the ratio approaches 1:1, or 100%.[60,61]

Functional Assessment

Instabilities produced on the examining table are easily produced functionally, especially in athletes who participate in activities such as vigorous cutting and jumping or rapid deceleration, which produce high physiological joint loads. Functional tests and numerous numerical knee rating systems have been developed for the knee, many of them for specific populations (e.g., athletes) or to assess outcomes after surgery or for specific conditions. The examiner must pick the appropriate test or scale, realizing that each has advantages and disadvantages.[62,63]

If the active, passive, and resisted isometric movements are performed with little difficulty, the examiner may put the patient through a series of **functional tests** to see whether these sequential activities produce pain or other symptoms. These tests may be scored by the time taken to do the test or by the distance or height attained when doing the test. If the results are so measured, three measurements should be taken and averaged. In some cases, the results of different tests may be combined. Fonseca and coworkers[64] found that the time ratio of figure-of-eight running to straight running was one of the most effective ways of differentiating patients with anterior cruciate ligament deficiencies from normal patients (Figure 12-36).

These functional activities, which are provided as examples, must be geared to the individual patient. Squatting reveals limitations of flexion and may cause impingement

Sequential Functional Tests for the Knee

- Walking
- Ascending and descending stairs (walking → running)
- Squatting (both knees should flex symmetrically)
- Squatting and then bouncing at the end of the squat (again, the two knees should act symmetrically)
- Running straight ahead
- Running straight ahead and stopping on command
- Vertical jump
- Running and twisting (figure-of-eight running, carioca)
- Jumping and going into a full squat
- Hard cuts, twists, pivots

with meniscal lesions. Duck waddle, if attempted, can demonstrate increased symptoms in meniscal and ligamentous lesions. Older patients should not be expected to accomplish the last five or six (see above) movements unless they have been doing these or similar activities in the recent past. Daniel and coworkers[65] outlined different functional and intensity levels that are useful especially for getting an indication of functional activities from a patient's perspective (Table 12-5). Functional strength tests for sedentary individuals are shown in Table 12-6.

Strobel and Stedtfeld[66] put forward the **one-leg hop** test. The patient stands and does a "long jump" hop on one leg while landing on the same leg. This is a **single-leg hop for distance** (Figure 12-37A).[67,68] Noyes and associates[67] considered symmetry of less than 85% between the legs to be abnormal. The test is repeated three times alternately with each leg. If instability is evident, the distance for the affected leg is less than that for the normal leg. Juris et al.[69] advocated doing a **maximal controlled leap** in addition to the one-leg hop test. For this test, which is said to test force absorption, the patient stands on one foot and "leaps forward" to land on the opposite

Table 12-5

Patient Activity Scale

Functional Levels	
Level I	Activities of daily living (ADL)
Level II	Straight running; sports that do not involve lower-limb agility activities; occupations involving heavy lifting
Level III	Activities that require lower-limb agility but not involving jumping, hard cutting, or pivoting
Level IV	Activities involving jumping, hard cutting, or pivoting
Intensity	
W	Work related or occupational
LR	Light recreational
VR	Vigorous recreational
C	Competitive

Exposure

Number of hours per year of participation at any given functional level and intensity

From Daniel D et al, editors: *Knee ligaments: structure, injury and repair*, p. 522, New York, 1990, Raven Press.

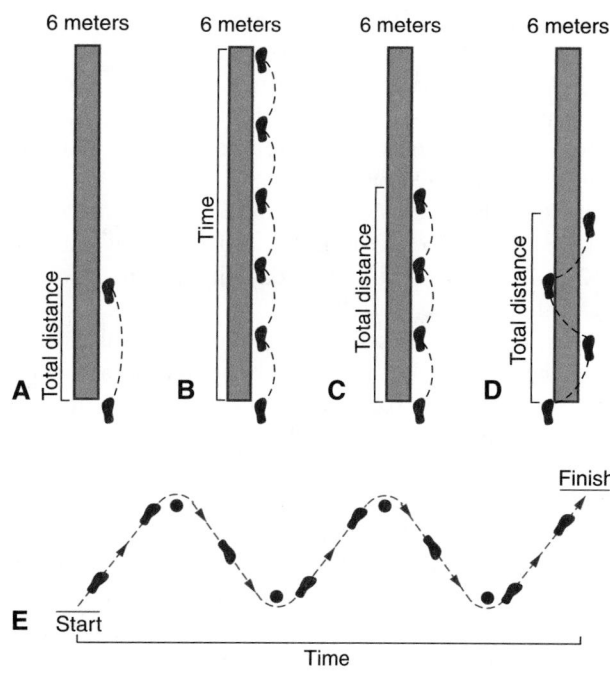

Figure 12-37

Hop tests. **A**, Single hop for distance. **B**, Timed hop. **C**, Triple hop for distance. **D**, Crossover hop for distance. **E**, 30-m agility hop test.

foot. Patients should be instructed to maintain the flexed hip/knee position during takeoff and extend the leg for landing. Patients must "stick" on landing with no movement of the landing foot and must be upright with hands on hips within 1 second. The distance is measured and the test repeated with the opposite start leg.

Table 12-6

Functional Testing of the Knee

Starting Position	Action	Functional Test
Standing	1. Walking backward 2. Running forward 20° (knee flexion)	6–8 m: functional 3–6 m: functionally fair 1–3 m: functionally poor 0 m: nonfunctional
Standing	1. Squat 20° to 30° 2. Jump, lifting body off floor	5 to 6 repetitions: functional 3 to 4 repetitions: functionally fair 1 to 2 repetitions: functionally poor 0 repetitions: nonfunctional

Data from Palmar ML, Epler M: *Clinical assessment procedures in physical therapy*, pp. 275–276, Philadelphia, 1990, JB Lippincott.

Since the advent of the single-leg hop, modifications have been developed. Each test is usually repeated three times, and the average of the three scores is used as the measured value. These modifications include the following:

1. **Single-leg hop for time**. With this test, the patient is assessed for the time taken to hop 6 m (20 ft) on one leg (Figure 12-37B). The good leg is tested first, followed by the injured leg.[67,68,70]

2. **Triple hop**. With this test, the patient is asked to hop as far as possible, taking three hops. The distance for the good leg is compared with that for the injured leg (Figure 12-37C).[67,68,70]

3. **Crossover hop**. A straight line is marked on the floor. The patient is asked to take three consecutive hops on one foot, crossing over the straight line each time (Figure 12-37D). The good limb is tested, followed by the injured limb, and the average distances attained with each leg are compared.[67] Risberg and Ekeland[71] modified this test and called it the **side jump test**. For this test, two 6-m parallel lines are placed 30 cm (12 inches) apart on the floor. Outside one line, 10 marks are made at 60-cm (24-inch) intervals. Outside the other line, marks are made at 60-cm (24-inch) intervals but starting at 30 cm (12 inches), so that the marks are staggered from one side to the other. The patient is asked to hop from marker to marker on each line. The good leg is timed, followed by the injured leg.

4. **Agility hop**. This hop test requires a space of 30 m (100 ft). Cones are placed 6 m (20 ft) apart (Figure 12-37E). The patient is then timed as he or she hops through the cones. The good limb is tested, followed by the injured limb, and the average times attained with each leg are compared.[70]

5. **Stairs hop test (stairs hopple test)**.[71] The patient is timed as he or she hops up and down several steps (20 to 25 steps recommended), first on the good leg and then on the injured leg.

These functional tests are for active persons and can be quite demanding. Losee[72] mentioned several additional tests. For example, in the **deceleration test**, the patient is asked to run at full speed and to stop suddenly on command.[26] The test is positive for rotary instability if the patient stops without using the quadriceps or decelerates in a crouched position (more than 30° flexion of the knee). The effect of the test can be accentuated by having the patient turn away from the affected leg just as he or she is about to stop.[73] As the patient does the test, the examiner should watch to ensure that the patient uses the affected leg to help stop. With instability problems, the patient uses only the good leg to stop, "hopping through" with the injured leg.

For the **"disco test,"** the patient stands on one leg with the knee flexed 10° to 20°. The patient is asked to rotate or twist left and right while holding the flexed position (Figure 12-38).[26] Apprehension during the test or refusal to do the test is a positive sign for rotary instability. If pain is felt on the joint line, it may indicate meniscus pathology, in which case it is called **Merke's sign**.[66] Pain on medial rotation along the joint line implies medial meniscus pathology, and pain on lateral rotation implies lateral meniscus pathology.

Larson[74] advocated the **leaning hop test**. For this test, the patient hops up and down on one leg while abducting the opposite leg. A positive test is apprehension during the test or refusal to do the test and is a positive sign for rotary instability.

Numerical rating systems are commonly done to determine the state of the knee. Most of these measures combine clinical (e.g., ROM) and functional (e.g., stair climbing) measures. Many of these scoring systems have not been tested on normal subjects and show possible interviewer bias, nor are the values given to each measure explained. In addition, there may be male and female differences.[75,76]

Noyes and colleagues[77–79] developed the Cincinnati Knee Rating System (Figure 12-39), which deals with pain, swelling, stability, and activity level and is a good functional rating system for active persons. Irrgang and associates[80] use two scales, an Activities of Daily Living Scale[81] and a Sports Activity Scale (Figures 12-40 and 12-41), to detect clinically significant changes over time. The Knee Society[82] also has a rating scale (Figure 12-42). The Knee Society advocates keeping knee rating and

Figure 12-38

Losee disco test. Flexion, compression, and rotation may lead to shift of femur on tibia, causing rotary instability.

functional assessment separate. This knee-rating scale deals first with pain, ROM, and stability, giving positive points up to 100 and grouping deductions that can take away from the overall value. Function is dealt with separately on the scale.

Lysholm and Gillquist[83] developed a frequently used scale primarily designed to score clinical instability that may also be used for chondral lesions of the knee[84] (Table 12-7). The International Knee Documentation Committee[85,86] has also developed a knee scale (Figure 12-43). Table 12-8 shows an example of a patellofemoral joint evaluation scale that can be used to assess functional levels in patients with patellofemoral syndrome after surgery or nonsurgery.[87,88] Similar scales used to measure patellofemoral dysfunction also exist.[89–92] Other scales, such as the Western Ontario and McMaster University Osteoarthritis Index (WOMAC), Knee Injury and Osteoarthritis Outcome Score (KOOS), and Lequesne Index, have been developed to determine the outcome of arthroplasties in osteoarthritis (see Chapter 11).[93–103] Each of these knee-rating scales is slightly different. The scale that works best for the examiner and the examiner's clientele should be used. Other knee-rating scales are also available.[83,104–108]

Cincinnati Knee Rating System

Symptoms (50 points):

Left	Right			Left	Right	
			1. Pain			*Location of pain:*
☐	☐	20	No pain, normal knee, performs 100%.	☐	☐	Medial (inner side)
☐	☐	16	Occasional pain with strenuous sports or heavy work, knee not entirely normal, some limitations, but minor and tolerable.	☐	☐	Anterior-patellar (front/knee cap)
				☐	☐	Posterior (back of knee)
☐	☐	12	Occasional pain with light recreational sports or moderate work activities, frequently brought on by vigorous activities, running, heavy labor, strenuous sports.	☐	☐	Diffuse (all over)
						Pain occurs on:
☐	☐	8	Pain, usually brought on by sports, light recreational activities, or moderate work. Occasionally occurs with walking, standing, or light work.	☐	☐	Stairs
				☐	☐	Sitting
				☐	☐	Kneeling
☐	☐	4	Pain is a significant problem with activities as simple as walking. Relieved by rest. Unable to do sports.	☐	☐	Standing
						Type of pain:
☐	☐	0	Pain present all the time, occurs with walking, standing and at nighttime. Not relieved with rest.	☐	☐	Sharp
				☐	☐	Aching
				☐	☐	Throbbing
☐	☐		I do not know what my pain level is. I have not tested my knee.	☐	☐	Burning

Intensity of pain:
☐ Mild ☐ Moderate ☐ Severe
Frequency: ☐ Intermittent ☐ Constant

Left	Right		
			2. Swelling
☐	☐	10	No swelling, normal knee, 100% activity.
☐	☐	8	Occasional swelling with strenuous sports or heavy work. Some limitations but minor and tolerable.
☐	☐	6	Occasional swelling with light recreational sports or moderate work activities, frequently brought on by vigorous activities, running, heavy labor, strenuous sports.
☐	☐	4	Swelling limits sports and moderate work. Occurs infrequently with simple walking activities or light work (about 3 times/year).
☐	☐	2	Swelling brought on by simple walking activities and light work. Relieved with rest.
☐	☐	0	Severe problem all of the time, with simple walking activities.
☐	☐		I do not know what my swelling level is. I have not tested my knee.

If swelling occurs it is: (check one box on each line)
Intensity: ☐ Mild ☐ Moderate ☐ Severe
Frequency: ☐ Intermittent ☐ Constant

Left	Right		
			3. Giving-way.
☐	☐	20	No giving-way, normal knee, performs 100%.
☐	☐	16	Occasional giving-way with strenuous sports or heavy work. Can participate in all sports but some guarding or limitations are still present.
☐	☐	12	Occasional giving-way with light recreational activities or moderate work. Able to compensate, limits vigorous activities; sports or heavy work; not able to cut or twist suddenly.
☐	☐	8	Giving-way limits sports and moderate work; occurs infrequently with walking or light work (about 3 times/year).
☐	☐	4	Giving-way with simple walking activities and light work. Occurs once per month. Requires guarding.
☐	☐	0	Severe problem with simple walking activities; cannot turn or twist while walking without giving-way.
☐	☐		I do not know my level of giving-way. I have not tested my knee.

4. Other Symptoms (unscored)

Left	Right	Knee stiffness			Kneecap grinding			Knee locking
☐	☐	None	☐	☐	None	☐	☐	None
☐	☐	Occasional	☐	☐	Mild	☐	☐	Occasional
☐	☐	Frequent	☐	☐	Moderate	☐	☐	Frequent
			☐	☐	Severe			

Figure 12-39

Cincinnati Knee Rating System. (From Noyes FR et al: Functional disability in the anterior cruciate insufficient knee syndrome, *Sports Med* 1:287–288, 1984.)

Continued

Cincinnati Knee Rating System (*Continued*)

Function (50 points):

			5. Overall activity level
☐	☐	20	No limitation, normal knee, able to do everything including strenuous sports or heavy labor.
☐	☐	16	Perform sports including vigorous activities, but at a lower performance level, involves guarding or some limits to heavy labor.
☐	☐	12	Light recreational activities possible with rare symptoms, more strenuous activities cause problems. Active but in different sports, limited to moderate work.
☐	☐	8	No sports or recreational activities possible. Walking activities possible with rare symptoms, limited to light work.
☐	☐	4	Walking, activities of daily living cause moderate symptoms, frequent limitation.
☐	☐	0	Walking, activities of daily living cause severe problems, persistent symptoms.
☐	☐		I do not know what my real activity level is, I have not tested my knee, or I have given up strenuous sports.

			6. Walking
☐	☐	10	Normal, unlimited.
☐	☐	8	Slight/mild problem.
☐	☐	6	Moderate problem: smooth surface possible up to 800 m.
☐	☐	4	Severe problem: only 2–3 blocks possible.
☐	☐	2	Severe problem: requires cane, crutches.

			7. Stairs
☐	☐	10	Normal, unlimited.
☐	☐	8	Slight/mild problem.
☐	☐	6	Moderate problem: only 10–15 steps possible.
☐	☐	4	Severe problem: requires bannister, support.
☐	☐	2	Severe problem: only 1–5 steps possible.

			8. Running activity
☐	☐	5	Normal, unlimited: fully competitive, strenuous.
☐	☐	4	Slight/mild problem: run half-speed.
☐	☐	3	Moderate problem: only 2–4 km possible.
☐	☐	2	Severe problem: only 1–2 blocks possible.
☐	☐	1	Severe problem: only a few steps.

			9. Jumping or twisting activities
☐	☐	5	Normal, unlimited, fully competitive, strenuous.
☐	☐	4	Slight/mild problem: some guarding, but sports possible.
☐	☐	3	Moderate problem: gave up strenuous sports; recreational sports possible.
☐	☐	2	Severe problem: affects all sports, must constantly guard.
☐	☐	1	Severe problem: only light activity possible (golf, swimming).

Total: Left [ ] Right [ ] (Maximum: 100 points)

Figure 12-39 cont'd ▮▬▬▬▬▬▬▬

Ligament Stability

Because the knee, more than any other joint in the body, depends on its ligaments to maintain its integrity, it is imperative that the ligaments be tested. The ligaments of the knee joint act as primary stabilizers and guide the movement of the bones in proper relation to one another. Depending on the motion being tested, the ligaments act as primary or secondary restraints (Table 12-9). For example, the anterior cruciate ligament is the primary restraint to anterior tibial displacement and a secondary restraint to varus-valgus motion in full extension and rotation.[80,109] If the primary restraint is injured, pathological motion occurs. If the secondary restraint is injured but the primary restraint is not, pathological motion in that direction does not occur.

If both primary and secondary restraints are injured, the pathological motion is greater.[80] There are several ligaments around the knee, but four deserve special mention (Figure 12-44).

Collateral and Cruciate Ligaments

Collateral Ligaments. The **medial (tibial) collateral ligament** lies more posteriorly than anteriorly on the medial aspect of the tibiofemoral joint. It is made up of two layers, one superficial and one deep. The deep layer is a thickening of the joint capsule that blends with the medial meniscus; it is sometimes called the medial capsular ligament. The superficial layer is a strong, broad triangular strap. It starts distal to the adductor tubercle and extends to the medial surface of the tibia, approximately 6 cm (2.4 inches) below the joint line. It blends with the

Text continued on page 758

Instructions:

The following questionnaire is designed to determine the symptoms and limitations that you experience because of your knee while you perform your usual *daily activities.* Please answer each question by ***checking the statement that best describes you over the last 1 to 2 days.*** For a given question, more than one of the statements may describe you, but please mark ONLY the statement which best describes you during your usual daily activities.

Symptoms

1. To what degree does pain in your knee affect your daily activity level?
   ___ I never have pain in my knee.
   ___ I have pain in my knee but it does not affect my daily activity.
   ___ Pain affects my activity slightly.
   ___ Pain affects my activity moderately.
   ___ Pain affects my activity severely.
   ___ Pain in my knee prevents me from performing all daily activities.

2. To what degree does grinding or grating of your knee affect your daily activity level?
   ___ I never have grinding or grating in my knee.
   ___ I have grinding or grating in my knee, but it does not affect my daily activity.
   ___ Grinding or grating affects my activity slightly.
   ___ Grinding or grating affects my activity moderately.
   ___ Grinding or grating affects my activity severely.
   ___ Grinding or grating in my knee prevents me from performing all daily activities.

3. To what degree does stiffness in your knee affect your daily activity level?
   ___ I never have stiffness in my knee.
   ___ I have stiffness in my knee, but it does not affect my daily activity.
   ___ Stiffness affects my activity slightly.
   ___ Stiffness affects my activity moderately.
   ___ Stiffness affects my activity severely.
   ___ Stiffness in my knee prevents me from performing all daily activities.

4. To what degree does swelling in your knee affect your daily activity level?
   ___ I never have swelling in my knee.
   ___ I have swelling in my knee, but it does not affect my daily activity.
   ___ Swelling affects my activity slightly.
   ___ Swelling affects my activity moderately.
   ___ Swelling affects my activity severely.
   ___ Swelling in my knee prevents me from performing all daily activities.

5. To what degree does slipping of your knee affect your daily activity level?
   ___ I never have slipping of my knee.
   ___ I have slipping of my knee, but it does not affect my daily activity.
   ___ Slipping of my knee affects my activity slightly.
   ___ Slipping of my knee affects my activity moderately.
   ___ Slipping of my knee affects my activity severely.
   ___ Slipping of my knee prevents me from performing all daily activities.

6. To what degree does buckling of your knee affect your daily activity level?
   ___ I never have buckling of my knee.
   ___ I have buckling of my knee, but it does not affect my daily activity level.
   ___ Buckling of my knee affects my activity slightly.
   ___ Buckling of my knee affects my activity moderately.
   ___ Buckling of my knee affects my activity severely.
   ___ Buckling of my knee prevents me from performing all daily activities.

7. To what degree does weakness or lack of strength of your leg affect your daily activity level?
   ___ My leg never feels weak.
   ___ My leg feels weak, but it does not affect my daily activity.
   ___ Weakness affects my activity slightly.
   ___ Weakness affects my activity moderately.
   ___ Weakness affects my activity severely.
   ___ Weakness of my leg prevents me from performing all daily activities.

Functional Disability with Activities of Daily Living

8. How does your knee affect your ability to walk?
   ___ My knee does not affect my ability to walk.
   ___ I have pain in my knee when walking, but it does not limit my ability to walk.
   ___ My knee prevents me from walking more than 1 mile.
   ___ My knee prevents me from walking more than 1/2 mile.
   ___ My knee prevents me from walking more than 1 block.
   ___ My knee prevents me from walking.

9. Because of your knee, do you walk with crutches or a cane?
   ___ I can walk without crutches or a cane.
   ___ My knee causes me to walk with one crutch or a cane.
   ___ My knee causes me to walk with two crutches.
   ___ Because of my knee, I cannot walk, even with crutches.

10. Does your knee cause you to limp when you walk?
   ___ I can walk without a limp.
   ___ Sometimes my knee causes me to walk with a limp.
   ___ Because of my knee, I cannot walk without a limp.

11. How does your knee affect your ability to go up stairs?
   ___ My knee does not affect my ability to go up stairs.
   ___ I have pain in my knee when going up stairs, but it does not limit my ability to go up stairs.
   ___ I am able to go up stairs normally, but I need to rely on use of a railing.
   ___ I am able to go up stairs one step at a time with the use of a railing.
   ___ I have to use crutches or a cane to go up stairs.
   ___ I cannot go up stairs.

Figure 12-40 ▬▬▬

Activities of Daily Living Scale of the Knee Outcome Survey. (From Irrgang JJ et al: ligamentous and meniscal injuries. In Zachazewski JE et al, editors: *Athletic injuries and rehabilitation*, pp. 683–684, Philadelphia, 1996, WB Saunders.)

Continued

Activities of Daily Living Scale of the Knee Outcome Survey (Continued)

12. How does your knee affect your ability to go down stairs?
    ___ My knee does not affect my ability to go down stairs.
    ___ I have pain in my knee when going down stairs, but it does not limit my ability to go down stairs.
    ___ I am able to go down stairs normally, but I need to rely on use of a railing.
    ___ I am able to go down stairs one step at a time with the use of a railing.
    ___ I have to use crutches or a cane to go down stairs.
    ___ I cannot go down stairs.

13. How does your knee affect your ability to stand?
    ___ My knee does not affect my ability to stand. I can stand for unlimited amounts of time.
    ___ I have pain in my knee when standing, but it does not limit my ability to stand.
    ___ Because of my knee, I cannot stand for more than 1 hour.
    ___ Because of my knee, I cannot stand for more than 1/2 hour.
    ___ Because of my knee, I cannot stand for more than 10 minutes.
    ___ I cannot stand because of my knee.

14. How does your knee affect your ability to kneel on the front of your knee?
    ___ My knee does not affect my ability to kneel on the front of my knee. I can kneel for unlimited amounts of time.
    ___ I have pain when kneeling on the front of my knee, but it does not limit my ability to kneel.
    ___ I cannot kneel on the front of my knee for more than 1 hour.
    ___ I cannot kneel on the front of my knee for more than 1/2 hour.
    ___ I cannot kneel on the front of my knee for more than 10 minutes.
    ___ I cannot kneel on the front of my knee.

15. How does your knee affect your ability to squat?
    ___ My knee does not affect my ability to squat. I can squat all the way down.
    ___ I have pain when squatting, but I can still squat all the way down.
    ___ I cannot squat more than 3/4 of the way down.
    ___ I cannot squat more than halfway down.
    ___ I cannot squat more than 1/4 of the way down.
    ___ I cannot squat at all.

16. How does your knee affect your ability to sit with your knee bent?
    ___ My knee does not affect my ability to sit with my knee bent. I can sit for unlimited amounts of time.
    ___ I have pain when sitting with my knee bent, but it does not limit my ability to sit.
    ___ I cannot sit with my knee bent for more than 1 hour.
    ___ I cannot sit with my knee bent for more than 1/2 hour.
    ___ I cannot sit with my knee bent for more than 10 minutes.
    ___ I cannot sit with my knee bent.

17. How does your knee affect your ability to rise from a chair?
    ___ My knee does not affect my ability to rise from a chair.
    ___ I have pain when rising from the seated position, but it does not affect my ability to rise from the seated position.
    ___ Because of my knee, I can only rise from a chair if I use my hands and arms to assist.
    ___ Because of my knee, I cannot rise from a chair.

18. How would you rate your current level of knee function during your *usual daily activities* on a scale from 0 to 100, with 100 being your level of knee function prior to your injury?

    _____

19. How would you rate the *overall function* of your knee during your *usual daily activities*?
    _____ normal
    _____ nearly normal
    _____ abnormal
    _____ severely abnormal

20. As a result of your knee injury, how would you rate your *current level of daily activity*?
    _____ normal
    _____ nearly normal
    _____ abnormal
    _____ severely abnormal

21. Since initiation of treatment for your knee, how would you describe your progress?
    _____ greatly improved
    _____ somewhat improved
    _____ neither improved/worsened
    _____ somewhat worse
    _____ greatly worse

Changes in Daily Activity Level

Please use the following scale to answer questions A–C below.

1 = I was able to perform *unlimited physical work,* which included lifting and climbing.
2 = I was able to perform *limited physical work,* which included lifting and climbing.
3 = I was able to perform *unlimited light activities,* which included walking on level surfaces and stairs.
4 = I was able to perform *limited light activities,* which included walking on level surfaces and stairs.
5 = I was *unable to perform light activities,* which included walking on level surfaces and stairs.

A. ___ *Prior to your knee injury,* how would you describe your usual daily activity? Please indicate only the **HIGHEST** level of activity that described you before your knee injury.

B. ___ *Prior to surgery or treatment* of your knee, how would you describe your usual daily activity? Please indicate only the **HIGHEST** level of activity that described you prior to surgery or treatment to your knee.

C. ___ How would you describe your *current level* of daily activity? Please indicate only the **HIGHEST** level of activity that describes you over the last 1 to 2 days.

Figure 12-40 cont'd

Sports Activity Scale of the Knee Outcome Survey

Instructions:

The following questionnaire is designed to determine the symptoms and limitations that you experience because of your knee while you participate in sports activities. Please answer each question by checking the statement that best describes you over the last 1 to 2 days. For a given question, more than one of the statements may describe you, but please mark ONLY the statement which best describes you when you participate in sports activities.

Symptoms

1. To what degree does pain in your knee affect your sports activity level?
   ___ I never have pain in my knee.
   ___ Knee pain does not affect my activity.
   ___ Slightly.
   ___ Moderately.
   ___ Severely.
   ___ Prevents me from performing all sports activities.

2. To what degree does grinding or grating of your knee affect your sports activity level?
   ___ I never have grinding or grating in my knee.
   ___ Grinding/grating does not affect my activity.
   ___ Slightly.
   ___ Moderately.
   ___ Severely.
   ___ Prevents me from performing all sports activities.

3. To what degree does stiffness in your knee affect your sports activity level?
   ___ I never have stiffness in my knee.
   ___ Knee stiffness does not affect my activity.
   ___ Slightly.
   ___ Moderately.
   ___ Severely.
   ___ Prevents me from performing all sports activities.

4. To what degree does swelling in your knee affect your sports activity level?
   ___ I never have swelling in my knee.
   ___ Knee swelling does not affect my activity.
   ___ Slightly.
   ___ Moderately.
   ___ Severely.
   ___ Prevents me from performing all sports activities.

5. To what degree does partial giving way or slipping of your knee affect your sports activity level?
   ___ I never have partial giving way or slipping of my knee.
   ___ Partial giving way does not affect my activity.
   ___ Slightly.
   ___ Moderately.
   ___ Severely.
   ___ Prevents me from performing all sports activities.

6. To what degree does complete giving way or buckling of your knee affect your sports activity level?
   ___ I never have complete giving way or buckling in my knee.
   ___ Knee buckling does not affect my activity.
   ___ Slightly.
   ___ Moderately.
   ___ Severely.
   ___ Prevents me from performing all sports activities.

Functional Disability with Sports Activities

1. How does your knee affect your ability to run straight ahead?
   ___ I am able to run straight ahead full speed without limitations.
   ___ I have pain in my knee but it does not affect my ability.
   ___ Slightly.
   ___ Moderately.
   ___ Severely.
   ___ Prevents me from running.

2. How does your knee affect your ability to jump and land on your involved leg?
   ___ I am able to jump and land on my involved leg without limitations.
   ___ I have pain in my knee but it does not affect my ability.
   ___ Slightly.
   ___ Moderately.
   ___ Severely.
   ___ Prevents me from jumping and landing.

3. How does your knee affect your ability to stop and start quickly?
   ___ I am able to start and stop quickly without limitations.
   ___ I have pain in my knee but it does not affect my ability.
   ___ Slightly.
   ___ Moderately.
   ___ Severely.
   ___ Prevents me from stopping and starting quickly.

4. How does your knee affect your ability to cut and pivot on your involved leg?
   ___ I am able to cut and pivot on my involved leg without limitations.
   ___ I have pain in my knee but it does not affect my ability.
   ___ Slightly.
   ___ Moderately.
   ___ Severely.
   ___ Prevents me from jumping and landing.

Figure 12-41

Sports Activity Scale of the Knee Outcome Survey. (From Irrgang JJ et al: ligamentous and meniscal injuries. In Zachazewski JE et al, editors: *Athletic injuries and rehabilitation*, pp. 683–685, Philadelphia, 1996, WB Saunders.)

Knee Society Knee Score

Patient category
A. Unilateral or bilateral (opposite knee successfully replaced)
B. Unilateral, other knee symptomatic
C. Multiple arthritis or medical infirmity

Pain	Points	Function	Points
None	50	Walking	50
Mild or occasional	45	Unlimited	40
Stairs only	40	>10 blocks	30
Walking and stairs	30	5–10 blocks	20
Moderate		<5 blocks	10
Occasional	20	Housebound	0
Continual	10	Unable	
Severe	0	Stairs	
		Normal up and down	50
Range of Motion		Normal up; down with rail	40
(5° = 1 point)	25	Up and down with rail	30
		Up with rail; unable down	15
Stability (maximum		Unable	0
movement in any position)			
		Subtotal	
Anteroposterior			
<5 mm	10	Deductions (minus)	
5–10 mm	5	Cane	5
10 mm	0	Two canes	10
Mediolateral		Crutches or walker	20
<5°	15		
6°–9°	10	**Total deductions**	
10°–14°	5		
15°	0	**Function score**	

Subtotal

Deductions (minus)

Flexion contracture	
5°–10°	2
10°–15°	5
16°–20°	10
>20°	15
Extension lag	
<10°	5
10°–20°	10
>20°	15
Alignment	
5°–10°	0
0°–4°	3 points each degree
11°–15°	3 points each degree
Other	20

Total deductions

Pain score
(if total is a minus number, score is 0)

Figure 12-42

Knee Society knee score. (From Insall JN et al: Rationale of the Knee Society clinical rating system, *Clin Orthop* 248:14, 1989.)

posterior capsule and is separated from the capsule and the medial meniscus by a bursa.

The entire medial collateral ligament is tight throughout the full ROM, although there is varying stress placed on different parts of the ligament as it moves through the full range because of the shape of the femoral condyles.

All of its fibers are taut on full extension. In flexion, the anterior fibers are the most taut; in mid range, the posterior fibers are the most taut.[110]

The **lateral (fibular) collateral ligament** is round and lies under the tendon of the biceps femoris muscle. It runs from the lateral epicondyle of the femur to the

Table 12-7

Lysholm Scoring Scale

	Points
Limp (5 points)	
None	5
Slight or periodic	3
Severe and constant	0
Support (5 points)	
Full support	5
Stick or crutch	3
Weight bearing impossible	0
Stair Climbing (10 points)	
No problems	10
Slightly impaired	6
One step at a time	2
Unable	0
Squatting (5 points)	
No problems	5
Slightly impaired	4
Not past 90°	2
Unable	0
Walking, Running, and Jumping (70 points)	
Instability	
Never giving way	30
Rarely during athletic or other severe exertion	25
Frequently during athletic or other severe exertion (or unable to participate)	20
Occasionally in daily activities	10
Often in daily activities	5
Every step	0
Pain	
None	30
Inconstant and slight during severe exertion	25
Marked on giving way	20
Marked during severe exertion	15
Marked on or after walking more than 2 km	10
Marked on or after walking less than 2 km	5
Constant and severe	0
Swelling	
None	10
With giving way	7
On severe exertion	5
On ordinary exertion	2
Constant	0
Atrophy of Thigh (5 points)	
None	5
1–2 cm	3
More than 2 cm	0
Total Score	100

Modified from Lysholm J, Gillquist J: Evaluation of knee ligament surgery results with special emphasis on use of a scoring scale, *Am J Sports Med* 10:150–154, 1982.

fibular head. It also lies more posteriorly than anteriorly. This ligament is tight in extension and loosens in flexion, especially after 30° flexion. As the knee flexes, it provides protection to the lateral aspect of the knee. It is not attached to the lateral meniscus but rather is separated from it by a small fat pad.[110]

Cruciate Ligaments. The cruciate ligaments cross each other and are the primary rotary stabilizers of the knee.[111] These strong ligaments are named in relation to their attachment to the tibia and are intracapsular but extrasynovial. Each ligament has an anteromedial and a posterolateral portion. The anterior cruciate ligament has, in addition, an intermediate portion.

The **anterior cruciate ligament** extends superiorly, posteriorly, and laterally, twisting on itself as it extends from the tibia to the femur. Its main functions are to prevent anterior movement of the tibia on the femur, to check lateral rotation of the tibia in flexion, and, to a lesser extent, to check extension and hyperextension at the knee. It also helps to control the normal rolling and gliding movement of the knee. The anteromedial bundle is tight in both flexion and extension, whereas the posterolateral bundle is tight on extension only. As a whole, the ligament has the least amount of stress on it between 30° and 60° flexion.[110–113]

The **posterior cruciate ligament** extends superiorly, anteriorly, and medially from the tibia to the femur. This strong, fan-shaped ligament, the stoutest ligament in the knee, is a primary stabilizer of the knee against posterior movement of the tibia on the femur, and it checks extension and hyperextension. In addition, the ligament helps to maintain rotary stability and functions as the knee's central axis of rotation. Along with the anterior cruciate ligament, it acts as a rotary guide to the "screwing home" mechanism of the knee.[110,113] For the posterior cruciate ligament, the bulk of the fibers are tight at 30° flexion, but the posterolateral fibers are loose in early flexion.

With lateral rotation of the tibia, both collateral ligaments become more taut, and the cruciate ligaments become relaxed (Figure 12-45). With medial rotation of the tibia, the reverse action occurs: the collateral ligaments become more relaxed, and the cruciate ligaments become tighter.[110,114]

Testing of Ligaments

When testing the ligaments of the knee, the examiner must watch for four one-plane instabilities and four rotational instabilities (Table 12-10 and Figure 12-46).

There are a number of tests for each type of instability. The examiner should use the one or two tests that he or she believes gives the best results. It is not essential to do all of the tests discussed. The techniques chosen must be practiced diligently so that the examiner becomes proficient at doing them; only with practice will the examiner be able to determine which structures are injured. It is

Guidelines for Evaluating Outcome of Knee Ligament Injury or Surgery

Name: _____ First name: _____ DOB: ___/___/___ med. rec. #:_____

Examiner: _____ Date of examination: __/__/__ Date of injury/ies: __/__/__ ; __/__/__ Date of surgeries: __/__/__

Causes of injury: □ ADL*[2]　□ traff.　□ non-pivoting non-contact sports　□ pivoting non-contact sp.　□ contact sp. □ work

Time inj. to surg.: _____ (months)　□ acute (0-2 weeks)　□ subacute (2-8 weeks)　□ chronic (>8 weeks)

Knee involved: □ r. □ l.　opposite knee: □ norm.　□ injured　exam. under anesthes.: □ yes　□ no

Postop. diagnosis: _____

Surgical proced.: _____

Status menisci: norm. □ med. □ lat.　1/3 removed: □ med. □ lat.　2/3 removed: □ med. □ lat.　compl. rem. □ med. □ lat.

Morphotype:　□ lax　□ normal　□ tight　□ varus　□ valgus

Activ. level*[3]:　preinjury: □ I □ II □ III □ IV　pretreatment: □ I □ II □ III □ IV

present: □ I □ II □ III □ IV　Eventual change knee-related: □ yes □ no

GROUPS (PROBLEM AREA)	QUALIFICATION WITHIN GROUPS　*[4]				GROUP QUALIFIC.			
	A: normal	B: nearly norm.	C: abnormal	D: sev. abnorm.	A	B	C	D*[4]
1. PATIENT SUBJECTIVE ASSESSMENT								
How does your knee function?	□ normally	□ nearly norm.	□ abnormally	□ sev. abnorm.				
On a scale of 0 to 3 how does your knee affect your activity level?	□ 0	□ 1	□ 2	□ 3	□	□	□	□
2. SYMPTOMS (absence of significant symptoms, at highest activity level known by patient) *[5]								
No pain at activity level *[3]	□ I	□ II	□ III	□ IV or worse				
No swelling at activity level *[3]	□ I	□ II	□ III	□ IV or worse				
No partial giving way at activity level *[3]	□ I	□ II	□ III	□ IV or worse				
No complete giving way at activity level *[3]	□ I	□ II	□ III	□ IV or worse	□	□	□	□
3. RANGE OF MOTION: Flex./ext.: documented side: __/__/__ opposite side: __/__/__ *[6]								
Lack of extension (from zero anatomic)	□ <3°	□ 3-5°	□ 6-10°	□ >10°				
△ *[7] lack of flexion	□ 0-5°	□ 6-15°	□ 16-25°	□ >25°	□	□	□	□
4. LIGAMENT EXAMINATION *[8]		3 to 5mm or	6 to 10mm					
△ *[7] Lachman (in 25°. flex.) *[9]	□ −1 to 2mm	□ −1 to −3mm[10]	□ or <−3mm	□ >10mm				
idem (alternative measurement, optional)	□ −1 to 2mm	□ 3-5/−1 to −3mm	□ 6-10/<−3mm	□ >10mm				
Endpoint: □ firm □ soft								
△ *[7] total a.p.transl. in 70° flex. *[9]	□ 0 to 2mm	□ 3 to 5mm	□ 6 to 10mm	□ >10mm				
idem (alternative measurement, optional)	□ 0 to 2mm	□ 3 to 5mm	□ 6 to 10mm	□ >10mm				
△ *[7] post. sag in 70° flex.	□ 0 to 2mm	□ 3 to 5mm	□ 6 to 10mm	□ >10mm				
△ *[7] med. joint opening (valgus rotation)	□ 0 to 2mm	□ 3 to 5mm	□ 6 to 10mm	□ >10mm				
△ *[7] lat. joint opening (varus rotation)	□ 0 to 2mm	□ 3 to 5mm	□ 6 to 10mm	□ >10mm				
Pivot shift *[11]	□ neg.	□ + (glide)	□ ++ (clunk)	□ +++ (gross)				
△ *[7] reversed pivot shift	□ equal (neg.)	□ slight	□ marked	□ gross				
	□ equal (pos.)				□	□	□	□
5. COMPARTMENTAL FINDINGS *[12]								
△ *[7] Crepitus patellofemoral	□ none/equal	□ moderate	□ painful	□ severe				
△ *[7] Crepitus medial compartment	□ none	□ moderate	□ painful	□ severe				
△ *[7] Crepitus lateral compartment	□ none	□ moderate	□ painful	□ severe				
6. HARVEST SITE PATHOLOGY *[13]								
Tenderness, irritation, numbness	□ none	□ slight	□ moderate	□ severe				
7. X-RAY FINDINGS (DEGENERATIVE JOINT DISEASE) *[14]								
Patellofemoral cartilage space	□ normal	□ >4mm	□ 2-4mm	□ <2mm				
Medial compartment cartilage space	□ normal	□ >4mm	□ 2-4mm	□ <2mm				
Lateral compartment cartilage space	□ normal	□ >4mm	□ 2-4mm	□ <2mm				
8. FUNCTIONAL TEST *[15]								
△ One leg hop (percent of opposite side)	□ 90-100%	□ 76-90%	□ 50-75%	□ <50%				
FINAL EVALUATION					□	□	□	□

Figure 12-43 ▮▮▮▮

International Knee Documentation Committee guidelines for evaluating outcome after knee ligament injury and/or surgery. (From Hefti F, Mullen W, Jakob RP et al: Evaluation of knee ligament injuries with the IKDC form, *Knee Surg Sports Traumatol Arthrosc* 1:226–234, 1993. © Springer-Verlag.)

Table 12-8

Patellofemoral Joint Evaluation Scale*

	Points
Limp	
None	5
Slight or episodic	3
Severe	0
Assistive Devices	
None	5
Cane or brace	3
Unable to bear weight	0
Stair Climbing	
No problem	20
Slight impairment	15
Very slowly	10
One step at a time, always same leg first	5
Unable	0
Crepitation	
None	5
Annoying	3
Limits activities	2
Severe	0
Inability, "Giving Way"	
Never	20
Occasionally with vigorous activities	10
Frequently with vigorous activities	8
Occasionally with daily activities	5
Frequently with daily activities	2
Every day	0
Swelling	
None	10
After vigorous activities only	5
After walking or mild activities	2
Constant	0
Pain	
None	35
Occasionally with vigorous activities	30
Marked with vigorous activities	20
Marked with walking 1 mile or mild to moderate rest pain	15
Marked with walking <1 mile	10
Constant and severe	0

From Karlsson J et al: Eleven year follow up of patellofemoral pain syndromes, *Clin J Sport Med* 6:23, 1996.

*Functional results were assessed according to the patellofemoral scoring scale. Excellent results equal 90–100 points, good 80–89, fair 60–79, and poor <60 points.

also important to understand that the direction of instability does not imply that only structures in that direction are injured. For example, with anterolateral rotary instability, it is not necessarily structures on the anterolateral side of the knee that are injured. In fact, posterior structures are often commonly injured as well. With anterolat-

---

Instabilities about the Knee

- One-plane medial instability
- One-plane lateral instability
- One-plane anterior instability
- One-plane posterior instability
- Anteromedial rotary instability
- Anterolateral rotary instability
- Posteromedial rotary instability
- Posterolateral rotary instability

---

eral rotary instability, the posterolateral capsule and the arcuate-popliteus complex may also be injured.[26]

When testing for ligament stability of the knee, the examiner should keep the following points in mind:

1. The normal knee is tested first to establish a baseline and to show the patient what to expect. This action helps to gain the patient's confidence by showing what the test involves.

2. When one is comparing the normal and injured limbs, the test must be the same for both limbs. The examiner must use the same initial starting position and the same amount of force, apply the same force at the same point or throughout the range, and note the position at which the displacement occurs.[115]

3. The muscles must be relaxed if the tests are to be valid. Maximum laxity would be demonstrated with the patient under anesthesia.

4. The appropriate stress should be applied gently.

5. The stress is repeated several times and increased to the point of pain to demonstrate maximum laxity without causing muscle spasm.

6. It is not only the degree of opening but also the quality of the opening (i.e., the end feel) that is of concern. Left-right differences of 3 mm or more are classified as pathological.[115]

7. If the ligament is intact, there should be an abrupt stop or end feel when the ligament is stressed. A soft or indistinct end feel usually signifies ligamentous injury.[116]

8. Ligaments of the knee tend to act in concert to maintain stability, and individual ligaments are difficult to isolate in terms of their function. Therefore more than one test may be found to be positive when assessing for the different instabilities. For example, a patient may exhibit a one-plane medial and one-plane anterior instability as well as an anteromedial and/or anterolateral rotary instability, depending on the severity of the injury to the various ligamentous structures.

Table 12-9

Primary and Secondary Restraints of the Knee

Tibial Motion	Primary Restraints	Secondary Restraints
Anterior translation	ACL	MCL, LCL; middle third of mediolateral capsule; popliteus corner, semimembranosus corner, iliotibial band
Posterior translation	PCL	MCL, LCL; posterior third of mediolateral capsule; popliteus tendon; anterior and posterior meniscofemoral ligaments
Valgus rotation (medial gapping)	MCL	ACL, PCL; posterior capsule when knee fully extended, semimembranosus corner
Varus rotation (lateral gapping)	LCL	ACL, PCL; posterior capsule when knee fully extended, popliteus corner
Lateral rotation	MCL, LCL	Popliteus corner
Medial rotation	ACL, PCL	Anteroposterior meniscofemoral ligaments, semimembranosus corner

Modified from Zachazewski JE et al, editors: *Athletic injuries and rehabilitation*, p. 627, Philadelphia, 1996, WB Saunders.
ACL, Anterior cruciate ligament; *LCL*, lateral collateral ligament; *MCL*, medial collateral ligament; *PCL*, posterior cruciate ligament.

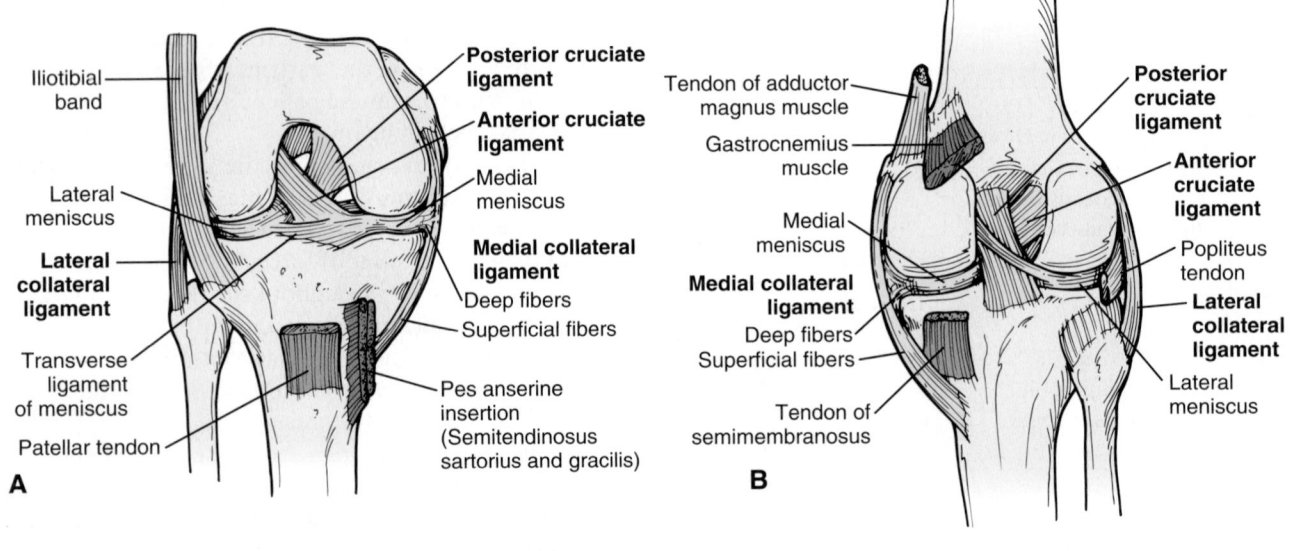

Figure 12-44
Anterior and posterior views of knee. **A,** Anterior view. The patellar tendon is removed, and the knee is flexed. Note that the cruciate ligament rises in front of the anterior tibial spine, not from it. Note also that the medial meniscus is firmly attached to the medial collateral ligament. **B,** Posterior view with the knee extended and the posterior ligament removed. The two layers of the medial collateral ligament are shown, as is the tibial portion of the lateral collateral ligament. The posterior cruciate ligament rises behind the tibia, not on its upper surface. Note the femoral attachment of the anterior cruciate ligament on the back of the notch.

9. Tests for ligament instability are more accurate for assessment of a chronic injury than for assessment of an acute injury in the unanesthetized knee because of the presence of muscle spasm and swelling in the acutely injured knee.

10. For the tests involving rotary instability in which the tibia is moved in relation to the femur, if the movement is into extension, subluxation of the tibia relative to the femur occurs in a positive test. If the movement is into flexion, reduction of the tibia relative to the femur occurs in a positive test.

11. Positive rotational tests should not be repeated too frequently because they may lead to articular cartilage damage, further meniscal tearing, or further damage to injured ligaments.

12. Because the ligamentous tests are subjective tests, the more experience the examiner has in doing them, the more accurate will be the interpretation of the test.

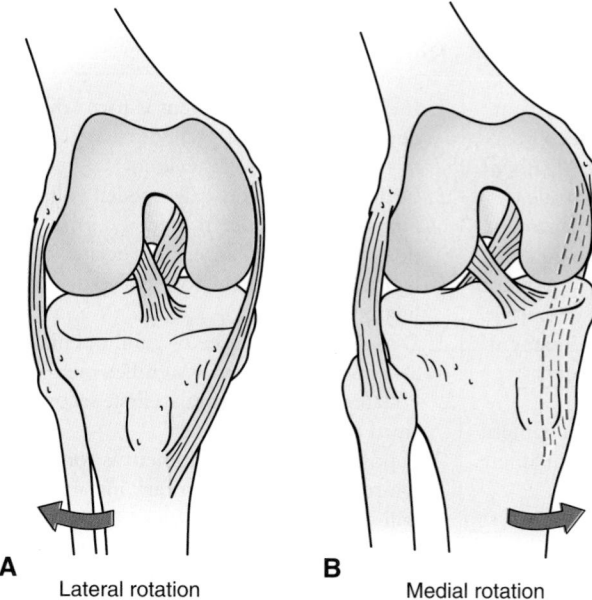

A Lateral rotation   **B** Medial rotation

Figure 12-45

Effect of tibial rotation on cruciate and collateral ligaments.
A, The collateral ligament is taut; the cruciate ligament is lax.
B, The collateral ligament is lax; the cruciate ligament is taut.

Ligamentous Tests Commonly Performed on the Knee	
One-plane medial instability:	Valgus stress at 0° and 30° Hughston's valgus stress at 0° and 30°
One-plane lateral instability:	Varus stress at 0° and 30° Hughston's varus stress at 0° and 30°
One-plane anterior instability:	Lachman test or its modifications Drawer test Active drawer test
One-plane posterior instability:	Posterior sag Drawer test Active drawer test Godfrey test
Anteromedial rotary instability:	Slocum test
Anterolateral rotary instability:	Pivot shift test Losee test Jerk test of Hughston Slocum ARLI test Crossover test Noyes flexion-rotation drawer test
Posteromedial rotary instability:	Hughston's posteromedial drawer test Posteromedial pivot shift test
Posterolateral rotary instability:	Hughston's posterolateral drawer test Jakob test External rotation recurvatum Loomer's posterolateral rotary instability test Tibial external rotation test

The examiner should select only one or two from each group of tests and learn to do them well rather than learn all of the tests and risk doing them poorly.

Tests for One-Plane Medial Instability

The **abduction (valgus stress) test** is an assessment for one-plane (straight) medial instability, which means that the tibia moves away from the femur (i.e., gaps) on the medial side (Figure 12-47). The examiner applies a valgus stress (pushes the knee medially) at the knee while the ankle is stabilized in slight lateral rotation either with the hand or with the leg held between the examiner's arm and trunk. The knee is first in full extension, and then it is slightly flexed (20° to 30°) so that it is "unlocked."

It has been advocated that resting the test thigh on the examining table enables the patient to relax more and is easier for the examiner. The knee rests on the edge of the table; the lower leg is controlled by the examiner's stabilizing the thigh on the table, and the lower leg is abducted, applying a valgus stress to the knee (Figure 12-48).[28] Similarly, a varus stress may be applied to stress the lateral structures.

Hughston[28] advocates a third way to do this test **(Hughston's valgus stress test)**. The patient is positioned as above, and the examiner faces the patient's foot, placing his or her body against the patient's thigh to help stabilize the upper leg in combination with one hand, which can also palpate the joint line. With the other hand, the examiner grasps the patient's big toe and applies a valgus stress, allowing any natural rotation of the tibia (Figure 12-49). Similarly, a varus stress may be applied to test the lateral structures, but in this case, the examiner grasps the lateral aspect of the foot near the fifth and fourth toes. A varus stress is then applied to the knee. Doing the test in this fashion often allows the patient to relax more and is less likely to lead to muscle spasm limiting movement.

If the test is positive (i.e., the tibia moves away from the femur an excessive amount when a valgus stress is applied) when the knee is *in extension*, the following structures may have been injured to some degree:

1. Medial collateral ligament (superficial and deep fibers)
2. Posterior oblique ligament
3. Posteromedial capsule
4. Anterior cruciate ligament
5. Posterior cruciate ligament
6. Medial quadriceps expansion
7. Semimembranosus muscle

Table 12-10

Tests for Ligamentous Instability around the Knee

Instability	Tests Used to Determine Instability	Structures Injured to Some Degree if Test Positive*	Notes
One-plane medial (straight medial)	1. Abduction (valgus) stress with knee in full extension	1. Medial collateral ligament (superficial and deep fibers) 2. Posterior oblique ligament 3. Posteromedial capsule 4. Anterior cruciate ligament 5. Posterior cruciate ligament 6. Medial quadriceps expansion 7. Semimembranosus muscle	1. If either cruciate ligament is torn (third-degree sprain) or stretched, rotary instability will also be evident 2. Order of injury is usually medial collateral ligament, then posteromedial corner, posterior capsule, anterior cruciate ligament, and finally posterior cruciate ligament
	2. Abduction (valgus) stress with knee slightly flexed (20° to 30°)	1. Medial collateral ligament (superficial and deep fibers) 2. Posterior oblique ligament 3. Posterior cruciate ligament	1. Depending on degree of pain, opening, and end feel, primarily signifies medial collateral ligament sprain (first, second, or third degree) 2. If posterior cruciate ligament is torn (third-degree sprain), rotary instability will also be evident 3. Opening of 12° to 15° signifies injury to posterior cruciate ligament 4. If tibia is laterally rotated, stress is taken off posterior cruciate ligament 5. If tibia is medially rotated, stress is increased on cruciate ligaments while medial collateral ligament relaxes
One-plane lateral (straight lateral)	1. Adduction (varus) stress with knee in full extension	1. Lateral collateral ligament 2. Posterolateral capsule 3. Arcuate-popliteus complex 4. Biceps femoris tendon 5. Anterior cruciate ligament 6. Posterior cruciate ligament 7. Lateral gastrocnemius muscle	1. If either cruciate ligament is torn (third-degree sprain) or stretched, rotary instability will also be evident 2. Order of injury is lateral collateral ligament, arcuate-popliteus complex, anterior cruciate ligament, posterior cruciate ligament 3. With severe injury (third degree), common peroneal nerve and circulation may be affected
	2. Adduction (varus) stress with knee slightly flexed (20° to 30°) and tibia laterally rotated	1. Lateral collateral ligament 2. Posterolateral capsule 3. Arcuate-popliteus complex 4. Iliotibial band 5. Biceps femoris tendon	1. Depending on degree of pain, opening, and end feel, primarily signifies lateral collateral ligament sprain (first, second, or third degree) 2. If tibia is not laterally rotated, maximum stress will not be placed on lateral collateral ligament 3. Lateral rotation of tibia results in relaxation of both cruciate ligaments 4. With flexion, the iliotibial band lies over the center of the lateral joint line 5. If tibia is medially rotated, stress is increased on both cruciate ligaments while lateral collateral ligament relaxes 6. Order of injury is lateral collateral ligament, arcuate-popliteus complex, and iliotibial band and/or biceps femoris
One-plane anterior	1. Lachman test (20° to 30° knee flexion) or its modifications	1. Anterior cruciate ligament 2. Posterior oblique ligament 3. Arcuate-popliteus complex	1. Medial collateral ligament and iliotibial band lax in this position 2. Tests primarily posterolateral bundle of anterior cruciate ligament 3. Primarily tests anterior cruciate ligament but with severe injury (third degree), structures in posteromedial and posterolateral corners may also be injured

Table 12-10—cont'd

Instability	Tests Used to Determine Instability	Structures Injured to Some Degree if Test Positive*	Notes
	2. Anterior drawer sign (90° knee flexion) 3. Active drawer test	1. Anterior cruciate ligament 2. Posterolateral capsule 3. Posteromedial capsule 4. Medial collateral ligament 5. Iliotibial band 6. Posterior oblique ligament 7. Arcuate-popliteus complex	1. Tests primarily anteromedial bundle of anterior cruciate ligament 2. If anterior cruciate ligament and medial or lateral structures are torn (third-degree sprain) or stretched, rotary instability will also be evident 3. Be sure posterior cruciate has not been injured, giving possible false-positive test
One-plane posterior	1. Posterior drawer sign (90° knee flexion) 2. Posterior sag sign 3. Active drawer test 4. Reverse Lachman test 5. Godfrey test	1. Posterior cruciate ligament 2. Arcuate-popliteus complex 3. Posterior oblique ligament 4. Anterior cruciate ligament	1. If posterior cruciate ligament and medial or lateral structures are torn (third-degree sprain) or stretched, rotary instability will also be evident 2. With severe injury (third degree), collateral ligaments may also be injured
Anteromedial rotary	1. Slocum test (foot laterally rotated 15°) 2. Lemaire's anteromedial jolt test 3. Dejour test	1. Medial collateral ligament (superficial and deep fibers) 2. Posterior oblique ligament 3. Posteromedial capsule 4. Anterior cruciate ligament	1. Test must not be done in extreme lateral rotation of tibia because passive stabilizing will result from "coiling" to maximum rotation
Anterolateral rotary	1. Slocum test (foot medially rotated 30°) 2. Losee test 3. Jerk test of Hughston 4. Active pivot shift 5. Nakajima test	1. Anterior cruciate ligament 2. Posterolateral capsule 3. Arcuate-popliteus complex 4. Lateral collateral ligament 5. Iliotibial band	1. Tests bring about anterior *subluxation* of the tibia on femur, causing patient to experience "giving way" sensation 2. Tests go from flexion to extension 3. Slocum test must not be done in extreme medial rotation of tibia because passive stabilization will result from "coiling" to maximum rotation 4. Shift may be "slip" (second degree) or "jerk" (third degree), depending on degree of sprain or injury
	1. Lateral pivot shift test of Macintosh 2. Slocum ALRI test 3. Crossover test 4. Flexion-rotation drawer test 5. Flexion-extension valgus test 6. Martens test	1. Anterior cruciate ligament 2. Posterolateral capsule 3. Arcuate-popliteus complex 4. Iliotibial band	1. Tests cause *reduction* of anterior subluxated tibia on femur 2. Tests go from extension to flexion 3. Shift may be "slip" (second degree) or "jerk" (third degree), depending on degree of sprain or injury
Posteromedial rotary	1. Hughston's posteromedial drawer sign 2. Posteromedial pivot shift test	1. Posterior cruciate ligament 2. Posterior oblique ligament 3. Medial collateral ligament (superficial and deep fibers) 4. Semimembranosus muscle 5. Posteromedial capsule 6. Anterior cruciate ligament	1. Watch for changing position of tibial tubercle relative to femoral condyles
Posterolateral rotary	1. Hughston's postero-lateral drawer sign 2. Jakob test (reverse pivot shift maneuver) 3. External rotational recurvatum test 4. Dynamic posterior shift test 5. Loomer's test 6. Active posterolateral drawer sign	1. Posterior cruciate ligament 2. Arcuate-popliteus ligament 3. Lateral collateral ligament 4. Biceps femoris tendon 5. Posterolateral capsule 6. Anterior cruciate ligament	1. Watch for changing position of tibial tubercle relative to femoral condyles

*The amount of displacement gives an indication of how badly and how much of the structures are injured (i.e., first-, second-, or third-degree sprain).

Figure 12-46

Instabilities about the knee. *PCL*, Posterior cruciate ligament; *POL*, posterior oblique ligament; *MCL*, medial collateral ligament; *ACL*, anterior cruciate ligament; *ITB*, iliotibial band; *LCL*, lateral collateral ligament; *PT*, popliteal tendon, *S*, sartorius; *G*, gracilis; *SM*, semimembranosus; *ST*, semitendinosus; *MG*, medial gastrocnemius; *LG*, lateral gastrocnemius.

Figure 12-47

Abduction (valgus stress) test. **A**, "Gapping" on the medial aspect of the knee. **B**, Positioning for testing the medial collateral ligament (extended knee).

Figure 12-48

Applying a valgus stress with thigh supported on examining table.

A positive finding on full extension is classified as a major disruption of the knee. The examiner usually finds that one or more of the rotary tests are also positive. If the examiner applies lateral rotation to the foot when performing the test in extension and finds excessive lateral rotation on the affected side, it is a sign of possible anteromedial rotary instability.

If the test is positive when the knee is *flexed* to 20° to 30°, the following structures may have been injured to some degree:

1. Medial collateral ligament
2. Posterior oblique ligament
3. Posterior cruciate ligament
4. Posteromedial capsule

This flexed part of the valgus stress test would be classified as the true test for one-plane medial instability.

If a stress radiograph is taken when the test is performed in full extension, a 5-mm opening indicates a grade 1 injury; up to 10 mm, a grade 2 injury; and more than 10 mm, a grade 3 injury.[110,117]

Figure 12-49

Hughston's valgus stress test.

Tests for One-Plane Lateral Instability

The **adduction (varus stress) test** is an assessment for one-plane lateral instability (i.e., the tibia moves away from the femur an excessive amount on the lateral aspect of the leg). The examiner applies a varus stress (pushes the knee laterally) at the knee while the ankle is stabilized (Figure 12-50). The test is first done with the knee in full extension and then with the knee in 20° to 30° of flexion. If the tibia is laterally rotated in full extension before the test, the cruciate ligaments will be uncoiled, and maximum stress will be placed on the collateral ligaments.

As previously mentioned (see Tests for One-Plane Medial Instability), **Hughston's varus stress test** may be used. In this case, the examiner grasps the fifth and fourth toes and applies a varus stress to the knee in extension and slightly (20° to 30°) flexed.

If the test is positive (i.e., the tibia moves away from the femur when a varus stress is applied) *in extension*, the following structures may have been injured to some degree:

1. Fibular or lateral collateral ligament
2. Posterolateral capsule
3. Arcuate-popliteus complex
4. Biceps femoris tendon
5. Posterior cruciate ligament
6. Anterior cruciate ligament
7. Lateral gastrocnemius muscle
8. Iliotibial band

The examiner usually finds that one or more rotary instability tests are also positive. A positive test indicates major instability of the knee.

If the test is positive when the knee is *flexed* 20° to 30° with lateral rotation of the tibia, the following structures may have been injured to some degree:

1. Lateral collateral ligament
2. Posterolateral capsule
3. Arcuate-popliteus complex

4. Iliotibial band
5. Biceps femoris tendon

This flexed part of the varus stress test is classified as the true test for one-plane lateral instability.

If a stress radiograph is taken when the test is performed in full extension, a 5-mm opening indicates a grade 1 injury; up to 8 mm, a grade 2 injury; and more than 8 mm, a grade 3 injury to the lateral ligaments of the knee.[110,117]

Both varus and valgus stress testing (**varus-valgus test**) can be performed at the same time while the examiner palpates the joint line. The examiner holds the ankle between the examiner's waist and forearm while the patient lies supine with the knee extended and then flexed. At the same time, the examiner palpates the medial and lateral joint lines with the fingers. Varus and valgus stresses are applied with the heels of the examiner's hands (Figure 12-51).[66]

Tests for One-Plane Anterior Instability

Some clinicians[26,28] believe that the posterior cruciate ligament should be tested (see Tests for One-Plane Posterior Instability) or observed for a posterior sag before the anterior cruciate ligament is tested to rule out false-positive tests for anterior translation. In either case, the examiner should be aware that a torn posterior cruciate can lead to a false-positive anterior translation test if the patient is tested in supine position with the knee flexed, because gravity causes the tibia to sag posteriorly.

Lachman Test. The Lachman test, which may also be referred to as the **Ritchie, Trillat,** or **Lachman-Trillat test**, is the best indicator of injury to the anterior cruciate ligament, especially the posterolateral band,[118–123] although this has been questioned.[124] It is a test for one-plane anterior instability. The patient lies supine with the involved leg beside the examiner. The examiner holds the patient's knee between full extension and 30° of flexion. This position is close to the functional

A **B**

Figure 12-50
Adduction (varus stress) test. **A,** One-plane lateral instability "gapping" on the lateral aspect. **B,** Positioning for testing lateral collateral ligament in extension.

Figure 12-51
Varus-valgus test. **A,** Knee flexed. **B,** Knee extended.

position of the knee, in which the anterior cruciate ligament plays a major role. The patient's femur is stabilized with one of the examiner's hands (the "outside" hand) while the proximal aspect of the tibia is moved forward with the other ("inside") hand (Figure 12-52). Frank[125] reported that to achieve the best results, the tibia should be slightly laterally rotated and the anterior tibial translation force should be applied from the posteromedial aspect. Therefore the hand on the tibia should apply the translation force. A positive sign is indicated by a "mushy" or soft end feel when the tibia is moved forward on the femur (increased anterior translation with medial rotation of the tibia) and disappearance of the infrapatellar tendon slope.[123] A false-negative test may occur if the femur is not properly stabilized, if a meniscus lesion blocks translation, or if the tibia is medially rotated.[125] A positive sign indicates that the following structures may have been injured to some degree:

1. Anterior cruciate ligament (especially the posterolateral bundle)
2. Posterior oblique ligament
3. Arcuate-popliteus complex

Other ways of doing the Lachman test have also been advocated. The method that works for the examiner and

Figure 12-52
Hand position for classic Lachman test.

that the examiner can use competently should be selected. Another method (**modification 1**) has the patient sitting with the leg over the edge of the examining table. The examiner sits facing the patient and supports the foot of the test leg on the examiner's thigh so that the patient's knee is flexed 30°. The examiner stabilizes the thigh with one hand and pulls the tibia forward with the other hand (Figure 12-53). Abnormal forward motion is considered to be a positive test.[126]

For examiners with small hands, the **stable Lachman test (modification 2)** is recommended. The patient lies supine with the knee resting on the examiner's knee (Figure 12-54). One of the examiner's hands stabilizes the femur against the examiner's thigh, and the other hand applies an anterior stress.[66,127] Adler and associates[128] described a modification of this method, which they called the **drop leg Lachman test (modification 3)**. The patient lies supine, and the leg to be examined is abducted off the side of the examining table and the knee is flexed to 25°. One of the examiner's hands stabilizes the femur against the table while the patient's foot is held between the examiner's knees. The examiner's other hand is then free to apply the anterior translation force (Figure 12-55). They found there was greater anterior laxity demonstrated when doing the test this way than when doing it the classical way.[128]

Modification 4 has the patient lying supine while the examiner stabilizes the foot between the examiner's thorax and arm. Both hands are placed around the tibia, the knee is flexed 20° to 30°, and an anterior drawer movement is performed.[66] This technique allows gravity to control movement of the femur, which may not be sufficient to show a good positive test (Figure 12-56).

Another way of doing the test (**modification 5**) is for the patient to lie supine while the examiner stands beside the leg to be tested with the eyes level with the knee. The examiner grasps the femur with one hand and the tibia with the other hand.[66] The tibia is pulled forward, and any abnormal motion is noted (Figure 12-57). As with the regular Lachman test, the examiner may have difficulty stabilizing the femur if the examiner has small hands.

To perform the **prone Lachman test (modification 6)**,[129,130] the patient lies prone, and the examiner stabilizes the foot between the examiner's thorax and arm and places one hand around the tibia. The other hand stabilizes the femur (Figure 12-58). Gravity assists anterior movement with this method, but it is more difficult to determine the quality of the end feel.

Figure 12-54
Stable Lachman test (modification 2).

Figure 12-53
Lachman test (modification 1).

Figure 12-55
Drop leg Lachman test (modification 3).

Figure 12-56
Lachman test (modification 4).

Figure 12-57
Lachman test (modification 5).

Figure 12-58
Prone Lachman test (modification 6).

For the **active (no touch) Lachman test (modification 7)**,[66,131,132] the patient lies supine with the knee over the examiner's forearm so that the knee is flexed approximately 30° (Figure 12-59). The patient is asked to actively extend the knee, and the examiner watches for anterior displacement of the tibia relative to the unaffected side. The test may also be carried out with the foot held down on the table to increase the pull of the quadriceps. In this case, the test has been called the **maximum**

quadriceps test (modification 8).[66] The examiner must be certain that there is no posterior sag before performing the test.

The Lachman test may be graded with a stress radiograph: a 3- to 6-mm anterior movement of the tibia relative to the femur is classified as a grade 1 injury; 6 to 9 mm, grade 2; 10 to 16 mm, grade 3; and 16 to 20 mm, grade 4.[66]

Drawer Sign. The drawer sign is a test for one-plane anterior and one-plane posterior instabilities.[133] The difficulty with this test is in determining the neutral starting position if the ligaments have been injured. The patient's knee is flexed to 90°, and the hip is flexed to 45°. In this position, the anterior cruciate ligament is almost parallel with the tibial plateau. The patient's foot is held on the table by the examiner's body with the examiner sitting on the patient's forefoot and the foot in neutral rotation. The examiner's hands are placed around the tibia to ensure that the hamstring muscles are relaxed (Figures 12-60 and 12-61). The tibia is then drawn forward on the femur. The normal amount of movement that should be present is approximately 6 mm. This part of the test assesses one-plane anterior instability. If the test is positive (i.e., the tibia moves forward more than 6 mm on the femur), the following structures may have been injured to some degree:

Figure 12-59

A, Active Lachman (maximum quadriceps) test (modification 8). **B,** No-touch Lachman test (modification 7). Open arrow shows where the examiner watches for shift.

1. Anterior cruciate ligament (especially the antero-medial bundle)
2. Posterolateral capsule
3. Posteromedial capsule
4. Medial collateral ligament (deep fibers)
5. Iliotibial band
6. Posterior oblique ligament
7. Arcuate-popliteus complex

If only the anterior cruciate ligament is torn, the test is negative, because other structures (posterior capsule and posterolateral and posteromedial structures) limit movement. In addition, hemarthrosis, a torn medial meniscus (posterior horn) wedged against the medial femoral condyle, or hamstring spasm may result in a false-negative test. Hughston[28] points out that tearing of the coronary or meniscotibial ligament can allow the tibia to translate forward more than normal, even in the presence of an intact anterior cruciate ligament. In this case, when the anterior drawer test is performed, anteromedial rotation (subluxation) of the tibia occurs.

When performing this test, the examiner must ensure that the posterior cruciate ligament is not torn or injured.

Figure 12-60

Position for drawer sign.

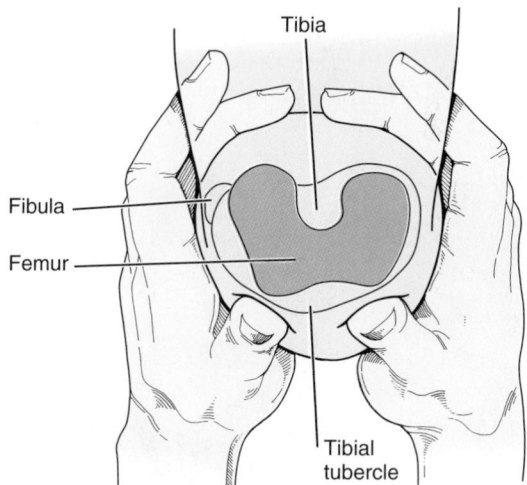

Figure 12-61

This view of the knee from above shows the inside of the knee joint during performance of the anterior drawer test in flexion. The hands are in place, and the overlay of the femur on the tibia demonstrates that the anterior and posterior motions are normal. The index fingers are ensuring that the hamstrings are relaxed. If, on pulling or pushing tibia, rotation of tibial plateau occurs, the examiner should check for rotary instabilities. (Redrawn from Hughston JC: *Knee ligaments: injury and repair,* p 111, St Louis, 1993, Mosby.)

If it has been torn, it will allow the tibia to drop or slide back on the femur, and when the examiner pulls the tibia forward, a large amount of movement will occur, giving a false-positive sign (see Posterior Sag Sign). Therefore the test should be considered positive only if it is shown that the posterior sag is not present.

Weatherwax[134] described a modified way of testing the anterior drawer (**90-90 anterior drawer**). The patient lies supine. The examiner flexes the patient's hip and knee to 90° and supports the lower leg between the examiner's trunk and forearm. The examiner places the hands around the tibia, as with the standard test, and applies sufficient force to slowly lift the patient's buttock off the table (Figure 12-62).

If, when doing the anterior drawer test, there is an audible snap or palpable jerk (**Finochietto jumping sign**) when the tibia is pulled forward and the tibia moves forward excessively, a meniscus lesion is probably accompanying the torn anterior cruciate ligament.[66]

After the anterior movement of the tibia on the femur, the posterior movement of the tibia on the femur should be completed. In this part of the test, the tibia is pushed back on the femur. This phase is a test for one-plane posterior instability. If the test is positive or a posterior sag is evident, the following structures may have been injured to some degree:

1. Posterior cruciate ligament
2. Arcuate-popliteus complex
3. Posterior oblique ligament
4. Anterior cruciate ligament

If the arcuate-popliteus complex remains intact, a positive posterior drawer sign may not be elicited.[135] If, when the tibia is pushed backward, the examiner forcefully rotates the tibia laterally and excessive movement occurs, the test is positive for posterolateral instability. Warren[136] calls this maneuver the **arcuate spin test**.

Feagin[129] advocated doing the drawer test with the patient sitting with the leg hanging relaxed over the end of the examining table (**sitting anterior drawer test**). The examiner places the hands as with the standardized test and slowly draws the tibia first forward and then backward to test the anterior and posterior drawer (Figure 12-63). The examiner uses the thumbs to palpate the tibial plateau movement relative to the femur. The examiner may also note any rotational deformity. The advantage of doing the test this way is that the posterior sag is eliminated because the effect of gravity is eliminated.

Active Drawer Test. The patient is positioned as for the normal drawer test. The examiner holds the patient's foot down. The patient is asked to try to straighten the leg, and the examiner prevents the patient from doing so (isometric test). Muller[110] advocated allowing the foot to

Figure 12-62
Anterior drawer test in 90° flexion with the hip flexed 90°.

Figure 12-63
Anterior drawer test in sitting position. Examiner feels anterior shift with thumbs.

be free and noting when the foot is lifted off the table, which occurs only after the tibia has shifted forward and stabilized. If the anterior cruciate ligament or posterior cruciate ligament is torn, the anterior contour of the knee changes as the tibia is drawn forward. If the posterior cruciate ligament is torn, a posterior sag is evident before the patient contracts the quadriceps. Contraction of the quadriceps causes the tibia to shift forward to its normal position, indicating a positive test for a torn posterior cruciate ligament.[137,138] If there is no posterior sag present and if the tibia shifts forward more on the injured side than the noninjured side, it is a positive test for anterior cruciate ligament disruption (Figure 12-64).[137] A second part of the test may be instituted by having the patient contract the hamstrings isometrically so that the tibial plateau moves posteriorly. This part of the test accentuates the posterior sag for posterior cruciate insufficiency, if present, and ensures maximum movement for anterior cruciate insufficiency if a quadriceps contraction is tried a second time.[66] The active drawer test is a better expression of posterior cruciate insufficiency than of anterior cruciate insufficiency.[139]

With the drawer sign or test, if the anterior or posterior cruciate ligament is torn (third-degree sprain), some rotary instability will be evident when the appropriate ligamentous tests are performed.

Tests for One-Plane Posterior Instability[140,141]

Posterior Sag Sign (Gravity Drawer Test). The patient lies supine with the hip flexed to 45° and the knee flexed to 90°. In this position, the tibia "drops back," or sags back, on the femur because of gravity if the posterior cruciate ligament is torn (Figure 12-65). Posterior tibial displacement is more noticeable when the knee is flexed 90° to 110° than when the knee is only slightly flexed. It is a test for one-plane posterior instability. Normally, the medial tibial plateau extends 1 cm anteriorly beyond the femoral condyle when the knee is flexed 90°. If this "step" is lost, which is what occurs with a positive posterior sag caused by a torn posterior cruciate ligament, this **step-off test** or **thumb sign** is considered positive.[33,43,139,140] The examiner must be careful because the position could result in a false-positive anterior drawer test for the anterior cruciate ligament if the sag remains unnoticed. If there is minimal or no swelling, the sag is evident because of an obvious concavity distal to the patella. If the posterior sag sign is present, the following structures may have been injured to some degree:

Figure 12-65

Sag sign. **A,** Illustration of posterior sag sign. **B,** Note profile of two knees; the left (nearer) sags backward compared with the normal right knee, indicating posterior cruciate defect. (From O'Donoghue DH: *Treatment of injuries to athletes,* ed 4, p 450, Philadelphia, 1984, WB Saunders.)

Figure 12-64

Active anterior drawer test. Examiner watches for anterior shift.

1. Posterior cruciate ligament
2. Arcuate-popliteus complex
3. Posterior oblique ligament
4. Anterior cruciate ligament

If it appears that the patient has a positive posterior sag sign, the patient should carefully extend the knee while the examiner holds the hip in 90° to 100° of flexion. This action is sometimes called the **voluntary anterior drawer sign**, and the results are similar to those of the active anterior drawer test. As the patient does this slowly, the tibial plateau moves or shifts forward to its normal position, indicating that the tibia was previously posteriorly subluxated (posterior cruciate tear) on the femur.

Reverse Lachman Test.[66] The patient lies prone with the knee flexed to 30°, and the examiner grasps the tibia with one hand while fixing the femur with the other hand (Figure 12-66). The examiner ensures that the hamstring muscles are relaxed. The examiner then pulls the tibia up (posteriorly), noting the amount of movement and the quality of the end feel. It is a test for the posterior cruciate ligament. The examiner should be wary of a false-positive test if the anterior cruciate ligament has been torn, because gravity may cause an anterior shift. This test is not as accurate for the posterior cruciate ligament as the posterior drawer test, because when the posterior cruciate ligament is torn, the greatest posterior displacement is at 90°.

Drawer Sign or Test. This test has been described previously. Veltri and Warren[138] report that the posterior drawer test is one of the most effective means of clinically diagnosing posterior cruciate and posterolateral (popliteus) corner injuries.

Active Drawer Test. This test has been described previously.

Godfrey (Gravity) Test.[66] The patient lies supine, and the examiner holds both legs while flexing the patient's hips and knees to 90° (Figure 12-67). If there

Figure 12-66
Reverse Lachman test.

Figure 12-67
Godfrey test. Examiner watches for posterior shift, which is not evident in this case.

is posterior instability, a posterior sag of the tibia is seen. If manual posterior pressure is applied to the tibia, posterior displacement may increase.

Tests for Anteromedial Rotary Instability

For these rotary tests, the examiner is watching for abnormal tibial motion. In this case, the examiner watches the medial side of the tibia to see if it rotates anteriorly more than the uninjured side.

Slocum Test. The Slocum test assesses both anterior rotary instabilities.[142] The patient's knee is flexed to 80° or 90°, and the hip is flexed to 45°. The foot is first placed in 30° medial rotation (Figure 12-68). The examiner then sits on the patient's forefoot to hold the foot in position and draws the tibia forward; if the test is positive, movement occurs primarily on the lateral side of the knee. This movement is excessive relative to the unaffected side and indicates anterolateral rotary instability. It also indicates that the following structures may have been injured to some degree:

1. Anterior cruciate ligament
2. Posterolateral capsule
3. Arcuate-popliteus complex
4. Lateral collateral ligament
5. Posterior cruciate ligament
6. Iliotibial band

Figure 12-68
Slocum test.

A   **B**

Figure 12-69
Slocum test with the patient in the sitting position. Examiner rotates foot one way (i.e., medially or laterally) and then pushes the tibia backwards (**A**) or pulls it forward (**B**), comparing the amount of rotation and anterior and posterior movement in each knee.

If the examiner finds anterolateral instability during this first position of the Slocum test, the second part of the test, which assesses anteromedial rotary instability in this position, is of less value.[143]

In the second part of the test, the foot is placed in 15° of lateral rotation, and the tibia is drawn forward by the examiner. This part of the test is sometimes referred to as **Lemaire's T drawer test**. If the test is positive, the movement occurs primarily on the medial side of the knee. This movement is excessive relative to the unaffected side and indicates anteromedial rotary instability. It also indicates that the following structures may have been injured to some degree:

1. Medial collateral ligament (especially the superficial fibers, although the deep fibers may also be affected)
2. Posterior oblique ligament
3. Posteromedial capsule
4. Anterior cruciate ligament

For the Slocum test, it is imperative that the examiner medially or laterally rotate the foot to the degrees shown. If the examiner rotates the tibia as far as it will go, the test will be negative for movement, because this action tightens all of the remaining structures.

If a stress radiograph is taken during the test, minimal or no movement indicates a negative test; 1 mm or less,

a grade 1 injury; 1 to 2 mm, a grade 2 injury; and more than 2 mm, a grade 3 injury.[117]

The test may also be performed with the patient sitting with the knees flexed over the edge of the examining table (Figure 12-69).[110] The examiner applies an anterior or a posterior force while holding the foot medially or laterally rotated. If this procedure is used, the examiner must remember that use of the anterior force tests for anterior rotary instability, whereas use of the posterior force tests for posterior rotary instability (see Hughston's Posteromedial and Posterolateral Drawer Sign in later sections). The examiner should note whether the movement is excessive on the medial or on the lateral side of the knee relative to the normal knee. Excessive movement indicates a positive test.

Dejour Test.[26] The patient lies supine. The examiner holds the patient's leg with one arm against the body and the hand under the calf to lift the tibia while applying a valgus stress. The other hand pushes the femur down (Figure 12-70). In extension, this action causes anteromedial subluxation in the pathological knee. If the knee is then flexed, the tibial plateau reduces suddenly, indicating a positive test. If the jolt is painful, it indicates that the medial meniscus has been injured. If it is not painful, the posteromedial corner has been injured.

Figure 12-70
Dejour test.

Tests for Anterolateral Rotary Instability

When performing these tests, the examiner is looking for abnormal (excessive) anterior rotation of the tibia on the lateral side relative to the femur.

Slocum Test. This test has been described previously.

Lateral Pivot Shift Maneuver (Test of MacIntosh). This is the primary test used to assess anterolateral rotary instability of the knee and is an excellent test for ruptures (third-degree sprains) of the anterior cruciate ligament.144–147 Like most provocative tests, it does have a disadvantage, however. In the apprehensive patient, because of the forces applied during the test, protective muscle contraction may lead to a false-negative test.[26] During this test, the tibia moves away from the femur on the lateral side (but rotates medially) and moves anteriorly in relation to the femur (Figure 12-71).

Normally, the knee's center of rotation changes constantly through its ROM as a result of the shape of the femoral condyles, ligamentous restraint, and muscle tension. The path of movement of the tibia on the femur is described as a combination of rolling and sliding, with rolling predominating when the instant center is near the joint line and sliding predominating when the instant center shifts distally from the contact area. The MacIntosh test is a duplication of the anterior subluxation-reduction phenomenon that occurs during the normal gait cycle when the anterior cruciate ligament is torn. Therefore it illustrates a **dynamic subluxation**. This shift occurs between 20° and 40° of flexion (0° being full extension). It is this phenomenon that gives the patient the clinical description of feeling the knee "give way" (Figure 12-72).

The patient lies supine with the hip both flexed and abducted 30° and relaxed in slight medial rotation (20°). The examiner holds the patient's foot with one hand while the other hand is placed at the knee, holding the leg in slight medial rotation. This is done by placing the heel of the hand behind the fibula and over the lateral head of the gastrocnemius muscle with the tibia medially rotated, causing the tibia to subluxate anteriorly as the knee is taken into extension (Figure 12-73). Bach and colleagues[148] modified the position to slight lateral rotation, because they believed that lateral tibial rotation gives a more pronounced pivot shift when the test is positive. In slight flexion, the secondary restraints (i.e., hamstrings, lateral femoral condyle, lateral meniscus) are less efficient than in full flexion. It is important to realize that in full extension subluxation does not occur, because

Figure 12-71
Anterolateral rotary instability.

Figure 12-72
Anterior shift of the tibia during the lateral pivot shift test.

Figure 12-73
Lateral pivot shift test.

iliotibial band has also been torn, the test does not work (the subluxation will be evident, but the "jog" will not occur). In addition, if either meniscus has been torn, it may limit or prevent the subluxation reduction motion seen in the test.

If the patient is tense or apprehensive, the test can be modified; this is called the **soft pivot shift test** (Figure 12-75). The patient lies supine, and the examiner supports the test foot with one hand while placing the other hand over the calf muscle 10 to 20 cm (4 to 8 inches) distal to the knee joint. The examiner flexes and extends the knee slowly and gently. After three to five cycles, the examiner applies axial compression while the other hand over the calf exerts an anterior pressure. In a positive test, the tibia subluxates and reduces, but not with the same apprehensive, jerky feeling.[66] Kennedy[117] advocated pushing on the fibular head with the thumb when performing this maneuver. Because hip abduction and adduction have an effect on the iliotibial band, hip position plays an important role in the test. Subluxation is most obvious when the hip is abducted and least obvious when it is adducted. In addition, lateral rotation of the tibia allows greater subluxation because, like abduction, it decreases the stress on the iliotibial band.[66] If the test is positive, the following structures have probably been injured to some degree:

1. Anterior cruciate ligament
2. Posterolateral capsule
3. Arcuate-popliteus complex
4. Lateral collateral ligament
5. Iliotibial band

Active Pivot Shift Test.[149] The patient sits with the foot on the floor in neutral rotation and the knee flexed 80° to 90°. The patient is asked to isometrically contract the quadriceps while the examiner stabilizes the foot. A positive test is indicated by anterolateral subluxation of the lateral tibial plateau and is indicative of anterolateral instability (Figure 12-76).

of the "locking home" of the tibia on the femur.[26] With slight flexion, however, the secondary restraints are less restrictive, and subluxation occurs. The examiner then applies a valgus stress to the knee while maintaining a medial rotation torque on the tibia at the ankle. The leg is then flexed, and at approximately 30° to 40° the tibia reduces or "jogs" backward. The patient says that that is what the "giving way" feels like, indicating a positive test. The reduction of the tibia on the femur is caused by the change in position of the iliotibial band when it switches from an extensor function to a flexor function, pulling the tibia back into its normal position (Figure 12-74). The test involves two phases: first subluxation and then reduction. The iliotibial band must be intact for the test to work. In cases of anterolateral instability in which the

Figure 12-74
Biomechanics of the pivot shift. Three phases occur during the pivot shift maneuver. Under load transmission in the lateral compartment, the tibia rolls from a reduced position in neutral rotation to anterior subluxation and some medial rotation. Under increasing flexion to 20°, the condyle becomes jammed behind the posterior slope of the lateral plateau. The iliotibial band, especially the femorotibial portion, becomes tight until, at 30° to 40°, it is gliding behind the flexion axis, initiating reduction in more flexion and some lateral rotation.

Figure 12-75

Soft pivot shift test. Examiner watches for anterior shift.

With active contraction of quadriceps, tibia rotates or is pulled forward

Figure 12-76

Active pivot shift test.

Losee Test. This test is a clinical duplication of the anterolateral rotary instability mechanism of injury. The patient lies supine while relaxed.[150] The examiner holds the patient's ankle and foot so that the leg is laterally rotated and braced against the examiner's abdomen. The knee is then flexed to 30°, and the examiner ensures that the hamstring muscles are relaxed (Figure 12-77). The lateral rotation ensures that the subluxation of the knee is reduced at the beginning of the test. With the examiner's other hand positioned so that the fingers lie over the patella and the thumb is hooked behind the fibular head, a valgus force is applied to the knee; the examiner uses the abdomen as a fulcrum while extending the patient's knee and applying forward pressure behind the fibular head with the thumb.

The valgus stress compresses the structures in the lateral compartment and makes the anterior subluxation, if present, more noticeable. At the same time, the foot and ankle are allowed to drift into medial rotation. If the foot and ankle are not allowed to rotate medially, the anterior subluxation of the lateral tibial plateau may be prevented. Just before full extension of the knee, there will be a "clunk" forward if the test is positive, and the patient must recognize the movement as the instability that was previously experienced. This clunk means that the tibia has subluxated anteriorly and indicates injury to the same structures as those indicated by a positive pivot shift maneuver. Kocher et al.[151] reported that the test could be used as a good check of functional instability after surgical reconstruction.

Figure 12-77

The Losee test begins with the knee in flexion and the tibia in lateral rotation and valgus stress. As the knee is extended, the foot is allowed to medially rotate, and the previously subluxated tibia reduces as the knee approaches full extension. A palpable "clunk" correlates with anterior cruciate ligament tear. (Redrawn from Scott WN, editor: *Ligament and extensor mechanism injuries of the knee: diagnosis and treatment*, p. 96, St Louis, 1991, Mosby.)

Jerk Test of Hughston.[152] This test is similar to the pivot shift maneuver. The positioning of the patient and the examiner is the same, except that the patient's hip is flexed to 45°. With this test, the knee is first flexed to 90°. The leg is then extended, maintaining medial rotation and a valgus stress (Figure 12-78). At approximately 20° to 30° of flexion, the tibia shifts forward, causing a subluxation of the lateral tibial plateau with a jerk if the test is positive. If the leg is carried into further extension, it spontaneously reduces. A positive jerk test indicates that the same structures are injured as indicated by a positive pivot shift maneuver and assesses anterolateral

rotary instability. According to the literature,[110] this test is not as sensitive as the pivot shift test.

Slocum ALRI Test. Anterolateral rotary instability (ALRI) is also assessed by the Slocum ALRI test.[110,143] The patient is in the side-lying position (approximately 30° from supine). The bottom leg is the uninvolved leg. The knee of the uninvolved leg is flexed to add stability (Figure 12-79). The foot of the involved leg rests and is stabilized on the examining table with the patient's foot in medial rotation and the knee in extension and valgus. This position helps to eliminate hip rotation during the test. The examiner applies a valgus stress to the

A   **B**   **C**

Figure 12-78

Jerk test of Hughston. **A,** The knee is flexed to 90°, and the heel of one hand is placed behind the fibular head to produce medial rotation of the tibia. **B,** At 20° to 30°, the lateral tibial plateau subluxates anteriorly. **C,** At full extension, the lateral tibial plateau is reduced. (Redrawn from Irrgang JJ et al: The knee: ligamentous and meniscal injuries. In Zachazewski JE et al, editors: *Athletic injuries and rehabilitation,* pp. 683–644, Philadelphia, 1996, WB Saunders.)

(1) Inward stress

(2) Knee flexion

Stabilize

Figure 12-79

Slocum anterolateral rotary instability test.

knee while flexing the knee. The subluxation of the knee reduces at between 25° and 45° of flexion if the test is positive. A positive test indicates injury to the same structures as indicated in the pivot shift maneuver. The main advantage of this test is that it aids in relaxation of the patient's hamstring muscles and is easier to perform on heavy or tense patients.

Crossover Test of Arnold. The patient is asked to cross the uninvolved leg in front of the involved leg (Figure 12-80). The examiner then carefully steps on the patient's involved foot to stabilize it and instructs the patient to rotate the upper torso away from the injured leg approximately 90° from the fixed foot. When this position is achieved, the patient contracts the quadriceps muscles, producing the same symptoms and testing the same structures as in the lateral pivot shift test.

Noyes Flexion-Rotation Drawer Test. Described by Noyes et al.,[153] this test is a modification of the pivot shift maneuver. It can be used in the acutely injured knee and is felt by some[11] to be more sensitive than the other antero-lateral rotary instability tests. The patient lies supine, and the examiner holds the patient's ankle between the examiner's trunk and arm with the hands around the tibia (Figure 12-81). The examiner flexes the patient's knee to 20° to 30° while maintaining the tibia in neutral rotation. The tibia is then pushed posteriorly, as in a posterior drawer test. This posterior movement reduces the subluxation of the tibia, indicating a positive test for antero-lateral rotary instability. If the tibia is alternately pushed posteriorly and released and the femur is allowed to rotate freely, the reduction and subluxation are seen and felt as the femur rotates medially and laterally.

Lemaire's Jolt Test.[26] The patient is in side-lying position with the test leg uppermost. For the test to work, the patient must be relaxed. With one hand, the examiner medially rotates the tibia by grasping the foot and medially rotating it with the knee in extension. The back of the other hand pushes lightly against the biceps tendon and head of the fibula while the hand on the foot flexes and extends the knee (Figure 12-82). In a positive test, at about 15° to 20° of flexion, a "jolt" occurs with displacement of the tibia, indicating a positive test for anterolateral instability.

Flexion-Extension Valgus Test. The patient lies supine, and the examiner holds the patient's leg as in the Noyes test. The examiner palpates the joint line with the thumb and fingers of both hands, and a valgus stress and axial compression are applied while the knee is flexed and extended (Figure 12-83). If the anterior cruciate ligament is torn, the examiner feels the reduction and subluxation. The tibia is not rotated, so the subluxation is easily felt.[154]

Nakajima Test.[66] The patient lies supine, and the examiner stands on the side of the test leg. The patient's foot is held with one hand, which medially rotates the tibia. The knee is flexed to 90°. The examiner's other hand is placed over the lateral femoral condyle with the thumb behind the head of the fibula, pushing it forward. The examiner slowly extends the knee while pushing the head of the fibula forward, noting whether subluxation occurs, which indicates a positive test.

Martens Test.[66] The patient and examiner are positioned as for the Noyes test. The examiner grips the patient's leg distal to the knee joint with one hand and pushes the femur posteriorly with the other hand. A valgus

Figure 12-80
Crossover test.

Test leg

Figure 12-81

Flexion-rotation drawer test combines elements of Lachman test and lateral pivot shift. Flexion from *A* to *B* results in posterior reduction of subluxated tibia and medial rotation of femur. Positive test results correlate with anterior cruciate ligament disruption. (Redrawn from Scott WN, editor: *Ligament and extensor mechanism injuries of the knee: diagnosis and treatment*, p. 94, St Louis, 1991, Mosby.)

stress is applied to the knee as the knee is flexed until the tibia reduces, indicating a positive test (Figure 12-84).

Tests for Posteromedial Rotary Instability[155-157]

When performing these tests, the examiner is looking for abnormal (excessive) posterior rotation of the medial side of the tibia relative to the femur. A note of caution: if the leg is positioned so that gravity may affect the relation of the tibia to the femur (e.g., supine-lying position, hip at 45°, knee at 90°), the medial side of the tibia may "drop back" into excessive posterior rotation just

by positioning. In this case, if the examiner is not aware of this abnormal position, a false-positive test for anteromedial rotary instability may occur if testing for anteromedial rotary instability when in fact the real problem is posteromedial rotation instability.

Hughston's Posteromedial and Posterolateral Drawer Sign. The patient lies supine with the knee flexed to 80°

Figure 12-82

Lemaire's jolt test for anterolateral rotary instability.

Figure 12-83

Flexion-extension valgus test. Arrow shows compression. (Redrawn from Hanks GA et al: Anterolateral instability of the knee, *J Sports Med* 9:226, 1981.)

Figure 12-84
Martens test.

to 90° and the hip flexed to 45° (Figure 12-85).[158] The examiner medially rotates the patient's foot slightly and sits on the foot to stabilize it. The examiner then pushes the tibia posteriorly. If the tibia moves or rotates posteriorly on the medial aspect an excessive amount relative to the normal knee, the test is positive and indicates posteromedial rotary instability. A positive test indicates that the following structures have probably been injured to some degree:

1. Posterior cruciate ligament
2. Posterior oblique ligament
3. Medial collateral ligament (superficial and deep fibers)
4. Semimembranosus tendon
5. Posteromedial capsule
6. Anterior cruciate ligament
7. Medial meniscus

The medial tubercle rotates posteriorly around the posterior cruciate ligament when the tibia is in mild medial rotation. If the posterior cruciate ligament is also torn, the posteromedial movement is greater, and the tibia subluxates posteriorly (Figure 12-86).

The test may also be done with the patient sitting with the knee flexed over the edge of the examining table. The examiner pushes posteriorly while holding the patient's leg in medial rotation, watching for the same excessive movement.

Figure 12-85
Posteromedial and posterolateral drawer test, anterior view. **A,** Starting position for posterolateral drawer test. **B,** Positive posterolateral drawer test with posterior and lateral rotation of the lateral tibial condyle.

Figure 12-86
Posterolateral drawer test. **A,** If the posterior cruciate ligament is intact, the tibia rotates posterolaterally. **B,** If the posterior cruciate ligament is torn, the tibia rotates posterolaterally and subluxates posteriorly.

Posterolateral rotary instability may be tested in a similar fashion.[158] The patient and examiner are in the same position, but the patient's foot is slightly laterally rotated. If the tibia rotates posteriorly on the lateral side an excessive amount relative to the uninvolved leg when the examiner pushes the tibia posteriorly, the test is positive for posterolateral rotary instability. The test is positive only if the posterior cruciate ligament and lateral collateral ligaments are torn.[159] The examiner may palpate the fibula while doing the movement to feel for excessive movement.

Posteromedial Pivot Shift Test.[160] The patient lies relaxed in the supine position. The examiner passively flexes the knee more than 45° while applying a varus stress, compression, and medial rotation of the tibia; in a "positive" knee, these movements cause subluxation of the medial tibial plateau posteriorly. The examiner then takes the knee into extension. At about 20° to 40° of flexion, the tibia shifts into the reduced position. A positive test indicates that the following structures are injured:

1. Posterior cruciate ligament
2. Medial collateral ligament
3. Posterior oblique ligament

Tests for Posterolateral Rotary Instability[159,161–164]

The examiner is looking for abnormal (excessive) posterior rotation of the lateral side of the tibia when performing these tests. As with the posteromedial rotation, the examiner must always be aware that positioning the leg (gravity may cause the lateral tibia to "drop back") may lead to a false-positive anterolateral rotary instability when, in fact, the problem is actually a posterolateral instability problem.

Hughston's Posteromedial and Posterolateral Drawer Sign. This test has been described previously. For posterolateral instability to occur, the following structures must have been injured to some degree:

1. Posterior cruciate ligament
2. Arcuate-popliteus complex
3. Lateral collateral ligament
4. Biceps femoris tendon
5. Posterolateral capsule
6. Anterior cruciate ligament

Jakob Test (Reverse Pivot Shift Maneuver). This is a test for posterolateral rotary instability,[110,165] and it can be performed in two ways. In the first method, the patient stands and leans against a wall with the uninjured side adjacent to the wall and the body weight distributed equally between the two feet (Figure 12-87). The examiner's hands are placed above and below the involved knee, and a valgus stress is exerted while flexion of the patient's knee is initiated. If there is a jerk in the knee or the tibia shifts posteriorly and the "giving way" phenomenon occurs during this maneuver, it indicates injury to the lateral collateral ligament, arcuate-popliteus complex, and mid third of the lateral capsule.[159]

Figure 12-87
Jakob test (method 1, showing valgus stress and flexion).

In the second method, the patient lies in the supine position with the hamstring muscles relaxed. The examiner faces the patient, lifts the patient's leg, and supports the leg against the examiner's pelvis. The examiner's other hand supports the lateral side of the calf with the palm on the proximal fibula. The knee is flexed to 70° to 80° of flexion, and the foot is laterally rotated, causing the lateral tibial plateau to subluxate posteriorly (Figure 12-88A). The knee is taken into extension by

A **B**

Figure 12-88
Reverse pivot shift test, method 2. **A,** Flexed position with lateral rotation causes lateral tibial tubercle to subluxate. **B,** As the extended position is approached, the lateral tibial tubercle reduces.

its own weight while the examiner leans on the foot to impart a valgus stress to the knee through the leg. As the knee approaches 20° of flexion, the lateral tibial tubercle shifts forward or anteriorly into the neutral rotation and reduces the subluxation, indicating a positive test (Figure 12-88B). The leg is then flexed again, and the foot falls back into lateral rotation and posterior subluxation.

External Rotation Recurvatum Test. There are two methods for performing this test. In the first method, the patient lies in the supine position with the lower limbs relaxed. The examiner gently grasps the big toe of each foot and lifts both feet off the examining table (Figure 12-89).[158,161,166] The patient is told to keep the quadriceps muscles relaxed (i.e., it is a passive test). While elevating the legs, the examiner watches the tibial tuberosities. With a positive test, the affected knee goes into relative hyperextension on the lateral aspect because of the force of gravity, with the tibia and tibial tuberosity rotating laterally. The affected knee has the appearance of a relative genu varum. It is a test for posterolateral rotary instability in extension.

In the second method, the patient lies supine and the examiner's hand holds the patient's heel or foot and flexes the knee to 30° to 40° (Figure 12-90).[158] The examiner's other hand holds the posterolateral aspect of the patient's knee and slowly extends it. With the hand on the knee, the examiner feels the relative hyperextension and lateral rotation occurring in the injured limb compared with the uninjured limb.

Loomer's Posterolateral Rotary Instability Test.[166,167] The patient lies supine and flexes both hips and both knees to 90°. The examiner then grasps the feet and maximally laterally rotates both tibias (Figure 12-91).

The test is considered positive if the injured tibia laterally rotates excessively and there is a posterior sag of the affected tibial tubercle; both signs must be present for a positive test. This test is similar to the **Bousquet external hypermobility test.**[26]

Veltri and associates[168–170] describe a modification of Loomer's test that is called the **tibial lateral rotation test** or **dial test** (Figure 12-92). This test is designed to show loss of the posterolateral support structures of the knee. The patient may be placed supine or prone. The examiner

Figure 12-89
External rotational recurvatum test (method 1).

Figure 12-90

External recurvatum test (method 2). The test is begun by holding the knee in flexion *(left)*. As the knee is slowly extended, the hand at the knee feels the lateral rotation and recurvatum at the posterolateral aspect of the knee.

Figure 12-91

Loomer's test.

flexes the knee to 30°, extends the foot over the side of the examining table, and stabilizes the femur on the table.[171] The examiner then laterally rotates the tibia on the femur and compares the amount of rotation with that on the good side. If the test is done in supine position, the examiner can observe the amount of tibial tubercle movement and compare. The test is then repeated with the knee flexed to 90° and the thigh still on the examining table. If the tibia rotates less at 90° than at 30°, an isolated posterolateral (popliteus corner) injury is more likely. If the knee rotates more at 90°, injury to both the popliteus corner and posterior cruciate injury are more likely.[138,159,161–163]

Dynamic Posterior Shift Test.[172] The patient lies supine, and the examiner flexes the hip and knee of the test leg to 90° with the femur in neutral rotation. One hand of the examiner stabilizes the anterior thigh while the other hand extends the knee. If the test is positive, the tibia reduces anteriorly with a clunk as extension is reached. The test is positive for posterior and posterolateral instabilities. If the knee is painful before extension is accomplished, the hip flexion may be decreased, but the hamstrings must be kept tight (Figure 12-93).

Active Posterolateral Drawer Sign.[173] The patient sits with the foot on the floor in neutral rotation. The knee is flexed to 80° to 90°. The patient is asked to isometrically contract the hamstrings, primarily the lateral one (biceps femoris), while the examiner stabilizes the foot. A positive test for posterolateral instability is posterior subluxation of the lateral tibial plateau (Figure 12-94).

Standing Apprehension Test.[174] The patient stands on the affected knee. The examiner then pushes anteriorly and medially on the anterolateral part of the lateral femoral condyle crossing the joint line. The patient is then asked to slightly flex the knee while the examiner pushes with the thumb (Figure 12-95). Condylar movement and a "giving way" sensation are considered positive signs for posterolateral instability.

Text continued on page 787

Figure 12-92
Tibial external rotation test or dial test in supine position. **A,** At 30° flexion. **B,** At 90° flexion.

Figure 12-93
Dynamic posterior shift test. **A,** Starting position in flexion. **B,** Extended position in which posterior shift occurs.

Figure 12-94
Active posterolateral drawer sign or test. Examiner watches for posterolateral shift.

Ligament Testing Devices

Ligament testing devices for the knee have been developed to help quantify the displacement occurring in the knee and how this displacement is modified when ligaments are injured. Most commonly, these devices test anteroposterior displacement, although more expensive ones may test other displacements. These devices are used primarily to assist in diagnosing ligament injuries (third-degree sprains) by detecting abnormal (pathological) motion, to provide a quantified measurement of motion, and to measure the amount of motion after surgery (e.g., whether normal motion limits were reestablished).[175-178]

The most commonly used ligament testing devices are the KT-1000 arthrometer, which measures anteroposterior displacement; the Genucom, which measures anteroposterior, mediolateral, and rotation displacement; and the Stryker knee laxity tester. Of the three, the KT-1000 is most commonly used. Other units have been developed but are not commonly used.[26,179-182] These devices should be considered adjuncts to clinical assess-

ment and should be used primarily to confirm a clinical diagnosis.[28]

Each of these devices works on the principle of positioning the limb in a specific manner, applying a force that causes displacement, and subsequently measuring the amount of displacement or translation caused by the applied force.[175,183,184] The measurements obtained depend on the experience and ability of the examiner, the joint position, muscle activity or inactivity, the constraints present in the joint and those imposed by the testing systems, the amount of displacing force, and the measurement system used.[175] The greatest sources of error when using the arthrometer are the inability to stabilize the patellar sensor pad and lack of muscle relaxation.[185]

Because the KT-1000 arthrometer is the most commonly used testing device for anteroposterior displacement, it is briefly described here. More detailed descriptions of its use are found elsewhere[80,183-185] and should be consulted if the examiner plans to use this device. The arthrometer is placed on the anterior aspect of the tibia and is held in place with two Velcro straps (Figures 12-96 and 12-97). A thigh support and foot support help to hold the leg in proper alignment, with straps if necessary. There are two sensor pads, one on the tibial tubercle and one on the patella. Because the patella is one of the sensor points, knees that are swollen and demonstrate a ballotable patella should not be tested unless the knee is aspirated to minimize false-positive readings.[186] These pads detect relative movement. Forces to translate the tibia are applied through a force-sensing handle.

After the device is properly positioned and the leg is properly relaxed, several tests may be performed, first on the good knee and then on the injured knee.

Quadriceps Neutral Test. The patient's knee is flexed to 90°, and the arthrometer is positioned on the leg. A 9-kg (20-lb) posterior force is applied through the apparatus to establish a reference position. The patient is then asked to perform an isolated quadriceps contraction. If the tibia shifts forward, the knee angle is altered until there is no movement of the tibia when the quadriceps contracts. This position is called the **quadriceps neutral angle** or **quadriceps active position**, and it usually occurs at about 70° flexion (see Figure 12-128). This position is found on the good knee and is used as a reference or starting position for the injured knee. If, when the injured knee is tested in this position, the anterior displacement is greater than 1 mm, the translation is abnormal and probably indicates a posterior cruciate ligament sprain.[175,185]

Test in Quadriceps Active Position. With the patient's leg positioned at the quadriceps neutral angle, the examiner applies a 9-kg (20-lb) anterior force, followed by a 9-kg (20-lb) posterior force. The results for the good and injured knee are compared.[175,185]

A   **B**

Figure 12-95

Standing apprehension test for posterolateral instability. **A,** Starting position. **B,** With knee flexed.

Figure 12-96

KT-1000 arthrometer. A posterior *(2)* or anterior *(3)* force is applied. A constant force *(1)* is applied to stabilize the patellar sensor pad. *A,* Force handle; *B,* patellar sensor pad; *C,* tibial sensor pad; *D,* Velcro straps; *E,* arthrometer body; *F,* displacement dial; *G,* thigh support; *H,* foot support. (From Daniel D, Akeson W, O'Conner J, editors: *Knee ligaments: structure, injury and repair,* p. 428, New York, 1990, Raven Press.)

Test in 30° Flexion. With the patient's leg positioned as shown in Figure 12-96, five tests are performed:
1. 9-kg (20-lb) posterior displacement
2. 7-kg (15-lb) anterior (Lachman) displacement
3. 9-kg (20-lb) anterior (Lachman) displacement
4. Maximum anterior (Lachman) displacement, usually 14 to 18 kg (30 to 40 lb)
5. Quadriceps active anterior displacement

The difference between the 7-kg and the 9-kg anterior displacement tests is called the **compliance index.**

For the maximum anterior displacement test, the examiner manually pulls or translates the tibia forward on the femur, using a pull of approximately 14 to 18 kg (30 to 40 lb). For the quadriceps active test, the patient is asked to lift the heel slowly off the table; displacement as the heel leaves the table is noted. Differences of more than 3 mm between the good and injured legs are considered diagnostic for injury to the anterior cruciate or posterior cruciate.[175,185] Force displacement curves (Figure 12-98) and frequency distribution curves (Figure 12-99)

Flex knee (20-30°) to engage patella in femoral trochlea

Support thigh to place patella facing up

Apply pressure to stabilize patella

Figure 12-97

The knee is supported in a flexed position to engage the patella in the femoral trochlea. In some patients, the thigh support must be raised an additional 3 to 6 cm to provide sufficient knee flexion to engage the patella in the femoral trochlea. This may be done by placing a board under the thigh support. The thigh should be supported so that the patella is facing up. Occasionally, a thigh strap is used to accomplish this task. The examiner stabilizes the patellar sensor with manual pressure. The stabilizing hand should rest against the lateral thigh and should apply 1 to 2.25 kg (2 to 5 lb) of pressure on the patellar sensor pad. The hand position, patellar sensor position, and patellar sensor pressure must remain constant throughout the test. Variation of the pressure on the patellar sensor pad and rotation of the pad is a common cause of measurement error. (From Daniel D et al, editors: *Knee ligaments: structure, injury and repair*, p. 428, New York, 1990, Raven Press.)

Figure 12-98

Force-displacement curves for normal knees and for knees with anterior cruciate ligament (ACL) deficit. The compliance index is obtained by measuring the displacement between the 67- and 89-N anterior-force levels. On this curve, the compliance index for the normal knee is 1 mm; for the knee with an ACL deficit, it is 3 mm. (From Daniel D et al, editors: *Knee ligaments: structure, injury and repair*, p. 433, New York, 1990, Raven Press.)

Displacement | Side to Side Difference

20 lb.

Compliance Index

Manual Maximum

Quadriceps Active

Millimeters

Figure 12-99

Frequency distribution curves of anterior laxity in normal knee in 30° of flexion and in knees with unilateral chronic anterior cruciate ligament disruption. (From Daniel DM, Stone ML: Diagnosis of knee ligament injury: test and measurements of joint laxity. In Feagin JA, editor: *The crucial ligaments*, p. 298, New York, 1988, Churchill Livingstone.)

demonstrate differences between the normal and pathological knees. Tests involving larger translation forces have been found to be more responsive to translation differences.[187]

It is important to realize that the accuracy of the readings for these devices depends very much on positioning, muscle relaxation, and the experience of the operator. Reliability of any of these measuring devices may be greatly affected if these factors are not controlled.[175,179,180,184,188–195]

Special Tests

Although most special tests on the knee are done only if the examiner suspects certain pathologies and wants to do a confirming test, tests for swelling should always be performed. The reliability, validity, specificity, and sensitivity of many of the special/diagnostic tests used in the knee are outlined in Appendix 12-1.

Tests for Meniscus Injury

Although there are several tests for a meniscus injury, none can be considered definitive without considerable experience on the part of the examiner. Even with experience, the examiner must do a thorough history and examination since a positive test is more likely to be found if one suspects the condition is present.[196,197]

Special Tests Commonly Performed on the Knee

Meniscus lesions:	McMurray test
	Apley's test
	"Bounce home" test
Plica lesions:	Mediopatellar plica test
	Plica "stutter" test
	Hughston's plica test
Swelling:	Brush test
	Indentation test
	Patellar tap test
Patellofemoral syndrome:	Clarke's sign
	McConnell test
Quadriceps pull:	Q-angle
	Tubercle sulcus angle
Osteochondritis dissecans:	Wilson test
Patellar instability:	Apprehension test
Iliotibial band friction syndrome:	Noble compression test
Leg length:	Leg length tests

Because the menisci are avascular and have no nerve supply on their inner two thirds, an injury to the meniscus can result in little or no pain or swelling, making diagnosis even more difficult. Often, a combination of tests and clinical signs is needed to have a high level of

---

Signs and Symptoms of Meniscus Injury

- Joint line pain
- Loss of flexion (>10°)
- Loss of extension (>5°)
- Swelling (synovial)
- Crepitus
- Positive special test

---

suspicion of meniscus injury.[198] In some cases, however, joint line pain or tenderness, if the ligaments have been ruled out as causes of the pain, is the result of meniscus pathology. It has been found, however, that only about 50% of meniscus injuries have joint line pain or tenderness, especially with anterior cruciate tears, so this finding should not be used in isolation for diagnosis.[199]

McMurray Test. The patient lies in the supine position with the knee completely flexed (the heel to the buttock).[200,201] The examiner then medially rotates the tibia and extends the knee (Figure 12-100). If there is a loose fragment of the lateral meniscus, this action causes a snap or click that is often accompanied by pain. By repeatedly changing the amount of flexion and then applying the medial rotation to the tibia followed by extension, the examiner can test the entire posterior aspect of the meniscus from the posterior horn to the middle segment. The anterior half of the meniscus is not as easily tested because the pressure on the meniscus is not as great. To test the medial meniscus, the examiner performs the same procedure with the knee laterally rotated. Kim and colleagues[202] reported that meniscus lesions may be found on the medial side with medial rotation and on the lateral side with lateral rotation.

The test may be modified by medially rotating the tibia, extending the knee, and moving through the full ROM to test the lateral meniscus. The process is repeated several times. The tibia is then laterally rotated, and the process is repeated to test the medial meniscus. Both methods are described by McMurray.[200]

Apley's Test.[203] The patient lies in the prone position with the knee flexed to 90°. The patient's thigh is then anchored to the examining table with the examiner's knee (Figure 12-101). The examiner medially and laterally rotates the tibia, combined first with distraction, while noting any restriction, excessive movement, or discomfort. Then the process is repeated using compression instead of distraction. If rotation plus distraction is more painful or shows increased rotation relative to the normal side, the lesion is probably ligamentous. If the rotation plus compression is

Figure 12-100

McMurray test. **A,** Medial meniscus test. **B,** Lateral meniscus test.

more painful or shows decreased rotation relative to the normal side, the lesion is probably a meniscus injury.

"Bounce Home" Test. The patient lies in the supine position, and the heel of the patient's foot is cupped in the examiner's hand (Figure 12-102). The patient's knee is completely flexed, and the knee is passively allowed to extend. If extension is not complete or has a rubbery end feel ("springy block"), there is something blocking full extension. The most likely cause of a block is a torn meniscus. Oni[204] reported that if the knee is allowed to quickly extend in one movement or jerk and the patient experiences a sharp pain on the joint line, which may radiate up or down the leg, the test is positive for a meniscus lesion.

Figure 12-101
Apley's test. **A,** Distraction. **B,** Compression.

Figure 12-102
Bounce home test.

Thessaly Test.[205] The patient stands flat footed on one leg while the examiner provides his or her hands for balance. The patient then flexes the knee to 20° and rotates the femur on the tibia medially and laterally three times while maintaining the 20° flexion. The patient tests first the good leg and then the injured leg. The test is considered positive for a meniscus tear if the patient experiences medial or lateral joint line discomfort. The patient may also have a sense of locking or catching in the knee.

O'Donohue's Test. If a patient experiences pain along the joint line, the patient is asked to lie in the supine position. The examiner flexes the knee to 90°, rotates it medially and laterally twice, and then fully flexes and rotates it both ways again. A positive sign is indicated by increased pain on rotation in either or both positions and is indicative of capsular irritation or a meniscus tear.

Modified Helfet Test.[206] In the normal knee, the tibial tuberosity is in line with the midline of the patella when the knee is flexed to 90°. When the knee is extended, however, the tibial tubercle is in line with the lateral border of the patella (Figure 12-103). If this change does not occur with the change in movement, rotation is blocked, indicating that there is injury to the meniscus, there is a possible cruciate injury, or the quadriceps muscles have insufficient strength to "screw home" the knee.

Flexed knee   Extended knee

Figure 12-103
Modified Helfet test (negative test shown).

Test for Retreating or Retracting Meniscus. The patient sits on the edge of the examining table or lies in the supine position with the knee flexed to 90°.[206] The examiner places one finger over the joint line of the patient's knee anterior to the medial collateral ligament, where the curved margin of the medial femoral condyle approaches the tibial tuberosity (Figure 12-104). The patient's leg and foot are then passively laterally rotated, and the meniscus normally disappears. The leg is medially and laterally rotated several times, with the meniscus appearing and disappearing. The knee must be flexed and the muscles relaxed to do the test. If the meniscus does not appear, a torn meniscus is indicated because rotation of the tibia is not occurring. The examiner must palpate carefully, because a distinct structure is difficult to palpate. If the examiner medially and laterally rotates the unaffected leg several times first, the meniscus can be felt pushing against the finger on medial rotation, and it disappears on lateral rotation.

Steinman's Tenderness Displacement Test. Steinman's sign is indicated by point tenderness and pain on the joint line that appears to move anteriorly when the knee is extended and moves posteriorly when the knee is flexed. It indicates a possible meniscus tear. Medial pain is elicited on lateral rotation, and lateral pain is elicited on medial rotation.

Payr's Test. The patient lies supine with the test leg in the figure-four position (Figure 12-105). If pain is elicited on the medial joint line, the test is considered positive for a meniscus lesion, primarily in the middle or posterior part of the meniscus.[66]

Bohler's Sign. The patient lies in the supine position, and the examiner applies varus and valgus stresses to the knee. Pain in the opposite joint line (valgus stress for lateral meniscus) on stress testing is a positive sign for meniscus pathology.[66]

Figure 12-105
Payr's sign for a meniscus lesion.

Bragard's Sign. The patient lies supine, and the examiner flexes the patient's knee. The examiner then laterally rotates the tibia and extends the knee (Figure 12-106). Pain and tenderness on the medial joint line indicate medial meniscus pathology. If the examiner then medially rotates the tibia and flexes the knee, the pain and tenderness will decrease.[66] Both of these symptoms indicate medial meniscus pathology.

Kromer's Sign. This test is similar to Bohler's sign except that the knee is flexed and extended while the varus and valgus stresses are applied.[66] A positive test is indicated by the same pain on the opposite joint line.

Childress' Sign. The patient squats and performs a "duck waddle."[66] Pain, snapping, or a click is considered positive for a posterior horn lesion of the meniscus.

Anderson Medial-Lateral Grind Test.[207] The patient lies supine. The examiner holds the test leg between the trunk and the arm while the index finger and thumb of the opposite hand are placed over the anterior joint line (Figure 12-107). A valgus stress is applied to the knee as it is passively flexed to 45°; then a varus stress is applied to the knee as it is passively extended, producing a circular motion to the knee. The motion is repeated, increasing the varus and valgus stresses with each rotation. A distinct grinding is felt on the joint line if there is meniscus pathology. The test may also show a pivot shift if the anterior cruciate ligament has been torn.

Passler Rotational Grind Test.[66] The patient sits with the test knee extended and held at the ankle between the examiner's legs proximal to the examiner's knees. The examiner places both thumbs over the medial joint line and moves the knee in a circular fashion, medially and laterally rotating the tibia while the knee is rotated through

Figure 12-104
Test for a retreating meniscus.

Figure 12-106

Bragard's sign for a meniscus lesion. **A,** Medial meniscus test. **B,** Lateral meniscus test.

Figure 12-107

Anderson medial-lateral grind test. **A,** Flexion and valgus stress. **B,** Extension and varus stress.

various flexion angles. Simultaneously, the examiner applies a varus or a valgus stress (Figure 12-108). Pain elicited on the joint line indicates a meniscus lesion.

Cabot's Popliteal Sign.[66] The patient lies supine, and the examiner positions the test leg in the figure-four position. The examiner palpates the joint line with the thumb and forefinger of one hand and places the other hand proximal to the ankle of the test leg. The patient is asked to isometrically straighten the knee while the examiner resists the movement. A positive test, signifying a meniscus lesion, is indicated by pain on the joint (Figure 12-109).

Figure 12-108

Passler rotational grind test for meniscus pathology.

Figure 12-109
Cabot's popliteal sign for a meniscus lesion.

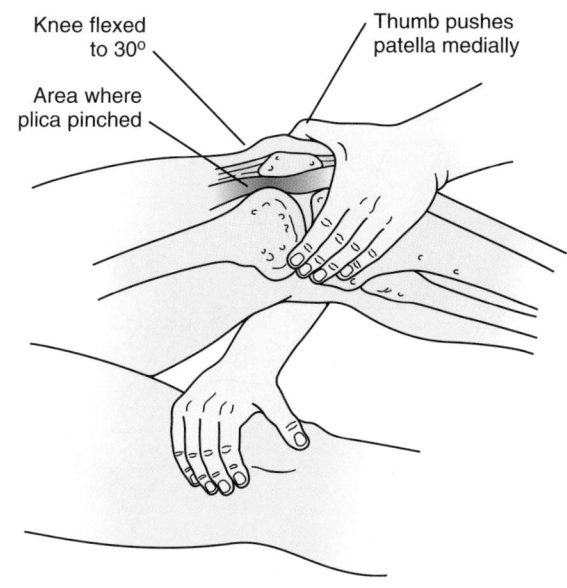

Knee flexed to 30°
Area where plica pinched
Thumb pushes patella medially

Figure 12-110
Test for mediopatellar plica.

Plica Tests

In the knee, plica are embryological remnants that have remained in some people after birth.[208-210] Normally, they are reabsorbed by the time of birth although remnants may be present in 20% to 50% of knees.[211-213] Because an abnormal plica can mimic meniscus pathology, it is essential that the plica tests be performed as well as the meniscus tests if a meniscus or plica injury is suspected.

Mediopatellar Plica Test (Mital-Hayden Test). The patient lies in the supine position with the affected knee flexed to 30° resting on a support or the examiner's arm (Figure 12-110). The examiner then pushes the patella medially with the thumb. If the patient complains of pain or a click, it indicates a positive test caused by pinching of the edge of the plica between the medial femoral condyle and the patella. The pain may indicate a mediopatellar plica.[214]

Plica "Stutter" Test. The patient is seated on the edge of the examining table with both knees flexed to 90°. The examiner places a finger over one patella to palpate during movement. The patient is then instructed to slowly extend

the knee. If the test is positive, the patella stutters or jumps somewhere between 60° and 45° of flexion (0° being straight leg) during an otherwise smooth movement. The test is effective only if there is no joint swelling.

Hughston's Plica Test. The patient lies in the supine position, and the examiner flexes the knee and medially rotates the tibia with one arm and hand while pressing the patella medially with the heel of the other hand and palpating the medial femoral condyle with the fingers of the same hand (Figure 12-111). The patient's knee is passively flexed and extended while the examiner feels for "popping" of the plica band under the fingers. The popping indicates a positive test.[152]

Patellar Bowstring Test.[51] The patient lies on his or her side with the test leg uppermost. Using the heel of one hand, the examiner pushes the patella medially and holds it there. The examiner then flexes the patient's knee and medially rotates the tibia with the other hand. The patient's knee is then extended (Figure 12-112) while the examiner feels for any sounds.

Tests for Swelling

When assessing swelling, the examiner must determine the type and amount of swelling that are present. Although the tests for swelling are listed under Special Tests, the examiner should always be testing for swelling when examining the knee. In addition, the examiner must differentiate between swelling and synovial thickening. With swelling, the knee assumes its resting position of 15° to 25° of flexion, which allows the synovial cavity the maximum capacity for holding fluid. If the injury is sufficiently severe, the fluid extravasates into the soft

Figure 12-111

Examination for suprapatellar plica. The foot and tibia are held in medial rotation. The patella is displaced slightly medially with the fingers over the course of the plica. The knee is passively flexed and extended, eliciting a "pop" of the plica and associated tenderness. (Redrawn from Hughston JC, Walsh WM, Puddu G: *Patellar subluxation and dislocation*, p 29, Philadelphia, 1984, WB Saunders.)

tissue surrounding the joint as a result of torn structures (i.e., ligaments, capsule, synovium). Therefore lack of effusion should not lull the examiner into thinking the injury is a minor one.

If the swelling consists of blood that results in a hemarthrosis (within the joint), it may be caused by a ligament tear, osteochondral fracture, or peripheral meniscus tear. "Blood" swelling comes on very quickly (within 1 to 2 hours), and the skin becomes very taut. On palpation, it has a "doughy" feeling and is relatively hard to the touch. The joint surface feels warm. Usually, excess blood should be aspirated, or osteoarthritis may result from irritation of the cartilage. Blood swelling in the form of ecchymosis may also be seen around the knee, but commonly this blood will begin to "track" down the leg because of gravity as it becomes visible (see Figure 1-8).

Normally, synovial fluid swelling caused by joint irritation occurs in 8 to 24 hours. The feeling within the joint is a fluctuating or "boggy" feeling. The joint surface feels warm and tender. Swelling usually occurs with activity and disappears after a few days of inactivity.

The third type of joint swelling is purulent or pus swelling, in which the joint surface is hot to the touch. Often it is red, and the patient has general signs of infection or pyrexia.

Brush, Stroke, or Bulge Test. Also called the **wipe test**, this test assesses minimal effusion. The examiner commences just below the joint line on the medial side of the patella, stroking proximally toward the patient's hip as far as the suprapatellar pouch two or three times with the palm and fingers (Figure 12-113). With the opposite hand, the examiner strokes down the lateral side of the patella. A wave of fluid passes to the medial side of the joint and bulges just below the medial distal portion or border of the patella. The wave of fluid may take up to 2 seconds to appear. Normally, the knee contains 1 to 7 mL of synovial fluid. This test shows as little as 4 to 8 mL of extra fluid within the knee.

A   **B**

Figure 12-112

Bowstring test for plica. **A,** Using the heel of one hand, the examiner pushes the patella medially and holds it there. The examiner then flexes the patient's knee and medially rotates the tibia with the other hand. **B,** The patient's knee is then extended while the examiner feels for any sounds.

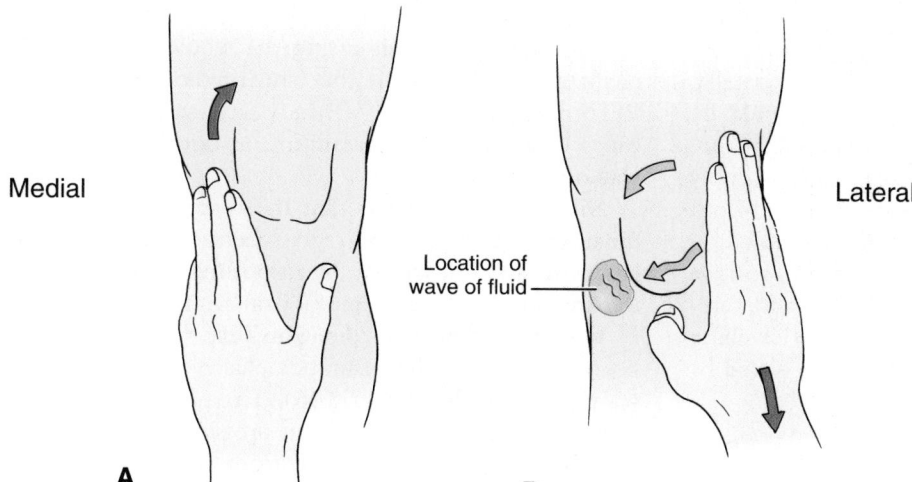

Medial

Lateral

Location of wave of fluid

A   B

Figure 12-113
Brush test for swelling. **A,** Hand strokes up. **B,** Hand strokes down.

Indentation Test.[215] The patient lies supine. The examiner passively flexes the good leg, noting an indentation on the lateral side of the patellar tendon (Figure 12-114). The good knee is fully flexed, and the indentation remains. The injured knee is then slowly flexed while the examiner watches for the disappearance of the indentation. At that point, knee flexion is stopped. The disappearance of the indentation is caused by swelling and indicates a positive test. The angle at which the indentation disappears depends on the amount of swelling. The greater the swelling, the sooner the indentation disappears. If the thumb and finger are placed on each side of the patellar tendon, the fluid can be made to fluctuate back and forth. This method, like the brush test, can detect minimal levels of swelling.

Peripatellar Swelling Test.[216] The patient lies supine with the knee extended. The examiner carefully milks fluid from the suprapatellar pouch distally. With the opposite hand, the examiner palpates adjacent to the patellar tendon (usually on the medial side) for fluid accumulation or a wave of fluid passing under the fingers. Reider[41] calls this a **palpable fluid wave**. If less swelling is evident, Reider[41] suggests the **visible** fluid wave. The examiner strokes the fluid into the suprapatellar pouch. With one hand, the examiner then squeezes or pushes down on the suprapatellar pouch while watching the hollows on each side of the patella for a wave of fluid to pass. This test is similar to the brush test.

Fluctuation Test. The examiner places the palm of one hand over the suprapatellar pouch and the palm of the other hand anterior to the joint with the thumb and index finger just beyond the margins of the patella (Figure 12-115). By pressing down with one hand and then the other, the examiner may feel the synovial fluid fluctuate under the hands and move from one hand to the other, indicating significant effusion.

Figure 12-114
Indentation test. Arrow indicates where to watch for filling of indentation.

Figure 12-115
Hand positioning for fluctuation test. First one hand is pushed down *(arrow 1);* then the other hand is pushed down *(arrow 2).* The examiner will feel fluid shifting back and forth under one hand and then the other.

Patellar Tap Test ("Ballotable Patella"). With the patient's knee extended or flexed to discomfort, the examiner applies a slight tap or pressure over the patella. When this is done, a floating of the patella should be felt. This is sometimes called the **"dancing patella"** sign. A modification of this test calls for the examiner to apply the thumb and forefinger of one hand lightly on both sides of the patella. The examiner then strokes down on the suprapatellar pouch with the other hand.[66] A positive test is indicated by separation of the thumb and forefinger. This test can detect a large amount of swelling (40 to 50 mL) in the knee, which can also be noted by observation.

Tests for Patellofemoral Dysfunction

Patellofemoral dysfunction (patellofemoral pain syndrome [PFPS]) implies there is some pathology affecting the patellofemoral joint.[217] This pathology may be the result of biomechanical factors or pathophysiological processes or loss of tissue homeostasis resulting in synovitis and an inflamed fat pad.[218] Commonly, patients with patellofemoral problems experience pain when climbing or descending stairs, when stepping up or down, with prolonged sitting **(movie sign)**, when squatting, or when getting up from a chair. The examiner should consider assessing the whole lower kinetic chain and its effect on the patellofemoral joint when PFPS is suspected.[45–50,219,220] In some cases, the pain may cause reflex inhibition, resulting in buckling or giving way of the knee.[221]

Nijs et al.[222] reported that the vastus medialis coordination test, the patellar apprehension test, and the eccentric step test had the most positive likelihood ratio in patients with patellofemoral pain syndrome.

Vastus Medialis Coordination Test.[222,223] The patient lies supine while the examiner places a fist under the patient's knee (Figure 12-116). The patient is asked to slowly extend the knee without pressing into the examiner's fist or lifting the leg away from the fist while trying to achieve full extension. The test is considered positive if the patient cannot fully extend the knee or has difficulty achieving full extension smoothly or tries to use the hip flexors or extensors to accomplish the task.

Clarke's Sign (Patellar Grind Test). This test assesses the presence of patellofemoral dysfunction. The examiner presses down slightly proximal to the upper pole or base of the patella with the web of the hand as the patient lies relaxed with the knee extended (Figure 12-117). Reider[41] recommends pushing down on the patella directly. The patient is then asked to contract the quadriceps muscles while the examiner pushes down. If the patient can complete and maintain the contraction without pain, the test is considered negative. If the test causes retropatellar pain and the patient cannot hold a contraction, the test is considered positive. Because the examiner can achieve a positive test on anyone if sufficient pressure is applied to the patella, the amount of pressure that is applied must be carefully controlled. The best way to do this is to repeat the procedure several times, increasing the pressure each time and comparing the results with those of the unaffected side. To test different parts of the patella, the knee should be tested in 30°, 60°, and 90° of flexion as well as in full extension.

Some Factors that MAY Contribute to Patellofemoral Pain Syndrome*

- Patellar dysplasia (e.g., patella alta or baja)
- Tight patellar retinaculum (especially lateral)
- Abnormal patellar tracking
- Abnormal patellar tilt or rotation
- Abnormal patellar alignment relative to the femur (e.g., Q-angle outside the normal 13° to 18°)
- Crossover gait
- Excessive genu valgum/varum
- Muscle weakness (e.g., vastus medialis obliquus, hip abductor and lateral rotators, ankle dorsiflexors)
- Muscle imbalance (e.g., quadriceps/hamstrings ratio)
- Excessive tibial torsion (especially medial)
- Foot malalignment (e.g., rearfoot varus or valgus, excessive pronation/supination of the foot)
- Muscle hypomobility (e.g., quadriceps, hamstrings, gastrocnemius, iliotibial band, hip adductors)
- Trauma to patella (e.g., dislocation, direct blow)
- Abnormal repetitive stress to patella (e.g., running on the same side of road or sidewalk continually [camber of road or sidewalk affects foot-knee mechanics])
- Training shoes worn (e.g., control shoe versus cushioning shoe, shoes "broken down")
- Excessive pelvic tilt (anterior/posterior, medial/lateral)

*Patellofemoral pain syndrome may be the result of any or all of the above. In reality, the definitive cause of patellofemoral pain syndrome is unknown.

Figure 12-116
Vastus medialis coordination test.

Figure 12-117
Clarke's sign.

McConnell Test for Chondromalacia Patellae. The patient is sitting with the femur laterally rotated. The patient performs isometric quadriceps contractions at 120°, 90°, 60°, 30°, and 0°, with each contraction held for 10 seconds. If pain is produced during any of the contractions, the patient's leg is passively returned to full extension by the examiner. The patient's leg is then fully supported on the examiner's knee, and the examiner pushes the patella medially. The medial glide is maintained while the knee is returned to the painful angle, and the patient performs an isometric contraction, again with the patella held medially. If the pain is decreased, the pain is patellofemoral in origin. Each angle is tested in a similar fashion.[224]

Active Patellar Grind Test.[41] The patient sits on the examining table with the knee flexed 90° over the edge of the table. While the patient slowly straightens the knee, the examiner places a hand over the patella to feel for crepitus. Where in the ROM that pain occurs will give an indication of what part of the patella is demonstrating pathology (see Figure 12-2). Greater force can be applied through the patella by asking the patient to step up and step down on a small stool while the examiner gently palpates the patella for crepitus and pain **(step up–step down test).**[41]

Step Up Test.[221] The patient stands beside a stool that is 25 cm (10 inches) high. The examiner asks the patient to step up sideways onto the stool using the good leg. The test is repeated with the other leg. Normally, the patient should have no difficulty doing the test and have no pain. Inability to do the test may indicate patellofemoral arthralgia, weak quadriceps, or an inability to stabilize the pelvis (Figure 12-118, *A*).

Eccentric Step Test.[107,108,222] The patient stands on a 15-cm (6 inch)–high step or stool while keeping the hands on the hips. The patient steps down, first leading with the injured leg (this tests the good leg first) as slowly and smoothly as he or she can (Figure 12-118B). The test is considered positive if pain is felt by the patient during the test.

Waldron Test. This test also assesses the presence of patellofemoral syndrome and functions in a similar fashion to the two tests above.[42] The examiner palpates the patella while the patient performs several slow deep knee bends (these may be unilateral squats or bilateral for easier comparison) (Figure 12-118, *C*). As the patient goes through the ROM, the examiner should note the amount of crepitus (significant only if accompanied by pain), where it occurs in the ROM, the amount of pain, and whether there is "catching" or poor tracking of the patella (see Figure 12-28) throughout the movement. If pain and crepitus occur together during the movement, it is considered a positive sign.[42]

Passive Patellar Tilt Test. The patient lies supine with the knee extended and the quadriceps relaxed. The examiner stands at the end of the examining table and lifts the lateral edge of the patella away from the lateral femoral condyle. The patella should not be pushed medially or laterally but rather should remain in the femoral trochlea.[225] The normal angle is 15°, although males may have an angle 5° less than that of females (Figure 12-119). Patients with angles less than this are prone to patellofemoral syndrome. Watson et al.[226] have questioned the reliability of this test, especially when performed by inexperienced examiners.

Lateral Pull Test. The patient lies supine with the leg extended. The patient contracts the quadriceps while the examiner watches the movement of the patella.[225] Normally, the patella moves superiorly, or superiorly and laterally in equal proportions (Figure 12-120). If lateral movement is excessive, the test is positive for lateral overpull of the quadriceps, resulting in a patellofemoral arthralgia. Watson et al.[226] have questioned the reliability of this test especially when performed by inexperienced examiners.

Zohler's Sign.[66] The patient lies supine with the knees extended. The examiner pulls the patella distally and holds it in this position. The patient is asked to contract the quadriceps (Figure 12-121). Pain indicates a positive test for chondromalacia patellae. However, the test may be positive (false positive) in a large proportion of the normal population.

Frund's Sign. The patient is in the sitting position. The examiner percusses the patella in various positions of knee flexion. Pain indicates a positive test and may signify chondromalacia patellae.

Other Tests

Q-Angle or Patellofemoral Angle. The Q-angle (quadriceps angle) is defined as the angle between the quadriceps muscles (primarily the rectus femoris) and the patellar tendon and represents the angle of quadriceps muscle force (Figure 12-122).[227] The angle is obtained

Figure 12-118

Step tests. **A,** Step up test. **B,** Eccentric step test. **C,** Waldron test.

by first ensuring that the lower limbs are at a right angle to the line joining the two anterior superior iliac spines (ASISs). A line is then drawn from the ASIS to the midpoint of the patella on the same side and from the tibial tubercle to the midpoint of the patella. The angle formed by the crossing of these two lines is called the Q-angle. The foot should be placed in a neutral position in regard to supination and pronation and the hip in a neutral position in regard to medial and lateral rotation, because it has been found that different foot and hip positions alter the Q-angle.[228]

Normally, the Q-angle is 13° for males and 18° for females when the knee is straight (Figure 12-123) although Grelsamer et al.[229] reported male and female values are similar when patient height is considered. Any angle less than 13° may be associated with chondromalacia patellae or patella alta. An angle greater than 18° is often associated with chondromalacia patellae, subluxing patella, increased femoral anteversion, genu valgum, lateral displacement of tibial tubercle, or increased lateral

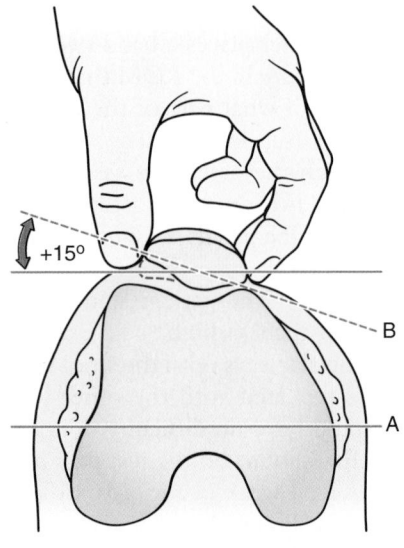

Figure 12-119

Passive patellar tilt test. (Redrawn from Kolowich PA, Paulos LE, Rosenberg TD et al: Lateral release of the patella: indications and contraindications, *Am J Sports Med* 18:361, 1990.)

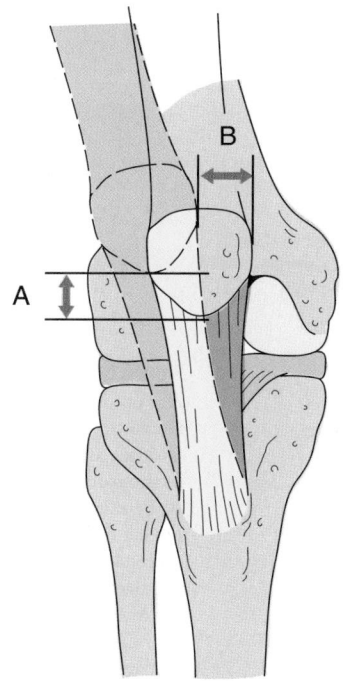

Figure 12-120
Lateral pull test. Normally, A > B or A = B; with lateral overpull of the quadriceps, B > A. (From Kolowich PA, Paulos LE, Rosenberg TD et al: Lateral release of the patella: indications and contraindications, *Am J Sports Med* 18:361, 1990.)

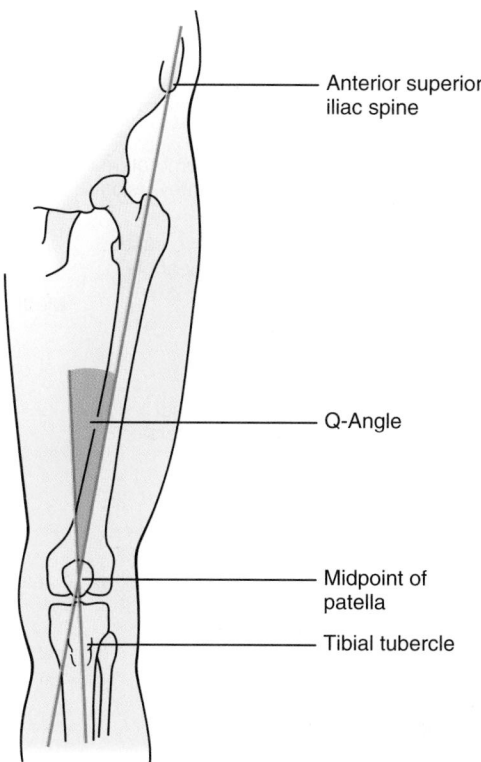

Figure 12-122
Quadriceps angle (Q-angle).

Anterior superior iliac spine

Q-Angle

Midpoint of patella

Tibial tubercle

Figure 12-121
Zohler's sign for chondromalacia patellae.

tibial torsion. During the test, which may be done either with radiographs or physically on the patient, the quadriceps should be relaxed. If measured with the patient in the sitting position, the Q-angle should be 0° (Figure 12-124). While the patient is in a sitting position, the presence of the **"bayonet sign,"** which indicates an abnormal alignment of the quadriceps musculature, patellar tendon, or tibial shaft, should be noted (Figure 12-125).

Hughston et al.[152] advocate doing the test with the quadriceps contracted. If measured with the quadriceps contracted and the knee fully extended, the Q-angle should be 8° to 10°. Any angle greater than 10° is considered abnormal. The examiner must ensure that a standardized measurement procedure is used to ensure consistent values.[230]

Tubercle Sulcus Angle (Q-Angle at 90°).[28,224] This measurement is also used to measure the angle of quadriceps pull. A vertical line is drawn from the center of the patella to the center of the tibial tubercle. A second horizontal line is drawn through the femoral epicondyle (Figure 12-126). Normally the lines are perpendicular. Angles greater than 10° from the perpendicular are considered abnormal. Lateral patellar subluxation may affect the results.

Another measurement, which is similar to the Q-angle, is the **A-angle**, which measures the relation of the patella to the tibial tubercle. This measurement, which is not as commonly used as the Q-angle, consists of a vertical line that divides the patella into two halves and a line drawn from the tibial tubercle to the apex of the inferior pole of the patella. The resulting angle is the A-angle (Figure 12-127).[231,232] Some have questioned the reliability of this measurement because of the difficulty in consistently finding appropriate landmarks.[233]

Figure 12-123

A, Femoral neck anteversion and lateral tibial torsion increase the Q-angle and lead to lateral tracking of the patella on the femoral sulcus. **B,** Femoral neck retroversion and medial tibial torsion decrease the Q-angle and tend to centralize the tracking of the patella. (Redrawn from Tria AJ, Palumbo RC: Conservative treatment of patellofemoral pain, *Semin Orthop* 5:116–117, 1990.)

Figure 12-124
Q-angle in flexed position. Exaggerated Q-angle in the patient's right knee is seen as residual positive Q-angle with the knee flexed. Normally, the Q-angle in flexion should be 0°. (Redrawn from Hughston JC, Walsh WM, Puddu G: *Patellar subluxation and dislocation*, p. 24, Philadelphia, 1984, WB Saunders.)

Daniel's Quadriceps Neutral Angle Test.[234] The patient lies supine, and the unaffected leg is tested first. The patient's hip is flexed to 45°, and the knee is flexed to 90° with the foot flat on the examining table. The patient is asked to extend the knee isometrically while the examiner holds down the foot. If tibial displacement is noted, knee flexion is decreased (posterior tibial displacement) or increased (anterior tibial displacement). The process is repeated until the angle at which there is no tibial displacement is reached (Figure 12-128). This angle, the quadriceps neutral angle, averages 70° (range, 60° to 90°). The injured knee is placed in the same neutral angle position, and the patient is asked to contract the quadriceps. Any anterior displacement indicates posterior cruciate ligament insufficiency. The quadriceps neutral angle is primarily used for machine testing of laxity (e.g., KT-1000 arthrometer, Stryker knee laxity test apparatus).

Wilson Test. This is a test for **osteochondritis dissecans.**[235] The patient sits with the knee flexed over the examining table. The knee is then actively extended with the tibia medially rotated. At approximately 30° of flexion (0° being straight leg), the pain in the knee increases, and the patient is asked to stop the flexion movement. The patient is then asked to rotate the tibia laterally, and the pain disappears. This finding means a positive test, which is indicative of osteochondritis dissecans of the femoral condyle. The test is positive only if the lesion is at the classic site for osteochondritis dissecans of the knee, namely, the medial femoral condyle near the intercondylar notch (Figure 12-129).

Fairbank's Apprehension Test. This is a test for **dislocation of the patella.**[152,236] The patient lies in the supine position with the quadriceps muscles relaxed

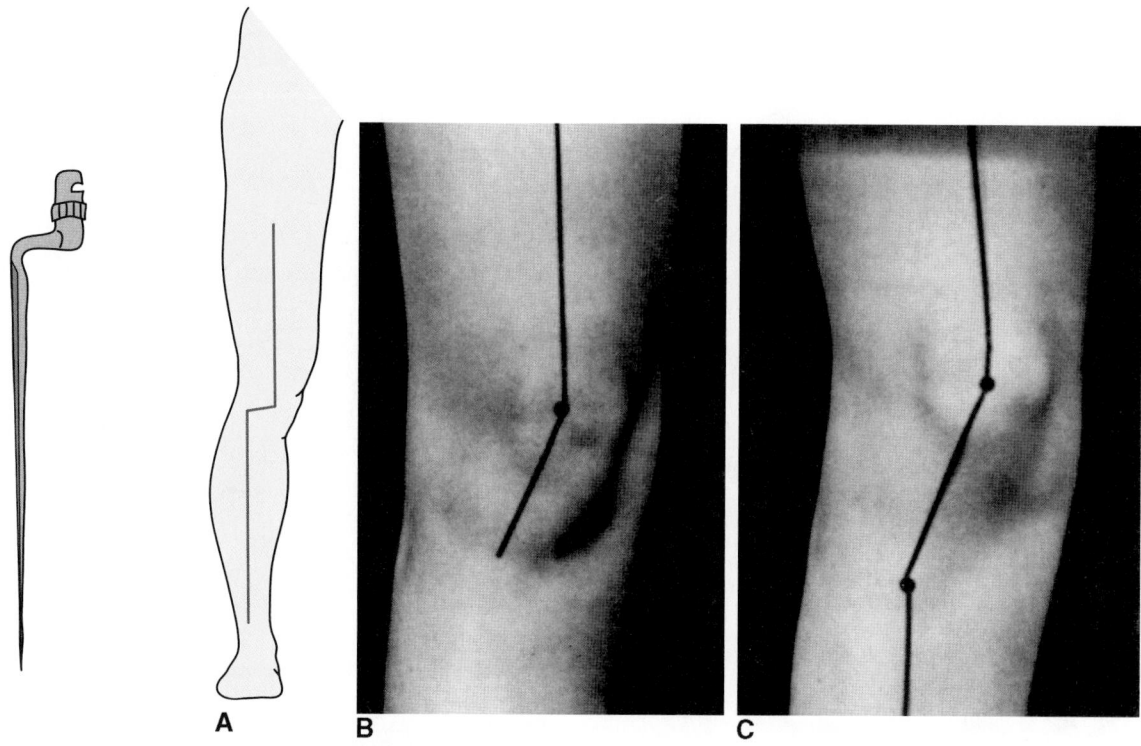

Figure 12-125

Increased Q-angle. **A,** Bayonet sign. Tibia vara of proximal third causes a markedly increased Q-angle. Alignment of the quadriceps, patellar tendon, and tibial shaft resembles a French bayonet. **B,** Q-angle with the knee in full extension is only slightly increased over normal. **C,** However, with the knee flexed at 30°, there is failure of the tibia to derotate normally and failure of the patellar tendon to line up with the anterior crest of the tibia. This is not an infrequent finding in patients with patellofemoral arthralgia. Increased medial femoral torsion (anteversion) combined with increased lateral tibial torsion will cause the same bayonet sign. (**A** from Hughston JC et al: *Patellar subluxation and dislocation,* p. 26, Philadelphia, 1984, WB Saunders; **B** and **C** from Ficat RP, Hungerford DS: *Disorders of the patello-femoral joint,* p. 117, Baltimore, 1977, Williams & Wilkins.)

and the knee flexed to 30° while the examiner carefully and slowly pushes the patella laterally (Figure 12-130). Tanner et al.[237] believed the patella should be pushed laterally and distally to make the test more sensitive. If the patient feels the patella is going to dislocate, the patient will contract the quadriceps muscles to bring the patella back "into line." This action indicates a positive test. The patient will also have an apprehensive look.

Noble Compression Test. This is a test for **iliotibial band friction syndrome**.[238] The patient lies in the supine position, and the examiner flexes the patient's knee to 90°, accompanied by hip flexion (Figure 12-131). Pressure is then applied to the lateral femoral epicondyle, or 1 to 2 cm (0.4 to 0.8 inch) proximal to it, with the thumb. While the pressure is maintained, the patient's knee is passively extended. At approximately 30° of flexion (0° being straight leg), the patient experiences severe pain over the lateral femoral condyle. Pain indicates a positive test. The patient states that it is the same pain that occurs with activity.

Functional Test for Quadriceps Contusion. The patient lies in the prone position while the examiner passively flexes the knee as much as possible. If passive knee flexion is 90° or more, it is only a mild contusion. If passive knee flexion is less than 90°, the contusion is moderate to severe, and the patient should not be allowed to bear weight. Normally, the heel-to-buttock distance should not exceed 10 cm (4 inches) in men and 5 cm (2 inches) in women. This test may also be used to test tightness of the quadriceps (vasti) muscles. If the range is limited and the end feel is muscle stretch, the vastus medialis, lateralis, and/or intermedius is tight. Testing for a tight rectus femoris is described in the hip chapter (Chapter 11).

Test for Knee Extension Contracture (Heel Height Difference).[239] The patient lies prone with the thighs supported and the legs relaxed. The examiner measures the difference in heel height (Figure 12-132). One centimeter of difference approximates 1°, depending on leg length. The test, along with the accompanying end feel, would be used to test for joint contracture (tissue stretch)

Figure 12-126
Tubercle sulcus angle of 90°. With the knee flexed to 90°, the transepicondylar line is assessed. The axis of the patellar tendon is compared with a perpendicular to the transepicondylar line. (Modified from Kolowich PA et al: Lateral release of the patella: indications and contraindications, *Am J Sports Med* 18:361, 1990.)

Figure 12-127
Location of landmarks of the A-angle. (Redrawn from Ehrat M et al: Reliability of assessing patellar alignment: the A-angle, *J Orthop Sports Phys Ther* 19:23, 1994.)

and possibly tight hamstrings (muscle stretch). Swelling may also cause a positive test.

Tests for Hamstring Tightness. These tests are described in Chapter 11.

Measurement of Leg Length. The patient lies in the supine position with the legs at a right angle to a line joining the two ASISs. With a tape measure, the examiner obtains the distance from one ASIS to the lateral or medial malleolus on that side, placing the metal end of the tape measure immediately distal to and up against the ASIS (Figure 12-133). The tape is stretched so that the other hand pushes the tape against the distal aspect of the medial (or lateral) malleolus, and the reading on the

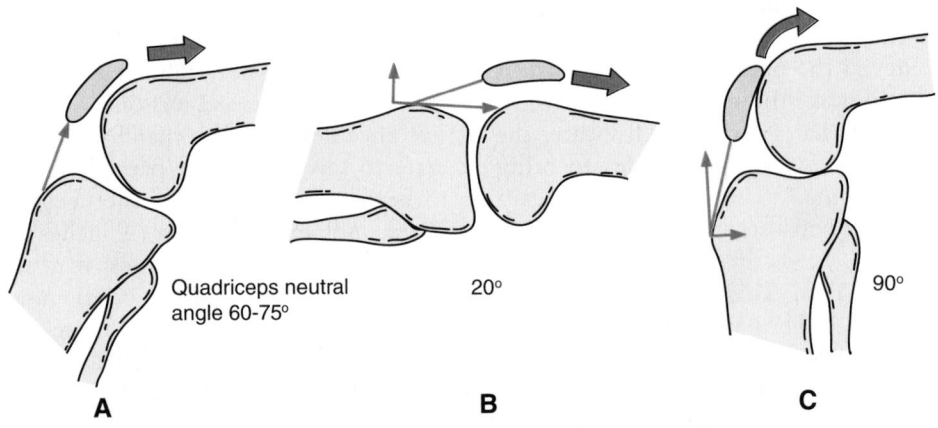

Figure 12-128
During open chain knee extension, tibial translation is a function of the shear force produced by the patellar tendon. **A,** Quadriceps neutral position. The patellar tendon force is perpendicular to the tibial plateaus and results in compression of the joint surfaces without shear force. **B,** At flexion angles less than the angle of the quadriceps neutral position, orientation of the patellar tendon produces anterior shear of the tibia. **C,** At angles greater than the angle of the quadriceps neutral position, patellar tendon force causes a posterior shear of the tibia. (From Daniel DM P et al: Use of the quadriceps active test to diagnose posterior cruciate ligament disruption and measure posterior laxity of the knee, *J Bone Joint Surg Am* 70:386–391, 1988.)

Figure 12-129
Classic site of osteochondritis dissecans.

Figure 12-130
Apprehension test. (Redrawn from Hughston JC et al: *Patellar subluxation and dislocation*, p. 29, Philadelphia, 1984, WB Saunders.)

Figure 12-131
Noble compression test.

tape measure is noted. The other side is tested similarly. A difference between the two sides of as much as 1.0 to 1.5 cm is considered normal. However, the examiner must remember that even this difference may result in pathological symptoms. If there is a difference, the examiner can determine its site of occurrence by measuring from the high point on the iliac crest to the greater trochanter (for coxa vara), from the greater trochanter to the lateral knee joint line (for femoral shaft length), and from the medial knee joint line to the medial malleolus (for tibial length). The two legs are then compared. The examiner must also remember that torsion deformities to the femur or tibia can alter leg length.

Functional Leg Length. The patient stands in the normal relaxed stance. The examiner palpates the ASISs and then the posterior superior iliac spines (PSISs) and notes any differences. The examiner then positions the patient so that the patient's subtalar joints are in neutral while bearing weight (see Chapter 13). While the patient holds this position with the toes straight ahead and the knee straight, the examiner repalpates the ASISs and the PSISs. If the previously noted differences remain, the pelvis and sacroiliac joints should be evaluated further. If the previously noted differences disappear, the examiner should suspect a functional leg length difference caused by hip, knee, ankle, or foot problems—primarily ankle or foot problems.

Measurement of Muscle Bulk (Anthropometric Measurements for Effusion and Atrophy). The examiner selects areas where muscle bulk or swelling is greatest and measures the circumference of the leg. It is important to note on the patient's chart how far above or below the apex or base of the patella one is measuring and whether the tape measure is placed above or below that mark. The following are common measurement points:

1. 15 cm (6 inches) below the apex of the patella
2. Apex of the patella or joint line
3. 5 cm (2 inches) above the base of the patella
4. 10 cm (4 inches) above the base of the patella
5. 15 cm (6 inches) above the base of the patella
6. 23 cm (9 inches) above the base of the patella

Hughston[43] advocated using the lateral joint line rather than the patella for the beginning point of measurement; he believed that the joint line was more constant. The examiner must also note, if possible, whether swelling or muscle bulk is being measured and remember that there is no correlation between muscle bulk and strength.

Reflexes and Cutaneous Distribution

Having completed the ligamentous and other tests of the knee, if a scanning examination has not been carried out, the examiner next determines whether the reflexes

Figure 12-132

Heel height difference. The patient lies prone on the examining table with the lower limbs supported by the thighs. The difference in heel height is measured. The conversion of heel height difference to degrees of extension lost depends on the leg length. The tangent of angle θ is the heel height difference (HHD) divided by the lower-leg segment length (LLSL). The LLSL is proportional to patient height. (From Daniel D, Akeson W, O'Conner J, editors: *Knee ligaments: structure, injury and repair,* p 32, New York, 1990, Raven Press.)

around the knee joint are normal, especially if neurological involvement is suspected (Figure 12-134). The patellar (L3-L4) and medial hamstring (L5-S1) reflexes should be checked for differences between the two sides.

The examiner must keep in mind the dermatome patterns of the various nerve roots (Figure 12-135) as well as the cutaneous distribution of the peripheral nerves

Figure 12-133

Measuring leg length (to the lateral malleolus).

(Figure 12-136). To test for altered sensation, a sensation scanning examination should be performed using relaxed hands and fingers to cover all aspects of the thigh, knee, and leg. Any differences in sensation should be noted and can be mapped out further with the use of a pinwheel, pin, cotton batting, or soft brush.

True knee pain tends to be localized to the knee, but it may also be referred to the hip or ankle (Figure 12-137). In a similar fashion, pain may be referred to the knee from the lumbar spine, hip (e.g., slipped capital femoral epiphysis in children), and ankle. Sometimes a lesion of the medial meniscus leads to irritation of the infrapatellar branch of the saphenous nerve. The result is a hyperaesthetic area the size of a quarter on the medial side of the knee. This finding is called **Turner's sign**.[66] Muscles about the knee and their pain referral pattern are shown in Table 12-11.

Peripheral Nerve Injuries about the Knee

Common Peroneal Nerve (L4 through S2). This nerve is vulnerable to injury in the posterolateral knee and as it winds around the head of the fibula. It has also been reported that the nerve may be stretched as a result

A **B**

Figure 12-134
Reflexes of the knee. **A,** Patellar (L3). **B,** Medial hamstrings (L5).

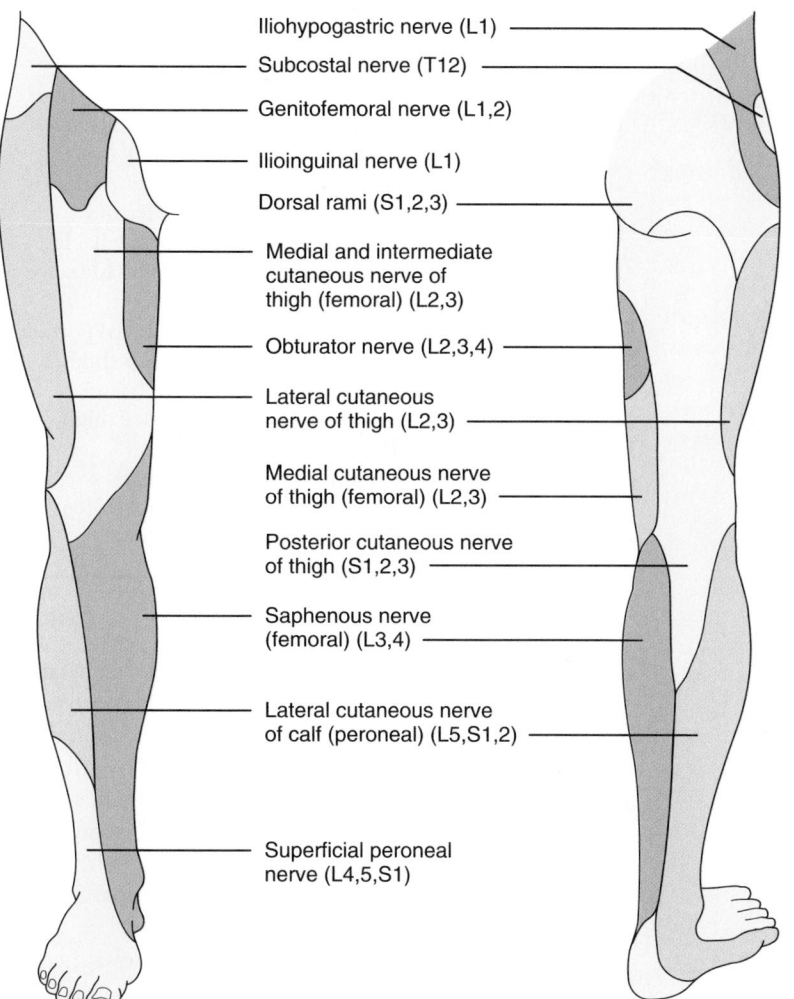

Iliohypogastric nerve (L1)

Subcostal nerve (T12)

Genitofemoral nerve (L1,2)

Ilioinguinal nerve (L1)

Dorsal rami (S1,2,3)

Medial and intermediate
cutaneous nerve of
thigh (femoral) (L2,3)

Obturator nerve (L2,3,4)

Lateral cutaneous
nerve of thigh (L2,3)

Medial cutaneous nerve
of thigh (femoral) (L2,3)

Posterior cutaneous nerve
of thigh (S1,2,3)

Saphenous nerve
(femoral) (L3,4)

Lateral cutaneous nerve
of calf (peroneal) (L5,S1,2)

Superficial peroneal
nerve (L4,5,S1)

Figure 12-135
Peripheral nerve sensory distribution about the knee.

Figure 12-136
Dermatomes about the knee.

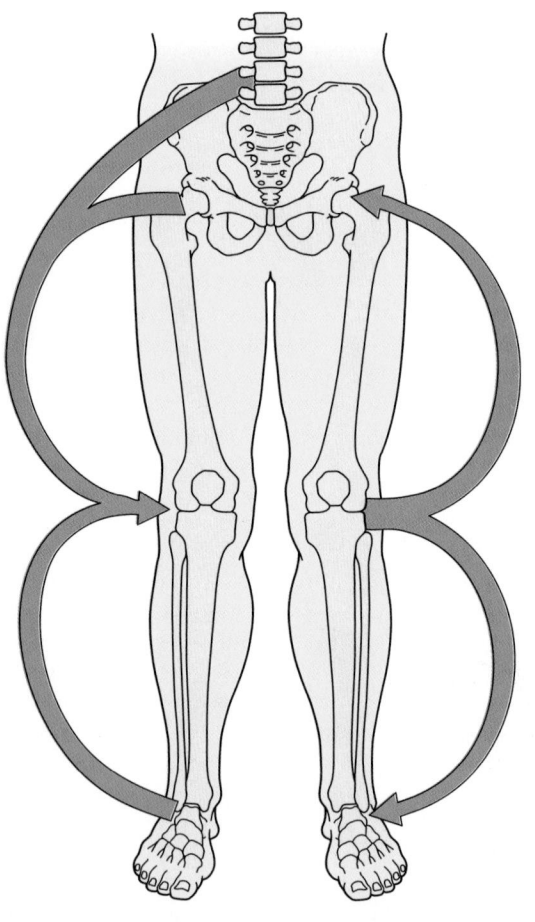

Figure 12-137
Patterns of referred pain to and from the knee.

Table 12-11
Knee Muscles and Referral of Pain

Muscle	Referral Pattern
Tensor fasciae latae	Lateral aspect of thigh
Sartorius	Over course of muscle (anterior thigh)
Quadriceps	Anterior thigh, patella, lateral thigh and knee (vastus lateralis)
Adductor longus and brevis	Superior anterolateral thigh, anterior thigh, proximal to patella and sometimes down anteromedial leg
Adductor magnus	Medial thigh from groin to adductor tubercle
Gracilis	Medial thigh (primarily the mid portion)
Semimembranosus and semitendinosus	Ischial tuberosity, posterior thigh, and posteromedial calf
Biceps femoris	Posterior knee up posterior thigh
Popliteus	Posterior knee
Gastrocnemius	Posterior knee, posterolateral calf, and posteromedial calf to foot instep
Plantaris	Posterior knee and calf

of pulling on the peroneus longus muscle in a lateral ankle sprain,[239-241] direct trauma, injury to the posterolateral corner, or a varus stress to the knee.[28,164] The result is weakness or paralysis of muscles supplied by the deep and superficial peroneal nerves, the two branches of the common peroneal nerve (Table 12-12). This causes an inability to dorsiflex the foot (drop foot), resulting in a steppage gait and an inability to evert the foot. Sensory loss is as shown in Figure 12-138.

Saphenous Nerve (L2 through L4). The saphenous nerve is a sensory branch of the femoral nerve that arises

Table 12-12

Peripheral Nerve Injuries (Neuropathy) about the Knee

Nerve	Muscle Weakness	Sensory Alteration	Reflexes Affected

Common peroneal nerve	Tibialis anterior (DP)
	Extensor digitorum brevis (DP)
	Extensor digitorum longus (DP)
	Extensor hallucis longus (DP)
	Peroneus tertius (DP)
	Peroneus longus (SP)
	Peroneus brevis (SP)
		Area around head of fibula
		Web space between first and
		  second toes (DP)
		Lateral aspect of leg and
		  dorsum of foot (SP)
			No common reflexes affected

Saphenous nerve	None	Medial side of knee, may
		  extend down medial side of
		  leg to medial malleolus
			None

DP, Deep peroneal branch; *SP*, superficial peroneal branch.

Anterior view

Posterior view

Figure 12-138

Common peroneal nerve.

near the inguinal ligament and passes down the leg to supply the skin on the medial side of the knee and calf. The nerve is sometimes injured during surgery or trauma, or it may be entrapped as it passes between the vastus medialis and adductor magnus muscles. Entrapment may lead to medial knee pain (burning) that is aggravated by walking, standing, and quadriceps exercises.[242-244] Sensory loss after surgery or trauma is shown in Figure 12-135.

Joint Play Movements

For joint play movements on the knee, the patient is placed in the supine position (Figure 12-139). The movement on the affected side is compared with that on the normal side.

Joint Play Movements of the Knee Complex

- Backward glide of tibia on femur
- Forward glide of tibia on femur
- Medial translation of tibia on femur
- Lateral translation of tibia on femur
- Medial displacement of patella
- Lateral displacement of patella
- Depression of patella
- Anteroposterior movement of fibula on tibia

Backward and Forward Movements of Tibia on Femur

The patient is asked to lie in the supine position with the test knee flexed to 90° and the hip flexed to 45°. The examiner then places the heel of the hand over the tibial tuberosity while stabilizing the patient's limb with the other hand and pushing backward with the heel of the hand. The end feel of the movement is normally tissue stretch. To perform the forward movement, the examiner places both hands around the posterior aspect of the tibia. Before performing the joint play movement, the examiner must ensure that the hamstrings and gastrocnemius muscles are relaxed. The tibia is then drawn forward on the femur. The examiner feels the quality of the movement, which normally is tissue stretch. These joint play movements are similar to those used in the anterior and posterior drawer tests for ligamentous stability.

Medial and Lateral Translation of Tibia on Femur

The patient lies supine, and the patient's leg is held between the examiner's trunk and arm. To test medial translation, the examiner puts one hand on the lateral side of the tibia and one hand on the medial side of the femur. The tibia is then pushed or translated medially on the femur. Excessive movement may indicate a

torn anterior cruciate ligament (Figure 12-140). To test lateral translation, the examiner puts one hand on the medial side of the tibia and one hand on the lateral side of the femur. The tibia is then pushed or translated laterally on the femur. Excessive movement may indicate a torn posterior cruciate ligament. The normal end feel of each movement is tissue stretch.[66] Liorzou[26] reports that Galway did a similar test with the knee flexed to 90° and the foot on the examining table. If the tibial plateau bulges laterally, Wrisberg's ligament or the lateral meniscus may be injured.

Medial and Lateral Displacements of Patella

The patient is in the supine position with the knee slightly flexed on a pillow or over the examiner's knee (30° flexion). The examiner's thumbs are placed against the medial or lateral edge of the patella, and a force is applied to the side of the patella, with the fingers used for stabilization. The process is then repeated, with pressure applied to the other side of the patella. The other knee is tested as a comparison.

This joint play is similar to the passive movements of the patella; as in the passive test, the patella can be displaced by approximately half of its width medially and laterally. The examiner must do the movements slowly and carefully to ensure that the patella is not prone to dislocation.

Depression (Distal Movement) of Patella

The patient is in a supine position with the knee slightly flexed. The examiner then places one hand over the patient's patella so that the pisiform bone rests over the base of the patella. The other hand is placed so that the finger and thumb can grasp the medial and lateral edges of the patella to direct its movement. The examiner then rests the first hand over the second hand and applies a caudal force to the base of the patella, directing the caudal movement with the second hand so that the patella does not grind against the femoral condyles.

Anteroposterior Movement of Fibula on Tibia

The patient is supine with the knee flexed to 90° and the hip to 45°. The examiner then sits on the patient's foot and places one hand around the patient's knee to stabilize the knee and leg. The mobilizing hand is placed around the head of the fibula. The fibula is drawn forward on the tibia, and the movement and end feel are tested. The fibula then slides back to its resting position of its own accord. The movement is tested several times and compared with that of the other side. Care must be taken when performing this test because the common peroneal nerve, which winds around the head of the fibula, may be easily compressed, causing pain. If the superior tibiofibular joint is stiff or hypomobile, the test

Figure 12-139

Joint play movements of the knee. **A,** Anterior movement of the tibia on the femur. **B,** Posterior movement of the tibia on the femur. **C,** Patellar movement, distally. **D,** Patellar movement, medially. **E,** Anterior movement of the superior tibiofibular joint.

A   **B**

Figure 12-140
Medial and lateral shift of tibia on femur. **A,** Medial translation for anterior cruciate pathology. **B,** Lateral translation for posterior cruciate pathology.

itself will cause discomfort. In most cases, foot dorsiflexion will cause lateral knee pain if the superior tibiofibular joint is hypomobile.

Palpation

The patient lies supine with the knee slightly flexed. It is wise to put the knee in several positions during palpation. For example, meniscal cysts are best palpated at 45°, whereas the joint line is easiest to palpate at 90°. When palpating, the examiner looks for abnormal tenderness, swelling, nodules, or abnormal temperature. The following structures should be palpated (Figure 12-141).

Anterior Palpation with Knee Extended

Patella, Patellar Tendon, Patellar Retinaculum, Associated Bursa, Cartilaginous Surface of the Patella, and Plica. The patella can easily be palpated over the anterior aspect of the knee. The base of the patella lies superiorly, and the apex lies distally. After palpating the apex of the patella (for possible jumper's knee), the examiner moves distally, palpating the patellar tendon (for paratenonitis or tendinosis) and the overlying infrapatellar bursa (for Parson's knee) as well as the fat pad that lies behind the tendon. When the knee is extended, the fat pad often extends beyond the sides of the tendon. Moving distally, the examiner comes to the tibial tuberosity, which should be palpated for enlargement (possible Osgood-Schlatter disease).

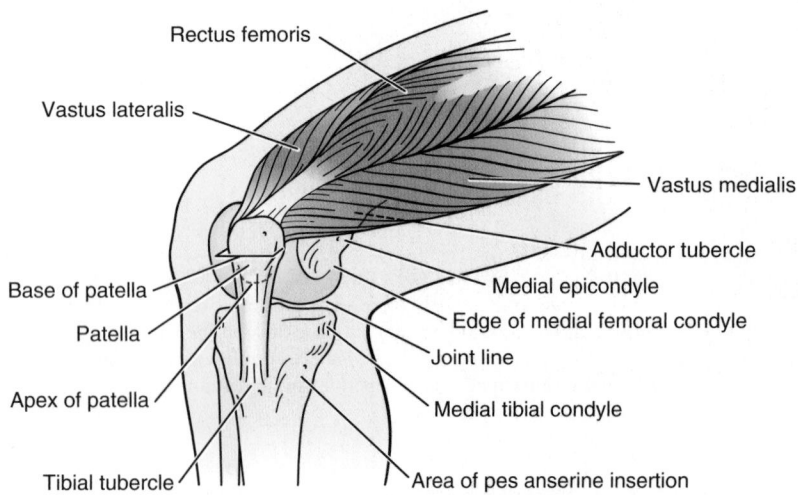

Rectus femoris
Vastus lateralis
Vastus medialis
Adductor tubercle
Base of patella
Medial epicondyle
Patella
Edge of medial femoral condyle
Apex of patella
Joint line
Medial tibial condyle
Tibial tubercle
Area of pes anserine insertion

Figure 12-141
Landmarks of the knee.

Returning to the patella, the examiner can palpate the skin lying over the patella for pathology (prepatellar bursitis or housemaid's knee) and then extend medially and laterally to palpate the patellar retinaculum on both sides of the patella. With the examiner pushing down on the lateral aspect of the patella, the medial retinaculum can be brought under tension and then palpated for tender areas. The lateral retinaculum can be palpated in a similar fashion, with the examiner pushing down on the medial aspect of the patella. By stressing the retinaculum, the examiner is separating the retinaculum from the underlying tissue.

With the quadriceps muscles relaxed, the articular facets of the patella are palpated for tenderness (possible chondromalacia patellae), as shown in Figure 12-142. This palpation is often facilitated by carefully pushing the patella medially to palpate the medial facets and laterally to palpate the lateral facet.

As the medial edge of the patella is palpated, the examiner should carefully feel for the presence of a mediopatellar plica. The plica, if pathological, may be palpated as a thickened ridge medial to the patella. To help confirm the presence of the plica, the examiner flexes the patient's knee to 30° and pushes the patella medially. If the plica is present and pathological, this maneuver often causes pain.

Suprapatellar Pouch.   Returning to the anterior surface of the patella and moving proximally beyond the base of the patella, the examiner's fingers will lie over the suprapatellar pouch. The examiner then lifts the skin and underlying tissue between the thumb and fingers (Figure 12-143). In this way, the synovial membrane of the suprapatellar pouch, which is continuous with that of the knee joint, can be palpated as a very slippery surface normally. The examiner should feel for any thickness, tenderness, or nodules, the presence of which may indicate pathology.

Quadriceps Muscles (Vastus Medialis, Vastus Intermedius, Vastus Lateralis, Rectus Femoris) and Sartorius.   After palpating the suprapatellar pouch, the examiner palpates the quadriceps for tenderness (possible first- or second-degree strain), defects (third-degree strain), atonia, or hard masses (myositis ossificans).

Medial Collateral Ligament.   If the examiner moves medially from the patella so that the fingers lie over the medial aspect of the tibiofemoral joint, the fingers will lie over the medial collateral ligament, which should be palpated along its entire length for tenderness (possible sprain) or other pathology (e.g., Pellegrini-Stieda syndrome—bone development in the medial collateral ligament).

Pes Anserinus.   Medial and slightly distal to the tibial tuberosity, the examiner may palpate the pes anserinus (the common aponeurosis of the tendons of gracilis, semitendinosus, and sartorius muscles) for tenderness. Any associated swelling may indicate pes anserine bursitis.

Tensor Fascia Lata (Iliotibial Band and Head of Fibula).   As the examiner moves laterally from the tibial tuberosity, the head of the fibula can be palpated. Medial and slightly superior to the fibula, the examiner palpates the insertion of the iliotibial band into the lateral condyle of the tibia. When the knee is extended, it stands out as a strong, visible ridge anterolateral to the knee joint. As the examiner moves proximally, the iliotibial band is palpated along its entire length.

Figure 12-142
Checking for patellar medial and lateral facet tenderness. Note that tenderness may be related to structures other than patellar surfaces beneath the examining finger. (Redrawn from Hughston JC et al. *Patellar subluxation and dislocation*, p 28, Philadelphia, 1984, WB Saunders.)

Figure 12-143
Palpation of the suprapatellar pouch.

Anterior Palpation with Knee Flexed

Tibiofemoral Joint Line and Meniscal Cysts. The patient's knee is flexed at 45°, and the examiner palpates the joint line, especially on the lateral aspect, for any evidence of swelling (possible meniscal cyst), tenderness, or other pathology.[245]

Tibiofemoral Joint Line, Tibial Plateau, Femoral Condyles, and Adductor Muscles. The patient's knee is flexed to 90°. If the examiner returns to the patella, palpates the apex of the patella, and moves medially or laterally, the fingers will lie on the tibiofemoral joint line, which should be palpated along its entire length. As the joint line is palpated, the examiner should also palpate the tibial plateau (for possible coronary ligament sprain) medially and laterally, as well as the femoral condyles.

Both condyles should be palpated carefully for any tenderness (e.g., osteochondritis dissecans). Beginning at the superior aspect of the femoral condyles, the examiner should note that the lateral condyle extends farther anteriorly (i.e., higher) than the medial condyle. The trochlear groove between the two condyles can then be palpated. As the medial condyle is palpated, a sharp edge appears on the condyle medially. If the edge is followed posteriorly, the adductor tubercle can be palpated on the posteromedial portion of the medial femoral condyle. After palpating the adductor tubercle, the examiner moves proximally, palpating the adductor muscles of the hip for tenderness or other signs of pathology.

Anterior Palpation with Foot of Test Leg Resting on Opposite Knee

Kennedy[117] has advocated palpation of the lateral collateral ligament by having the patient in the sitting or lying position (Figure 12-144). The patient's knee is flexed to 90°, and the hip is laterally rotated so that the ankle of the test leg rests on the knee of the other leg (figure-four position). The examiner then places the knee into a varus position, and the ropelike ligament stands out if the ligament is intact.

Posterior Palpation with the Knee Slightly Flexed

Posterior Aspect of Knee Joint. The soft tissue on the posterior aspect of the knee should be palpated for tenderness or swelling (e.g., Baker's cyst). In some patients, the popliteal artery (pulse) may be palpated by running the hand down the center of the posterior knee.

Posterolateral Aspect of Knee Joint. The posterolateral corner of the knee is sometimes called the **popliteus corner**. The examiner should attempt to palpate the arcuate-popliteus complex, the lateral gastrocnemius muscle, the biceps femoris muscle, and possibly the lateral meniscus in this area. A sesamoid bone is sometimes found inserted in the tendon of the lateral head of the gastrocnemius muscle. This bone, referred to as the **fabella**, may be interpreted as a loose body in the posterolateral aspect of the knee by an unwary examiner (see Figure 12-159).

Posteromedial Aspect of Knee Joint. The posteromedial corner of the knee joint is sometimes referred to as the **semimembranosus corner**. The examiner should attempt to palpate the posterior oblique ligament, the semimembranosus muscle, the medial gastrocnemius muscle, and possibly the medial meniscus in this area for tenderness or pathology.

Hamstring and Gastrocnemius Muscles. After the various parts of the posterior aspect of the knee have been palpated, the tendons and muscle bellies of the hamstring muscle group (biceps femoris, semitendinosus, semimembranosus) proximally and of the gastrocnemius muscle distally should be palpated for tenderness, swelling, or other signs of pathology.

Diagnostic Imaging

Plain Film Radiography

For evaluation of knee injuries, anteroposterior and lateral views are most commonly obtained. Depending on the suspected pathology, other views may be taken as well. Usually, the anteroposterior view is taken with the patient bearing weight. Imaging should not be used indiscriminately but should be considered an adjunct to examination; it is used primarily to confirm a diagnosis obtained by careful assessment.[246-248] Stiell and associates[249] have developed the **Ottawa knee rules** for the use of radiography in acute knee injuries.[141,250] They believed knee radiography was only necessary in acute knee injuries if the patient is 55 years of age or older or had isolated tenderness of the patella, tenderness at the head of the fibula, inability to flex the knee to 90°, or an inability to walk four steps (bearing weight). The use of the Ottawa knee rules in children is supported by some[251,252] and questioned by others.[253]

Palpate lateral collateral ligament

Figure 12-144
Palpation of the lateral (fibular) collateral ligament.

Anteroposterior View. When looking at radiographs of the knee (Figure 12-145), the examiner should note any possible fractures (e.g., osteochondral, fibular head), diminished joint space (possible osteoarthritis; Figures 12-146 and 12-147), epiphyseal damage, lipping (see Figure 12-147), loose bodies, alterations in bone texture, abnormal calcification, ossification (e.g., Pellegrini-Stieda syndrome; Figure 12-148) or tumors, accessory ossification centers, varus or valgus deformity, patellar position, patella alta (Figures 12-149 and 12-150) or baja, and asymmetry of femoral condyles.[254,255] Weight-bearing radiographs of knees in 30° flexion are recommended for cases of suspected arthritis or degeneration.[256] Stress, non–weight-bearing radiographs of this view illustrate excessive gapping medially or laterally, indicating ligamentous instability (Figure 12-151). The examiner should also remember the possible presence of the fabella, which is seen in 20% of the population. Epiphyseal fractures (Figure 12-152) and osteochondritis dissecans (Figure 12-153) may also be seen in this view.[257,258] The presence of the **Segund sign** or **lateral capsular sign**, which is an avulsion fracture, often indicates severe lateral capsular injury and probably anterior cruciate ligament disruption (Figure 12-154).[11,259–261]

Figure 12-145

Normal radiographs of the knee. **A,** Anteroposterior view. **B,** Lateral view. **C,** Tunnel view. **D,** Skyline view. (From Reilly BM: *Practical strategies in outpatient medicine*, p. 1188, Philadelphia, 1991, WB Saunders.)

Figure 12-146

Anteroposterior x-ray showing degenerative arthritis of the knee. Note the loss of joint space caused by loss of cartilage (both sides) and meniscus (on medial side).

Figure 12-148

Pellegrini-Stieda syndrome. Note calcium formation within the substance of the medial collateral ligament *(arrow)*.

Figure 12-147

Osteoarthritis of the knee: femorotibial compartment abnormalities. Radiograph of a coronal section of a cadaveric knee indicates osteoarthritis changes that are more prominent in the medial femorotibial compartment. Findings include joint space narrowing related to cartilage erosion, subchondral bony sclerosis, osteophytosis *(open arrow)*, and sharpening of the tibial spines *(arrowheads)*. Degeneration of both the medial meniscus and the lateral meniscus is evident. (From Resnick D, Kransdorf MJ: *Bone and joint imaging*, p 386, Philadelphia, 2005, WB Saunders.)

Lateral View. With this view,[152,254,262] the examiner should note the same structures as seen with the anteroposterior view (Figures 12-155 and 12-156). This view is usually done in side-lying position with the knee flexed to 45°.[263] To determine the normal positioning of the patella, the standing, weight-bearing lateral view is used to determine the ratio of patellar length to patellar tendon length (Figure 12-157); several methods are possible.[264–266] Berg and associates[267] reported that the Blackburne-Peel method was the most consistent. This view also illustrates Osgood-Schlatter disease (Figure 12-158), the presence of the fabella (Figure 12-159), the arcuate sign (avulsion fracture of the arcuate complex leading to posterolateral instability; Figure 12-160),[164,268] myositis ossificans (Figures 12-161 and 12-162), and avulsion of the anterior cruciate insertion (Figure 12-163). Stress radiographs of this view can be used to show complete tears (+8 mm) of the posterior cruciate ligament.[269]

Intercondylar Notch (Tunnel View X-ray). With this view (patient prone, knee flexed from 45° to 90°) (Figure 12-164), the tibia and intercondylar attachments of the cruciate ligaments can be examined as well as the width of the intercondylar notch, which is less in women.[270] This narrower notch can put the anterior cruciate at greater risk of tearing.[270] Also, any loose bodies or possibility of osteochondritis dissecans, subluxation, patellar tilt (lateral or medial), or dislocation should be noted.

VIEW	KNEE FLEXION	PATIENT POSITION	MEASUREMENT		MISCELLANEOUS
AP	0 degrees	Standing, feet straight ahead	Normal	Greater than 20 mm abnormal	— Hypoplastic patella — Lateral subluxation of patella — Bipartite patella — Asymmetry of femoral condylar (abnormal femoral anteversion or femoral rotation)
Lateral	90 degrees	Supine	Normal	Patella alta	— Patella infera — Patellar fracture
	Approx. 30 degrees	Supine	P / PT	Ratio of P:PT = 1.0 More than 20% variation is abnormal	
	30 degrees	Supine		Blumensaat's line (see text)	

Figure 12-149

Summary of radiographic findings in patella alta. (From Carson WG Jr et al: Patellofemoral disorders: physical and radiographic evaluation. I. Physical examination, *Clin Orthop* 185:179, 1984.)

Figure 12-150

Anteroposterior view of the knee. **A,** Normal patellar position. **B,** Patella alta. **C,** Patella baja. (From Hughston JC et al: *Patellar subluxation and dislocation*, p. 50, Philadelphia, 1984, WB Saunders.)

Figure 12-151

This valgus stress radiograph shows the patient's knee in full extension. Note the gapping on the medial side *(arrow)*. (From Mital MA, Karlin LI: Diagnostic arthroscopy in sports injuries, *Orthop Clin North Am* 11:775, 1980.)

Figure 12-152

A Salter-Harris type III injury *(arrow)* of the growth plate and epiphysis. Main attention should be directed toward restitution of the joint surface. (From Ehrlich MG, Strain RE: Epiphyseal injuries about the knee, *Orthop Clin North Am* 10:93, 1979.)

Axial (Skyline) View. This 30° tangential view (Figure 12-165) is primarily used for suspected patellar problems, such as patellar subluxation and dysplasia (Figure 12-166).[47,255,262,271,272] It may be taken at different angles, as shown in Figures 12-167 to 12-169, or it may be used to determine the type of patella present, as shown in Figure 12-170. Figure 12-171 illustrates abnormal patellar forms. Other patellofemoral measurements include lateral patellar displacement (see Figure 12-168) and the lateral/medial trochlear ratio or sulcus angle (see Figure 12-169).[262,273]

Arthrography

Arthrograms of the knee are used primarily to diagnose tears in the menisci (Figure 12-172) and plica

Figure 12-153

A, Osteochondritis dissecans—actually an osteochondral fracture *(arrow)* of the femoral condyle—with almost the entire femoral attachment of the posterior cruciate ligament remaining attached to the fragment. **B,** Three months after repair of posterior cruciate to femur. Excellent function is restored. Complete filling in of this defect is unlikely at this age. (From O'Donoghue DH: *Treatment of injuries to athletes,* ed 4, p. 575, Philadelphia, 1984, WB Saunders.)

Figure 12-154

Segund sign. Note avulsion fracture adjacent to lateral tibial plateau *(arrow)*. This lateral capsular injury often signifies an anterior cruciate ligament tear.

Figure 12-155

Lateral view at 90° shows the normal position of the patella. (From Hughston JC et al: *Patellar subluxation and dislocation*, p. 52, Philadelphia, 1984, WB Saunders.)

(Figure 12-173) although their use is being replaced by arthroscopy. Double-contrast arthrograms are also used (Figure 12-174). Arthrograms combined with computed tomography (CT) scans (CT arthrograms) are useful for assessing meniscus tears, articular cartilage, meniscal and popliteal cysts, and synovial plica.[274]

Arthroscopy

The arthroscope is being used increasingly to diagnose lesions of the knee and to repair many of them surgically.[275–277] By using various approaches (portals) to the knee, the surgeon is able to view all of the structures to determine whether they have been injured (Figure 12-175).

Figure 12-156

Lateral view of the patella at 45°. **A,** Normal patellar position in relation to the intercondylar notch. **B,** Patella alta. (From Hughston JC et al: *Patellar subluxation and dislocation*, p. 52, Philadelphia, 1984, WB Saunders.)

Figure 12-157

Indices for measurement of patellar height. **A,** Insall-Salvati. **B,** Modified Insall-Salvati. **C,** Blackburne.
D, de Carvalho. **E,** Caton. (From Grelsamer RP, Meadows S: The modified Insall-Salvati ratio for assessment
of patellar height, *Clin Orthop* 282:172, 1992.)

Computed Tomography

CT scans are often used to view soft tissue as well as bone
(Figure 12-176).

Magnetic Resonance Imaging

Magnetic resonance imaging (MRI) is advantageous
because of its ability to show soft tissue as well as bone

tissue while providing no exposure to ionizing radiation.[278] It has largely replaced CT scans for evaluation of
the knee.[279] MRI has been found to be useful in diagnosing lesions of the tendon (Figure 12-177), bone bruises
(Figure 12-178), menisci (Figures 12-179 and 12-
180), plica (Figure 12-181), collateral ligaments (Figure
12-182), cruciate ligaments (Figure 12-183), Baker's cyst

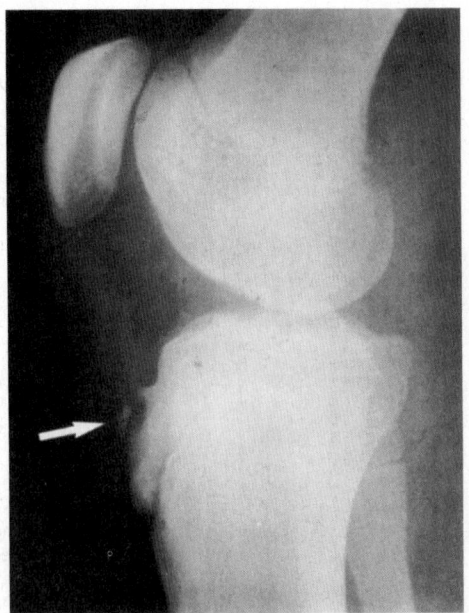

Figure 12-158

Osgood-Schlatter disease, showing epiphysitis of the entire epiphysis
(arrow), with irregularity of the epiphyseal line. Because this
epiphyseal cartilage is continuous with that of the upper tibia, it
should not be disturbed. If surgery is used, exposure should be
superficial to the epiphyseal cartilage. (From O'Donoghue DH:
Treatment of injuries to athletes, ed 4, p. 574, Philadelphia, 1984, WB
Saunders.)

Figure 12-159

Sesamoid bone (fabella) in the gastrocnemius muscle.

Figure 12-160

Arcuate sign or fibular styloid fracture on lateral radiograph, **A,** with comparative diagram, **B**. The arcuate sign is pathognomonic of posterolateral corner injuries. It is an avulsion fracture of the arcuate complex. The fracture (*denoted by arrow*) is small and posteriorly located with minimal displacement. Circles denote the insertions of the arcuate complex. (From Bahk MS, Cosgarea AJ: Physical examination and imaging of the lateral collateral ligament and posterolateral corner of the knee, *Sports Med Arthrosc Rev* 14:16, 2006. **B** modified from Laprade RF et al: The posterolateral attachments of the knee: a qualitative and quantitative morphologic analysis of the fibular collateral ligament, popliteus tendon, popliteofibular ligament, and lateral gastrocnemius tendon, *Am J Sports Med* 31[6]:856, 2003.)

Figure 12-161

Myositis ossificans traumatica: maturing ossification. In this 11-year-old boy who fell from the steps of a swimming pool, lateral radiographs of the femur 1 month, **A,** and 5 months, **B,** after the injury show maturation of the ossifying process. Initially separated from the bone, the process subsequently merged with the anterior femoral surface. (From Resnick D, Kransdorf MJ: *Bone and joint imaging,* p. 1361, Philadelphia, 2005, WB Saunders. Courtesy of G Greenway, MD, Dallas.)

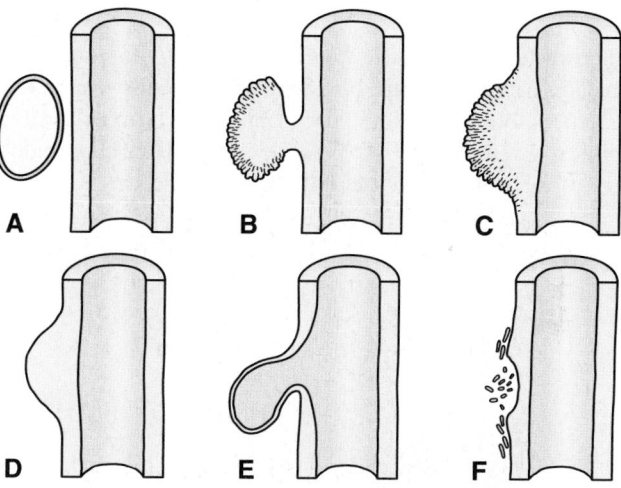

Figure 12-162

Myositis ossificans traumatica: differential diagnosis. **A,** Myositis ossificans traumatica. The shell-like configuration of the ossification, with a clear zone between it and the underlying bone, is typical of this condition. In some cases, there may be a cortical bridge. **B,** Parosteal osteosarcoma. These lesions appear as central ossifying foci with irregular outlines and may be connected to the underlying bone by a stalk. **C,** Periosteal osteosarcoma. These tumors arise in the cortex of the diaphysis of a tubular bone and produce cortical thickening and speculated osteoid matrix. **D,** Osteoma. Characteristic of this lesion is a localized excrescence that produces bulging of the cortical contour. **E,** Osteochondroma. An exostosis protrudes from the cortical surface. Its medullary and cortical bone is continuous with that of the underlying osseous structure. **F,** Juxtacortical (periosteal) chondroma. These periosteal lesions produce localized excavation of the cortex, with periostitis. They may contain calcification. (Redrawn from Resnick D, Kransdorf MJ: *Bone and joint imaging,* p. 1361, Philadelphia, 2005, WB Saunders.)

Figure 12-163
Avulsion fracture of the tibial insertion of the anterior cruciate ligament.

Figure 12-165
Positioning for the patellofemoral (skyline) view. (Redrawn from Larson RL, Grana WA, editors: *The knee: form, function, pathology and treatment*, p. 107, Philadelphia, 1993, WB Saunders.)

(Figure 12-184), muscle strains (Figure 12-185), chondromalacia patellae (Figure 12-186), patellar tendon tears, and fractures, but it should be used only to confirm or clarify a clinical diagnosis.[73,261,280–291] Sanders and Miller[282] provide a good overview of the use of MRI about the knee.

Xeroradiography

Xeroradiography may be used to delineate the edge of bone (Figure 12-187).

Text continued on page 832

Figure 12-164
Position for intercondylar notch view. (Redrawn from Larson RL, Grana WA, editors: *The knee: form, function, pathology and treatment*, p. 106, Philadelphia, 1993, WB Saunders.)

Figure 12-166
Skyline (sunrise) view of patellofemoral joints. Note the lateral displacement of both patellae, especially the one on the right. Note also the alpine hunter's cap shape of patella.

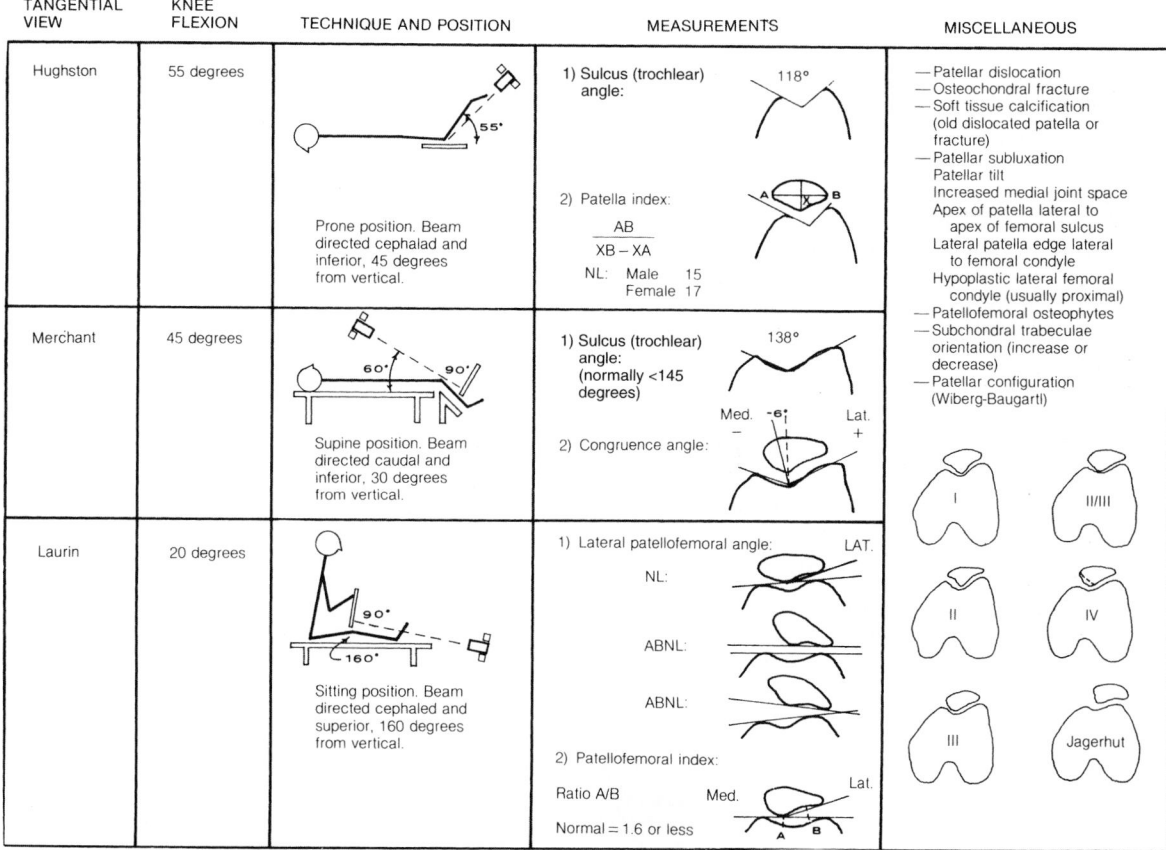

TANGENTIAL VIEW	KNEE FLEXION	TECHNIQUE AND POSITION	MEASUREMENTS	MISCELLANEOUS
Hughston	55 degrees	Prone position. Beam directed cephalad and inferior, 45 degrees from vertical.	1) Sulcus (trochlear) angle: 118° 2) Patella index: $$\frac{AB}{XB - XA}$$ NL: Male 15 / Female 17	— Patellar dislocation — Osteochondral fracture — Soft tissue calcification (old dislocated patella or fracture) — Patellar subluxation Patellar tilt Increased medial joint space Apex of patella lateral to apex of femoral sulcus Lateral patella edge lateral to femoral condyle Hypoplastic lateral femoral condyle (usually proximal) — Patellofemoral osteophytes — Subchondral trabeculae orientation (increase or decrease) — Patellar configuration (Wiberg-Baugartl)
Merchant	45 degrees	Supine position. Beam directed caudal and inferior, 30 degrees from vertical.	1) Sulcus (trochlear) angle: (normally <145 degrees) 138° 2) Congruence angle: Med. −6 Lat.	
Laurin	20 degrees	Sitting position. Beam directed cephaled and superior, 160 degrees from vertical.	1) Lateral patellofemoral angle: LAT. NL: ABNL: ABNL: 2) Patellofemoral index: Ratio A/B Med. Lat. Normal = 1.6 or less	

Figure 12-167
Summary of radiographic findings, tangential view. (From Carson WG Jr et al: Patellofemoral disorders: physical and radiographic evaluation. I. Physical examination, *Clin Orthop* 185:182, 1984.)

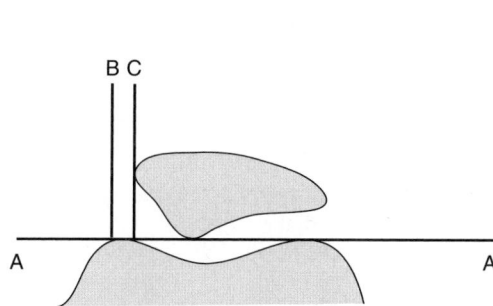

Figure 12-168
Lateral patellar displacement. A line is drawn through the highest points of the medial and lateral femoral condyles *(AA)*. A perpendicular to that line, at the medial edge of the medial femoral condyle *(B)*, normally lies 1 mm or less medial to the patella *(line C)*. (From Laurin CA, Dussault R, Levesque HP: The tangential x-ray investigation of the patellofemoral joint, *Clin Orthop* 144:16, 1979.)

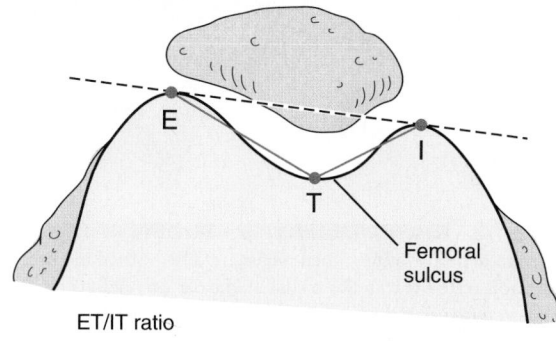

Figure 12-169
The lateral/medial trochlear ratio is the ratio between the external and internal segments (ET and IT) joining the highest points of the femoral condyles to the deepest point of the trochlear groove. It measures the dysplasia of the medial aspect of the trochlea. (Redrawn from Beaconsfield T et al: Radiographic measurements in patellofemoral disorders, *Clin Orthop* 308:22, 1994.)

Figure 12-170
Examples of patellar variations. **A,** Wilberg type I. **B,** Wilberg type II. **C,** Wilberg type III. (From Ficat RP, Hungerford DS: *Disorders of the patello-femoral joint*, p. 53, Baltimore, 1977, Williams & Wilkins.)

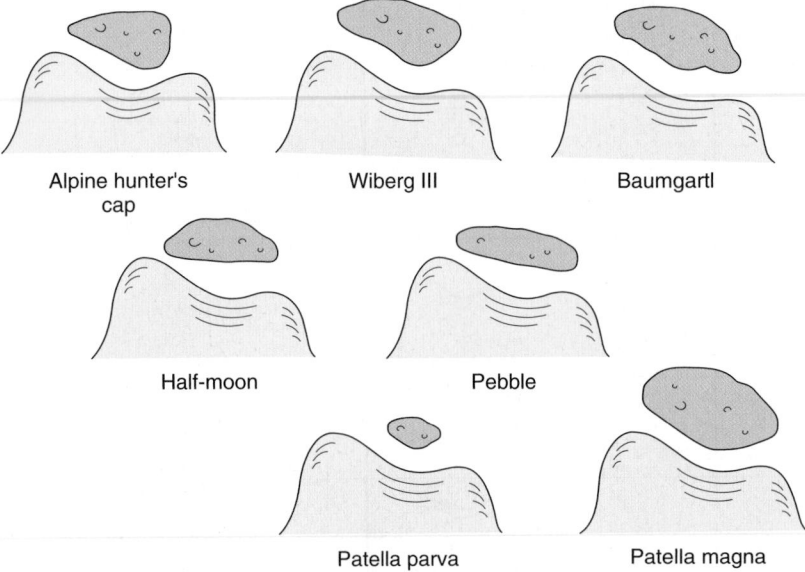

Alpine hunter's cap

Wiberg III

Baumgartl

Half-moon

Pebble

Patella parva

Patella magna

Figure 12-171

Variations in patellar form that are considered dysplastic. (Redrawn from Ficat RP, Hungerford DS: *Disorders of the patello-femoral joint*, p. 55, Baltimore, 1977, Williams & Wilkins.)

Figure 12-172

Arthrogram demonstrating a torn meniscus. The normal meniscus on the lateral side, **A,** is compared with the easily demonstrated tear in the medial meniscus *(arrow)* in the same patient, **B.** (From Reilly BM: *Practical strategies in outpatient medicine*, p. 1198, Philadelphia, 1991, WB Saunders.)

Figure 12-173

Tangential patellar view after arthrography, showing thinning and slight roughening of the patellar cartilage, especially medially. The mediopatellar plica *(p)* is markedly thickened. (From Weissman BNW, Sledge CB: *Orthopedic radiology*, p. 536, Philadelphia, 1986, WB Saunders.)

Figure 12-174
Double-contrast arthrogram. **A,** The anteroposterior view demonstrates the menisci and articular cartilage.
B, The lateral projection illustrates the extent of the joint space. (From Forrester DM, Brown JC:
The radiology of joint disease, ed 3, p. 200, Philadelphia, 1987, WB Saunders.)

Figure 12-175
Arthroscopy of the knee. (From Patel D: Superior lateral-medial
approach to arthroscopic meniscectomy, *Orthop Clin North Am*
13:301, 1982.)

Figure 12-176
Muscular anatomy as shown on computed tomography scan;
images through the upper femur, **A,** and lower third of femur,

Continued

Figure 12-176 cont'd

B, are shown. *AB,* Adductor brevis; *AL,* adductor longus; *AM,* adductor magnus; *B,* biceps femoris; *Gr,* gracilis; *n,* tibial and common peroneal nerves; *RF,* rectus femoris; *S,* sartorius; *Sm,* semimembranosus; *St,* semitendinosus; *V,* deep femoral vein and artery; *VI,* vastus intermedius; *VL,* vastus lateralis; *VM,* vastus medialis. (From Weissman BNW, Sledge CB: *Orthopedic radiology,* p. 504, Philadelphia, 1986, WB Saunders.)

Figure 12-177

A, A lateral plain radiograph and, **B,** a T1-weighted MRI scan of an injured knee show a normal contour of the intact patella tendon *(broad arrow)* and infrapatellar fat pad *(narrow arrow).* **C,** A lateral plain radiograph and, **D,** a T2-weighted MRI scan of an injured knee show disruption of the patella tendon *(broad arrow)* and infrapatellar fat pad *(narrow arrow)* at the inferior pole with associated patella alta. (From Chin KR, Sodl JF: Infrapatellar fat pad disruption—a radiographic sign of patellar tendon rupture, *Clin Orthop Relat Res* 440:224–225, 2005.)

Figure 12-178

Bone bruise from patellar dislocation-relocation injury. Transverse fat-suppressed intermediate-weighted (TR/TEeff, 3500/12) fast spin echo MR image. A high-signal-intensity contusion (*arrow*) is apparent in the lateral femoral condyle. Also note the torn medial patellofemoral ligament (*arrowheads*) (From Resnick D, Kransdorf MJ: *Bone and joint imaging*, p 121, Philadelphia, 2005, WB Saunders.)

Figure 12-179

Recurrent meniscal tear after partial medial meniscectomy. Sagittal fat-suppressed T1-weighted (TR/TE, 800/15) spin echo MR image after a knee arthrogram performed with a dilute gadolinium mixture. Injected contrast enters the substance of a new meniscal tear (*arrow*) in the remnant of the posterior horn. Also note the degenerative cartilage loss along the medial femoral surface (*arrowheads*). (From Resnick D, Kransdorf MJ: *Bone and joint imaging*, p. 126, Philadelphia, 2005, WB Saunders.)

Figure 12-180

Magnetic resonance image showing lesion of the posterior horn of the medial meniscus, **A.** In some cases, contrast can be enhanced by the intra-articular injection of gadolinium diethylenetriamene penta-acetic acid (DTPA). **B,** Inferior longitudinal tear with an associated horizontal tear. (From Strobel M, Stedtfeld HW: *Diagnostic evaluation of the knee*, p. 240, Berlin, 1990, Springer-Verlag.)

Figure 12-181

Magnetic resonance image of mediopatellar plica. **A,** Sagittal, T2-weighted image located medial to the patella demonstrates an effusion present within the knee joint that appears white. The vertical linear band seen within the joint *(open arrows)* represents the medial plica. **B,** Transaxial STIR image through the patellofemoral joint again demonstrates the effusion *(arrowheads)*, which appears bright and surrounds a tonguelike extension of tissue arising from the medial joint line and located between the patella *(P)* and the femur *(F)*. This tissue represents a medial plica. In this location, plicae can become hypertrophied and lead to symptoms and signs of internal derangement. (From Kursunoglu-Brahme S, Resnick D: Magnetic resonance imaging of the knee, *Orthop Clin North Am* 21:571, 1990.)

Figure 12-182

Injuries of the medial collateral ligament: complete tear. Coronal intermediate-weighted (TR/TE, 1500/12), **A,** and T2-weighted (TR/TE, 1500/80), **B,** spin echo MR images show complete disruption *(arrows)* of the fibers of the medial collateral ligament. Note the increase in signal intensity in the ligament and soft tissues in **B**. A joint effusion is present. Additional injuries in this patient included tears of the lateral meniscus and anterior cruciate ligament. (From Resnick D, Kransdorf MJ: *Bone and joint imaging*, p. 959, Philadelphia, 2005, WB Saunders. Courtesy V Chandnani, MD, Pittsburgh.)

Figure 12-183

Magnetic resonance image showing intact posterior cruciate ligament *(arrow)*. (From Strobel M, Stedtfeld HW: *Diagnostic evaluation of the knee*, p. 243, Berlin, 1990, Springer-Verlag.)

Figure 12-184

Baker's cyst. Transverse T2-weighted (TR/TE, 2500/80) spin echo MR image of the knee. Fluid distends the semimembranosus-gastrocnemius recess, **B**. The neck of the popliteal cyst is located between the tendons of the medial gastrocnemius *(curved arrow)* and semimembranosus *(straight arrow)* tendons. (From Resnick D, Kransdorf MJ: *Bone and joint imaging*, p. 124, Philadelphia, 2005, WB Saunders.)

Figure 12-185

Magnetic resonance (MR) images showing tendon rupture in a 22-year-old athlete who pulled his hamstring on two occasions and was unable to run. Seven centimeters above the patella, **A,** axial T1-weighted (TR, 600 msec; TE, 20 msec) and, **B,** T2-weighted (TR, 2000 msec; TE, 85 msec) MR images show abnormally high signal intensity of the right semitendinosus muscle *(arrows)* compared with the normal left side. **C,** Sagittal T2-weighted MR image (TR, 2000 msec; TE, 85 msec) discloses that retracted semitendinosus muscle *(asterisk)* has an abnormally high signal intensity. The arrow indicates a torn musculotendinous junction. (From Bassett LW, Gold RH: Magnetic resonance imaging of the musculoskeletal system: an overview, *Clin Orthop* 244:20, 1989.)

Figure 12-186

Chondromalacia patellae. **A,** Bone scan shows a focal area of increased uptake in the medial aspect of the left patellofemoral joint *(arrows)*.

Figure 12-186 cont'd
B, Intermediate-weighted spin echo MR image shows abnormal signal and erosion in the medial aspect of the patellar cartilage *(arrows)*. (From Resnick D, Kransdorf MJ: *Bone and joint imaging*, p. 112, Philadelphia, 2005, WB Saunders.)

Figure 12-187
Xeroradiography of the knee. **A,** Anteroposterior view. **B,** Lateral view. *F,* Infrapatellar fat pad; *G,* gastrocnemius; *H,* hamstrings; *MCL,* medial collateral ligament; *PL,* peroneus longus; *QT,* quadriceps tendon; *T,* patellar tendon; *VL,* vastus lateralis; *VM,* vastus medialis. (From Weissman BNW, Sledge CB: *Orthopedic radiology*, p. 504, Philadelphia, 1986, WB Saunders.)

Précis of the Knee Assessment*

History
Observation
Examination
Active movements
  Knee flexion
  Knee extension
  Medial rotation of the tibia on the femur
  Lateral rotation of the tibia on the femur
Passive movements (as in active movements)
Resisted isometric movements
  Knee flexion
  Knee extension
  Ankle plantar flexion
  Ankle dorsiflexion
Tests for ligament stability
  Test for one-plane medial instability
  Test for one-plane lateral instability
  Tests for one-plane anterior and posterior instabilities
  Tests for anteromedial and anterolateral rotary instabilities
  Tests for posteromedial and posterolateral rotary instabilities
Functional assessment
Special tests
  Tests for meniscus injury

  Plica tests
  Tests for swelling
  Other tests
Reflexes and cutaneous distribution
Joint play movements
  Backward and forward movements of the tibia on the femur
  Medial and lateral translation of the tibia on the femur
  Medial and lateral displacements of the patella
  Depression of the patella
  Anteroposterior movement of the fibula on the tibia
Palpation
Diagnostic imaging
After any examination, the patient should be warned of the possibility of exacerbation of symptoms as a result of the assessment.

*Although examination of the knee may be carried out with the patient in the supine position, some of the tests may require the patient to move to other positions (e.g., standing, lying, prone, sitting). When these tests are used, the examination should be planned in such a way that the movement and therefore the discomfort experienced by the patient are kept to a minimum. The sequence should be from standing to sitting, to supine lying, to side lying, and finally, to prone lying.

Case Studies

When doing these case studies, the examiner should list the appropriate questions to be asked and why they are being asked, what to look for and why, and what things should be tested and why. Depending on the answers of the patient (and the examiner should consider different responses), several possible causes of the patient's problem may become evident (examples are given in parentheses). A differential diagnosis chart should be made. The examiner can then decide how different diagnoses may affect the treatment plan. For example, a 16-year-old female volleyball player comes to you with knee pain (Table 12-13). Her knee is painful when she plays, and she sometimes feels a clicking when going up and down stairs. Describe your assessment plan for this patient (meniscus pathology versus plica syndrome).

1. A 59-year-old man presents to you with moderate pain and swelling of 4 months' duration in his right knee. There is no history of trauma. The pain and swelling have become worse during the past month. Describe your assessment plan for this patient (osteoarthritis versus meniscus pathology).

2. A 24-year-old male football player is referred to you for treatment after a surgical repair to the anterior cruciate and medial collateral ligaments of the right knee. He is still in a splint, but the surgeon says the splint can be removed for treatment. Describe your assessment plan for this patient.

3. A 54-year-old man comes to you for treatment. He has difficulty walking and pain in the left hamstrings that is referred into the area of the gluteal fold. There is ecchymosis evident in the posterior knee and a small amount in the superior calf area. Describe your assessment plan for this patient (hamstring strain versus sciatica).

4. An 18-year-old woman presents to your clinic with anterior knee pain. Design your assessment plan for this patient (chondromalacia patellae versus plica syndrome).

5. A 17-year-old male soccer player comes to you saying that his knee feels unstable. He says he was playing soccer, twisted to challenge a player, and felt a pop in his knee. Describe your assessment plan for this patient (osteochondral fracture versus anterior cruciate sprain).

Continued

Case Studies—cont'd

6. A 10-year-old boy is brought to you by his parents. He is experiencing anterior knee pain. Describe your assessment plan for this patient (Osgood-Schlatter syndrome versus chondromalacia patellae).

7. A 20-year-old female rugby player comes to you with lateral knee pain that is sometimes referred down the leg. The knee hurts when she walks. She vaguely remembers being kicked in the knee while playing rugby 10 days earlier. Describe your assessment plan for this patient (superior tibiofibular joint subluxation versus common peroneal nerve neuropraxia).

8. An 18-year-old female swimmer presents to you with medial knee pain. She has just increased her training to 10,000 m per day. Describe your assessment plan for this patient (medial collateral ligament sprain versus chondromalacia patellae).

Table 12-13

Differential Diagnosis of Meniscus and Mediopatellar Plica Syndrome

	Medial Meniscus	Mediopatellar Plica Syndrome
History	Mechanism of injury: rotation, flexion, and valgus stress (may be acute or insidious) while weight bearing	Mechanism of injury: flexion, rotation (usually insidious onset)
Pain	Joint line	May be joint line but also superomedial to joint line
Swelling	May be present	May be present
Locking or giving way	Locking more likely	Giving way more likely
Active movement	May be limited	Usually full but extremes of motion may be painful, catching may occur on movement
Passive movement	Pain at extremes	Pain possible at extreme of flexion
Resisted isometric movement	Normal	Normal unless pinching causes pain and reflex inhibition
Ligament tests	Negative	Negative
Special tests	McMurray may be positive, Apley's test may be positive	Mediopatellar plica test positive, plica "stutter" test positive, Hughston's plica test positive
Palpation	Joint line tenderness	Plica may demonstrate thickening and be bandlike

References

To enhance this text and add value for the reader, all references have been incorporated into a CD-ROM that is provided with this text. The reader can view the reference source and access it online whenever possible. There are a total of 351 cited references and other general references for this chapter.

APPENDIX 12-1

RELIABILITY, VALIDITY, SPECIFICITY, AND SENSITIVITY OF SPECIAL/DIAGNOSTIC TESTS USED IN THE KNEE

6-MIN WALK

Sensitivity	Validity
• r = 0.87[103]	• Concurrent validity with time on treadmill ($r = -0.34$, with VO_{2max} r = -0.26, knee strength $r = -0.15$)[103]

ANTERIOR DRAWER SIGN

Sensitivity
• Chronic 79.6%[292]

ANTERIOR DRAWER TEST

Specificity	Sensitivity	Odds Ratio
• 92%[293]	• 27%[303] 56%[293]	• Positive likelihood ratio 6.7, negative likelihood ratio 0.5
• 100%[294]	• 41%[294] 91%[295]	• Positive likelihood ratio 5, negative likelihood ratio 0.6
• 100%[295]	• 9%[304] 70%[305]	• Positive likelihood ratio 33.3, negative likelihood ratio 0.1
• 50%[296]	• 18%[306] 58%[296]	• Positive likelihood ratio 1.2, negative likelihood ratio 0.8
• 100%[297]	• 95%[307] 78%[297]	• Positive likelihood ratio 87.9, negative likelihood ratio 0.2
• 96%[298]	• 61%[308] 25%[298]	• Positive likelihood ratio 5.9, negative likelihood ratio 0.8
• 87%[299]	• 76%[299] 39%[300]	• Positive likelihood ratio 5.6, negative likelihood ratio 0.3
• 97%[300]	• 52%[120] 71%[301]	• Positive likelihood ratio 11.2, negative likelihood ratio 0.6
• 100%[120]	• Whole group 55%, acute 49%, chronic 92%[302]	• Positive likelihood ratio 82.5, negative likelihood ratio 0.5
• 77%[301]		• Positive likelihood ratio 3.095, negative likelihood ratio 0.4
• Whole group 92%, acute 58%, chronic 91%[302]		• Positive likelihood ratio: whole group 7.3, acute 1.4, chronic 8.9; negative likelihood ratio: whole group 0.48, acute 0.88, chronic 0.08

ANTERIOR KNEE PAIN

Reliability	Responsiveness
• Test-retest ICC = 0.95[309]	• Responsiveness is as 100-point scale and needs a change of 14 points to reflect true change—area under the curve ROC 0.77[309]

ASSOCIATION OF AT LEAST TWO OF THESE TESTS FOR MENISCAL INJURY (TENDERNESS ON PALPATION OF THE JOINT LINE, BOHLER TEST, MCMURRAY'S TEST, STEINMANN TEST, APLEY'S GRIPPING TEST, PAYR TEST)

Specificity	Sensitivity	Odds Ratio
• Medial meniscus 76%, lateral meniscus 98%, overall 87%[310]	• Medial meniscus 100%, lateral meniscus 92%, overall 96.5%[310]	• Positive likelihood ratio: medial meniscus 4.16, lateral meniscus 46, overall 7.42; negative likelihood ratio: medial meniscus 0, lateral meniscus 0.08, overall 0.04

CAR (GETTING IN AND OUT OF A CAR)

Reliability	Validity
• r = 0.88[103]	• Concurrent validity with time on treadmill (r = -0.33, with VO_{2max} r = -0.29, knee strength r = -0.22)[103]

CHAIR-SIT

Reliability
• r = 0.62[103]

CINCINNATI KNEE RATING SYSTEM

Reliability	Validity	Responsiveness
• Test-retest ICC = 0.97 (analog score ICC = 0.96)[311] • Test-retest uninjured population: ICC > 0.71 for subscales, ACL reconstructed ICC > 0.75[79]	• Content validity (no floor effect and limited ceiling effect), item-discriminant validity (subscales and quadriceps strength r < −0.23, hamstring strength r < −0.30, age r < −0.26, anteroposterior displacement KT-1000 r < −0.38, patellofemoral crepitus r < 0.19, flexion r < 0.29, extension r < 0.26)[79] • Construct validity (p = 0.001 for higher values on the scale for subjects with chronic injury, deterioration of cartilage, prior failed ACL reconstruction, fair or poor patient perception of follow-up, surgical complications, symptoms with no sports, symptoms with no work, injured at work)[79]	• Effect size for subscales: pain 1.40, swelling 1.18, partial giving way 1.87, full giving way 1.49, symptoms average 1.74, ADL function average 0.69, sports function average 1.91, overall rating score 3.49[79]

CLARKE'S TEST

Odds Ratio

• Positive likelihood ratio 1.94, negative likelihood ratio 0.69[222]

CROSSOVER HOP

Reliability

• Intrarater ICC = 0.94, SEM = 28.8, CM 95%, CI 56.5[312]
• Test-retest ICC = 0.96, SEM = 15.95[313]
• Test-retest ICC = 0.93, SEM = 17.74[314]
• Test-retest uninjured ICC = 0.95, ACL reconstructed ICC = 0.98[311]
• Test-retest ICC = 0.90[315]

ECCENTRIC STEP TEST

Odds Ratio

• Positive likelihood ratio 2.34, negative likelihood ratio 0.71[222]

END FEEL KNEE EXTENSION

Reliability

• Intrarater k = 1, interrater k = 0.25[316]

END FEEL KNEE FLEXION

Reliability

• Intrarater k = 0.64, interrater k = 0.02[316]

ENG (FOR PATELLOFEMORAL SYNDROME)

Reliability	Validity
• Test-retest ICC = 0.92, SEM = 4.8[90]	• Correlation with Kujala −0.52, Flandry 0.66, FIQ 0.55, VAS for worst pain 0.39, VAS for usual pain 0.43[90]

Continued

APPENDIX 12-1—cont'd

FIQ (FUNCTIONAL INDEX QUESTIONNAIRE)

Reliability	Validity	Responsiveness
• Test-retest ICC = 0.49[317] • Test-retest ICC = 0.94, SEM = 1[90]	• Correlation with Kujala 0.58, Flandry –0.66, ENG –0.55, VAS for worst pain –0.43, VAS for usual pain –0.45[90]	• Effect size for patellofemoral pain 0.32[318]

FLANDRY (FOR PATELLOFEMORAL SYNDROME)

Reliability	Validity
• Test-retest ICC = 0.95, SEM = 120[90]	• Correlation with Kujala –0.54, ENG 0.66, FIQ –0.66, VAS for worst pain 0.54, VAS for usual pain 0.57[90]

FLEXION-ROTATION DRAWER TEST (NOYES)

Sensitivity

• Acute 56%, subacute 93%, chronic 88%, overall 72%[319]

FUNCTIONAL TESTS

Test	Reliability
• Anterior lunge	• ICC = 0.82, SEM = 0.38[320]
• Balance and reach	• ICC = 0.83, SEM = 0.68[320]
• Bilateral squat	• ICC = 0.79, SEM = 0.47[320]
• Single-leg press	• ICC = 0.82, SEM = 0.56[320]
• Step down	• ICC = 0.94, SEM = 0.53[320]

INCLINED SQUAT STRENGTH TEST PROTOCOL

Reliability

• Test-retest 50 (squat rep ICC = 0.80, 20 sec rep ICC = 0.89)[321]

JERK TEST OF HUGHSTON

Sensitivity

• Acute 23%, subacute 33%, chronic 61%, overall 34%[319]
• Chronic 89.8%[292]

KNEE INJURY AND OSTEOARTHRITIS OUTCOME SCORE (KOOS)

Reliability	Validity	Responsiveness
• Pain ICC = 0.85, symptoms ICC = 0.93, ADL ICC = 0.75, sports and recreation ICC = 0.81, knee-related quality of life ICC = 0.86[101]	• Construct validity—correlation SF-36 (subscales r < 0.68)[101]	• Effect size for pain 0.84, for symptoms 0.87, for ADL 0.94, for sports and recreation 1.16, for knee quality of life 1.65[101]

KT-1000

Reliability	Specificity	Sensitivity	Odds Ratio
• Intrarater SEM < 0.64 (expert ICC > 0.96, novice ICC > 0.90), interrater SEM < 1.59 (expert ICC = 0.79, novice ICC = 0.65)[322] • Intrarater (anterior: 15 lb r = 0.63, 20 lb r = 0.69, 30 lb r = 0.73; posterior: 15 lb r = 0.15, 20 lb r = 0.34), interrater (anterior: 15 lb r = 0.78, 20 lb r = 0.81, 30 lb r = 0.84; posterior: 15 lb r = 0.72, 20 lb r = 0.77)[323] • Intrarater ICC = 0.83, interrater ICC = 0.62 (for posterior laxity)[195] • Intertester (15 lb ICC = 0.75, SEM = 2; 20 lb ICC = 0.75, SEM = 2; 30 lb ICC = 0.67, SEM = 2.5)[324] • Interrater (67 newtons: injured knee ICC = 0.79, SEM = 1; noninjured ICC = 0.77, SEM = 0.8; 89 newtons: injured ICC = 0.78, SEM = 0.9; maximal manual injured ICC = 0.88, SEM = 1.2; noninjured ICC = 0.77, SEM = 1.5)[325] • Error sources for 90% confidence interval (1.9 mm) normal subjects[189] • Mean error of 0.13 mm, SD = 0.12 mm, greatest error = 0.6 mm[193] • Intrarater uninvolved limb ICC = 0.69, involved limb ICC = 0.91[326] • Interrater no anesthesia ICC = 0.55, with anesthesia ICC = 0.60[327]	• 70% no anesthesia, 70% with anesthesia[327]	• 50% no anesthesia, 60% with anesthesia[327]	• Positive likelihood ratio: no anesthesia 1.6, with anesthesia 2; negative likelihood ratio: no anesthesia 0.71, with anesthesia 0.57

KUJALA (FOR PATELLOFEMORAL SYNDROME)

Reliability	Validity
• Test-retest ICC = 0.90, SEM = 4.7[90]	• Correlation with Flandry –0.54, ENG –0.52, FIQ 0.58, VAS for worst pain –0.37, VAS for usual pain –0.34[90]

LACHMAN TEST (RITCHIE, TRILLAT, LACHMAN-TRILLAT)

Reliability	Validity	Specificity	Sensitivity	Odds Ratio
• Intrarater kappa percent agreement (pos/neg k = 0.51, PA = 76%; end feel k = 0.33, PA = 55%); interrater (pos/neg k = 0.19, PA = 60%)[124] • Kappa test retest (k = 0.29, interrater k = 0.23)[328]	• Predictive value positive = 47%; predictive value negative = 64%[124]	• 95%[329] • 46%[124] • 90%[293] • 60%[294] • 94%[330] • 100%[297] • 100%[299] • 97%[230] • 100%[120] • Whole group 94%, acute 97%, chronic 90%[302]	• Chronic 98.6%[292] • 75%[329] • 71%[124] • 91%[303] • 63%[293] • 86%[294] • 100%[331] • 80%[304] • 99%[305] • 74%[306] • 97%[307] • 68%[330] • 91%[297] • 95%[308] • 96%[299] • 48%[300] • 96%[120] • Whole group 94%, acute 97%, chronic 90%[302]	• Positive likelihood ratio 15, negative likelihood ratio 0.26 • Positive likelihood ratio 1.31, negative likelihood ratio 0.63 • Positive likelihood ratio 6.5, negative likelihood ratio 0.4 • Positive likelihood ratio 2.2, negative likelihood ratio 0.2 • Positive likelihood ratio 10.7, negative likelihood ratio 0.3 • Positive likelihood ratio 102.1, negative likelihood ratio 0.1 • Positive likelihood ratio 58.2, negative likelihood ratio 0.1 • Positive likelihood ratio 13.8, negative likelihood ratio 0.5 • Positive likelihood ratio 6.5, negative likelihood ratio 0.4 • Positive likelihood ratio 151.7, negative likelihood ratio 0 • Positive likelihood ratio: whole group 10.2, acute 9.4, chronic 7.1; negative likelihood ratio: whole group 0.2, acute 0.1, chronic 0.2

Continued

APPENDIX 12-1—cont'd

LATERAL PIVOT SHIFT TEST OF MACINTOSH

Sensitivity

- Acute 25%, subacute 40%, chronic 52%, overall 36%[319]

LEQUESNE INDEX FOR KNEE OSTEOARTHRITIS

Reliability	Validity
• Test-retest k = 0.95[100] • Test-retest ICC = 0.95[99]	• Convergent validity (VAS pain r = 0.45, VAS handicap r = 0.38), divergent validity (score anxiety r = 0.15, score depression r = 0.30, score of Kellgren r = 0.11, circumference of thigh r = 0.17)[100] • Convergent validity (WOMAC sec A r = 0.56, sec B r = 0.48, sec C r = 0.78, VAS pain r = 0.46, VAS handicap r = 0.40, VAS Dw r = 0.65), divergent validity (score of anxiety r = 0.16, score of depression r = 0.28, score of Kellgren r = 0.13, circumference of thigh r = 0.18)[99]

LIFT/CARRY A WEIGHT

Reliability	Validity
• r = 0.92[103]	• Concurrent validity with time on treadmill (r = −0.32, with VO_{2max} r = −0.26, knee strength r = −0.47)[103]

LOSEE TEST

Sensitivity

- Acute 29%, subacute 33%, chronic 61%, overall 40%[319]

LOWER EXTREMITY FUNCTIONAL SCALE

Reliability	Validity	Responsiveness
• Test-retest ICC = 0.98[309] • Chronbach alpha 0.93, SEM 3.4, test-retest reliability 0.85[332]	• Cross-sectional validity = correlation with time up and go 0.51, time stairs 0.47, FIM ambulation 0.45, FIM stairs 0.16, pain intensity 0.33, pain limitation 0.51, 6-min walk 0.53, pooled index 0.68[332] • There was a statistically significant difference between patients receiving home care and not; p = 0.016[332] • Longitudinal validity = time up and go 0.22, time stairs 0.46, FIM ambulation 0.07, FIM stairs 0.13, pain intensity 0.30, pain limitation 0.49, 6-min walk 0.59, pooled index 0.64[332]	• Responsiveness is as 80-point scale and needs a change of 8 points to reflect true change—area under the curve ROC 0.69[309]

LYSHOLM KNEE SCORING SCALE

Reliability	Validity	Sensitivity	Responsiveness
• 1–3 days r = 0.75, 1–14 days r = 0.69, 3–14 days r = 0.68[333] • Test-retest ICC > 0.70[84] • Test-retest overall ICC = 0.93, pain ICC = 0.73, instability ICC = 0.87, locking ICC = 0.67, stair- climbing ICC = 0.81, limping ICC = 0.76, swelling ICC = 0.75, squatting ICC = 0.86[334]	• Internal consistency Cronbach alpha = 0.65; content validity—acceptable ceiling and floor effect > 30%; criterion validity—p < 0.05 for physical functioning, roles: physical and body pain domains of the SF-12 and pain, stiffness, and function domains of the WOMAC scale and the Tegner activity scale; construct validity— p < 0.01 for the Lysholm scale and patients with lower activity level, greater number of chondral surfaces with Outerbridge grade 4, patients with full-thickness chondral defects, patients with chondral effects associated with meniscus more than with subjects with isolated chondral defects, patient with more difficulty with ADL, patients with more difficulty at work because of the knee problem, patients with previous injury, patients with poorer assessment of the overall knee function[84] • Concurrent validity: Lysholm with hospital for special surgery p < 0.001, Lysholm with Cincinnati knee ligament p < 0.003[62] • Cronbach alpha 0.73; content validity: acceptable floor and ceiling effects (<30%); criterion validity: correlation with physical component of the SF-12 (r = 0.55); construct validity: the hypotheses were significant; had lower scores: patients with lower activity levels, acute injury, worker's compensation claim, more difficulty with ADL, more difficulty working, more difficulty doing sports, patients who assessed their overall knee function as abnormal or severely abnormal, degenerative or complex tear (p < 0.01)[334]	• Is not sensitive for the ACL injury[333]	• Effect size for isolated lesion 1.2 (SRM = 0.97), combined lesions 1.2 (SRM = 1.13)[334]

MCCONNELL TEST FOR CHONDROMALACIA PATELLAE

Reliability

• Intrarater k = –0.6—0.35, interrater k ICC = -0.02—0.19 (alignment)[335]

MCCONNELL TEST FOR MEDIOLATERAL PATELLA ROTATION

Reliability	Validity
• Intertester r = 0.91 for the medial distance, r = 0.94 for the lateral distance[336]	• Criterion validity with MRI *r* = 0.90[336]

Continued

APPENDIX 12-1—cont'd

MCMURRAY TEST

Reliability	Specificity	Sensitivity	Odds Ratio
• Intrarater SEM < 0.64 (expert ICC > 0.96, novice ICC > 0.90), interrater SEM < 1.59 (expert ICC = 0.79, novice ICC = 0.65)[322] • Intrarater (anterior: 15 lb r = 0.63, 20 lb r = 0.69, 30 lb r = 0.73; posterior: 15 lb r = 0.15, 20 lb r = 0.34), interrater (anterior: 15 lb r = 0.78, 20 lb r = 0.81, 30 lb r = 0.84; posterior: 15 lb r = 0.72, 20 lb r = 0.77)[323] • Intrarater ICC = 0.83, interrater ICC = 0.62 (for posterior laxity)[195] • Intertester (15 lb: ICC = 0.75, SEM = 2; 20 lb: ICC = 0.75, SEM = 2; 30 lb: ICC = 0.67, SEM = 2.5)[324] • Interrater (67 newtons: injured knee ICC = 0.79, SEM = 1; noninjured ICC = 0.77, SEM = 0.8; 89 newtons: injured ICC = 0.78, SEM = 0.9; maximal manual injured ICC = 0.88, SEM = 1.2; noninjured ICC = 0.77, SEM = 1.5)[325] • Error sources for 90% confidence interval (1.9 mm) normal subjects[189] • Mean error of 0.13 mm, SD = 0.12, millimeter greatest error = 0.6 mm[193] • Intrarater uninvolved limb ICC = 0.69, involved limb ICC = 0.91[326] • Interrater no anesthesia ICC = 0.55, with anesthesia ICC = 0.60[327]	• Medial 93.2%, lateral 93.5%, both 93.4%[337] • 65% negative predictive value, 98% sensitivity for medial thud and medial meniscus tear[201]	• Medial 64.7%, lateral 51.6%, both 58.5%[337] • 83% positive predictive value, 16% sensitivity for medial thud and medial meniscus tear[201]	• Positive likelihood ratio: medial 9.51, lateral 7.94, both 8.86; negative likelihood ratio: medial 0.38, lateral 0.52, both 0.44 • Positive likelihood ratio for medial thud and medial meniscus tear 8, negative likelihood ratio for medial thud and medial meniscus tear 0.86

MRI FOR MENISCUS INJURY

Specificity	Sensitivity	Odds Ratio
• Medial meniscus 71%, lateral meniscus 100%, overall 85.5%[310]	• Medial meniscus 96%, lateral meniscus 100%, overall 98%[310]	• Positive likelihood ratio: medial meniscus 3.31, lateral meniscus 100, overall 6.76; negative likelihood ratio: medial meniscus 0.06, lateral meniscus 0, overall 0.02

MRI TO MEASURE CARTILAGE THICKNESS AND VOLUME

Reliability

• Intraexaminer—global cartilage ICC > 0.958, compartments ICC > 0.974, condyles ICC > 0.943[338]
• Test retest within reader Pearson correlation r > 0.978[338]

PALPATION TO DETECT PATELLAR TENDINOPATHY

Reliability	Specificity	Sensitivity	Odds Ratio
• r = 0.82[339]	• In symptomatic subjects 9% (palpation to determine tenderness 47%)[339]	• In symptomatic subjects 68% (palpation to determine tenderness 56%)[339]	• Positive likelihood ratio for symptomatic subjects 0.74 (palpation to determine tenderness 1.06); negative likelihood ratio for symptomatic subjects 3.55 (palpation to determine tenderness 0.94)

PATELLAR ALIGNMENT WITH MRI

Reliability

- Intertester for the bony angles (sulcus angle r = 0.94, congruence angle r = 0.98, lateral patellofemoral angle r = 0.93), for the cartilage surface (sulcus angle r = 0.83, congruence angle r = 0.99, lateral patellofemoral angle r = 0.81)[340]

PATELLAR APPREHENSION TEST

Odds Ratio

- Positive likelihood ratio 2.26, negative likelihood ratio 0.79[222]

PIVOT DRAWER TEST

Sensitivity

- Acute 60%, subacute 87%, chronic 91%, overall 75%[319]

PIVOT SHIFT TEST

Specificity	Sensitivity	Odds Ratio
• 97%[293] • 100%[294] • 89%[299] • 100%[300] • 100%[120] • Whole group 98%, acute • 100%, chronic 97%[302]	• 42%[303] • 31%[293] • 9%[294] • 9%[304] • 35[305] • 29%[306] • 71%[308] • 93%[299] • 6%[300] • 9%[120] • Whole group 24%, acute • 32%, chronic 40%[302]	• Positive likelihood ratio 8.8, negative likelihood ratio 0.7 • Positive likelihood ratio 1.3, negative likelihood ratio 1 • Positive likelihood ratio 8.5, negative likelihood ratio 0.1 • Positive likelihood ratio 7.1, negative likelihood ratio 0.9 • Positive likelihood ratio 14.4, negative likelihood ratio 0.9 • Positive likelihood ratio: whole group 8.5, acute 1.3, chronic 7.7; negative likelihood ratio: whole group 0.9, acute 1.0, chronic 0.8

Q-ANGLE OR PATELLOFEMORAL ANGLE

Reliability	Validity
• Interrater (full extension ICC = 0.20, 20° flexion ICC = 0.17), intrarater (full extension ICC = 0.22, 20° flexion ICC = 0.14)[341]	• Correlation with radiographs (full extension ICC = 0.32, 20° flexion ICC = 0.13)[341]

RADIOGRAPHIC MEASUREMENT OF FEMOROTIBIAL ROTATION IN WEIGHT BEARING

Reliability

- Test retest—rotation of the femur and tibia and Q-angle 2° to 3° of SD and for patellar translation about 3 mm SD[342]

RHEUMATOID AND ARTHRITIS OUTCOME SCORES (RAOSS)

Reliability	Validity	Responsiveness
• Test retest (subscales): pain ICC = 0.87, symptoms ICC = 0.85, ADL ICC = 0.92, sports and recreation ICC = 0.76, QOL ICC = 0.92[343]	• Construct validity (RAOS daily living × SF-36 r = 0.65, RAOS sports recreation × SF-36 r = 0.63, RAOS ADL × HAQ r = −0.72, RAOS sports and recreation × HAQ r = −0.64)[343]	• Effect size (subscales): pain 0.40, symptoms 0.41, ADL 0.44, sports recreation 0.42, QOL 0.3[343]

SINGLE HOP FOR DISTANCE LATERAL

Reliability

- Test-retest ICC = 0.91, SEM = 6[344]

Continued

APPENDIX 12-1—cont'd

SINGLE HOP FOR DISTANCE MEDIAL

Reliability

- Test-retest ICC = 0.87, SEM = 7[344]

SINGLE-LEG HOP TEST FOR DISTANCE

Reliability	Validity
• Intrarater ICC = 0.92 dominant leg, 0.96 nondominant leg, 0.89 both legs[345] • Test-retest ICC = 0.92, SEM = 4.61[314] • Test-retest ICC = 0.96, SEM = 4.56[313] • Test-retest ICC > 0.82 for the injured leg ACL, ICC > 0.80 for the noninjured leg[346] • Intratester ICC = 0.88[326] • Test-retest ICC = 0.96[347] • Test-retest ICC = 0.93[315]	• Correlation with standing balance with eyes open on a stable surface r = −0.37, eyes open on a foam surface r = −0.46, eyes closed on a stable surface r = −0.63, landing from maximal hop r = −0.53[348]

SINGLE-LEG HOP FOR TIME

Reliability

- Test-retest ICC = 0.92[315]

6-M HOP TEST FOR TIME

Reliability

- Test-retest ICC = 0.92, SEM = 0.06[314]
- Test-retest ICC = 0.66, SEM = 0.13[313]
- Intrarater ICC = 0.90[326]
- Test-retest uninjured ICC = 0.95, ACL reconstructed ICC = 0.96[311]
- Test-retest ICC = 0.90[315]

SLOCUM TEST

Sensitivity

- Acute 40%, subacute 53%, chronic 64%, overall 50%[319]

STAIR CLIMB

Reliability	Validity
• r = 0.93[103] • Interrater kappa = 0.66[349]	• Concurrent validity with time on treadmill (r = −0.31, with VO_{2max} r = −0.31, knee strength r = −0.51)[103]

STAIRS HOP TEST (STAIRS HOPPLE TEST)

Reliability

- Test-retest uninjured ICC = 0.96, ACL reconstructed ICC = 0.96[311]

STEP UP TEST

Reliability	Responsiveness
• ICC = 0.63[318]	• Effect size for patellofemoral pain 0.65 for all the subjects[318]

TEGNER ACTIVITY SCALE

Reliability	Validity	Responsiveness
• Test-retest ICC = 0.82[334]	• Content validity: acceptable floor and ceiling effects (<30%); criterion validity: correlation with physical component of the SF-12 ($r = 0.46$); construct validity: the hypotheses were significant, had lower scores for patients with lower activity levels, acute injury, worker's compensation claim, more difficulty with ADL, more difficulty working, more difficulty doing sports, patients who assessed their overall knee function as abnormal or severely abnormal, degenerative or complex tear ($p < 0.01$)[334]	• Effect size for the group with isolated lesions 0.61 (SRM = 0.60), combined lesions 0.83 (SRM = 0.70)[334]

TRIPLE HOP

Reliability

- Test-retest ICC = 0.97, SEM = 11.17[314]
- Test-retest ICC = 0.95, SEM = 14.44[313]
- Test-retest ICC = 0.94[315]

ULTRASOUND FOR ACL RUPTURE

Specificity	Sensitivity	Odds Ratio
• 98%[350]	• 96%[350]	• Positive likelihood ratio 48, negative likelihood radio 0.04

VALGUS STRESS TEST

Reliability

- Interrater measure in kappa (k) and percent of agreement (PA) (motion k = 0.1, 6 PA = 56%; pain k = 0.33, PA = 60%; end feel k = 0.38, PA = 80%)[351]

VAS FOR USUAL PAIN ON PATELLOFEMORAL SYNDROME

Reliability	Validity
• Test-retest ICC = 0.77, SEM = 1.2[90]	• Correlation with Kujala –0.34, Flandry 0.57, ENG 0.43, FIQ –0.45, VAS for worst pain 0.63[90]

VAS FOR WORST PAIN ON PATELLOFEMORAL SYNDROME

Reliability	Validity
• Test-retest ICC = 0.79, SEM = 1.1[90]	• Correlation with Kujala –0.37, Flandry 0.54, ENG 0.39, FIQ –0.43, VAS for usual pain 0.63[90]

VASTUS MEDIALIS COORDINATION TEST

Odds Ratio

- Positive likelihood ratio 2.26, negative likelihood ratio 0.90[222]

VERTICAL JUMP (Hop)

Reliability

- Intrarater ICC = 0.97[326]
- Test-retest uninjured ICC = 0.92, ACL reconstructed ICC = 0.94[311]
- Test-retest ICC = 0.85[315]

WALDRON TEST

Odds Ratio

- Positive likelihood ratio: test I 1.41, test II 1.05; negative likelihood ratio: test I 0.81, test II 0.99[222]

CHAPTER 13

LOWER LEG, ANKLE, AND FOOT

At least 80% of the general population has foot problems, but these problems can often be corrected by proper assessment, treatment, and, above all, care of the feet. Lesions of the ankle and foot can alter the mechanics of gait and, as a result, cause stress on other lower limb joints, which in turn may lead to pathology in these joints.

The foot and ankle combine flexibility with stability because of the many bones, their shapes, and their attachments. The lower leg, ankle, and foot have two principal functions: propulsion and support. For propulsion, they act like a flexible lever; for support, they act like a rigid structure that holds up the entire body.

Functions of the Foot

- Acts as a support base that provides the necessary stability for upright posture with minimal muscle effort
- Provides a mechanism for rotation of the tibia and fibula during the stance phase of gait
- Provides flexibility to adapt to uneven terrain
- Provides flexibility for absorption of shock
- Acts as a lever during push-off

Although the joints of the lower leg, ankle, and foot are discussed separately, they act as functional groups, not as isolated joints. As the terminal part of the lower kinetic chain, the lower leg, ankle, and foot have the ability to distribute and dissipate the different forces (e.g., compressive, shearing, rotary, tensile) acting on the body through contact with the ground.[1] This is especially evident during gait. In the foot, the movement occurring at each individual joint is minimal. However, when combined, there normally is sufficient range of motion (ROM) in all of the joints to allow functional mobility as well as functional stability. For ease of understanding, the joints of the foot are divided into three sections: hindfoot (rearfoot), midfoot, and forefoot.

Applied Anatomy

Hindfoot (Rearfoot)

Tibiofibular Joint. The inferior (distal) tibiofibular joint is a fibrous or syndesmosis type of joint. It is supported by the anterior tibiofibular, posterior tibiofibular, and inferior transverse ligaments as well as the interosseous ligaments (Figure 13-1). The movements at this joint are minimal but allow a small amount of spread (1 to 2 mm) at the ankle joint during dorsiflexion. This same action allows the fibula to move up and down during dorsiflexion and plantar flexion. Dorsiflexion at the ankle joint causes the fibula to move superiorly, putting stress on both the inferior tibiofibular joint at the ankle and the superior tibiofibular joint at the knee. The fibula carries more of the axial load when it is dorsiflexed. On average, the fibula carries about 17% of the axial loading.[2] The joint is supplied by the deep peroneal and tibial nerves.

Talocrural (Ankle) Joint. The talocrural joint is a uniaxial, modified hinge, synovial joint located between the **talus**, the **medial malleolus** of the tibia, and the **lateral malleolus** of the fibula. The talus is shaped so that in dorsiflexion it is wedged between the malleoli, allowing little or no inversion or eversion at the ankle joint. The talus is approximately 2.4 mm (0.1 inch) wider anteriorly than posteriorly. The medial malleolus is shorter, extending halfway down the talus, whereas the lateral malleolus extends almost to the level of the subtalar joint. The joint is supplied by branches of the tibial and deep peroneal nerves.

Figure 13-1

Ligaments of the hindfoot and midfoot. **A,** Medial view. **B,** Lateral view.

Continued

Figure 13-1 cont'd ▰▰▰▰
C, Posterior view. **D,** Coronal section through the left talocrural and talocalcanean joints. **E,** Superior view of ligaments on the lateral aspect. **F,** Superior view of deep deltoid ligament on the medial aspect.

The talocrural joint is designed for stability, especially in dorsiflexion. In plantar flexion, it is much more mobile. This joint is responsible for the anterior-posterior (dorsiflexion-plantar flexion) movement that occurs in the ankle-foot complex. Its close packed position is maximum dorsiflexion, and its capsular pattern is more a limitation of plantar flexion than of dorsiflexion. This joint is most stable in the dorsiflexed position. The resting position is 10° of plantar flexion, midway between maximum inversion and maximum eversion. The talocrural joint has one degree of freedom, and the movements possible at this joint are dorsiflexion and plantar flexion.

On the medial side of the joint, the major ligament is the **deltoid** or **medial collateral ligament**, which consists of four separate ligaments: the tibionavicular, tibiocalcanean, and posterior tibiotalar ligaments superficially, all of which resist talar abduction, and the anterior tibiotalar ligament, which lies deep to the other three ligaments and resists lateral translation and lateral rotation of the talus. On the lateral aspect, the talocrural joint is supported by the anterior talofibular ligament, which provides stability against excessive inversion of the talus; the posterior talofibular ligament, which resists ankle dorsiflexion, adduction ("tilt"), medial rotation, and medial translation of the talus; and the calcaneofibular ligament, which provides stability against maximum inversion at the ankle and subtalar joints. The anterior talofibular ligament is the ligament most commonly injured by a lateral ankle sprain, followed by the calcaneofibular ligament.

Subtalar (Talocalcanean) Joint. The subtalar joint is a synovial joint having three degrees of freedom and a close packed position of supination. Supporting the subtalar joint are the lateral talocalcanean and medial talocalcanean ligaments. In addition, the interosseous talocalcanean and cervical ligaments limit eversion.

The movements possible at the subtalar joint are gliding and rotation. With injury to the area (e.g., sprain, fracture), this joint and the talocrural joint often become hypomobile, partially because the talus has no muscles attaching to it. Medial rotation of the leg causes a valgus (outward) movement of the calcaneus, whereas lateral rotation of the leg produces a varus (inward) movement of the calcaneus. The axis of the joint is at an angle of 40° to 45° inclined vertically and 15° to 18° to the sagittal plane.

Midfoot (Midtarsal Joints)

In isolation, the midtarsal joints allow only a minimal amount of movement. Taken together, however, they allow significant movement to enable the foot to adapt to many positions without putting undue stress on the joints. **Chopart's joint** refers collectively to the midtarsal joints between the talus-calcaneus and the navicular-cuboid.

Talocalcaneonavicular Joint. The talocalcaneonavicular joint is a ball-and-socket synovial joint with three degrees of freedom. Its close packed position is supination, and the dorsal talonavicular ligament, bifurcated ligament, and plantar calcaneonavicular (spring) ligament support the joint (see Figure 13-1; Figure 13-2). Movements possible at this joint are gliding and rotation.

Cuneonavicular Joint. The cuneonavicular joint is a plane synovial joint with a close packed position of supination. The movements possible at this joint are slight gliding and rotation.

Cuboideonavicular Joint. The cuboideonavicular joint is fibrous, its close packed position being supination. The movements possible at this joint are slight gliding and rotation.

Intercuneiform Joints. The intercuneiform joints are plane synovial joints with a close packed position of supination. The movements possible at these joints are slight gliding and rotation.

Joints of the Hindfoot

Tibiofibular Joint

Resting position:	Plantar flexion
Close packed position:	Maximum dorsiflexion
Capsular pattern:	Pain on stress

Talocrural (Ankle) Joint

Resting position:	10° plantar flexion, midway between inversion and eversion
Close packed position:	Maximum dorsiflexion
Capsular pattern:	Plantar flexion, dorsiflexion

Subtalar Joint

Resting position:	Midway between extremes of range of motion
Close packed position:	Supination
Capsular pattern:	Varus, valgus

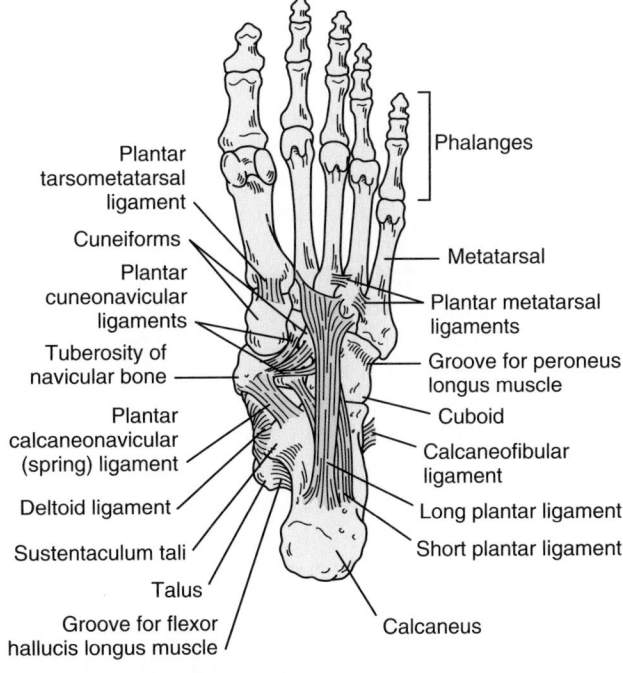

Figure 13-2
Ligaments on plantar aspect of foot.

Cuneocuboid Joint. The cuneocuboid joint is a plane synovial joint with a close packed position of supination. The movements of slight gliding and rotation are possible at this joint.

Calcaneocuboid Joint. The calcaneocuboid joint is saddle shaped with a close packed position of supination. Supporting this joint are the bifurcated ligament, the calcaneocuboid ligament, and the long plantar ligaments. The movement possible at this joint is gliding with conjunct rotation.

Joints of the Midfoot (Midtarsal Joints)	
Resting position:	Midway between extremes of range of motion
Close packed position:	Supination
Capsular pattern:	Dorsiflexion, plantar flexion, adduction, medial rotation

Joints of the Forefoot	
Tarsometatarsal Joints	
Resting position:	Midway between extremes of range of motion
Close packed position:	Supination
Capsular pattern:	None
Metatarsophalangeal Joints	
Resting position:	Midway between extremes of range of motion (10° extension)
Close packed position:	Full extension
Capsular pattern:	Big toe: extension, flexion
Second to fifth toe: variable	
Interphalangeal Joints	
Resting position:	Slight flexion
Close packed position:	Full extension
Capsular pattern:	Flexion, extension

Forefoot

Tarsometatarsal Joints. The tarsometatarsal joints are plane synovial joints with a close packed position of supination. The movement possible at these joints is gliding. Taken together, these joints are referred to as **Lisfranc's joint.**[3]

Intermetatarsal Joints. The four intermetatarsal joints are plane synovial joints with a close packed position of supination. The movement possible at these joints is gliding.

Metatarsophalangeal Joints. The five metatarsophalangeal joints are condyloid synovial joints with two degrees of freedom. Their close packed position is full extension. Their capsular pattern is variable for the lateral four joints and more limitation of extension than flexion for the hallux (big toe); their resting position is 10° of extension. The movements possible at these joints are flexion, extension, abduction, and adduction.

Interphalangeal Joints. The interphalangeal joints are synovial hinge joints with one degree of freedom. The close packed position is full extension, and the capsular pattern is more limitation of flexion than of extension. The resting position of the distal and proximal interphalangeal joints is slight flexion. The movements possible at these joints are flexion and extension.

Patient History

It is important to take a detailed and complete history when assessing the lower leg, ankle, and foot. In addition to the questions listed under Patient History in Chapter 1 the examiner should obtain the following information from the patient:

1. *What is the patient's occupation?* Whether the patient stands a great deal and the types of surfaces on which the patient usually stands may have bearing on what is causing the problem.

2. *What was the mechanism of injury?* What was the position of the foot at the time of the injury? Ankle sprains occur most often when the foot is plantar flexed, inverted, and adducted, with injury to the anterior talofibular ligament, anterolateral capsule, and possibly the distal tibiofibular ligament.[4,5] This same mechanism can lead to a malleolar or talar dome fracture and sinus tarsi syndrome.[6] Figure 13-3 outlines some of the common mechanisms of injury to the ankle. With injury to the lateral ligaments, the structures (articular surfaces) may be damaged on the medial side owing to compression leading to medial as well as lateral pain.[7] In fact, if the lateral ligaments are completely torn and the capsule disrupted, medial pain may predominate. Achilles tendinosis or paratenonitis often arises as the result of overuse, increased activity, or change in a high-stress training program. A dorsiflexion injury, accompanied by a snapping and pain on the lateral aspect that rapidly diminishes, may indicate a tear of the peroneal retinaculum.[8] Taunton et al. list some causes of overuse injuries in the lower limb.[9]

3. *Did the patient notice a transient or fixed deformity of the foot or ankle at the time of injury?* Was there any transitory locking (e.g., loose body, muscle spasm)? An affirmative answer may indicate a fracture causing immediate swelling that decreased as it spread into the surrounding tissue.

Figure 13-3

A, Supination-lateral rotation injury. Lateral rotation forces applied to a supinated foot initially result in rupture of the anterior tibiofibular ligament (stage I). As the forces continue, a short oblique fracture of the distal portion of the fibula occurs (stage II). Stage III involves a fracture of the posterior aspect of the tibia. Stage IV is a fracture of the medial malleolus. **B,** Supination-adduction injury. Adduction forces applied to a supinated foot initially result in a traction or avulsion fracture of the distal portion of the fibula or rupture of the lateral ligaments (stage I). As forces continue, fracture of the medial malleolus or rupture of the deltoid ligament occurs (stage II). The fibular fracture is typically transverse, and that of the medial malleolus is oblique or nearly vertical. **C,** Pronation-lateral rotation injury. Forces of lateral rotation applied to a pronated foot initially result in rupture of the deltoid ligament or fracture of the medial malleolus (stage I). As forces continue, the anterior tibiofibular ligament is ruptured (stage II). A high fibular fracture (stage III) and fracture of the posterior tibial margin (stage IV) are the final stages in this mechanism of injury. **D,** Pronation-abduction injury. The first two stages of this injury are identical to those of the pronation-external rotation fracture complex. Stage III is a transverse supramalleolar fibular fracture that may be comminuted laterally. (Redrawn from Resnick D, Kransdorf MJ: *Bone and joint imaging*, pp. 867–868, Philadelphia, 2005, WB Saunders.)

Causes of Overuse Injuries to the Lower Limb

- Prolonged training season
- Impact force of activity
- Training or competing on hard surfaces
- Change of training surface
- Downhill running
- Lack of flexibility
- Individual muscle weakness or poor reciprocal muscle strength
- Overstriding
- Poor posture
- High mileage or sudden change in mileage
- Too much, too soon
- Overtraining
- Anatomical factors (e.g., malalignment)
- Wrong type of footwear
- Road or sidewalk camber

From Taunton J et al: Leg, foot and ankle injuries. In Zachazewski JE et al: *Athletic injuries and rehabilitation*, p. 730, Philadelphia, 1996, WB Saunders.

4. *Was the patient able to continue the activity after the injury?* If so, the injury is probably not too severe, provided there is no loss of stability. Inability to bear weight, severe pain, and rapid swelling indicate a severe injury.[8]

Walking is compatible with a second-degree sprain; pain with running usually indicates a first-degree injury.[10]

5. *Was there any swelling or bruising (ecchymosis)* (Figure 13-4, *A*)? How quickly and where did it develop? This question can elicit some idea of the type of swelling (e.g., blood, synovial, purulent) and whether it is intracapsular or extracapsular. Figure 13-4, *B*, shows "skate bite" in which there is swelling over the extensor tendons of the foot caused by irritation from doing up stiff ice skates too tight.

6. *Are symptoms improving, becoming worse, or staying the same?* It is important to know the type of onset (macrotrauma, microtrauma) and the duration and intensity of symptoms (acute, subacute, chronic). Edwards et al. outlined some of the chronic causes of leg pain in athletes.[11]

7. *What are the sites and boundaries of pain or abnormal sensation?* The examiner should note whether the pattern is one of a dermatome, a peripheral nerve, or another painful structure.

8. *What is the patient's usual activity or pastime?* Answers to this question should give some idea of the stresses placed on the lower leg, ankle, and foot; how frequently they are applied; and whether the patient is suffering from a repetitive stress injury.

9. *Does activity make a difference?* Pain after activity suggests overuse. For example, with overuse injuries, pain initially comes on after the activity. As the injury

A

B

Figure 13-4

A, Ecchymosis following fracture of small toe. **B,** "Skate bite." Swelling over extensor tendons.

Differential Diagnosis of Chronic Leg Pain in the Athlete

Bone Periosteum
- Medial tibial stress syndrome ("shin splints")*
- Stress fracture*

Vascular
- Popliteal artery entrapment syndrome
- Intermittent claudication

Referred Pain
- Nerve entrapment
  - Peripheral
  - Spinal/radiculopathy
- Referred pain
  - Knee abnormality
  - Hip abnormality (especially in young patients)

Muscle/Tendon
- Chronic exertional compartment syndrome
- Muscle strains
- Tendinitis/tendinosis

Neoplasm

Infection

Modified from Edwards PH et al: A practical approach for the differential diagnosis of chronic leg pain in the athlete, *Am J Sports Med* 33:1244, 2005. *These two conditions are commonly different stages of the same pathological continuum.

---

progresses, pain or soreness is present at the beginning of the activity, then goes away during the activity only to return afterward. In later stages of the problem, the pain is constantly present. Pain during the activity suggests stress on the injured structure.

10. *Where is the pain?* Does the patient indicate a specific location or area? For example, with shin splints (**medial tibial stress syndrome**) or a compartment syndrome (acute or chronic type), the patient usually indicates a diffuse area.[12–15] With a stress fracture, the area of pain tends to be more specific. Anterolateral ankle impingement demonstrates anterolateral ankle joint tenderness, anterolateral ankle joint swelling (extracapsular), pain with force dorsiflexion and eversion, pain with single leg squat, pain with activities and possible absence of ankle instability.[16] Peroneal tendon problems show posterolateral pain and may be associated with lateral ankle instability.[17]

11. *Does walking on various terrains make a difference in regard to the foot problem?* If so, which terrains cause the most obvious problem? For example, walking on grass (an uneven surface) may bother the patient more than walking on a sidewalk (a relatively even surface), or the patient may find walking on a relatively soft surface (e.g., grass) easier than walk-

ing on a hard surface (e.g., cement). Prepared surfaces such as sidewalks, roads, and playing fields often have a camber to allow water runoff. This camber can cause problems in some cases of overuse.

12. *What types of shoes does the patient wear?* What kind of heel do the shoes have? Are the shoes in good condition? Does the patient make use of orthoses? If so, are they still functional? When an appointment is being made for an assessment, the patient should be told not to wear new shoes, so the examiner can use the shoes to determine the patient's usual shoe wear pattern. The examiner should also note whether the shoes offer proper support. The patient should bring any orthoses he or she is using to the assessment.

13. *Is there a history of previous injury, affliction or surgery?* For example, poliomyelitis may lead to a pes cavus. Systemic conditions such as diabetes, gout, psoriasis, and collagen diseases may manifest themselves first in the foot. If there was previous surgery, did the pain resolve following surgery? Is the pain the same as before surgery? Is it new pain?

14. For active people, especially runners or joggers, the following questions should also be considered:[18]

   a. *How long has the patient been running or jogging?*

   b. *On what type of terrain and surface does the patient train?*

   c. *In what types of workouts does the patient participate?* Have the workouts changed lately? How many workouts are done per week? How far does the patient run per week? (Joggers run approximately 2 to 30 km [1.2 to 18.6 miles] per week at a pace of 5 to 10 minutes/km, and sports runners run 30 to 65 km [18.6 to 40 miles] per week at a pace of 5 to 6 minutes/km. Long-distance runners run 60 to 180 km [37 to 112 miles] per week at a pace of 4 to 5 minutes/km. Elite runners run 100 to 270 km [62 to 168 miles] per week at a pace of 3.3 to 4 minutes/km.)

   d. *What types of warmup, stretching, and postexercise routines does the patient do?* The answers give the examiner some idea of whether the warmup and stretching activities are static or ballistic and whether these activities could be detrimental.

   e. *What types and styles of athletic shoes does the patient wear?* (The patient should have the shoes at the examination.) Are they "control" or "cushioning" shoes? People with a cavus foot are more likely to need a cushioning shoe, whereas those with a planus foot are more likely to need a control shoe. The examiner should be able to tell if the shoes fit properly.

   f. *Does the patient wear socks while training?* If so, what kind (e.g., cotton, wool, nylon) and how many pairs?

   g. *When was the patient's last race? How long was it? When is the patient's next race?* The answers give the examiner some idea of how long the problem has been present and how long it will be until maximum stress is again placed on the joints.

Observation

Observation of the foot is extensive. Because of the stresses the foot is subjected to and because it, like the hand, can project signs of systemic problems and disease, the examiner should carefully and meticulously inspect the foot.

When performing the observation, the examiner should remember to compare the weight-bearing (closed-chain) with the non-weight-bearing (open-chain) posture of the foot.[19] During open-chain motion, the talus is considered fixed; during closed-chain motion, the talus moves to help the foot and leg adapt to the terrain and to the stresses that are applied to the foot. Even though the calcaneus is touching a surface in closed-chain movement, for descriptive purposes, it is still considered to be moving. The weight-bearing stance of the foot shows how the body compensates for structural abnormalities (Figure 13-5). The non-weight-bearing posture shows functional and structural abilities without compensation (Figure 13-6). The observation includes looking at the patient from the front, from the side, and from behind in the weight-bearing (standing) position and from the

Figure 13-6

A, Open-chain (non-weight-bearing) supination of the subtalar joint (right foot). When the non-weight-bearing foot is moved at the subtalar joint in the direction of supination, the talus is stable, and the calcaneus and foot move around the talus. The calcaneus and foot invert, plantar flex, and adduct. These positional changes, associated with subtalar joint supination, are readily visible when compared with the pronated position of the subtalar joint. **B,** Open-chain (non-weight-bearing) pronation of the subtalar joint (right foot). When the subtalar joint is moved into a pronated position in the non-weight-bearing foot, the foot abducts, everts, and dorsiflexes around the stable talus. The positional variances can best be appreciated by comparing this illustration with the supinated position of the subtalar joint. (Redrawn from Root ML et al: *Normal and abnormal function of the foot*, p. 29, Los Angeles, 1977, Clinical Biomechanics.)

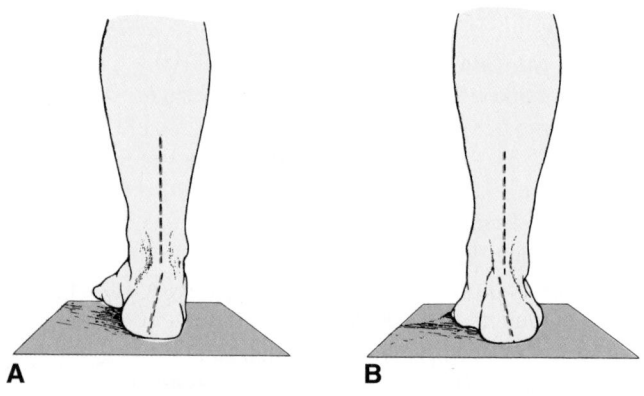

Figure 13-5

A, Closed-chain (weight-bearing) supination of the subtalar joint (right foot). Supination of the subtalar joint in the weight-bearing foot results in motion of both the calcaneus and the talus. The calcaneus moves in the frontal plane, and the talus moves in the transverse and sagittal planes. The calcaneus inverts, and the talus simultaneously abducts and dorsiflexes relative to the calcaneus. The leg follows the motion of the talus in the transverse plane and laterally rotates. The leg also follows the sagittal plane motion of the talus to some degree. The dorsiflexion motion of the talus on the calcaneus, therefore, tends to impart a slight extension motion to the knee. **B,** Closed-chain (weight-bearing) pronation of the subtalar joint (right foot). Pronation of the subtalar joint in the weight-bearing foot results in eversion of the calcaneus; the talus adducts and plantar flexes relative to the calcaneus. The leg follows the talus in a transverse plane and medially rotates. In a sagittal plane, the leg also moves to some extent with the talus. As the talus plantar flexes, the proximal aspect of the tibia moves forward to flex the knee slightly. (Redrawn from Root M et al: *Normal and abnormal function of the foot*, p. 30, Los Angeles, 1977, Clinical Biomechanics.)

front, from the side, and from behind in the sitting position with the legs and feet not bearing weight. The examiner should note the patient's willingness and ability to use the feet. The bony and soft-tissue contours of the foot should be normal, and any deviation should be noted. Often, painful callosities may be found over abnormal bony prominences. The examiner should note any scars or sinuses.

Weight-Bearing Position, Anterior View

With the patient in a standing position, the examiner should observe whether the patient's hips and trunk are in normal position. Excessive lateral rotation of the hip or rotation of the trunk away from the opposite hip elevates the medial longitudinal arch of the foot, whereas medial rotation of the hip or trunk rotation toward the opposite hip tends to flatten the arch (Figure 13-7). Medial rotation of the hip can also cause pigeon toes, a condition more commonly associated with medial tibial torsion or rotation. If the iliotibial band is tight, the tightness may cause eversion and lateral rotation of the foot.

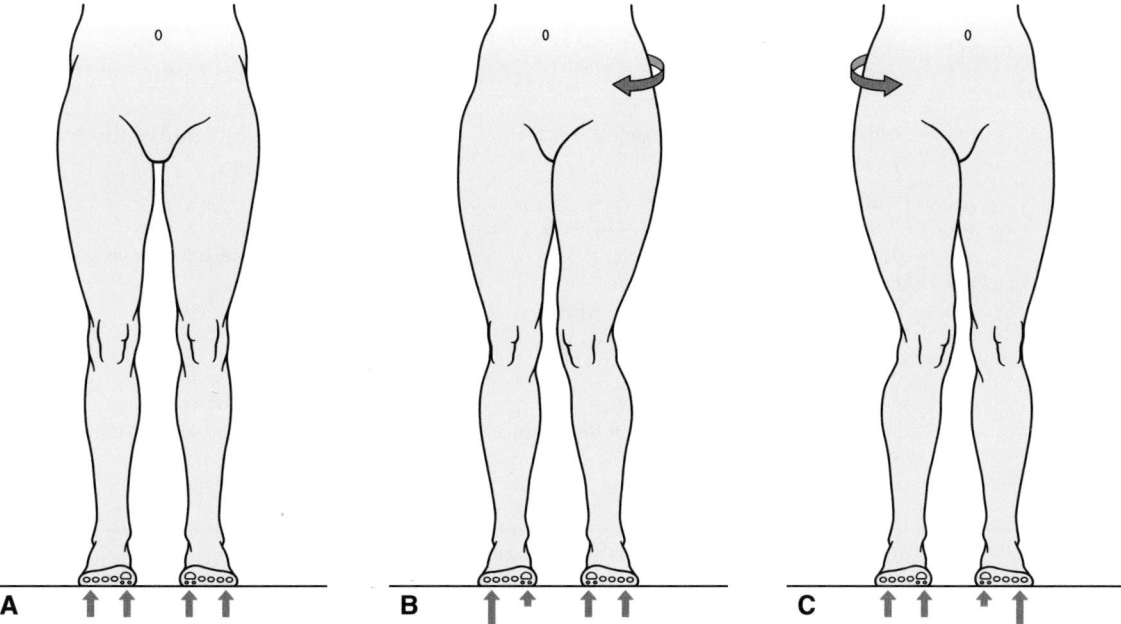

Figure 13-7

A, During static stance, ground reaction forces *(arrows)* directed upward against the plantar aspects of both feet maintain the transverse plane equilibrium and stability of the lower extremities and pelvis. Equal ground reaction forces are exerted on the lateral and medial plantar surfaces of both feet. **B,** When the trunk is rotated to the right, the right foot supinates and the left pronates. The right forefoot inverts from the ground; vertical ground reaction forces are greater against the lateral side of the forefoot *(large arrow)* and less against the medial side of the forefoot *(small arrow)*. The left forefoot remains flat on the ground, and vertical ground reaction forces are distributed evenly against the forefoot *(equal arrows)*. **C,** When the trunk is rotated to the left, ground reaction exerts unequal forces against the left forefoot and equal forces against the right forefoot. (Redrawn from Root ML et al: *Normal and abnormal function of the foot*, p. 102, Los Angeles, 1977, Clinical Biomechanics.)

Figure 13-8

Swelling within the talocrural and subtalar joint capsule.

The examiner should also look at the tibia to note any local or general bone swelling (Figure 13-8). Does the tibia have a normal shape, or is it bowed? Is there any torsional deformity? The medial malleolus usually lies anterior to the lateral malleolus. Pigeon toes, or toe-in deformity, results from a medial tibial torsion deformity; it does not constitute a foot deformity (Table 13-1).

Figure 13-9 shows the anterosuperior view of the feet in the weight-bearing stance. The examiner should note whether there is any asymmetry, malalignment (Table 13-2), or excessive supination or pronation of the foot. **Supination** of the foot involves inversion and outward rotation of the heel, adduction of the forefoot with inward rotation at the tarsometatarsal joints to maintain contact with the ground and outward rotation at the midtarsal joints, and plantar flexion at the subtalar joint and midtarsal joints so that the medial longitudinal arch is accentuated (Figure 13-10, *A*). In addition, along with lateral rotation of the talus, there is lateral rotation of the leg in relation to the foot (Figure 13-11). Supination of the foot causes the proximal aspect of the tibia to move posteriorly. It is required during propulsion to give rigidity to the foot and requires less muscle work than pronation.

Table 13-1

Causes of Toeing-In and Toeing-Out in Children

Level of Affection	Toe In	Toe Out
Feet-ankles	Pronated feet (protective toeing-in)	Pes valgus from contracture of triceps surae muscle
	Metatarsus varus	Talipes calcaneovalgus
	Talipes varus and equinovarus	Congenital convex pes planovalgus
Leg-knee	Tibia vara (Blount's disease) and developmental genu varum	Lateral tibial torsion
	Abnormal medial tibial torsion	Congenital absence of hypoplasia of the fibula
	Genu valgum—developmental (protective toeing-in to shift body center of gravity medially)	
Femur-hip	Abnormal femoral antetorsion	Abnormal femoral retroversion
	Spasticity of medial rotators of hip (cerebral palsy)	Flaccid paralysis of medial rotators of hip
Acetabulum	Maldirected—facing anteriorly	Maldirected—facing posteriorly

From Tachdjian MO: *Pediatric orthopedics*, p. 2817, Philadelphia, 1990, WB Saunders.

Figure 13-9

Anterosuperior view of the feet (weight-bearing position).

Pronation of the foot involves eversion and inward rotation of the heel, abduction of the forefoot with outward rotation at the tarsometatarsal joints and inward rotation at the midtarsal joints, and medial rotation of the talus causing medial rotation of the leg in relation to the foot, and dorsiflexion of the subtalar and midtarsal joints (Figure 13-12), resulting in a decrease in the medial longitudinal arch (Figure 13-10, *B*). This movement causes the proximal aspect of the tibia to move anteriorly. The

pronated foot has greater subtalar motion than the supinated foot and requires more muscle work to maintain stance stability than the supinated foot. The foot is much more mobile in this position.

The definitions used in this chapter are the ones preferred by orthopedists and podiatrists. Anatomists and kinesiologists such as Kapandji refer to inversion as a combination of adduction and supination and to eversion as a combination of abduction and pronation.[20] Lipscomb and Ibrahim[21] as well as Williams and Warwick[22] have defined supination and pronation as opposite the terms just mentioned. Because of the confusion in terminology concerning the terms supination and pronation, readers of books and articles on the foot must be careful to discern exactly what each author means.

In the infant, the foot is normally pronated. As the child matures, the foot begins to supinate, accompanied by development of the medial longitudinal arch. The foot also appears to be more pronated in the infant because of the fat pad in the medial longitudinal arch.

The examiner should note how the patient stands and walks. Normally, in standing, 50% to 60% of the weight is taken on the heel and 40% to 50% is taken by the metatarsal heads. The foot assumes a slight toe-out position. This angle (the **Fick angle**) is approximately 12° to 18° from the sagittal axis of the body, developing from 5° in children (Figure 13-13).[23] During movement, the foot is subjected to high loading, and pathology may cause the gait to be altered. The cumulative force to which each foot is subjected during the day is the equivalent of 639 metric tons in a person who weighs approximately 90 kg, or the equivalent of walking 13 km per day.

Table 13-2

Malalignment about the Foot and Ankle

Malalignment	Possible Correlated Motions or Postures	Possible Compensatory Motions or Postures
Ankle equinus		Hypermobile first ray Subtalar or midtarsal excessive pronation Hip or knee flexion Genu recurvation
Rearfoot varus Excessive subtalar supination (calcaneal varus)	Tibial; tibial and femoral; or tibial femoral, and pelvic lateral rotation	Excessive medial rotation along the lower quarter chain Hallux valgus Plantar flexed first ray Functional forefoot valgus Excessive or prolonged midtarsal pronation
Rearfoot valgus Excessive subtalar pronation (calcaneal valgus)	Tibial; tibial and femoral; or tibial, femoral, and pelvic medial rotation Hallux valgus	Excessive lateral rotation along the lower quarter chain Functional forefoot varus
Forefoot varus	Subtalar supination and related rotation along the lower quarter	Plantar flexed first ray Hallux valgus Excessive midtarsal or subtalar pronation or prolonged pronation Excessive tibial; tibial and femoral; or tibial, femoral, and pelvic medial rotation, or all with contralateral lumbar spine rotation
Forefoot valgus	Hallux valgus Subtalar pronation and related rotation along the lower quarter	Excessive midtarsal or subtalar supination Excessive tibial; tibial and femoral; or tibial, femoral, and pelvic lateral rotation, or all with ipsilateral lumbar spine rotation
Metatarsus adductus	Hallux valgus Medial tibial torsion Flatfoot Toeing-in	
Hallux valgus	Forefoot valgus Subtalar pronation and related rotation along the lower quarter	Excessive tibial; tibial and femoral; or tibial, femoral, and pelvic lateral rotation, or all with ipsilateral lumbar spine rotation

From Riegger-Krugh C, Keysor JJ: Skeletal malalignment of the lower quarter: Correlated and compensatory motions and postures, *J Orthop Sports Phys Ther* 23:166, 1996.

Foot Loading during Gait

Walking:	1.2 times the body weight
Running:	2 times the body weight
Jumping (from height of 60 cm [2 feet]):	5 times the body weight

When weight bearing, if the relation of the foot to the ankle is normal, all of the metatarsal bones bear weight, and all of the metatarsal heads lie in the same transverse plane. The forefoot and hindfoot should be parallel to each other and to the floor. The midtarsal joints are in maximum pronation, and the subtalar joint is in neutral position. The subtalar and talocrural joints should be parallel to the floor. Finally, the posterior bisection of the calcaneus and distal one third of the leg should form two vertical, parallel lines.[24]

If the examiner has noted any asymmetry in standing, the examiner should place the talus (or foot) in neutral (see Special Tests) to see if the asymmetry disappears. If the asymmetry is present in normal standing, it is a **functional asymmetry**. If it is still present when the foot is in neutral, it is also an **anatomical or structural asymmetry**, in which case a structural deformity is probably causing the asymmetry. Leg-heel and forefoot-heel alignment (see Special Tests) may also be checked, especially if asymmetry is present.

Figure 13-10
Supination (**A**) and pronation (**B**) of the (non-weight-bearing) foot.

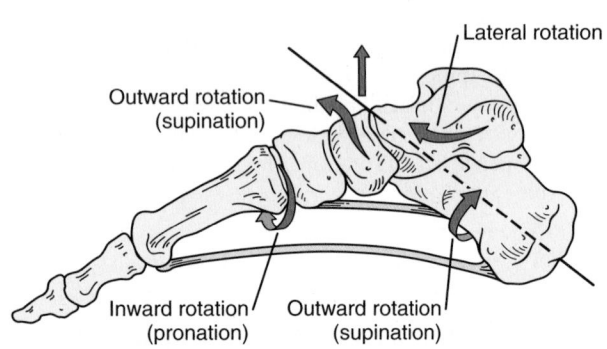

Figure 13-11
Supination of the foot produced by lateral rotation of the tibia. The rear foot and midfoot outwardly rotate (supinate) and the forefoot inwardly rotates (pronates) on the midfoot. As foot is plantar flexed, plantar fascia becomes tight along with ligaments to provide stable foot for push off. (Modified from Richardson JK, Iglarsh ZA, editors: *Clinical orthopedic physical therapy*, p. 513, Philadelphia, 1994, WB Saunders.)

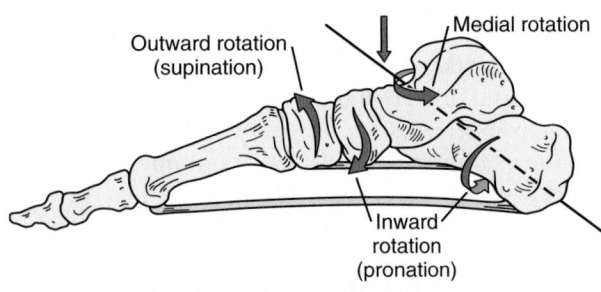

Figure 13-12
Pronation of the foot produced by medial rotation of the tibia. The rear foot and midfoot inwardly rotate (pronate) and the forefoot outwardly rotates (supinates) on the midfoot. Plantar fascia and plantar ligaments become taut as they absorb the ground reaction forces. (Modified from Richardson JK, Iglarsh ZA, editors: *Clinical orthopedic physical therapy*, p. 513, Philadelphia, 1994, WB Saunders.)

Figure 13-13
Fick angle.

The examiner should note whether the patient uses a cane or other walking aid. Use of a cane in the opposite hand diminishes the stress on the ankle joint and foot by approximately one third.

Any prominent bumps or exostoses should be noted, as should any splaying (widening) of the forefoot. Splaying of the forefoot and metatarsus primus varus is more evident in weight bearing. There are three types of forefoot,[25] based on the length of the metatarsal bones (Figure 13-14):

1. **Index Plus Type.** The first metatarsal (1) is longer than the second (2), with the others (3, 4, and 5) of progressively decreasing lengths, so that 1>2>3>4>5. This can result in an Egyptian type foot (Figure 13-15).

2. **Index Plus-Minus Type.** The first metatarsal is equal in length to the second metatarsal, with the others progressively diminishing in length, so that 1 = 2>3>4>5. This results in a squared type foot (see Figure 13-15).

3. **Index Minus Type.** The second metatarsal is longer than the first and third metatarsals. The fourth and fifth metatarsals are progressively shorter than the third, so that 1<2>3>4>5. This results in a Morton's or Greek type foot (see Figure 13-15).

The examiner should note whether the toenails appear normal. Older individuals have more brittle nails. The

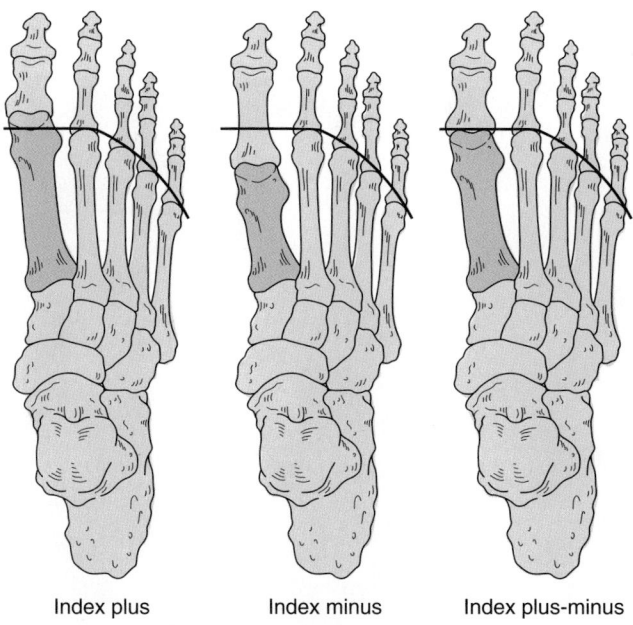

Figure 13-14
Metatarsal classifications.

Index plus   Index minus   Index plus-minus

Squared foot
9%

Mortons or
Greek foot
22%

Egyptian foot
69%

Figure 13-15
Types of feet seen in the general population.

examiner should look for warts, calluses, and corns. Warts are especially tender to the pinch (but not to direct pressure), but calluses are not. Plantar warts also tend to separate from the surrounding tissues, but calluses do not. Corns are similar to calluses but have a central nidus. They may be hard (on outside or upper aspect of toes) or soft (between toes) because of moisture.

Any swelling or pitting edema within the Achilles tendon, ankle, and foot should be noted (Figure 13-16). If there is any swelling, the examiner should note whether it is intracapsular or extracapsular. Swelling above the lateral malleolus may be related to a fibular fracture or disruption of the syndesmosis ("high" ankle sprain).[26,27] This injury takes a long time to heal and may involve the

A   **B**

Figure 13-16
Ankle sprain. **A,** Note pattern of pitting edema on top of the left foot. **B,** The swelling is intracapsular, as indicated by swelling on both sides of the left Achilles tendon.

Continued

Figure 13-16 cont'd

C, Extracapsular swelling. **D,** Midtarsal swelling. **E,** Synovial thickening (not swelling) because of repeated ankle sprains. **F,** Achilles swelling.

Table 13-3

Classification of Ankle Sprains

Severity	Pathology	Signs and Symptoms	Disability
Grade I (mild) stable	Mild stretch No instability Single ligament involved (usually anterior talofibular ligament)	No hemorrhage Minimal swelling Point tenderness No anterior drawer sign No varus laxity	No or little limp Minimal functional loss Difficulty hopping Recovery 8 days (range, 2–10)
Grade II (moderate) stable	Large spectrum of injury Mild to moderate instability Complete tearing of anterior talofibular ligament or partial tearing of anterior talofibular plus calcaneofibular ligaments	Some hemorrhage Localized swelling (margins of Achilles tendon less defined) Anterior drawer sign may be present No varus laxity	Limp with walking Unable to toe raise Unable to hop Unable to run Recovery 20 days (range, 10–30)
Grade III (severe) two-ligament, unstable	Significant instability Complete tear of anterior capsule, anterior talofibular and calcaneofibular ligaments	Diffuse swelling on both sides of Achilles tendon, early hemorrhage Possible tenderness medially and laterally Positive anterior drawer sign Positive varus laxity	Unable to bear weight fully Significant pain inhibition Initially almost complete loss of range of motion Recovery 40 days (range, 30–90)

From Reid DC: *Sports injury assessment and rehabilitation*, p. 226, New York, 1992, Churchill Livingstone.

anterior and/or posterior tibiofibular ligament as well as the ligaments of the talocrural joint. Swelling posterior to the lateral malleolus may indicate peroneal retinacular injury. Lateral ankle sprains initially swell distal to the lateral malleolus, but swelling may spread into the foot if the capsule has been torn (Table 13-3).[8] The examiner should also check the patient's gait for the position of the foot at heel strike, at foot flat, and at toe off. The gait cycle is described in greater detail in Chapter 14.

Any vasomotor changes should be recorded, including loss of hair on the foot, toenail changes, osteoporosis as seen on radiographs, and possible differences in temperature between the limbs. Systemic diseases such as diabetes can also lead to foot problems as a result of altered sensation, which facilitates injury.

The examiner should look for any circulatory impairment or presence of varicose veins. Brick-red color or cyanosis when the limb is dependent is an indication of impairment. Does this condition change to rapid blanching, or does it stay normal on elevation of the limbs? Change indicates circulatory impairment.

Weight-Bearing Position, Posterior View

From behind, the examiner compares the bulk of the calf muscles and notes any differences. Variation may be caused by peripheral nerve lesions, nerve root problems, or atrophy resulting from disuse after injury. The Achilles

tendons on each side should be compared (see Figure 13-16, *F*). If a tendon appears to curve out (Figure 13-17), it may indicate a fallen medial longitudinal arch, resulting in a pes planus (flatfoot) condition **(Helbing's sign)**.[28]

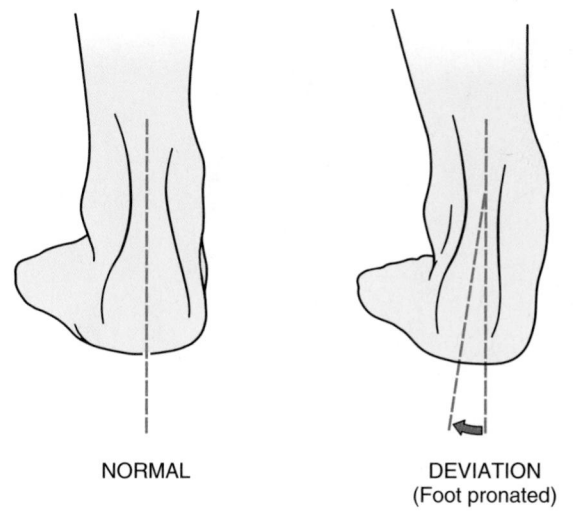

NORMAL   DEVIATION
(Foot pronated)

Figure 13-17

Normal and deviated Achilles tendon. The deviation is often seen with pes planus (flatfoot) and when the medial longitudinal arch is lower or has "dropped."

The examiner observes the calcaneus for normality of shape and position. Runners often build up bone and a callus on the heel, producing a "pump bump" **(Haglund's deformity)** as a result of pressure on the heel (Figure 13-18).[29,30]

The malleoli are compared for positioning. Normally, the lateral malleolus extends farther distally than the medial malleolus; however, the medial malleolus extends farther anteriorly.

Weight-Bearing Position, Lateral View

With the side view, the examiner is primarily observing the longitudinal arches of the foot (Figure 13-19). The examiner should note whether the medial arch is higher than the lateral arch (as would be expected). Differences in the arches may often be determined by looking at the footprint patterns (Figure 13-20). The footprint pattern can be established by putting a light film of baby oil and then powder on the patient's foot and asking the patient to step down on a piece of colored paper.

The arches of the feet (Figure 13-21) are maintained by three mechanisms:[31] (1) wedging of the interlocking tarsal and metatarsal bones; (2) tightening of the ligaments on the plantar aspect of the foot; and (3) the intrinsic and extrinsic muscles of the foot and their tendons, which help to support the arches. The longitudinal arches form a cone as a result of the angle of the metatarsal bones in relation to the floor. With the medial longitudinal arch being more evident, this angle is greater on the medial side. The angle formed by each of the metatarsals with the floor is shown in Figure 13-22.

Figure 13-18
"Pump bumps" from tight ice skates.

Normal   Pes Planus   Pes Cavus

Figure 13-20
Footprint patterns.

Figure 13-19
Lateral and medial views of the feet showing longitudinal arches.

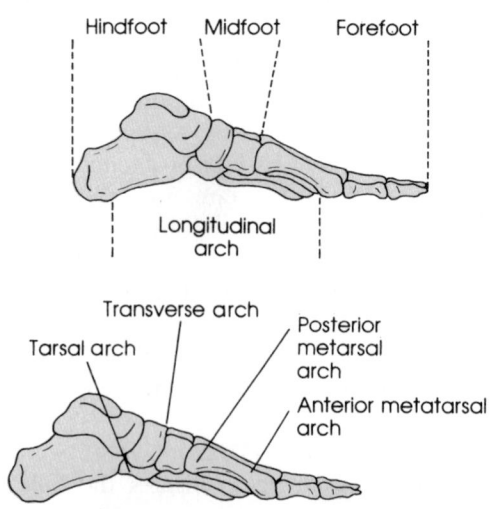

Hindfoot   Midfoot   Forefoot

Longitudinal arch

Transverse arch

Posterior metarsal arch

Tarsal arch

Anterior metatarsal arch

Figure 13-21
Divisions and arches of the foot (medial view).

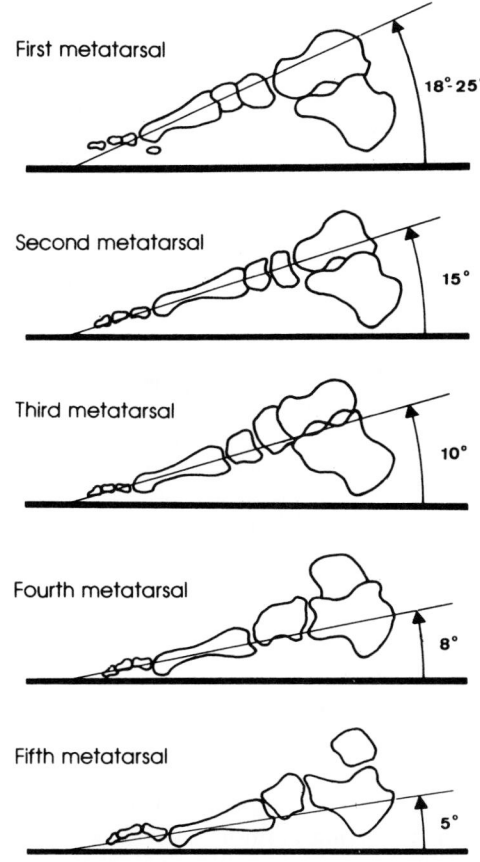

Figure 13-22
Angle formed by each metatarsal with the floor. (Modified from Jahss MH: *Disorders of the foot*, p. 1231, Philadelphia, 1991, WB Saunders.)

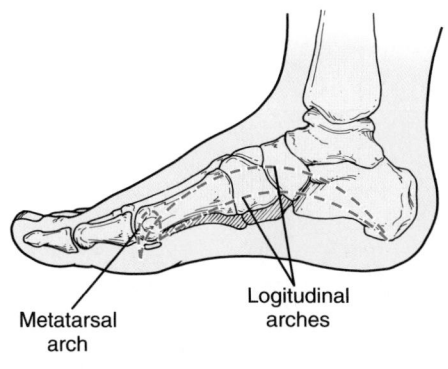

Figure 13-24
Arches of the foot (medial view).

The **medial longitudinal arch** consists of the calcaneal tuberosity, the talus, the navicular, three cuneiforms, and the first, second, and third metatarsal bones (Figures 13-23 and 13-24). This arch is maintained by the tibialis anterior, tibialis posterior, flexor digitorum longus, flexor hallucis longus, abductor hallucis, and flexor digitorum brevis muscles; the plantar fascia or aponeurosis; and the plantar calcaneonavicular ligament. The plantar aponeurosis plays a major role during the stance and push-off phases of gait, which helps to distribute Achilles tendon forces under the forefoot to the metatarsal heads and phalanges.[32]

The calcaneus, cuboid, and fourth and fifth metatarsal bones make up the **lateral longitudinal arch** (Figure 13-25). This arch is more stable and less adjustable than the medial longitudinal arch. The arch is maintained by the peroneus longus, peroneus brevis, peroneus tertius, abductor digiti minimi, and flexor digitorum brevis muscles; the plantar fascia; the long plantar ligament; and the short plantar ligament.[31]

The **transverse arch** is maintained by the tibialis posterior, tibialis anterior, and peroneus longus muscles and the plantar fascia (Figure 13-26). This arch consists of the navicular, cuneiforms, cuboid, and metatarsal bones. The arch is sometimes divided into three parts: tarsal, posterior metatarsal, and anterior metatarsal. A loss of

Figure 13-23
Supports of the medial longitudinal arch of the foot.

Figure 13-25
Supports of the lateral longitudinal arch of the foot: plantar aponeurosis (including the abductor digiti minimi and the flexor digitorum brevis IV and V); long plantar ligament; short plantar ligament.

the anterior metatarsal arch results in callus formation under the heads of the metatarsal bones (especially the second and third metatarsal heads). The metatarsophalangeal joints are slightly extended when the patient is in the normal standing position because the longitudinal arches of the foot curve down toward the toes.[31]

Non-Weight-Bearing Position

With the patient in a supine, non-weight-bearing position, the examiner should look for abnormalities such as callosities, plantar warts, scars, and sinuses or pressure sores on the soles of the feet as well as swelling which is more prominent on the dorsum of the foot. In addition, by looking at the foot from anterior to posterior, as shown in Figure 13-27, the examiner can observe whether the patient has a "fallen" metatarsal arch. Normally, in the non-weight-bearing position, the arch is visible. If the arch falls, callosities are often found over the metatarsal heads. The arch may be reversed, or it may fall because of an equinus forefoot, pes cavus, rheumatoid arthritis, short heel cord, or hammertoes. Abnormal width of one ankle in relation to the other (**Keen's sign**) may be caused by swelling, loss of integrity of the syndesmosis, or a malleolar fracture.

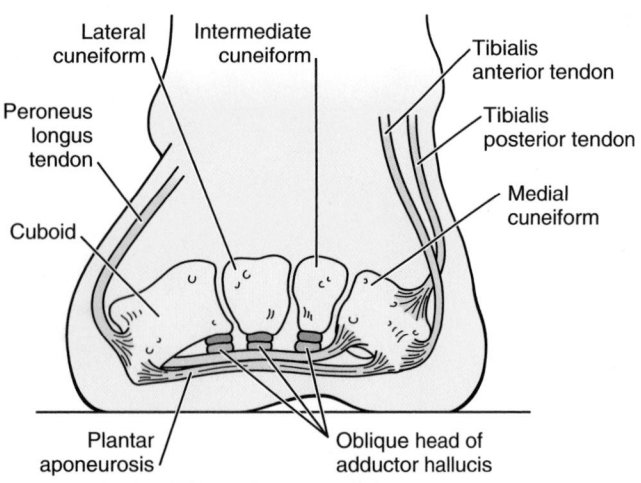

Figure 13-26
Supports of the transverse arch of the foot.

Figure 13-27
Fallen metatarsal arch.

A   **B**

Figure 13-28

Talipes equinovarus (clubfoot) in a child aged 4 months. **A,** Anterior view. **B,** Posterior view. (From Klenerman L: *The foot and its disorders,* p. 64, Boston, 1982, Blackwell Scientific.)

Young children should be assessed for clubfoot deformities, the most common of which is talipes equinovarus (Figures 13-28 and 13-29; Table 13-4). These types of deformities are often associated with other anomalies, such as spina bifida.

Common Deformities, Deviations, and Injuries

Equinus Deformity (Talipes Equinus). This deformity is characterized by limited dorsiflexion (less than 10°) at the talocrural joint, usually as a result of contracture of the gastrocnemius or soleus muscles or Achilles tendon. It may also be caused by structural bone deformity (primarily in the talus), trauma, or inflammatory disease. The deformity causes increased stress to the forefoot, which may lead to a rocker-bottom foot and excessive pronation at the subtalar joint. This deviation can contribute to conditions such as plantar fasciitis, metatarsalgia, heel spurs, and talonavicular pain.[18]

Clubfoot. This congenital deformity is relatively common and can take many forms, the most common of which is **talipes equinovarus**. Its cause is unknown, but there are probably multifactorial genetic causes modified by environmental factors.[33] It sometimes coexists with other congenital deformities, such as spina bifida and cleft palate. The flexible form is easily treated, but the resistant type often requires surgery. On assessment, the ROM is limited and the foot has abnormal form (see Figure 13-29).

Figure 13-29

Components of talipes equinovarus.

Table 13-4

Differential Diagnosis of Postural Clubfoot and Talipes Equinovarus

	Postural Clubfoot	Talipes Equinovarus
Etiology	Intrauterine malposture	Primary germ plasm defect
		Defective cartilaginous anlage of the talus
Pathological Anatomy		
Head and neck of talus	Normal	Medial and plantar tilt
	Declination angle of talus normal (150° to 155°)	Declination angle of talus decreased (115° to 135°)
Talocalcaneonavicular joint	Normal	Subluxed or dislocated medially and plantarward
Effect of manipulation in fetal specimens	Normal alignment of foot can be restored	Talocalcaneonavicular subluxation cannot be reduced unless ligaments connecting navicular to calcaneus, talus, and tibia are sectioned and posterior capsule and ligaments divided
Clinical Features		
Severity of deformity	Mild and flexible	Marked and rigid
Heel	Normal size	Small, drawn up
Relation between navicular and medial malleolus	Normal space between two bones; can insert finger	Navicular abuts medial malleolus: finger cannot be inserted between two bones
Lateral malleolus	Normal position	Posteriorly displaced with anterior part of talus very prominent in front of it
Skin creases on:		
Dorsolateral aspect of foot	Present; normal	Thin or absent
Medial and plantar aspects of foot	No furrowed skin	Furrowed skin
Posterior aspect of ankle	Normal	Deep crease
Calf and leg atrophy	None or very minimal	Moderate to marked
Treatment	Passive manipulation followed by retention by adhesive strapping, splint, or cast	Primary open reduction of talocalcaneonavicular joint often required; surgery is conservative
		Closed methods of reduction often unsuccessful
		Prolonged retentive apparatus essential
Prognosis	Excellent; result is normal foot	Poor with closed methods
		Prolonged cast immobilization results in smaller foot and atrophied leg

From Tachdjian MO: *The child's foot*, p. 163, Philadelphia, 1985, WB Saunders.

Hindfoot Varus (Subtalar or Rearfoot Varus). This structural deviation involves inversion of the calcaneus when the subtalar joint is in the neutral position. The hindfoot is mildly rigid with calcaneal eversion; therefore, pronation is limited. It may contribute to the appearance of a pes cavus foot, making the medial longitudinal arch appear accentuated. It may be the result of tibia varus (genu varum), and, because of the extra subtalar pronation necessary at the beginning of stance, normal supination during early propulsion may be prevented. This deviation can contribute to conditions such as retrocalcaneal exostosis (pump bumps), shin splints, plantar fasciitis, hamstring strains, and knee and ankle pathology (Figure 13-30).[18]

Hindfoot Valgus (Subtalar or Rearfoot Valgus). This structural deformity involves eversion of the calcaneus

Figure 13-30

Hindfoot deformities (right foot). **A,** Hindfoot varus (heel appears inverted). **B,** Hindfoot valgus (heel appears everted).

when the subtalar joint is in the neutral position. The hindfoot is mobile, which may lead to excessive pronation and limited supination. It may result from genu valgum (knock knees) and may contribute to the appearance of a pes planus foot, with the medial longitudinal arch appearing flattened. Because of the increased mobility, it is less likely to cause problems than hindfoot varus. It is often associated with tibia valgus (see Figure 13-30) and has been associated with posterior tibial tendon insufficiency.[34]

Forefoot Valgus. This structural midtarsal deviation involves eversion of the forefoot on the hindfoot when the subtalar joint is in the neutral position because the normal valgus tilt (35° to 45°) of the head and neck of the talus to its trochlea has been exceeded. With this deformity, during the weight-bearing phase of gait, the midtarsal joint is supinated so that the lateral aspect of the foot is brought into contact with the ground. Like hindfoot valgus, it contributes to decreasing the medial longitudinal arch and therefore clinically resembles a planus foot. The prolonged supination can contribute to conditions such as lateral ankle sprains, iliotibial band syndrome, plantar fasciitis, anterior tarsal tunnel syndrome, toe deformities, sesamoiditis, and leg and thigh pain (Figure 13-31).[18,35]

Forefoot Varus. This structural midtarsal joint deviation involves inversion of the forefoot on the hindfoot when the subtalar joint is in the neutral position. It occurs because the normal valgus tilt (35° to 45°) of the head and neck of the talus to its trochlea has not

been achieved.[18,35,36] Clinically, it contributes to decreasing the medial longitudinal arch and therefore resembles pes planus. With this deformity, during the weight-bearing phase of gait, the midtarsal joint is completely pronated in an attempt to bring the first metatarsal head in contact with the ground. The prolonged rotation that results can contribute to conditions such as tibialis posterior paratenonitis, patellofemoral syndrome, toe deformities, ligamentous stress (medially), shin splints, plantar fasciitis, postural fatigue, and Morton's neuroma (see Figure 13-31).

Metatarsus Adductus (Hooked Forefoot). This deformity is the most common foot deviation in children. It may be seen at birth but often is not noticed until the child begins to stand. The foot appears to be adducted and supinated (kidney shaped with medial deviation), and the hindfoot may or may not be in valgus.[37] It may be associated with hip dysplasia. Eighty-five to 90% of cases resolve spontaneously.[33]

Pes Cavus ("Hollow Foot" or Rigid Foot). A pes cavus may be caused by a congenital problem; a neurological problem such as spina bifida, poliomyelitis, or Charcot-Marie-Tooth disease; talipes equinovarus; or muscle imbalance. There may also be a genetic factor, because it tends to run in families.

The longitudinal arches are accentuated (Figure 13-32), and the metatarsal heads are lower in relation to the hindfoot so that there is a dropping of the forefoot on the hindfoot at the tarsometatarsal joints (Figure 13-33). The soft tissues of the sole of the foot are abnormally short, which gives the foot a shortened appearance. If the deformity persists, the bones eventually alter their shape, perpetuating the deformity. The heel is normal, at least initially. Claw toes are often associated with the condition because of the dropping of the forefoot combined with the pull of the extensor tendons. The examiner often finds painful callosities beneath the metatarsal heads that are caused by the loss of the metatarsal arch and tenderness along the deformed toes. There is pain in the tarsal region after time because of osteoarthritic changes in these joints.

The longitudinal arches are high on both the medial and lateral aspects, so that a lateral longitudinal arch occurs in some severe cases, and the forefoot is thickened and splayed (Table 13-5). The metatarsal heads are prominent on the sole of the foot, and the toes do not touch the ground, even on active or passive movement. This type of deformity leads to a rigid foot with little ability to absorb shock and adapt to stress. People with this deformity have difficulty doing repetitive stress activity (e.g., long-distance running, ballet) and require a cushioning shoe. In severe cases, the cavus foot is often associated with neurological disorders.[33]

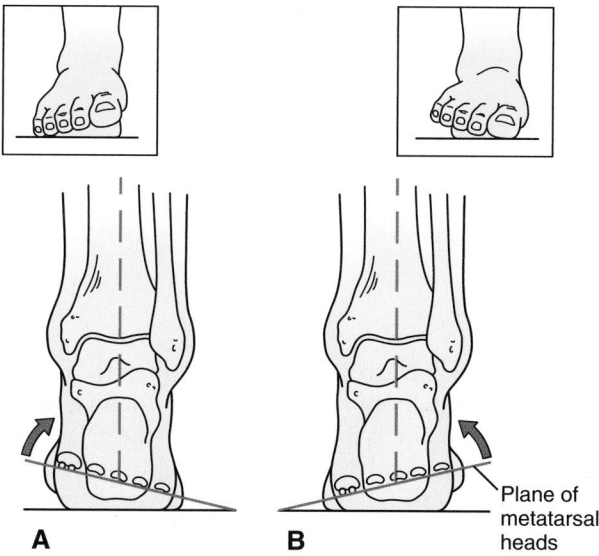

Figure 13-31 ▬▬▬▬▬

Forefoot deformities (right foot). **A,** Forefoot varus (metatarsal heads raised on medial side). **B,** Forefoot valgus (metatarsal heads raised on lateral side).

Figure 13-32

Pes cavus ("hollow foot"). Note the high medial longitudinal arch, early clawing of the big toe, and the heel in varus. (From Klenerman L: *The foot and its disorders*, p. 72, Boston, 1982, Blackwell Scientific.)

Pes Planus

Neutral

Pes Cavus

Figure 13-33

Talometatarsal angle used to define pes planus, neutral, and pes cavus foot types. (Redrawn from Jahss MH, editor: *Disorders of the foot and ankle: medical and surgical management*, ed 2, vol 1, Philadelphia, 1991, WB Saunders.)

Table 13-5

Pes Cavus Classification

Classification	Features
1. Mild	Longitudinal arch appears high NWB
	Longitudinal arch almost normal WB
	Toes clawed NWB
	Toes may be normal WB
	May have hindfoot varus
2. Moderate	Longitudinal arch high NWB and WB
	Claw toes evident NWB and WB
	Calluses under prominent metatarsal heads
	Dorsiflexion may be limited
	Forefoot plantar flexed on hindfoot
3. Severe	Calcaneus cannot pronate past 5° varus
	Heel in varus, foot in valgus
	Decreased ROM in foot

NWB = non-weight-bearing; *WB* = weight bearing; *ROM* = range of motion.

Pes Planus (Flatfoot or Mobile Foot). Flatfoot may be congenital, or it may result from trauma, muscle weakness, ligament laxity, dropping of the talar head, paralysis, or a pronated foot. For example, a traumatic flatfoot may follow fracture of the calcaneus. It may also be caused by a postural deformity, such as medial rotation of the hips or medial tibial torsion. It is a relatively common foot deformity that often causes little or no problem. Therefore, the examiner should not necessarily assume that a flat, mobile foot needs to be treated.

Because the foot is mobile, patients with flatfoot function well without treatment and often need only a control shoe to avoid problems in prolonged stress situations.

It must be remembered that all infants have flatfeet up to approximately 2 years of age. This appearance in part results from the fat pad in the longitudinal arch and in part from the incomplete formation of the arches. With pes planus, the medial longitudinal arch is reduced, so that on standing its borders are close to or in contact with the ground. This results from the hindfoot dropping in relation to the forefoot (see Figure 13-33). If the condition persists into adulthood, it may become a permanent structural deformity, leading to a defect or alteration of the tarsal bones and the talonavicular joints.

There are two types of flatfoot deformities. The first type (**rigid** or **congenital flatfoot**) is relatively rare. The calcaneus is found in a valgus position, whereas the midtarsal region is in pronation. The talus faces medially and downward, and the navicular is displaced dorsally and laterally on the talus. There are accompanying soft-tissue contractures and bony changes. The second type is **acquired** or **flexible flatfoot** (Figure 13-34). In this case, the deformity is similar to the rigid flatfoot, but the foot is mobile (Table 13-6) and there are few, if any, soft-tissue contractures and bony changes. It is usually caused by hereditary factors and is sometimes called a **hypermobile flatfoot**. Flexible flatfoot may result from tibial or femoral torsion, coxa vara, or a defect in the subtalar joint. If the arch appears when the patient stands on tiptoes, the patient may have a mobile flatfoot. This type of flatfoot seldom needs treatment.

Rocker-Bottom Foot. In the rocker-bottom foot deformity, the forefoot is dorsiflexed on the hindfoot. This results in a "broken midfoot," so that the medial and longitudinal arches are absent and the foot appears to be bent the wrong way (i.e., convex to the floor instead of the normal concave).

Figure 13-34
Pes planus (flatfoot).

Table 13-6
Pes Planus Classification

Classification	Features
1. Mild	4° to 6° hindfoot valgus
	4° to 6° forefoot valgus
2. Moderate	6° to 10° hindfoot valgus
	6° to 10° forefoot varus
	Poor shock absorption at heel strike
3. Severe	10° to 15° hindfoot valgus
	8° to 10° forefoot varus
	Equinus deformity may be present

Splay Foot. This deformity, which is broadening of the forefoot, is often caused by weakness of the intrinsic muscles and associated weakness of the inter-metatarsal ligament and dropping of the anterior metatarsal arch.

Morton's Metatarsalgia (Interdigital Neuroma). Morton's metatarsalgia refers to the formation of an interdigital neuroma as a result of injury to one of the digital nerves (Figure 13-35). Usually, it is the digital nerve between the third and fourth toes, so the examiner must take care to differentially diagnose the condition from a stress fracture of one of the metatarsals in the same area (**march fracture**). (A stress fracture will be more painful when the bone is palpated and a bone scan would be positive.) While walking or running, the patient is suddenly seized with an agonizing pain on the outer border of the forefoot. The pain is often intermittent, like a cramp, shooting up the side and to the tip of the affected toe or the adjacent two toes. Squeezing the metatarsal bones together elicits pain because of the pressure on the digital nerve. On palpation, pain is more likely to be between the bones rather than on the bone. The condition tends to occur more frequently in women than in men.

Exostosis (Bony Spur). Exostosis is an abnormal bony outgrowth extending from the surface of the bone (Figure 13-36). It is actually an increase in the bone mass at the site of an irritative lesion in response to overuse, trauma, or excessive pressure. The common areas of occurrence in the foot are on the dorsal aspect of the tarsometatarsal joint, the head of the fifth metatarsal bone, the calcaneus (where it is often called a pump bump or runner's bump), the insertion of the plantar fascia, and the superior aspect of the navicular bone. Most often these exostoses are the result of poorly fitting footwear that leads to undue pressure on the bone.

Figure 13-35

The applied anatomy of Morton's metatarsalgia. The interdigital nerve to the space between the third and fourth digits has been divided 2 cm above the neuroma and is reflected downward. The plantar digital vessels are shown entering the neuroma. The end of the flat dissector is on the upper margin of the transverse ligament. The end of the probe points to the intermetatarsophalangeal bursa. (From Klenerman L: *The foot and its disorders*, p. 143, Boston, 1982, Blackwell Scientific.)

Figure 13-36

Common areas of exostosis formation in the foot.

Hallux Valgus. Hallux valgus is a relatively common condition in which there is medial deviation of the head of the first metatarsal bone in relation to the center of the body and lateral deviation of the head in relation to the center of the foot (Figure 13-37). The cause of hallux valgus is varied. It may result from a hereditary factor and is often familial. Women tend to be affected more than men. Trying to keep up with fashion may be a contributing factor if the patient wears tight or pointed shoes, tight stockings, or high-heeled shoes.[38]

A   B

Figure 13-37

A, An example of congruous hallux valgus. **B,** Pathological hallux valgus with bilateral bunions and overlapped toes. Note how the deviating big toe (hallux) rotates and pushes under the second toe. (**B** from Gartland JJ: *Fundamentals of orthopedics*, p. 401, Philadelphia, 1987, WB Saunders.)

As the metatarsal bones move medially, the base of the proximal phalanx is carried with it, and the phalanx pivots around the adductor hallucis muscle that inserts into it, causing the distal end as well as the distal phalanx to deviate laterally in relation to the center of the body. The long flexor and extensor muscles then have a bowstring effect as they are displaced to the lateral side of the joint, which can lead to increased stress on the proximal phalanx.[39]

A callus develops over the medial side of the head of the metatarsal bone, and the bursa becomes thickened and inflamed; excessive bone (exostosis) forms, resulting in a **bunion** (Figure 13-38).[9,40] These three changes—callus, thickened bursa, and exostosis—make up the bunion, a condition separate from hallux valgus, although it is the result of hallux valgus.

In normal persons, the **metatarsophalangeal angle** (the angle between the longitudinal axis of the metatarsal bone and the proximal phalanx) is 8° to 20° (Figure 13-39). This angle is increased to varying degrees in hallux valgus.

The first type **(congruous hallux valgus)** is a simple exaggeration of the normal relation of the metatarsal to the phalanx of the big toe. The deformity does not progress, and the valgus deformity is between 20° and 30°. The opposing joint surfaces are congruent. It requires little treatment, and often the biggest problem is cosmetic.

The second type **(pathological hallux valgus)** is a potentially progressive deformity, increasing from 20°

Figure 13-39
Metatarsophalangeal (hallux valgus) angle.

to 60°. The joint surfaces are no longer congruent, and some may even go to subluxation. This type may occur in deviated (early) and subluxed (later) stages.

When looking at the foot, the examiner may find that there is a widening gap between the first and second metatarsal bones (increased **intermetatarsal angle**) and a lateral deflection of the phalanx at the metatarsophalangeal joint. The joint capsule lengthens on the medial aspect and is contracted on the lateral aspect. The toes rotate on the long axis so that the toenail faces medially because of the pull of the adductor hallucis muscle. Sometimes, the big toe deviates so far that it lies over or under the second toe.

Figure 13-38
A, Bunions apparent on both feet. **B,** Schematic line drawing of a bunion.

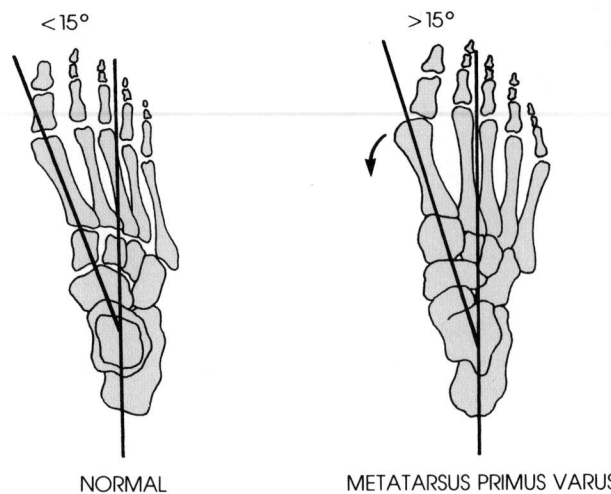

NORMAL   METATARSUS PRIMUS VARUS

Figure 13-40

Normal foot and metatarsus primus varus. (Note increased intermetatarsal angle.)

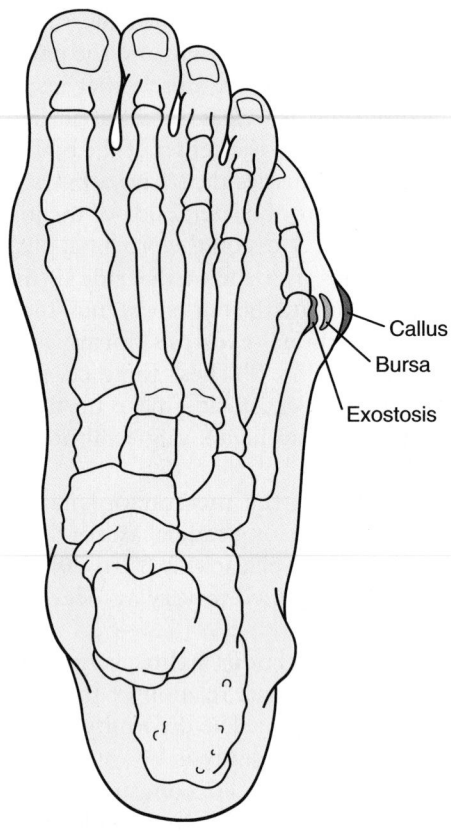

Figure 13-41

A bunionette or tailor's bunion.

Of all hallux valgus cases, 80% are caused by **metatarsus primus varus**, in which the intermetatarsal or metatarsal angle is increased to more than 15° (Figure 13-40).[41,42] Metatarsus primus varus is an abduction deformity of the first metatarsal bone in relation to the tarsal and other metatarsal bones so that the medial border of the forefoot is curved. Normally, this angle is between 0° and 15°.

Bunionette (Tailor's Bunion). This deformity is characterized by prominence of the lateral aspect of the fifth toe metatarsal head (Figure 13-41).[43] If associated with hallux valgus, it results in a splayed foot. It is often associated with a pronated foot.

Hallux Rigidus. Hallux rigidus is a condition in which dorsiflexion or extension of the big toe is limited because of osteoarthritis of the first metatarsophalangeal joint.[44] Hallux rigidus may also be caused by an anatomical abnormality of the foot, an abnormally long first metatarsal bone (index plus type forefoot; see Figure 13-14), pronation of the forefoot, or trauma. There are two types: acute and chronic.

The acute, or adolescent, type occurs primarily in young people with long, narrow, pronated feet and occurs more frequently in boys than in girls. Pain and stiffness in the big toe come on quickly; the pain is described as constant, burning, throbbing, or aching. Tenderness may be palpated over the metatarsophalangeal joint, and the toe is initially held stiff because of muscle spasm. The first metatarsal head may be elevated, large, and tender. The weight distribution pattern in the gait is shown in Figure 13-42.

The second (chronic) type of hallux rigidus is much more common and occurs primarily in adults—again, in men more frequently than in women. It is frequently bilateral and is usually the result of repeated minor trauma resulting in osteoarthritic changes to the metatarsophalangeal joint of the big toe. The toe stiffens gradually, and the pain, once established, persists. The patient complains primarily of pain at the base of the big toe on walking.

Plantar Flexed First Ray. This structural deformity occurs when the first ray (big toe) lies lower than the other four metatarsal bones, so that the forefoot is everted when the metatarsal bones are aligned. If present congenitally, it is indicative of a cavus foot. In its acquired form, it occurs as compensation for tibia varum (genu varum) with limited calcaneal eversion. This deformity can contribute to the same conditions seen with forefoot valgus.[18] The neutral position of the first ray is the position in which the first metatarsal head lies in the same transverse plane as the second through fourth metatarsal heads when they are maximally dorsiflexed.[45]

A   B   C

Figure 13-42
Weight-bearing patterns in hallux rigidus. **A,** Hallux rigidus gait pattern. **B,** Normal gait pattern. **C,** Shoe develops oblique creases with hallux rigidus. (**C** redrawn from Jahss MH: *Disorders of the foot*, p. 60, Philadelphia, 1991, WB Saunders.)

Turf Toe. Turf toe is a hyperextension injury (sprain) combined with compressive loading to the metatarsophalangeal joint of the hallux. It can cause a significant functional disability, especially in sports, where the hallux is put under high loads. It is often related to the use of flexible footwear and artificial turf.[46,47]

Morton's (Atavistic or Grecian) Foot. With a Morton's foot, the second toe is longer than the first. The length difference may be due to different lengths of the metatarsals (see Figure 13-14). Increased stress is put on this longer toe, and the big toe tends to be hypomobile. There is often hypertrophy of the second metatarsal bone because more stress is put through the second toe. In fact, the second metatarsal can become as large as the first metatarsal. People with this deformity often have difficulty putting on tight-fitting footwear (e.g., skates, ski boots) or dancing (e.g., en pointe in ballet). The different types of feet and their proportional representations in the population are shown in Figure 13-15.

Claw Toes. A claw-toe deformity results in hyperextension of the metatarsophalangeal joints and flexion of the proximal and distal interphalangeal joints (Figure 13-43, *A*). Claw toes usually result from the defective actions of lumbrical and interosseus muscles that cause the toes to become functionless. This condition may be unilateral or bilateral and may be associated with pes cavus, fallen metatarsal arch, spina bifida, or other neurological problems.

Hammer Toe. A hammer toe deformity consists of an extension contracture at the metatarsophalangeal joint and flexion contracture at the proximal interphalangeal joint; the distal interphalangeal joint may be flexed, straight, or hyperextended (Figure 13-43, *B*).[40,48] The interosseus muscles are unable to hold the proximal phalanx in the neutral position and therefore lose their flexion effect.

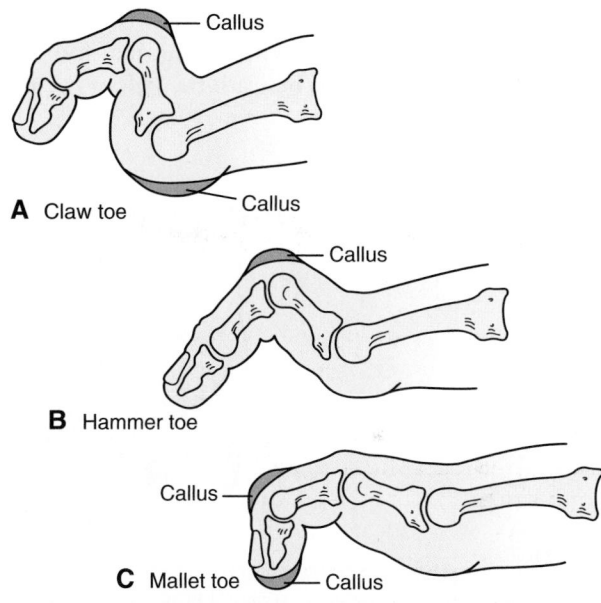

Figure 13-43
Toe deformities. **A,** Claw toe. Note that the proximal and distal interphalangeal joints are hyperflexed and the metatarsophalangeal joint is dorsally subluxated. **B,** Hammer toe. Note the flexion deformity of the proximal interphalangeal joints. The distal interphalangeal joint is in neutral position or slight flexion. **C,** Mallet toe. There is flexion contracture of the distal interphalangeal joint. The proximal interphalangeal and metatarsophalangeal joints are in neutral position.

This results in clawing of the toe by the long flexors and extensors leading to and accentuating the deformity. The causes of hammertoe include an imbalance of the synergic muscles, hereditary factors, and mechanical factors such as poorly fitting shoes or hallux valgus. It is usually seen only in one toe—the second toe. Often, there is a callus or corn over the dorsum of the flexed joint. The condition is often asymptomatic, especially if the hammertoe is flexible or semiflexible. The rigid type of hammertoe is likely to cause the greatest problems.

Mallet Toe. Mallet toe is associated with a flexion deformity of the distal interphalangeal joint (Figure 13-43, C).[40,48] It can occur on any of the four lateral toes. Often, a corn or callus is present over the dorsum of the affected joint. The condition is usually asymptomatic. It is commonly seen with ill-fitting or poorly designed footwear.[43]

Polydactyly. This developmental anomaly is characterized by the presence of an extra digit or toe. It may be seen in isolation or with other anomalies such as polydactyly of the hands and **syndactyly** (webbing) of the toes. The primary concern with this anomaly is cosmesis.[49]

Shoes

The examiner looks at the patient's shoes, both inside and outside, for weight-bearing and wear patterns (Figures 13-44 and 13-45). With the normal foot, the greatest wear on the shoe is beneath the ball of the foot

Figure 13-44

Pes planus (flatfoot) or calcaneus in valgus can lead to misshapen shoes. Note the prominence of the talar head.

Head of talus

and slightly to the lateral side and the posterolateral aspect of the heel. If shoes are too small or too narrow, they may pinch the feet, causing deformities and affecting normal growth. If shoes are worn out, they offer little support. If shoes are stiff, they limit proper movement of the foot.

Platform-type or high-heeled shoes often cause painful knees because the patient wearing these shoes usually walks with the knees flexed, which may increase the stress on the patella. Continuous wearing of high-heeled shoes may cause the calf muscles to contract and may lead to sore knees and a painful back, because the lumbar spine goes into increased lordotic posture to maintain the center of gravity in its normal position. In addition, these shoes increase the potential for ankle sprains and fractures because a raised center of gravity puts the wearer off balance.

High-heeled and pointed shoes often contribute to hallux valgus, bunions, march fractures, and Morton's metatarsalgia that may result because the toes are being pushed together. Shoes with a negative heel may lead to hyperextension of the knees and patellofemoral syndrome. High-cut or high-top shoes that cover the medial and lateral malleoli offer more support than low-cut shoes or those that do not cover the malleoli.

Excessive bulging on the medial side of the shoe suggests a valgus or everted foot, whereas excessive bulging on the lateral side suggests an inverted foot. Drop foot resulting from musculature weakness scuffs the toe of the shoe. Oblique forefoot creases in the shoe indicate possible hallux rigidus; absence of forefoot creases indicates no toe-off action during gait.

Examination

As with any assessment, the examiner must compare one side with the other and note any asymmetry. This comparison is necessary because of individual differences among normal people.

Figure 13-45

Misshapen shoes caused by severely pronated feet. (From Gartland JJ: *Fundamentals of orthopedics*, p. 398, Philadelphia, 1987, WB Saunders.)

Active Movements

The first movements tested during the examination are active, with painful movements being tested last. These movements should be done in both weight-bearing (Figures 13-46 and 13-47) and non-weight-bearing (long leg sitting or supine lying; Figure 13-48) positions, and the examiner should note any differences because foot deformities and deviations in addition to decreased ROM can lead to injury.[50] Lindsjo and colleagues advocated testing weight-bearing ROM by putting the test foot on a 30-cm (12-inch) stool for ease of measurement and flexing the knee.[51]

Plantar Flexion

Plantar flexion of the ankle is approximately 50° (see Figure 13-48, *A*), and the patient's heel normally inverts when the movement is performed in weight bearing (Figure 13-49). If heel inversion does not occur, the foot is unstable, or there is tibialis posterior weakness or tightness.[29,52,53] The tibialis posterior muscle and tendon balance the pull of the peroneal muscles, protect the spring ligament, and invert and stabilize the hindfoot during toe off.[54] Pain in the spring ligament as well as the medial midfoot and hindfoot ligaments, hindfoot valgus, plantar flexed talar head, and forefoot abduction should lead the examiner to assessing the tibialis posterior for proper function.[29]

Dorsiflexion

Dorsiflexion of the ankle is usually 20° past the anatomical position (plantigrade), which is with the foot at 90° to the bones of the leg (see Figure 13-48, *B*). For normal locomotion, 10° of dorsiflexion and 20° to 25° of plantar flexion at the ankle are required.

Supination and Pronation

Supination is 45° to 60° and pronation is 15° to 30°, although individuals vary (see Figure 13-48, *C* and *D*). It is more important to compare the movement with that of the patient's normal side (Figures 13-50 and 13-51).

Weight-Bearing Active Movements of the Lower Leg, Ankle, and Foot

- Plantar flexion (flexion), standing on the toes
- Dorsiflexion (extension), standing on the heels
- Supination, standing on the lateral edge of the foot
- Pronation, standing on the medial edge of the foot
- Toe extension
- Toe flexion
- Combined movements (if necessary)
- Sustained positions (if necessary)
- Repetitive movements (if necessary)

Non-Weight-Bearing Active Movements of the Lower Leg, Ankle, and Foot

- Plantar flexion (flexion), 50°
- Dorsiflexion (extension), 20°
- Supination, 45° to 60°
- Pronation, 15° to 30°
- Toe extension, lateral four toes (MTP, 40°; PIP, 0°; DIP, 30°) and great toe (MTP, 70°; IP, 0°)
- Toe flexion, lateral four toes (MTP, 40°; PIP, 35°; DIP, 60°) and great toe (MTP, 45°; IP, 90°)
- Toe abduction
- Toe adduction
- Combined movements (if necessary)
- Sustained positions (if necessary)
- Repetitive movements (if necessary)

DIP = distal interphalangeal joint; *MTP* = metatarsophalangeal joint; *PIP* = proximal interphalangeal joint.

Supination combines the movements of inversion, adduction, and plantar flexion; pronation combines the movements of eversion, abduction, and dorsiflexion of the foot and ankle. As the patient does the movement, the examiner should watch for the possibility of subluxation of various tendons. The peroneal tendons are especially prone to subluxation, and their subluxation is evident on eversion (Figure 13-52). If tibialis anterior is weak, supination will be affected. If the peronei are weak or the tendons sublux, pronation will be affected.

Toe Extension and Flexion

Movement of the toes occurs at the metatarsophalangeal and proximal and distal interphalangeal joints (see Figure 13-48, *E* and *F*). Extension of the great toe occurs primarily at the metatarsophalangeal joint (70°); there is minimal or no extension at the interphalangeal joint. For the great toe, 45° flexion occurs at the metatarsophalangeal joint, and 90° occurs at the interphalangeal joint.

For the lateral four toes, extension occurs primarily at the metatarsophalangeal (40°) and distal interphalangeal joints (30°). Extension at the proximal interphalangeal joints is negligible. For the lateral four toes, 40° flexion occurs at the metatarsophalangeal joints, 35° occurs at the proximal interphalangeal joints, and 60° occurs at the distal interphalangeal joints.

Toe Abduction and Adduction

Abduction and adduction of the toes are measured with the second toe as midline. Although the range of motion of abduction can be measured, this is not usually done. The common practice is to ask the patient to spread the toes and then bring them back together (see Figure 13-48, *G* and *H*). The amount and quality of movement are compared with those of the unaffected side.

Figure 13-46
Active movements (weight-bearing posture). **A,** Plantar flexion. **B,** Dorsiflexion. **C,** Supination. **D,** Pronation. **E,** Toe extension. **F,** Toe flexion.

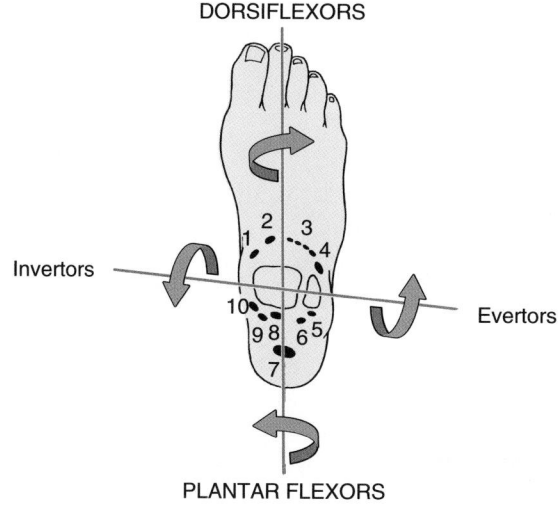

DORSIFLEXORS

Invertors

Evertors

PLANTAR FLEXORS

Figure 13-47

Motion diagram of the ankle. *1* = tibialis anterior; *2* = extensor hallucis longus; *3* = extensor digitorum longus; *4* = peroneus tertius; *5* = peroneus brevis; *6* = peroneus longus; *7* = Achilles tendon (soleus and gastrocnemius); *8* = flexor hallucis longus; *9* = flexor digitorum longus; *10* = tibialis posterior.

If the history has indicated that weight-bearing or non-weight-bearing combined or repetitive movements or sustained postures result in symptoms, these movements should also be tested. The examiner should ask the patient to walk on the toes, heels, and outer and inner borders of the feet. These actions indicate the patient's muscle power and control and the functional ROM. With a third-degree strain (rupture) of the Achilles tendon, the patient is not able to walk on the toes. Lack of dorsiflex-ion makes it difficult for the patient to walk on the heels. When the patient walks on the inner or outer borders of the feet, pain and difficulty are experienced in the presence of a subtalar lesion.

The examiner should also check the efficiency of the toes. Are the toes straight and parallel? Is the patient able to flex, extend, adduct, and abduct the toes? The toes have a primarily ambulatory function, although, with training, they can develop a prehensile function. The toes extend the weight-bearing area forward and, by so doing, reduce the load on the metatarsal heads. The great toe also has a primary function of pushing off during gait.

When assessing the active movements, the examiner must remember that peripheral nerve injuries may alter the pattern of movement. For example, the common peroneal nerve may be injured as it winds around the head of the fibula, resulting in altered nerve conduction to the peroneus longus and brevis muscles (superficial peroneal nerve) or the tibialis anterior, extensor digitorum longus, and extensor hallucis longus (deep peroneal nerve).[55] In such cases, the movements controlled by these muscles are altered. In addition, there are sensory changes that must be noted.

Passive Movements

The passive movements of the lower leg, ankle, and foot are performed with the patient in a non-weight-bearing position (Figure 13-53). As with other joints, if the active ROM is full, overpressure can be applied to test end feel during the active, non-weight-bearing movements to negate the need to do passive movements.

A

B

Figure 13-48

Active movements (non-weight-bearing posture). **A,** Plantar flexion. **B,** Dorsiflexion.

Continued

Figure 13-48 cont'd

C, Supination. **D,** Pronation. **E,** Toe extension. **F,** Toe flexion. **G,** Toe abduction. **H,** Toe adduction.

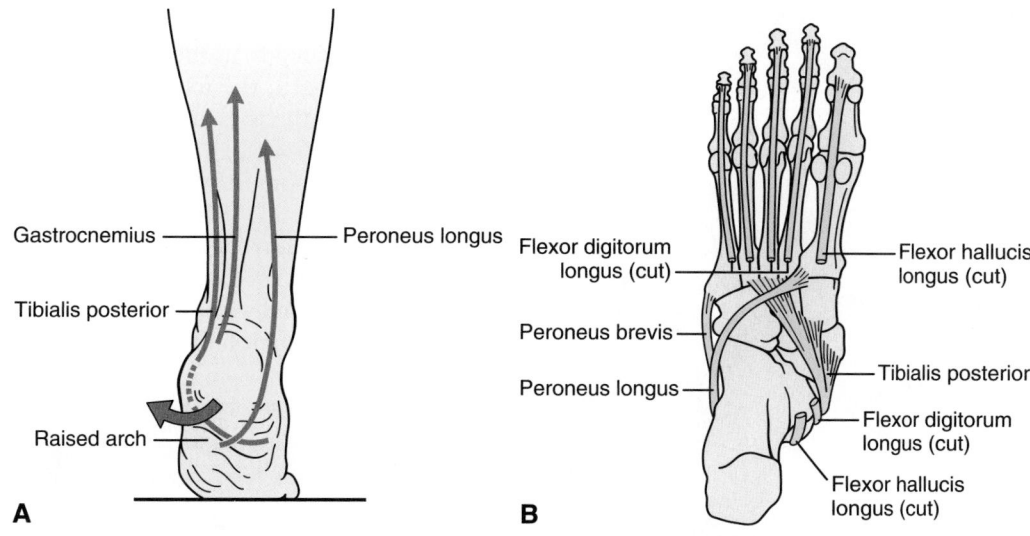

Figure 13-49

A, Inversion of heel while standing on toes (plantar flexion of ankle). Note that peroneus longus and tibialis posterior support the medial longitudinal and transverse arches. **B,** Plantar view of the right foot shows the distal course of the tendons of the peroneus longus, peroneus brevis, and tibialis posterior. The tendons of the flexor digitorum longus and flexor hallucis longus are cut. Note the force couple relationship between the two peroneal muscles and tibialis posterior to control inversion and eversion along with the long flexors and extensors (**B** redrawn from Neumann DA: *Kinesiology of the musculoskeletal system: foundations for physical rehabilitation*, p. 511, St. Louis, 2002, Mosby.)

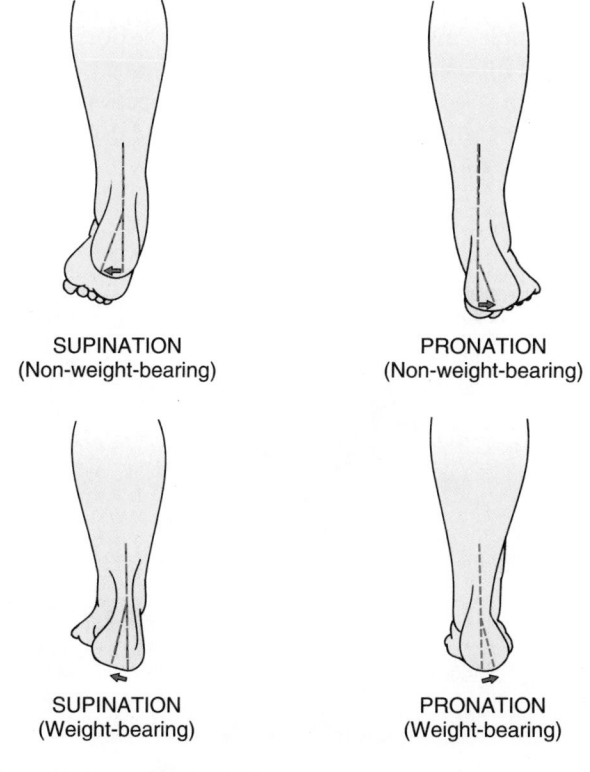

Figure 13-50

Supination and pronation of the foot in weight-bearing and non-weight-bearing postures (posterior views of the right limb).

Figure 13-51

Anterior view of the foot in pronation and supination (weight-bearing stance).

Each movement should be carefully checked, especially if deformities or asymmetries have been noticed during the observation. These deformities or asymmetries may cause problems in other areas of the lower kinetic chain. For example, limited dorsiflexion or tight heel cords may lead to anterior knee pain or ankle injuries.[56] Because the gastrocnemius is a two-joint muscle, dorsiflexion should be tested with the knee straight to test this muscles for

Figure 13-52
Habitual subluxation of the peroneal tendons. The peroneal tendons pass anterior to the retrofibular sulcus but not anterior to the distal fibula, in contradistinction to traumatic subluxation. (From Kelikian H, Kelikian AS: *Disorders of the ankle*, p. 765, Philadelphia, 1985, WB Saunders.)

greater mobility and flexibility in the Achilles tendon in a baby or young child than there is in an adult. For example, in the newborn, the foot can readily be dorsiflexed passively so that the toes and dorsum of the foot touch the skin over the tibia. In the adult, however, dorsiflexion is limited to 20° more than plantigrade. If the patient can only attain plantigrade (90°), then the gastrocnemius or soleus is tight. If gastrocnemius is tight, the ankle ROM is limited with the knee extended. If soleus is tight, the ankle ROM is limited with the knee flexed. If tibialis posterior is tight, supination of the foot will be limited.

> ### Passive Movements of the Lower Leg, Ankle, and Foot and Normal End Feel
>
> - Plantar flexion at the talocrural joint (tissue stretch)
> - Dorsiflexion at the talocrural joint (tissue stretch)
> - Inversion at the subtalar joint (tissue stretch)
> - Eversion of the subtalar joint (tissue stretch)
> - Adduction at the midtarsal joints (tissue stretch)
> - Abduction at the midtarsal joints (tissue stretch)
> - Flexion of the toes (tissue stretch)
> - Extension of the toes (tissue stretch)
> - Adduction of the toes (tissue stretch)
> - Abduction of the toes (tissue stretch)

tightness. Testing with the knee bent to 90°, isolates soleus. Stovitz and Coetzee recommended testing the Achilles tendon and its associated muscles with the subtalar joint in neutral with a lateral force applied to the talar neck to lock the foot during testing.[53] This eliminates calcaneal eversion or forefoot dorsiflexion from contributing to an apparent normal Achilles tendon. There is

Some movements may be tested in combination to more closely approximate what occurs functionally. For example, instead of testing plantar flexion, adduction, and inversion separately, supination, as a combined movement, may be tested. Similarly, pronation may be tested as a combined movement, instead of dorsiflexion, abduction, and eversion.

A

B

Figure 13-53
Passive movements of the ankle. **A,** Plantar flexion. **B,** Dorsiflexion.

Continued

Figure 13-53 cont'd
C, Inversion. D, Eversion. E, Abduction and adduction. F, Toe flexion and extension. G, Toe abduction.

During passive movements of the ankle and foot, any capsular patterns should be noted. The capsular pattern of the talocrural joint is more limitation of plantar flexion than of dorsiflexion; the subtalar joint capsular pattern shows more limitation of varus range than of valgus ROM. The midtarsal joint capsular pattern is dorsiflexion most limited, followed by plantar flexion, adduction, and medial rotation. The first metatarsophalangeal joint has a capsular pattern in which extension is most limited, followed by flexion. The pattern for the second through fifth metatarsophalangeal joints is variable. The capsular pattern of the interphalangeal joints is flexion most limited, followed by extension.

Resisted Isometric Movements

The resisted isometric movements are performed to test the contractile tissue around the foot, ankle, and lower leg. The patient is in the sitting or supine lying position, and the patient's foot is placed in the anatomical position (plantigrade or 90°; Figure 13-54). Table 13-7 shows the muscles acting over the foot and ankle. Strength results may very depending on age and sex.[57]

Resisted Isometric Movements of the Lower Leg, Ankle, and Foot

- Knee flexion
- Plantar flexion
- Dorsiflexion
- Supination
- Pronation
- Toe extension
- Toe flexion

Dorsiflexion is sometimes tested with the patient's hip flexed to 45° and the knee flexed to 90°, as illustrated in Figure 13-54, *B*. Testing with the patient in this position enables the examiner to exert a greater isometric force. Resisted isometric knee flexion must be performed, because the triceps surae (gastrocnemius and soleus muscles together) act on the knee as well as on the ankle and foot.

If the history has indicated that eccentric, concentric, or econcentric muscle action has caused symptoms, these movements should also be tested, but only after the isometric tests have been completed.

Functional Assessment

If the patient is able to do the movements already described with little difficulty, functional tests may be performed to see whether these sequential activities produce pain or other symptoms. Full ROM is often not necessary for the patient to lead a functional life.

These activities, which are examples only, must be geared to the individual patient. Older patients should not be expected to do some of the activities unless they have been doing these or similar ones in the recent past (Table 13-8). Because the functional tests place a stress on the other lower limb joints (e.g., knee, hip, sacroiliac, lumbar joints), the examiner must ensure that these joints exhibit no pathology before all of the tests are completed.

Functional Activities of the Lower Leg, Ankle, and Foot (in Sequential Order)

- Squatting (both ankles should dorsiflex symmetrically)
- Standing on toes (both ankles should plantar flex symmetrically)
- Squatting and bouncing at the end of a squat
- Standing on one foot at a time
- Standing on the toes, one foot at a time
- Going up and down stairs
- Walking on the toes
- Running straight ahead
- Running, twisting, and cutting
- Jumping
- Jumping and going into a full squat

A   **B**

Figure 13-54

Resisted isometric movements of the lower leg, ankle, and foot. **A,** Knee flexion. **B,** Dorsiflexion.

Continued

Figure 13-54 cont'd
C, Plantar flexion. **D,** Supination. **E,** Pronation. **F,** Toe extension.

On the other hand, functional tests for other joints in the lower limb (e.g., hop test for the knee) may not be sensitive enough to test ankle function.[58] However, Wikstrom et al. felt a modified hop test (jump test) was an effective way to determine functional ankle instability.[59] The test involves standing on two feet, jumping forward half the height of the patient's vertical jump and landing on one leg (good leg first).

Conditions such as vascular intermittent claudication and anterior compartment syndrome that occur within a specific time frame must also be considered in an assessment and when considering function.[60,61]

Balance and proprioception are tested by asking the patient to stand on the unaffected leg and then on the affected leg, first with the eyes open and then with the eyes closed. Any differences in balance time or difficulty in balancing give an idea of proprioceptive ability, especially differences that occurred when the patient's eyes were closed (Figure 13-55).[62]

Kaikkonen and colleagues developed a numerical scoring system to evaluate functional outcome after ankle injury[63] (Table 13-9). The Ankle Joint Functional Assessment Tool and the Foot Functional Index (Figure 13-56),[64,65,66] which was developed for an elderly outpatient population, are two other functional tests. Other scales have been developed for specific pathologies (e.g., fractures) about the ankle or can be applied to injuries in any part of the lower limb (e.g., LEF scale; see Chapter 11).[67–72]

Special Tests

When assessing the lower leg, ankle, and foot, it is important to always assess the neutral position of the

---

Range of Motion Necessary at the Foot and Ankle for Selected Locomotion Activities

Descending stairs:	Full dorsiflexion (20°)
Walking:	Dorsiflexion (10°); plantar flexion (20° to 25°)

Table 13-7

Muscles of the Lower Limb, Ankle, and Foot: Their Actions, Nerve Supply, and Nerve Root Derivation (Peripheral Nerves)

Action	Muscles Acting	Nerve Supply	Nerve Root Derivation
Plantar flexion (flexion) of ankle	1. Gastrocnemius*	Tibial	S1-S2
	2. Soleus*	Tibial	S1-S2
	3. Plantaris	Tibial	S1-S2
	4. Flexor digitorum longus	Tibial	S2-S3
	5. Peroneus longus	Superficial peroneal	L5, S1-S2
	6. Peroneus brevis	Superficial peroneal	L5, S1-S2
	7. Flexor hallucis longus	Tibial	S2-S3
	8. Tibialis posterior	Tibial	L4-L5
Dorsiflexion (extension) of ankle	1. Tibialis anterior	Deep peroneal	L4-L5
	2. Extensor digitorum longus	Deep peroneal	L5, S1
	3. Extensor hallucis longus	Deep peroneal	L5, S1
	4. Peroneus tertius	Deep peroneal	L5, S1
Inversion	1. Tibialis posterior	Tibial	L4-L5
	2. Flexor digitorum longus	Tibial	S2-S3
	3. Flexor hallucis longus	Tibial	S2-S3
	4. Tibialis anterior	Deep peroneal	L4-L5
	5. Extensor hallucis longus	Deep peroneal	L5, S1
Eversion	1. Peroneus longus	Superficial peroneal	L5, S1-S2
	2. Peroneus brevis	Superficial peroneal	L5, S1-S2
	3. Peroneus tertius	Deep peroneal	L5, S1
	4. Extensor digitorum longus	Deep peroneal	L5, S1
Flexion of toes	1. Flexor digitorum longus	Tibial	S2-S3
	2. Flexor hallucis longus	Tibial	S2-S3
	3. Flexor digitorum brevis	Tibial (medial plantar branch)	S2-S3
	4. Flexor hallucis brevis	Tibial (medial plantar branch)	S2-S3
	5. Flexor accessorius (Quadratus plantae)	Tibial (lateral plantar branch)	S2-S3
	6. Interossei	Tibial (lateral plantar branch)	S2-S3
	7. Flexor digiti minimi brevis	Tibial (lateral plantar branch)	S2-S3
	8. Lumbricals (metatarsophalangeal joints)	Tibial (first by medial plantar branch; second through fourth by lateral plantar branch)	S2-S3
Extension of toes	1. Extensor digitorum longus	Deep peroneal	L5, S1
	2. Extensor hallucis longus	Deep peroneal	L5, S1
	3. Extensor digitorum brevis	Deep peroneal (lateral terminal branch)	S1-S2
	4. Lumbricals (interphalangeal joints)	Tibial (first by medial plantar branch; second through fourth by lateral plantar branch)	S2-S3
Abduction of toes	1. Abductor hallucis	Tibial (medial plantar branch)	S2-S3
	2. Abductor digiti minimi	Tibial (lateral plantar branch)	S2-S3
	3. Dorsal interossei	Tibial (lateral plantar branch)	S2-S3
Adduction of toes	1. Adductor hallucis	Tibial (lateral plantar branch)	S2-S3
	2. Plantar interossei	Tibial (lateral plantar branch)	S2-S3

*The gastrocnemius and soleus muscles are sometimes grouped together as the triceps surae muscles.

talus in both weight-bearing and non-weight-bearing situations. This will help the examiner to differentiate functional from structural deformities. Other tests that should be carried out include alignment, functional leg length, and tibial torsion tests. Of the other tests, only those that the examiner wishes to use as confirming tests need be performed. Special tests should never be used in isolation but can be used to confirm clinical findings.

Table 13-8

Functional Testing of the Foot and Ankle

Starting Position	Action	Functional Test
Standing on one leg*	Lift toes and forefeet off ground (dorsiflexion)	10 to 15 Repetitions: Functional 5 to 9 Repetitions: Functionally fair 1 to 4 Repetitions: Functionally poor 0 Repetitions: Nonfunctional
Standing on one leg*	Lift heels off ground (plantar flexion)	10 to 15 Repetitions: Functional 5 to 9 Repetitions: Functionally fair 1 to 4 Repetitions: Functionally poor 0 Repetitions: Nonfunctional
Standing on one leg*	Lift lateral aspect of foot off ground (ankle eversion)	5 to 6 Repetitions: Functional 3 to 4 Repetitions: Functionally fair 1 to 2 Repetitions: Functionally poor 0 Repetitions: Nonfunctional
Standing on one leg*	Lift medial aspect of foot off ground (ankle inversion)	5 to 6 Repetitions: Functional 3 to 4 Repetitions: Functionally fair 1 to 2 Repetitions: Functionally poor 0 Repetitions: Nonfunctional
Seated	Pull small towel up under toes or pick up and release small object (i.e., pencil, marble, cotton ball) (toe flexion)	10 to 15 Repetitions: Functional 5 to 9 Repetitions: Functionally fair 1 to 4 Repetitions: Functionally poor 0 Repetitions: Nonfunctional
Seated	Lift toes off ground (toe extension)	10 to 15 Repetitions: Functional 5 to 9 Repetitions: Functionally fair 1 to 4 Repetitions: Functionally poor 0 Repetitions: Nonfunctional

Data from Palmer ML, Epler M: *Clinical assessment procedures in physical therapy*, pp. 308–310, Philadelphia, 1990, JB Lippincott.
*Hand may hold something for balance only.

The reliability, validity, specificity, and sensitivity of some of the special/diagnostic tests used in the lower leg, ankle and foot are outlined in Appendix 13-1.

Tests for Neutral Position of the Talus

The neutral position of the talus is often referred to as the neutral or balanced position of the foot. This so-called neutral position is an ideal position that, in reality, is not commonly found in people in normal weight bearing.[19]

> **Special Tests Commonly Performed on the Lower Leg, Ankle, and Foot**
>
> • Neutral position of the talus (weight bearing and non-weight-bearing)
> • Leg-heel alignment
> • Forefoot-heel alignment
> • Tests for tibial torsion
> • Anterior drawer sign of the ankle
> • Talar tilt
> • Leg length
> • Thompson test

For most patients, the subtalar joint is normally in slight valgus, with the forefoot in slight varus and the calcaneus in slight valgus. The tibia is in slight varus,[73] so each joint slightly compensates for the adjacent one. The neutral position is used as a starting position to determine foot and leg deviations. Functional asymmetry may occur in the lower limb in normal standing; the examiner should then put the talus in the neutral position to see whether the asymmetry remains. If it does, there is **anatomical or structural asymmetry** as well as **functional asymmetry**. If the asymmetry disappears, there is only functional asymmetry, which is often easier to treat.

Neutral Position of the Talus (Weight-Bearing Position). The patient stands with the feet in a relaxed standing position so that the base width and Fick angle are normal for the patient. Usually, only one foot is tested at a time. The examiner palpates the head of the talus on the dorsal aspect of the foot with the thumb and forefinger of one hand (Figure 13-57). The patient slowly rotates the trunk to the right and then to the left, which causes the tibia to medially and laterally rotate so that the talus supinates and pronates. If the foot is positioned so that the talar head does not appear to bulge to either side, then the subtalar joint will be in its neutral position

A   **B**

Figure 13-55
Balance and proprioception. **A,** One leg, with eyes open. **B,** One leg, with eyes closed.

in weight bearing.[36] Mueller et al.[74] described a progression of the neutral talus position in standing called the **navicular drop test** to quantify midfoot mobility and its effect on other parts of the kinetic chain.[75] Using a small rigid ruler, the examiner first measures the height of the navicular from the floor in the neutral talus position using the most prominent part of the navicular tuberosity and then measures the height of the navicular in normal relaxed standing. The difference is called the navicular drop and indicates the amount of foot pronation or flattening of the medial longitudinal arch during standing (Figure 13-58).[75,76] Any measurement greater than 10 mm is considered abnormal. Experience in measuring is necessary to ensure reliable measures.[77]

Neutral Position of the Talus (Supine). The patient lies supine with the feet extending over the end of the examining table. The examiner grasps the patient's foot over the fourth and fifth metatarsal heads, using the thumb and index finger of one hand. The examiner palpates both sides of the head of the talus on the dorsum of the foot with the thumb and index finger of the other hand (Figure 13-59). The examiner then gently, passively dorsiflexes the foot until resistance is felt. While the examiner maintains the dorsiflexion, the foot is passively moved through an arc of supination (talar head bulges laterally) and pronation (talar head bulges medially). If the foot is positioned so that the talar head does not appear to bulge to either side, the subtalar joint will be in its neutral non-weight-bearing position.[24,36,45,78] This supine test position is best for determining the relation of the forefoot to the hindfoot.

Table 13-9

Scoring Scale for Subjective and Functional Follow-up Evaluation after Ankle Injury*

I	**Subjective Assessment of the Injured Ankle**[†]	
	No symptoms of any kind	15
	Mild symptoms	10
	Moderate symptoms	5
	Severe symptoms	0
II	**Can You Walk Normally?**	
	Yes	15
	No	0
III	**Can You Run Normally?**	
	Yes	10
	No	0
IV	**Climbing Down Stairs**[‡]	
	Less than 18 seconds	10
	18 to 20 seconds	5
	Longer than 20 seconds	0
V	**Rising on Heels With Injured Leg**	
	More than 40 times	10
	30 to 39 times	5
	Fewer than 30 times	0
VI	**Rising on Toes with Injured Leg**	
	More than 40 times	10
	30 to 39 times	5
	Fewer than 30 times	0
VII	**Single-Limbed Stance with Injured Leg**[§]	
	Longer than 55 seconds	10
	50 to 55 seconds	5
	Less than 50 seconds	0
VIII	**Laxity of the Ankle Joints (ADS)**	
	Stable (≤5 mm)	10
	Moderate instability (6–10 mm)	5
	Severe instability (>10 mm)	0
IX	**Dorsiflexion Range of Motion, Injured Leg**	
	≥10°	10
	5°–9°	5
	<5°	0

From Kaikkonen A et al: A performance test protocol and scoring scale for the evaluation of ankle injuries, *Am J Sports Med* 22:465, 1994.

*Total: Excellent, 85–100; good, 70–80; fair, 55–65; poor, ≤50.
†Pain, swelling, stiffness, tenderness, or giving way during activity (mild, only one of these symptoms is present; moderate, two to three of these symptoms are present; severe, four or more of these symptoms are present).
‡Two levels of staircase (length, 12 m) with 44 steps (height, 13 cm; depth, 22 cm).
§On square beam (10 cm×10 cm×30 cm).
ADS = anterior drawer sign.

Neutral Position of the Talus (Prone). The patient lies prone with the foot extended over the end of the examining table (Figure 13-60). The examiner grasps the patient's foot over the fourth and fifth metatarsal heads with the index finger and thumb of one hand. The examiner palpates both sides of the talus on the dorsum of the foot, using the thumb and index finger of the other hand. The examiner then passively and gently dorsiflexes the foot until resistance is felt (Figure 13-61). While maintaining the dorsiflexed position, the examiner moves the foot back and forth through an arc of supination (talar head bulges laterally) and pronation (talar head bulges medially). As the arc of movement is performed, there is a point in the arc at which the foot appears to fall off to one side or the other more easily. This point is the neutral, non-weight-bearing position of the subtalar joint.[24,36,45,78] This prone test position is best for determining the relation of the hindfoot to the leg.

Tests for Alignment

Alignment tests are used to determine the relation of the leg to the hindfoot and the relation of the hindfoot to the forefoot.[79] These tests are used to differentiate functional from anatomical (structural) deformities or asymmetries.

Leg-Heel Alignment. The patient lies in the prone position with the foot extending over the end of the examining table. The examiner places a mark over the midline of the calcaneus at the insertion of the Achilles tendon. The examiner makes a second mark approximately 1 cm distal to the first mark and as close to the midline of the calcaneus as possible. A **calcaneal line** is then made to join the two marks. Next, the examiner makes two marks on the lower third of the leg in the midline. These two marks are joined, forming the **tibial line**, which represents the longitudinal axis of the tibia. The examiner then places the subtalar joint in the prone neutral position. While the subtalar joint is held in neutral, the examiner looks at the two lines. If the lines are parallel or in slight varus (2° to 8°), the leg-to-heel alignment is considered normal.[78] If the heel is inverted, the patient has hindfoot varus; if the heel is everted, the patient has hindfoot valgus (Figure 13-62).

Forefoot-Heel Alignment. The patient lies supine with the feet extending over the end of the examining table. The examiner positions the subtalar joint in supine neutral position. While maintaining this position, the examiner pronates the midtarsal joints maximally and then observes the relation between the vertical axis of the heel and the plane of the second through fourth metatarsal heads (Figure 13-63). Normally, the plane is perpendicular to the vertical axis. If the medial side of the foot is raised, the patient has a forefoot varus; if the lateral side of the foot is raised, the patient has a forefoot valgus.[24,78]

Coleman Block Test[80]**.** This test differentiates a hindfoot varus resulting from a forefoot valgus from a hindfoot varus resulting from a tight tibialis posterior. If the patient is found to have a hindfoot varus in standing, the examiner places a lift or block under the lateral side of the forefoot. If the hindfoot varus is corrected,

A. Foot Pain Subscale

The line below each item represents the amount of pain you had during the past week performing an activity because of your foot condition. On the far left is "no pain," and on the far right is "worst pain imaginable." Place a vertical mark on the line to indicate how much pain you had performing each activity because of your feet during the past week. If you did not perform an activity during the past week, mark that item N/A.

How severe is your foot pain?

Foot pain at worst:
No pain _____ Worst pain imaginable

Foot pain in morning:
No pain _____ Worst pain imaginable

Pain walking barefoot:
No pain _____ Worst pain imaginable

Pain standing barefoot:
No pain _____ Worst pain imaginable

Pain walking with shoes:
No pain _____ Worst pain imaginable

Pain standing with shoes:
No pain _____ Worst pain imaginable

Pain walking with orthotics:
No pain _____ Worst pain imaginable

Pain standing with orthotics:
No pain_____ Worst pain imaginable

Foot pain end of day:
No pain _____ Worst pain imaginable

B. Foot Function Index Disability Subscale

The line below each item represents the amount of difficulty you had during the past week performing an activity because of your foot condition. On the far left is "no difficulty," and on the far right is "so difficult unable." Place a vertical mark on the line to indicate how much difficulty you had performing each activity because of your feet during the past week. If you did not perform an activity during the past week, mark that item N/A.

How much difficulty did you have?

Walking around the house:
No difficulty _____ So difficult unable

Walking outside on uneven ground:
No difficulty _____ So difficult unable

Walking four or more blocks:
No difficulty _____ So difficult unable

Climbing stairs:
No difficulty _____ So difficult unable

Descending stairs:
No difficulty _____ So difficult unable

Standing on tip toe:
No difficulty _____ So difficult unable

Getting out of a chair:
No difficulty _____ So difficult unable

Climbing up or down curbs:
No difficulty _____ So difficult unable

Walking fast or running:
No difficulty _____ So difficult unable

Figure 13-56 ▬▬▬
Foot function index.

C. Activity Limitation Subscale

The line below each item represents the amount of activity that you were able to do during the past week relative to several questions. On the far left is "no restriction," and on the far right is "no activity." Place a vertical mark on the line to indicate how much your foot enabled you to do during the past week in response to each of the questions. If a particular question does not apply, mark that item N/A.

Stayed inside all day because of feet:
No restriction _____ No activity

Stayed in bed all day because of feet:
No restriction _____ No activity

Limited activities because of feet:
No restriction _____ No activity

Used assistive device indoors:
No restriction _____ No activity

Used assistive device outdoors:
No restriction _____ No activity

Data from Budiman-Mak E et al: The foot function index: a measure of foot pain and disability, *J Clin Epidemiol* 44:561–570, 1991.

Figure 13-56 cont'd
Foot function index.

Figure 13-57
Determining the neutral position of the subtalar joint in standing (weight bearing).

it indicates the hindfoot is flexible and the hindfoot varus is due to a plantar flexed first ray or a valgus forefoot (Figure 13-64). If it does not correct, the tibialis posterior is tight.

Tests for Tibial Torsion

When testing for tibial torsion, the examiner must realize that some lateral tibial torsion (13° to 18° in adults, less in children) is normally present.[81] If tibial torsion is more than 18°, it is referred to as a toe-out position. If tibial torsion is less than 13°, it is referred to as a toe-in position. Excessive toeing-in is sometimes referred to as pigeon toes and may be caused by medial tibial torsion, medial femoral torsion, or excessive femoral anteversion (see Table 13-1).

Tibial Torsion (Sitting). Tibial torsion is measured by having the patient sit with the knees flexed to 90° over the edge of the examining table (Figure 13-65). The examiner places the thumb of one hand over the apex of one malleolus and the index finger of the same hand over the apex of the other malleolus. Next, the examiner visualizes the axes of the knee and of the ankle. The lines are not normally parallel but instead form an angle of 12° to 18° owing to lateral rotation of the tibia.[18]

Navicular drop

Navicular height standing with talus in neutral

Navicular height with normal relaxed standing

Figure 13-58
Illustration of two different foot positions required for navicular drop measurement.

Figure 13-59

Determining the neutral position of the subtalar joint in supine position.

Figure 13-60

Prone lying with legs in figure-4 position to assess neutral position of the subtalar joint.

Tibial Torsion (Supine). The patient lies supine. The examiner ensures that the femoral condyle lies in the frontal plane (patella facing straight up). The examiner palpates the apex of both malleoli with one hand and draws a line on the heel representing a line joining the two apices. A second line is drawn on the heel parallel to the floor. The angle formed by the intersection of the two lines indicates the amount of lateral tibial torsion.

Tibial Torsion (Prone). The patient lies prone with the knee flexed to 90°. The examiner views from above the angle formed by the foot and thigh (Figure 13-66) after the subtalar joint has been placed in the neutral position, noting the angle the foot makes with the tibia.[82] This method is most often used in children because it is easier to observe the feet from above.

"Too Many Toes" Sign. The patient stands in a normal relaxed position while the examiner views the patient from behind. If the heel is in valgus, the forefoot abducted, or the tibia laterally rotated more than normal (tibial torsion), the examiner can see more toes on the affected side than on the normal side (Figure 13-67).[83] Similarly, lateral femoral torsion could cause the "too many toes" test to be positive. If the talus is positioned in neutral and the calcaneus is in neutral, the "too many toes" sign means the forefoot is adducted on the rearfoot and may be seen with excessive pronation (hyperpronation).[53,84] Hyperpronation is often associated with metatarsalgia, plantar fasciitis, hallux valgus, and posterior tibial tendon pathology.[53]

Tests for Ligamentous Instability

Anterior Drawer Test of the Ankle. This test is designed primarily to test for injuries to the anterior talofibular ligament, the most frequently injured ligament in the ankle.[85–87] The patient lies supine with the foot relaxed. The examiner stabilizes the tibia and fibula, holds the patient's foot in 20° of plantar flexion, and draws the talus forward in the ankle mortise (Figure 13-68).[88–90] Sometimes, a dimple appears over the area of the anterior talofibular ligament on anterior translation (**dimple** or **suction sign**) if pain and muscle spasm are minimal.[91–93] In the plantar-flexed position, the anterior talofibular ligament is perpendicular to the long axis of the tibia. By adding inversion, which gives an anterolateral stress, the examiner can increase the stress on the anterior talofibular ligament and the calcaneofibular ligament. A positive anterior drawer test may be obtained with a tear of only the anterior talofibular ligament, but anterior translation is greater if both ligaments are torn, especially if the foot is tested in dorsiflexion.[94] If straight anterior movement or translation occurs (Figure 13-69, *B*), the test indicates both medial and lateral ligament insufficiencies. This bilateral finding, which is often more evident in dorsiflexion, means that the superficial and deep deltoid ligaments, as well as the anterior talofibular

Figure 13-61

Determining the neutral position of the subtalar joints in the prone position. **A,** Side view. **B,** Superior view.

Figure 13-62

Alignment of leg and heel.

ligament and anterolateral capsule, have been torn. If the tear is on only one side, only that side would translate forward. For example, with a lateral tear, the lateral side would translate forward, causing medial rotation of the talus and resulting in anterolateral rotary instability (Figure 13-69, *C*), which is increasingly evident with growing plantar flexion of the foot.[23,25,95–97]

Ideally, the knee should be placed in 90° of flexion to alleviate tension on the Achilles tendon. The test should be performed in plantar flexion and in dorsiflexion to test for straight and rotational instabilities.

The test may also be performed by stabilizing the foot and talus and pushing the tibia and fibula posteriorly on the talus (see Figure 13-68, *B*). In this case, excessive posterior movement of the tibia and fibula on the talus indicates a positive test.

Prone Anterior Drawer Test[98]. The patient lies prone with the feet extending over the end of the examining table. With one hand, the examiner pushes the heel steadily forward (Figure 13-70). Excessive anterior movement and a sucking in of the skin on both sides of the Achilles tendon indicate a positive sign. The test, like the previous one, indicates ligamentous instability, primarily the anterior talofibular ligament.

Figure 13-63
Alignment of forefoot and heel (superior view).

Talar Tilt. The patient lies in the supine or side lying position with the foot relaxed (Figure 13-71).[23,99] The patient's gastrocnemius muscle may be relaxed by flexion of the knee. This test is to determine whether the calcaneofibular ligament is torn.[86,94] The normal side is tested first for comparison. The foot is held in the anatomical (90°) position, which brings the calcaneofibular ligament perpendicular to the long axis of the talus. If the foot is plantar flexed, the anterior talofibular ligament is more likely to be tested (**inversion stress test**).[93] The talus is then tilted from side to side into adduction and abduction. Adduction tests the calcaneofibular ligament and, to some degree, the anterior talofibular ligament by increasing the stress on the ligament.[10] Abduction stresses the deltoid ligament, primarily the tibionavicular, tibiocalcaneal, and posterior tibiotalar ligaments. On a radiograph, the talar tilt may be measured by obtaining the angle between the distal aspect of the tibia and the proximal surface of the talus (see the discussion of stress radiographs presented later in the chapter).

Squeeze Test of the Leg. The patient lies supine. The examiner grasps the lower leg at midcalf and squeezes the tibia and fibula together (Figure 13-72). The examiner then applies the same load at more distal locations moving toward the ankle. Pain in the lower leg may indicate a syndesmosis injury, provided that fracture, contusion, and compartment syndrome have been ruled out.[8,87,100–103] Brosky and associates called this test the **distal tibiofibular compression test** and applied the compression over the malleoli rather than the shaft of the tibia and fibula (Figure 13-73).[104] Nussbaum et al. reported that the "length of tenderness" above the lateral malleolus indicates severity.[105]

External Rotation Stress Test (Kleiger Test)[87,93,101,102,104–108]. The patient is seated with the leg hanging over the examining table with the knee at 90°. The examiner stabilizes the leg with one hand. With the other hand, the examiner holds the foot in plantigrade (90°) and applies a passive lateral rotation stress to the foot and ankle. The test is positive for a syndesmosis ("high ankle") injury if pain is produced over the anterior or posterior tibiofibular ligaments and the interosseous membrane (Figure 13-74). If the patient has pain medially and the examiner feels the talus displace from the medial malleolus, it may indicate a tear of the deltoid ligament. On a stress radiograph, if the medial clear space is increased, it suggests rupture of the ligament (see the discussion presented later in the chapter) if the lateral malleolus is intact.

Point (Palpation) Test[27,101,108]. The patient is positioned in sitting or supine. The examiner then applies a gradual pressure over the anteroinferior tibiofibular ligament (anterior aspect of the distal tibia fibular syndesmosis) using the index finger (Figure 13-75). Pain in the syndesmosis area indicates a positive test.

Cotton Test[64,102,109]. This test is also used to assess for syndesmosis instability caused by separation of the tibia and fibula (diastasis). The two bones are normally held together by four ligaments (the tibiofibular interosseous ligament, anteroinferior tibiofibular ligament, posteroinferior tibiofibular ligament, and transverse tibiofibular ligament).[110] The examiner stabilizes the distal tibia and fibula with one hand and applies a medial and lateral translation force (not an inversion/eversion force) with the other hand to the foot.[64] Any lateral translation (>3 to 5 mm) or clunk indicates syndesmotic instability.[64,111]

Dorsiflexion Maneuver[101,108,112]. The patient sits on the edge of the table. The examiner stabilizes the patient's leg with one hand and with the other hand passively and forcefully dorsiflexes the foot by holding onto the heel and using the forearm to dorsiflex the foot (Figure 13-76). Pain on forced dorsiflexion indicates a positive test.

Dorsiflexion Compression Test[101,108]. While in bilateral weight-bearing, the patient is asked to move his

Figure 13-64

Coleman block test. **A,** On initial examination, the hindfoot is in varus. **B,** The patient stands with a book or block under the lateral side of the forefoot, and the hindfoot is reexamined. Heel varus correction indicates that the hindfoot deformity is flexible and that the varus position is secondary to the plantarflexed first ray, or valgus position of the forefoot.

or her ankle into extreme dorsiflexion (Figure 13-77, *A*). The patient is asked to note whether this maneuver is painful while the examiner notes the end range of motion. The patient then assumes a normal standing position again. The examiner applies a compression force using two hands surrounding the malleoli of the injured leg. While this compression is maintained, the patient is asked to move into dorsiflexion again (Figure 13-77, *B*). A decrease in pain on dorsiflexion or an increase in dorsiflexion range indicates a positive test.

Crossed Leg Test[108,113]. The patient sits in a chair with the affected leg crossed over the opposite knee so the midpoint of the fibula is resting on the opposite knee (Figure 13-78). The examiner then applies a gentle force to the medial aspect of the knee of the injured leg. If the patient experiences pain in the area of the distal syndesmosis, it indicates a positive test.

Heel Thump Test[108,114]. The patient is in sitting or lying. The examiner uses one hand to stabilize the leg. With the other hand, the examiner applies a firm thump on the heel with the fist so that the force is applied to the center of the heel and in line with the long axis of the tibia (Figure 13-79). A positive test (i.e., pain) in the area of the ankle indicates a syndesmosis injury. Pain along the shaft of the tibia may indicate a stress fracture.

Other Tests

Functional Leg Length[115]. The patient stands in the normal relaxed stance (Figure 13-80). The examiner palpates the anterior superior iliac spines and then the pos-

Figure 13-65

Determination of tibial torsion in sitting (superior view). The torsion angle determined by the intersection of the knee axis and the ankle axis. (Modified from Hunt GC, editor: *Physical therapy of the foot and ankle*, Clinics in Physical Therapy, p. 80, New York, 1988, Churchill Livingstone.)

Figure 13-67

"Too-many-toes" sign signifying lateral foot or tibial rotation. Two-and-one-half toes shown on the left foot, four toes on the abnormal right foot. (Redrawn from Baxter DE, editor: *The foot and ankle in sport*, p. 45, St. Louis, 1995, Mosby.)

Figure 13-66

Measurement of tibial torsion in the prone position.

A

B

Figure 13-68

Anterior drawer test. **A,** Method 1—drawing the foot forward. **B,** Method 2—pushing the leg back.

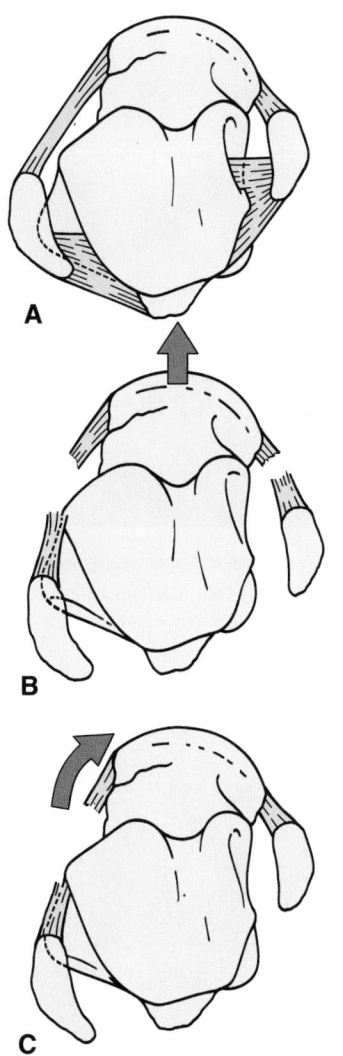

Figure 13-69
Anterior drawer test. **A,** Normal relation between talus and malleoli.
B, Straight anterior translation (one-plane anterior instability).
C, Lateral rotary translation (anterolateral rotary instability).

Figure 13-70
Prone anterior drawer test.

Figure 13-71
Talar tilt test.

Figure 13-72
Squeeze test for stress fracture or ankle syndesmosis pathology.

terior superior iliac spines and notes any differences. The examiner then positions the patient so that the patient's subtalar joints are in neutral position while weight bearing. The patient maintains this position with the toes straight ahead and the knees straight, and the examiner repalpates the anterior and the posterior superior iliac spines. If the previously noted differences remain, the pelvis and sacroiliac joints should be evaluated further. If the previously noted differences disappear, the examiner should suspect a functional leg length difference resulting from hip, knee, or ankle and foot problems—primarily, ankle and foot problems (Tables 13-10 and 13-11). The examiner must then determine what is causing the difference. For example, foot pronation is often

Figure 13-73
Distal tibiofibular compression test.

Figure 13-75
Point (palpation) test. The examiner applies pressure over the anterior aspect of the distal tibiofibular syndesmosis.

Figure 13-74
External rotation stress test.

Figure 13-76
Dorsiflexion maneuver. The examiner stabilizes the leg with one hand and passively moves the foot toward dorsiflexion with the other hand using the forearm.

seen with forefoot or hindfoot varus, tibial varus, tight muscles (e.g., calf, hamstrings, hip flexors), or weak muscles (e.g., ankle invertors, piriformis).

Thompson's (Simmonds') Test (Sign for Achilles Tendon Rupture). The patient lies prone or kneels on a chair with the feet over the edge of the table or chair (Figure 13-81). While the patient is relaxed, the examiner squeezes the calf muscles. The absence of plantar flexion when the muscle is squeezed indicates a positive test and a ruptured Achilles tendon (third-degree strain).[116–119]

A   **B**

Figure 13-77

Dorsiflexion compression test. **A,** Step 1: Patient dorsiflexes feet while standing. **B,** Step 2: Patient dorsiflexes feet while examiner squeezes malleoli together.

One should be careful not to assume that the Achilles tendon is not ruptured if the patient is able to plantar flex the foot while not bearing weight. The long flexor muscles can perform this function in the non-weight-bearing stance even with a rupture of the Achilles tendon.

Figure-8 Ankle Measurement for Swelling[120–123]. The patient is positioned in long sitting with the ankle and lower leg beyond the end of the examining table with the ankle in plantigrade (90°). Using a 6 mm (one-quarter-inch) wide plastic tape measure, the examiner places the end of the tape measure midway between the tibialis anterior tendon and the lateral malleolus, drawing the tape medially across the instep just distal to the navicular tuberosity. The tape is then pulled across the arch of the foot just proximal to the base of the fifth metatarsal, across the tibialis anterior tendon, and then around the ankle joint just distal to the tip of the medial malleolus, across the Achilles tendon, and just distal to the lateral malleolus, returning to the starting position (Figure 13-82). The measurement is repeated three times and an average taken.

Test for Peroneal Tendon Dislocation[124]. The patient is placed in prone on the examining table with the knee flexed to 90°. The posterolateral region of the ankle is inspected for swelling. The patient is then asked to actively dorsiflex and plantar flex the ankle along with eversion against the examiner's resistance (Figure 13-83). If the tendon subluxes from behind the lateral malleolus, the test is positive.

Patla Tibialis Posterior Length Test[52]. The patient is in prone lying with the knee flexed to 90° and the calcaneus held in eversion and the ankle in dorsiflexion with one hand (Figure 13-84). With the other hand, the examiner's thumb contacts the plantar surface of the bases of the second, third, and fourth metatarsals while the index and middle fingers contact the plantar surface of the navicular. The examiner then determines the end feel by pushing dorsally on the navicular and metatarsal heads. The end feel is compared with the normal side. A reproduction of the patient's symptoms indicates a positive test.

Swing Test for Posterior Tibiotalar Subluxation[125]. The patient sits with feet dangling over the edge of

Figure 13-78

Crossed-leg test. The patient sits in a chair, with the injured leg resting across the knee of the uninjured leg. The examiner applies a gentle force on the medial knee of the injured leg.

Figure 13-79

Heel thump test. The examiner holds the patient's leg with one hand and with the other hand applies a gentle but firm thump on the heel with the fist.

the examining table (Figure 13-85). The examiner places the hands around the dorsum of the foot using the fingers to keep the feet parallel to the floor. With the thumbs, the examiner palpates the anterior portion of the talus. The examiner then passively plantar flexes and dorsiflexes the foot and compares the quality and degree of movement between feet, especially into dorsiflexion. Resistance to normal dorsiflexion in the injured ankle indicates a positive test for posterior tibiotalar subluxation.

Feiss Line[24]. The examiner marks the apex of the medial malleolus and the plantar aspect of the first metatarsophalangeal joint while the patient is not bearing weight. The examiner then palpates the navicular tuberosity on the medial aspect of the foot, noting where it lies relative to a line joining the two previously made points. The patient then stands with the feet 8 to 15 cm (3 to 6 inches) apart. The two points are checked to ensure that they still represent the apex of the medial malleolus and the plantar aspect of the metatarsophalangeal joint. The navicular tubercle is again palpated (Figure 13-86). The navicular tubercle nor-

mally lies on or close to the line joining the two points. If the tubercle falls one third of the distance to the floor, it represents a first-degree flatfoot; if it falls two thirds of the distance, it represents a second-degree flatfoot; if it rests on the floor, it represents a third-degree flatfoot (see Figure 3-33, *A*).

Hoffa's Test. The patient lies prone with the feet extended over the edge of the examining table. The examiner palpates the Achilles tendon while the patient plantar flexes and dorsiflexes the foot. If one Achilles tendon (the injured one) feels less taut than the other one, the test is considered positive for a calcaneal fracture. Passive dorsiflexion on the affected side is also greater.

Tinel's Sign at the Ankle (Percussion Sign). Tinel's sign may be elicited in two places around the ankle. The anterior tibial branch of the deep peroneal nerve may be percussed in front of the ankle (Figure 13-87, *A*). The posterior tibial nerve may be percussed as it passes behind the medial malleolus (Figure 13-87, *B*). In both cases, tingling or paresthesia felt distally is a positive sign.

Table 13-10

Functional Limb Length Difference

Joint	Functional Lengthening	Functional Shortening
Foot	Supination	Pronation
Knee	Extension	Flexion
Hip	Lowering	Lifting
	Extension	Flexion
	Lateral rotation	Medial rotation
Sacroiliac	Anterior rotation	Posterior rotation

Modified from Wallace LA: Lower quarter pain: mechanical evaluation and treatment. In Grieve GP, editor: *Modern manual therapy of the vertebral column*, p. 467, Edinburgh, 1986, Churchill Livingstone.

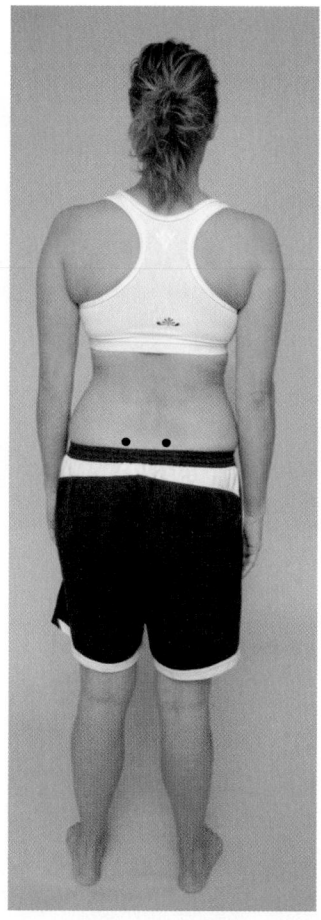

Figure 13-80

Functional leg length in standing position (subtalar joint in neutral). Dots on back indicate posterior superior iliac spines.

Duchenne Test[28]. The patient lies supine with the legs straight. The examiner pushes up on the head of the first metatarsal through the sole, pushing the foot into dorsiflexion. The test is positive for a lesion of the superficial peroneal nerve or a lesion of L4, L5, or S1 nerve root if, when the patient is asked to plantar flex the foot, the medial border dorsiflexes and offers no resistance while the lateral border plantar flexes.

Morton's Test[28]. The patient lies supine. The examiner grasps the foot around the metatarsal heads and squeezes the heads together. Pain is a positive sign for stress fracture or neuroma.

Homans' Sign. The patient's foot is passively dorsiflexed with the knee extended. Pain in the calf indicates a positive Homans' sign for deep vein thrombophlebitis (Figure 13-88). Tenderness is also elicited on palpation of the calf. In addition to these findings, the examiner may find pallor and swelling in the leg and a loss of the dorsalis pedis pulse.

Buerger's Test. This test is designed to test the arterial blood supply to the lower limb.[28] The patient lies supine while the examiner elevates the patient's leg to 45° for at least 3 minutes. If the foot blanches or the prominent veins collapse shortly after elevation, the test is positive for poor arterial blood circulation. The examiner

Table 13-11

Dynamic Limb Length Evaluation

Asymmetric Shoe Wear	Asymmetric Callus	Asymmetric Posture	Asymmetric Alignment or Movement
Shoe upper	Medial first distal interphalangeal	Foot	Toe-out
Heel counter	Medial first metatarsal	Ankle	Toe-grasp
Varus or valgus	Second and third metatarsal heads	Knee	Patellar alignment over foot
		Hip	Knee flexion
Shoe sole	Fourth and fifth metatarsal heads	Pelvis	Hip drop
Posterior lateral heel	Calcaneus		Propulsion
Posterior central heel	Lateral		
Posterior medial heel	Central		
	Medial		

Modified from Wallace LA: Limb length difference and back pain. In Grieve GP, editor: *Modern manual therapy of the vertebral column*, p. 469, Edinburgh, 1986, Churchill Livingstone.

Figure 13-81

Thompson's test for Achilles tendon rupture. **A,** Prone lying position. **B,** Kneeling position. In each case, foot plantar flexes *(arrow)* if the test result is negative.

Figure 13-82

Figure-8 ankle measurement for swelling.

then asks the patient to sit with the legs dangling over the edge of the bed. If it takes 1 to 2 minutes for the limb color to be restored and the veins to fill and become prominent, the test is confirmed positive.

Reflexes and Cutaneous Distribution

The examiner must be aware of the sensory distribution of the various peripheral nerves in the foot, especially the superficial peroneal, deep peroneal, and saphenous nerves,

Figure 13-83

Test for peroneal tendon dislocation. Arrow indicates where to look for subluxing tendon.

Figure 13-84
Patla tibialis posterior length test.

Figure 13-85
Swing test for posterior tibiotalar subluxation.

A

B

Figure 13-86
A, Feiss line in nonweight bearing. Navicular is in normal position.
B, Feiss line in weight bearing. Navicular is slightly below line (within normal limits).

and the branches of the tibial nerve (sural, medial calcaneal, medial plantar, and lateral plantar; Figure 13-89).

The examiner must also differentiate between the peripheral nerve sensory distribution and the sensory nerve root distribution or dermatomes (Figure 13-90). Although dermatomes vary among individuals, their pattern is never identical to the peripheral nerve distribution, which tends to be more consistent among patients.

The examiner should test the patient's sensation by running his or her hands over the anterior, lateral, medial, and posterior surfaces of the patient's leg below the knee, foot, and toes (sensation scanning examination). Any difference in sensation should be noted and can be mapped out in more detail with a pinwheel, pin, cotton batten, or brush.

The examiner must test the patient's reflexes. Commonly checked in this region are the Achilles reflex[126] (S1-S2; Figure 13-91) and the posterior tibial reflex (L4-L5; Figure 13-92). These reflexes may be affected by age and may be absent in older normal individuals.[126]

Figure 13-87
Tinel's sign. **A,** Anterior tibial branch of deep peroneal nerve.
B, Posterior tibial nerve.

Figure 13-88
Homans' sign for thrombophlebitis. **A,** Test. **B,** Palpation for
tenderness in thrombophlebitis.

The examiner may also wish to test for pyramidal tract (upper motor neuron) disease. There are various methods for testing the pathological reflexes, including the Babinski, Chaddock, Oppenheim, and Gordon reflexes (Figure 13-93). A positive sign in all of these tests is extension of the big toe. The Babinski reflex also causes fanning of the second through fifth toes. The most common and reliable test is the Babinski test.[127]

The examiner must remember that pain may be referred to the lower leg, ankle, or foot from the lumbar spine, sacrum, hip, or knee (Figure 13-94). Conversely, pain from a lesion in the lower leg, ankle, or foot may be transmitted to the hip or knee. Table 13-12 shows the muscles of the lower leg, ankle, and foot, and their patterns of pain referral.

Peripheral Nerve Injuries of the Lower Leg, Ankle, and Foot

Deep Peroneal Nerve (L4 through S2). The deep peroneal nerve, a branch of the common peroneal nerve, which is itself a branch of the sciatic nerve (Figures 13-95 and 13-96), is most commonly injured (compressed) in **anterior compartment syndrome** in the leg, and where it passes under the extensor retinaculum **(anterior tarsal tunnel syndrome)**.[83,128–134] Compression may be caused by trauma, tight shoelaces, a ganglion, or pes cavus.[130] Motor loss (Table 13-13) includes an inability to dorsiflex the foot **(drop foot)**, which results in a high steppage gait and an inability to control ankle movement. Because the deep peroneal nerve is primarily motor, there is minimal sensory loss, but this loss can be aggravating, especially in anterior tarsal tunnel syndrome (see Figure 13-96). The sensory loss is a small triangular area between the first and second toes. Pain is often accentuated by plantar flexion.[130] With the tunnel syndrome, muscle weakness is minimal (extensor digitorum brevis); there is burning pain between the first and second toes that is sometimes referred to the dorsum of the foot.

Superficial Peroneal Nerve (L4 through S2). Injuries to the superficial peroneal nerve, a branch of the common peroneal nerve (Figure 13-97; see Figure 13-95), are rare but they have been reported to be associated with lateral ankle (inversion) sprains causing stretching of the nerve, or the nerve may be entrapped as it pierces the deep fascia to become subcutaneous about 10 to 13 cm (4 to 5 inches) above the lateral malleolus (Figure 13-98).[52,84,129,132,133,135–138] Motor loss with the high lesion near the head of the fibula is primarily loss of foot eversion and loss of ankle stability. With both lesions, the sensory loss is the same. The superficial peroneal nerve has a greater sensory role than the deep branch; it supplies the lateral side of the leg and dorsum of the foot (see Figure 13-97). This sensory alteration is often greater with activity. If the examiner plantar flexes and inverts the foot while applying pressure over the distal site, symptoms usually result.[139]

Pahor and Toppenberg reported that the slump test (see Chapter 9) combined with plantar flexion and inversion of the foot can be performed to rule out neurological injury to the nerve following lateral ankle sprains.[140]

Tibial Nerve (L4 through S3). The tibial nerve, a branch of the sciatic nerve (Figures 13-99 and 13-100), has a major role to play in the lower leg, ankle, and foot because it supplies all the muscles in the posterior leg and on the sole of the foot. The nerve may be injured in the popliteal area at the knee from trauma (e.g., dislocation, blow) or from entrapment as it passes over the popliteus and under the soleus. **Popliteal entrapment** syndrome or injury may accompany an ankle sprain.[136] At the ankle, the nerve may be compressed as it passes through the tarsal tunnel, which is formed by the medial malleolus,

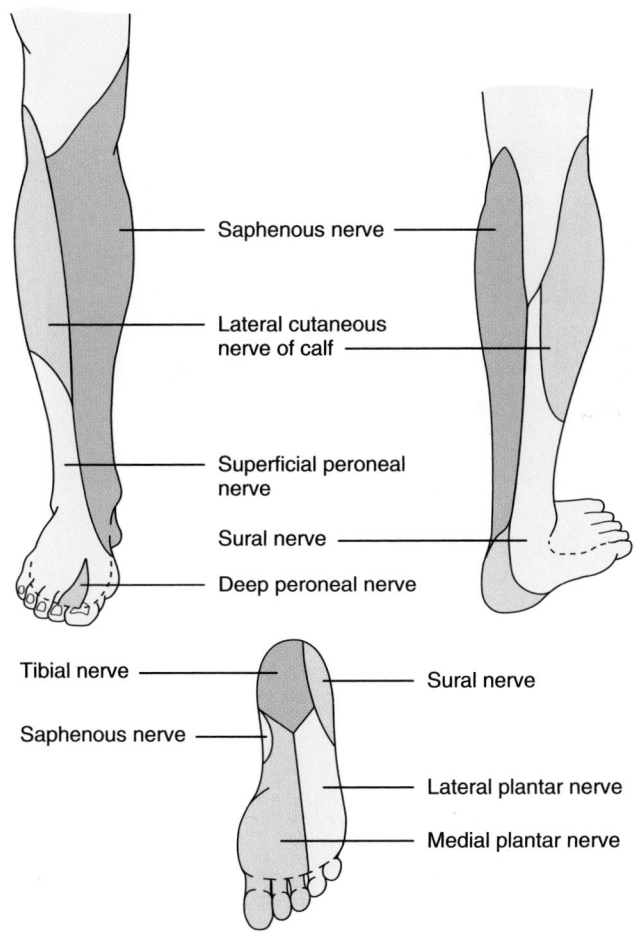

Figure 13-89
Peripheral nerve distribution in the lower leg, ankle, and foot.

Figure 13-90
Dermatomes of the lower leg, ankle, and foot.

Figure 13-91
Test of Achilles reflex (S1-S2). **A,** Prone lying. **B,** Kneeling.

Figure 13-92
Tibialis posterior reflex.

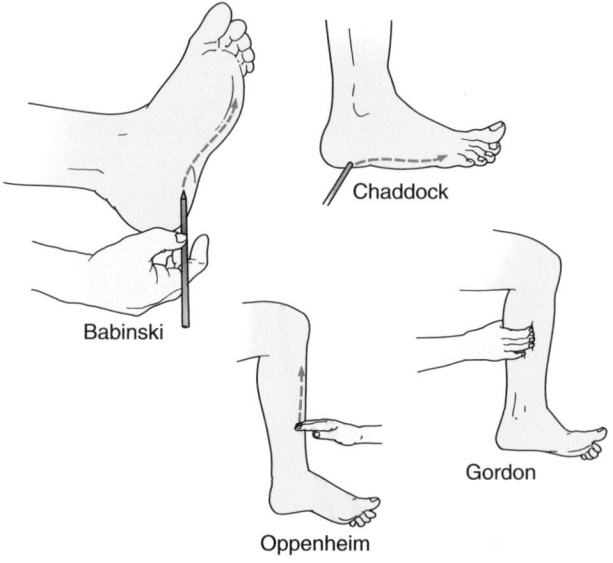

Figure 13-93
Pathological reflexes for pyramidal tract disease.

calcaneus, and talus on one side and the deltoid ligament (primarily the tibiocalcanean ligament) on the other. This compression is referred to as **tarsal tunnel syndrome** (see Figure 13-100).[129,134,141,142]

Injury to the nerve at the knee causes a major functional disability. Functionally, the patient is unable to plantar flex and invert the foot, which has a major effect on gait. In addition, the patient is unable to flex, abduct, or adduct the toes. Sensory loss involves primarily the sole of the foot, lateral surface of the heel, and plantar surfaces of the toes. With popliteal entrapment syndrome, the popliteal artery is often compressed with the nerve, leading to vascular symptoms (e.g., numbness, tingling, intermittent cramping, weakened dorsalis pedis pulse) and neurological signs.

Compression in the tarsal tunnel may be caused by swelling after trauma, a space-occupying lesion (e.g., ganglion), inflammation (e.g., paratenonitis), valgus deformity,

Figure 13-94
Pattern of referred pain to and from the ankle.

or chronic inversion.[49,131–133,143–150] Sammarco and associates reported the possibility of **double crush injury** in the lower limb involving the sciatic nerve (L4 through S3) and one of its branches.[151] The examiner must always keep this possibility in mind when assessing for nerve pathology in the lower limb, especially in patients who do not appear to be recovering. Pain and paresthesia into the sole of the foot are often present and are worse after long periods of standing or walking or at night.[129] The pain may be localized or may radiate over the medial side of the ankle distal to the medial malleolus. The condition is sometimes misdiagnosed as plantar fasciitis (Table 13-14).[152] In long-standing cases, motor weakness may become evident in the muscles of the sole of the foot that are supplied by the terminal branches of the tibial nerve (i.e., the medial and lateral plantar nerves).

The **sural nerve** (L5 through S2) is a sensory branch of the tibial nerve supplying the skin on the posterolateral aspect of the lower one third of the leg and the lateral aspect of the foot (Figure 13-101). Injury can result from a blow, trauma (e.g., fracture), or stretching (e.g., accompanying an ankle sprain).[49,84,132,150] Shooting pain and paresthesia in its sensory distribution are diagnostic signs.[129]

The **medial plantar nerve** (Figure 13-102), another branch of the tibial nerve that is found in the foot, may be entrapped in the longitudinal arch, causing aching in the arch, burning pain in the heel, and altered sensation in the sole of the foot behind the hallux. This condition is associated with hindfoot valgus and may be referred to as **jogger's foot**.[129,134,153,154]

Table 13-12

Muscles of the Lower Leg, Ankle, and Foot and Referral of Pain

Muscle	Referral Pattern
Tibialis anterior	Anterior lower leg, medial dorsum of foot to hallux
Peroneus longus	Superolateral aspect of lower leg
Peroneus brevis	Lower lateral leg, over lateral malleolus and lateral aspect of foot
Peroneus tertius	Lower lateral leg, anterior to lateral malleolus and onto dorsum of foot, or behind lateral malleolus to lateral heel
Gastrocnemius	Behind knee, posterior leg to instep of foot
Soleus	Posterior leg to heel and sometimes to sole of foot
Plantaris	Posterior knee to upper half of posterior leg
Tibialis posterior	Posterior leg, Achilles tendon, heel and sole of foot
Extensor digitorum longus	Anterolateral leg to dorsum of foot
Extensor hallucis longus	Anterior leg to dorsomedial foot
Flexor digitorum longus	Posteromedial leg, over medial malleolus, distal sole of foot
Flexor hallucis longus	Plantar aspect of hallux
Extensor digitorum brevis and extensor hallucis brevis	Dorsum of foot
Abductor hallucis	Medial heel and instep
Abductor digiti minimi	Sole of foot over fifth metatarsal
Flexor digitorum brevis	Over metatarsal head
Quadratus plantae (flexor accessorius)	Plantar aspect of heel
Adductor hallucis	Sole of foot over metatarsals
Flexor hallucis brevis	Dorsal and plantar aspect of first metatarsal and hallux
Interossei	Dorsum and plantar aspect of equivalent metatarsal and toe

Figure 13-95

Superficial peroneal nerve travels in the lateral compartment of the leg and can be entrapped as it pierces the fascia 8 to 12 cm proximal to the tip of the lateral malleolus. The deep peroneal nerve can be compressed as it pierces the intermuscular septum to travel in the anterior compartment and under the retinaculum.

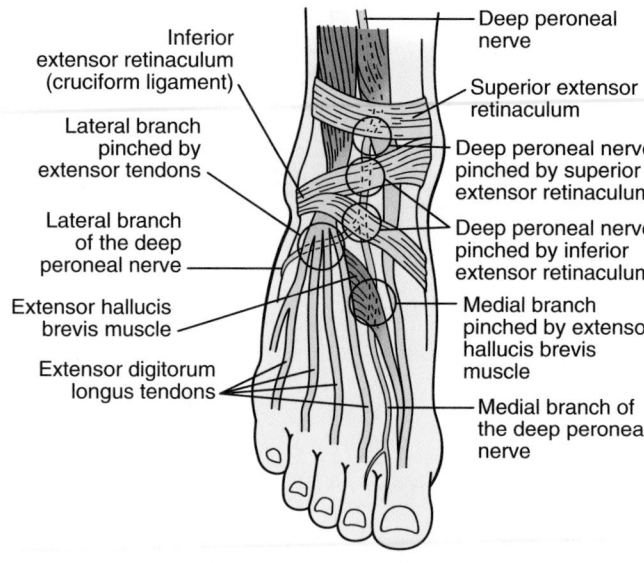

Figure 13-96

Compression of deep peroneal nerve by the extensor retinaculum or other structures.

Similarly, the **lateral plantar nerve** may be entrapped between the deep fascia of the abductor hallucis and the quadratus plantae (flexor accessorius) muscles (Figure 13-103).[129,155] The patient complains of chronic, dull, aching heel pain that is accentuated by walking and running. There is no complaint of numbness. The condition is accentuated by excessive foot pronation.[155]

Saphenous Nerve. This nerve is a sensory branch of the femoral nerve. If it is injured, sensation on the medial side of the leg and foot is affected.[156] More details are given in Chapter 12.

Joint Play Movements

The joint play movements (Figures 13-104 through 13-107) are performed with the patient in the supine or side lying position, depending on which movement is being performed. A comparison of movement between the normal or unaffected side and the injured side should be made.

Long-Axis Extension

Long-axis extension is performed by stabilizing the proximal segment and applying traction to the distal segment. For example, at the ankle, the examiner stabilizes the tibia and fibula by using a strap or just allowing the leg to relax. Both hands are then placed around the ankle, distal to the malleoli, and a longitudinal distractive force is applied. At the metatarsophalangeal and interphalangeal joints, the examiner stabilizes the metatarsal bone or proximal phalanx and applies a longitudinal distractive force to the proximal or distal phalanx, respectively.

Joint Play Movements of the Lower Leg, Ankle, and Foot	
Talocrural (ankle joint)	Long-axis extension (traction) Anteroposterior glide
Subtalar joint	Talar rock Side tilt medially and laterally
Midtarsal joints	Anteroposterior glide Rotation
Tarsometatarsal joints	Anteroposterior glide Rotation
Metatarsophalangeal and interphalangeal joints	Long-axis extension (traction) Anteroposterior glide Lateral or side glide Rotation

Table 13-13

Peripheral Nerve Injuries (Neuropathy) of the Lower Leg, Ankle, and Foot

Nerve	Muscle Weakness	Sensory Alteration	Reflexes Affected
Deep peroneal nerve (L4 through S2)	Tibialis anterior Extensor digitorum longus Extensor digitorum brevis Extensor hallucis longus Peroneus tertius	Triangular area between the first and second toes	None
Superficial peroneal nerve (L4 through S2)	Peroneus longus Peroneus brevis	Lateral aspect of leg and dorsum of foot	None
Tibial nerve (L4 through S3)	Gastrocnemius Soleus Plantaris Tibialis posterior Flexor digitorum longus Flexor hallucis longus Flexor accessorius (quadratus plantae) Abductor digiti minimi Flexor digiti minimi Lumbricals Interossei Adductor hallucis Abductor hallucis Flexor digitorum brevis Flexor hallucis brevis	Sole of foot except medial border, plantar surface of toes	Achilles (S1-S2) Tibialis posterior (L4-L5)

Figure 13-97

Common peroneal nerve and its branches, the superficial and deep peroneal nerves.

Figure 13-98

Stretching of the superficial peroneal nerve as a result of inversion of ankle.

L4
L5
S1
S2
S3

Sciatic nerve

Biceps,
long head

Semitendinosus

Semimembranosus

Adductor magnus,
posterior part

Tibial nerve

Plantaris

Gastrocnemius

Popliteus

Soleus

Flexor
hallucis
longus

Flexor
digitorum
longus

Tibialis
posterior

Biceps
short head

**Common
peroneal nerve**

**Deep
peroneal nerve**
(going anterior)

Peroneus
longus

Peroneus brevis

**Superficial
peroneal nerve**

Posterior view

Medial sural
cutan. and sural

Lateral
plantar

Medial
plantar

Medial
calcaneal

Adductor
hallucis

All plantar
interossei

All dorsal
interossei

Three lateral
lumbricals

Flexor digiti
minimi brevis

Abductor
digiti minimi

Quadratus
plantae

**Lateral
plantar nerve**

Flexor
hallucis
brevis

First
lumbrical

Flexor digiti
torum brevis

Adductor
hallucis

**Medial
plantar
nerve**

Plantar view

Figure 13-99
Distribution of the branches of the sciatic
nerve with tibial nerve highlighted.

Anteroposterior Glide

Anteroposterior glide at the ankle joint is performed by stabilizing the tibia and fibula and drawing the talus and foot forward. To test the posterior movement, the examiner pushes the talus and foot back on the tibia and fibula. There is a difference in the arc of movement between the two actions in tests of joint play. During the anterior movement, the foot should move in an arc into plantar flexion; during the posterior movement, the foot should move in an arc into dorsiflexion. Although similar to the anterior drawer test, the movements are not the same.

Anteroposterior glide at the midtarsal and tarsometatarsal joints is performed in a fashion similar to that used to test the carpal bones at the wrist. For the midtarsal joints, the examiner stabilizes the navicular, talus, and calcaneus with one hand by grasping the bones in the web space, thumb, and fingers. The other hand is placed around the distal row of tarsal bones (cuneiforms and cuboid). If the hands are positioned properly, they should touch each other, as in Figure 13-105. An anteroposterior gliding movement of the distal row of tarsal bones is applied while the proximal row of tarsal bones is stabilized. The examiner's hands are then moved distally so that the stabilizing hand rests over the distal row of tarsal bones and the mobilizing hand rests over the proximal aspect of the metatarsal bones. Again, the hands should be positioned so that they touch each other. An anteroposterior gliding movement of the metatarsal bones is applied while the distal row of tarsal bones is stabilized.

Anteroposterior glide of the metatarsophalangeal and interphalangeal joints is performed by stabilizing the proximal bone (metatarsal or phalanx) and moving the distal bone (phalanx) in an anteroposterior gliding motion in relation to the stabilized bone.

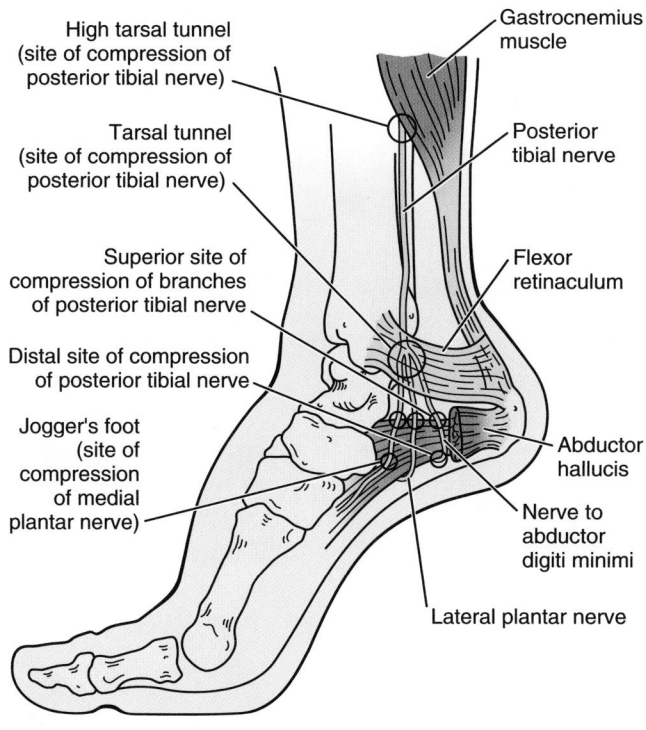

Figure 13-100
Tarsal tunnel syndrome.

Talar Rock

Talar rock is the only joint play movement performed with the patient in the side lying position.[99] Both the hip and knee are flexed. The examiner sits with his or her back to the patient, as illustrated in Figure 13-105, *A*, and places both hands around the ankle just distal to the malleoli. A slight distractive force is applied to the ankle, and a rocking movement forward and backward (plantar flexion-dorsiflexion) is applied to the foot. Normally, the examiner should feel a clunk at the extreme of each movement. As with all joint play movements, the movement is compared with that of the unaffected side.

Figure 13-101
Sural nerve travels between the two heads of the gastrocnemius muscle and then becomes superficial in the distal third of the leg. The common peroneal nerve may become entrapped as it courses anteriorly between the fibular head and the peroneus longus. The tibial nerve may be entrapped as it passes through soleus and in the tarsal tunnel.

Table 13-14

Differential Diagnosis of Plantar Fasciitis and Tarsal Tunnel Syndrome

	Plantar Fasciitis	**Tarsal Tunnel Syndrome**
Cause	Overuse	Trauma, space occupying lesion, inflammation, inversion, pronation, valgus deformity
Pain	Plantar aspect of foot, anterior calcaneus	Medial heel and medial longitudinal arch
	Worse with walking, running, and in the morning (sometimes improves with activity)	Worse with standing, walking, and at night
Electrodiagnosis	Normal	Prolonged motor and sensory latencies
Active movements	Full range of motion	Full range of motion
Passive movements	Full range of motion	May have pain on pronation
Resisted isometric movements	Normal	Weakness of foot intrinsics may be present
Sensory deficits	No	Possible
Reflexes	Normal	Normal

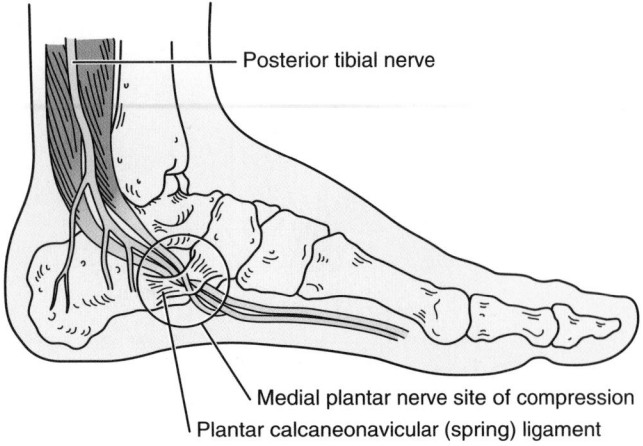

Figure 13-102

Jogger's foot (entrapment of the medial plantar nerve).

A

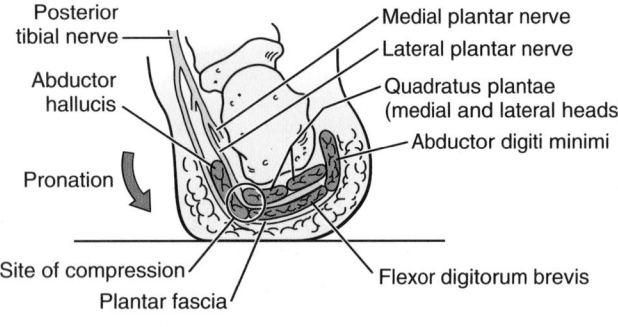

B

Figure 13-103

Entrapment of the lateral plantar nerve as it changes direction. **A,** Medial view. **B,** Posterior view.

Side Tilt

Side tilt at the subtalar joint is performed by placing both hands around the calcaneus (see Figure 13-105, *B*). The wrists are flexed and extended, tilting the calcaneus medially

A

B

Figure 13-104

Joint play movements at the talocrural joint. **A,** Long-axis extension. **B,** Anteroposterior glide at the talocrural joint.

and laterally on the talus. The examiner keeps the patient's foot in the anatomical position while performing the movement. The movement is identical to that used to test the calcaneofibular ligament in the talar tilt test.

Rotation

Rotation at the midtarsal joints is performed in a similar fashion to the anteroposterior glide at these joints. The proximal row of tarsal bones (navicular, calcaneus, and talus) is stabilized, and the mobilizing hand is placed

Figure 13-105
Joint play movements at the subtalar joint. **A,** Talar rock with slight traction applied. Talus is rocked anterior and posteriorly. **B,** Side tilt.

Figure 13-106
Joint play movements in the midtarsal and tarsometatarsal joints. **A,** Anteroposterior glide. **B,** Rotation.

around the distal tarsal bones (cuneiforms and cuboid). The distal row of bones is then rotated on the proximal row of bones. Rotation at the tarsometatarsal joints is performed in a similar fashion. Rotation at the metatarsophalangeal and interphalangeal joints is performed by stabilizing the proximal bone with one hand, applying slight traction, and rotating the distal bone with the other hand.

Side Glide

Side glide at the metatarsophalangeal and interphalangeal joints is performed by stabilizing the proximal bone with one hand. The examiner then uses the other hand to apply slight traction to the distal bone and moves the distal bone sideways (right and left) in relation to the stabilized bone without causing torsion motion at the joint.

Tests for Tarsal Bone Mobility

In addition to testing of the tarsal bones as a group, the bones should be tested individually, especially if symptoms resulted from group testing. The examiner may test these individual bones using whatever method is desired realizing that the amount of movement normally is minimal. An example of individual tarsal bone testing was put forward by Kaltenborn,[157] who advocates 10 tests to determine the mobility of the tarsal bones.

Palpation

The examiner palpates for any swelling, noting whether it is intracapsular or extracapsular. Extracapsular swelling around the ankle is indicated by swelling on only one side of the Achilles tendon, whereas intracapsular swelling is indicated by swelling on both sides (see Figure 13-16).

Kaltenborn's 10 Tests for Tarsal Mobility

1. Fixate the second and third cuneiforms, and mobilize the second metatarsal bone
2. Fixate the second and third cuneiform bones, and mobilize the third metatarsal bone
3. Fixate the first cuneiform bone, and mobilize the first metatarsal bone
4. Fixate the navicular bone, and mobilize the first, second, and third cuneiform bones
5. Fixate the talus, and mobilize the navicular bone
6. Fixate the cuboid bone, and mobilize the fourth and fifth metatarsal bones
7. Fixate the navicular and third cuneiform bones, and mobilize the cuboid bone
8. Fixate the calcaneus, and mobilize the cuboid bone
9. Fixate the talus, and mobilize the calcaneus
10. Fixate the talus, and mobilize the tibia and fibula

Pitting edema, if present, should be noted. If swelling is present at the end of the day and absent after a night of recumbency, venous insufficiency, caused by a weakening or insufficiency of the action of the muscle pump of the lower leg muscles, may be implied. Swelling in the ankle may persist for many weeks after injury as a result of this insufficiency.

The examiner should also notice the texture of the skin and nails. The skin of an ischemic foot shows a loss of hair and becomes thin and inelastic. In addition, the nails become coarse, thickened, and irregular. Many of the nail changes seen in the hand (see Chapter 7) in the presence of systemic disease are also seen in the foot. With poor circulation, the foot will also feel colder. The foot is palpated in the non-weight-bearing and long leg sitting or supine positions. The following structures, including the joints between them, should be palpated.

Figure 13-107

Joint play movements at the metatarsophalangeal and interphalangeal joints. **A,** Long-axis extension. **B,** Anteroposterior glide. **C,** Side glide. **D,** Rotation.

Figure 13-108

Bones of the ankle and foot. **A,** Dorsal view. **B,** Plantar view.

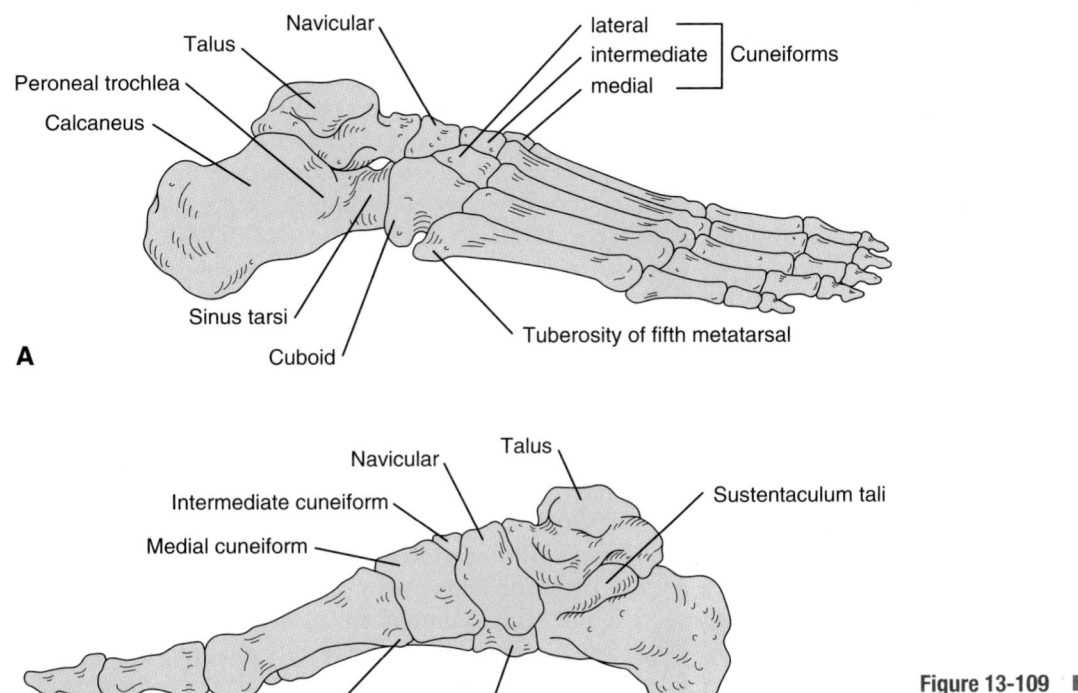

Figure 13-109

Bones of the foot from the lateral **A,** and medial **B,** sides.

Palpation Anteriorly and Anteromedially

Toes and Metatarsal, Cuneiform, and Navicular Bones. Starting on the medial side, the great toe and its two phalanges are easily palpated. Moving proximally, the examiner comes to the first metatarsal bone (Figure 13-108). The head of the first metatarsal should be palpated carefully. On the medial aspect of the foot, the examiner palpates for any evidence of a bunion (exostosis, callus, and inflamed bursa), which is often associated with hallux valgus. On the plantar aspect, the two sesamoid bones just proximal to the head of the first metatarsal may be palpated.[158] The examiner then palpates the first metatarsal bone along its length to the first cuneiform bone and notes any tenderness, swelling, or signs of pathology. While moving proximally past the first cuneiform on its medial aspect, the examiner will feel a bony prominence, the tubercle of the navicular bone. The examiner then returns to the first cuneiform bone and moves laterally on the dorsal and plantar surface, palpating the second and third cuneiforms (Figure 13-109). Like the first cuneiform, the navicular and second and third cuneiform bones should be palpated on their dorsal and plantar aspects for signs of pathology such as fracture, exostosis, or **Köhler's bone disease** (osteochondritis of the navicular bone).

Moving laterally, the examiner palpates the three phalanges of each of the lateral four toes. Each of the lateral four metatarsals is palpated proximally to check for conditions such as **Freiberg's disease** (osteochondrosis of the second metatarsal head). Under the heads of the second and third metatarsals on the plantar aspect, the examiner should feel for any evidence of a callus, which may indicate a fallen metatarsal arch. Care must be taken to palpate the base of the fifth metatarsal (styloid process) and adjacent cuboid bone for signs of pathology. Also, the lateral aspect of the head of the fifth metatarsal may demonstrate a bunion similar to that seen on the first toe; this is called a tailor's bunion (see Figure 13-41).

In addition to palpating the metatarsal bones, the examiner palpates between the bones for evidence of pathology (e.g., interdigital neuroma) as well as the intrinsic muscles of the foot.

Medial Malleolus, Medial Tarsal Bones, and Posterior Tibial Artery. The examiner stabilizes the patient's heel by holding the calcaneus with one hand and palpates the distal edges of the medial malleolus for tenderness or swelling with the other hand. Moving from the distal extent of the medial malleolus along a line joining the navicular tubercle, the examiner moves along the talus until the head of the talus is reached. As the head of the talus is palpated, the examiner may evert and invert the foot, feeling the movement between the talar head and navicular bone. Eversion causes the talar head to become more prominent, as does pes planus. At the same time, the tibialis posterior tendon may be palpated where it inserts into the navicular and cuneiform bones. Rupture (third-degree strain) of this tendon leads to a valgus foot. The four ligaments that make up the deltoid ligament may also be palpated for signs of pathology.

Returning to the medial malleolus at its distal extent, the examiner moves further distally (approximately one finger width) until he or she feels another bony prominence, the sustentaculum tali of the calcaneus. This bony prominence is often small and difficult to palpate. Moving further posteriorly, the examiner palpates the medial aspect of the calcaneus for signs of pathology (e.g., sprain, fracture, tarsal tunnel syndrome). As the examiner moves to the plantar aspect of the calcaneus, the heel fat pad, intrinsic foot muscles, and plantar fascia are palpated for signs of pathology (e.g., heel bruise, plantar fasciitis, bone spur).

The examiner then returns to the medial malleolus and palpates along its posterior surface, noting the movement of the tibialis posterior and long flexor tendons (and checking for paratenonitis) during plantar flexion and dorsiflexion and noting any swelling or crepitus. At the same time, the posterior tibial artery, which supplies blood to 75% of the foot, may be palpated as it runs posterior to the medial malleolus. This pulse is often difficult to palpate in individuals with "plump" ankles and in the presence of edema or synovial thickening.

Anterior Tibia, Neck of Talus, and Dorsalis Pedis Artery. The examiner moves to the anterior aspect of the medial malleolus and follows its course laterally onto the distal end of the tibia. As the examiner moves distally, the fingers will rest on the talus. If the ankle is then plantar flexed and dorsiflexed, the anterior aspect of the articular surface of the talus can be palpated for signs of pathology (e.g., osteochondritis dissecans, talar dome fracture). As the examiner moves further distally, the fingers can follow the course of the neck of the talus to the talar head. Moving distally from the tibia, the examiner should be able to palpate the long extensor tendons, the tibialis anterior tendon, and, with care, the extensor retinaculum (Figure 13-110). If the examiner moves further distally over the cuneiforms or between the first and second metatarsal bones, the dorsalis pedis pulse (branch of the anterior tibial artery) may be palpated. It may be found between the tendons of extensor digitorum longus and extensor hallucis longus over the junction of the first and second cuneiform bones. If an anterior compartment syndrome is suspected, this pulse should be palpated and compared with that of the opposite side. It should be remembered, however, that this pulse is normally absent in 10% of the population.

Palpation Anteriorly and Anterolaterally

Lateral Malleolus, Calcaneus, Sinus Tarsi, and Cuboid Bone. The lateral malleolus is palpated at the distal extent of the fibula. It should be noted that the lateral malleolus extends further distally and lies more posterior than the medial malleolus. The examiner then stabilizes the calcaneus with one hand and palpates with the other hand, as done previously. As the examiner moves distally from the lateral malleolus, the fingers lie along the lateral edge of the calcaneus, which is palpated with care. At the same time, the peroneal tendons can be palpated as they angle around the lateral malleolus to their insertion in the foot and up to their origin in the peroneal muscles of the leg. The peroneal retinaculum, which holds the peroneal tendons in place as they angle around the lateral malleolus, is also palpated for tenderness (see Figure 13-110). While palpating the retinaculum, the examiner should ask the patient to invert and evert the foot. If the peroneal retinaculum is torn, the peroneal tendons will often slip out of their groove or dislocate on eversion (see Figure 13-53). While the lateral malleolus is being palpated,

the lateral ligaments (anterior talofibular, calcaneofibular, and posterior talofibular) should be palpated for tenderness and swelling (see Figure 13-1).

Returning to the lateral malleolus, the examiner palpates its anterior surface and then moves anteriorly to the extensor digitorum brevis muscle, the only muscle on the dorsum of the foot. By palpating carefully and deeply through the muscle, the examiner can feel a depression (the sinus tarsi) (Figure 13-111). If the fingers are left in the depression and the foot is inverted, the examiner will feel the neck of the talus, and the fingers will be pushed deeper into the depression. Tenderness in this area may indicate a sprain to the anterior talofibular ligament (see Figure 13-111), the most frequently injured ligament in the lower leg, ankle, and foot.

The cuboid bone may be palpated in two ways. The examiner may move further distally from the sinus tarsi (approximately one finger width) so that the fingers lie over the cuboid bone. Or the styloid process at the base of the fifth metatarsal bone may be palpated, and, as the examiner moves slightly proximally, the fingers will lie over the cuboid bone. In either case, the cuboid should be palpated on its dorsal, lateral, and plantar surfaces for signs of pathology.

Inferior Tibiofibular Joint, Tibia, and Muscles of the Leg. Starting at the lateral malleolus and following its anterior border, the examiner should note any signs of pathology. The inferior tibiofibular joint is almost impossible to feel; however, it lies between the tibia and fibula and just superior to the talus. The examiner then follows the shin, or crest, of the tibia superiorly, observing for

- Superior extensor retinaculum
- Tibialis anterior tendon
- Inferior extensor retinaculum
- Dorsalis pedis artery
- Extensor digitorum longus tendons
- Extensor hallucis longus tendon

A

- Tibialis anterior tendon
- Extensor digitorum longus tendons
- Superior extensor retinaculum
- Peroneus brevis tendon
- Peroneus longus tendon
- Inferior extensor retinaculum
- Superior peroneal retinaculum
- Inferior peroneal retinaculum

B

Figure 13-110 ▬▬▬
Retinaculum of the ankle. **A,** Anterior view. **B,** Lateral view.

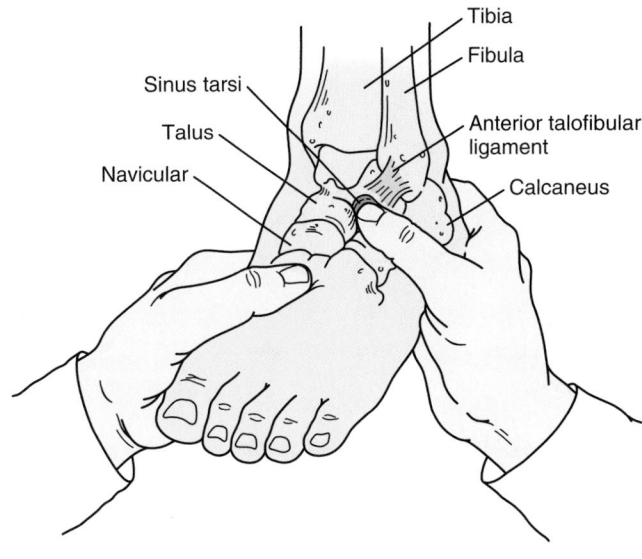

- Tibia
- Fibula
- Sinus tarsi
- Talus
- Navicular
- Anterior talofibular ligament
- Calcaneus

Figure 13-111 ▬▬▬
Palpation of the sinus tarsi and the anterior talofibular ligament.

signs of pathology (e.g., shin splints, anterior compartment syndrome, stress fracture). At the same time, the muscles of the lateral compartment (peronei) and anterior compartment (tibialis anterior and long extensors) should be carefully palpated for tenderness or swelling.

Palpation Posteriorly

The patient is then asked to lie in the prone position with the feet over the end of the examining table. The examiner palpates the following structures.

Calcaneus and Achilles Tendon. The examiner palpates the calcaneus and surrounding soft tissue for swelling (i.e., retrocalcaneal bursitis), exostosis (e.g., pump bump—Haglund's deformity), or other signs of pathology. In children, care should be taken in palpating the calcaneal epiphysis for evidence of **Sever's disease** (calcaneal apophysitis; Figure 13-112). Moving proximally, the examiner palpates the Achilles tendon, noting any swelling or thickening (e.g., paratenonitis,

retro-Achilles bursitis) or crepitation on movement. Any swelling caused by an intracapsular sprain of the ankle would also be evident posteriorly. Proximal to the Achilles tendon, the dome or superior surface of the calcaneus may also be palpated.

Posterior Compartment Muscles of the Leg. Moving further proximally, the examiner palpates the superficial (triceps surae) and deep posterior compartment muscles (tibialis posterior and long flexors) of the leg along their lengths for signs of pathology (e.g., strain, thrombosis).

Diagnostic Imaging

Plain Film Radiography

When viewing any radiograph, the examiner should look for changes and differences between the right and left lower legs, ankles, and feet, such as osteoporosis or alterations in soft tissue, joint space, and alignment. Both weight-bearing and non-weight-bearing views should be taken. Routinely, anteroposterior, lateral, and mortise views are taken.[8,159,160] However, x-rays should not be used indiscriminately and findings should be considered in conjunction with other clinical signs and symptoms.[161] Stiell and others have developed rules **(Ottawa ankle rules)** for the proper use of x-rays after ankle or foot injuries (Figure 13-113).[162–165] Leddy and

Figure 13-112

In Sever's disease (calcaneal apophysitis), there is fragmentation of the posterior apophysis off the calcaneus, causing achillodynia.
A, Lateral roentgenogram of a 10-year-old boy with pain around the insertion of the Achilles tendon. **B,** Axial view of the calcaneus. **C** and **D,** Representations of films A and B, respectively. (From Kelikian H, Kelikian AS: *Disorders of the ankle*, p. 121, Philadelphia, 1985, WB Saunders.)

Figure 13-113

Ottawa rules for ankle and foot radiographic series in ankle injury patients. Radiographic series are needed only if there is bone tenderness at **A, B, C,** or **D**; inability to bear weight, and malleolar or midfoot pain. Gray shaded areas show Buffalo modification.

associates modified these rules with the **Buffalo modification**.[166] In addition to the Ottawa rules, the Buffalo modification includes the crest (midportion) of the malleolus, proximal to the ligament attachments (see Figure 13-113). Ottawa ankle rules do not apply to people under the age of 18, in the presence of multiple painful injury, head injury, intoxication, pregnancy, or neurological deficit.[93] Concern must also be given for the mechanism of injury. For example, snowboarders commonly fracture the lateral process of the talus. Thus, a history of falling while snowboarding with tenderness below the lateral malleolus would indicate the

need for an x-ray.[54] To be viewed properly, individual radiographs must be made of the ankle, lower leg, and foot (Figure 13-114).[8,24,167–170]

Ottawa Rules for Ankle X-rays (with Buffalo Modifications)

- Tenderness over lateral malleolus to 6 cm proximally
- Tenderness over medial malleolus to 6 cm proximally
- Tenderness over navicular
- Tenderness over base of fifth metatarsal

Kager's triangle

Figure 13-114

Radiographs of normal ankle. **A,** Anteroposterior view. Note tibiofibular overlap *(between arrows)*. **B,** Internal oblique (mortise) view. Arrow demonstrates alignment of lateral talus with posterior cortex of tibia. **C,** Lateral view. Note the presence of Kager's triangle with an intact Achilles tendon. (From Weissman BNW, Sledge CB: *Orthopedic radiology,* pp. 590-591, Philadelphia, 1986, WB Saunders.)

Anteroposterior View of the Ankle. The examiner notes the shape, position (whether the medial clear space is normal), and texture of the bones and determines whether there is any fractured or new subperiosteal bone. The **medial clear space** is the space between the talus and medial malleolus (Figure 13-115). It is normally 2 to 3 mm wide, and values greater than this indicate a lateral talar shift with disruption of the ankle mortise (e.g., fibular fracture)[110,161] with disruption of the deltoid and tibiofibular ligaments[171] and therefore of the tibiofibular syndesmosis.[8,102,108,172] The **tibiofibular overlap** or **tibiofibular clear space** (see Figure 13-114, *A*) should be at least 6 mm, and greater than 1 mm in the mortise view although any alteration and related injury has been questioned.[110,171,173] In addition, the configuration, congruity, and inclination of the talar dome in relation to the tibial vault above it should be noted, because it may indicate osteochondritis dissecans (Figure 13-116).[23] If epiphyseal plates are present, the examiner should note whether they appear normal. Any increase or decrease in joint space, greater reduction of the tibial overlap, widening of the interosseus space, and greater visibility of the digital fossa should also be noted.

Mortise View of the Ankle. With this view, the ankle mortise and distal tibiofibular joint can be visualized. To obtain this view, which is a modification of the anteroposterior view, the foot and leg are medially rotated 15° to 30°.

Figure 13-115

Syndesmotic radiographic criteria. A finding outside any of these criteria indicates a syndesmosis injury. **A,** Anteroposterior view. **B,** Mortise view. *A* = lateral border of posterior tibial malleolus; *B* = medial border of fibula; *C* = lateral border of anterior tibial tubercle.

Figure 13-116

Osteochondritis dissecans of the talus: medial lesion. **A,** Note the lucent lesion of the medial talar dome (*arrow*), the site of an osteochondral fragment. **B,** Corresponding coronal, volume gradient (TR/TE, 28/7; flip angle, 25 degrees) MR image shows the nondisplaced fragment. (From Resnick D, Kransdorf MJ: *Bone and joint imaging*, p. 808, Philadelphia, 2005, WB Saunders.)

Lateral View of Leg, Ankle, and Foot. With this view, the examiner notes the shape, position, and texture of bones, including the tibial tubercle (Figure 13-117). Any fracture, new subperiosteal bone, or bone spurs should be noted (Figure 13-118). The examiner must note whether the epiphyseal lines are normal and whether there is any increase or decrease in joint space. Although this view clearly shows the talus and calcaneus, there is overlap of the midtarsal, metatarsal, and phalangeal structures. On the lateral x-ray, the presence or absence of **Kager's triangle** (see Figure 13-114, *C*) may be used to

Criteria for Syndesmosis Injury[24,174]	
Medial clear space	>4 mm
Tibiofibular overlap	<2.1 mm ♀
	<5.7 mm ♂
Clear space between fibula and peronea incisura of tibia	<5.2 mm ♀
	<6.5 mm ♂
Medial clear space	>Superior clear space

Figure 13-117

Lateral view of the foot. **A,** Weight-bearing posture. The soft-tissue pads are flattened beneath the heel and in the forepart of the foot, and the first metatarsal head is elevated by the sesamoids beneath it. **B,** Non-weight-bearing posture. The bony alignment and configuration are satisfactory, but the lack of resistance from the floor to the body weight permits variations, which make such views unsatisfactory for determining foot contours. (From Jahss MH: *Disorders of the foot*, pp 68, 72, Philadelphia, 1991, WB Saunders.)

diagnose a ruptured Achilles tendon.[175] When viewing lateral films, the examiner must also be aware of Sever's disease and Köhler's disease (Figure 13-119). The presence of a **Haglund deformity** (abnormally enlarged posterosuperior aspect of calcaneus) or "pump bump" (abnormally large calcaneal protuberance as a result of retrocalcaneal bursitis and thickened Achilles tendon) can be determined by measuring parallel pitch lines (Figure 13-120).[29,30] Fowler and Phillip also used the posterior calcaneal angle to determine the same measurement (see Figure 13-120, *B*).[29,30,176]

Dorsoplanar View of the Foot. The dorsoplanar view is used primarily to project the forefoot. As with the previous views, the examiner should note the position, shape, and texture of the bones of the foot (Figure 13-121). The presence of a metatarsus primus varus or a condition such as Köhler's disease should be noted.

Medial Oblique View of the Foot. This view is often taken because it gives the clearest picture of the tarsal bones and joints and the metatarsal shafts and bases (Figures 13-122 and 13-123). The medial oblique view shows any pathology in the calcaneocuboid joint as well as the presence of a calcaneonavicular bar (Figures 13-124 and 13-125).

Stress Oblique View. The examiner should note whether there is a calcaneonavicular bar or abnormality of the calcaneus or navicular bones.

Stress Film. The stress radiograph is used to compare the two ankles for integrity of the ligaments (Figures 13-126 and 13-127).[95,143,177–181] Anteroposterior views are most commonly used. With the application of an eversion or abduction stress, tilting of the talus by more than 10° is considered pathological.[182] An increase in the medial clear space (space between medial malleolus and talus) of more than 2 to 3 mm is considered pathological and usually indicates insufficiency of the deltoid ligament, especially the tibiotalar ligament. Instability may also be demonstrated by widening of the syndesmosis (the mortise between the tibia and fibula). An inversion or adduction stress causing 8° to 10° more movement on one ankle than the other is considered pathological and is indicative of torn lateral ligaments. If the talus has not moved, or if it is fixed but its distal end is unduly prominent, subtalar instability is suggested.

Measurements on Plain Radiographs. Plain radiographs may be used to measure different angles and axes. For example, Figure 13-128 shows the ankle joint axis, and Figure 13-129 shows the subtalar joint axis. Figures 13-130 and 13-131 show various angles measured in the ankle and foot. These angles may change during development, so in some cases serial radiographs may be of benefit.[183]

Abnormal Ossicles or Accessory Bones. The foot often exhibits abnormal ossicles, and their presence may lead to incorrect interpretation of radiographic films (Figure 13-132). These bones are pieces of the prominences of

Figure 13-118

A, Talotibial spurs. **B,** Impingement occurs when foot is dorsiflexed. **C,** Heel spur. (**A** and **B** from O'Donoghue DH: *Treatment of injuries to athletes*, ed 4, p. 627, Philadelphia, 1984, WB Saunders.)

various tarsal bones that for some reason (e.g., fracture, secondary ossification center) are separated from the normal bone (e.g., os trigonum; Figure 13-133).[28,184] A sesamoid bone, on the other hand, is incorporated into the substance of a tendon, with one surface articulat-

ing with the adjacent bones. A sesamoid bone moves with the tendon and is found over bony prominences or where the tendon makes a change in direction. In addition to the normal sesamoid bones under the big toe, sesamoid bones may also be found in the tendons of peroneus longus and tibialis posterior. Abnormal ossicles are more likely to occur in the foot than anywhere else in the body.

Films Showing Bone Development. Like the bones of the hand, the bones of the foot form within a certain time period (Figure 13-134). However, because the foot is subjected to greater forces and environmental effects than the hand, it is not usually used to determine skeletal age. X-rays of the foot often show the developing bone deformities seen in clubfoot (Figure 13-135). Although not all of the bones are present at birth, a series of films will show differences when compared with films of normal feet.

Text continued on page 923

A **B**

Figure 13-119
Radiographs of the foot. **A,** Bilateral involvement with condensation in the early stage of Köhler's disease.
B, Same foot 2 years later shows restoration of contour on the way to completion. (From Jahss MH: *Disorders of the foot*, p. 608, Philadelphia, 1991, WB Saunders.)

A **B**

Figure 13-120
Quantitative evaluation of the shape and pitch of the os calcis. **A,** The parallel pitch lines (PPL) determine the prominence of the bursal projection *(BP)*. The lower PPL *(PPL₁)* is the base line, constructed as for the posterior calcaneal angle. A perpendicular *(d)* is constructed between the posterior lip of the talar articular facet *(T)* and the base line. The upper PPL *(PPL₂)* is drawn parallel to the base line at distance *d*. A bursal projection touching or below the PPL₂ is normal, not prominent, a −PPL. The pitch angle *(y)* is formed by the intersection of the base line *(PPL₁)* with the horizontal. **B,** The posterior calcaneal angle *(x)* of Fowler and Philip is that angle formed by the intersection of the base line tangent to the anterior tubercle **A,**[176] and the medial tuberosity *(M)* with the line tangent to the posterior surface of the bursal project *(BP)* and the posterior tuberosity *(P)*.

Continued

Figure 13-120 cont'd

C, Haglund syndrome is diagnosed on the lateral view of the heel by a +PPL; a cortically intact bursal projection; loss of the retrocalcaneal recess, indicating retrocalcaneal bursitis; thickening of the Achilles tendon, measuring over 9 mm at 2 cm above the bursal projection; loss of the sharp interface between the Achilles tendon and the pre-Achilles fat pad, indicating Achilles tendonitis; and convexity of the posterior soft tissues at the level of the Achilles tendon insertion, indicating superficial tendo Achilles bursitis. Clinically, this latter finding presents as a pump-bump. **D,** Patient with hypertrophic osteoarthritic spurring of the bursal projection. This bony projection displaces the Achilles tendon and adjacent soft tissues posteriorly and creates a pump-bump, which is prone to trauma if improper shoes are worn. Although this patient clinically had a pump-bump, it was produced by the posterior displacement of normal tissues at the level of a prominent bursal projection. (From Pavlov H et al: The Haglund deformity: initial and differential diagnosis, *Radiology* 144:85–86, 1982.)

Figure 13-121

Dorsoplanar view of the foot. **A,** Weight-bearing posture. The cuneiform-first metatarsal joint is clearly shown (*arrow*), as are the transverse intertarsal joints, in contrast to the non-weight-bearing radiographs.
B, Non-weight-bearing posture. The joint between the medial and middle cuneiforms is clearly shown; the other midtarsal joints are obscure.

C

Figure 13-121 cont'd
C, In this patient, note the subtle displacement of the second through fifth metatarsal bases. The medial edge of the second metatarsal base *(solid arrow)* is not aligned with the medial edge of the second cuneiform *(arrowhead)*. Fractures of the base of the second metatarsal bone and cuboid are evident *(open arrows)*. (**A** and **B** from Jahss MH: *Disorders of the foot*, pp 69, 71, Philadelphia, 1991, WB Saunders. **C** from Resnick D, Kransdorf MJ: *Bone and joint imaging*, p. 873, Philadelphia, 2005, WB Saunders.)

A   **B**

Figure 13-122
Metatarsals and phalanges. **A,** With the beam centered directly over the foot, the metatarsal bases and adjacent tarsal bones are shown much more clearly than in part B. **B,** Both feet are examined with the beam centered between the feet (right foot shown). Marked overlap of metatarsal bases and adjacent tarsal bones is shown. The midtarsal joint can be seen as a continuous line or cyma. (From Klenerman L: *The foot and its disorders*, p. 306, Boston, 1982, Blackwell Scientific.)

Figure 13-123
Fracture of the base of the fifth metatarsal. All fractures in this region have generally been referred to as "Jones fractures" after the original description put forth in 1902 by Sir Robert Jones, who personally sustained this fracture while dancing. Unfortunately, the persistence of this eponym has resulted in significant confusion in the management of these fractures, because at least two distinct fracture patterns occur at the base of the fifth metatarsal: avulsion fracture of the tuberosity at the attachment of the peroneus brevis, and transverse fracture of the proximal diaphysis, as shown here *(arrow)*. The management of these two types of fractures is distinctly different, because of the healing potential of the diaphyseal fracture is diminished and the rate of fibrous union or subsequent refracture is high. Inadequate initial treatment may contribute to nonunion or delayed union of the diaphyseal fracture, and thus this fracture must be distinguished from the less complicated, more proximal avulsion fracture. (From McKinnis LN: *Fundamentals of musculoskeletal imaging*, p. 397, Philadelphia, 2005, FA Davis.)

Figure 13-124

Diagrammatic representation of the types of union. **A,** Fibrous. **B,** Cartilaginous. **C,** Osseous. **D,** Prominent process on the calcaneus. **E,** Prominent process on the navicular. **F,** Separate calcaneonavicular ossicle (calcaneum secondarium). (From Klenerman L: *The foot and its disorders*, p. 336, Boston, 1982, Blackwell Scientific.)

Figure 13-125

Calcaneonavicular coalition or bar. **A,** Total bony union, as well as bony breaks on the upper surfaces of the navicular and talus. The head of the talus may well be small. **B,** Fibrous or cartilaginous, rather than osseous, union between the bones is shown with osteoarthritic changes of the opposing bone surfaces and an enlarged navicular. (From Klenerman L: *The foot and its disorders*, p. 340, Boston, 1982, Blackwell Scientific.)

Figure 13-126

Positive findings on diagrammatic stress radiographs. **A,** Abduction stress. **B,** Adduction stress. **C,** Increased (2 to 3 mm) medial clear space (lateral rotary stress).

Common Ossicles in the Foot

- Os trigonum (separate posterior talar tubercle)
- Os tibiale externum (separate navicular tuberosity)
- Bipartite medial cuneiform (separated into upper and lower halves)
- Os vesalianum (separate tuberosity of the base of the fifth metatarsal)
- Os sustentaculi (separate part of the sustentaculum tali)
- Os supranaviculare (dorsum of the talonavicular joint)

Arthrography

Arthrograms of the ankle are indicated whenever there is acute ligament injury, chronic ligament laxity, or indications of loose body or osteochondritis dissecans (Figures 13-136 and 13-137).[8,23,185,186] Leakage of the contrast medium indicates tearing of the joint capsule or capsular ligaments. Normally, the talocrural joint admits only about 6 mL of contrast medium.

Figure 13-127

Abnormal stress views: anterior talofibular and calcaneofibular ligament tears. Anteroposterior (**A**) and lateral (**B**) views of the right ankle showing hypertrophic lipping from the anterior tibia and talus. The syndesmosis is slightly wide. Comparison varus stress views of the right (**C**) and left (**D**) ankles show abnormal talar tilt on the right, particularly when compared with the normal left side. This is diagnostic of an anterior talofibular ligament tear on the right, with or without a calcaneofibular ligament tear. The anterior drawer test is abnormal on the right

Continued

Figure 13-127 cont'd

(E) compared with the left (F). Comparison can be made by noting the anterior shift of the midtalus in relation to the midtibia *(arrows)* on each side, the loss of parallelism of the subchondral cortices on the right, or the marked widening of the posterior joint space *(lines)* on the abnormal as compared with the normal side. This is consistent with an anterior talofibular ligament tear on the right. (From Weissman BNW, Sledge CB: *Orthopedic radiology*, p. 600, Philadelphia, 1986, WB Saunders.)

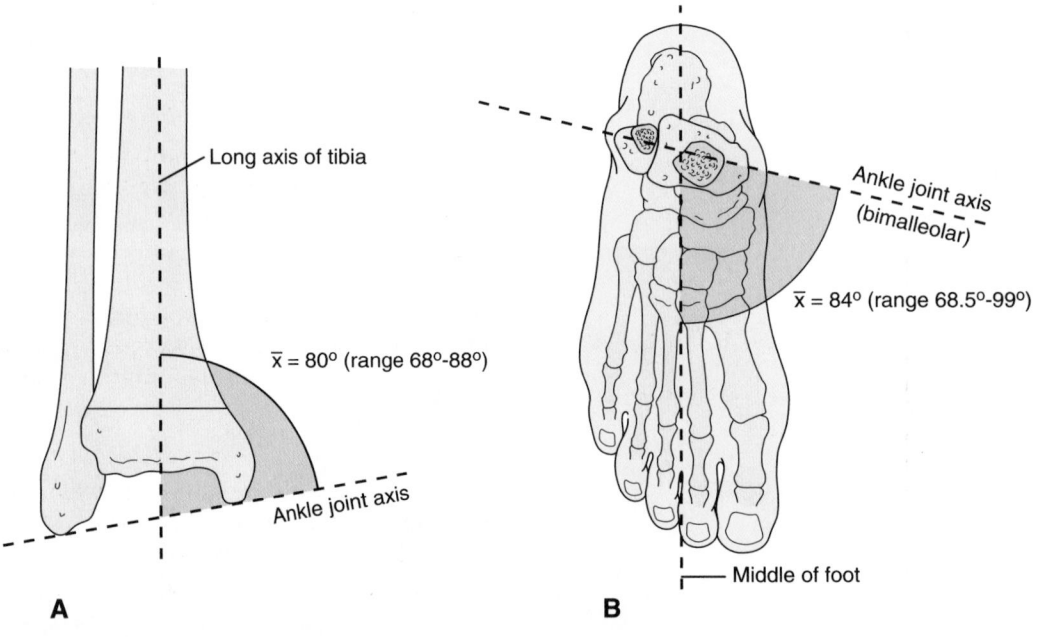

Figure 13-128

Orientation of the ankle joint axis. Mean values measure (A) 80° from a vertical reference and (B) 84° from the longitudinal reference of the foot. (Adapted from Hunt GC, editor: *Physical therapy of the foot and ankle*, New York, 1988; Churchill Livingstone; and Isman RE, Inman VT: *Anthropometric studies of the human foot and ankle: technical report No. 58*, San Francisco, 1968, University of California.)

Computed Tomography

Computed tomography scans are useful for determining the relation among the bones and for giving a view of the relation between bony and soft tissues (Figures 13-138 and 13-139).

Magnetic Resonance Imaging

Magnetic resonance imaging (MRI) is an especially useful, although sometimes overused, technique for delineating bony and soft tissues around the ankle and foot (Figures 13-140 to 13-143).[16] MRI may be used to diagnose

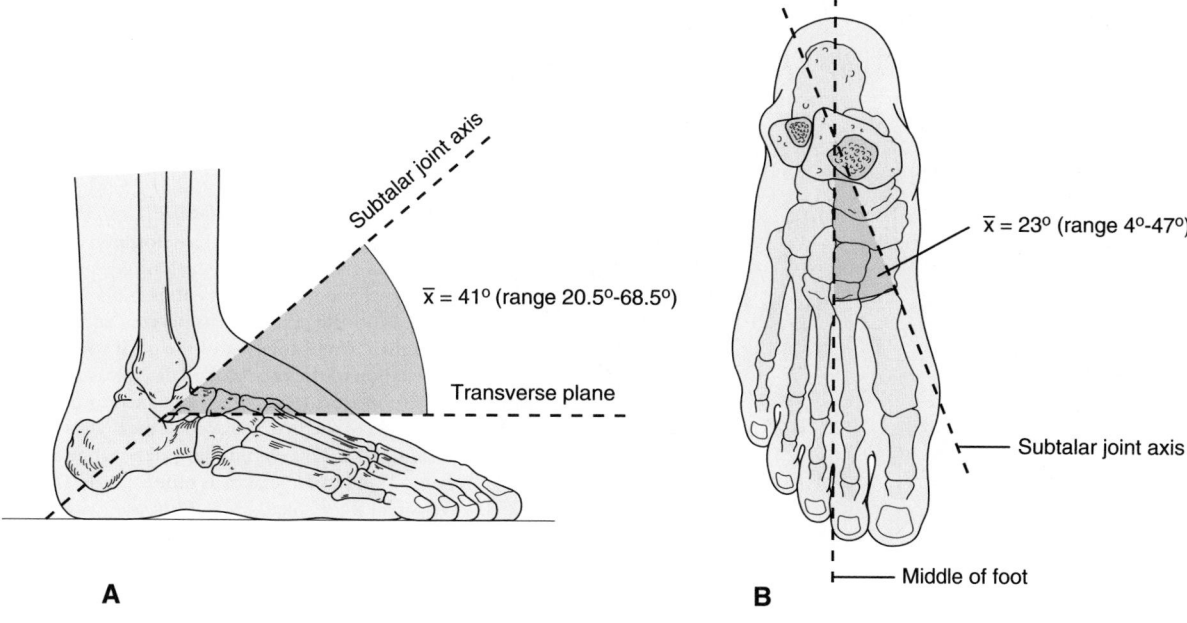

Figure 13-129

Orientation of the subtalar joint axis. Mean values measure **(A)** 41° from the transverse plane and **(B)** 23° medially from the longitudinal reference of the foot. (Adapted from GC Hunt, editor: *Physical therapy of the foot and ankle*, New York, 1988, Churchill Livingstone; and Isman RE, Inman VT: *Anthropometric studies of the human foot and ankle: technical report no. 58*, San Francisco, 1968, University of California.)

ruptured tendons (e.g., Achilles, peroneal), ligament tears (Figure 13-144), and fractures (e.g., osteochondral fractures, osteonecrosis).[187-195]

Bone Scans

Bone scans are used in the lower limb, ankle, and foot to diagnose stress fractures, primarily those of the tibia (Figures 13-145 and 13-146) and metatarsal bones.

Ultrasonography

This technique makes use of the ultrasonic waves to determine possible tissue injury. With an experienced operator, it may show injury to growth plates in the presence of a normal radiograph or prenatal pathology.[196,197]

Text continued on page 935

Figure 13-130

Angles of the foot. *1* = lateral talocalcaneal angle; *2* = calcaneal inclination angle; *3* = talar declination angle; *4* = talocalcaneal angle (two methods).

Figure 13-131

Measurement of hallux valgus deformity. On the left, the angle of intersection of the long axes of the proximal phalangeal and the first metatarsal shafts *(dotted lines)* is 40°. Normally, this angle is no greater than 10°. On the right, there is rotation of the great toe and lateral subluxation of the proximal phalanx, leaving about one half of the articular surface of the metacarpal uncovered. The angle of the first and second metatarsal shafts *(solid lines)* is 22°. On standing views, angles of greater than 10° indicate metatarsus primus varus. (From Weissman BNW, Sledge CB: *Orthopedic radiology*, p. 657, Philadelphia, 1986, WB Saunders.)

Figure 13-132

Accessory tarsal bones. *1* = os sesamoideum tibialis anterior; *2* = os cuneometatarsale I tibiale; *3* = os cuneometatarsale I plantare; *4* = os intermetatarsale I; *5* = os cuneometatarsale II dorsale; *6* = os unci; *7* = os intermetatarsale IV; *8* = os vesalianum; *9* = os paracuneiforme; *10* = os naviculocuneiforme I dorsale; *11* = os intercuneiforme; *12* = os sesamoideum tibialis posterior (according to Trolle, this may be the same as 15); *13* = os cuboideum secundarium; *14* = os peroneum; *15* = os tibiale (externum); *16* = os talonaviculare dorsale; *17* = os calcaneus secundarius; *18* = os supertalare; *19* = os trochleae; *20* = os talotibiale dorsale; *21* = os in sinu tarsi; *22* = os sustentaculi proprium; *23* = calcaneus accessorius; *24* = os talocalcaneare posterior; *25* = os trigonum; *26* = os aponeurosis plantaris; *27* = os supracalcaneum; *28* = os subcalcaneum; *29* = os tendinis Achilles. (Redrawn from Klenerman L: *The foot and its disorders*, p. 361, Boston, 1982, Blackwell Scientific.)

Figure 13-133
Lateral view of the ankle, showing the os trigonum (**A**) and
Stieda's process (**B**). (Redrawn from Brodsky AE, Khalil MA: Talar
compression syndrome, *Foot Ankle* 7:338-344, 1987.)

Figure 13-134
Anteroposterior diagram of the foot showing the times of appearance
(in months) of the centers of ossification for boys (and for girls, in
parentheses). (Redrawn from Hoerr NL et al: *Radiographic atlas
of skeletal development of the foot and ankle*, Springfield, Ill, 1962,
Charles C Thomas, with kind permission of Charles C Thomas,
Springfield, Ill.)

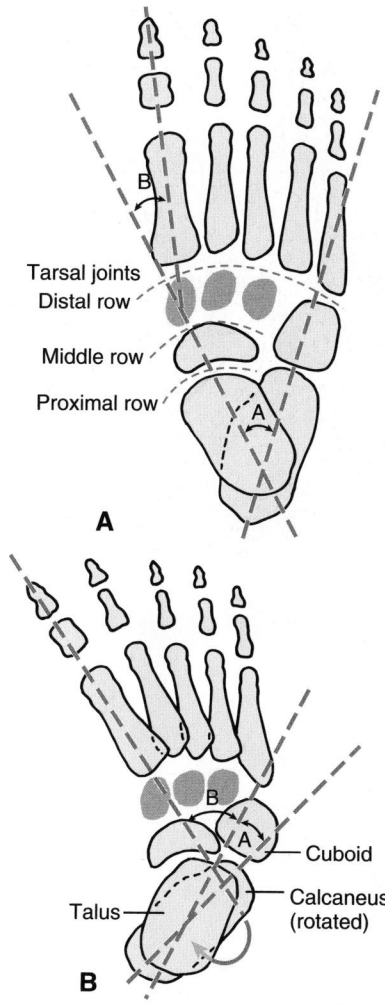

Figure 13-135
Representations of the foot as seen on radiographs. **A,** Representation
of the normal foot. The cuboid blocks medial movement of the
foot at the middle row of tarsal joints because of its unique location.
It alone occupies a position in both rows of tarsal joints. The
talocalcaneal angle (angle A) is measured by drawing lines through
the long axes of the talus and calcaneus. One should attempt to be as
accurate as possible in making these measurements. The normal range
for this measurement is 20° to 40° in the young child. The talus-first
metatarsal angle (angle B) is measured by drawing lines through
the long axis of the talus and along the long axis of the first metatarsal.
The normal range is 0° to −20°. **B,** Hindfoot varus, as manifested by a
decreased talocalcaneal angle (angle A), and talonavicular subluxation,
as manifested by a talocalcaneal angle of less than 15° and a talus-
first metatarsal angle (angle B) of more than 15°. Talonavicular
subluxation occurs through the medial movement of three bones,
which move as a unit. The navicular, cuboid, and calcaneus move
medially through the combined movements of medial translation and
supination of the proximal tarsal bones, whereas the calcaneus inverts
beneath the talus. (Redrawn from Simons GW: Analytical radiography
and the progressive approach in talipes equinovarus, *Orthop Clin
North Am* 9:189, 1978.)

Figure 13-136

Normal positive-contrast ankle arthrogram. Anteroposterior (A), internal oblique or mortise
B, and lateral **C,** views and a tomogram **D,** in the internal oblique projection show contrast agent
coating the articular surfaces and filling normally present anterior *(white arrows)*, posterior *(open arrow)*,
and syndesmotic *(black arrows)* recesses. There is no extension of contrast medium into the soft tissue
medially or laterally. (From Weissman BNW, Sledge CB: *Orthopedic radiology*, p. 596, Philadelphia, 1986,
WB Saunders.)

Figure 13-137

Contrast arthrography showing acute tear of the anterior tibiofibular ligament. **A,** Anteroposterior arthrogram of the right ankle 14 hours after the injury showing extravasation of contrast medium in front and around the lateral aspect of the fibula. **B,** Lateral view of the same. **C** and **D,** Illustrations of arthrograms A and B, respectively. (Modified from Kelikian H, Kelikian AS: *Disorders of the ankle*, p. 143, Philadelphia, 1985, WB Saunders.)

Figure 13-138

Normal anatomy of the ankle and foot as seen on computed tomography scans. **A,** Coronal section through the ankle and subtalar joint. T = talus, C = calcaneus, F = fibula. **B,** Farther anteriorly, the sustentaculum tali (S), the site of insertion of the talocalcaneal ligament (X), the subtalar joint (ST), and the mid-talocalcaneonavicular joint (t) are shown. **C,** Anterior to the sustentaculum tali, the talus (T) and the calcaneus C, are shown. **D,** The peroneus brevis (PB), peroneus longus (PL), posterior tibial (TP), and flexor digitorum longus (FDL) muscles are shown. AHL = abductor hallucis longus, FDB = flexor digitorum brevis, QP = quadratus plantae, AD = abductor digiti quinti pedis. This scan is at the level of the posterior aspect of the sustentaculum tali. (From Weissman BNW, Sledge CB: *Orthopedic radiology*, p. 632, Philadelphia, 1986, WB Saunders.)

Figure 13-139

Coronal computed tomographic view showing talocalcaneal coalition on the right. (From Rettig AC, et al: Radiographic evaluation of foot and ankle injuries in the athlete, *Clin Sports Med* 6:914, 1987.)

Figure 13-140

Sagittal and coronal magnetic resonance images of the ankle. **A,** Sagittal projection. Note the white bone marrow (BM) and subcutaneous fat (F), black tendons (T) and ligaments, gray muscles (M) and articular cartilage (C), and black cortical bone (B). **B,** Coronal projection. Note the black appearance of the deltoid ligament *(white arrow)* and interosseous ligament *(black arrowhead)* between the talus and calcaneus. (From Kingston S: Magnetic resonance imaging of the ankle and foot, *Clin Sports Med* 7:19, 1988.)

Figure 13-141

Magnetic resonance images showing partial Achilles tendon tear. Sagittal, proton-density (**A**) and T2-weighted magnetic resonance images (**B**) reveal a large tear at the Achilles insertion with intratendinous fluid *(long arrow)* and fraying and thickening of the distal tendon *(short arrow)*.

Continued

Figure 13-141 cont'd
C, Complete Achilles tendon tear. Sagittal, proton-density magnetic resonance image reveals disruption of the Achilles tendon *(long arrows)* and thickening of its distal portion *(short arrow)*. **D,** On an axial, T1-weighted magnetic resonance image, only gray granulation tissue is shown within the paratenon *(short arrow)*. The intact plantaris tendon passes along the medial border of the paratenon *(long arrow)*. (From Kerr R, et al: Magnetic resonance imaging of foot and ankle trauma, *Orthop Clin North Am* 21:593, 1990.)

Figure 13-142
Morton's neuroma. **A,** Coronal T1-weighted (TR/TE, 600/20) spin echo MR image shows a mass *(arrow)* of low signal intensity between the third and fourth metatarsal heads. **B,** This mass *(arrow)* has high signal intensity on a coronal fat-suppressed fast spin echo (TR/TE, 3500/50) MR image. A small amount of fluid may be present in the intermetatarsal bursa *(arrowhead)*. (From Resnick D, Kransdorf MJ: *Bone and joint imaging*, p. 1051, Philadelphia, 2005, WB Saunders.)

Figure 13-143

Appearance of normal ankle ligaments. **A,** The intact anterior talofibular ligament *(arrowheads)* is of low signal intensity on this T1-weighted transaxial image. Note the elliptical shape of the talus and the presence of the lateral malleolar fossa. **B,** Intact anterior *(arrowheads)* and posterior *(arrows)* tibiofibular ligaments are of uniform low signal intensity. The medial border of the lateral malleolus is flattened, indicating that this is the level of the tibiofibular ligaments. **C,** Intact tibiotalar component of the deltoid *(arrowheads)*. Note the osteochondral defect of the lateral talar dome. **D,** Posterior talofibular ligaments *(arrowheads)* on T1-weighted coronal image. The deltoid and posterior talofibular ligaments have a striated appearance rather than a homogeneous low-signal-intensity appearance like the anterior talofibular ligament. (© 2001 American Academy of Orthopaedic Surgeons. Reprinted from the *Journal of the American Academy of Orthopaedic Surgeons*, vol 9(3), pp. 187–199, with permission.)

Figure 13-144
Chronic tear of the anterior talofibular ligament. This transaxial T2-weighted image demonstrates the absence of the anterior talofibular ligament, with high-signal-intensity fluid *(arrows)* filling the expected location of the ligament. (© 2001 American Academy of Orthopaedic Surgeons. Reprinted from the *Journal of the American Academy of Orthopaedic Surgeons*, vol 9(3), pp. 187–199, with permission.)

Figure 13-145
Bone scan of whole body. Arrow indicates area of increased isotope uptake ("hot spot") in the right tibia, which is consistent with a stress-related lesion.

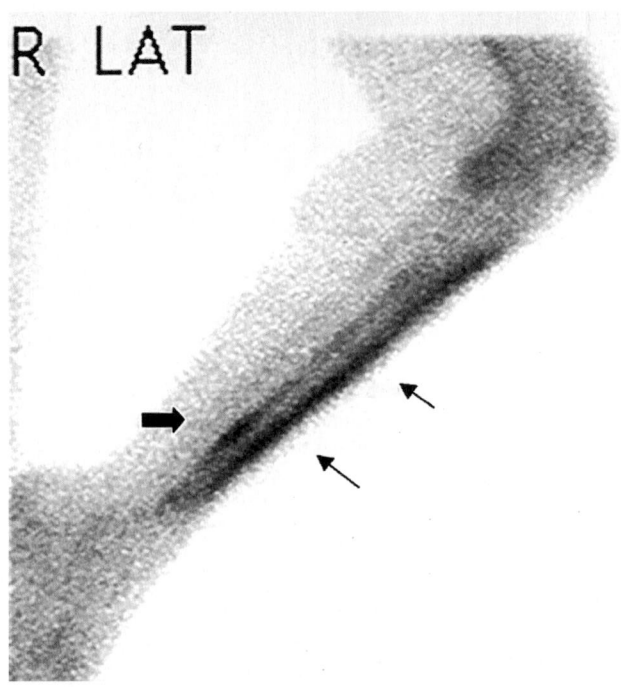

Figure 13-146
Stress fracture of the tibia and anterior shin splint. A short fusiform area of increased uptake in the posterior aspect of the distal shaft of the tibia represents a stress fracture *(large arrow)*. A long longitudinal area of increased uptake in the anterior aspect of the tibial shaft is consistent with a shin splint *(small arrows)*. (From Resnick D, Kransdorf MJ: *Bone and joint imaging*, p. 103, Philadelphia, 2005, WB Saunders.)

Précis of the Lower Leg, Ankle, and Foot Assessment*

History
Observation
Examination
  Active movements, weight-bearing (standing)
    Plantar flexion
    Dorsiflexion
    Supination
    Pronation
    Toe extension
    Toe flexion
  Active movements, non-weight-bearing (sitting or supine lying)
    Plantar flexion
    Dorsiflexion
    Supination
    Pronation
    Toe extension
    Toe flexion
    Toe abduction
    Toe adduction
  Special tests (sitting)
    Tibial torsion
  Passive movements (supine lying)
    Plantar flexion at the talocrural (ankle) joint
    Dorsiflexion at the talocrural joint
    Inversion at the subtalar joint
    Eversion at the subtalar joint
    Adduction at the midtarsal joints
    Abduction at the midtarsal joints
    Flexion of the toes
    Extension of the toes
    Adduction of the toes
    Abduction of the toes
  Resisted isometric movements (supine lying)
    Knee flexion
    Plantar flexion

    Dorsiflexion
    Supination
    Pronation
    Toe extension
    Toe flexion
  Special tests (supine lying)
    Neutral position of talus
    Anterior drawer sign
    Talar tilt
    Leg length
  Reflexes and cutaneous distribution (supine lying)
  Joint play movements (supine and side lying)
    Long-axis extension
    Anteroposterior glide
    Talar rock
    Side tilt
    Rotation
    Side glide
    Tarsal bone mobility
  Palpation (supine lying and prone lying)
  Special tests (prone lying)
    Neutral position of talus
    Leg heel alignment
    Foot-heel alignment
    Tibial torsion
    Thompson test
  Functional assessment (standing)
  Special tests (standing)
    Neutral position of talus
  Diagnostic imaging

---

*The précis is shown in an order that limits the amount of moving that the patient has to do but ensures that all necessary structures are tested. It does not follow the order of the text. After any examination, the patient should be warned of the possibility that symptoms will exacerbate as a result of the assessment.

Case Studies

When doing these case studies, the examiner should list the appropriate questions to be asked and why they are being asked, identify what to look for and why, and specify what things should be tested and why. Depending on the patient's answers (and the examiner should consider different responses), several possible causes of the patient's problem may become evident (examples are given in parentheses). A differential diagnosis chart should be made (see Table 13-15 as an example). The examiner can then decide how different diagnoses may affect the treatment plan.

1. A 38-year-old man ruptured his Achilles tendon 4 weeks earlier and had it surgically repaired. The cast has been removed. Describe your assessment plan for this patient.

2. A 24-year-old woman presents at your clinic with a painful left foot. There is no history of trauma; however, the pain has been present for approximately 6 years and has become worse in the past year. Describe your assessment plan for this patient (Morton's neuroma versus plantar fasciitis).

3. A 59-year-old man comes to you complaining of pain in his right calf and some numbness in his right foot. He also complains of some stiffness in his back. Describe your assessment plan for this patient (lumbar spondylosis versus tibial nerve palsy).

4. A 10-year-old boy recently had a triple arthrodesis for talipes equinovarus. The cast has now been removed. Describe your assessment plan for this patient.

5. A 16-year-old female volleyball player comes to you complaining of left ankle pain and difficulty

Case Studies—cont'd

walking after she stepped on another player's foot and went over on her ankle. The injury occurred 30 minutes earlier, and her ankle is swollen. Describe your assessment plan for this patient (malleolar fracture versus ligament sprain).

6. A 25-year-old woman tells you that she is training for a marathon but that every time she increases her mileage, her right foot hurts. Some time ago, someone told her she had a cavus foot. Describe your assessment plan for this patient.

7. Parents bring a 2-year-old boy to you and express concern that the child appears to have flat feet and "pigeon toes." Describe your assessment plan for this patient.

8. A 32-year-old woman comes to you complaining of ankle pain. She states that she sprained it 9 months earlier and thought it was better. However, she has now returned to training, and the ankle is bothering her. Describe your assessment plan for this patient (proprioceptive loss versus instability).

Table 13-15

Differential Diagnosis of Lower Leg Compartment Syndrome

	Compartment Syndrome	Shin Splints*	Stress Fracture*	Tumor
Pain (type)	Severe cramping, diffuse pain, and tightness	Diffuse along medial two thirds of tibial border	Deep, nagging localized with minimal radiation	Deep, nagging (bone) with some radiation
Pain with rest	Decreases or disappears	Decreases or disappears	Present, especially night pain	Present, often night pain
Pain with activity	Increases	Increases	Present (may increase)	Present
Pain with warm-up	May increase or become present	May disappear	Unilateral	Unaltered
Range of motion	Limited in acute phase	Limited	Normal	Normal
Onset	Gradual to sudden	Gradual	Gradual	?
Altered sensation	Sometimes	No	No	Sometimes
Muscle weakness or paralysis	Maybe	No	No	Not usually
Stretching	Increases pain	Increases pain	Minimal pain alteration	No increase in pain
Radiography	Normal	Normal	Early, negative; late, positive (?)	Usually positive
Bone scan	Negative	Periosteal uptake	Positive	Positive
Pulse	Affected sometimes	Normal	Normal	Normal
Palpation	Tender, tight compartment	Diffuse tenderness	Point tenderness	Point or diffuse tenderness
Cause	Muscle expansion	Overuse	Overuse	?
Duration and recovery	None without surgery	None without rest	Up to 3 months	None without treatment

From Magee DJ: *Sports physiotherapy manual*, Edmonton, 1988, University of Alberta Bookstore.
*These two conditions are different stages of tibial stress syndrome.

References

To enhance this text and add value for the reader, all references have been incorporated into a CD-ROM that is provided with this text. The reader can view the reference source and access it online whenever possible. There are a total of 210 cited references and other general references for this chapter.

APPENDIX 13-1

Reliability, Validity, Specificity, and Sensitivity of Special/Diagnostic Tests Used in the Lower Leg, Ankle and Foot

ANKLE METER (ANTERIOR DRAWER)

Validity

- Radiography and ATD measurements r = 0.91[198]

ARCH INDEX

Reliability	**Validity**
- Test-retest ICC = 0.99[199]	- Validity correlation with radiographic measurements r = 0.514 – 0.708[199]

DERIFIELD-THOMPSON TEST

Reliability

- Intrarater (differences in mean values <1.46 mm); interrater (differences in mean values <2 mm)[200]

DISTAL TIBIOFIBULAR COMPRESSION TEST

Reliability

- Interrater k = 0.50[101]

EXTERNAL ROTATION STRESS TEST

Reliability

- Interrater k = 0.75[101]

FIGURE-OF-EIGHT METHOD (FOR EDEMA)

Reliability

- Interrater ICC = 0.99, intrarater ICC = 0.99[120]

FOOT POSTURE INDEX

Reliability	**Validity**
- Test-retest ICC = 0.61[199]	- Validity correlation with radiographic measurements r = 0.360 – 0.593[199]

FOREFOOT-HEEL ALIGNMENT

Reliability

- Intrarater ICC = 0.88, interrater ICC = 0.86[201]

FUNCTIONAL ANKLE INSTABILITY QUESTIONNAIRE (FAI)

Validity

- FAI ankle had significantly greater AP displacement than uninjured (P = 0.040) and also had significantly greater anterior displacement in the radiography (P = 0.045)[202]

FUNCTIONAL LEG LENGTH

Reliability

- Standing intrarater ICC = 0.86, interrater ICC = 0.67[201]

Continued

APPENDIX 13-1—cont'd

LEG-HEEL ALIGNMENT (REARFOOT)

Reliability

- Intrarater ICC = 0.86[203]

MORTON'S TEST

Reliability	**Validity**
• Intrarater ICC = 0.06–0.47[204]	• Criterion validity – agreement between measurements with ruler and equipment ICC < 0.06[204]

MRI ANTERIOR TALOFIBULAR

Sensitivity

- 100%[205]

MRI POSTERIOR FIBULAR

Sensitivity

- 88%[205]

MRI POSTERIOR TALOFIBULAR

Sensitivity

- 100%[205]

MRI FOR LIGAMENT RUPTURE

Reliability

- Interrater k = 0.4, intrarater k = 0.6[205]

NAVICULAR DROP TEST

Reliability

- Intrarater ICC = 0.6 SEM = 2.57, interrater ICC = 0.57 SEM = 2.72[206]
- Intrarater ICC = 0.78 SEM = 1.68[74]
- Interrater subtalar joint neutral ICC = 0.77 (SEM = 3.33), relaxed standing foot posture ICC = 0.86 (SEM = 3.23), relaxed standing position with repalpation ICC = 0.90 (SEM = 3.06), single limb stance ICC = 0.84 (SEM = 3.20), as reported in the literature ICC = 0.71 (SEM = 2.62), with account of skin marking error ICC = 0.79 (SEM = 2.93), difference between bilateral standing in subtalar neutral position and single limb stance in relaxed standing posture ICC = 0.67 (SEM = 3.20)[75]
- Intrarater subtalar joint neutral ICC = 0.84 (SEM = 1.61), relaxed standing foot posture ICC = 0.92 (SEM = 2.09), relaxed standing position with repalpation ICC = 0.94 (SEM = 1.85), single limb stance ICC = 0.95 (SEM = 1.57), as reported in the literature ICC = 0.94 (SEM = 1.25), with account of skin marking error ICC = 0.90 (SEM = 1.89), difference between bilateral standing in subtalar neutral position and single limb stance in relaxed standing posture ICC = 0.87 (SEM = 2.04)[75]

NAVICULAR HEIGHT RADIOGRAPH

Reliability	**Validity**
• Test-retest ICC = 0.99[199]	• Validity correlation with radiographic measurements r = 0.437 – 0.792[199]

NEUTRAL POSITION OF THE TALUS

Reliability

- Interrater ICC = 0.76[207]
- Interrater ICC = 0.60[208]

NEUTRAL POSITION OF THE TALUS IN PRONE

Reliability

- Intrarater ICC = 0.06 SEM = 2.29, interrater ICC = 0 SEM = 2.51[206]
- Intrarater ICC = 0.77, interrater ICC = 0.25[209]
- Intrarater ICC = 0.67 SEM = 1.26[74]

NEUTRAL POSITION OF THE TALUS IN WEIGHT-BEARING POSITION

Reliability

- Intrarater ICC = 0.14 SEM = 2.46, interrater ICC = 0.15 SEM = 2.43[206]
- Intrarater ICC = 0.85 SEM = 1.1, interrater ICC = 0.79 SEM = 1.3[210]

NORMALIZED NAVICULAR HEIGHT RADIOGRAPH

Reliability	Validity
- Test-retest ICC = 0.98[199]	- Validity correlation with radiographic measurements r = 0.454 – 0.777[199]

CHAPTER 14

ASSESSMENT OF GAIT

Walking is the simple act of falling forward and catching oneself. One foot is always in contact with the ground, and within a cycle, there are two periods of single-leg support and two periods of double-leg support. With running, there is a period of time during which neither foot is in contact with the ground, a period called "double float."

Winter felt walking gait performs five main functions.[1] First, it helps to support of the head, arms, and trunk by maintaining a semirigid lower limb. Second, it helps to maintain upright posture and balance. Third, it controls the foot to allow it to clear obstacles and enables gentle heel or toe landing through eccentric muscle action. Fourth, it generates mechanical energy by concentric muscle contraction to initiate, maintain, and, if desired, increase forward velocity. Finally, through eccentric action of the muscles, it provides shock absorption and stability and decreases forward velocity of the body.

The locomotion pattern tends to be variable and irregular until about the age of 7 years.[2] Several functional tasks are involved in gait, including forward progression, which is executed in a stepping movement in a wide range of rapid and comfortable walking speeds. Second, the body must be balanced alternately on one limb and then the other; this is accompanied by repeated adjustments of limb length. Finally, there is support of the upright body.

Gait assessment or analysis takes a great deal of time, practice, and technical skill combined with standardization for the clinician to develop the necessary skills.[3–5] Most gait analysis today is performed with force platforms to measure ground reaction forces, electromyography to measure muscle activity, and high-speed video motion analysis systems to measure movement. Discussion of these techniques, however, is beyond the scope of this book. This chapter gives only a brief overview of a complex task, assessment of normal and pathological gait; detailed assessment of gait is left to other authors.[6–14] The various terms commonly used to describe gait, the normal pattern of gait, the assessment of gait, and common abnormal gaits are reviewed.

Definitions[5–10]

Gait Cycle

The **gait cycle** is the time interval or sequence of motions occurring between two consecutive initial contacts of the same foot (Figure 14-1). For example, if heel strike is the initial contact, the gait cycle for the right leg is from one heel strike to the next heel strike on the same foot. The gait cycle is a description of what happens in one leg. The same sequence of events is repeated with the other leg, but it is 180° out of phase.[8] Neumann clearly described the terminology that applies to the gait cycle events[15] (Figure 14-2). Table 14-1 demonstrates the periods or phases of the gait cycle, the function of each phase, and what is happening in the opposite limb.[8] The gait cycle consists of two phases for each foot: **stance phase,** which makes up 60% to 65% of the walking cycle, and **swing phase,** which makes up 35% to 40% of the walking cycle. In addition, there are two periods of double support and one period of single-leg stance during the gait cycle.

As the velocity of the cycle increases, the cycle length or stride length decreases. For example, in jogging, the gait cycle is 70% of the walking cycle, and in running,

Figure 14-1
Gait cycle, stride length, and step length.

the gait cycle is 60% that of walking.[16] In addition, as the speed of movement increases, the function of the muscles changes somewhat, and their electromyographic activity may increase or decrease. Generally, gait velocity decreases with age.[17] Montero-Odasso et al. found the gait velocity (<0.8 m/sec) could be used to determine mobility impairment in the elderly.[18]

Stance Phase

The stance phase of gait occurs when the foot is on the ground and bearing weight (Figure 14-3). It allows the lower leg to support the weight of the body and, by so doing, acts as a shock absorber while allowing the body to advance over the supporting limb.[16] Normally, this phase makes up 60% of the gait cycle and consists of five subphases, or instants.

Stages (Instants) of Stance Phase

- Initial contact (heel strike)
- Load response (foot flat)
- Midstance (single-leg stance)
- Terminal stance (heel off)
- Preswing (toe off)

The **initial contact** instant is the **weight-loading** or **weight acceptance period** of the stance leg, which accounts for the first 10% of the gait cycle. During this period, one foot is coming off the floor while the other foot is accepting body weight and absorbing the shock of initial contact. Because both feet are in contact with the floor, it is a period of **double support** or **double-leg stance**.

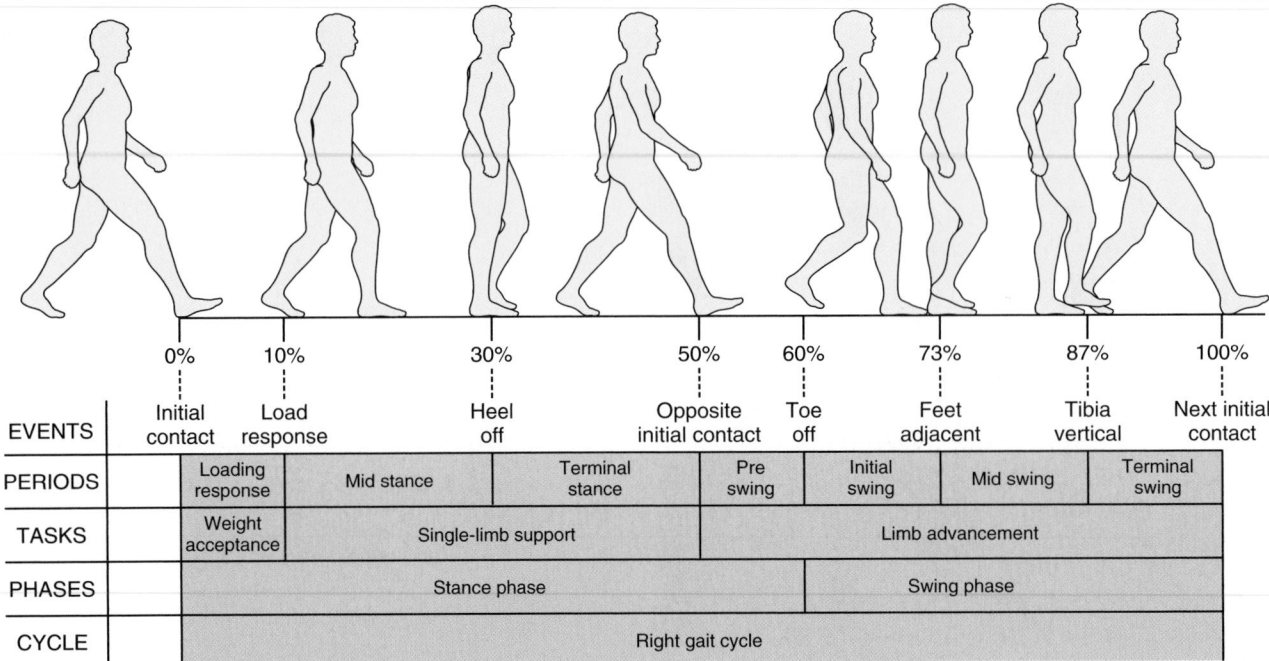

Figure 14-2

Terminology to describe the events of the gait cycle. *Initial contact* corresponds to the beginning of stance when the foot first contacts the ground at 0% of gait cycle. *Load response* occurs when the contralateral foot leaves the ground at 10% of gait cycle. *Heel off* corresponds to the heel lifting from the ground and occurs at approximately 30% of gait cycle. *Opposite initial contact* corresponds to the foot contact of the opposite limb, typically at 50% of gait cycle. *Toe off* occurs when the foot leaves the ground at 60% of gait cycle. *Feet adjacent* takes place when the foot of the swing leg is next to the foot of the stance leg at 73% of gait cycle. *Tibia vertical* corresponds to the tibia of the swing leg being oriented in the vertical direction at 87% of gait cycle. The final event is, again, initial contact, which in fact is the start of the next gait cycle. These eight events divide the gait cycle into seven periods. *Loading response*, between initial contact and opposite toe off, corresponds to the time when the weight is accepted by the lower extremity, initiating contact with the ground. *Midstance* is from opposite toe off to heel rise (10% to 30% of gait cycle). *Terminal stance* begins when the heel rises and ends when the contralateral lower extremity touches the ground, from 30% to 50% of gait cycle. *Preswing* takes place from foot contact of the contralateral limb to toe off of the ipsilateral foot, which is the time corresponding to the second double-limb support period of the gait cycle (50% to 60% of gait cycle). *Initial swing* is from toe off to feet adjacent, when the foot of the swing leg is next to the foot of the stance leg (60% to 73% of gait cycle). *Midswing* is from feet adjacent to when the tibia of the swing leg is vertical (73% to 87% of gait cycle). *Terminal swing* is from a vertical position of the tibia to immediately before heel contact (87% to 100% of the gait cycle). The first 10% of the gait cycle corresponds to a task of weight acceptance—when body mass is transferred from one lower extremity to the other. Single-limb support, from 10% to 50% of the gait cycle, bears the weight of the body as the opposite limb swings forward. The last 10% of stance phase and the entire swing phase advance the limb forward to a new location. (Modified from Neumann DA: *Kinesiology of the musculoskeletal system: foundations of physical rehabilitation*, St. Louis, p 532, 2002, Mosby.)

Table 14-1

Gait Cycle: Periods and Functions

Period	Percentage of Cycle	Function	Contralateral Limb
Initial double limb support	0–12	Loading, weight transfer	Unloading and preparing for swing (preswing)
Single limb support	12–50	Support of entire body weight: center of mass moving forward	Swing
Second double limb support	50–62	Unloading and preparing for swing (preswing)	Loading, weight transfer
Initial swing	62–75	Foot clearance	Single limb support
Midswing	75–85	Limb advances in front of body	Single limb support
Terminal swing	85–100	Limb deceleration, preparation for weight transfer	Single limb support

From Sutherland DH et al: Kinematics of normal human walking. In Rose J, Gamble JG, editors: *Human locomotion*, p 27, Baltimore, 1994, Williams & Wilkins.

| Initial contact | Loading response | Midstance (single-leg stance) | Terminal stance | Pre-swing |

Figure 14-3

Stance phase of gait.

The **load response** and **midstance** instants consist of the **single support** or **single-leg stance,** which accounts for the next 40% of the gait cycle. During this period, one leg alone carries the body weight while the other leg goes through its swing phase. The stance leg must be able to hold the weight of the body, and the body must be able to balance on the one leg. In addition, lateral hip stability must be exhibited to maintain balance, and the tibia of the stance leg must advance over the stationary foot.

The **terminal stance** and **preswing** instants make up the **weight-unloading period,** which accounts for the next 10% of the gait cycle. During this period, the stance leg is unloading the body weight to the contralateral limb and preparing the leg for the swing phase. As with the first two instants, both feet are in contact, so double support occurs for the second time during the gait cycle.

Swing Phase

The swing phase of gait occurs when the foot is not bearing weight and is moving forward (Figure 14-4). The swing phase allows the toes of the swing leg to clear the floor and allows for leg length adjustments. In addition, it allows the swing leg to advance forward. It makes up approximately 40% of the gait cycle and consists of three subphases.

| Initial swing (acceleration) | Midswing | Terminal swing (deceleration) |

Figure 14-4

Swing phase of gait.

Subphases (Instants) of Swing Phase

- Initial swing (acceleration)
- Midswing
- Terminal swing (deceleration)

Acceleration occurs when the foot is lifted off the floor. During normal gait, rapid knee flexion and ankle dorsiflexion occur to allow the swing limb to accelerate forward. In some pathological conditions, loss or alteration of knee flexion and ankle dorsiflexion leads to alterations in gait.

The **midswing** instant occurs when the swing leg is adjacent to the weight-bearing leg, which is in midstance.

During the final instant (**terminal swing** or **deceleration**), the swinging leg slows down in preparation for initial contact with the floor. With normal gait, active quadriceps and hamstring muscle actions are required. The quadriceps muscles control knee extension, and the hamstrings control the amount of hip flexion.

During running or with increased velocity, the stance phase decreases and a **float phase** or **double unsupported phase** occurs while the double support phase disappears (Figure 14-5).[16,19] Although the single-leg stance phase decreases, the load increases two or three times.[20] The motion occurring at each of the joints (pelvis, hip, knee, ankle) is similar for walking and for running, but the required range of motion (ROM) increases with the speed of the activity. For example, hip flexion in walking is about 40° to 45°, whereas in running it is 60° to 75°.[21]

Double-Leg Stance

Double-leg stance is that phase of gait in which parts of both feet are on the ground. In normal gait, it occurs twice during the gait cycle and represents about 25% of the cycle. This percentage increases the more slowly one walks; it becomes shorter as walking speed increases (Figure 14-6) and disappears in running.

WALKING

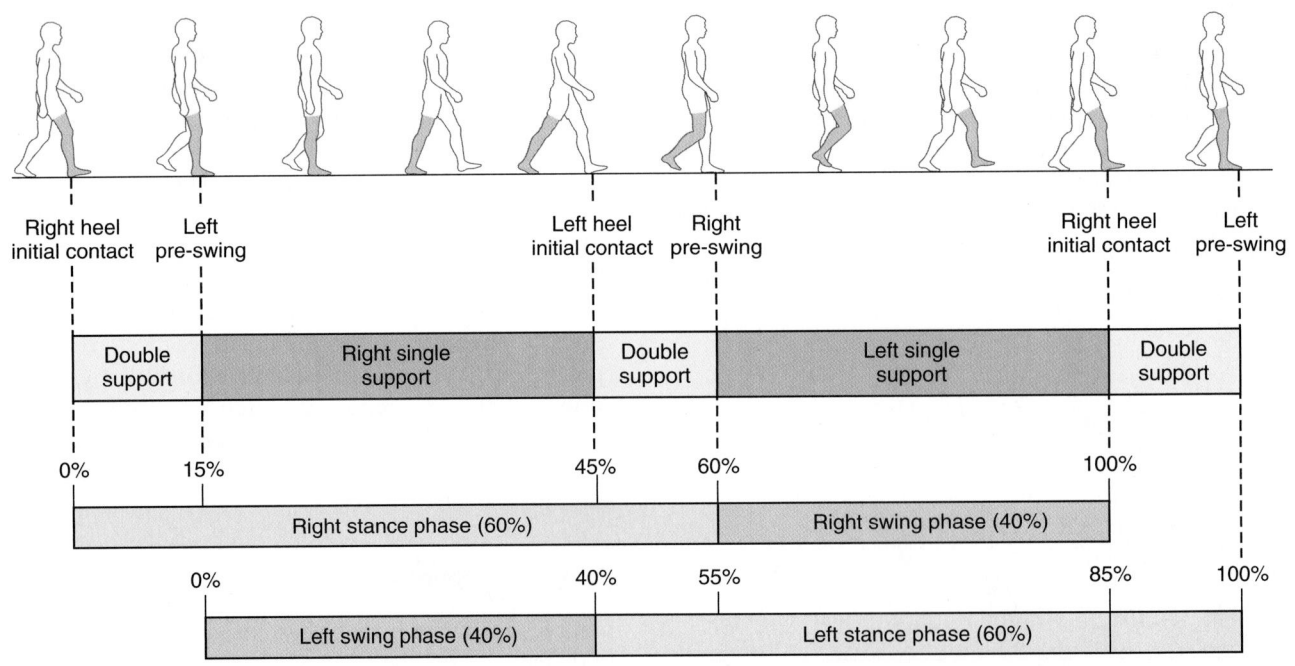

| Stance (65%) | | Swing (35%) |

Right heel strike · Mid stance · Foot off · Left heel strike

Right heel strike · Mid stance · Toe off · Double limb un-supported · Left heel strike · Mid stance · Double limb un-supported · Right heel strike

| Stance (40%) | Float (15%) | Swing (30%) | Float (15%) |

RUNNING

Figure 14-5

Comparison of the phases of the walking and running cycles.

Right heel initial contact · Left pre-swing · Left heel initial contact · Right pre-swing · Right heel initial contact · Left pre-swing

| Double support | Right single support | Double support | Left single support | Double support |

0% · 15% · 45% · 60% · 100%

| Right stance phase (60%) | Right swing phase (40%) |

0% · 40% · 55% · 85% · 100%

| Left swing phase (40%) | Left stance phase (60%) |

Time, percent of cycle

Figure 14-6

Time dimensions of the walking cycle. (Adapted from Inman VT, Ralston HJ, Todd F: *Human walking*, p. 26, Baltimore, 1981, Williams & Wilkins.)

Single-Leg Stance

The single-leg stance phase of gait occurs when only one leg is on the ground; this occurs twice during the normal gait cycle and takes up approximately 30% of the cycle.

Normal Parameters of Gait[7–11,22]

The parameters that follow and their values are considered normal for a population between the ages of 8 and 45 years. It should be pointed out, however, that a relatively normal gait pattern is seen in persons as young as 3 years of age.[2] There are, however, differences between individuals of the same sex and between men and women.[23] For the majority of the population outside of these ages, there are alterations caused by neurological development, balance control, aging, changes in limb length, and maturation.[2] For example, with maturity, walking velocity and step length increase, and cadence decreases.[24] It is also important to evaluate gait on the basis of normal gait for someone the same age. This is especially true for children.

> **Gait Parameters That are Significantly Decreased in Women Compared with Men[22]**
>
> - Velocity
> - Stride and step length
> - Proportional distance of center of gravity from ground
> - Sagittal hip motion
> - Knee flexion in initial swing
> - Width of base of support
> - Vertical head excursion
> - Lateral head excursion
> - Shoulder sagittal motion
> - Elbow flexion

Base (Step) Width

The normal base width, which is the distance between the two feet, is 5 to 10 cm (2 to 4 inches; Figure 14-7). If the base is wider, the examiner may suspect some pathology (e.g., cerebellar or inner ear problems) that results in poor balance, a condition such as diabetes or peripheral neuropathy that may indicate a loss of sensation, or

5-10 cm

Figure 14-7
Normal base width.

a musculoskeletal problem (e.g., tight hip abductors). In the first two cases, the patient tends to have a wider base to maintain balance. With increased speed, the base width normally decreases to zero, and in some cases, **crossover** occurs, in which one foot lands where the other should and vice versa. Such crossover can lead to gait alterations and other problems.[25]

Step Length

Step length, or gait length, is the distance between successive contact points on opposite feet (see Figure 14-1). Normally, this distance is about 72 cm (28 inches) being relatively constant for each individual (i.e., step length is commonly related to preferred walking speed)[15,26] and should be equal for both legs. It varies with age and sex, with children taking smaller steps than adults and females taking smaller steps than males.[20] Height also has an effect: a taller person takes larger steps. Step length tends to decrease with age, fatigue, pain, and disease. If step length is normal for both legs, the **rhythm of walking** will be smooth. If there is pain in one limb, the patient attempts to take weight off that limb as quickly as possible, altering the rhythm.

Normal Gait Parameters	
• Base width:	5-10 cm
• Step length:	approximately 72 cm
• Stride length:	approximately 144 cm
• Cadence:	90-120 steps/min
• Gait speed:	approximately 1.4 m/sec

Stride Length

Stride length is the linear distance in the plane of progression between successive points of foot-to-floor contact of the same foot. The stride length is normally about 144 cm (56 inches) and in reality is one gait cycle.[15] Stride length, like step length, decreases with age, pain, disease, and fatigue.[17,27] The age changes are often the result of decreased walking pace or speed.[27,28]

Lateral Pelvic Shift (Pelvic List)

Lateral pelvic shift, or pelvic list, is the side-to-side movement of the pelvis during walking. It is necessary to center the weight of the body over the stance leg for balance (Figure 14-8). The lateral pelvic shift is normally 2.5 to 5 cm (1 to 2 inches). It increases if the feet are farther apart. The pelvic list causes relative adduction of

Figure 14-8
Pelvic shift. Numbers indicate that one lateral or vertical shift occurs and then the other; they do not occur at the same time. *1* = right lateral shift; *2* = left lateral shift; *3* = right vertical shift; *4* = left vertical shift.

the weight-bearing limb, facilitating the action of the hip adductors. If these muscles are weak, a **Trendelenburg's gait** results (see Figure 14-18).

Vertical Pelvic Shift

Vertical pelvic shift keeps the center of gravity from moving up and down more than 5 cm (2 inches) during normal gait. By means of a vertical pelvic shift, the high point occurs during midstance and the low point during initial contact; the height of these points may increase during the swing phase if the knee is fused or does not bend because of protective spasm or swelling. The head is never higher during normal gait than it is when the person is standing on both feet. Therefore, if a person can stand in an opening, he or she should be able to move through the opening without hitting the head.[7] On the swing phase, the hip is lower on the swing side, and the patient must flex the knee and dorsiflex the foot to clear the toe. This action shortens the extremity length at midstance and decreases the center of gravity rise.

Figure 14-9
Pelvic rotation. Left forward pelvic rotation is illustrated.

Pelvic Rotation

Pelvic rotation is necessary to lessen the angle of the femur with the floor, and, in so doing, it lengthens the femur (Figure 14-9). The rotation decreases the amplitude of displacement along the path traveled by the center of gravity and thereby decreases the center-of-gravity dip. There is a total of 8° pelvic rotation, with 4° forward on the swing leg and 4° posteriorly on the stance leg. To maintain balance, the thorax rotates in the opposite direction. When the pelvis rotates clockwise, the thorax rotates counterclockwise, and vice versa. These concurrent rotations provide counterrotation forces and help regulate the speed of walking.

In the lower limb, rotation is evident at each joint. The farther the joint is from the trunk, the greater the amount of rotation. For example, rotation in the tibia is three times greater than rotation in the pelvis.[7]

Center of Gravity

Normally, in the standing position, the center of gravity is 5 cm (2 inches) anterior to the second sacral vertebra; it tends to be slightly higher in men than in women because men tend to have a greater body mass in the shoulder area. The vertical and horizontal displacements

of the center of gravity describe a figure eight, occupying a 5-cm (2-inch) square within the pelvis during walking. The vertical displacement, which describes a smooth sinusoidal curve during walking, can be observed from the side. The patient's head descends during weight-loading and weight-unloading periods and rises during single-leg stance.

Normal Cadence

The normal cadence is between 90 and 120 steps per minute.[29–31] The cadence of women is usually 6 to 9 steps per minute higher than that of men.[31] With age, the cadence decreases. Figure 14-10 illustrates the cadence of normal gait from heel strike to toe off showing the changing weight distribution. With pathology or deformity (e.g., a cavus foot), this weight-bearing pattern may be altered. As the pace of walking increases, the stride width increases, and the toeing-out angle decreases. Gait speed is about 1.4 m/sec (3 mph).[15]

Normal Pattern of Gait[6–11,15,29,32,33]

Stance Phase

As previously mentioned, there are five instants involved during the stance phase of gait. These are now described in order of occurrence. This phase is the **closed kinetic chain** phase of gait. The action occurring at the various joints causes a chain reaction because of the stresses put on the joints and supporting structures with weight bearing. The foot becomes the fixed stable segment, and alterations occur from the foot up, with the joints of the foot adapting first, followed by those of the ankle, knee, hip, pelvis, spine, and finally the upper limb, which acts as a counterbalance to movement in the lower limb.[34] The relations between the joints are constantly changing. Table 14-2 summarizes the movement at the hip, knee, ankle, and foot during the stance phase.[35]

Initial Contact (Heel Strike)
Initial contact occurs when the limb first strikes the ground. Normally, this occurs when the heel strikes and the limb is being prepared to take weight. During the initial contact, the pelvis is level and medially rotated on the side of initial contact, whereas the trunk is aligned between the two lower limbs. The hip is flexed 30° to 49° and is medially rotated; the knee is slightly flexed or extended; the tibia is laterally rotated; the ankle is at 90° with the foot supinated; and the hindfoot is everted. At this instant, there is little force going through the limb.

If pain occurs in the heel at this time, it may be caused by a heel spur, bone bruise, heel fat-pad bruise, or bursitis. This pain may cause increased flexion of the knee, with early plantar flexion to relieve the stress or pressure

Figure 14-10

The cadence of gait. **A,** Normal foot. **B,** Cavus foot. (From Viladot A: *Patologia del Antepié,* Barcelona, 1975, Ediciones Toray, SA.)

Table 14-2

Summary of Joint Motions at the Hip, Knee, Tibia, Foot, and Ankle during the Stance Phase of Gait

		Hip	
		Kinetic Motion	
Phase	**Kinematic Motion**	**External Forces**	**Internal Forces**
Heel strike	20° to 40° of hip flexion moving toward extension; slight adduction and lateral rotation	Reaction force in front of joint; flexion moment moving toward extension; forward pelvic rotation	Gluteus maximus and hamstrings working eccentrically to resist flexion moment; erector spinae working eccentrically to resist forward bend
Foot flat	Hip moving into extension, adduction, medial rotation	Flexion moment	Gluteus maximus and hamstrings contracting concentrically to bring hip into extension; erector spinae resisting trunk flexion
Midstance	Moving through neutral position; pelvis rotating posteriorly	Reaction force posterior to hip joint; extension moment	Iliopsoas working eccentrically to resist extension; gluteus medius contracting in reverse action to stabilize opposite pelvis
Heel off	10° to 15° extension of hip abduction, lateral rotation	Extension moment decreasing after double-limb support begins	Iliopsoas activity continuing
Toe off	Moving toward 10° extension, abduction, lateral rotation	Decrease of extension moment	Adductor magnus working eccentrically to control or stabilize pelvis; iliopsoas activity continuing

Table 14-2—cont'd

	Knee and Tibia			
	Kinematic Motion		**Kinetic Motion**	
Phase	**Knee**	**Tibia**	**External Forces**	**Internal Forces**
Heel strike	In full extension before heel contact; flexing as heel strikes floor	Slight lateral rotation	Rapidly increasing reaction forces behind knee joint causing flexion moment	Quadriceps femoris contracting eccentrically to control rapid knee flexion and to prevent buckling
Foot flat	In 20° flexion moving toward extension	Medial rotation	Flexion moment	After foot is flat, quadriceps femoris activity becoming concentric to bring femur over tibia
Midstance	In 15° flexion moving toward extension	Neutral	Maximum flexion moment	Quadriceps femoris activity decreasing; gastrocnemius working eccentrically to control excessive knee extension
Heel off	In 4° flexion moving toward extension	*Lateral rotation*	Reaction forces moving anterior to joint; extension moment	Gastrocnemius beginning to work concentrically to start knee flexion
Toe off	Moving from near full extension to 40° flexion	Lateral rotation	Reaction forces moving posterior to joint as knee flexes; flexion moment	Quadriceps femoris contracting eccentrically

	Foot and Ankle			
	Kinematic Motion		**Kinetic Motion**	
Phase	**Foot**	**Ankle**	**External Forces**	**Internal Forces**
Heel strike	Supination (rigid) at heel contact	Moving into plantar flexion	Reaction forces behind joint axis; plantar flexion moment at heel strike	Dorsiflexors (tibialis anterior, extensor digitorum longus, and extensor hallucis longus) contracting eccentrically to slow plantar flexion
Foot flat	Pronation, adapting to support surface	Plantar flexion to dorsiflexion over a fixed foot	Maximum plantar flexion moment; reaction forces beginning to shift anterior, producing a dorsiflexion moment	Dorsiflexion activity decreasing; tibialis posterior, flexor hallucis longus, and flexor digitorum longus working eccentrically to control pronation
Midstance	Neutral	3° of dorsiflexion	Slight dorsiflexion moment	Plantar flexor muscles (gastrocsoleus and peroneal muscles), activated to control dorsiflexion of the tibia and fibula over a fixed foot, contracting eccentrically
Heel off	Supination as foot becomes rigid for push-off	15° dorsiflexion toward plantar flexion	Maximal dorsiflexion moment	Plantar flexor muscles beginning to contract concentrically to prepare for push off
Toe off	Supination	20° plantar flexion	Dorsiflexion moment	Plantar flexor muscles at peak activity but becoming inactive as foot leaves ground

Modified from Giallonardo LM: Gait. In Myers RS, editor: *Saunders manual of physical therapy practice*, pp 1108–1109, Philadelphia, 1995, WB Saunders.

on the painful tissues. If the knee is weak, the patient may extend the knee by using the hand or may hit the heel hard on the ground to whip the knee into extension. A patient may do this because of weakness of the muscles (e.g., reflex inhibition, poliomyelitis, an internal derangement of the knee, a nerve root lesion [L2, L3, or L4], femoral neuropathy). In the past, this instant was referred to as "heel strike"; however, with some pathological gaits, heel strike may not be the first instant. Instead, the toes, the forefoot, or the entire foot may initially contact the ground. If the dorsiflexor muscles are weak, the foot drops, slaps, or flops down. The weakness may be caused by a peroneal neuropathy or nerve root lesion (L4). A knee flexion contracture or spasticity may cause the same alteration.

Load Response (Weight Acceptance or Foot Flat)

Load response is a critical event in that the person subconsciously decides whether the limb is able to bear the weight of the body. The trunk is aligned with the stance leg. The pelvis drops slightly on the swing leg side and medially rotates on the same side. The flexed and laterally rotated hip moves into extension, and the knee flexes 15° to 25°. The tibia is medially rotated and begins to move forward over the fixed foot as the body swings over the foot. The ankle is plantar flexed, and the hindfoot is inverted. The foot moves into pronation, because this position unlocks the foot and enables it to adapt to different terrains and postures. The forefoot is pronated, unlocking the subtalar and metatarsal joints to enable them to absorb the shock more effectively, and the plantar aspect is in contact with the floor.

Abnormal responses include excessive or no knee motion as a result of weak quadriceps, plantar flexor contractures, or spasticity.[9]

Midstance (Single-Leg Support)

The midstance instant is a period of stationary foot support. Normally, the weight of the foot is evenly distributed over the entire foot. The trunk is aligned over the stance leg, and the pelvis shows a slight drop to the swing leg side.

During this stage, there is maximum extension of the hip (10° to 15°) with lateral rotation, and the greatest force is on the hip. Painful hip, knee, or ankle conditions cause this phase to be shortened as the patient hurries through the phase to decrease the pain. If the gluteus medius (L5 nerve root) is weak, Trendelenburg's sign is present. The knee flexes, and the ankle is locked at 5° to 8° of dorsiflexion, rolling forward on the forefoot (roll-off). The foot is in contact with the floor; the forefoot is pronated, and the hindfoot is inverted. This instant is a critical event for the ankle. If pain is elicited during this period, the phase will be shortened and the heel may lift off early. This pain is commonly caused by conditions such as arthritis, rigid pes planus, fallen metatarsal or longitudinal arches, plantar fasciitis, or Morton's metatarsalgia. Therefore, pathology at the hip, ankle, or knee can modify the gait in this phase.

Terminal Stance (Heel Off)

In the final stages, the trunk is initially aligned over the lower limbs and moves toward the stance leg. The pelvis is initially level and posteriorly rotated and then dips to the swing leg side, remaining posteriorly rotated. The heel is in neutral and slight medial rotation; the knee is extended with the tibia laterally rotated. At the ankle, plantar flexion occurs as the critical event. This action helps to smooth the pathway of the center of gravity. The forefoot is initially in contact with the floor, and then the weight on the foot moves forward with plantar flexion so that only the big toe is in contact with the floor. At the same time, the forefoot moves from inversion to eversion.

Preswing (Toe Off)

The preswing phase is the acceleration phase as the toe pushes the leg forward. The trunk remains erect, the pelvis remains posteriorly rotated, and the hip is extended and slightly medially rotated. The knee flexes to 30° to 35° (critical event), and the ankle is plantar flexed. Because the center of gravity is anterior to the hip, the hip can be accelerated forward in initial swing.

If pain is elicited during this instant, it may be caused by a hallux rigidus, turf toe, or any other pathology involving the great toe (hallux), especially the metatarsophalangeal joint of the hallux. With injury to the joint, the patient is unable to push off on the medial aspect of the foot; instead, the patient pushes off on the lateral aspect of the foot to compensate for the painful metatarsophalangeal joint or, in some cases, a painful metatarsal arch resulting from increased pressure on the metatarsal heads. If the plantar flexors are weak (e.g., S1-S2 nerve root pathology), push-off may be absent. During this phase, the foot pronates so that there is a rigid base for better push-off.

During walking, a cane can be used to decrease the load on the limb. Lyu and associates have shown that using a cane in the contralateral upper limb,[36] if the cane tip touches the ground at the same time as the heel, can reduce the force at heel strike by 34%, by 25% at midstance, and about 30% at toe off.

Swing Phase

The swing phase of gait involves the lower limb in an **open kinetic chain;** the foot is not fixed on the ground, and the stresses on the limb are therefore less and easier to dissipate. During this phase, alterations occur from the spine down through the pelvis, hip, ankle, and foot. The

Table 14-3

Summary of Joint Motion and Forces during Swing Phase: Acceleration to Midswing and Midswing to Deceleration

Joint	Acceleration to Midswing		Midswing to Deceleration	
	Kinematic Motion	Kinetic Motion	Kinematic Motion	Kinetic Motion
Hip	Slight flexion (0° to 15°) moving to 30° flexion and lateral rotation to neutral	Hip flexors working concentrically to bring limb through; contralateral gluteus medius concentrically contracting to maintain pelvis position	Continued flexion at about 30° to 40°	Gluteus maximus contracting eccentrically to slow hip flexion
Knee	30° to 60° knee flexion and lateral rotation of tibia moving toward neutral	Hamstrings concentrically contracting	Moving to near full extension and slight lateral tibial rotation	Quadriceps femoris contracting concentrically and hamstrings contracting eccentrically
Ankle and foot	20° dorsiflexion and slight pronation	Dorsiflexors contracting concentrically	Ankle in neutral; foot in slight supination	Dorsiflexors contracting isometrically

From Giallonardo LM: Gait. In Myers RS, editor: *Saunders manual of physical therapy practice*, p. 1110, Philadelphia, 1995, WB Saunders.

pelvis and hip provide the most stability in the lower limb during the non-weight-bearing phase. Table 14-3 summarizes the motions occurring in the lower limb during the swing phase.

The three instants composing the swing phase of gait are now described in order of occurrence.

Initial Swing

During the first subphase of acceleration (Figure 14-11), flexion and medial rotation of the hip and flexion of the knee occur. The pelvis medially rotates and dips to the swing leg side. The trunk is aligned with the stance leg. In addition, the ankle continues to plantar flex. The foot is not in contact with the floor. The forefoot continues supinating, and the hindfoot continues everting. The dorsiflexor muscles of the ankle contract to allow the foot to clear the ground, and the knee exhibits its maximum flexion during gait of about 60°. If the quadriceps muscles are weak, the trunk muscles thrust the pelvis forward to provide forward momentum to the leg.

Midswing

During the midswing instant, the hip continues to flex and medially rotate, and the knee continues to flex. The ankle is in the anatomical or plantigrade position (90°) for the first 25% of the stance phase to permit the foot and midtarsal joints to unlock so that the foot can adapt to uneven terrain when it begins weight bearing. The forefoot is supinated, and the hindfoot is everted. The pelvis and trunk are in the same position as during the previous stage. If the ankle dorsiflexor muscles are weak

(e.g., drop foot), the patient demonstrates a **steppage gait** (see Figure 14-24). In such a gait, the hip flexes excessively so that the toes can clear the ground.

Terminal Swing (Deceleration)

During the final subphase, the hip continues to flex and medially rotate, and the knee reaches its maximum extension. At the ankle, dorsiflexion has occurred. The forefoot is supinated, and the hindfoot is everted. The trunk and pelvis maintain the same position as before. The hamstring muscles contract during the terminal phase to slow the swing; if the hamstrings are weak (e.g., S1-S2 nerve root lesion), heel strike may be excessively harsh to lock the knee in extension.

Joint Motion during Normal Gait

Although there is a tendency to talk about gait as action around joints, the examiner must not forget that muscles play a significant role in what happens at the joints. Table 14-4 illustrates the actions of some of the muscles used during gait.[37]

Hip. The function of the hip is to extend the leg during the stance phase and flex the leg during the swing phase. The ligaments of the hip help to stabilize it in extension. The hip extensors help to initiate movement, as do the hip flexors; both groups of muscles work phasically.[38] The hip flexors (primarily the iliopsoas muscle) contract to slow extension; the hip extensors (primarily the hamstring muscles) contract to slow flexion. In this way, they work eccentrically. The abductor muscles provide stability during single-leg support, a critical event for the hip.[38]

RANGE OF MOTION SUMMARY

	Weight Acceptance		Single Limb Support		Swing Limb Advancement			
Reference Limb	IC	LR	MSt	TSt	PSw	ISw	MSw	TSw
Opposite Limb	PSw	PSw	ISw/MSw	TSw	IC/LR	MSt	MSt	TSt
TRUNK	Erect →							
PELVIS	5° Fwd Rotation	5° Fwd Rotation	0°	5° Bkwd Rotation	5° Bkwd Rotation	5° Bkwd Rotation	0°	5° Fwd Rotation
HIP	25° Flex	25° Flex	0°	20° Apparent Hyperext	0°	15° Flex	25° Flex	25° Flex
KNEE	0°	15° Flex	0°	0°	40° Flex	60° Flex	25° Flex	0°
ANKLE	0°	10° Plantar Flex	5° Dorsiflex	10° Dorsiflex	20° Plantar flex	10° Plantar flex	0°	0°
TOES	0°	0°	0°	30° MTP Ext	60° MTP Ext	0°	0°	0°

Figure 14-11
Normal range of motion during gait cycle. IC = initial contact; LR = load response; MSt = midstance; TSt = terminal stance; PSw = preswing; ISw = initial swing; MSw = midswing; TSw = terminal swing. (Copyright 1991 LAREI, Rancho Los Amigos Medical Center, Downey, Calif 90242; from The Pathokinesiology Service and The Physical Therapy Department, Rancho Los Amigos Medical Center: Observational Gait Analysis. Downey, Calif, Los Amigos Research and Educational Institute, Inc., 1996, p. 30.)

Table 14-4

Muscle Actions during Gait Cycle

Phase of Gait	Mechanical Goals	Active Muscle Groups	Examples
Stance Phase			
Initial contact	Position foot, begin deceleration	Ankle dorsiflexors, hip extensors, knee flexors	Anterior tibialis, gluteus maximus, hamstrings
Loading response	Accept weight, stabilize pelvis, decelerate mass	Knee extensors, hip abductors, ankle plantar flexors	Vasti, gluteus medius, gastrocnemius, soleus
Midstance	Stabilize knee, preserve momentum	Ankle plantar flexors (isometric)	Gastrocnemius, soleus
Terminal stance	Accelerate mass	Ankle plantar flexors (concentric)	Gastrocnemius, soleus
Swing Phase			
Preswing	Prepare for swing	Hip flexors	Iliopsoas, rectus femoris
Initial swing	Clear foot, vary cadence	Ankle dorsiflexors, hip flexors	Tibialis anterior, iliopsoas, rectus femoris
Midswing	Clear foot	Ankle dorsiflexors	Tibialis anterior
Terminal swing	Decelerate shank, decelerate leg, position foot, prepare for contact	Knee flexors, hip extensors, ankle dorsiflexors, knee extensors	Hamstrings, gluteus maximus, tibialis anterior, vasti

From Rab GT: Muscle. In Rose J, Gamble JG, editors: *Human locomotion*, p. 113, Baltimore, 1994, Williams & Wilkins.

If there is loss of movement of the hip, the compensatory mechanisms are increased mobility of the knee on the same side and increased mobility of the contralateral hip. In addition, the lumbar spine shows increased mobility.

Knee. When the knee is in flexion during the first three instants of the stance phase of gait, it acts as a shock absorber. Painful knees are not able to do this. One of the critical events of the knee is extension. The functions of the knee during gait are to bear weight, absorb shock, extend the stride length, and allow the foot to move through its swing. The quadriceps muscles use only 4% to 5% of their maximum voluntary contraction to extend the knee, but in so doing, they help to control weight acceptance. The hamstring muscles flex the knee and slow the leg in the swing phase, working eccentrically.

If the knee has a flexion deformity, the hip is flexed and therefore loses its extension power, which is a critical event for the hip. Pathological conditions such as patellofemoral syndrome also cause deviations from normal gait. For example, patients with patellofemoral syndrome show less knee flexion during the single-leg stance phase, combined with lateral femoral rotation during the swing phase.[39] On heel strike to foot flat, the femur then medially rotates, and if this compensating medial rotation is too great, it causes excessive pronation, which then stresses the medial aspect of the patellofemoral joint.

Gastrocnemius and Soleus. The gastrocnemius and soleus muscles are important in gait. They use 85% of their maximum voluntary contraction during normal walking. These muscles help to restrain the body's forward momentum during forward movement. They also contribute to knee and ankle stability, restrain forward rotation of the tibia on the talus during the stance phase, and minimize the vertical pelvic shift, thereby conserving energy.[40] To accomplish these functions during gait, the triceps surae work eccentrically and concentrically.

Foot and Ankle. The foot and ankle play major roles in gait in that the various joints allow the foot to accommodate to the ground. The joints of the foot and ankle work interdependently during normal gait. When the heel contacts the ground, the lower limb becomes a closed kinetic chain, and movements and stresses must be absorbed by the structures of the lower limb.

When looking at the ankle, the examiner should observe immediate plantar flexion at initial contact. Loss of this plantar flexion (e.g., tibial nerve neuropathy) results in an inability to transfer weight to the anterior foot, increased ankle dorsiflexion, and increased knee flexion. In addition, the duration of single-leg stance on the affected side decreases, and the step length on the opposite side decreases. Furthermore, quadriceps action at the knee increases because of the lack of knee stability caused by the loss of the triceps surae, with the end result being that walking velocity decreases.[40] The foot then dorsiflexes through midstance or single-leg stance, with maximum dorsiflexion being reached just before heel off. The examiner should note whether there is sufficient plantar flexion during push-off.

Overview and Patient History

The assessment of a patient's gait should be included in any assessment of the lower limb. The examiner must keep in mind that the posture of the head, neck, thorax, and lumbar spine can affect gait even if no pathology is evident in the lower limb. The examiner must be able to identify the action of each body segment and note any deviation from normal during the individual phases of gait. For this reason, it is important to understand the normal parameters of gait and the mechanism of gait as it occurs. With this knowledge, the ways in which the gait is altered under pathological conditions can be better understood.

Musculoskeletal pathology tends to modify gait because of muscle weakness, pain, or altered ROM, so the examiner should watch closely for these factors when observing gait. Many patients can adapt automatically to these changes, provided they have normal sensation and can develop selective control.[9] Patients with upper motor neuron lesions have greater alterations and cannot easily adapt because, in addition to the musculoskeletal problems, they also present with spasticity, control problems, and sensory disturbances.[9] It is important that the examiner read the patient's chart and take a history from the patient regarding any disease or injury, past or present, that may be causing gait problems.

Observation

The examiner should first perform a general overview of the patient's posture, looking for any asymmetry, and then observe the patient's gait, looking at stride length, step frequency, time of swing, speed of walking, and duration of the complete walking cycle. This is normally done with the patient in shorts, wearing no shoes or socks. If gait is observed wearing shoes, the same shoes should be used for each test.[41] A steady gait pattern is usually established within three steps; it is initiated by the body's becoming unbalanced so that the patient can lift one foot off the ground to take the first step.[42] After this overview is completed, the examiner can look at specific parts of the gait in terms of phases and what happens at each joint during these phases.

Because gait constantly changes as one stops and starts, hurries, dawdles, and walks with others, it is important to remember whether the movements the patient is capable of are normal and whether the speeds, phases, strides, and durations of the cycles occur in normal combinations. In addition to observing walking at a normal speed, the patient's slow and fast gait speeds should be examined to see whether these changes affect the gait. The examiner must watch the upper limbs and trunk, as well as the lumbar spine, pelvis, hips, knees, feet, and ankles during these changes. Female patients should be in a bra and briefs, and male patients should be in shorts. The patient should walk barefoot. In this way, the motions of the toes, feet, legs, pelvis, trunk, and upper limbs can properly be observed.

The examiner should ask the patient to walk in the usual manner, using any aids necessary (e.g., parallel bars,

crutches, walker, canes). While the patient is walking, the examiner makes an initial general observation of any obvious limp or deformity.

The examiner should observe the gait from the front, from behind, and from the side, in each instance observing from proximal to distal and watching the pelvis and lumbar spine down to the ankle and foot as well as from the foot up. For example, in the swing phase (open kinetic chain) movement starts proximally and moves distally. In the stance phase (closed kinetic chain), movement is reversed, starting in the foot and moving proximally. The examiner should observe the movements in the trunk and upper limbs, which normally are in the opposite direction to those of the lower limbs. This method provides a sequential, thorough manner of assessment. Rancho Los Amigos Medical Center has developed a useful gait analysis chart (Figure 14-12). By using the chart during observation, the examiner can determine deviations and their effect on gait in an easily used and easily retained method of recording. The dark gray boxes indicate what normally should occur; the lighter gray and white boxes indicate minor and major deviations from the normal, respectively. Minor deviations imply that the functional task of walking is not affected. Major deviations imply that the mechanics of walking are affected adversely.[43]

Anterior View

When observing from the front as the patient walks, the examiner should note whether any lateral tilt of the pelvis occurs, whether there is any sideways swaying of the trunk, whether the pelvis rotates on a horizontal plane, whether the trunk and upper extremity rotate in the opposite direction to the pelvis, and whether reciprocal arm swing is present. Usually, the trunk and upper extremity rotation is approximately 180° out of phase with the pelvis—that is, as the pelvis and lower limb rotate one way, the trunk and upper limb rotate in the opposite direction. This action helps provide a balancing effect and smoothes the forward progression of the body. The examiner may also note movements at the hip (rotation and abduction-adduction), knee (rotation and abduction-adduction), and ankle and foot (amount of toe-out and toe-in, dorsiflexion-plantar flexion, supination-pronation). The examiner should note any bowing of the femur or the tibia, any medial or lateral rotation of the hips, femur, or tibia, and the position of the feet as the patient goes through the gait cycle (Figure 14-13). This view is best used to examine the weight-loading period of the gait cycle. The examiner should also note whether there is any abduction or circumduction of the swing leg, whether there is atrophy of the musculature of the anterior thigh and leg, and whether the base width is normal.

GAIT ANALYSIS: FULL BODY

RANCHO LOS AMIGOS MEDICAL CENTER
PHYSICAL THERAPY DEPARTMENT

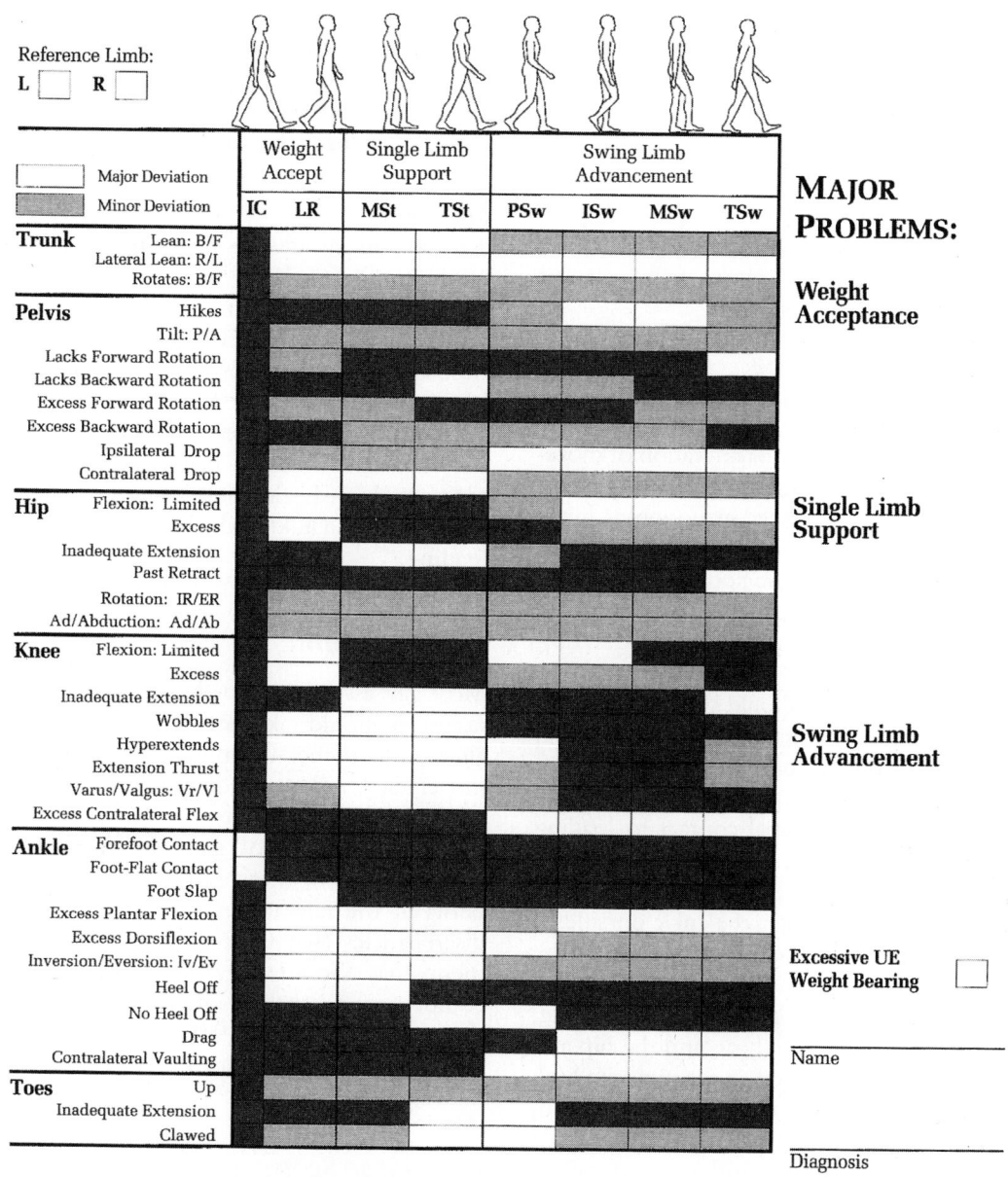

Figure 14-12

Gait analysis of the full body. (Copyright 1996 LAREI, Rancho Los Amigos Medical Center, Downey, Calif 90242; from the Pathokinesiology Service and the Physical Therapy Department, Rancho Los Amigos Medical Center: Observational Gait Analysis. Downey, Calif, Los Amigos Research and Educational Institute, Inc., 1996, p. 64.)

Lateral View

From the side, the examiner should observe rotation of the shoulder and thorax during the gait cycle, as well as reciprocal arm swing. Spinal posture (e.g., lordosis), pelvic rotation, and movements in the joints of the lower limbs should be noted. These movements include flexion-extension at the hip, flexion-extension at the knee, and dorsiflexion-plantar flexion at the ankle. From the lateral aspect, the examiner may also observe step length, stride length, cadence, and the other time dimensions of gait (see Figure 14-6).[33] This view allows observation of the interactions between the walking surface and the various body parts.

During stance and gait, the toes angle out 5° to 18° (Fick angle).

The examiner must remember that there may be some compensation by the lumbar spine for limitation of movement in the hip. The patient should be observed to determine whether there is sufficient knee extension at initial contact, followed almost immediately by slight flexion until the foot makes contact with the floor; whether there is control of the slightly flexed knee during load response and midstance; and whether there is sufficient flexion during preswing and initial swing. Also, any hyperextension of the knee during the gait cycle should be noted. Finally, the examiner should note whether there is coordination of movement among the hip, knee, and ankle; even or uneven gait length; and even or uneven duration of steps.

As the patient moves from initial contact to loading response, the foot flexes immediately, and the knee flexes until the foot is flat on the floor. During this period, the hip is also flexed. During midstance, the ankle dorsiflexes as the body pivots in an arc over the stationary foot. At the same time, the hip and knee extend, lengthening the leg. As the patient moves from terminal stance to preswing, the ankle plantar flexes to raise the heel, and the hip and knee flex as the weight is transferred to the opposite leg.

During the initial swing, the ankle is plantar flexed, and the hip and knee are maximally flexed. As the leg progresses to midswing, the ankle dorsiflexes, and the hip and knee begin to extend. As the patient moves from midswing to terminal swing, the ankle remains in the neutral position while the hip and knee continue extending. As the leg moves from terminal swing to initial contact, the knee reaches maximum extension; the ankle remains in neutral, and no further hip extension occurs at this stage.

Posterior View

When observing the gait cycle from behind, the examiner should notice the same structures that were viewed from the front. Rotation of the shoulders and thorax, reciprocal arm swing, and pelvic list and rotation may be noted

posteriorly, as well as hip, knee, ankle, and subtalar joint movement. Heel rise and base of support (base width) are easier to view posteriorly. Any abnormal abduction or adduction movements or lateral displacement of the body segments should be noted. This view is best to examine the weight-unloading period of the gait cycle. The examiner can note whether heel rise is equal for both feet and whether the heels turn in or out. The observation should also include lateral movement of the spine and the musculature of the back, buttocks, posterior thigh, and calf.

Footwear

The patient should be asked to walk in normal footwear as well as in bare feet. The examiner should take time to observe the patient's footwear and observe any wearing down of the heels or socks, the condition of the shoe uppers, creases, and so on. The feet should also be examined for callus formations, blisters, corns, and bunions. Different shoes can modify a patient's gait and the amount of energy necessary to perform gait. For example, high-heeled shoes alter movement, especially at the knee and ankle, which in turn increases the vertical loading.[44]

Examination

Most gait assessment involves observation. However, the examiner should take time, especially if he or she notices altered gait, to measure muscle strength (active and resisted movement) and range of movement (active and passive movement) at each joint involved in the gait cycle.

The parameters of gait (see normal parameters of gait) may also be measured to see if there are differences between the left and right gait cycles.[45,46] Leg length discrepancies (see Chapter 11 for leg length measurement) may also affect gait. Children tend to have better compensation mechanisms for leg length discrepancies than do adults.[47] Table 9-7 gives functional causes of leg length differences. Tables 11-10, 12-2, and 13-2 outline malalignments that may also affect gait.

Locomotion Scores

In addition to the detailed assessment of gait, locomotion scales or grading systems have been developed that include subjective and objective scores, which are combined for a total score. Figure 14-14 is a locomotion scoring scale that was developed for rheumatoid arthritis.[48] Figure 14-15 shows the modified Gait Abnormality Scale (GARS-M) for elderly people who may be at high risk to falling.[49–51] In addition to including all aspects of locomotion, it gives an overall estimation of functional disability for patients with rheumatoid arthritis. Wolf and associates reported on the Emory Functional Ambulation Profile and established its reliability and validity.[52,53] The profile

Detailed and Total Locomotion Score in Chronic Arthritis

UPPER EXTREMITIES

A.   Subjective score (max. 100 points)

1.   **Pain (max. 33 points)**   ___
   33   None at ordinary activity
   25   Mild, inconstant, unilaterally, not interfering with normal activity
   17   Mild bilateral or moderate unilateral, constant use of analgesics
   10   Moderate pain despite large doses of analgesics, affecting activity
   5   Severe pain despite large doses of analgesics, affecting activity
   0   Severe bilateral, unable to work and use walking supports, prevents physical activity

2–4.   **Pain score reduction**   ___
   −10%   Unilateral hand pain
   −25%   Bilateral hand pain
   −25%   Severe pain from both lower extremities or neck

   Sum: ___

ABILITY (max. 67 points)

Degree of disability

General (max. 20 points)	None	Mild	Moderate	Severe or unable	
5–6. Manage work, household routines, shopping, child care (min. 3 of 4)	8☐	6☐	3☐	0☐	R 5 / L 6
7–8. ADL (home and kitchen chore, personal care, dressing, etc.)	7☐	5☐	2☐	0☐	R 7 / L 8
9–10. Drive a car or use public transportation	5☐		2☐	0☐	R 9 / L 10

Special (max. 47 points)					
11–12. Feeding (hold knife, cup, open milk pack)	10☐	7☐	4☐	0☐	R 11 / L 12
13–14. Carry 3 kg burden	5☐		2☐	0☐	R 13 / L 14
15–18. Use telephone	5☐		2☐	0☐	R 15 / L 16
17–18. Comb hair, brush teeth, shave	5☐		2☐	0☐	R 17 / L 18
19–20. Wash the axillas	5☐		2☐	0☐	R 19 / L 20
21–22. Reach things over shoulder level	5☐		2☐	0☐	R 21 / L 22
23–24. Use of walking support(s)	12☐	7☐	4☐	0☐	R 23 / L 24

Sum: right ___   left ___   Both (R/2 + L/2) ___

SUBJECTIVE SCORE: (pain: ___, ability: ___)   _____

B.   Objective score—physical signs (max. 100 points)

		Right	Left
Shoulder (max. 35 points)			
25–26. Flexion:	>90° = 10p, 45-90° = 5 p, <45° = 0p	☐25	☐26
27–28. Extension:	>20° = 5p, 0-20° = 3p, 0° = 0p	☐27	☐28
29–30. Abduction:	>90° = 10p, 45-90° = 5p, <45° = 0p	☐29	☐30
31–32. Medial rot.:	>15° = 5p, <15° = 0p	☐31	☐32
33–34. Lateral rot.:	>10° = 5p, <10° = 0p	☐33	☐34
Elbow (max. 35 points)			
35–36. Flexion (from 90°):	>120° = 10p, 100-120° = 7p, 90-100° = 4p, 0° = 0p	☐35	☐36
37–38. Extension defect:	0-30° = 10p, 30-60° = 7p, 60-90° = 4p, 90° = 0p	☐37	☐38
39–40. Deformity: none + stable = 5p, rigid deformity = 2p, laxid = 0p		☐39	☐40
41–42. Varus-valgus: <5° = 10p, 5-10° = 7p stressed varus-valgus >15° = 3p, >25° = 0p		☐41	☐42
Wrist (max. 15 points)			
43–44. Deformity (rigid, laxid): none = 15p, mild = 10p, moderate = 5p, severe = 0p		☐43	☐44
Hand (max. 15 points)			
45–46. Deformity (rigid, laxid): none = 15p, mild = 10p, moderate = 5p, severe = 0p		☐45	☐46

Sum: right ___   left ___   Both (R/2 + L/2) ___

OBJECTIVE SCORE: ___   **SUBJ. + OBJ. SCORE:** ☐ **(a)**
                                  (upper extremities)

Figure 14-14 ▐▬▬▬▬▬▬▬▬▬

Locomotion scoring scale. (Modified from Larsson SE, Jonsson B: Locomotion score in rheumatoid arthritis, *Acta Orthop Scand* 60:272, 1989. © Munksgaard International Publishers, Ltd., Copenhagen, Denmark.)

Continued

measures different tasks and surfaces for stroke patients and can differentiate between those suffering from a stroke and normals. The profile does time trials and measures such things as a 5-meter (16.4 feet) walk on bare floor and carpeted floor, an "up and go" task, negotiating an obstacle course, and stair climbing. Other functional tests include the Get Up and Go Test,[54] the Functional Ambulatory Classification Scale,[55,56] and the Performance Oriented Balance and Mobility Assessment (POMA).[57]

Compensatory Mechanisms

The examiner must try to determine the primary cause of gait faults and the compensatory factors used to main-tain an energy-saving gait. The patient tries to use the most energy-saving gait possible.[58] Speed of walking can also modify many of the normal parameters of gait.[59] Therefore, not only the gait pattern but also the speed of the activity and its effects must be noted. This type of assessment allows the examiner to set appropriate goals and plan a logical approach to treatment.

Abnormal Gait

Gait deviations can occur for three reasons. First, they may occur because of pathology or injury in the specific joint (Table 14-5). Second, they may occur as compensations for injury or pathology in other joints on the same or ipsilateral

Detailed and Total Locomotion Score in Chronic Arthritis—(Cont'd)

LOWER EXTREMITIES

C. Subjective score (max. 100 points)

47. **Pain (max. 44 points)** ___
   44 None at ordinary activity
   40 Slight, occasional ache or awareness of pain, not influencing activity
   30 Mild bilateral or moderate unilateral, may take analgesics
   20 Moderate, affecting ordinary activities and work, consistent use of analgesics.
   10 Severe pain in spite of optimal medication
   0 Severe, preventing most of activity or patient bedridden

48–50. **Pain score reduction** ___
   −25% Moderate or severe pain from more than one ipsilateral joint
   −50% Moderate or severe pain from more than one contralateral joint
   −10% Severe pain from upper extremities or neck

Sum: ___

ABILITY (max. 56 points)

Walk (max. 36 points)

51. Limp: none = 12p, slight = 8p, moderate = 5p, severe =0p ☐

52. Support: none = 12p, cane for long walks = 8p, cane most of time = 5p
   one crutch or can't use = 3p, two canes = 2p
   two crutches or can't walk = 0p ☐

53. Distance: unlimited = 12p, >400m = 8p, <400m = 5p
   indoors only = 2p, bed or chair = 0p ☐

Special (max. 20 points)

54. Climb stairs: without difficulty = 6p ☐
   with difficulty or by using banister = 3p
   with great difficulty or unable = 0p

55. Shoes and socks: without difficulty = 6p, with difficulty = 3p, unable = 0p ☐

56. Sitting: without difficulty = 6p, only short time or on high chair = 3p, unable to use any chair = 0p ☐

57. Transportation: can use public transportation = 2p, unable = 0p ☐

Sum: pain: ___, **ability:** ___ (walk: ___, special: ___)

SUBJECTIVE SCORE: ___

D. Objective score—physical signs (max. 100 points)

			Right	Left
Hip (max. 35 points)				
58–59. Flexion:	>90° = 10p, 60–90° = 5p, <60° = 0p		☐58	☐59
60–61. Extension defect:	0-10° = 10p, 10–30° = 5p, >30° = 0p		☐60	☐61
62–63. Abduction/adduction:	>10° = 10p, −10–10° = 5p, <−10° = 0p		☐62	☐63
64–65. Rotation:	>0° = 5p, 0° = 0p		☐64	☐65
Knee (max. 35 points)				
66–67. Flexion:	>100° = 10p, 80–100° = 8p, 60–80° = 5p		☐66	☐67
68–69. Extension defect:	0° = 10p, 0–10° = 8p, 10–20° = 5p			
	20-30° = 2p, >30° = 0p		☐68	☐69
70–71. Varus-valgus:	<7° = 10p, 7–15° = 8p stressed v/v 15–30° = 5p, >30° = 0p		☐70	☐71
72–73. Deformity:	none + stable = 5p, rigid = 2p, laxid = 0p		☐72	☐73
Ankle (max. 15 points)				
74–75. Deformity (rigid, laxid): none = 15p, mild = 10p, moderate = 5p, severe = 0p			☐74	☐75
Feet (max. 15 points)				
76–77. Deformity (rigid, laxid): None = 15p, mild = 10p, moderate = 5p, severe = 0p			☐76	☐77

SUM: right: ___ **left:** ___ **Both (R/2 + L/2):** ___

OBJECTIVE SCORE: ___   **SUBJ. + OBJ. SCORE:** ☐ (b)
(lower extremities)

TOTAL LOCOMOTION SCORE: (a + b) ___

Figure 14-14 cont'd

side. Finally, they may occur as compensations for injury or pathology on the opposite or contralateral limb (Table 14-6).[15] Some of the more common gait abnormalities are discussed next, but this list is by no means inclusive.

Antalgic (Painful) Gait

The antalgic or painful gait is self-protective and is the result of injury to the pelvis, hip, knee, ankle, or foot. The stance phase on the affected leg is shorter than that on the nonaffected leg, because the patient attempts to remove weight from the affected leg as quickly as possible; therefore, the amount of time on each leg should be noted. The swing phase of the uninvolved leg is decreased. The result is a shorter step length on the uninvolved side, decreased walking velocity, and decreased cadence.[33] In addition, the painful region is often supported by one

hand, if it is within reach, and the other arm, acting as a counterbalance, is outstretched. If a painful hip is causing the problem, the patient also shifts the body weight over the painful hip. This shift decreases the pull of the abductor muscles, which decreases the pressure on the femoral head from more than two times the body weight to approximately body weight, owing to vertical instead of angular placement of the load over the hip. Flynn and Widmann have outlined some of the causes of a painful limp in children[60] (Table 14-7).

Arthrogenic (Stiff Hip or Knee) Gait

The arthrogenic gait results from stiffness, laxity, or deformity, and it may be painful or pain free. If the knee or hip is fused or the knee has recently been removed from a cylinder cast, the pelvis must be elevated by exaggerated

Text continued on page 964

MODIFIED GAIT ABNORMALITY RATING SCALE (GARS-M)

NAME _____ NO. _____ VISIT _____ DATE _____

1. VARIABILITY – A MEASURE OF INCONSISTENCY AND ARRHYTHMICITY OF STEPPING AND OF ARM MOVEMENTS

   0 = fluid and predictably paced limb movements
   1 = occasional interruptions (changes in velocity), approximately 25% of time
   2 = unpredictability of rhythm approximately 25%-75% of time
   3 = random timing of limb movements

2. GUARDEDNESS – HESITANCY, SLOWNESS, DIMINISHED PROPULSION, AND LACK OF COMMITMENT IN STEPPING AND ARM SWING

   0 = good forward momentum and lack of apprehension in propulsion
   1 = center of gravity of head, arms, and trunk (HAT) projects only slightly in front of push-off, but still good arm-leg coordination
   2 = HAT held over anterior aspect of foot, and some moderate loss of smooth reciprocation
   3 = HAT held over rear aspect of stance-phase foot, and great tentativity in stepping

3. STAGGERING – SUDDEN AND UNEXPECTED LATERALLY DIRECTED PARTIAL LOSSES OF BALANCE

   0 = no losses of balance to side
   1 = a single lurch to side
   2 = two lurches to side
   3 = three or more lurches to side

4. FOOT CONTACT – THE DEGREE TO WHICH THE HEEL STRIKES THE GROUND BEFORE THE FOREFOOT

   0 = very obvious angle of impact of heel on ground
   1 = barely visible contact of heel before forefoot
   2 = entire foot lands flat on ground
   3 = anterior aspect of foot strikes ground before heel

5. HIP ROM – THE DEGREE OF LOSS OF HIP RANGE OF MOTION SEEN DURING A GAIT CYCLE

   0 = obvious angulation of thigh backward during double support (10 degrees)
   1 = just barely visible angulation backward from vertical
   2 = thigh in line with vertical projection from ground
   3 = thigh angled forward from vertical at maximum posterior excursion

6. SHOULDER EXTENSION – A MEASURE OF THE DECREASE OF SHOULDER ROM

   0 = clearly seen movement of upper arm anterior (15 degrees) and posterior (20 degrees) to vertical axis of trunk
   1 = shoulder flexes slightly anterior to vertical axis
   2 = shoulder comes only to vertical axis, or slightly posterior to it during flexion
   3 = shoulder stays well behind vertical axis during entire excursion

7. ARM-HEEL STRIKE SYNCHRONY – THE EXTENT TO WHICH THE CONTRALATERAL MOVEMENTS OF AN ARM AND LEG ARE OUT OF PHASE

   0 = good temporal conjunction of arm and contralateral leg at apex of shoulder and hip excursions all of the time
   1 = arm and leg slightly out of phase 25% of the time
   2 = arm and leg moderately out of phase 25%-50% of the time
   3 = little or no temporal coherence of arm and leg

ROM = range of motion.

Figure 14-15

Modified Gait Abnormality Rating Scale (GARS-M). (From Dutton M: *Orthopedic examination, evaluation and intervention*, p. 389, New York, 2004, McGraw-Hill.)

Table 14-5

Gait Deviations Secondary to Specific Impairments*

Gait Deviations at the Hip/Pelvis/Trunk Secondary to Specific Hip/Pelvis/Trunk Impairments*

Observed Gait Deviation at the Hip/Pelvis/Trunk	Likely Impairment	Selected Pathological Precursors	Mechanical Rationale and/or Associated Compensations
Backward trunk lean during loading response	Weak hip extensors	Paralysis of poliomyelitis	This action moves the line of gravity of the trunk behind the hip and reduces the need for hip extension torque
Lateral trunk lean toward the stance leg; because this movement compensates for a weakness, it is often called a "compensated" Trendelenburg gait and is referred to as a waddling gait if bilateral	Marked weakness of the hip abductors	Guillain-Barré or poliomyelitis	Shifting the trunk over the supporting limb reduces the demand on the hip abductors
	Hip pain	Arthritis	Shifting the trunk over the supporting lower extremity reduces compressive joint forces associated with the action of hip abductors
Excessive downward drop of the contralateral pelvis during stance (referred to as a positive Trendelenburg sign if present during single-limb standing)	Mild weakness of the gluteus medius of the stance leg	Guillain-Barré or poliomyelitis	Whereas the Trendelenburg sign may be observed in single-limb standing, a compensated Trendelenburg gait often occurs when there has been severe weakness of the hip abductors
Forward bending of the trunk during mid and terminal stance, as the hip is moved over the foot	Hip flexion contracture	Hip osteoarthritis	Forward trunk lean is used to compensate for lack of hip extension; an alternate adaptation could be excessive lumbar lordosis
	Hip pain	Hip osteoarthritis	Keeping the hip at 30 degrees of flexion minimizes intraarticular pressure
Excessive lumbar lordosis in terminal stance	Hip flexion contracture	Arthritis	Lack of hip extension in terminal stance is compensated for by increased lordosis
Trunk lurches backward and toward the unaffected stance leg from heel off to mid swing	Hip flexor weakness	L2-L3 nerve compression	Hip flexion is passively generated by a backward movement of the trunk
Posterior tilt of the pelvis during initial swing	Hip flexor weakness	L2-L3 nerve compression	Abdominals are used during initial swing to advance the swing leg
Hip circumduction: semicircle movement of the hip during swing—combining hip flexion, hip abduction, and forward rotation of the pelvis	Hip flexor weakness	L2-L3 nerve compression	Hip abductors are used as flexors

Gait Deviations at the Knee Secondary to Specific Knee Impairments*

Observed Gait Deviation at the Knee	Likely Impairment	Selected Pathological Precursors	Mechanical Rationale and/or Associated Compensations
Rapid extension of the knee (knee extensor thrust) immediately after initial contact	Spasticity of the quadriceps	Upper motor neuron lesion	Depending on the status of the posterior structures of the knee, may occur with or without knee hyperextension

Observed Gait Deviation	Likely Impairment	Selected Pathological Precursors	Mechanical Rationale and/or Associated Compensations
Knee remains extended during the loading response, but there is no extensor thrust	Weak quadriceps	Femoral nerve palsy, L3-L4 compression neuropathy	Knee remains fully extended throughout stance. An associated anterior trunk lean in the early part of stance moves the line of gravity of the trunk, slightly anterior to the axis of rotation of the knee, which keeps the knee extended without action of the knee extensors; this gait deviation may lead to an excessive stretching of the posterior capsule of the knee and eventual knee hyperextension (genu recurvatum) during stance
	Knee pain	Arthritis	Knee is kept in extension to reduce the need for quadriceps activity and associated compressive forces; it may be accompanied by an antalgic gait pattern characterized by a reduced stance time and shorter step length
Genu recurvatum (hyperextension) during stance	Knee extensor weakness (see the two previously described gait deviations)	Poliomyelitis	Secondary to progressive stretching of the posterior capsule of the knee
Varus thrust during stance	Laxity of the posterior and lateral ligamentous joint structures of the knee	Traumatic injury or progressive laxity	Rapid varus deviation of the knee during mid stance, typically accompanied by knee hyperextension
Flexed position of the knee during stance and lack of knee extension in terminal swing	Knee flexion contracture >10° (genu flexum) Hamstring overactivity (spasticity)	Upper motor neuron lesion	Associated increase in hip flexion and ankle dorsiflexion during stance
	Knee pain and joint effusion	Trauma or arthritis	Knee is kept in flexion since this is the position of lowest intraarticular pressure
Reduced or absent knee flexion during swing	Spasticity of knee extensors Knee extension contracture	Upper motor neuron lesion Immobilization (cast, brace) or surgical fusion	Compensatory hip hiking and/or hip circumduction could be noted

Gait Deviations at the Ankle/Foot Secondary to Specific Ankle/Foot Impairments*

Observed Gait Deviation at the Ankle/Foot	Likely Impairment	Selected Pathological Precursors	Mechanical Rationale and/or Associated Compensations
"Foot slap": rapid ankle plantar flexion occurs following heel contact; the name foot slap is derived from the characteristic noise made by the forefoot hitting the ground	Mild weakness of ankle dorsiflexors	Common peroneal nerve palsy and distal peripheral neuropathy	Ankle dorsiflexors have sufficient strength to dorsiflex the ankle during swing but not enough to control ankle plantar flexion after heel contact
Entire plantar aspect of the foot touches the ground at initial contact,† followed by normal, passive ankle dorsiflexion during the rest of stance	Marked weakness of ankle dorsiflexors	Common peroneal nerve palsy and distal peripheral neuropathy	Sufficient strength of the dorsiflexors to partially, but not completely, dorsiflex the ankle during swing; normal dorsiflexion occurs during stance as long as the ankle has normal range of motion
Initial contact with the ground is made by the forefoot followed by the heel region; normal passive ankle dorsiflexion occurs during stance	Severe weakness of ankle dorsiflexors	Common peroneal nerve palsy and distal peripheral neuropathy	No active ankle dorsiflexion is possible during swing; normal dorsiflexion occurs during stance as long as the ankle has normal range of motion

Continued

Table 14-5—cont'd

Observed Gait Deviation at the Ankle/Foot	Likely Impairment	Selected Pathological Precursors	Mechanical Rationale and/or Associated Compensations
Initial contact is made with the forefoot, but the heel never makes contact with the ground during stance	Heel pain Plantar flexion contracture (pes equinus deformity) or spasticity of ankle plantar flexors	Calcaneal fracture, plantar fasciitis Upper motor neuron lesion/ cerebral palsy, cerebrovascular accident (CVA)	Purposeful strategy to avoid weight bearing on the heel To maintain the weight over the foot, the knee and hip are kept in flexion throughout stance, leading to a "crouched gait"
Initial contact is made with the forefoot, and the heel is brought to the ground by a posterior displacement of the tibia	Plantar flexion contracture (pes equinus deformity) or spasticity of ankle plantar flexors	Upper motor neuron lesion (cerebral palsy, CVA) Ankle fusion in a plantar flexed position	Knee hyperextension occurs during stance owing to the inability of the tibia to move forward over the foot; hip flexion and excessive forward trunk lean during terminal stance occur to shift the weight of the body over the foot
Premature elevation of the heel in midstance	Lack of ankle dorsiflexion	Congenital or acquired muscular tightness of ankle plantar flexors	Characteristic bouncing gait pattern
Heel remains in contact with the ground late in terminal stance	Weakness or flaccid paralysis of plantar flexors with or without a fixed dorsiflexed position of the ankle (pes calcaneus deformity)	Peripheral or central nervous system disorders Excessive surgical lengthening of the Achilles tendon	Excessive ankle dorsiflexion results in prolonged heel contact, reduced push off, and a shorter step length
Supinated foot position and weight bearing on the lateral aspect of the foot during stance	Pes cavus deformity	Congenital structural deformity	A high medial longitudinal arch is noted with reduced midfoot mobility throughout swing and stance
Excessive foot pronation occurs during stance with failure of the foot to supinate in mid stance; normal medial longitudinal arch noted during swing	Rearfoot varus and/or forefoot varus	Congenital or acquired structural deformity	Excessive foot pronation and associated flattening of the medial longitudinal arch may be accompanied by a general internal rotation of the lower extremity during stance
Excessive foot pronation with weight bearing on the medial portion of the foot during stance; the medial longitudinal arch remains absent during swing	Weakness (paralysis) of ankle invertors Pes planus deformity	Upper motor neuron lesion Congenital structural deformity	An overall excessive internal rotation of the lower extremity during stance is possible
Excessive inversion and plantar flexion of the foot and ankle occur during swing and at initial contact	Pes equinovarus because of spasticity of the plantar flexors and invertors	Upper motor neuron lesion (cerebral palsy, CVA)	Contact with the ground is made with the lateral border of the forefoot Weight bearing on the lateral border of the foot during stance
Ankle remains plantar flexed during swing and can be associated with dragging of the toes, typically called drop foot	Weakness of dorsiflexors and/ or pes equinus deformity	Common peroneal nerve palsy	Hip hiking, hip circumduction, or excessive hip and knee flexion of the swing leg or vaulting of the stance leg may be noted to lift the toes off the ground and prevent the toes from dragging during swing

From Neumann DA: *Kinesiology of the musculoskeletal system: foundations of physical rehabilitation*, pp 562-564, 566, St. Louis, 2002, Mosby.
*An impairment is a loss or an abnormality in physiological, psychological, or anatomical structure or function.
†Initial contact is often used instead of heel contact to reflect the fact that with many gait deviations the heel is not the section of the foot that makes initial contact with the ground.

Table 14-6

Gait Deviations as a Compensation for a Lower Extremity Impairment

Gait Deviations Observed at the Hip/Pelvis/Trunk as a Compensation for an Impairment of the Ipsilateral Ankle, Ipsilateral Knee, or Contralateral Lower Extremity

Observed Gait Deviation at the Hip/Pelvis/Trunk	Likely Impairment	Mechanical Rationale
Forward bending of the trunk during the loading response	Weak quadriceps	Trunk is brought forward to move the line of gravity anterior to the axis of rotation of the knee, thereby reducing the need for knee extensors
Forward bending of the trunk during mid and terminal stance	Pes equinus deformity	Lack of ankle dorsiflexion during stance results in knee hyperextension and forward trunk lean to move the weight of the body over the stance foot
Excessive hip and knee flexion during swing	Often caused by the lack of ankle dorsiflexion of the swing leg; may also be caused by a functionally or anatomically short contralateral stance leg	Used to clear the toes of the swing leg
Hip circumduction during swing	Lack of shortening of the swing leg secondary to reduced hip flexion, reduced knee flexion, and/or lack of ankle dorsiflexion	Used to lift the foot of the swing leg off the ground and provide toe clearance
Hip hiking (elevation of the ipsilateral pelvis during swing)	Lack of shortening of the swing leg secondary to reduced hip flexion, reduced knee flexion, and/or lack of ankle dorsiflexion Functionally or anatomically short stance leg	Used to lift the foot of the swing leg off the ground and provide toe clearance
Excessive backward horizontal rotation of the pelvis on the side of the stance leg in terminal stance	Ankle plantar flexor weakness	Ankle plantar flexor weakness leads to prolonged heel contact and lack of push off; an increased pelvic horizontal rotation is used to lengthen the limb and maintain adequate step length

Gait Deviations Observed at the Knee as a Compensation for an Impairment of the Ipsilateral Ankle, Ipsilateral Hip, or Contralateral Lower Extremity

Observed Gait Deviation at the Knee	Likely Impairment	Mechanical Rationale
Knee is kept in flexion during stance despite the knee having normal range of motion on examination	Impairments at the ankle or the hip including a pes calcaneus deformity, plantar flexor weakness, and hip flexion contracture	Exaggerated ankle dorsiflexion or hip flexion during stance forces the knee in a flexed position; the contralateral (healthy) swing leg shows exaggerated hip and knee flexion to clear the toes owing to the functionally shorter stance leg
Hyperextension of the knee (genu recurvatum) from initial contact to pre swing	Ankle plantar flexion contracture (pes equinus deformity) or spasticity of ankle plantar flexors	Knee must hyperextend to compensate for the lack of forward displacement of the tibia during stance
Antalgic gait	Painful stance leg	This is characterized by a shorter step length and stance time on the side of the painful lower extremity; it may be accompanied by ipsilateral trunk lean; if hip pain, contralateral trunk lean occurs with knee and foot pain
Excessive knee flexion in swing	Lack of ankle dorsiflexion of the swing leg or a short stance leg	Strategy to increase toe clearance of the swing leg and is typically accompanied by increased hip flexion

Continued

Table 14-6—cont'd

Gait Deviations Seen at the Knee as a Compensation for an Impairment of the Ipsilateral Ankle, Ipsilateral Hip, or Contralateral Lower Extremity

Observed Gait Deviation at the Ankle/Foot	Likely Impairment	Mechanical Rationale
Vaulting: compensatory mechanism demonstrated by exaggerated ankle plantar flexion during mid stance; leads to excessive vertical movement of the body	Any impairment of the contralateral lower extremity that reduces hip flexion, knee flexion, or ankle dorsiflexion during swing	Strategy used to allow the foot of a functionally long, contralateral lower extremity to clear the ground during swing
Excessive foot angle during stance that is called toeing-out	Retroversion of the neck of the femur or tight hip external rotators	Foot is in excessive toeing-out because of excessive external rotation of the lower extremity
Reduction of the normal foot ankle during stance that is called toeing-in	Excessive femoral anteversion or spasticity of the hip adductors and/or hip internal rotators	General internal rotation of the lower extremity

From Neumann DA: *Kinesiology of the musculoskeletal system: foundations of physical rehabilitation*, pp 563, 565, 567, St. Louis, 2002, Mosby.

Table 14-7

Differential Diagnosis of Antalgic Gait

<4 Years	4 to 10 Years	>10 Years
Toddler's fracture (tibia or foot)	Fracture (especially physeal)	Stress fracture (femur, tibia, foot, pars interarticularis)
Osteomyelitis, septic arthritis, discitis	Osteomyelitis, septic arthritis, discitis	Osteomyelitis, septic arthritis, discitis
Arthritis (juvenile rheumatoid arthritis, Lyme disease)	Legg-Calvé-Perthes disease	Slipped capital femoral epiphysis
Discoid lateral meniscus	Transient synovitis	Osgood-Schlatter disease or Sinding-Larsen-Johansson syndrome
Foreign body in the foot	Osteochondritis dissecans (knee or ankle)	Osteochondritis dissecans (knee or ankle)
Benign or malignant tumor	Discoid lateral meniscus	Chondromalacia patellae
	Sever's apophysitis (calcaneus)	Arthritis (Lyme disease, gonococcal)
	Accessory tarsal navicular	Accessory tarsal navicular
	Foreign body in the foot	Tarsal coalition
	Arthritis (juvenile rheumatoid arthritis, Lyme disease)	Benign or malignant tumor
	Benign or malignant tumor	

© 2001 American Academy of Orthopaedic Surgeons. Reprinted from the *Journal of the American Academy of Orthopaedic Surgeons*, vol 9(2), pp 89–98.

plantar flexion of the opposite ankle and circumduction of the stiff leg (**circumducted gait**) to provide toe clearance. The patient with this gait lifts the entire leg higher than normal to clear the ground because of a stiff hip or knee (Figure 14-16). The arc of movement helps to decrease the elevation needed to clear the affected leg. Because of the loss of flexibility in the hip, knee, or both, the gait lengths are different for the two legs. When the stiff limb is bearing weight, the gait length is usually smaller.

Ataxic Gait

If the patient has poor sensation or lacks muscle coordination, there is a tendency toward poor balance and a broad base (Figure 14-17). The gait of a person with cerebellar ataxia includes a lurch or stagger, and all movements are exaggerated. The feet of an individual with sensory ataxia slap the ground because they cannot be felt. The patient also watches the feet while walking. The resulting gait is irregular, jerky, and weaving.

Contracture Gaits

Joints of the lower limb may exhibit contracture if immobilization has been prolonged or pathology to the joint has not been properly cared for. Hip flexion contracture often results in increased lumbar lordosis and extension of the trunk combined with knee flexion to get the foot

Figure 14-16
Arthrogenic (stiff knee or hip) gait. **A,** Excessive plantar flexion. **B,** Circumduction.

Figure 14-17
Ataxic gait. (Redrawn from Judge RD. Zuidema GD, Fitzgerald FT: *Clinical diagnosis: a physiological approach*, p. 438, Boston, 1982, Little, Brown.)

on the ground. With a knee flexion contracture, the patient demonstrates excessive ankle dorsiflexion from late swing phase to early stance phase on the uninvolved leg and early heel rise on the involved side in terminal stance. Plantar flexion contracture at the ankle results in knee hyperextension (midstance of affected leg) and forward bending of the trunk with hip flexion (midstance to terminal stance of affected leg). Heel rise on the affected leg also occurs earlier.[33]

Equinus Gait (Toe Walking)

This childhood gait is seen with talipes equinovarus (club foot) (Table 14-8). Weight bearing is primarily on the dorsolateral or lateral edge of the foot, depending on the degree of deformity. The weight-bearing phase on the affected limb is decreased, and a limp is present. The pelvis and femur are laterally rotated to partially compensate for tibial and foot medial rotation.[2]

Gluteus Maximus Gait

If the gluteus maximus muscle, which is a primary hip extensor, is weak, the patient thrusts the thorax posteriorly at initial contact (heel strike) to maintain hip extension of the stance leg. The resulting gait involves a characteristic backward lurch of the trunk (Figure 14-18).

Table 14-8

Differential Diagnosis of a Nonantalgic Limp

Equinus Gait (Toe-Walking)	Trendelenburg Gait	Circumduction Gait/ Vaulting Gait	Steppage Gait
Idiopathic tight Achilles tendon	Legg-Calvé-Perthes disease	Limb-length discrepancy	Cerebral palsy
Clubfoot (residual or untreated)	Developmental dysplasia of the hip	Cerebral palsy	Myelodysplasia
Cerebral palsy	Slipped capital femoral epiphysis	Any cause of ankle or knee stiffness	Charcot-Marie-Tooth disease
Limb-length discrepancy	Muscular dystrophy		Friedreich's ataxia
	Hemiplegic cerebral palsy		Tibial nerve palsy
	Weak gluteus medius		

© 2001 American Academy of Orthopaedic Surgeons. Reprinted from the *Journal of the American Academy of Orthopaedic Surgeons*, vol 9(2), pp 89–98.

Gluteus Medius (Trendelenburg's) Gait

If the hip abductor muscles (gluteus medius and minimus) are weak, the stabilizing effect of these muscles during stance phase is lost, and the patient exhibits an excessive lateral list in which the thorax is thrust laterally to keep the center of gravity over the stance leg (Figure 14-19). A positive Trendelenburg's sign is also exhibited (i.e., the contralateral side droops because the ipsilateral hip abductors do not stabilize or prevent the droop). If there is bilateral weakness of the gluteus medius muscles, the gait shows accentuated side-to-side movement, resulting in a wobbling gait or "chorus girl swing." This gait may also be seen in patients with congenital dislocation of the hip and coxa vara (see Table 14-8).

Figure 14-18
Gluteus maximus gait.

Figure 14-19
Gluteus medius (Trendelenburg's) gait.

Hemiplegic or Hemiparetic Gait

The patient with hemiplegic or hemiparetic gait swings the paraplegic leg outward and ahead in a circle (circumduction) or pushes it ahead (Figure 14-20). In addition, the affected upper limb is carried across the trunk for balance. This is sometimes referred to as a **neurogenic** or **flaccid gait.**

Parkinsonian Gait

The neck, trunk, and knees of a patient with parkinsonian gait are flexed. The gait is characterized by shuffling or short rapid steps (marche à petits pas) at times. The arms are held stiffly and do not have their normal associative movement (Figure 14-21). During the gait, the patient may lean forward and walk progressively faster as though unable to stop **(festination).**[61]

Plantar Flexor Gait

If the plantar flexor muscles are unable to perform their function, ankle and knee stability are greatly affected. Loss of the plantar flexors results in decrease or absence

Figure 14-21

Parkinsonian gait. (Redrawn from Judge RD, Zuidema GD, Fitzgerald FT: *Clinical diagnosis: a physiological approach*, p. 496, Boston, 1982, Little, Brown.)

Figure 14-20

Hemiplegic (hemiparetic) gait. (Redrawn from Judge RD, Zuidema GD, Fitzgerald FT: *Clinical diagnosis: a physiological approach*, p. 438, Boston, 1982, Little, Brown.)

of push-off. The stance phase is less, and there is a shorter step length on the unaffected side.[33]

Psoatic Limp

The psoatic limp is seen in patients with conditions affecting the hip, such as Legg-Calvé-Perthes disease. The patient demonstrates a difficulty in swing-through, and the limp may be accompanied by exaggerated trunk and pelvic movement.[33] The limp may be caused by weakness or reflex inhibition of the psoas major muscle. Classic manifestations of this limp are lateral rotation, flexion, and adduction of the hip (Figure 14-22). The patient exaggerates movement of the pelvis and trunk to help move the thigh into flexion.

Quadriceps Avoidance Gait

If the quadriceps muscles have been injured (e.g., femoral nerve neuropathy, reflex inhibition, trauma −3°strain), the patient compensates in the trunk and lower leg. Forward flexion of the trunk combined with strong ankle plantar flexion causes the knee to extend (hyperextend). The knee may be held extended by using the iliotibial

Figure 14-22

Psoatic limp. Note lateral rotation, flexion, and abduction of affected hip.

Figure 14-23

Scissors gait. (Redrawn from Judge RD, Zuidema GD, Fitzgerald FT: *Clinical diagnosis: a physiological approach*, p. 439, Boston, 1982, Little, Brown.)

band. If the trunk, hip flexors, and ankle muscles cannot perform this movement, the patient may use a hand to extend the knee.[33]

Scissors Gait

This gait is the result of spastic paralysis of the hip adductor muscles, which causes the knees to be drawn together so that the legs can be swung forward only with great effort (Figure 14-23). This is seen in spastic paraplegics and may be referred to as a **neurogenic** or **spastic gait.**

Short Leg Gait

If one leg is shorter than the other or there is a deformity in one of the bones of the leg, the patient may demonstrate a lateral shift to the affected side, and the pelvis tilts down on the affected side, creating a limp (Figure 14-24). The patient may also supinate the foot on the affected side to try to "lengthen" the limb. The joints of the unaffected limb may demonstrate exaggerated flexion, or hip hiking may occur during the swing phase to allow the foot to clear the ground.[33] The weight-bearing period may be the same for the two legs. How a patient

Figure 14-24

Short leg gait.

adapts for leg length difference has wide variability.[62,63] With proper footwear, the gait may appear normal. This gait may also be termed **painless osteogenic gait.**

Steppage or Drop Foot Gait

The patient with a steppage gait has weak or paralyzed dorsiflexor muscles, resulting in a drop foot. To compensate and avoid dragging the toes against the ground, the patient lifts the knee higher than normal (Figure 14-25). At initial contact, the foot slaps on the ground because of loss of control of the dorsiflexor muscles resulting from injury to the muscles, their peripheral nerve supply, or the nerve roots supplying the muscles (see Table 14-8).[64]

Table 14-9 lists common gait pathologies that can modify gait and the phase in which the deviation occurs.[35]

Figure 14-25
Steppage or drop foot gait. (Redrawn from Judge RD, Zuidema GD, Fitzgerald FT: *Clinical diagnosis: a physiological approach*, p. 438, Boston, 1982, Little, Brown.)

Table 14-9
Common Gait Pathologies

Deviation	Phase	Cause
Excessive foot pronation	Midstance through toe off	Compensated forefoot or rearfoot varus deformity; uncompensated forefoot valgus deformity; pes planus; decreased ankle dorsiflexion; increased tibial varum; long limb; uncompensated medial rotation of tibia or femur; weak tibialis posterior
Excessive foot supination	Heel strike through midstance	Compensated forefoot valgus deformity; pes cavus; short limb, uncompensated lateral rotation of tibia or femur; limited calcaneal eversion; plantar flexed first ray; upper motor neuron muscle balance
Excessive calcaneal eversion	Initial contact through midstance	Excessive tibia vara; forefoot varus; tibialis posterior weakness; excessive lower extremity medial rotation (because of muscle imbalances, femoral anteversion)
Excessive varus	Heel strike to toe off	Contracture; overactivity of muscles on medial aspect of foot
Excessive valgus	Heel strike to toe off	Weak invertors; foot hypermobility
Bouncing or exaggerated plantar flexion	Midstance through toe off	Heel cord contracture; increased tone of gastrocnemius and soleus

Continued

Table 14-9—cont'd

Deviation	Phase	Cause
Excessive dorsiflexion	Heel strike to toe off	Compensation for knee flexion contracture; inadequate plantar flexor strength; adaptive shortening of dorsiflexors; increased muscle tone of dorsiflexors; pes calcaneus deformity
Insufficient push off	Midstance through toe off	Gastrocnemius and soleus weakness; Achilles tendon rupture; metatarsalgia; hallux rigidus
Foot slap	Heel strike to foot flat	Dorsiflexor weakness; lack of lower limb sensation
Steppage gait (exaggerated hip and knee flexion to clear foot)	Acceleration through deceleration	Dorsiflexor weakness or paralysis; functional leg length discrepancy
Excessive knee flexion	Heel strike through toe off	Hamstring contracture; decreased range of motion in ankle dorsiflexion; plantar flexor muscle weakness; lengthened limb; hip flexion contracture
Excessive knee extension/inadequate knee flexion	Heel strike to foot flat and swing	Pain; anterior trunk deviation/bending; weakness of quadriceps, hyperextension is a compensation and places body weight vector anterior to knee; spasticity of the quadriceps, noted more during the loading response and during initial swing intervals; joint deformity
Genu recurvatum (knee hyperextension)	Heel strike through midstance	Quadriceps femoris weak or short; compensated hamstring weakness; Achilles tendon contracture; habit
Abnormal internal hip rotation (toe-in gait)		Adaptive shortening of iliotibial band; weakness of hip external rotators; femoral anteversion; adaptive shortening of hip internal rotators
Abnormal external hip rotation (toe-out gait)		Adaptive shortening of hip external rotators; femoral retroversion; weakness of hip internal rotators
Increased hip adduction (scissors gait)	Heel strike to toe off	Spasticity or contracture of ipsilateral hip adductors; ipsilateral hip adductor weakness; coxa vara
Decreased hip swing through (psoatic limp)		Legg-Calvé-Perthes disease; weakness or reflex inhibition of psoas major muscle; pain
Excessive medial or lateral femur rotation (femoral torsion)	Heel strike through toe off	Medial or lateral hamstrings tight, respectively; opposite muscle group weakness; anteversion or retroversion, respectively
Increased base of support (>4 inches/10 cm)	Heel strike through toe off	Abductor muscle contracture; instability; genu valgum; leg length discrepancy; fear of losing balance
Decreased base of support (<2 inches/5 cm)	Heel strike through toe off	Adductor muscle contracture; genu varum
Circumduction	Acceleration through deceleration	Increased limb length; abductor muscle shortening or overuse; stiff hip or knee
Hip hiking	Acceleration through deceleration	Increased limb length; hamstring weakness; inadequate hip or knee flexion or ankle dorsiflexion; quadratus lumborum shortening

Table 14-9—cont'd

Deviation	Phase	Cause
Vaulting (ground clearance of swinging leg will increase if subject goes up on toes of stance period leg)	Foot flat to toe off	Functional leg-length discrepancy; vaulting occurs on shorter limb side
Inadequate hip flexion	Acceleration through heel strike	Hip flexor muscle weakness; hip extensor muscle shortening; increased limb length; hip joint arthrosis
Inadequate hip extension (causes trunk forward bending, increased lordosis)	Midstance through toe off	Hip flexion contracture; hip extensor muscle weakness; iliotibial band contracture; hip flexor spasticity; pain
Increased lumbar lordosis	Foot flat to toe off	Inability to extend hip; hip flexion contracture or hip ankylosis
Excessive trunk back bending (gluteus maximus gait)	Heel strike through midstance	Hip extensor or flexor muscle weakness; hip pain; decreased range of motion of knee
Excessive trunk forward bending	Deceleration through midstance	Quadriceps femoris and gluteus maximus weakness; decreased ankle dorsiflexion; hip flexion contracture
Excessive trunk lateral flexion (compensated Trendelenburg's gait)	Foot flat through heel off	Gluteus medius weakness; hip pain; unequal leg length; hip pathology; wide base
Pelvic drop	Foot flat through heel off	Contralateral gluteus medius weakness; adaptive shortening of quadratus lumborum; contralateral hip adductor spasticity
Excessive pelvic rotation	Heel strike to toe off	Adaptively shortened/spasticity of hip flexors on same side; limited hip joint flexion
Slower cadence than expected for person's age		Generalized weakness; pain; joint motion restrictions; poor voluntary motor control
Shorter stance phase on involved side and decreased swing phase on uninvolved side (shorter stride length on uninvolved side, decrease lateral sway over involved stance limb, decrease in cadence, decrease in velocity, use of assistive device)		Antalgic gait resulting from painful injury to lower limb and pelvic region
Stance phase longer on one side		Pain; lack of trunk and pelvic rotation; weakness of lower limb muscles; restrictions in lower limb joints; poor muscle control; increased muscle tone

Adapted from Giallonardo LM: Gait. In Myers RS, editor: *Saunders manual of physical therapy practice*, p 1112, Philadelphia, 1995, WB Saunders; and Dutton M: *Orthopedic examination, evaluation and intervention*, New York, 2004, McGraw-Hill.

References

To enhance this text and add value for the reader, all references have been incorporated into a CD-ROM that is provided with this text. The reader can view the reference source and access it online whenever possible. There are a total of 64 cited references and other general references for this chapter.

CHAPTER 15

ASSESSMENT OF POSTURE

Postural Development

Through evolution, human beings have assumed an upright erect or bipedal posture. The advantage of an erect posture is that it enables the hands to be free and the eyes to be farther from the ground so that the individual can see farther ahead. The disadvantages include an increased strain on the spine and lower limbs and comparative difficulties in respiration and transport of the blood to the brain.

Posture, which is the relative disposition of the body at any one moment, is a composite of the positions of the different joints of the body at that time. The position of each joint has an effect on the position of the other joints. Classically, ideal static postural alignment (viewed from the side) is defined as a straight line (line of gravity) that passes through the earlobe, the bodies of the cervical vertebrae, the tip of the shoulder, midway through the thorax, through the bodies of the lumbar vertebrae, slightly posterior to the hip joint, slightly anterior to the axis of the knee joint, and just anterior to the lateral malleolus (Figure 15-1).[1] **Correct posture** is the position in which minimum stress is applied to each joint. Upright posture is the normal standing posture for humans. Although upright posture allows one to see farther and provides freedom to move the arms, it does have disadvantages. It places greater stress on the lower limbs, pelvis, and spine; reduces stability; and increases the work of the heart.[2] If the upright posture is correct, minimal muscle activity is needed to maintain the position.

Any static position that increases the stress to the joints may be called **faulty posture**. If a person has strong, flexible muscles, faulty postures may not affect the joints because he or she has the ability to change position readily so that the stresses do not become excessive. If the joints are stiff (hypomobile) or too mobile (hypermobile), or the muscles are weak, shortened, or lengthened, however, the posture cannot be easily altered to the correct alignment, and the result can be some form of pathology. The pathology may be the result of the cumulative effect of repeated small stresses (microtrauma) over a long period of time or of constant abnormal stresses (macrotrauma) over a short period of time. These chronic stresses can result in the same problems that are seen when a sudden (acute) severe stress is applied to the body. The abnormal stresses cause excessive wearing of the articular surfaces of joints and produce osteophytes and traction spurs, which represent the body's attempt to alter its structure to accommodate these repeated stresses. The soft tissue (e.g., muscles, ligaments) may become weakened, stretched, or traumatized by the increased stress. Thus postural deviations do not always cause symptoms, but over time, they may do so.[3] The application of an acute stress on the chronic stress may exacerbate the problem and produce the signs and symptoms that initially prompt the patient to seek aid.

At birth, the entire spine is concave forward, or flexed (Figure 15-2). Curves of the spine found at birth are called **primary curves**. The curves that retain this position, those of the thoracic spine and sacrum, are therefore classified as primary curves of the spine. As the child grows (Figure 15-3), **secondary curves** appear and are convex forward, or extended. At about the age of 3 months, when the child begins to lift the head, the cervical spine becomes convex forward, producing the cervical lordosis. In the lumbar spine, the secondary curve develops

ANATOMIC LANDMARKS

SURFACE LANDMARKS

Bilateral symmetry of
head and facial bones

Ear lobe

Bisects cervical vertebral bodies

Shoulder levels

Bisects sternum

Nipple levels

Arm-thoracic distance
Bisects vertebral bodies
Bisects umbilicus
Pelvic crest levels

ASIS levels
Levels of greater trochanter
Bisects pubic symphysis

Anterior line of reference

Joint line levels
Head of fibula levels

Malleoli levels

A

IDEAL LINE OF GRAVITY

Figure 15-1

Ideal postural alignment. **A,** Front view. On a typical patient (*photo*) note the difference in shoulder height and
nipple height and apparent arm length difference, arm-thorax difference, and difference in out-toeing.

Continued

slightly later (6 to 8 months), when the child begins to
sit up and walk. In old age, the secondary curves again
begin to disappear as the spine starts to return to a flexed
position as the result of disc degeneration, ligamentous
calcification, osteoporosis, and vertebral wedging.

In the child, the center of gravity is at the level of
the twelfth thoracic vertebra. As the child grows older,
the center of gravity drops, eventually reaching the level
of the second sacral vertebra in adults (slightly higher in
males). The child stands with a wide base to maintain
balance, and the knees are flexed. The knees are slightly
bowed (genu varum) until about 18 months of age. The
child then becomes slightly knock kneed (genu valgum)
until the age of 3 years. By the age of 6 years, the legs

ANATOMIC LANDMARKS

SURFACE LANDMARKS

- Posterior to coronal suture
- External auditory meatus
- Odontoid process
- Bodies of cervical vertebrae
- Head of humerus
- Midthorax
- Bodies of lumbar vertebrae
- High point of iliac crest
- ASIS to PSIS angle
- Greater trochanter of femur
- Gluteal fold
- Lateral line of reference
- Base of patella
- Joint line levels (apex of patella)
- Head of fibula levels
- Anterior to lateral malleolus
- Lateral malleolus

B

IDEAL LINE OF GRAVITY

Figure 15-1 cont'd

B, Side view. Typical patient (*photo*) with good lateral alignment.

should naturally straighten (Figure 15-4). The lumbar spine in the child has an exaggerated lumbar curve, or excessive lordosis. This accentuated curve is caused by the presence of large abdominal contents, weakness of the abdominal musculature, and the small pelvis characteristic of children at this age.

Initially, a child is flatfooted, or appears to be, as the result of the minimal development of the medial longitudinal arch and the fat pad that is found in the arch. As the child grows, the fat pad slowly decreases in size, making the medial arch more evident. In addition, as the foot develops and the muscles strengthen, the arches of the feet develop normally and become more evident.

During adolescence, posture changes because of hormonal influence with the onset of puberty and

ANATOMIC LANDMARKS

SURFACE LANDMARKS

- Bilateral symmetry of head
- Cervical spinal processes
- Shoulder height levels
- Acromion levels
- Normal scapular position
- Inferior angle of scapula levels
- Thoracic spinal processes
- Bilateral trunk symmetry
- Lumbar spinal processes
- Pelvic crest levels
- PSIS levels
- Greater trochanter levels
- Gluteal cleft levels
- Tibiofemoral joint spaces
- Knee creases levels
- Head of fibula levels
- Malleoli levels

C

IDEAL LINE OF GRAVITY

Figure 15-1 cont'd

C, Back view. On a typical patient (*photo*) note the difference in shoulder slope, shoulder height, height of inferior scapular angles, and rotation of arms. In this view, also note straight Achilles tendons.

musculoskeletal growth. Human beings go through two growth spurts, one when they are very young and a more obvious one when they are in adolescence. This second growth spurt lasts 2.5 to 4 years.[4] During this period, growth is accompanied by sexual maturation. Females develop quicker and sooner than males. Females enter puberty between 8 and 14 years of age, and puberty lasts about 3 years. Males enter puberty between 9.5 and 16

years of age, and it lasts up to 5 years.[2] It is during this period that body differences arise between males and females, with males tending toward longer leg and arm length, wider shoulders, smaller hip width, and greater overall skeletal size and height than females. Because of the rapid growth spurt, individuals, especially males, may appear ungainly, and poor postural habits and changes are more likely to occur at this age.

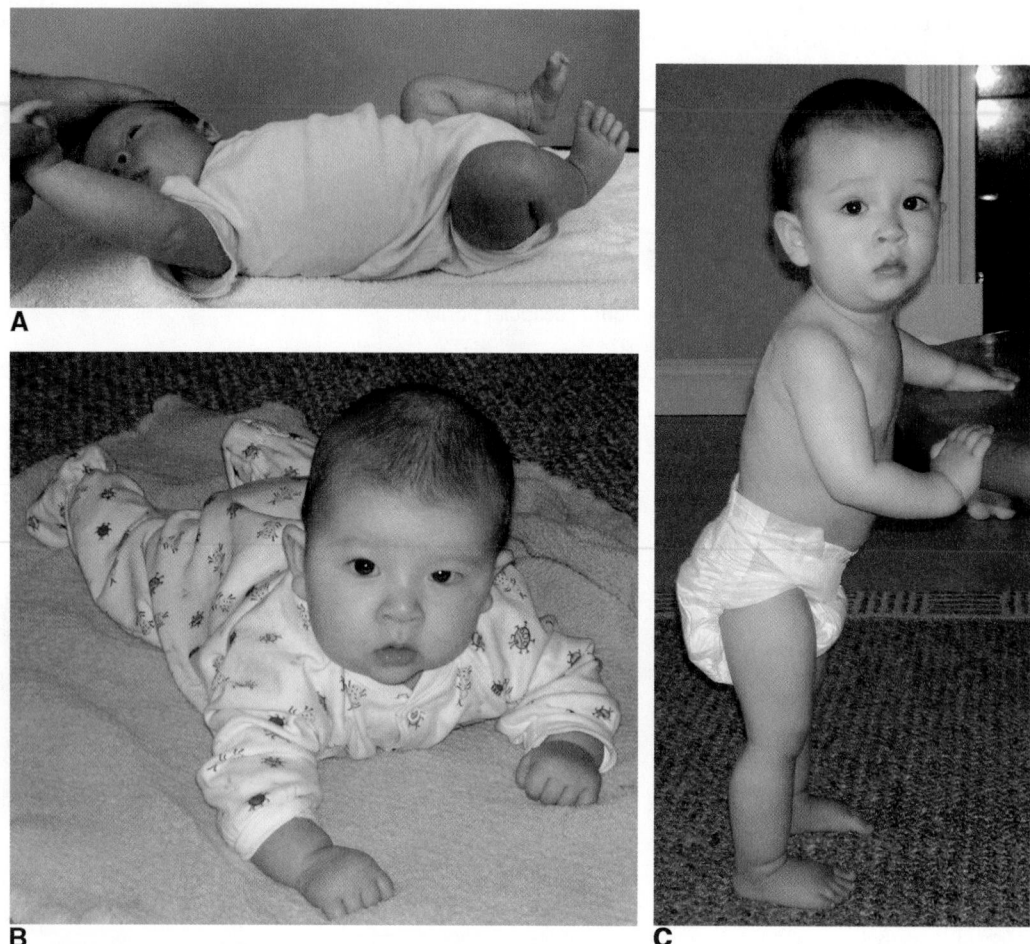

Figure 15-2

Postural development. **A,** Flexed posture in a newborn. **B,** Development of secondary cervical curve.
C, Development of secondary lumbar curve.

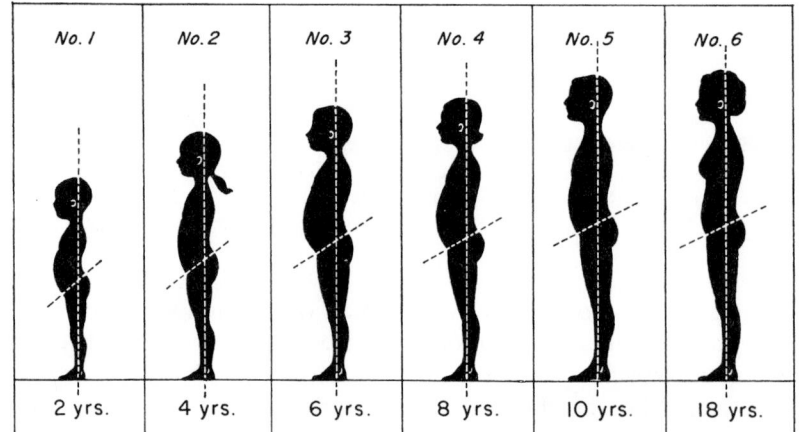

Figure 15-3

Postural changes with age. Apparent kyphosis at 6 and 8 years is caused by scapular winging. (From McMorris
RO: Faulty postures, *Pediatr Clin North Am* 8:214, 1961.)

Newborn-
moderate genu varum

6 months-
minimal genu varum

1 year, 7 months-
legs straight

2 years, 6 months-
physiological genu valgum

Protective toeing-in

4 to 6 years-
legs straight with normal
toeing-out

Figure 15-4

Physiological evolution of lower-limb alignment at various ages in infancy and childhood. (Redrawn from Tachdjian MO: *Pediatric orthopedics*, p. 1463, Philadelphia, 1972, WB Saunders.)

Factors Affecting Posture

Several anatomical features may affect correct posture. These features may be enhanced or cause additional problems when combined with pathological or congenital states, such as Klippel-Feil syndrome, Scheuermann's disease (juvenile kyphosis), scoliosis, or disc disease.

Causes of Poor Posture

There are many examples of poor posture (Figure 15-5). Some of the causes are postural (positional), and some are structural.

Postural (Positional) Factors

The most common postural problem is poor postural habit; that is, for whatever reason, the patient does not

---

Anatomical Factors Affecting Correct Posture

- Bony contours (e.g., hemivertebra)
- Laxity of ligamentous structures
- Fascial and musculotendinous tightness (e.g., tensor fasciae latae, pectorals, hip flexors)
- Muscle tonus (e.g., gluteus maximus, abdominals, erector spinae)
- Pelvic angle (normal is 30°)
- Joint position and mobility
- Neurogenic outflow and inflow

---

maintain a correct posture. This type of posture is often seen in the person who stands or sits for long periods and begins to slouch. Maintenance of correct posture requires muscles that are strong, flexible, and easily adaptable to

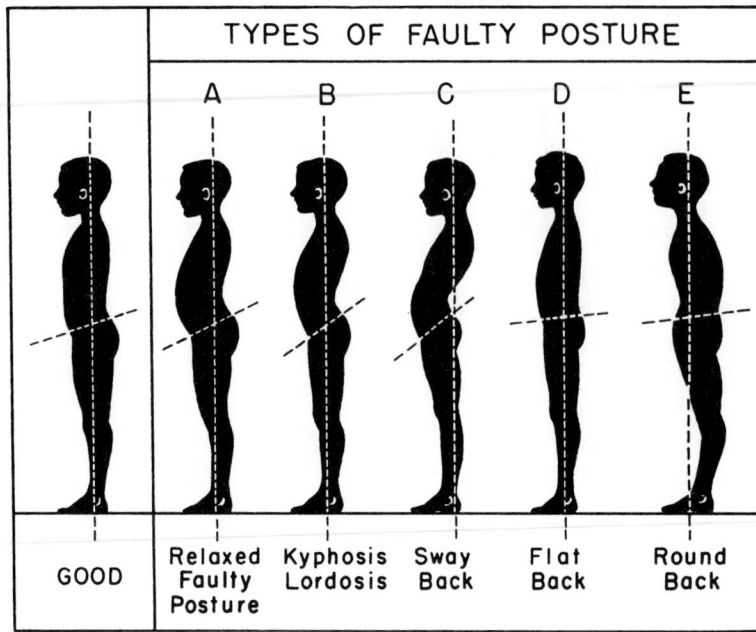

TYPES OF FAULTY POSTURE

| GOOD | A Relaxed Faulty Posture | B Kyphosis Lordosis | C Sway Back | D Flat Back | E Round Back |

Figure 15-5

Examples of faulty posture. (From McMorris RO: Faulty postures, *Pediatr Clin North Am* 8:217, 1961.)

environmental change. These muscles must continually work against gravity and in harmony with one another to maintain an upright posture.

Another cause of poor postural habits, especially in children, is not wanting to appear taller than one's peers. If a child has an early, rapid growth spurt there may be a tendency to slouch so as not to "stand out" and appear different. Such a spurt may also result in the unequal growth of the various structures, and this may lead to altered posture; for example, the growth of muscle may not keep up with the growth of bone. This process is sometimes evident in adolescents with tight hamstrings.

Muscle imbalance and muscle contracture are other causes of poor posture. For example, a tight iliopsoas muscle increases the lumbar lordosis in the lumbar spine.

Pain may also cause poor posture. Pressure on a nerve root in the lumbar spine can lead to pain in the back and result in a scoliosis as the body unconsciously adopts a posture that decreases the pain.

Respiratory conditions (e.g., emphysema), general weakness, excess weight, loss of proprioception, or muscle spasm (as seen in cerebral palsy or with trauma, as examples) may also lead to poor posture.

The majority of postural nonstructural faults are relatively easy to correct after the problem has been identified. The treatment involves strengthening weak muscles, stretching tight structures, and teaching the patient that it is his or her responsibility to maintain a correct upright posture in standing, sitting, and other activities of daily living.

Structural Factors

Structural deformities that are the result of congenital anomalies, developmental problems, trauma, or disease may cause an alteration of posture. For example, a significant difference in leg length or an anomaly of the spine, such as a hemivertebra, may alter the posture.

Structural deformities involve mainly changes in bone and therefore are not easily correctable without surgery. However, patients often can be relieved of symptoms by proper postural care instruction.

Common Spinal Deformities

Lordosis

Lordosis is an anterior curvature of the spine (Figure 15-6).[5-9] Pathologically, it is an exaggeration of the normal curves found in the cervical and lumbar spines. Causes of increased lordosis include (1) postural or functional deformity; (2) lax muscles, especially the abdominal muscles, in combination with tight muscles, especially hip flexors or lumbar extensors (Table 15-1); (3) a heavy abdomen, resulting from excess weight or pregnancy; (4) compensatory mechanisms that result from another deformity, such as kyphosis (Figure 15-7); (5) tight and commonly strong muscles (Table 15-1); (6) spondylolisthesis; (7) congenital problems, such as bilateral congenital dislocation of the hip; (8) failure of segmentation of the neural arch of a facet joint segment; or (9) fashion (e.g., wearing high-heeled shoes). There are two types of exaggerated lordosis, pathological lordosis and swayback deformity.

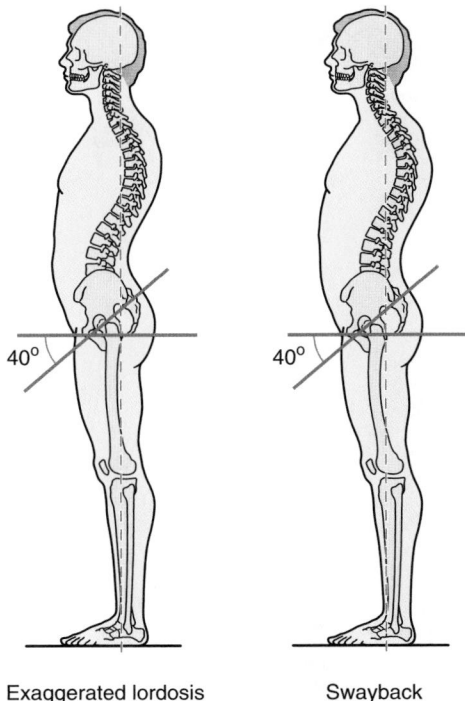

Exaggerated lordosis   Swayback

Figure 15-6
Examples of lordosis.

Table 15-1

Changes Associated with Pathological Lordosis

Body Segment Alignment	Pelvis anteriorly tilted with lordosis increased
	Knees hyperextended
	Ankle joints slightly plantar flexed
Muscles Commonly Elongated and Weak	Anterior abdominals
	Small muscles of lumbar spine (multifidus, rotators)
	Lower and middle trapezius
	Hamstrings may lengthen initially or shorten to compensate where posture has been present for some time
	Rhomboids?
	Upper (thoracic and cervical) erector spinae
	Hyoid muscles
Muscles Commonly Short and Strong	Lumbar erector spinae
	Hip flexors
	Upper trapezius
	Pectoralis major and minor
	Levator scapulae
	Sternocleidomastoid
	Scalene muscles
	Suboccipital muscles
Joints Commonly Affected	Lumbar spine
	Pelvic joints
	Hip joints
	Thoracic spine
	Scapulothoracic joints
	Glenohumeral joints
	Cervical spine
	Atlanto-occipital joints
	Temporomandibular joints

Adapted from Kendall FP, McCreary EK: *Muscles: testing and function*, Baltimore, 1983, Williams & Wilkins; Giallonardo LM: Posture. In Myers RS, editor: *Saunders manual of physical therapy practice*, Philadelphia, 1995, WB Saunders.

Pathological Lordosis. In the patient with pathological lordosis, one may often observe sagging shoulders (scapulae are protracted and arms are medially rotated), medial rotation of the legs, and poking forward of the head so that it is in front of the center of gravity (Figure 15-8). This posture is adopted in an attempt to keep the center of gravity where it should be. Deviation in one part of the body often leads to deviation in another part of the body in an attempt to maintain the correct center of gravity and the correct visual plane. This type of exaggerated lordosis is the most common postural deviation seen.

The pelvic angle, normally approximately 30°, is increased with lordosis. With excessive or pathological lordosis, there is an increase in the pelvic angle to approximately 40°, accompanied by a mobile spine and an anterior pelvic tilt. Exaggerated lumbar lordosis is usually accompanied by weakness of the deep lumbar extensors and tightness of the hip flexors and tensor fasciae latae combined with weak abdominals (see Table 15-1).[10]

Swayback Deformity. With a swayback deformity, there is increased pelvic inclination to approximately 40°, and the thoracolumbar spine exhibits a kyphosis (Figure 15-9). A swayback deformity results in the spine's bending back rather sharply at the lumbosacral angle. With this postural deformity, the entire pelvis shifts anteriorly, causing the hips to move into extension. To maintain the

center of gravity in its normal position, the thoracic spine flexes on the lumbar spine. The result is an increase in the lumbar and thoracic curves. Such a deformity may be associated with tightness of the hip extensors, lower lumbar extensors, and upper abdominals, along with weakness of the hip flexors, lower abdominals, and lower thoracic extensors (Table 15-2).[1]

Kyphosis

Kyphosis is a posterior curvature of the spine (Figures 15-10 and 15-11).[7,9,11-15] Pathologically, it is an exaggeration of the normal curve found in the thoracic spine. There are several causes of kyphosis, including tuberculosis, vertebral compression fractures, Scheuermann's disease,

Figure 15-7
Faulty posture illustrating exaggerated lordosis and kyphosis. (From Kendall FP, McCreary EK: *Muscles: testing and function*, p. 281, Baltimore, 1983, Williams & Wilkins.)

Figure 15-8
Pathological lordosis with compensatory forward head posture.

Figure 15-9
Faulty posture illustrating a swayback. (From Kendall FP, McCreary EK: *Muscles: testing and function*, p. 284, Baltimore, 1983, Williams & Wilkins.)

ankylosing spondylitis, senile osteoporosis, tumors, compensation in conjunction with lordosis, and congenital anomalies.[11] The congenital anomalies include a partial segmental defect, as seen in osseous metaplasia, or centrum hypoplasia and aplasia.[14,16,17] In addition, paralysis may lead to a kyphosis because of the loss of muscle action needed to maintain the correct posture combined with the forces of gravity.

Pathological conditions such as Scheuermann's vertebral osteochondritis may also result in a structural kyphosis (Figure 15-12). In this condition, inflammation of the bone and cartilage occurs around the ring epiphysis of the vertebral body. The condition often leads to an anterior wedging of the vertebra. It is a growth disorder that affects approximately 10% of the population, and in most cases several vertebrae are affected. The most common area for the disease to occur is between T10 and L2.

The four types of kyphosis are round back, humpback, flat back, and dowager's hump.

elvis the
egment, hip
of posture
nobile to

ttens
sterior tilt
yperextended
redominantly
ed down to

nger in

rs

d, gluteus
erior fibers)

oblique

nort but

, tensor
liotibial
side

Hip
Thoracic
Scapulothoracic joints
Glenohumeral joints
Cervical spine
Atlanto-occipital joints
Temporomandibular joints

Adapted from Kendall FP, McCreary EK: *Muscles: testing and function*, Baltimore, 1983, Williams & Wilkins; Giallonardo LM: Posture. In Myers RS, editor: *Saunders manual of physical therapy practice*, Philadelphia, 1995, WB Saunders.

Round Back. The patient with a round back has a long, rounded curve with decreased pelvic inclination (<30°) and thoracolumbar kyphosis. The patient often presents with the trunk flexed forward and a decreased lumbar curve (Figure 15-13). On examination, there are tight hip extensors and trunk flexors with weak hip flexors and lumbar extensors (Table 15-3).

| Flat back | Hump back | Round back |

Figure 15-10
Examples of kyphosis.

Figure 15-11
Faulty posture illustrating thoracic kyphosis. (From Moe JH et al: *Scoliosis and other spinal deformities*, p. 152, Philadelphia, 1978, WB Saunders.)

Figure 15-12

A classic x-ray appearance of the spine in a patient with Scheuermann's disease. Note the wedged vertebra *(1)*, Schmorl's nodules *(2)*, and marked irregularity of the vertebral end plates *(3)*. (From Moe JH et al: *Scoliosis and other spinal deformities*, p. 332, Philadelphia, 1978, WB Saunders.)

Table 15-3

Changes Associated with a Round Back Form of Kyphosis

Body Segment Alignment	Head held forward with cervical spine hyperextended
	Scapulae may be protracted
	Increased thoracic kyphosis
	Hips flexed, knees hyperextended
	Head usually most anteriorly placed body segment
Muscles Commonly Elongated and Weak	Neck flexors
	Upper erector spinae
	External oblique muscles
	If scapulae are protracted, middle and lower trapezius
	Thoracic erector spinae
	Rhomboids
Muscles Commonly Short and Strong	Neck extensors
	Hip flexors
	If scapulae are protracted, serratus anterior, pectoralis major and/or minor, upper trapezius, levator scapulae
	Upper abdominal muscles
	Intercostals
Joints Commonly Affected	Thoracic spine
	Scapulothoracic joints
	Glenohumeral joints

Adapted from Kendall FP, McCreary EK: *Muscles: testing and function*, Baltimore, 1983, Williams & Wilkins; Giallonardo LM: Posture. In Myers RS, editor: *Saunders manual of physical therapy practice*, Philadelphia, 1995, WB Saunders.

Figure 15-13

Round back form of kyphosis.

Humpback or Gibbus. With humpback, there is a localized, sharp posterior angulation in the thoracic spine (Figure 15-14). This is commonly a structural deformity as the result of a fracture or pathology.

Flat Back. A patient with flat back has decreased pelvic inclination to 20° and a mobile lumbar spine (Figure 15-15). Table 15-4 outlines the structures affected.

Dowager's Hump. Dowager's hump is often seen in older patients, especially women. The deformity commonly is caused by osteoporosis, in which the thoracic vertebral bodies begin to degenerate and wedge in an anterior direction, resulting in a kyphosis (Figure 15-16).

Kypholordotic Posture. In some cases, both the thoracic and lumbar spine may be affected. Figure 15-17 and Table 15-5 outline the changes seen with this posture.

Scoliosis

Scoliosis is a lateral curvature of the spine.[11,13,18-24] This type of deformity is often the most visible spinal deformity, especially in its severe forms. The most famous example of scoliosis is the "hunchback of Notre Dame."

Figure 15-14
Humpback or gibbus deformity.

Figure 15-15
Faulty posture illustrating flat back. (From Kendall FP, McCreary EK: *Muscles: testing and function*, p 285, Baltimore, 1983, Williams & Wilkins.)

Table 15-4

Changes Associated with a Flat Back Form of Kyphosis

Body Segment Alignment	Loss of lordosis with pelvis in posterior tilt
	Hip and knee joints hyperextended
	Forward head posture with increased flexion to upper thoracic spine
Muscles Commonly Elongated and Weak	One-joint hip flexors
	Lumbar extensors
	Local stabilizers (multifidus, rotators)
	Scapular protractors?
	Anterior intercostals
Muscles Commonly Short and Strong	Hamstrings
	Abdominals may be strong with back muscles slightly elongated
	Hip extensors
	Scapular retractors?
	Thoracic erector spinae
Joints Commonly Affected	Lumbar spine
	Pelvic joints
	Scapulothoracic joints?
	Thoracic spine
	Cervical spine?

Adapted from Kendall FP, McCreary EK: *Muscles: testing and function*, Baltimore, 1983, Williams & Wilkins; Giallonardo LM: Posture. In Myers RS, editor: *Saunders manual of physical therapy practice*, Philadelphia, 1995, WB Saunders.

In the cervical spine, a scoliosis is called a **torticollis**. There are several types of scoliosis, some of which are nonstructural (Figure 15-18) and some of which are structural. **Nonstructural** or **functional scoliosis** may be caused by postural problems, hysteria, nerve root irritation, inflammation, or compensation caused by leg length discrepancy or contracture (in the lumbar spine) (Table 15-6).[23] **Structural scoliosis** primarily involves bony deformity, which may be congenital or acquired, or excessive muscle weakness, as seen in a person with long-term quadriplegia. This type of scoliosis may be caused by wedge vertebra, hemivertebra (Figure 15-19), or failure of segmentation. It may be idiopathic (genetic) (Figure 15-20); neuromuscular, resulting from an upper or lower motor neuron lesion; or myopathic, resulting from muscular disease; or it may be caused by arthrogryposis, resulting from persistent joint contracture,[17] or by conditions such as neurofibromatosis, mesenchymal disorders, or trauma. It may accompany infection, tumors, and inflammatory conditions that result in bone destruction. Torticollis may occur because of neuromuscular problems, because of congenital problems (abnormal sternocleidomastoid muscle), or in conjunction with malocclusion of the temporomandibular joints or with ear problems (referred to the cervical spine).

AGE 20 75

7-9 cm

Figure 15-16

Loss of height resulting from osteoporosis leading to dowager's hump. Note the flexed head and protruding abdomen, which occur partially to maintain the center of gravity in its normal position.

Figure 15-17

Kypholordotic posture.

Table 15-5
Changes Associated with Kypholordotic Posture

Body Segment Alignment	Head held forward with cervical spine hyperextended
	Scapulae may be protracted
	Increased lumbar lordosis and increased thoracic kyphosis
	Pelvis anteriorly tilted
	Hip flexed, knee hyperextended
	Head usually most anteriorly placed body segment
Muscles Commonly Elongated and Weak	Neck flexors
	Upper erector spinae
	External oblique muscles
	If scapulae are protracted, middle and lower trapezius
	Thoracic erector spinae
	Middle and lower trapezius
	Rhomboids
Muscles Commonly Short and Strong	Neck extensors
	Hip flexors
	If scapulae are protracted, serratus anterior, pectoralis major and/or minor, upper trapezius
	Intercostals
Joints Commonly Affected	Thoracic spine
	Lumbar spine
	Scapulothoracic joints
	Glenohumeral joints

Adapted from Kendall FP, McCreary EK: *Muscles: testing and function*, Baltimore, 1983, Williams & Wilkins; Giallonardo LM: Posture. In Myers RS, editor: *Saunders manual of physical therapy practice*, Philadelphia, 1995, WB Saunders.

With structural scoliosis, the patient lacks normal flexibility, and side bending becomes asymmetrical. This type of scoliosis may be progressive, and the curve does not disappear on forward flexion. It is most commonly seen in the thoracic or thoracolumbar spine. With nonstructural scoliosis, there is no bony deformity; this type of scoliosis is not progressive. The spine shows segmental limitation, and side bending is usually symmetrical. The nonstructural scoliotic curve disappears on forward flexion. This type of scoliosis is usually found in the cervical, lumbar, or thoracolumbar area.

Idiopathic scoliosis accounts for 75% to 85% of all cases of structural scoliosis. The vertebral bodies rotate into the convexity of the curve, with the spinous processes going toward the concavity of the curve. There is a fixed rotational prominence on the convex side, which is best seen on forward flexion from the skyline view. This prominence is sometimes called a "razorback spine." The disc spaces are narrowed on the concave side and widened on the convex side. There is distortion of the vertebral body, and vital capacity is considerably lowered if the lateral curvature exceeds 60°; compression and malposition

Figure 15-18 ▰
Congenital muscular torticollis on the right in a 10-year-old boy. Note the contracted sternocleidomastoid muscle. (From Tachdjian MO: *Pediatric orthopedics*, p. 74, Philadelphia, 1972, WB Saunders.)

of the organs within the rib cage also occur. Examples of scoliotic curves are shown in Figure 15-21.

Patient History

As with any history, the examiner must ensure that the information obtained is as complete as possible. By listening to the patient, the examiner can often comprehend the problem. The information should include a history of the problem, the patient's general condition and health, and family history. If a child is being examined, the examiner must also obtain prenatal and postnatal his-

tories, including the health of or injuries experienced by the mother during pregnancy, any complications during pregnancy or delivery, and drugs taken by the mother during that period, especially during the first trimester, which is the period in which most of the congenital anomalies develop.

It should be remembered that it is unusual for a patient to present with just a postural problem. It is the symptoms produced by the pathology that is causing the postural abnormality that initiate the consultation. The examiner therefore must be cognizant of various underlying pathological conditions when assessing posture.

Table 15-6

Changes Associated with Postural Scoliosis

Body Segment Alignment	Spine curves to left or right May have single or double curve or one main curve and one or two compensatory curves Ribs may protrude on one side and be depressed (paravertebral valley) on the other side ("hump and hollow" on forward flexion because of vertebral rotation) May have short leg—pelvis tilted laterally—concave side high Shoulder/scapula may drop on concave side of curve
Muscles Commonly Elongated and Weak	Muscles on the convex side Hip abductor muscles on concave side Foot pronator muscles on the long side
Muscles Commonly Short and Strong	Muscles on concave side Hip adductors on convex side Foot supinators on short side
Joints Commonly Affected	Lumbar spine Thoracic spine Pelvic joints Hip joints Foot joints Scapulothoracic joints Glenohumeral joints Cervical spine (torticollis) Atlanto-occipital joints Temporomandibular joints

Adapted from Kendall FP, McCreary EK: *Muscles: testing and function*, Baltimore, 1983, Williams & Wilkins; Giallonardo LM: Posture. In Myers RS, editor: *Saunders manual of physical therapy practice*, Philadelphia, 1995, WB Saunders.

Figure 15-19

Scoliosis caused by hemivertebra. (From Moe JH, Bradford DS, Winter RB et al: *Scoliosis and other spinal deformities*, p. 134, Philadelphia, 1978, WB Saunders.)

The following questions should be asked:

1. *Was there any history of injury?* If so, what was the mechanism of injury? For example, lifting often causes lower spine problems, which may lead to altered posture.

2. *If there is a history of injury, had the patient experienced any back injury or pain previously?* If so, what caused that injury or pain? Was it a specific posture, sustained posture, or caused by repetitive movements? If so, what were the postures and/or movements?

3. *Are there any postures (e.g., standing with one foot on low stool, sitting with legs crossed) that give the patient relief or increase the patient's symptoms?*[25] The examiner can later test these postures to help determine the problem.

4. *Does the family have any history of back problems or other special problems?* Conditions such as hemiverte-bra, scoliosis, and Klippel-Feil syndrome may be congenital.

5. *Has the patient had any previous illnesses, surgery, or severe injuries?*

6. *Is there a history of any other conditions, such as connective tissue diseases, that have a high incidence of associated spinal problems?*

7. *Does footwear make a difference to the patient's posture or symptoms?* For example, high-heeled shoes often lead to excessive lordosis.[26]

8. *How old is the patient?* Many spinal problems begin in childhood or are the result of degeneration in the aged population.

9. *In the child, has there been a growth spurt?* If so, when did it begin? Growth spurts often lead to tight muscles and altered posture.

10. *For females, when did menarche begin?* Does back pain appear to be associated with menses? Menarche indicates the point at which approximately two thirds of the female adolescent growth spurt has been completed.

11. *For males, has there been a voice change?* If so, when? This question also gives an indication of maturity or onset of puberty.

12. *If a deformity is present, is it progressive or stationary?*

13. *Does the patient experience any neurological symptoms (e.g., a "pins and needles" feeling or numbness)?*

14. *What is the nature, extent, type, and duration of the pain?*

Figure 15-20
Idiopathic structural right thoracic scoliosis. Line drawing shows prominent features of scoliosis. (Photographs from Tachdjian MO: *Pediatric orthopedics*, p. 1200, Philadelphia, 1972, WB Saunders.)

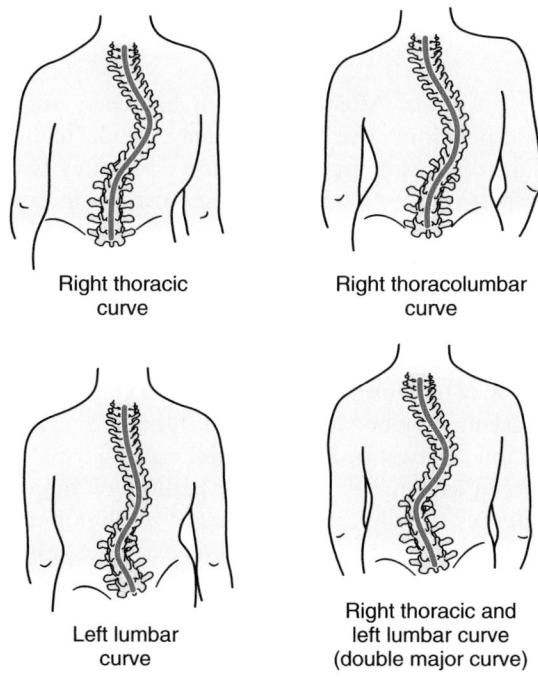

Right thoracic curve

Right thoracolumbar curve

Left lumbar curve

Right thoracic and left lumbar curve (double major curve)

Figure 15-21
Examples of scoliosis curve patterns.

15. *What positions or activities increase the pain or discomfort?*

16. *What positions or activities decrease the pain or discomfort?*

17. *For children, is there difficulty in fitting clothes?* For example, with scoliosis, the hem of a dress is usually uneven because of the spinal curvature.

18. *Does the patient have any difficulty breathing?* Structural deformities such as idiopathic scoliosis can lead to breathing problems in severe cases.

19. *Which hand is the dominant one?* Often, the dominant side shows a lower shoulder, with the hip slightly deviated to that side (Figure 15-22). The spine may deviate slightly to the opposite side, and the opposite foot is slightly more pronated.[7] The gluteus medius on the dominant side may also be weaker.

20. *Has there been any previous treatment?* If so, what was it? Was it successful?

Observation

Observation is the primary method of assessing posture and should be included in every assessment, looking for

Figure 15-22

Effect of handedness on posture. **A,** Right hand dominant. **B,** Left hand dominant. (From Kendall FP, McCreary EK: *Muscles: testing and function*, p. 294, Baltimore, 1983, Williams & Wilkins.)

asymmetrical changes that may contribute to or be the result of faulty posture. The following sections outline static posture, which forms the basis of dynamic posture (e.g., walking, running, lifting, throwing).[2]

To assess posture correctly, the patient must be adequately undressed. Male patients should be in shorts, and female patients should be in a bra and shorts. Ideally, the patient should not wear shoes or stockings. However, if the patient uses walking aids, braces, collars, or orthoses, they should be noted and may be used after the patient has been assessed in the "natural" state to determine the effect of the appliances.

The patient should be examined in the habitual, relaxed posture that is usually adopted. Often, it takes some time for the patient to adopt the usual posture because of tenseness, uneasiness, or uncertainty.

In the standing and sitting positions, the assessment is the same as the observation for the upper and lower limb scanning examinations of the cervical and lumbar spines. Assessment of posture should be carried out with the patient in the standing, sitting, and lying (supine and

prone) positions. After the patient has been examined in these positions, the examiner may decide to include other habitual, sustained, or repetitive postures assumed by the patient to see whether these postures increase or alter symptoms. The patient may also be assessed wearing different footwear to determine their effects on the posture and symptoms.

When observing a patient for abnormalities in posture, the examiner looks for asymmetry as a possible indication of what may be causing the postural fault (Figure 15-23). Some asymmetry between left and right sides is normal. The examiner must be able to differentiate normal deviations from asymmetry caused by pathology. Functional asymmetries usually refer to changes in alignment that occur with changes in posture. For example, nonstructural scoliosis may be present in standing because of a short leg but disappear on forward flexion. Anatomical or structural asymmetries are due to structural changes (e.g., idiopathic scoliosis).

As the examiner is watching for asymmetry, he or she should also note potential causes of asymmetry. For

POSTURE EVALUATION

| NAME: | AGE: | SEX: | HEIGHT: | WEIGHT: | DATE: |

Body type: Ectomorph / Mesomorph / Endomorph / Slight Build / Medium Build / Heavy Build

Uncorrected standing A   Corrected (talus in neutral) standing B   Postural Deformity Corrected C

ANTERIOR VIEW	Comments:
Head (aligned, forward, flexed, extended)	
Mandible (resting position, retracted)	
Shoulders (level, uneven)	
Rib cage (symmetric, asymmetric)	
Scoliosis (left, right, lumbar, thoracic, cervical)	
Pelvis (level, anterior/posterior tilt)	
Hips (coxa vara, coxa valga, anteversion, retroversion)	
Femurs (alignment, torsion)	
Knees (level, genu varum, genu valgum)	
Patellar position	
Tibias (alignment, torsions)	
Ankles (inversion, eversion)	
Rearfoot/forefoot alignment	
Feet (pes cavus, pes planus, supination/pronation)	
Toes (alignment, deformities)	
Leg length	

LATERAL VIEW	Comments:
Head (forward, flexed/extended)	
Mandible (resting, protracted/retracted)	
Scapulae (winging, elevation/depression)	
Thoracic kyphosis (increased/decreased)	
Lumbar lordosis (increased/decreased)	
Pelvis (anterior/posterior tilt)	
Knees (hyperextension/flexion)	
Feet (longitudinal arch)	

POSTERIOR VIEW	Comments:
Head (alignment, tilt)	
Shoulders (level)	
Scapulae (bilateral symmetry)	
Spine C-1 to sacrum (rotations, deviations)	
Pelvis (level, tilt)	
Sacrum (level at base and inferior lateral angles)	
Hips (level, uneven)	
Knees (creases level/uneven)	
Leg (rearfoot alignment)	
Ankles (inversion/eversion)	
Calcaneal position (inverted/everted)	

Pertinent Medical History:

Pertinent Radiographic Findings / Other Tests:

Figure 15-23

Example of standing posture evaluation form. Information is obtained by visual observation and palpation.
(Modified from Richardson JK, Iglarsh ZA: *Clinical orthopedic physical therapy*, Philadelphia, 1994, WB Saunders.)

example, the examiner should always watch for the presence of muscle wasting, soft tissue or bony swelling or enlargement, scars, and skin changes that may indicate present or past pathology.

Standing

The examiner should first determine the patient's body type (Figure 15-24).[25] The three body types are ectomorphic, mesomorphic, and endomorphic. The **ectomorph** is a person who has a thin body build characterized by a relative prominence of structures developed from the embryonic ectoderm. The **mesomorph** has a muscular or sturdy body build characterized by relative prominence of structures developed by the embryonic mesoderm. The **endomorph** has a heavy or fat body build characterized by relative prominence of structures developed from the embryonic endoderm.

Body Types

- Ectomorph
- Mesomorph
- Endomorph

In addition to body type, the examiner should note the emotional attitude of the patient. Is the patient tense, bored, or lethargic? Does the patient appear to be healthy, emaciated, or overweight? Answers to these questions can help the examiner determine how much must be done to correct any problems. For example, if the patient is lethargic, it may take longer to correct the problem than if he or she appears truly interested in correcting the problem. The examiner must remember that posture is in many ways an expression of one's personality, sense of well-being, and self-esteem.

Anterior View

When observing the patient from the front (Table 15-7; see Figure 15-1A), the examiner should note whether the following conditions hold true:

1. The head is straight on the shoulders (in midline). The examiner should note whether the head is habitually tilted to one side or rotated (e.g., torticollis) (Figure 15-25). The cause of altered head position must be established. For example, it may be the result of weak muscles, trauma, a hearing loss, temporomandibular joint problems, or the wearing of bifocal glasses.

Athletic   Asthenic   Pyknic

Athletic   Asthenic   Pyknic
(mesomorphic)   (ectomorphic)   (endomorphic)

Figure 15-24
Male and female body types. (From Debrunner HU: *Orthopedic diagnosis*, p. 86, London, 1970, E & S Livingstone.)

Table 15-7

Alignment in the Standing Posture: Anterior View

Body Segment	Line of Gravity Location	Observation
Head	Passes through middle of the forehead, nose, and chin	Eyes and ears should be level and symmetrical
Neck/shoulders		Right and left angles between shoulders and neck should be symmetrical; clavicles also should be symmetrical
Chest	Passes through the middle of the xiphoid process	Ribs on each side should be symmetrical
Abdomen/hips	Passes through the umbilicus (navel)	Right and left waist angles should be symmetrical
Hips/pelvis	Passes on a line equidistant from the right and left anterior superior iliac spines; passes through the symphysis pubis	Anterior superior iliac spines should be level
Knees	Passes between knees equidistant from medial femoral condyles	Patellae should be symmetrical and facing straight ahead
Ankles/feet	Passes between ankles equidistant from the medial malleoli	Malleoli should be symmetrical, and feet should be parallel
		Toes should not be curled, overlapping, or deviated to one side

From Levangie PK, Norkin CC: *Joint structures and function—a comprehensive analysis*, p. 498, Philadelphia, 2005, FA Davis.

Figure 15-25

Congenital torticollis in 18-year-old girl. Note the asymmetry of the face. (From Tachdjian MO: *Pediatric orthopedics*, p. 68, Philadelphia, 1972, WB Saunders.)

2. The posture of the jaw is normal. In the resting position, normal jaw posture is when the lips are gently pressed together, the teeth are slightly apart (freeway space), and the tip of the tongue is behind the upper teeth in the roof of the mouth. This position maintains the mandible in a good posture (i.e., slight negative pressure in the mouth reduces the work of the muscles). It also enables respiration through the nose and diaphragmatic breathing.

3. The tip of the nose is in line with the manubrium sternum, xiphisternum, and umbilicus. This line is the **anterior line of reference** used to divide the body into right and left halves (see Figure 15-1A). If the umbilicus is used as a reference point, the examiner should remember that the umbilicus is almost always slightly off center.

4. The upper trapezius neck line is equal on both sides. The muscle bulk of the trapezius muscles should be equal, and the slope of the muscles should be approximately equal. Because the dominant arm usually shows greater laxity by being slightly lower, the slope on the dominant side may be slightly greater.

5. The shoulders are level. In most cases, the dominant side is slightly lower.

6. The clavicles and acromioclavicular joints are level and equal. They should be symmetrical; any deviation should be noted. Deviations may be caused by subluxations or dislocations of the acromioclavicular or sternoclavicular joints, fractures, or clavicular rotation.

7. There is no protrusion, depression, or lateralization of the sternum, ribs, or costal cartilage. If there are changes, they should be noted.

8. The waist angles are equal, and the arms are equidistant from the waist. If a scoliosis is present, one arm hangs closer to the body than the other arm. The examiner should also note whether the arms are equally rotated medially or laterally.

9. The carrying angles at each elbow are equal. Any deviation should be noted. The normal carrying angle varies from 5° to 15°.

10. The palms of both hands face the body in the relaxed standing position. Any differences should be noted and may give an indication of rotation in the upper limb.

11. The "high points" of the iliac crest are the same height on each side (Figure 15-26). With a scoliosis, the patient may feel that one hip is "higher" than the other. This apparent high pelvis results from the lateral shift of the trunk; the pelvis is usually level. The same condition can cause the patient to feel that one leg is shorter than the other.

12. The anterior superior iliac spines (ASISs) are level. If one ASIS is higher than the other, there is a possibility that one leg is shorter than the other or that the pelvis is rotated more or shifted up or down more on one side.

13. The pubic bones are level at the symphysis pubis. Any deviation should be noted.

14. The patellae of the knees point straight ahead. Sometimes the patellae face outward ("frog eyes" patellae) or inward ("squinting" patellae). The position of the patella may also be altered by torsion of the femoral

A   **B**

Figure 15-26
Viewing height equality. **A,** Iliac crests. **B,** Anterior superior iliac spines.

neck (anteversion-retroversion), femoral shaft, or tibial shaft.

15. The knees are straight. The knees may be in genu varum or genu valgum. If the ankles are together and the knees are more than two finger-widths apart, the patient has some genu varum. If the knees are touching and the feet are apart, the patient has some genu valgum. Genu valgum is more likely to be seen in females. The examiner should note whether the deformity results from the femur, tibia, or both. In children, the knees go through a progression of being straight, going into genu varum (Figure 15-27), being straight, going into genu valgum (Figure 15-28), and finally being straight again during the first 6 years of life (see Figure 15-4).[13]

16. The heads of the fibulae are level.

17. The medial and lateral malleoli of the ankles are level. Normally, the medial malleoli are slightly anterior to the lateral malleoli, but the lateral malleoli extend farther distally.

18. Two arches are present in the feet and equal on the two sides. In this position, only the medial longitudinal arch is visible. The examiner should note any pes planus (flatfoot) or pronated foot, pes cavus ("hollow" foot) or supinated foot, or other deformities.

19. The feet angle out equally (this Fick angle is usually 5° to 18° [see Figure 14-13]; Figure 15-29). This finding means that the tibias are normally slightly laterally rotated (lateral tibial torsion). The presence of

Figure 15-27
Bilateral genu varum in mother and son. Note the associated medial tibial torsion. (From Tachdjian MO: *Pediatric orthopedics*, p. 1462, Philadelphia, 1972, WB Saunders.)

Figure 15-28
Bilateral genu valgum in an adolescent. (From Tachdjian MO: *Pediatric orthopedics*, p. 1467, Philadelphia, 1972, WB Saunders.)

Figure 15-29
Exaggerated lateral tibial torsion. In stance, with the patellae facing straight forward, the feet point outward. (From Tachdjian MO: *Pediatric orthopedics*, p 1461, Philadelphia, 1972, WB Saunders.)

pigeon toes usually indicates medial rotation of the tibias (medial tibial torsion), especially if the patellae face straight ahead. If the patellae face inward (squinting patellae) in the presence of "pigeon toes" or outward, the problem may be in the femur (abnormal femoral torsion or hip retroversion-anteversion problems).

20. There is no bowing of bone. Any bowing may indicate diseases such as osteomalacia or osteoporosis.

21. The bony and soft-tissue contours are equally symmetrical on the two halves of the body. Any indication of muscle wasting, muscle hypertrophy on one side, or bony asymmetry should be noted. Such a finding may indicate muscle or nerve pathology, or it may simply be related to the patient's job or recreational pursuits. For example, a rodeo bull rider will show hypertrophy of the muscles and bones on one side (the arm that he uses to hang on!).

In addition, the patient's skin is observed for abnormalities such as hairy patches (e.g., diastematomyelia), pigmented lesions (e.g., café au lait spots, neurofibromatosis), subcutaneous tumors, and scars (e.g., Ehlers-Danlos syndrome), all of which may lead to or contribute to postural problems (Figure 15-30). Table 15-8 shows some of the malalignment postures and their effect.[2,13,27,28] Changes in one body segment cause changes in other segments as the body attempts to compensate or adjust for the malignment.[2] Compensatory postures are those that represent the body's attempt to normalize appearance or improve function.[2]

A

B

Figure 15-30
Abnormal skin markings. **A,** Café au lait areas of pigmentation seen in neurofibromatosis. **B,** Lumbar hair patch seen in diastematomyelia. (From Moe JH, Bradford DS, Winter RB et al: *Scoliosis and other spinal deformities*, p. 20, Philadelphia, 1978, WB Saunders.)

Table 15-8

Malalignments Viewed Anteriorly[2,13,27,28]

Malalignment	Possible Correlated Motions or Postures	Possible Compensatory Motions or Postures
Torticollis	Rotation to same side limited	
	Side flexion to opposite side limited	
Scoliosis	Side flexion to convex side limited	
	Rotation to convex side limited	
	Rib hump on convex side	
Lateral pelvic tilt (pelvic drop—right leg stance)	Right hip adduction	Right lumbar lateral flexion
	Weak right abductors (positive Trendelenburg's)	Tight left adductors
Lateral pelvic tilt (pelvic hitch—right leg stance)	Right hip abduction	Left lumbar lateral flexion
	Weak left adductors	Tight right abductors
Forward rotation of one ilium on sacrum (right leg stance)	Right hip medial rotation	Left lumbar rotation
	Medial-facing patella	Scoliosis—concavity to left
	In-toeing	Knee flexion
	Pronation of foot	
	Long leg	
Excessive anteversion	Toeing-in	Lateral tibial torsion
	Subtalar pronation	Lateral rotation at knee
	Lateral patellar subluxation	Lateral rotation of tibia, femur, and/or pelvis
	Medial tibial torsion	Lumbar rotation on same side
	Medial femoral torsion	
Excessive retroversion	Toeing-out	Medial rotation at knee
	Subtalar supination	Medial rotation of tibia, femur, and/or pelvis
	Lateral tibial torsion	Lumbar rotation on opposite side
	Lateral femoral torsion	
Coxa vara	Pronated subtalar joint	Ipsilateral subtalar supination
	Medial rotation of leg	Contralateral subtalar pronation
	Short ipsilateral leg	Ipsilateral plantar flexion
	Anterior pelvic rotation	Contralateral genu recurvatum
		Contralateral hip and/or knee flexion
		Ipsilateral posterior pelvic rotation and ipsilateral lumbar rotation
Coxa valga	Supinated subtalar joint	Ipsilateral subtalar pronation
	Lateral rotation of leg	Contralateral subtalar supination
	Long ipsilateral leg	Contralateral plantar flexion
	Posterior pelvic tilt	Ipsilateral genu recurvatum
		Ipsilateral hip and/or knee flexion
		Ipsilateral anterior pelvic rotation and contralateral lumbar rotation
Medial femoral torsion	Excessive subtalar pronation	Excessive subtalar supination
	In-toeing	Functional forefoot valgus
	Medial facing or tilted patella ("squinting" patella)	
Lateral femoral torsion	Excessive subtalar supination	Excessive subtalar pronation
	Out-toeing	Functional forefoot varus
	Lateral-facing or tilted patella ("grasshopper eyes" or "frog eyes" patella)	
Genu valgum	Pes planus	Forefoot varus
	Excessive subtalar pronation	Excessive subtalar supination to allow the lateral heel to contact the ground
	Lateral tibial torsion	In-toeing to decrease lateral pelvic sway during gait
	Lateral patellar subluxation	Ipsilateral pelvic lateral rotation
	Excessive hip adduction	
	Ipsilateral hip excessive medial rotation	
	Lumbar spine contralateral rotation	

Continued

Table 15-8–cont'd

Malalignment	Possible Correlated Motions or Postures	Possible Compensatory Motions or Postures
Genu varum	Excessive lateral angulation of the tibia in the frontal plane; tibial varum Medial tibial torsion Ipsilateral hip lateral rotation Excessive hip abduction	Forefoot valgus Excessive subtalar pronation to allow the medial heel to contact the ground Ipsilateral pelvic medial rotation
Lateral tibial (malleolar) torsion	Out-toeing Excessive subtalar supination with related rotation along the lower quarter	Functional forefoot varus Excessive subtalar pronation with relaxed rotation along the lower quarter
Medial tibial (malleolar) torsion	In-toeing Metatarsus adductus Excessive subtalar pronation with related rotation along the lower quarter	Functional forefoot valgus Excessive subtalar supination with relaxed rotation along the lower quarter
Inadequate tibial retroflexion (bowing of the tibia)	Altered alignment of Achilles tendon causing altered associated joint motion	
Bowleg deformity of the tibia (tibial varum)	Medial tibial torsion	Forefoot valgus Excessive subtalar pronation
Ankle equinus		Hypermobile first ray Subtalar or midtarsal excessive pronation Hip or knee flexion Genu recurvatum
Forefoot valgus	Hallux valgus Subtalar pronation and related rotation along the lower quarter	Excessive midtarsal or subtalar supination Excessive tibial; tibial and femoral; or tibial, femoral, and pelvic lateral rotation, or all with ipsilateral lumbar spine rotation
Metatarsus adductus	Hallux valgus Medial tibial torsion Flatfoot Toeing-in	
Hallux valgus	Forefoot valgus Subtalar pronation and related rotation along the lower quarter	Excessive tibial; tibial and femoral; or tibial, femoral, and pelvic lateral rotation, or all with ipsilateral lumbar spine rotation
In-toeing	Pronated foot Medial tibial torsion Metatarsus varus Talipes varus or equinovarus Tibia or genu varum Medial femoral torsion Excessive femoral anteversion Tight medial hip rotators Acetabular dysplasia (facing anteriorly)	
Out-toeing	Tight Achilles Talipes calcaneovalgus Convex pes planovarus Lateral tibial torsion Hypoplastic (absence of) fibula Lateral femoral torsion Abnormal femoral retroversion Tight lateral rotators Flaccid medial rotators Acetabular dysplasia (facing posteriorly)	

Lateral View

From the side (Table 15-9; see Figure 15-1B), the examiner should note whether the following conditions hold true:

1. The earlobe is in line with the tip of the shoulder (acromion process) and the "high point" of the iliac crest. This line is the **lateral line of reference** dividing the body into front and back halves (see Figure 15-1B). If the chin pokes forward, an excessive lumbar lordosis may also be present. This compensatory change is caused by the body's attempt to maintain the center of gravity in the normal position.

2. Each spinal segment has a normal curve (Figure 15-31). Large gluteus maximus muscles or excessive fat may give the appearance of an exaggerated lordosis. The examiner should look at the spine in relation to the sacrum, not the gluteal muscles. Likewise, the scapulae may give the illusion of an increased kyphosis in the thoracic spine, especially if they are flat and the patient has rounded shoulders.

3. The shoulders are in proper alignment. If the shoulders droop forward (i.e., the scapulae protract), "rounded shoulders" are indicated. This improper alignment may be caused by habit or by tight pectoral muscles or weak scapular stabilizers.

4. The chest, abdominal, and back muscles have proper tone. Weakness or spasm of any of these muscles can lead to postural alterations.

5. There are no chest deformities, such as pectus carinatum (undue prominence of the sternum) or pectus excavatum (undue depression of the sternum).

6. The pelvic angle is normal (30°; Figure 15-32). The posterior superior iliac spine should be slightly higher than the anterior superior iliac spine.

7. The knees are straight, flexed, or in recurvatum (hyperextended). Usually, in the normal standing position, the knees are slightly flexed (0° to 5°). Hyperextension of the knees may cause an increase in lordosis in the lumbar spine. Tight hamstrings or gastrocnemius muscles can also cause knee flexion.

Figure 15-33 illustrates normal posture and some of the abnormal deviations seen when viewing the patient from the side. Table 15-10 shows some of the malalignment postures and their effect.[2,27,28]

Table 15-9

Alignment in the Standing Posture: Side View

Joints	Line of Gravity	External Moment	Passive Opposing Forces	Active Opposing Forces
Atlanto-occipital	Anterior (Anterior-to-transverse axis for flexion and extension)	Flexion	Ligamentum nuchae and alar ligaments; the tectorial, atlanto-axial, and posterior atlanto-occipital membranes	Rectus capitis posterior major and minor, semispinalis capitis and cervicis, splenius capitis and cervicis, and inferior and superior oblique muscles
Cervical	Posterior	Extension	Anterior longitudinal ligament, anterior anulus fibrosus fibers, and anterior zygapophyseal joint capsules	Anterior scalene, longus capitis and colli
Thoracic	Anterior	Flexion	Posterior longitudinal, supraspinous, and interspinous ligaments; posterior zygapophyseal joint capsules and posterior anulus fibrosus fibers	Ligamentum flavum, longissimus thoracis, iliocostalis thoracis, spinalis thoracis, and semispinalis thoracis
Lumbar	Posterior	Extension	Anterior longitudinal and iliolumbar ligaments, anterior fibers of the anulus fibrosus, and anterior zygapophyseal joint capsules	Rectus abdominis and external and internal oblique muscles
Sacroiliac joint	Anterior	Nutation	Sacrotuberous, sacrospinous, iliolumbar, and anterior sacroiliac ligaments	Transversus abdominis
Hip joint	Posterior	Extension	Iliofemoral ligament	Iliopsoas
Knee joint	Anterior	Extension	Posterior joint capsule	Hamstrings, gastrocnemius
Ankle joint	Anterior	Dorsiflexion		Soleus, gastrocnemius

From Levangie PK, Norkin CC: *Joint structures and function—a comprehensive analysis*, p. 493, Philadelphia, 2005, FA Davis.

Figure 15-31
Correct postural alignment. (From Kendall FP, McCreary EK: *Muscles: testing and function*, p. 280, Baltimore, 1983, Williams & Wilkins.)

Posterior View

When viewing from behind (Table 15-11; see Figure 15-1C), the examiner should note whether the following conditions hold true:

1. The shoulders are level, and the head is in midline. These findings should be compared with those from the anterior view.

2. The spines and inferior angles of the scapulae are level (Figure 15-34), and the medial borders of the scapulae are equidistant from the spine. If not, is there a rotational or winging deformity of one of the scapulae? Defects such as Sprengel's deformity should be noted (Figure 15-35).

3. The spine is straight or curved laterally, indicating scoliosis. A plumb line may be dropped from the spinous process of the seventh cervical vertebra (Figure 15-36).[29] Normally, the line passes through the gluteal cleft. This line is the **posterior line of reference** used to divide the body into right and left halves posteriorly (see Figure 15-1C). The dis-

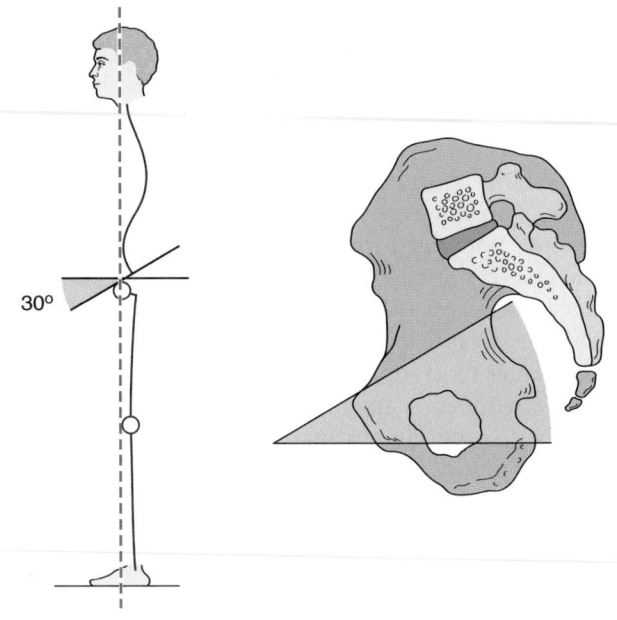

Figure 15-32
Normal pelvic angle.

tance from the vertical string to the gluteal cleft can be measured. This distance is sometimes used as a measurement of spinal imbalance, and it is noted whether the deviation is to the left or right. If a torticollis or cervicothoracic scoliosis is present, the plumb line should be dropped from the occipital protuberance.[11]

4. The ribs protrude or are symmetrical on both sides.

5. The waist angles are level.

6. The arms are equidistant from the body and equally rotated.

7. The posterior superior iliac spines (PSISs) are level (Figure 15-37). If one is higher than the other, one leg may be shorter or rotation of the pelvis may be present. The examiner should note how the PSISs relate to the ASISs. If the ASIS on one side and the PSIS on the other side are higher, there is a torsion deformity (anterior or posterior) at the sacroiliac joint. If the ASIS and PSIS on one side are higher than the ASIS and PSIS on the other side, there may be an up-slip at the sacroiliac joint on the high side.

8. The gluteal folds are level. Muscle weakness, nerve root problems, or nerve palsy may lead to asymmetry.

9. The knee joints are level. If they are not, it may indicate that one leg is shorter than the other (Figure 15-38).

10. Both of the Achilles tendons descend straight to the calcanei. If the tendons angle out, it may indicate a flatfoot deformity (pes planus).

11. The heels are straight or are angled in (rear-foot varus) or out (rear-foot valgus).

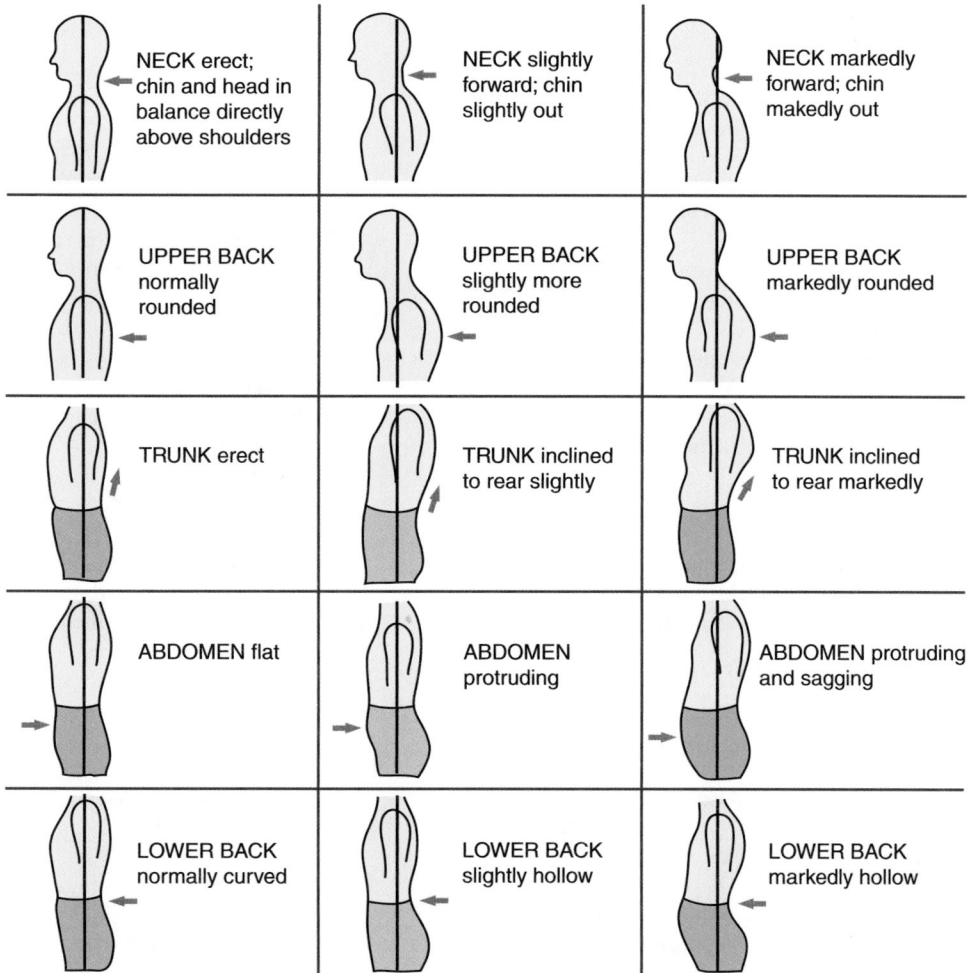

Figure 15-33
Postural deviations obvious from the side view. (Redrawn from Reedco Research, Auburn, NY.)

12. Bowing of femur or tibia is present or absent.

Figure 15-39 illustrates the normal posture and some of the abnormal deviations seen when viewing from behind. Table 15-12 highlights some of the malalignment postures and their effect.[2,13,27,28]

When viewing posture, the examiner should remember that the pelvis is usually the key to proper back posture. The normal pelvic angle is 30°, and the pelvis is held or balanced in this position by muscles. For the pelvis to "sit properly" on the femur, the following muscles must be strong, supple (mobile), and balanced: abdominals, hip flexors, hip extensors, superficial and deep back extensors, hip rotators, and hip abductors and adductors.

If the height of the patient is measured, especially in a child, the focal height of the child may be estimated by the use of a chart such as the one shown in Table 15-13.[30]

After the standing posture has been assessed, the examiner may decide to assess some additional postures (e.g., positional, sustained, or repetitive), especially if the patient has stated in the history that these different positions have caused problems or symptoms.

Forward Flexion

Having completed the assessment of normal standing, the examiner asks the patient to flex forward at the hips with the fingertips of both hands together so that the arms drop vertically (Figure 15-40). The feet should be together, and both knees should be straight. Any alteration from this posture will cause the spine to rotate, giving a false view.

From this position, using the anterior and posterior skyline views, the examiner can note the following:

1. Whether there is any asymmetry of the rib cage (e.g., rib hump); if a hump is present, a level and tape measure may be used to obtain the perpendicular distance between the hump and hollow (Figure 15-41)[11]
2. Whether there is any asymmetry in the spinal musculature

Table 15-10

Malalignments Viewed Laterally[2,27,28]

Malalignment	Possible Correlated Motions or Postures	Possible Compensatory Motions or Postures
Forward head posture	Extension of cervical spine Protracted scapula	Increased kyphosis in thoracic spine Increased lordosis in lumbar spine Medially rotated humerus
Round back	Extension of cervical spine Protracted scapula	Forward head posture Hips flexed Knees extended
Flat back	Posterior pelvic tilt	Hips extended Knees extended Forward head posture
Swayback	Pelvic neutral or posterior tilt	Pelvis slides anterior Kyphosis Hips extended Knees extended
Pathological lordosis	Pelvis anteriorly tilted Tight hip flexors	Knees extended Ankles plantar flexed
Anterior pelvic tilt	Hip flexion (tight hip flexors)	Lumbar extension (increased lordosis) Hyperextended knees Poking chin (cervical extension) Rounded shoulders (protracted scapula) Thoracic kyphosis Ankles plantar flexed
Posterior pelvic tilt	Hip extension	Lumbar flexion (flat back) Hips extended Knees extended Forward head posture
Backward rotation of one ilium on sacrum (right leg stance)	Right hip lateral rotation Lateral facing patella Out-toeing Supination of foot Short leg	Right lumbar rotation Scoliosis—concavity to right Knee extension
Genu recurvatum	Ankle plantar flexion Excessive anterior pelvic tilt	Posterior pelvic tilt Flexed trunk posture Excessive thoracic kyphosis
Excessive tibial retroversion (posterior slant of tibial plateaus)	Genu recurvatum	
Inadequate tibial retrotorsion (posterior deflection of proximal tibia because of hamstrings pull)	Flexed knee posture	

3. Whether a pathological kyphosis is present
4. Whether lumbar spine straightens or flexes as it normally should
5. Whether there is any restriction to forward bending, such as spondylolisthesis or tight hamstrings (Figures 15-42 and 15-43)

If, in the history, the patient said that sustained forward flexion caused symptoms, the examiner should ask the patient to assume the symptom-causing posture and maintain it for 15 to 30 seconds to determine whether symptoms arise or increase. Flexion has been found to decrease the stress on the facet joints, but it can increase the pressure in the nucleus pulposus.[31,32] Likewise, if repetitive forward flexion or combined movements (e.g., extension and rotation) have caused symptoms, the patient should be asked to do the repetitive or combined movements. Loading the spine by lifting an object may also cause symptoms and may be investigated if symptoms are not too great.

Table 15-11

Alignment in the Standing Posture: Posterior View

Body Segment	Line of Gravity Location	Observation
Head	Passes through middle of head	Head should be straight with no lateral tilting; angles between shoulders and neck should be equal
Arms		Arms should hang naturally so that the palms of the hands are facing the sides of the body
Shoulders/spine	Passes along vertebral column in a straight line, which should bisect the back into two symmetrical halves	Scapulae should lie flat against the rib cage, be equidistant from the line of gravity, and be separated by about 4 inches in the adult
Hips/pelvis	Passes through gluteal cleft of buttocks and should be equidistant from posterior superior iliac spines	The posterior superior iliac spines should be level; the gluteal folds should be level and symmetrical
Knees	Passes between knees equidistant from medial joint aspects	Look to see that the knees are level
Ankles/feet	Passes between ankles equidistant from the medial malleoli	The heel cords should be vertical, and the malleoli should be level and symmetrical

From Levangie PK, Norkin CC: *Joint structures and function—a comprehensive analysis*, p. 499, Philadelphia, 2005, FA Davis.

Figure 15-34

Correct postural alignment. (From Kendall FP, McCreary EK: *Muscles: testing and function*, p. 290, Baltimore, 1983, Williams & Wilkins.)

Figure 15-35

Sprengel's deformity. Note the small, high scapula on the right. (From Tachdjian MO: *Pediatric orthopedics*, p. 82, Philadelphia, 1972, WB Saunders.)

Sitting

With the patient seated on a stool so that the feet are on the ground and the back is unsupported, the examiner looks at the patient's posture (Figure 15-44). Sitting without a back support causes the patient to support

Figure 15-36

The patient is viewed from the back to evaluate the spine deformity. **A,** A typical right thoracic curve is shown. The left shoulder is lower, and the right scapula more prominent. Note the decreased distance between the right arm and the thorax, with the shift of the thorax to the right. The left iliac crest appears higher, but this is caused by the shift of the thorax, with fullness on the right and elimination of the waistline. The high hip is thus only apparent, not real. **B,** Plumb line dropped from the prominent vertebra of C7 (vertebra prominens) measures the decompensation of the upper thorax over the pelvis. The distance from the vertical plumb line to the gluteal cleft is measured in centimeters and is recorded, noting the direction of fall from the occipital protuberance (inion). (From Moe JH et al: *Scoliosis and other spinal deformities*, p. 14, Philadelphia, 1978, WB Saunders.)

his or her own posture and increases the amount of muscle activity needed to maintain the posture.[31] This observation is carried out, as in the standing position, from the front, back, and side. If any anteroposterior or lateral deviations of the spine are observed, the examiner should recall whether they were present when the patient was examined while standing. It should be noted whether the spinal curves increase or decrease when the patient is in the sitting position and how the curves change with different sitting postures.[33] From the front, it can be noted whether the knees are the same distance from the floor. If they are not, this may indicate a shortened tibia. From the side, it can be noted whether one knee protrudes farther than the other. If it does, this may indicate a shortened femur on the other side.

If the patient has stated in the history that going from standing to sitting or sitting to standing resulted in symptoms, the patient should be asked to repeat these maneuvers, provided the movements do not exacerbate the symptoms too much.

Supine Lying

With the patient in the supine-lying position, the examiner notes the position of the head and cervical spine as well as the shoulder girdle. The chest area is observed for any protrusion (e.g., pectus carinatum) or sunken areas (e.g., pectus excavatum).

The abdominal musculature should be observed to see whether it is strong or flabby, and the waist angles

Figure 15-37
Viewing height equality. **A,** Posterior superior iliac spines. **B,** Gluteal folds.

should be noted to see whether they are equal. As in the standing position, the ASISs should be viewed to see if they are level. Any extension in the lumbar spine should be noted. In addition, it should be noted whether bending the knees helps to decrease the lumbar curve; if it does, it may indicate tight hip flexors. The lower limbs should descend parallel from the pelvis. If they do not, or if they cannot be aligned parallel and at right angles to a line joining the ASISs, it may indicate an abduction or adduction contracture at the hip.

If, in the history, the patient has complained of symptoms on arising from supine lying or from going into the supine position, the examiner should ask the patient to repeat these movements, provided they do not exacerbate the symptoms.

Prone Lying

With the patient lying prone, the examiner notes the position of the head, neck, and shoulder girdle, as previously described. The head should be positioned so that it is not rotated, side flexed, or extended. Any condition such as Sprengel's deformity or rib hump should be noted, as should any spinal deviations. The examiner should determine whether the PSISs are level and should

Figure 15-38
A and **B,** Functional scoliosis resulting from short leg. **C** and **D,** The spinal position with short leg is corrected. (From Tachdjian MO: *Pediatric orthopedics*, p. 1192, Philadelphia, 1972, WB Saunders.)

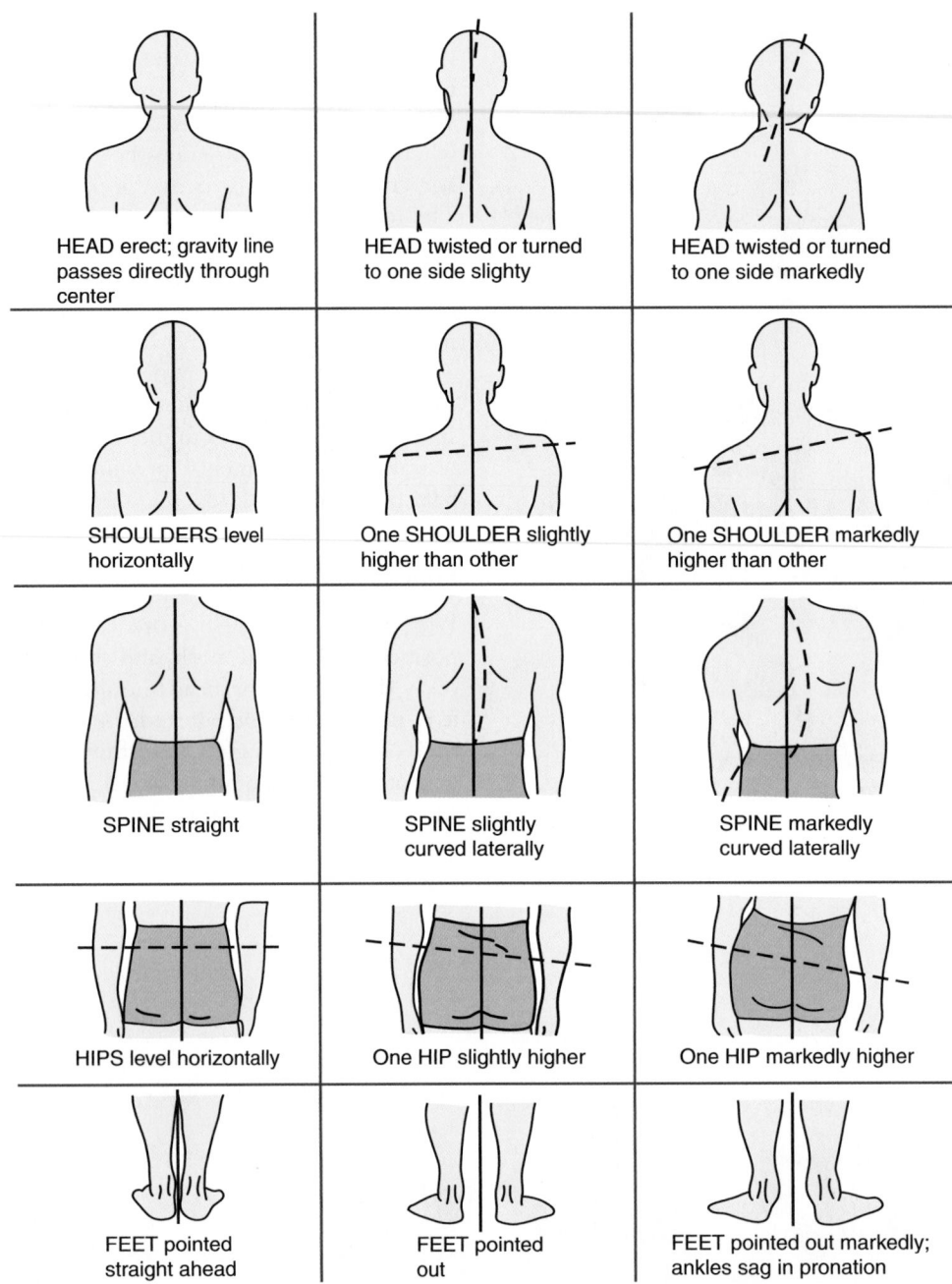

Figure 15-39
Postural deviations obvious from the posterior view. (Redrawn from Reedco Research, Auburn, NY.)

ensure that the musculature of the buttocks, posterior thighs, and calves is normal (Figure 15-45).

As with supine lying, if assuming the position or recovering from the position causes symptoms, the patient should be asked to repeat these movements, as long as symptoms are not made worse.

Examination

Assessment of posture primarily involves history and observation. If, on completing the history and observation, the examiner believes that a direct examination is necessary, the procedures outlined in this text for the

Table 15-12

Malalignments Viewed Posteriorly[*2,13,27,28]

Malalignment	Possible Correlated Motions or Postures	Possible Compensatory Motions or Postures
Scoliosis	Side flexion to convex side limited Rotation to convex side limited Rib hump on convex side	
Rear-foot varus Excessive subtalar supination (calcaneal varus)	Tibial; tibial and femoral; or tibial, femoral, and pelvic lateral rotation	Excessive medial rotation along the lower quarter chain Hallux valgus Plantar-flexed first ray Functional forefoot valgus Excessive or prolonged midtarsal pronation
Rear-foot valgus Excessive subtalar pronation (calcaneal valgus) Forefoot varus	Tibial; tibial and femoral; or tibial, femoral, and pelvic medial rotation Hallux valgus Subtalar supination and related rotation along the lower quarter	Excessive lateral rotation along the lower quarter chain Functional forefoot varus Plantar-flexed first ray Hallux valgus Excessive midtarsal or subtalar pronation or prolonged pronation Excessive tibial; tibial and femoral; or tibial, femoral, and pelvic medial rotation, or all with contralateral lumbar spine rotation

*Many of the posterior malalignments are also seen anteriorly.

Table 15-13

Percentage of Mature Height Attained at Different Ages

Chronological Age (yrs)	Percentage of Eventual Height	
	Boys	Girls
1	42.2	44.7
2	49.5	52.8
3	53.8	57.0
4	58.0	61.8
5	61.8	66.2
6	65.2	70.3
7	69.0	74.0
8	72.0	77.5
9	75.0	80.7
10	78.0	84.4
11	81.1	88.4
12	84.2	92.9
13	87.3	96.5
14	91.5	98.3
15	96.1	99.1
16	98.3	99.6
17	99.3	100.0
18	99.8	100.0

From Bayley N: The accurate prediction of growth and adult height, *Mod Probl Pediatr* 7:234–255, 1954.

various areas of the body should be followed. In addition, there are postural alignment measures such as the Flexicurve ruler and other measures that may be used to record postural alignments and changes.[34] With every postural assessment, however, the examiner should perform two tests: the leg length measurement[35–38] and the slump test.

Leg Length Measurement. The patient lies supine with the pelvis set square or "balanced" on the legs (i.e., the legs at an angle of 90° to a line joining the ASISs). The legs should be 15 to 20 cm (6 to 8 inches) apart and parallel to each other (Figure 15-46). The examiner then places one end of the tape measure against the distal aspect of the ASIS, holding it firmly against the bone. The index finger of the other hand is placed immediately distal to the medial or lateral malleolus and pushed against it. The thumbnail is brought down against the tip of the index fingers so that the tape measure is pinched between them. A reading is taken where the thumb and finger pinch together. A slight difference, up to 1.0 to 1.5 cm (0.4 to 0.6 inch), is considered normal but can still be relevant if pathology is present. Further information on measurement of true leg length may be found in Chapter 11.

Slump Test. The patient is seated on the edge of the examining table with the legs supported, the hips

Figure 15-40

Posture in forward flexion. **A,** Normal range of motion. Note reversal of lumbar curve. **B,** Excessive range of motion caused by excessive hip mobility.

Hump ———————

Hollow ———————

A

B

C

Figure 15-41

Rib hump in forward-bending test. **A,** Posterior view. **B,** Anterior view. The two sides are compared. Note the presence of a right thoracic prominence. **C,** Measurement of the prominence. The spirit level is positioned with the zero mark over the palpable spinous process in the area of maximal prominence. The level is made horizontal and the distance to the apex of the deformity (5 to 6 cm) noted. The perpendicular distance from the level to the hollow is measured at the same distance from the midline. A 2.4-cm right thoracic prominence is shown. (From Moe JH et al: *Scoliosis and other spinal deformities*, p. 17, Philadelphia, 1978, WB Saunders.)

Figure 15-42
Abnormal forward bending resulting from tight hamstrings in a patient with spondylolisthesis. (From Moe JH et al: *Scoliosis and other spinal deformities*, p. 19, Philadelphia, 1978, WB Saunders.)

Figure 15-43
Forward-bending position for viewing kyphosis (lateral view). **A,** Normal thoracic roundness is demonstrated with a gentle curve to the whole spine. **B,** An area of increased bending is seen in the thoracic spine, indicating structural changes, in a patient with Scheuermann's disease. (From Moe JH et al: *Scoliosis and other spinal deformities*, p. 18, Philadelphia, 1978, WB Saunders.)

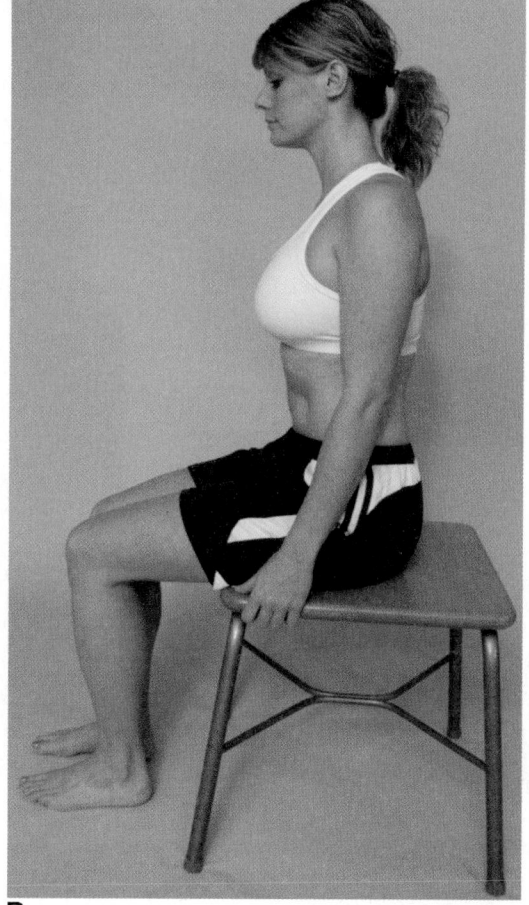

Figure 15-44
Posture in sitting position. **A,** Anterior view. **B,** Side view.

in neutral position (i.e., no rotation or abduction-adduction), and the hands behind the back (Figure 15-47). The examination is performed in several steps. First, the patient is asked to "slump" the back into thoracic and lumbar flexion. The examiner maintains the patient's chin in the neutral position to prevent neck and head flexion. The examiner then uses one arm to apply overpressure across the shoulders to maintain flexion of the thoracic and lumbar spines. While this position is held, the patient is asked to actively flex the cervical spine and head as far as possible (i.e., chin to chest). The examiner then applies overpressure to maintain flexion of all three parts of the spine (cervical, thoracic, lumbar), using the hand of the same arm to maintain overpressure in the cervical spine. With the other hand, the examiner then holds the patient's foot in maximum dorsiflexion. While the examiner holds these positions,

the patient is asked to actively straighten the knee as much as possible. The test is repeated with the other leg and then with both legs at the same time. If the patient is unable to fully extend the knee because of pain, the examiner releases the overpressure to the cervical spine and the patient actively extends the neck. If the knee extends farther, the symptoms decrease with neck extension, or the positioning of the patient increases the patient's symptoms, then the test is considered positive for increased tension in the neuromeningeal tract.[39-41] Further information on the slump test may be found in Chapter 9.

Additional Tests. Other tests may also be performed based on what the examiner has observed. For example, if the hip flexors appear tight, the Thomas test should be performed (see Chapter 11). Refer to Table 15-14 for a detailed presentation of good and faulty posture.

Text continued on page 1012

Figure 15-45
Structural kyphosis does not disappear on extension. (From Moe JH, Bradford DS, Winter RB et al: *Scoliosis and other spinal deformities*, p. 339, Philadelphia, 1978, WB Saunders.)

A   B

Figure 15-46
Measuring leg length. **A,** To medial malleolus. **B,** To lateral malleolus.

Figure 15-47

Sequence of subject postures in the slump test. **A,** Patient sits erect with hands behind back. **B,** Patient slumps lumbar and thoracic spine while either patient or examiner keeps head in neutral. **C,** Examiner pushes down on shoulders while patient holds head in neutral. **D,** Patient flexes head. Patient flexes head.

Continued

Figure 15-47 cont'd

E, Examiner carefully applies overpressure to cervical spine. **F,** Examiner extends patient's knee while holding the cervical spine flexed. **G,** While holding the knee extended and cervical spine flexed, the examiner dorsiflexes the foot. **H,** Patient extends head, which should relieve any symptoms. If symptoms are reproduced at any stage, further sequential movements are not attempted.

Table 15-14
Good and Faulty Posture: Summary Chart

Good Posture	Part	Faulty Posture
Head is held erect in a position of good balance.	Head	Chin up too high. Head protruding forward. Head tilted or rotated to one side.
Arms hang relaxed at the sides with palms of the hands facing toward the body. Elbows are slightly bent, so forearms hang slightly forward. Shoulders are level, and neither one is more forward or backward than the other when seen from the side. Scapulae lie flat against the rib cage. They are neither too close together nor too wide apart. In adults, a separation of approximately 10 cm (4 inches) is average.	Arms and shoulders	Holding the arms stiffly in any position forward, backward, or out from the body. Arms turned so that palms of hands face backward. One shoulder higher than the other. Both shoulders hiked up. One or both shoulders drooping forward or sloping. Shoulders rotated either clockwise or counterclockwise. Scapulae pulled back too hard. Scapulae too far apart. Scapulae too prominent, standing out from the rib cage ("winged scapulae").
A good position of the chest is one in which it is slightly up and slightly forward (while the back remains in good alignment). The chest appears to be in a position about halfway between that of a full inspiration and a forced expiration.	Chest	Depressed, or "hollow-chest," position. Lifted and held up too high, brought about by arching the back. Ribs more prominent on one side than on the other. Lower ribs flaring out or protruding.
In young children up to about the age of 10 yr, the abdomen normally protrudes somewhat. In older children and adults, it should be flat.	Abdomen	Entire abdomen protrudes. Lower part of the abdomen protrudes while the upper part is pulled in.
The front of the pelvis and the thighs are in a straight line. The buttocks are not prominent in back but instead slope slightly downward. The spine has four natural curves. In the neck and lower back, the curve is forward, and in the upper back and lowest part of the spine (sacral region), it is backward. The sacral curve is a fixed curve, whereas the other three are flexible.	Spine and pelvis (side view)	The low back arches forward too much (lordosis). The pelvis tilts forward too much. The front of the thigh forms an angle with the pelvis when this tilt is present. The normal forward curve in the low back has straightened out. The pelvis tips backward, and there is a slightly backward slant to the line of the pelvis in relation to the front of the hips (flat back). Increased backward curve in the upper back (kyphosis or round upper back). Increased forward curve in the neck. Almost always accompanied by round upper back and seen as a forward head. Lateral curve of the spine (scoliosis); toward one side (C curve), toward both sides (S curve).
Ideally, the body weight is borne evenly on both feet, and the hips are level. One side is not more prominent than the other as seen from front or back, nor is one hip more forward or backward than the other as seen from the side. The spine does not curve to the left or the right side. (A slight deviation to the left in right-handed individuals and to the right in left-handed individuals should not be considered abnormal. Also, because a tendency toward a slightly low right shoulder and slightly high right hip is frequently found in right-handed people, and vice versa for left-handed people, such deviations should not be considered abnormal.)	Hips, pelvis, and spine (back view)	One hip is higher than the other (lateral pelvic tilt). Sometimes it is not really much higher but appears so because a sideways sway of the body has made it more prominent. (Tailors and dressmakers often notice a lateral tilt because the hemline of skirts or length of trousers must be adjusted to the difference.) The hips are rotated so that one is farther forward than the other (clockwise or counterclockwise rotation).
Legs are straight up and down. Patellae face straight ahead when feet are in good position. Looking at the knees from the side, the knees are straight (i.e., neither bent forward nor "locked" backward).	Knees and legs	Knees touch when feet are apart (genu valgum). Knees are apart when feet touch (genu varum). Knees curves slightly backward (hyperextended knee) (genu recurvatum).

Continued

Table 15-14—cont'd

Good Posture	Part	Faulty Posture
In standing, the longitudinal arch has the shape of a half dome. Barefoot or in shoes without heels, the feet toe-out slightly. In shoes with heels, the feet are parallel. In walking with or without heels, the feet are parallel, and the weight is transferred from the heel along the outer border to the ball of the foot. In running, the feet are parallel or toe-in slightly. The weight is on the balls of the feet and toes because the heels do not come in contact with the ground.	Foot	Knee bends slightly forward, that is, it is not as straight as it should be (flexed knee). Patellae face slightly toward each other (medially rotated femurs). Patellae face slightly outward (laterally rotated femurs). Low longitudinal arch or flatfoot. Low metatarsal arch, usually indicated by calluses under the ball of the foot. Weight borne on the inner side of the foot (pronation). "Ankle rolls in." Weight borne on the outer border of the foot (supination). "Ankle rolls out." Toeing-out while walking or while standing in shoes with heels ("outflared" or "slue footed"). Toeing-in while walking or standing ("pigeon toed").
Toes should be straight, that is, neither curled downward nor bent upward. They should extend forward in line with the foot and not be squeezed together or overlap.	Toes	Toes bend up at the first joint and down at the middle and end joints so that the weight rests on the tips of the toes (hammer toes). This fault is often associated with wearing shoes that are too short. Big toe slants inward toward the midline of the foot (hallux valgus). This fault is often associated with wearing shoes that are too narrow and pointed at the toes.

Modified from Kendall FP, McCreary EK: *Muscles: testing and function*, Baltimore, 1983, Williams & Wilkins.

Précis of the Postural Assessment

History
Observation
  Standing (front, side, behind)
  Forward flexion (front, side, behind)
  Sitting (front, side, behind)
  Supine lying
  Prone lying
Examination
  Leg length measurement
  Slump test

Examination of specific joints (see appropriate chapter)
  As with any assessment, the patient must be warned that there may be some discomfort after the examination and that this discomfort is normal. Discomfort after any assessment should decrease within 24 hours. The examiner must keep in mind that several joints may be affected at the same time, either as the result of or as the cause of faulty posture. Therefore the examination of posture may be an extensive one, with observation both of the posture in general and of several specific joints in detail.

References

To enhance this text and add value for the reader, all references have been incorporated into a CD-ROM that is provided with this text. The reader can view the reference source and access it online whenever possible. There are a total of 41 cited references and other general references for this chapter.

ASSESSMENT OF THE AMPUTEE

An amputation is defined as the removal of part or all of a limb or some other outgrowth of the body. If fingers and partial nonmutilating hand injuries are excluded, lower-limb amputations are much more frequent than upper-limb amputations.[1] However, upper-limb amputations cause greater functional loss because the upper limbs are used more functionally and in many more diverse ways. There is also a greater functional sensory loss when an upper limb is involved. In addition, the upper-limb amputation causes a more obvious disfigurement and alteration of body image, which affects the actions and reactions of both the amputee and those with whom he or she interacts.[1,2] Amputations are considered to be a treatment of last resort when other methods, such as revascularization or reattachment, have failed or are not considered suitable treatment options.[2-5] Assessment of the amputee patient may involve assessing a patient before the amputation or after the amputation has taken place. In the first instance, the assessment is primarily carried out by one or more physicians deciding whether there is a need for such a procedure and then deciding the level at which the amputation should occur. In some cases, indexes or scores[6-19] may be used although some[20] have questioned their usefulness in the final outcome, especially in the case of trauma.

There are several indications for amputations.[21] The most common are trauma caused by compound fractures, blood vessel rupture, stab or gunshot injuries, compression injuries, severe burns, or cold injuries;[22] and vascular disease as the result of systemic problems, such as diabetes, arteriosclerosis, embolism, venous insufficiency, or peripheral vascular disease often aggravated by cigarette smoking.[23] About 75% of amputations in older patients fall within this second category.[24] The presence of suspected vascular disease may include more than the physical examination when considering whether to amputate. These other tests include blood tests, chest x-rays, electrocardiography, Doppler studies, arteriography, venograms, thermography, and transcutaneous PO_2 readings.[22] When trauma is the cause, the aim of the amputation is to restore maximum length with good soft-tissue covering.[22] In addition, amputations may be performed because of infections, tumors (both benign and more commonly, malignant types), neurological disorders (e.g., an anaesthetic limb from, for example, a complete plexus avulsion[25]), congenital deformity (e.g., partial or total absence of a limb), and amputations for cosmetic reasons (e.g., extra digit).[25-28] Younger people tend to experience more congenital, malignancy, and trauma-related amputations, whereas older people experience multiple pathophysiological mechanisms, as previously mentioned.

Causes of Amputation

- Trauma
- Vascular disease
- Infection
- Tumors
- Neurological disorders
- Congenital deformity

The examiner who has the opportunity to do a preoperative physical assessment of the patient who has been scheduled for an amputation should take the time to determine the patient's available muscle strength, range of motion (ROM), and functional mobility **bilaterally** to provide a baseline for future comparison if necessary. The size and position of any abnormal tissue degeneration or potential pressure areas should be recorded accurately, and functional levels should be assessed and recorded. If at all possible in this preoperative period, the patient should be given some instruction in bed mobility, as well as climbing in and out of bed with or without support. In addition, the examiner should ensure that the patient knows how to provide suitable care for pressure areas and preserve joint mobility to prevent any contractures from forming. If a lower-limb amputation is anticipated, the patient should be taught to use ambulatory aids such as crutches or wheelchair so that he or she can maintain as much mobility as possible after the amputation.

Levels of Amputation

Amputation surgery, whether performed to the upper limb or the lower limb, can occur at various levels (Figures 16-1 and 16-2).[29] For the most part, this chapter deals with assessment of the lower-limb amputee primarily because these amputations are more common. However, functional loss is usually greater for upper-limb amputees. Thus upper-limb amputee assessment deals much more with different functional demands than lower-limb

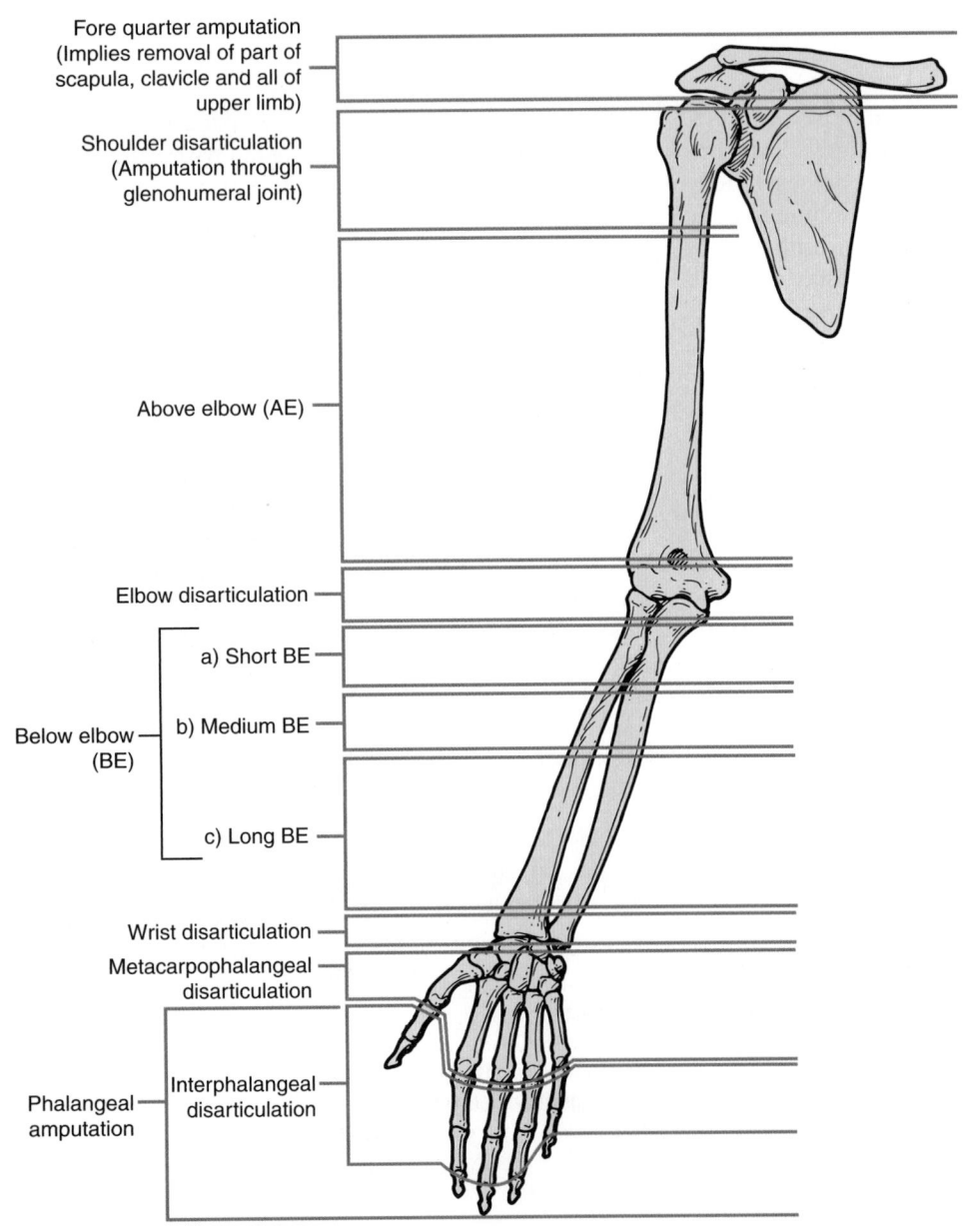

Fore quarter amputation
(Implies removal of part of
scapula, clavicle and all of
upper limb)

Shoulder disarticulation
(Amputation through
glenohumeral joint)

Above elbow (AE)

Elbow disarticulation

a) Short BE

Below elbow
(BE)

b) Medium BE

c) Long BE

Wrist disarticulation

Metacarpophalangeal
disarticulation

Interphalangeal
disarticulation

Phalangeal
amputation

Figure 16-1
Common levels of amputation—
upper limb.

Hemipelvecotomy
(Hindquarter amputation or
complete hip amputation)

Hip disarticulation
(Complete thigh amputation)
(Implies amputation through trochanters,
femoral neck or hip disarticulation)

a) Short AK (Upper thigh amputation)
3-4 inches below ischial tuberosity

Above knee (AK) amputation
(Partial thigh amputation)

b) Middle AK (Middle thigh amputation)
10-12 inches below ischial tuberosity

c) Supracondylar amputation
(Lower thigh amputation)

Knee disarticulation
(Compete leg amputation)

a) Very short BK
less than 2 inches below knee joint line
b) Short BK
(Upper leg amputation)
2-4 inches below knee joint

c) Medium BK
(Middle leg amputation)
5-8 inches below knee joint

Below Knee (BK) amputation
(Partial leg amputation)

d) Long BK
(Lower leg amputation)
8+ inches below knee joint

Syme amputation
(Amputation just above ankle)

Chopart disarticulation
(Partial tarsal amputation)
through midtarsal joints

Lisfranc's amputation
(Complete metatarsal amputation)
through tarsometatarsal joints

Transmetatarsal amputation
(Partial metatarsal amputation)
through metatarsal bones

Ankle disarticulation
(Complete tarsal amputation)

Toe amputation
(Compete phalangeal amputation)

Figure 16-2

Common levels of amputation—lower limb.

Figure 16-3

Amputation impairment. Percentage of impairments related to whole body, extremity, hand, or digit. *DIP*, Distal interphalangeal; *IP*, interphalangeal; *MP*, metacarpophalangeal; *PIP*, proximal interphalangeal. (Redrawn from Swanson AB et al: Evaluation of hand function. In Hunter JM et al, editors: *Rehabilitation of the hand*, p. 119, St Louis, 1990, Mosby.)

assessment. Figure 16-3 shows the percentage impairment caused by an upper-limb amputation.[30]

Amputation surgery may be one of two types—open or closed. Open, or primary, amputation is used in cases of infection in which the wound is left open after the amputated part is removed to allow clearance of infection. It requires a second procedure to close the wound. More commonly, a closed amputation is performed. This procedure is used when tissue viability is as normal as possible. At the time of the amputation, the skin flaps are closed, as is the wound. Commonly, the skin flaps are closed on the posterior and distal aspect of the stump because adhesions are less likely and an incision line is further from the bone, but other methods are also sometimes used.[31] The goal of amputation surgery is to create a dynamically balanced residual limb with good motor control and sensation.[32] The patient will need a well-healed, well-shaped residual stump with the greatest functional length possible in the limb.[32] The higher the level of the amputation, the greater the handicap.[25] In the lower limb, immediate prosthetic fitting helps facilitate early mobilization with more normal gait patterns.[26] Amputation should be considered to be a reconstructive

procedure leaving the patient with the best of possible alternatives.[33]

The second opportunity where the amputee patient may be assessed is following the surgery. This is more likely to be done by the physician or other health care professionals. In this case, the aim of the assessment is primarily to determine what functional deficits the patient has, to assess the fitting of the prosthesis, and to watch for complications. A good assessment enables the clinician to assist the patient in understanding and dealing with the specific physical and social limitations that the amputation has brought to his or her pattern of life.[34] It is this second scenario that will be described in the remainder of this chapter.

Patient History[34]

As with any assessment, the initial part of the examination will include the patient's history as it relates to the amputation, its cause, and any related factors. When doing the assessment of the amputee, it is important to determine the patient's past medical, surgical, preoperative ambulatory, and functional status for both upper and lower limbs, and preoperative symptoms. As part of this "past history," the examiner must develop some understanding of the patient's recreational activities, past psychiatric history (which may include information on alcohol or drug abuse), current stressors (including recent losses), pain tolerance, previous association with patients who have disabilities, and compliance with medical treatments.[24] In addition, information on family structure and possible support groups including family and friends must be discussed. Issues such as marital status, sexual history, family roles including familial support, strengths, and problems should be ascertained because they can impact greatly the outcome and how the patient ultimately functions as an amputee.[35,36]

Pertinent Information in Patient Assessment [24]

Relevant Patient Information
- Educational level
- Occupational history
- Avocational activities
- Psychiatric history, alcohol and drug use, problems with the law (it is important to have objective corroboration from the family)
- Current stressors, including recent losses
- Any pain sensitivity or tolerance
- Previous associations with patients having disabilities
- Compliance with medical treatment; obstacles to compliance

Family Structure
- Marital adjustment
- Sexual history
- Family roles; strengths and problem areas
- Health of others

The Patient's Perspective
- Current mood
- Anxieties and ideas associated with them
- What the patient imagines his or her future to be, that is, how the disability will change lifestyle, social relations, vocational future; self-concept
- The degree to which self-esteem is related to physique and physical skills
- Comfort in meeting a psychiatrist or psychologist
- How the patient thinks the adjustment is going
- The most pressing immediate concern
- The patient's understanding of the cause and probable course of disability
- How much the patient wants to know about the treatment as it progresses; how the patient prefers having a medical update

---

The examiner must determine and develop an understanding for any patient anxieties, why they are present, whether these anxieties can be dealt with by the examiner or if other health care specialists need to be involved, what the patient imagines his or her future to be, and how the disability will change his or her lifestyle, social rela-

tions, vocational future, and self-concept (Table 16-1). All these factors must be considered if the examiner hopes to have a successful outcome to treatment.

For the present medical history, the following questions should be asked:

1. *What is the patient's occupation?* Does the patient have any concerns about returning to his or her job? If so, what are the patient's future occupational plans? Is any vocational guidance or training required?

2. *What is the patient's present medical status?* For example, what was the reason for the amputation? Any systemic disease such as diabetes, cardiovascular or respiratory problems, arthritic joints, and lifestyle factors all have a bearing on successful treatment outcomes. Systemic disease or trauma may prolong the healing process, and the speed of recovery may be delayed.

3. *How long ago did the amputation occur?* In recent amputations, the initial concern is the healing of the stump and the prevention of complications. If the amputation surgery was a revision procedure, why was the revision necessary? Was the problem one of poor tissue viability, or was the procedure performed to enable the patient to obtain better functional results?

4. *If the amputation occurred some time ago (3 to 6 months or longer), has the patient experienced any complications over that period, such as tissue breakdown, ulcer formation, or blisters?*

5. *If the patient has a prosthesis, what does the patient think about the prosthesis, its fit, and its function?* How long has the prosthesis been worn (years? months?)? How long is the prosthesis worn each day? Is it worn every day? Is the suspension adequate? Are there any skin abrasions? Inadequacies in these areas will lead to patient frustration, to disappointment, and, ultimately, to the patient becoming discouraged about using the prosthesis and, in fact, may come to the state where the patient does not want to wear the prosthesis. If the prosthesis is uncomfortable or excessively noisy, it is unlikely the patient will use it or if it is used, it is unlikely the patient will use it properly. In the case of a lower-limb prosthesis, the patient may refuse to bear weight on the prosthesis. Cosmesis is another problem that is often of concern for amputees, especially for women, and when the amputation is in the upper limb the extremity is sometimes not covered with clothing. The examiner must differentiate between the discomfort of using something new and the discomfort caused by a specific prosthetic fault. In some cases, a prosthesis evaluation questionnaire[37] may be useful (Figure 16-4).

6. *Has the patient been looking after the stump properly, ensuring proper limb and sock hygiene?* Failure to do so easily leads to complications, such as skin breakdown, infection, and ulcers (see Table 16-1).[32]

Table 16-1
Patient Motivational and General Problems

Problem	Cause	Findings	Solution
Discouraged patient	Performance does not equal expectations	Does not wear prosthesis Complaints not related to physical findings	Sympathetic explanation of reasonably realistic goals Training
Failure to maintain good prosthetic habits	Lack of training New situations Poor motivation	Hip or knee flexion contracture Pressure sores Poor socket fit Abnormal gait patterns	Retraining Sympathetic encouragement
Poor hygiene	Poor motivation	Dermatitis Abscess formation Hidradenitis (inflammation of sweat glands)	Wash limb Clean socks Clean socket Antibiotics Surgical drainage
Rest pain	Phantom pain or sensation	Pain in missing segment of limb	Provide distracting sensation (a) Wrapping (b) Temperature changes (c) Activity with prosthesis (d) Transcutaneous nerve stimulation
	Neuroma Ischemia	Positive Tinel's sign Cramping pain aggravated by activity	Excise neuroma "Unweight" limb Stop smoking Revise amputation

Modified from Smith AG: Common problems of lower extremity amputees, *Orthop Clin North Am* 13:576, 1982.

Sample Items in the 10 Prosthesis Evaluation Questionnaire

(respondents are asked to rate the item over the past 4 weeks)

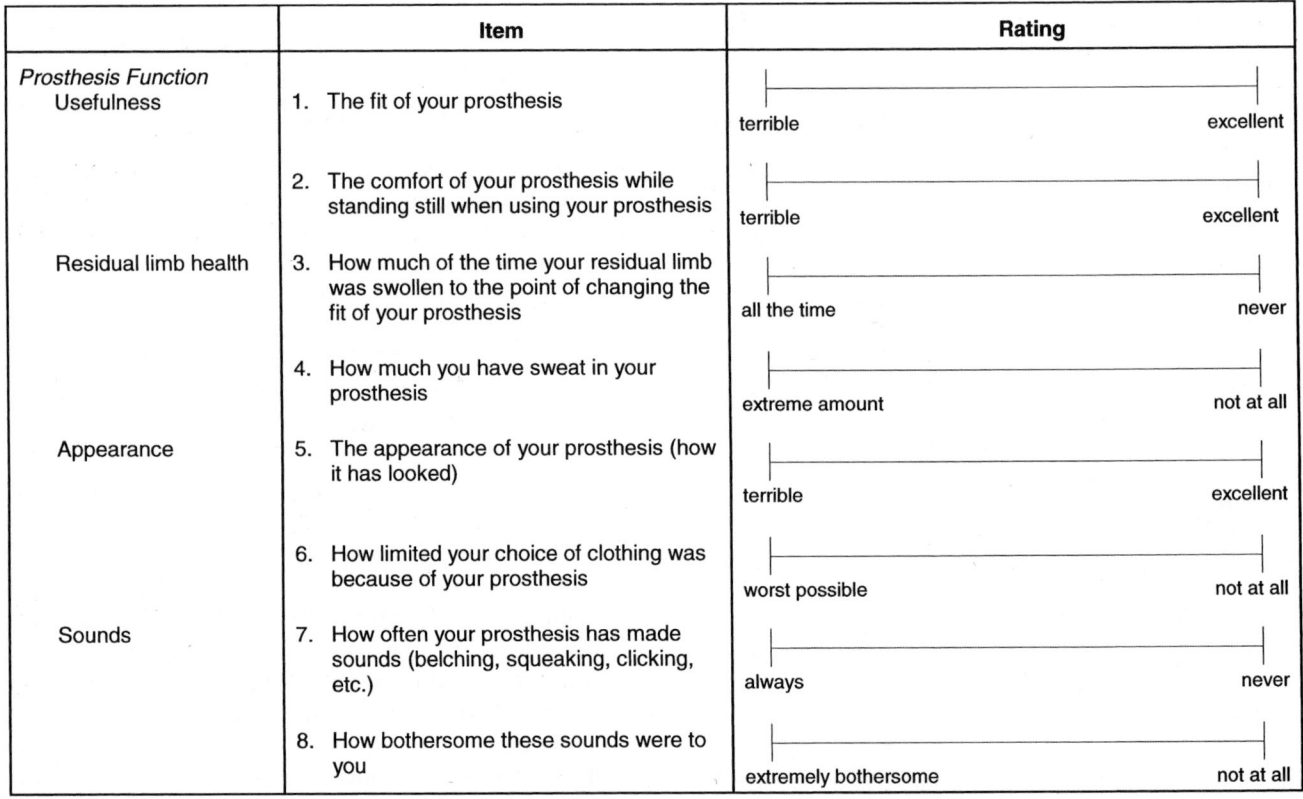

	Item	Rating
Prosthesis Function Usefulness	1. The fit of your prosthesis	terrible — excellent
	2. The comfort of your prosthesis while standing still when using your prosthesis	terrible — excellent
Residual limb health	3. How much of the time your residual limb was swollen to the point of changing the fit of your prosthesis	all the time — never
	4. How much you have sweat in your prosthesis	extreme amount — not at all
Appearance	5. The appearance of your prosthesis (how it has looked)	terrible — excellent
	6. How limited your choice of clothing was because of your prosthesis	worst possible — not at all
Sounds	7. How often your prosthesis has made sounds (belching, squeaking, clicking, etc.)	always — never
	8. How bothersome these sounds were to you	extremely bothersome — not at all

Figure 16-4

Sample items in the 10 prosthesis evaluation questionnaire (PEQ) scales. (Modified from Legro MW et al: Prosthetic evaluation questionnaire for persons with lower limb amputations: assessing prosthesis-related quality of life, *Arch Phys Med Rehabil* 79:934, 1998.)

	Item	Rating
Mobility Ambulation	9. Your ability to walk in close spaces when using your prosthesis	cannot —— no problem
	10. Your ability to walk on slippery surfaces (eg. wet tile, snow, a rainy street or boat deck) when using your prosthesis	cannot —— no problem
Transfers	11. Your ability to shower or bathe safely	cannot —— no problem
	12. Your ability to get in and out of a car when using your prosthesis	cannot —— no problem
Psychosocial Experience Perceived responses	13. How often the desire to avoid strangers' reactions to your prosthesis makes you avoid doing something you otherwise would have done	all the time —— never
	14. How a family member (other than your partner) has responded to your prosthesis	very poorly —— very well
Social burden	15. How much a burden your prosthesis has been on your partner or family member	extremely burdensome —— not at all
	16. Your ability to take care of someone else (eg. your partner, a child, a friend)	cannot —— no problem
Frustration	17. How frequently you were frustrated with your prosthesis	all the time —— never
	18. Think of the most frustrating event and rate what you felt at that time	extremely frustrated —— not at all
Well-being Well-being	19. How satisfied you have been with how things have worked out since your amputation	extremely dissatisifed —— extremely satisfied
	20. Your quality of life	worst possible life —— best possible life

Figure 16-4 cont'd

The remaining stump should be washed with care using mild soap. The stump sock should be changed and cleaned regularly, and the prosthesis socket should also be cleaned regularly with mild soap and water.[32]

7. *Does the patient have any pain or abnormal sensation?* Where is the pain or abnormal sensation? Is the pain intermittent or constant? What is the intensity of the pain (a visual analogue scale may be used—see Figure 1-4)? Where is the pain? What type of pain or abnormal sensation is it? **Phantom sensation** is an abnormal feeling the patient has for the limb, but the patient feels the sensation as being in the amputated part of the limb even though that part of the limb is not there.[22,38-40] This sensation is an almost universal consequence of limb amputation.[41,42] It may take numerous forms, including the feeling that someone is touching the amputated limb, pressure being applied to the

missing body part, cold, wetness, itching, tickle, pain, or fatigue. The intensity of these sensations may vary and may change over time. The sensations commonly have different meaning to different people. Phantom sensations are more commonly felt in the distal part of the excised extremity because the distal part of an extremity tends to be more richly innervated.[38]

Phantom pain is described as a painful sensation perceived in the missing body part in the case of an amputation, in the paralyzed part of a spinal cord injury patient, or following a nerve root avulsion in the case of a neurological injury.[22,38-41] Eighty percent of amputees experience some phantom pain sometime during the injury healing process. Phantom pain is relatively common, but it is unpredictable in terms of predisposing factors, severity, frequency, duration or character, aggravation by internal or external stimuli, or type of pain experienced.[38] Phantom pain is more likely to be seen in the upper-limb amputee than in the lower-limb amputee, and it tends to be more prolonged in the upper limb. Some patients report that the pain is of very high intensity, which may be evoked by some external or internal stimuli, whereas others report a dull, continuous aching or burning that does not seem to be episodic. Many amputees describe the pain as being knifelike, burning, sticking, shooting, prickling, throbbing, cramplike, squeezing, "like something trying to pull my leg off," or some type of electrical phenomenon (Figure 16-5).[39,41] Phantom pain generally begins within the first postsurgical week, and it commonly stabilizes after a few months but may occur several months or years after the amputation. It seems to decrease in frequency, duration, and severity during the first 6 months. Most commonly, phantom pain persisting beyond 6 months is very difficult to treat and usually does not change in character after that time. Some people, however, report that the intensity of pain will change with time. Prolonged healing or

Figure 16-5

Phantom limb pain. Some of the typical painful feelings that seem to stem from the missing limb. (Redrawn from Sherman RA: Stump and phantom limb pain, *Neurol Clin* 7:250, 1989.)

other complications such as fractures may cause phantom pain to persist for longer periods.

Stump pain is pain arising from the residual part of the body as opposed to phantom pain, which is felt in the missing part of the body.[22,38,39,41,42] It is commonly a sharp, sticking, or pressure feeling that, although diffuse, is localized to the end of the stump.[39] Stump pain is usually the result of six primary etiologies—prosthogenic, neurogenic, arthrogenic, sympathogenic, referred, and abnormal stump tissues.[38] The most common cause of stump pain is prosthogenic, which implies improper fitting of the prosthesis. The second type of stump pain is neurogenic, most commonly from the formation of a neuroma where the nerve was cut during surgery. Neuroma pain is usually characterized by sharp, shooting pain that can be evoked by light tapping over the neuroma (Tinel's sign). Third, stump pain may be arthrogenic or coming from an adjacent joint or surrounding tissues, usually as a result of changing stresses to the tissues or because sufficient time has not been allowed for the tissues to adapt to the new stresses being applied to them. For example, back pain is initially a common finding in above-knee amputees.[42] Fourth, stump pain may be sympathogenic or associated with the sympathetic nerve system. This pain is sometimes called causalgia, reflex sympathetic dystrophy, or, as some people now call it, sympathetically maintained pain. Fifth, the pain

---

Phantom Pain Sensations[39]

- Knifelike*†
- Sticking*
- Shooting
- Prickling
- Burning†
- Squeezing†
- Throbbing
- Pressing
- Cramplike
- Sawing
- Dull

*More common early
†More common after 6 months

may be referred. Nonradicular referred pain can come from the joints, muscles, or myofascial conditions. Last, abnormal tissue, such as bony exostosis, heterotrophic ossification, adherent scar, or sepsis (infection), can lead to pain in the remaining stump. Virtually every amputee will experience stump pain after amputation. Stump pain is a normal result of major surgery. However, it is frequently a shock to those patients who are not warned to expect it.[41] Stump pain is usually severe immediately after amputation and subsides quickly with healing. It tends to be more evident in patients who have nondecreasing phantom pain.[39] About 80% of amputees have functionally significant episodes of phantom or stump pain every year and may have almost constant, very low level, stump and phantom pain that they define as being over the threshold of nonpainful sensation.[41]

There is no evidence that phantom pain or stump pain is caused by psychological disorders although stress and psychological disturbances can exacerbate the pain.[41] They are both considered to be physiological phenomena.

Observation[34]

Following surgery, the examiner will observe the stump for any swelling and whether healing is occurring properly. The condition of the skin as well as the presence of joint contractures, especially if the amputation is close to a joint (e.g., below-knee [BK] amputation), should be noted. The amputee should be observed both without the prosthesis and while wearing the prosthesis. Generally, the lower-limb amputee is observed in three positions while wearing the prosthesis: standing, sitting, and walking.

To begin the observation of the amputee, the examiner first looks at the remaining good limb, noting sensation, pulses, temperature, and skin condition. The examiner takes time to observe the remaining limb that will have to take a greater functional role and often greater stresses because of the amputation to the other limb. If it is a lower-limb amputation, the remaining limb will have to take a greater load during gait. Are the skin and nails normal, or are trophic changes evident? Are there any sores or open areas? These changes may indicate circulatory impairment. What are the color and temperature of the remaining limb? Do they fall within normal limits? Are the pulses (e.g., femoral, tibial, dorsalis pedis) normal? Does the limb exhibit any deformity or swelling? Will the remaining limb be able to take the additional stress?

The examiner notes whether the patient is wearing the prosthesis or not. If the patient has the prosthesis on, then observation of the patient functioning with the prosthesis is first done with the patient standing, walking, and sitting. If the patient is not wearing the prosthesis, the examiner spends the initial period checking the stump and its condition, noting whether the wound is healing properly or whether there are any signs of drainage or weeping from the wound or evidence of tissue breakdown.[32] If the stump is covered with an elastic wrap or shrinker to assist in decreasing swelling, the examiner should note how it is applied, whether it fits smoothly or contains wrinkles, and whether the application is effective in reducing swelling. The examiner can then ask the patient to remove the wrap. At this stage, the examiner can ask the patient to demonstrate how he or she applies the wrap (if the patient does it himself or herself), or this may be left until later.

With the wrap off, the examiner then inspects the stump, noting its shape. The stump may be classed as cylindrical, conical, bony, bulbous, or edematous. The examiner looks for signs of unusual patterns of swelling (an indication the wrap has been applied incorrectly) (Figure 16-6); causes of residual limb edema (Figure 16-7); presence of skin abrasions, skin breakdown, or blisters (all of which may indicate poor prosthesis fit); or presence of infection (Table 16-2).[32] The examiner should note whether the scar is healing normally and whether the sutures have been removed or some remain. The scar may be classed as nontender, sensitive, invaginated, well healed, open, or adherent. The location of the scar and whether it will affect the fitting of the prosthesis should be noted. Any "dog ears" to the suture, which may interfere with the prosthesis, should also be noted. The mobility of the scar and tension of the skin and its mobility, especially over the distal end of the stump, should be observed. In addition, the color and temperature of the stump should be noted. Any potential weight-bearing areas (e.g., ischial tuberosity–above-knee [AK] amputation; patellar tendon–below-knee [BK] amputation) should also be inspected because these tissues will receive greater stress with the use of a prosthesis. The condition of the remaining joints and their supporting musculature (e.g., atrophied, fleshy, strong) should be noted.

If the patient has a prosthesis, the prosthesis is then inspected (Table 16-3). The examiner should note the socket type, the material used to construct it, and the type of suspension. The general workmanship of the prosthesis and whether it is satisfactory should be noted. The examiner should inspect the trim lines, the rivets, and other fastenings to see if they are neat and secure. Joint covers should shield mechanical joint heads to prevent damage to clothing. There should be no scratches or rough areas on the prosthesis. Plastic lamination should be uniform without appreciable missed areas.

Next, provided the patient is at the stage where the prosthesis has been fitted (in some cases, especially in the lower limb, the prosthesis may be fitted right after surgery; in other cases, the prosthesis is fitted after tissue healing is ensured), the patient is asked to put the prosthesis on while the examiner determines whether the patient can correctly and easily do this independently or only with help.

Figure 16-6
The effect of bad bandaging. **A,** An incorrectly applied bandage. **B,** The uneven residual limb contour produced by the incorrectly applied bandage. (From Engstrom B, Van de Ven C: *Therapy for amputees*, p. 53, Edinburgh, 1999, Churchill Livingstone.)

Figure 16-7
Causes of residual limb edema. (From Engstrom B, Van de Ven C: *Therapy for amputees*, p. 52, Edinburgh, 1999, Churchill Livingstone.)

Table 16-2

Amputation Problems

Problem	Cause	Findings	Solution
Limb shrinkage	Normal shrinkage with activity Weight loss	Limb too deep in socket Pressure areas on bony prominences Pressure on end of amputation Limb too short	Add stump socks Modify liners in socket New socket or prosthesis
Limb swelling	Edema Weight gain Failure to continue limb wrapping in recent amputee Failure to wear prosthesis for prolonged period without wrapping	Limb not fitting into socket Pressure on bony prominences Choking on end of stump Limb too long	Treat medical cause of edema Diet control Training in proper limb wrapping Socket relief Remove stump socks Wear stump shrinker
Joint contracture	Failure of preprosthetic training Lack of patient cooperation Patient does not wear prosthesis	Limb short Heel of prosthesis off floor Unstable gait Excessive knee and hip flexion when prosthesis off	Sympathetic encouragement Training Temporary prosthesis that is adjustable as contracture decreases

Modified from Smith AG: Common problems of lower extremity amputees, *Orthop Clin North Am* 13:570, 1982.

Table 16-3

Problems Related to the Prosthesis

Problem	Cause	Findings	Solution
Improper socket fit	Improper fabrication	Same as for limb swelling or shrinkage shortly after delivery	Socket relief New socket
Improper prosthetic alignment	Improper fabrication Patient changes height of shoe heel Joint contracture	Limb too long or too short with good socket fit Heel or toe off the floor Gait abnormalities Pressure areas on limb	Realign prosthesis Heel pads in shoe or shoes with original heel height Training to correct contracture
Inadequate suspension	Improper fabrication of suspension	Piston action of limb in socket Insecurity on weight bearing Abrasions Gait abnormality that is similar to findings when prosthesis is too long Prosthesis incorrectly rotated Restriction of joint motion	Readjust suspension

Modified from Smith AG: Common problems of lower extremity amputees, *Orthop Clin North Am* 13:574, 1982.

For the lower-limb amputee, once the prosthesis is fitted, the patient is first observed in standing position. As with the patient who is not an amputee, posture of the patient is assessed (see Chapter 15) and the examiner must determine if any deviations are structural or due to the prosthesis. In addition, the examiner notes the following:

1. Does the patient appear to be comfortable while standing, especially with the heels no more than 15 cm (6 inches) apart as seen in normal standing?
2. Is the patient able to "balance" on the prosthesis when standing on two legs or when weight shifting between the two legs? At the same time, the examiner should note whether the anteroposterior alignment of

the prosthesis is satisfactory so that the patient does not feel the knee is unstable or that the knee is being forced backward, in the case of a BK amputee. Also, the clinician should note whether the mediolateral alignment is satisfactory with the foot flat on the floor. There should be no uncomfortable pressure on the lateral or medial brim of the socket.

3. Is the prosthesis of correct length? When the patient rises on the prosthesis, is there any piston action of the stump in the prosthesis? Normally, there should be very little movement. Are the anterior, medial, and lateral walls of the prosthesis of adequate height? Do the medial and lateral walls of the stump contact the prosthesis in the correct places so that there is no weight on the end of the prosthesis? In the case of a joint disarticulation, weight bearing through the end of the stump may be allowed, at least partially.

4. Are the size, contours, and colors of the prosthesis approximately the same as those of the sound limb? Are the "joints" similarly placed to the normal limb? The prosthesis should be inspected from the front, back, and side to check this. The patient should be asked if he or she is satisfied with the appearance of the prosthesis.

5. Is the suspension, if present, adequate and fully supporting the prosthesis during weight bearing? Is the suspension adjustable if necessary?[43]

6. Does the patient consider the prosthesis satisfactory? This question will help to ensure that any items that may have been overlooked will be brought to the attention of the clinical team.

Next, the patient is observed seated while wearing the prosthesis. The examiner notes the following:

1. Can the patient sit comfortably with minimal bunching of the soft tissue around the prosthesis?

2. Does the socket remain securely on the stump? Is the patient able to sit comfortably with minimum functioning of the soft tissues around the prosthesis? Are the soft tissues and bony prominences free from excessive pressure? Does the prosthesis remain in good alignment?

The third phase of lower-limb amputee observation is to view the patient walking while wearing the prosthesis. During walking, the examiner should watch for hip or knee instability or abnormal gait. During this phase, the examiner observes the following:

1. Is the patient's performance and walking on a level surface satisfactory? Any gait deviation that requires attention should be noted. Gait deviations include an abducted or adducted gait, lateral trunk bending, circumduction, medial or lateral whip of the prosthesis, foot rotation on heel strike, uneven heel rise, foot slap, uneven step length, and vaulting. Also, the stump may be oversensitive and/or painful. A very short stump may fail to provide a sufficient lever arm for the pelvis. Finally, an abnormal gait pattern may develop because of a habitual pattern of movement.[22,44] A prosthesis aligned

in abduction may cause a wide base gait resulting in this abnormal gait pattern. Amputee balance may be difficult if an adduction contracture is present. An abducted gait is characterized by a very wide base with the prosthesis held away from the midline at all times. If the prosthesis is the cause of the abducted gait, it may be that the prosthesis is too large or that too much abduction may have been built into the prosthesis. A high medial wall may cause the amputee to hold the prosthesis away to avoid pressure on the pubic ramus. The pelvic band may be positioned too far away from the patient's body. This defective gait may also be caused by an abduction contracture or a poor habitual pattern of gait.[22,44]

Lateral bending of the trunk is characterized by excessive bending laterally, generally toward the prosthetic side, from the midline. If the prosthesis is the cause, it may be that it is too short or has an improperly shaped lateral wall that fails to provide adequate support for the femur. A high medial wall may cause the amputee to lean away to minimize the discomfort.

A circumduction gait is a swinging of the prosthesis laterally in a wide arc during the swing phase of gait. This defect may be due to the prosthesis being too long or the prosthesis having too much alignment stability or friction in the knee, making it difficult to bend the knee during the swing-through phase of gait. The amputee may have an abduction contracture of the stump or may lack confidence in flexing the prosthetic knee because of muscle weakness, or the amputee may fear stubbing the toe. Finally, this abnormal gait pattern may be the result of a habitually incorrect gait pattern.[22,44]

Medial or lateral whips are observed best when the patient walks away from the observer. A medial whip is present when the heel travels medially on initial flexion at the beginning of the swing phase, whereas a lateral whip exists with the heel moving laterally. If whipping occurs, then it is the fault of the prosthesis. Lateral whips are commonly seen from excessive medial rotation of the prosthetic knee. A medial whip may result from excessive lateral rotation of the knee. The socket may fit too tightly, thus reflecting stump rotation. Excessive valgus in the prosthetic knee may contribute to this defect. Also, a badly aligned toe break in the conventional foot may cause twisting at toe-off. Faulty walking habits by the amputee may also result in whips.[22,44]

Rotation of the prosthetic foot on heel strike is due to too much resistance to plantar flexion caused by the plantar flexor bumper or heel wedge.[22,44] If too much toe-out has been built into the prosthesis or if the socket fits too loosely, it may also cause a similar gait fault. If the amputee has poor stump muscle control or extends the stump too vigorously at heel strike, the same gait fault can occur.

If the amputee exhibits uneven arm swing, the altered gait may be due to poor balance, fear or insecurity, or a poor habitual pattern.

A long prosthetic step is seen when the amputee takes a longer step with the prosthesis than with the normal leg. If the prosthesis is at fault, it is usually due to insufficient initial flexion in the socket where a stump flexion contracture is present.[22,44]

Foot slap is a too rapid descent of the anterior portion of the prosthetic foot. It is commonly the result of plantar flexion resistance in the prosthesis being too soft, or the amputee may be driving the prosthesis into the walking surface too forcefully to ensure extension of the knee.[22,44]

Uneven heel rise is characterized by the prosthetic heel rising too much or too rapidly when the knee is flexed at the beginning of the swing phase. If the prosthesis is at fault, the knee joint may have insufficient friction and there may be an inadequate extension aid. The amputee may also be using more power than necessary to force the knee into flexion.[22,44]

Uneven timing is characterized by steps of unequal duration or length, usually by a very short stance phase on the prosthetic side. An improperly fitting socket may cause pain and a desire to shorten the stance phase on the prosthetic side. A weak extension aid or insufficient friction in the prosthetic knee can cause excessive heel rise and thus result in uneven timing because of a prolonged swing-through. Alignment stability may also be a factor if the knee buckles too easily. In addition, the amputee may have weak muscles in the stump and may not have developed good balance. Fear and insecurity may also contribute to this defect.[22,44]

Terminal swing impact is characterized by rapid forward movement of the shin piece allowing the knee to reach maximum extension with too much force before heel strike. If the prosthesis has insufficient knee friction or the knee extension aid is too strong, this gait fault may be seen. In addition, the amputee may be trying to assure himself or herself that the knee is in full extension by deliberately and forcefully extending the stump.[22,44]

The amputee who feels unstable at the prosthetic knee may develop a feeling of instability that could lead to the danger of falling. In this case, the prosthetic knee joint may be too far ahead of the TKA (thigh, knee, ankle) line and insufficient initial flexion may have been built into the socket. Plantar flexion resistance may also be too great, causing the knee to buckle at heel strike. Failure to limit dorsiflexion can lead to incomplete knee control. Also, the amputee may have weak hip extensor muscles or a severe hip flexion contracture leading to instability.[22,44]

Drop-off at the end of stance phase is characterized by a downward movement of the trunk as the body moves forward over the prosthesis. The prosthesis is at fault if there is inadequate limitation of dorsiflexion of the prosthetic foot. The keel of a SACH-type foot may be too short, or the toe break of the conventional foot may be too far posterior. The socket may have been placed too far anterior in relation to the foot.[22,44]

Excessive trunk extension during the stance phase in which the amputee creates an active lumbar lordosis may also be seen in some amputees. If the prosthesis is at fault, it may be due to an improperly shaped posterior wall causing forward rotation of the pelvis to avoid full weight bearing on the ischium. It may also be due to insufficient initial flexion being built into the socket. In addition, the amputee may demonstrate hip flexor tightness or weakness of the hip extensors and may be attempting to substitute with the lumbar erector spinae muscles. Weak abdominal muscles will contribute to this defect. The deviation may be due to a habitual pattern with the patient moving his or her shoulders backward in an effort to obtain better balance.[22,44]

Vaulting is characterized by rising on the toe of the normal foot to permit the amputee to swing the prosthesis through with little or no knee flexion. If the prosthesis is the cause, it may be too long or there may be inadequate socket suspension. Excessive alignment stability or some limitation of knee flexion, such as a knee lock or strong extension aid, may lead to altered gait. Vaulting is a fairly frequent habitual pattern that amputees develop. The amputee may also have fear of stubbing the toe, which could lead to this abnormal gait, or there may be some stump discomfort.[22,44]

The reader is referred to Lusardi et al.[44] and Engerstrom and Van de Ven[22] for further information on prosthetic gait. Normally, gait deviations observed in BK amputees will be fewer and less noticeable than in AK amputees.

2. Is the patient able to go up and down inclines and stairs satisfactorily? Is the patient able to kneel, bend down, and get up from kneeling?

3. Are the socket and suspension systems comfortable?

4. Does the prosthesis function quietly? Any noises coming from the prosthesis should be noted and the source of the noise determined. Occasionally, hissing may be heard as air enters and escapes from the socket as the amputee walks. This is associated with the piston action caused by inadequate suspension and poor socket fit or poor congruence between the socket and liner.[32,43]

After checking the gait while wearing the prosthesis, the prosthesis should be removed to check the patient's stump for tissue stress from the gait activity. At this stage, the examiner observes the following:

1. Does the patient's stump appear to be free of abrasions, discolorations, or excessive perspiration when the prosthesis is removed? Pressure discolorations and redness because of the prosthesis should normally disappear within 10 to 15 minutes. If they persist, then the causes of the irritation or pressure should be determined.

2. Is weight bearing distributed over the proper areas of the stump? For example, for a BK amputation with weight bearing on the patellar tendon, the medial-tibial flare, lateral distal, and posteroproximal aspects

of the stump should bear weight. An indication of the weight-bearing area sometimes may be obtained by noting the imprint of the stump sock on the skin of the stump. To determine the concentration and location of the distal pressure, it may be desirable to insert a piece of modeling clay in the bottom of the socket. Flattening of the clay will indicate distal contact.

Examination

Before the examination, the examiner should read the operative report to determine which muscles have been cut or how they have been stabilized along with the amputation since this will give the examiner some idea of the muscles available to move the limb and prosthesis and to provide stability during functional movement.

Measurements Related to Amputation

The examiner should note the length and circumference of the stump as well as scar length. Methods of measuring for prosthesis fitting are shown in the accompanying forms (Figures 16-8 and 16-9). Other measurements include the following:

1. Amputation type: short (10% to 33% of sound side length); medium (34% to 67% of sound side length); long (68% to 100% of sound side length)
2. Ulcer measurements (if present) and descriptions

Active Movements

When assessing the amputee, the examiner must determine the ability (strength and endurance) of the muscles to move the remaining joints in the remaining stump and the range of active motion available in those joints. Ideally, ROM at the remaining joints should be close to normal but may be affected by contractures or scarring. This is especially true for the hip and knee in lower-limb amputees. The ROM available will help determine the patient's ability to move and control the prosthesis as well as whether the muscles are able to control the available ROM and provide stability when the patient is in the prosthesis. In addition, the strength, endurance, and ROM of the opposite good limb must be assessed because greater stress will be placed on this limb, especially in the lower-limb amputee. In the case of an upper-limb amputee, if it has been the dominant limb that has experienced the amputation, the other limb will become the dominant limb of necessity, and new skills will have to be learned by that limb. In either case, a thorough assessment of the functional status of the remaining whole limb will be necessary, in addition to the examination of the amputated limb. The active movements performed would be the same as those listed for the individual joints in other chapters in this book.

Passive Movements

Passive movements of the amputated limb and remaining normal limb are necessary to ensure the necessary ROM is available and to prevent contractures or to restore ROM after contractures occur. For example, BK amputees are prone to hip flexion and knee flexion contractures, especially if the amputee spends long periods sitting in bed or in a wheelchair. The passive movements performed would be the same as those listed for the individual joints in other chapters in this book. Passive movements give the examiner an understanding of the end feel present so that if contractures occur, proper stretching treatment can be instituted. If laxity or instability is present, the patient can be instructed in proper stabilization exercises.

Resisted Isometric Movements

Resisted isometric movements should be performed on the muscles of the amputated limb as well as the remaining normal limb to ensure the patient has the strength and endurance (or exercise tolerance) that will enable the patient to use a prosthesis.[45] Resisted movements of all muscles of the remaining joints on both the amputated limb and the remaining limb must be tested. These resisted movements would be the same as those listed for the individual joints in other chapters in this book. In lower-limb amputations, the muscles of the hip and knee are especially important to check. In the upper limb, the muscles of the shoulder, which play a significant role in positioning the prosthesis, must be assessed. Such testing will enable the examiner to develop an exercise program to ensure maximum functionality of the patient.

Functional Assessment

For the amputee, functional assessment, for example, the Rivermead Mobility Index (RMI),[46] takes primary importance so the examiner must determine the amputee's level of function and independence both with and without a prosthesis. This assessment may involve the care of the remaining stump, ability to put on and take off the prosthetic device, and determining the patient's anticipated level of activity and whether this activity level can be realistically met given the patient's handicap.

For the lower-limb amputee, the examiner should determine the following:

1. The patient's gait and endurance when walking and whether external support (crutches, cane) is necessary.
2. The patient's bed mobility. That is, can the patient move easily in bed, or does he or she require assistance? Can the patient roll over, move from lying to sitting, or lie prone?
3. The patient's ability to transfer from sitting to standing and from bed to wheelchair.

Text continued on page 1030

UPPER-EXTREMITY PROSTHETIC MEASUREMENTS

Name of Patient_____Phone_____Date_____

Address_____City_____State/Zip_____

Male ☐   Female ☐   Date of Birth_____Height_____Weight_____

Type of Prosthesis_____Right_____Left_____

Figure 16-8

Upper-extremity prosthetic measurements. (Permission granted by the American Orthotic and Prosthetic Association, Alexandria, Va.)

LOWER-EXTREMITY PROSTHETIC MEASUREMENTS

Name of Patient _____ Phone _____ Date _____

Address _____ City _____ State _____

Age _____ Height _____ Weight _____

Type Prosthesis _____ Right _____ Left _____

Shoe Furnished: One ☐ Both ☐ None ☐

Shoe Lace Opening: Top ☐ Bottom ☐

Extra Light-Weight Limb: ☐

Extra Strong Limb: ☐

KB or BK Knee Joints: Size _____ Style _____

Angle Joint: Size _____ Style _____

KB or BK Thigh Lacing:

Eyelets ☐ Hooks ☐ Both ☐

Thigh Lacer Height: _____

Shoulder Loop Size: _____

Waist Belt Size: _____

Color: Caucasian ☐ Negroid ☐

Light Brown ☐ Medium ☐ Dark Brown ☐

Check Strap: Lace ☐ Leather Strap ☐

Measured by: _____

Shop Alterations

Lengthen Thigh _____ In. Shorten Thigh _____ In.

Lengthen Shin _____ In. Shorten Shin _____ In.

KB or BK Lace Opening: Top _ In. Bottom _ In.

Set BK Lacer on Joints:

Higher _____ In. Bottom _____ In.

Outside BK Joint Head:

Set In _____ In. Set Out _____ In.

Inside BK Joint Head:

Set In _____ In. Set Out _____ In.

Fit Foot In Shoe: Tight ☐ Loose ☐ Medium ☐

Make Heel Cushion: Soft ☐ Medium ☐ Firm ☐

Special Changes: _____

_____

_____

_____

Fitted By: _____

Finished BK Limb, Knee Center to Floor: _ In.

Finished AK Limb, Ischium to Floor: _____ In.

Weight of Finished Limb: _____ lbs. _____ oz.

Finish of Limb: Plastic Laminate ☐

Rawhide Enamel ☐

Special Features: _____

_____

_____

Date Completed: _____

BELOW KNEE

Stump Diameter at Level of Patella Tendon

M – L

A – P

IMPORTANT — Mark all Bony Prominences on Cast

Cast of Stump ( )

Limb Tracing ( )

M.T.P.

Length of Stump

Length of Tibia

ABOVE KNEE

A-P Dimension of Socket _____

Distance from Ischial Tuberosity to Adductor Longus Tendon _____

Reduced Socket Meas.	Dist. Below Ischium	Stump Meas.
	0	
	2	
	4	
	6	
	8	
	10	

Pelvic Circum.

Trochantor to Ant. Mid-Line

Ischial Tuber. to Floor

Femur Length

Stump Length

M – L Knee Diam.

Stump Sock Size

Forefoot to Heel

Shoe Size

Heel Height

Length of Foot

Knee Center

Tibial Plateau

Calf

Ankle

Measure from Floor Without Shoe

A

Figure 16-9

A, Lower-extremity prosthetic measurements. (*MTP*, Medial tibial plateau, the anatomical landmark of reference for establishing prosthetic build height and for starting circumferential measurements on the transtibial amputated residual limb.)

LOWER-EXTREMITY PROSTHETIC INFORMATION

Name of Patient _____

Site of Amputation _____ Right _____ Left _____

Clinic _____ Physician _____

(Show Location of Stump Details, Identify with Code Letters)

BELOW KNEE | | **ABOVE KNEE**

A = abrasion
B = boil or skin infection
Bu = bursa
Bs = bone spur
D = discoloration
E = edema
I = irritation
M = muscle bunching
P = pressure point
R = redundant tissue
S = scar
T = trigger point

Anterior   Posterior   Medial   Lateral (below knee)

Anterior   Posterior   Medial   Lateral (above knee)

BELOW-KNEE STUMP CHARACTERISTICS

Stump Shape: _____ Distal Padding: _____

Subcutaneous Tissue: Heavy ☐ Light ☐

Distal Pressure Tolerance: None ☐ Slight ☐ Good ☐

Condition of Thigh Musculature: Atrophy ☐ Normal ☐

Condition of Stump Musculature: Atrophy ☐ Normal ☐

Knee Stability: _____

Range of Knee Motion: _____

Degrees of Knee Contracture: _____

Condition of Cut Bones: Tibia _____ Fibula _____

Remarks: _____

_____

_____

_____

ABOVE-KNEE STUMP CHARACTERISTICS

Stump Musculature	Soft	Average	Hard
General _____			
Hamstring Group ____			
Gluteal Group ____			
Rectus Femorus ____			
Adductor Longus			

Subcutaneous Tissue: Heavy ☐ Light ☐

Ischium: Toughened ☐ Pressure Sensitive ☐

Muscle Padding _____ Prominent _____

Previous Ischial Bearing: Yes ☐ No ☐

Stump Lateral Convex   Concave
Contour: Out ☐   Flat ☐   In ☐
Degree of Contracture: Hip Flexion _____°
                            Abduction _____°

Stump Adduction _____° Remarks: _____

Prescription for Prosthesis

3 Foot Comp. Model	5 Knee Comp. Model	Socket Materials	Type of Symes	6 Hip-Joint Model Type
4 Ankle Comp. Model	Type of Socket	Shank Materials	Hip Disartic. Type	Type of Suspension

B

Figure 16-9 cont'd

B, Lower-extremity prosthetic information. (Permission granted by the American Orthotic and Prosthetic Association, Alexandria, VA.)

4. The patient's ability to balance in sitting and standing.
5. The patient's ability to get up from and down to different types of chairs.
6. The patient's ability to use aids (e.g., crutches, walker) for gait training. Can the patient manage a wheelchair?
7. The patient's ability to go up and down stairs and ramps and ability to move in confined spaces.
8. The patient's ability to get up from and down to the floor, as well as his or her ability to kneel, pick objects up from the floor, and do similar activities.

For the upper-limb amputee, the examiner should determine the following:

1. Whether the amputated part is from the dominant or nondominant limb
2. The patient's ability to perform functions of activities of daily living (ADL) and instrumental activities of daily living (IADL) (see Table 1-22)

Sensation Testing

The sensitivity of the stump must be tested to ensure normal sensation. Commonly, hypersensitive areas may be present that have to be desensitized. At the opposite extreme, some areas may have no sensation and require protection. In any case, sensation testing of the stump should involve, at a minimum, hot and cold sensation and light touch.

Psychological Testing

If necessary, psychological testing may be performed.[1,47] Some people have little difficulty adapting to the idea of losing a limb, whereas others have great difficulty accepting the fact that they have lost a limb. This acceptance may be related to how the patient lost the limb (trauma [suddenly] or from long-term problems, such as peripheral vascular disease), how active and independent the patient was before the amputation, or the patient's age (generally, children adapt much better to amputation and a prosthesis than adults). Sometimes, a psychological screening test, such as the Minnesota Multiphasic Personality Inventory (MMPI), may be used to determine the presence of depression, situational anxiety, and possible hysterical reaction to limb loss.[41]

Palpation

The examiner must take time during the examination to palpate the remaining stump of the limb. When palpating, the examiner is looking for normal mobility of the remaining tissues or any tissues that are adherent that may be amenable to treatment, any tissue tenderness, state of the overlying skin, tissue tension and texture, and any differences in tissue thickness, especially in "wear areas" where pressure is applied by the prosthesis. The uninvolved side should also be palpated for comparison.

Diagnostic Imaging

Although diagnostic imaging is not commonly a prerequisite for amputation surgery, especially in trauma cases, it may be used to evaluate the amputated stump. In this case, the examiner would be looking for the following:

1. The level of amputation to determine whether end-weight bearing is possible; for example, a joint disarticulation is more likely to allow end weight bearing.
2. The presence of deformity, bony spurs, or loose fragments.
3. The size and shape, especially of the end bone of the amputation.

Précis of the Amputee Assessment

History
Observation (with and without prosthesis on)
Standing (front, side, behind)
Sitting (front, side, behind)
Walking (front, side, behind) (watch for gait faults in lower-limb amputees)
Stump examination
Prosthesis examination
Examination
Stump measurements
Active movements
Passive movements
Resisted isometric movements
Functional assessment
Sensation testing
Psychological testing
Palpation
Diagnostic imaging

As with any assessment, the patient must be warned that there may be some discomfort after the examination and that this discomfort is normal. Discomfort after any assessment should decrease within 24 hours.

References

To enhance this text and add value for the reader, all references have been incorporated into a CD-ROM that is provided with this text. The reader can view the reference source and access it online whenever possible. There are a total of 47 cited references and other general references for this chapter.

APPENDIX 16-1

RELIABILITY, VALIDITY, SPECIFICITY AND SENSITIVITY OF FUNCTIONAL TESTS USED IN THE ASSESSMENT OF THE AMPUTEE

RIVERMEAD MOBILITY INDEX (RMI)	
Validity	**Responsiveness**
• Correlation with functional independence measure; subscale – motFIT (independence in daily activities r=0.83 and timed walking test – TWT (short-distance performance in walking) r=-0.70[46]	• Effect size=1.35[46]

CHAPTER 17

PRIMARY CARE ASSESSMENT

Although it would be ideal for a family physician who is familiar with the patient's and the family's history to perform a primary care assessment since he or she would more likely be aware of any congenital or developmental problems, the patient's immunization status, and any recent injuries or illnesses and therefore could provide continuity of care,[1–3] many people today do not have a family physician. As health care changes occur, more and more health care professionals are becoming involved in assessment of patients who come to them as first-level providers of medical care. This may involve nurse practitioners, physician assistants, and other health care providers, as well as physicians in primary care facilities, physical therapists with direct access in private practice, clinicians in sole-charge facilities, and sports therapists working and traveling with teams.[4–8] Thus it becomes important for clinicians to be able to evaluate and recognize the potential for health care problems, including systemic disease as a disease entity itself or a disease masquerading as neuromuscular dysfunction, that must be referred to the appropriate health professional.[9,10] Primary care assessment is a form of triage in which the clinician decides whether the patient's problem or problems fall within his or her scope of practice or should be referred to other health care professionals.[11–15]

In many ways, a primary care assessment is similar to a preparticipation examination used in sports because both assessments are used to clear patients of having certain problems that could affect activity and also to provide a mechanism in which problems can be referred to the appropriate health care professional.[16–22] This process involves an understanding of disease as well as an ability to distinguish what system may be affected through a detailed history, observation and examination, and an understanding of different levels of reporting ability of the patient.[9,23] It also requires the clinician to understand his or her limitations, the scope of practice of his or her chosen profession, and why the patient has come to see the clinician. For example, what is the patient's complaint? Is it related to how the patient feels? Is it related to his or her occupation? Is it related to a certain population, age, or gender?[18,24,25]

If the patient has symptoms, several questions should be asked that relate to the symptoms[26]:

1. Where is the symptom, and does it radiate?
2. What does the symptom feel like?
3. How bad is the symptom?
4. Where does (did) the symptom start?
5. How long does the symptom last?
6. How often does the symptom occur?
7. What brings the symptom on?
8. What makes the symptom better or worse?
9. Are there other symptoms associated with it?

Once these questions, and the ones discussed under the different systems as outlined later in the chapter, are answered, the examiner can decide to treat the patient or refer on to another health care professional, usually a physician. Goodman and Snyder[27] clearly outline cases in which referral to a physician is necessary (Table 17-1). This chapter is not meant to be all inclusive of conditions and systems that may need referral. Complete systems assessment is left to other sources.[26,27]

McKeag[28] has outlined five specific populations in which special areas of possible concern should be included in an examination. In the prepubescent patient (6 to 10 years of age), assessments should include examination for congenital abnormalities that may not have been diagnosed previously. In the pubescent patient (11 to 15 years

Table 17-1
Physician Referral

Immediate Medical Attention	Patient with anginal pain not relieved in 20 min Patient with angina who has nausea, vomiting, profuse sweating Diabetic patient demonstrating signs of confusion, lethargy, or changes in mental alertness and function Patient with bowel or bladder incontinence and/or saddle anesthesia secondary to cauda equina lesion Patient in anaphylactic shock
Medical Attention Necessary	***General Systemic*** Unknown cause Lack of significant objective neuromusculoskeletal signs and symptoms Lack of expected progress with physical therapy treatment Development of constitutional symptoms or associated signs and symptoms over the course of treatment Discovery of significant past medical history (PMH) unknown to physician Changes in health status that persist 7–10 days beyond expected time period Patient who is jaundiced and has not been diagnosed or treated Changes in size, shape, tenderness, and consistency of lymph nodes in more than one area, which persist more than 4 wk; painless, enlarged lymph nodes ***For Women*** Low back, hip, pelvic, groin, or sacroiliac symptoms without known etiology and in the presence of constitutional symptoms Symptoms correlated with menses Any spontaneous uterine bleeding after menopause For pregnant women: vaginal bleeding, elevated blood pressure, increased Braxton Hicks contractions during exercise ***Vital Signs (report these findings)*** Persistent rise or fall of blood pressure Blood pressure evaluation in any woman taking birth control pills (should be closely monitored by her physician) Pulse amplitude that fades with inspiration and strengthens with expiration Pulse increase more than 20 beats/min lasting more than 3 min after rest or changing position Difference between systolic and diastolic measurements of more than 4 mm Hg in pulse pressure Persistent low-grade (or higher) fever, especially associated with constitutional symptoms, most commonly sweats ***Cardiac*** Angina at rest Anginal pain not relieved in 20 min More than three sublingual nitroglycerin tablets required to gain relief Nitroglycerin does not relieve anginal pain Rest does not relieve angina Angina continues to increase in intensity after stimulus (e.g., cold, stress, exertion) has been eliminated Changes in pattern of angina Abnormally severe chest pain Patient has nausea, vomiting Anginal pain radiates to jaw or left arm Upper back feels abnormally cool, sweaty, or moist to touch Patient has any doubts about his or her condition ***Cancer*** Early warning sign or signs of cancer: seven early warning signs plus two additional signs pertinent to the physical therapy examination: proximal muscle weakness and change in deep tendon reflexes All soft-tissue lumps that persist or grow, whether painful or painless Any women presenting with chest, breast, axillary, or shoulder pain of unknown etiology, especially in the presence of a positive medical history (self or family) of cancer Bone pain, especially on weight bearing, that persists more than 1 wk and is worse at night

Continued

Table 17-1—cont'd

	Pulmonary
	Shoulder pain that is aggravated by supine positioning
	Shoulder, chest (thorax) pain that subsides with autosplinting (lying on the painful side)
	(For the patient with asthma): signs of asthma or bronchial activity during exercise
	Genitourinary
	Abnormal urinary constituents, e.g., change in color, odor, amount, flow of urine
	Any amount of blood in urine
	Musculoskeletal
	Symptoms that seem out of proportion to the injury, or symptoms persisting beyond the expected time for the nature of the injury
	Severe or chronic back pain accompanied by constitutional symptoms, especially fever
Precautions/ Contraindications to Therapy	Uncontrolled chronic heart failure or pulmonary edema
	Active myocarditis
	Resting heart rate > 120 or 130 beats/min*
	Resting systolic rate > 180–200 beats/min*
	Resting diastolic rate > 105–110 beats/min*
	Moderate dizziness, near-syncope
	Marked dyspnea
	Unusual fatigue
	Unsteadiness
	Loss of palpable pulse
	Postoperative posterior calf pain
	(For the patient with diabetes): chronically unstable blood sugar levels must be stabilized (normal: 80–120 mg/dl; "safe": 100–250 mg/dl)

From Goodman CC, Snyder TE: *Differential diagnosis in physical therapy*, pp 18-20, Philadelphia, 1995, WB Saunders.
*Unexplained or poorly tolerated by patient.

of age), the examination should include an evaluation of physical maturity and good health practices. The postpubescent or young adult group (16 to 30 years of age) has the widest variety of skills, levels, and motivation. For this group, the history of previous injuries and any sport-specific or activity-specific problems is particularly important. For the adult population (30 to 65 years of age), injury prevention (e.g., overuse), previous injury patterns, health concerns, and conditioning should be included in the examination. The final group consists of elderly patients (65 years of age or older), who require an examination based on individual requirements, because many of these people take up exercising or increased physical activity after a medical illness.[20] Age-related changes and their possible consequences are outlined in Table 17-2.

A primary care assessment may vary from a minimal medical examination or physical to rule out possible systemic problems to a very extensive examination involving laboratory tests, stress testing, profiling, x-rays, and other special protocols.[29] History, as well as a physical examination, plays a major role.[30-32] If the patient is going to be asked to do strenuous activity as part of his or her treatment program, various systems (e.g., heart, lungs) must be cleared to ensure the patient is capable of doing the activity.[33]

Characteristics of Systemic Symptoms

- No known cause or unknown etiology
- Gradual onset with progressive, cyclical course (worse/better/worse)
- Persist beyond expected time for that condition
- Constant
- Intense
- Bilateral symptoms (e.g., edema, nail bed changes, clubbing, numbness or tingling, weakness, skin pigmentation changes, or rash)
- Unrelieved by rest or change in position
- If relieved by rest or positional change, over time even these relieving factors no longer reduce symptoms
- Do not fit the expected mechanical or neuromusculoskeletal pattern; symptoms are out of proportion to the injury
- Symptoms cannot be altered (provoked, reproduced, alleviated, eliminated, aggravated) during examination
- Constitutional symptoms, especially fever and night sweats
- Disproportionate pain relief with aspirin (red flag for bone cancer)
- Night pain
- Pain described as knifelike, boring, deep, colicky, deep aching
- Pattern of pain coming and going like spasms

From Goodman CC, Snyder TE: *Differential diagnosis in physical therapy*, p16, Philadelphia, 1995, WB Saunders.

Table 17-2

Selected Age-Related Changes and Their Consequences

Organ/System	Age-Related Physiological Change*	Consequence of Age-Related Physiological Change	Disease, Not Age
General	↑ Body fat ↓ Total body water	↑ Volume of distribution for fat-soluble drugs ↓ Volume of distribution for water-soluble drugs	Obesity Anorexia
Eyes and ears	Presbyopia Lens opacification ↓ High-frequency acuity	↓ Accommodation ↑ Susceptibility to glare Difficulty discriminating words if background noise is present	Blindness Deafness
Endocrine	Impaired glucose tolerance ↓ Thyroxine clearance (and production) ↑ ADH, ↓ renin, and ↓ aldosterone ↓ Testosterone ↓ Vitamin D absorption and activation	↑ Glucose level in response to acute illness ↓ T_4 dose required in hypothyroidism — — Osteopenia	Diabetes mellitus Thyroid dysfunction ↓ NA⁺, ↑ K⁺ Impotence Osteoporosis Osteomalacia
Respiratory	↓ Lung elasticity and ↑ chest wall stiffness	Ventilation/perfusion mismatch and ↓ PO_2	Dyspnea Hypoxia
Cardiovascular	↓ Arterial compliance and ↑ systolic BP → LVH ↓ β-adrenergic responsiveness ↓ Baroreceptor sensitivity and ↓ SA node automaticity	Hypotensive response to ↑ HR, volume depletion, or loss of atrial contraction ↓ Cardiac output and HR response to stress Impaired blood pressure response to standing, volume depletion	Syncope Heart failure Heart block
Gastrointestinal	↓ Hepatic function ↓ Gastric acidity ↓ Colonic motility ↓ Anorectal function	Delayed metabolism of some drugs ↓ Ca⁺ absorption on empty stomach Constipation —	Cirrhosis Osteoporosis Vitamin B_{12} deficiency Fecal impaction Fecal incontinence
Hemotologic/immune system	↓ Bone marrow reserve (?) ↓ T-cell function ↑ Autoantibodies	— False-negative PPD response False-positive rheumatoid factor, antinuclear antibody	Anemia — Autoimmune disease
Renal	↓ Glomerular filtration rate ↓ Urine concentration/dilution (see also Endocrine)	Impaired excretion of some drugs Delayed response to salt or fluid restriction or overload; nocturia	↑ Serum creatinine ↑↓ Na⁺
Genitourinary	Vaginal/urethral mucosal atrophy Prostate enlargement	Dyspareunia Bacteriuria ↑ Residual urine volume	Symptomatic urinary tract infection Urinary incontinence Urinary retention
Musculoskeletal	↓ Lean body mass, muscle ↓ Bone density	— Osteopenia	Functional impairment Hip fracture
Nervous system	Brain atrophy ↓ Brain catechol synthesis ↓ Brain dopaminergic synthesis ↓ Righting reflexes ↓ Stage 4 sleep	Benign senescent forgetfulness — Stiffer gait ↑ Body sway Early wakening, insomnia	Dementia Delirium Depression Parkinson's disease Falls Sleep apnea

From Resnick N.: Geriatric medicine. In Isselbacher KJ et al, editors: *Harrison's principles of internal medicine*, ed 13, New York, 1994, McGraw-Hill.

ADH, Antidiuretic hormone; *BP*, blood pressure; *HR*, heart rate; *LVH*, left ventricular hypertrophy; *PPD*, purified protein derivative; *SA*, sinoatrial; T_4, thyroxine.

The table displays selected changes that occur normally with age and their physiological consequences. Changes as a result of disease rather than age are listed in the last column.

*Changes generally observed in healthy elderly subjects free of symptoms and detectable disease in the organ system studied. The changes are usually important only when the system is stressed or other factors are added (e.g., drugs, disease, or environmental challenge); they rarely result in symptoms otherwise.

Objectives of the Evaluation

Primary care evaluations have many useful purposes.[1,9,29,34,35] However, the examiner must remember that the primary purpose of the examination is to determine the patient's health problem and to either treat the patient or refer him or her to the appropriate health care professional.[1,9] As part of the examination, the examiner can **establish baseline values** for the patient. These may be compared with normal "textbook" values or used to determine change in the future. In other words, the assessment should not consist of simple "yes-no" questions. Instead, it must be very thorough to establish proper baseline levels.

Objectives of Primary Care Assessment

- Determine if disease is present
- Uncover preexisting conditions
- Determine unsuspected correctable conditions
- Determine health status
- Prevent injuries
- Avoid misinterpretation of findings
- Establish baseline values
- Act as a screening process
- Foster good health practices
- Develop rapport with the patient
- Establish guidelines
- Develop a musculoskeletal profile
- Counsel the patient
- Classify the patient
- Meet legal and insurance requirements
- Determine if referral is necessary

The primary care assessment is used to determine the health status of the patient. It also helps to prevent injuries through identification of any abnormalities, physical inadequacies, or poor conditioning that may put the patient at risk.[36] The examination may identify previously unsuspected conditions that are amenable to correction or that preclude participation in the desired activity. Similarly, the evaluation helps to avoid misinterpretation of findings that appear to be new but existed previously. For this reason, a review of previous health records, if possible, is also part of the primary care assessment.

The primary care assessment is also worthwhile to ensure that treatments have been carried out previously and that conditions previously diagnosed have been properly cared for. In this way, it acts as a screening process to ensure that treatment of potentially serious medical and surgical conditions has taken place. It also helps

to rule out potentially serious or threatening conditions that may temporarily preclude the patient from participation in work or recreational activities. For example, with infectious mononucleosis, contact sports may be precluded for a time because the patient's spleen is enlarged and is more easily injured or ruptured.

The assessment also gives the clinician an opportunity to foster good health practices and to promote optimum health and fitness. The assessment enables the health care provider to give proper health guidance and to determine the general state of health of the patient.

The assessment also gives the examiner a chance to develop a rapport with the patient. The examiner can learn what motivates the patient and, at the same time, help establish the patient's confidence in the health care staff. The examination may also be used to establish guidelines for the patient and health care team on questions of health, safety, and care. In addition, it provides an opportunity to counsel the patient.

Primary Care History

For a primary care assessment, the history plays a predominant role to ensure that questions related to the various systems are asked. A complete history can usually identify 60% to 75% of the problems affecting a patient.[22,29,37] For the young person or the patient with communication problems, both the patient and his or her parent or guardian should provide the history to ensure completeness. The rest of the assessment proceeds from the information determined in the history. The history provides details regarding health problems and injuries and enables the examiner to focus on any abnormalities that it brings out.[29] Generally, the history is completed by the patient's answering questions in a yes-no format (see Appendix 17-1 for a generic primary care assessment questionnaire). Using such a format decreases the chance of the patient forgetting something.[23] The "yes" answers then are investigated further in other parts of the assessment (see Appendix 17-2). It is important, however, that the "no" answers also be checked for accuracy. Ideally, oral histories, in which the health care professional asks the questions, are more accurate; but usually, because of time constraints, this is not possible. The history should include the patient's medical history as well as the family's medical history to rule out any congenital, hereditary, or injury problems. It is important that a complete health history be obtained, because the patient may leave out or hide information that may preclude the patient from taking part in a desired activity or because of possible secondary gain.[37]

Some general questions can be asked initially, and these can be used to cross-reference questions asked in specific areas of assessment:[29]

1. Have you ever been a patient in a hospital, emergency room, or clinic?

2. Have you ever seen a physician for an injury or illness?

3. Have you ever had x-rays?

4. Have you ever had an operation?

5. Are you presently taking any medication or pills?

6. Do you have any allergies (to medications, insects, food, or other things)?

7. When was your last vaccination? What was the vaccination for?

8. Have you ever been unable to work or participate in exercise or sports?

9. Have you ever experienced chest pain, dyspnea, or syncope during work, exercise, or activity?

10. Have you ever had a seizure?

11. Have you ever been told you had high blood pressure?

12. Have you ever been told you had high cholesterol?

13. Do you have trouble breathing or do you cough during or after activity?

These general questions cover wide areas, and the specific parts of the assessment should corroborate the answers given to these general questions. In addition, the examiner must consider the effect of psychosocial issues on both the patient and his or her reported symptoms. Haggman et al.[38] believed two questions were useful to screen for symptoms of depression:

1. During the past month, have you often been bothered by feeling down, depressed, or hopeless?

2. During the past month, have you been bothered by little interest or pleasure in doing things?

If the answer to both questions is yes, further psychological investigation may be warranted.[39,40] Waddell and Main[40] talked about illness behavior, a normal and reasonable behavior, which is what people do and say to communicate that they are ill. The examiner should always keep in mind the role psychosocial issues may have in anyone seeking primary care help.

The following assessment sections outline questions pertaining to specific body systems that may lead to further examination or testing and possible concerns or issues that must be dealt with if the patient is going to take part in a particular activity. The examiner may want to cover all of the systems or only those that appear pertinent to the problem.

Examination

The medical examination must be not only thorough but also applicable to the job, activity, exercise, or sport to which the person hopes to return or take part in. Health care professionals should always be alert for concealment, denial, or invention of problems on the part of the patient.

Parts of Primary Care Examination

- History
- Vital signs
  - Temperature
  - Blood pressure
  - Heart rate
  - Weight
- Head and face examination
- Neurological examination and convulsive disorders
- Musculoskeletal examination
- Cardiovascular examination
- Pulmonary examination
- Urogenital examination
- Gastrointestinal examination
- Dermatological examination
- Examination for heat illness
- Laboratory tests
- Physical fitness profile
  - Body composition
  - Maturity index
  - Flexibility
  - Strength, endurance, and power
  - Agility, balance, and reaction time
  - Cardiovascular fitness

Vital Signs

The initial part of the examination is performed to establish the patient's baseline physiological parameters and vital signs (see Chapter 1, Table 1-6), including pulse or heart rate, respiratory rate, blood pressure (systolic and diastolic), weight, and temperature (normal: 98.4°F [37°C], range: 96.5°F [35.8°C] to 99.4°F [37.4°C]). This part of the examination may be performed by any health care professional who has knowledge or an understanding of the techniques, and it is part of any primary care examination.[41,42]

Table 1-7 (see Chapter 1) outlines guidelines for blood pressure measurement.[43] High blood pressure values should be checked several times at 15- to 30-minute intervals, with the patient resting in between to determine whether a high reading is accurate or is being caused by anxiety ("white coat syndrome") or some similar reason. If three consecutive readings are high, the patient is said to have high blood pressure (hypertension) (see Chapter 1, Table 1-8). If the readings remain high, further investigation may be warranted.[1,43,44] Table 17-3 outlines the risk factors of hypertension.

Table 17-3

Risk Factors of Hypertension

Primary	Secondary
One or both parents with hypertension	Renal disease
Increased salt intake	Oral contraceptives
Excessive alcohol consumption	Cushing syndrome
Obesity	Sleep apnea syndrome
Race (blacks more commonly affected)	Endocrine (thyroid, parathyroid conditions)
Personality traits (tense, hostile)	Coarctation of aorta
Smoking	Renovascular disease
Diabetes	Adrenal cortex dysfunction
Physical inactivity	
Cholesterol >6.5 mmol/L or low-density lipoprotein cholesterol >4.0 mmol/L	

Complications of Hypertension

- Cardiovascular disease
- Heart failure
- Left ventricular hypertrophy
- Stroke
- Intracerebral hemorrhage
- Chronic renal insufficiency
- Renal disease

The following examination sections may be part of the primary care examination, but this will depend on what has been found from taking the history and vital signs. Only those sections that the examiner feels are relevant or are areas of concern would normally be investigated.

General Medical Problems

There are general systemic problems that the examiner must always keep in mind when doing an assessment. Some of the general medical (systemic) questions include the following:[13,27,45]

1. Have you ever been diagnosed with a systemic disease (e.g., diabetes)?
2. Have you ever been diagnosed with a progressive disease (e.g., muscular dystrophy, multiple sclerosis)?
3. Have you ever been told you have cancer?
4. Have you ever had anything similar to what you have now? How often?

5. Where exactly is your pain? What is the quality, frequency, and pattern of the pain?[46] What have you tried to do to alleviate the pain? On a scale of 1 (no pain) to 10 (pain is bad as it could possibly get), how would you rate your pain level?
6. Do you have any other symptoms?
7. Have you ever had any infections? How were they treated?
8. Do you have unexplained fatigue?
9. Have you ever had any unexplained weakness?
10. Do you bruise easily?

The presence of systemic disease (e.g., diabetes) does not rule out work or activity, but the examiner must ensure that there is either good control by the use of medication or that the disease will not cause undue risk to the patient or his or her well-being. It must also be determined whether the extent or intensity of the activity the patient has to do poses a significant threat to the patient's physical condition.[47] The examiner also has to be concerned about problems such as acute infection, malignancy, and progressive diseases such as multiple sclerosis.

Acute illnesses tend to be self-limiting and usually require only that the patient temporarily withdraw from work or activity, often to prevent spread to others.[29] Dehydration is made worse by febrile illness, which could, in certain circumstances, lead to heat disorders.

Head and Face

Eye Examination

Visual acuity is usually examined with the use of a Snellen or common eye chart. Peripheral vision and depth perception may also be tested. Questions related to the eye examination include the following:[29,48]

1. Have you had any problems with vision or your eyes?
2. Have you ever injured your eyes?
3. Do you wear glasses, contact lenses, or protective eyewear?
4. Are you color-blind?
5. Do you have a peripheral vision problem?
6. Have you ever used medications for an eye problem?
7. Have you ever had an eye infection?

Any abnormalities found or positive answers may require further examination. Uncorrected vision of less than 20/40 should be checked further.[34] Visual loss of 20/50 means that the patient can read at 20 feet what the average person can read at 50 feet. The health care professional should watch for problems that may preclude work, preclude participation in the chosen activity or sport, or affect the safety of the patient. Vision in only one eye results in lack of depth perception, which can be detrimental in certain activities. Patients with sight in only one eye should work at specific jobs or participate in physical activities only if they have an understanding of the dangers of participating and accept the risks. Such patients should not work or participate in sports for which there is no adequate eye protection.

Examples of Eye Conditions or Signs and Symptoms Requiring Further Examination

- Sudden vision loss
- Visual loss greater than 20/40
- Vision in one eye only
- Severe myopia
- Retinal detachment
- Retinal tear
- Corneal abrasion
- Iritis
- Conjunctivitis
- Proptosis (protrusion) of eye

If the patient wears glasses, the health care professional should ensure that the lenses are plastic, polycarbonate, or heat-treated (safety) glass to prevent them from shattering during work or activity.

Myopia, or nearsightedness, should be noted on the chart; such patients are more likely to suffer retinal degeneration, which increases the possibility of retinal detachment. Patients who have had a retinal detachment are sometimes excluded from contact sports or high-exertion jobs. People who have a retinal tear should be allowed to do strenuous activities only if cleared by a physician or specialist, and they should have a qualifying letter allowing them to return to work.

Pupil size should also be evaluated. In some patients, the pupils are of obvious different sizes (**anisocoria**). This difference should be noted in case the patient has to be evaluated for a head injury at a later date.[49] Assessment of the eyes is shown in Chapter 2.

Dental Examination

Questions to be asked concerning the patient's dental record include the following:[48]

1. When did you last see a dentist?
2. Have you ever had any problems with your teeth or gums?
3. Have you ever had any teeth knocked out, damaged, or extracted?
4. Do you wear a mouth guard?
5. Do you smoke or chew tobacco?
6. Have you ever had an injury to your face or jaws?

When looking for dental problems, which is usually done by a dentist, it is important to determine how many teeth the patient has and the last time he or she saw a dentist.

Ear Examination

Questions to be asked concerning the patient's ear problems include the following:

1. Do you have any problems with hearing?
2. Do you have an earache? (onset? duration?)
3. Is the earache associated with a cold, flu, or trauma?
4. Is there pain in the ear?
5. Is there any discharge from the ear?

Ear problems are commonly referred to a physician or an ear, nose, and throat specialist. Assessment of the ear is shown in Chapter 2.

Nose Examination

Questions to be asked concerning the patient's nose problems include the following:

1. What is the problem with your nose?
2. Can you breathe through the nose?
3. Do you have any discharge from the nose (e.g., blood, mucus)?
4. Do you use any medication through your nose (nose drops, nasal spray)?
5. Are both nostrils affected?

Assessment of the nose is shown in Chapter 2. Nose problems other than colds are commonly referred to a physician.

Neurological Examination and Convulsive Disorders (Including Head Injury)

The neurological examination is very important, especially in contact or collision activities or when there is a suspected head injury. Some of the more common questions asked in the neurological examination include the following[13,29]:

1. Have you ever been knocked out or been unconscious?
2. Have you ever had a head injury?
3. Have you had or do you have frequent or severe headaches?
4. Have you ever had a stinger or burner?
5. Have you ever had a time when one or more of your limbs went numb or "to sleep" during activity?
6. Have you ever fainted (syncope)?
7. Have you ever had a paralyzed limb?
8. Have you ever lost feeling or muscular control of your arms or legs?
9. Have you ever had a seizure?
10. Have you ever been in a motor vehicle accident or fallen and hit your head?

A positive answer to any of these questions could have a significant impact on what the patient is allowed to do and whether the patient is allowed to return to work or participate in contact or collision activities.

In the neurological examination, the examiner may assess the status of a head injury (see Chapter 2), perform a cranial nerve assessment (see Chapter 2) and sensation scan, and evaluate the different reflexes (see Chapter 1) if problems are suspected. The examiner must check for concussions and nerve palsies. Any positive neurological signs and symptoms uncovered in the examination, such as recurrent concussions or nerve palsies, should preclude strenuous activity until investigated further by a specialist before clearance to return to previous activities is given.

Examples of Neurological Conditions or Signs and Symptoms Requiring Further Examination

- More than one concussion
- Postconcussion syndrome
- Any history of head injury
- Expanding intracranial lesion
- Any history of seizure
- Neurological symptoms of undetermined cause
- Any history of stinger, burner, or neurapraxia
- Persistent weakness, numbness, or arm or leg pain
- Any history of transient quadriplegia
- Upper motor neuron symptoms
- Any history of nerve palsy

With convulsive disorders, the examiner needs to know the frequency of the episodes; how or whether control of the convulsions has been achieved; the use of routine medication; any circumstances that activate the convulsions; and whether the patient understands the disorder, its hazards, and its predisposing factors. Patients with epilepsy should be discouraged from activities such as skiing, scuba diving, parachuting, and climbing because of their inherent dangers.[29] If the activity involves water sports (e.g., swimming alone, scuba diving), auto racing, or any activity in which recurrent head trauma or unexpected falls may cause serious injury (e.g., mountain climbing, working at heights), then the patient with convulsive disorders should be discouraged from doing these activities. Patients whose activities should be restricted include those who experience daily or weekly seizures, those who display bizarre forms of psychomotor epilepsy, and those whose postconvalescent state is prolonged or typically includes marked abnormal behavior. It is important to understand whether the medication taken can maintain good control of the patient's condition, not only in everyday situations but also in stress situations. For example, hyperventilation may precipitate an epileptic seizure, and seizures tend to occur after exercise, not during the event. In addition, it is important to know whether the extent or intensity of the participation poses a significant threat to the patient's physical condition.

Musculoskeletal Examination

Like the neurological examination discussed previously, the musculoskeletal examination is often a very important part of an evaluation. Questions in the history related to this examination include the following:[31,50-54]

1. Have you ever pulled (strained) or hurt a muscle?
2. Have you ever torn (sprained) or stretched a ligament?
3. Have you ever subluxated or dislocated a joint or had a bone come out of joint?
4. Have you ever broken (fractured) a bone?
5. Have any of your joints ever swollen?
6. Have you ever had pain in the muscles or joints at work or during or after activity, exercise, or sports (Table 17-4)?
7. Have you ever had regular prolonged (>30 minutes) morning stiffness?
8. Have you ever had any rashes, eye infections, diarrhea associated with joint pains, and/or swelling?
9. Have you ever had any proximal weakness, excessive cramping, or muscle fasciculations?

Table 17-4

Comparison of Systemic and Musculoskeletal Joint Pain

Systemic	Musculoskeletal
Awakens at night	Decreases with rest
Deep aching, throbbing	Sharp
Reduced by pressure	Ceases when stressful action is stopped
Constant or waves/spasm	
Jaundice	Associated signs and symptoms
Migratory arthralgias	
Skin rash	Associated signs and symptoms
Fatigue	
Weight loss	Usually none
Low-grade fever	Trigger points may be accompanied by nausea, sweating
Muscular weakness	
Cyclical, progressive symptoms	
History of infection (hepatitis, streptococcosis, mononucleosis, measles)	

From Goodman CC, Snyder TE: *Differential diagnosis in physical therapy*, p 526, Philadelphia, 1995, WB Saunders.

A positive response to any of these questions requires further investigation.

The musculoskeletal examination begins with observation of the patient's posture (see Chapter 15), looking for any asymmetry. Asymmetry, combined with the history, may lead the examiner to do a detailed assessment of a specific joint (see Chapters 3 to 13). If no problems are noted, the examiner can do a quick **upper and lower scanning or screening examination** to check for potential problems and abnormal movement (e.g., hypomobility, hypermobility, capsular patterns, weakness, abnormal movement patterns, cheating movements).[41,55]

Upper and Lower Scanning Examination

- Cervical spine: flexion, extension, side flexion, rotation
- Shoulder shrug (resistance may be added)
- Shoulder: elevation through abduction, forward flexion and the plane of the scapula; medial and lateral rotation (resistance may be added)
- Elbow: flexion, extension, supination, pronation
- Wrist: flexion, extension, radial and ulnar deviation
- Fingers and thumb: open hands wide, make a tight fist
- Thoracic and lumbar spine: flexion (touch toes, knees straight—watch for spine versus hip movement), extension, side flexion, rotation
- Tighten quadriceps (quadriceps strength, symmetry)
- Test hamstring tightness
- Hip, knee, ankle, and foot: squat and bounce, heel-toe walking

---

If any deviation, weakness, or abnormality is found, or if the patient has reported a previous injury to a joint, a more detailed examination may be performed to assess active movements, passive movements, resisted isometric movements, special tests, functional tests, reflexes, sensation, myotomes, joint play, and palpation of that joint or associated joints.

When looking for musculoskeletal problems, it is important to consider whether the patient's job or what he or she wants to do will exacerbate an existing disease or injury, increase an existing deformity, or cause further bone or joint damage. When looking for musculoskeletal problems, the examiner may look at the patient's flexibility, strength, and endurance, as well as static and dynamic stability. Spinal instability (especially instability of the cervical or lumbar spine) or spondylolisthesis may preclude the patient from taking part in some activities. Maturation may also have to be considered when dealing with patients who are still growing, as may previous injuries, congenital problems, and growth abnormalities.

Examples of Musculoskeletal Conditions or Signs and Symptoms Requiring Further Examination

- Joint or spinal instability (static and dynamic)
- Joint swelling
- Unhealed muscle or ligament injury (especially 3° or if avulsion suspected)
- Possible fractures or dislocations/subluxations
- Unhealed or healing fracture
- Degenerative diseases
- Inflammatory diseases
- Unusual hypermobility or hypomobility
- Muscle weakness
- Growth or maturation disorders
- Repetitive stress disorders
- Myopathy
- Metabolic disease

Cardiovascular Examination

The cardiovascular examination should be performed in a quiet area because of the need to auscultate. In this part of the evaluation, the examiner looks for subtle but significant cardiac abnormalities so as to reduce the incidence of unexpected sudden death in sports or similar incidences at work.[2,32,56-61] In some cases, electrocardiograms (ECGs) or stress ECGs may be appropriate.[62] More than 90% of sudden deaths in exercise and sports among participants younger than 30 years of age involve the cardiovascular system.

The following questions should be asked in the history concerning the cardiovascular system:[9,13,27,29]

1. Have you ever had a heart attack?
2. Do you have a pacemaker or other device to assist your heart?
3. Have you ever had heart surgery?
4. Have you ever had frequent heartburn?
5. Have you ever experienced dizziness, fainting, or passing out during or after activity, exercise, or sports?
6. Have you ever experienced chest pain, tightness, crushing sensation, squeezing, or pressure in the chest at work or during or after activity, exercise, or sports (Table 17-5 and 17-6)?
7. When working or doing an activity, exercise, or sport, do you tire more quickly than others doing the same things?
8. Have you ever had high blood pressure?
9. Has your heart ever "raced" or skipped beats?
10. Have you ever been told you have a heart murmur?
11. Has anyone in your family ever had or died from heart problems?
12. Has anyone in your family died suddenly before the age of 50 years?

Table 17-5

Causes of Chest Pain

Systemic Causes	Neuromuscular Causes
Pulmonary	Tietze syndrome
Pulmonary embolism	Costochondritis
Spontaneous pneumothorax	Hypersensitive xiphoid
Pulmonary hypertension	Slipping rib syndrome
Cor pulmonale	Trigger points
Pleurisy with pneumonia	Myalgia
Cardiac	Rib fracture
Myocardial ischemia (angina)	Cervical spine disorders
Pericarditis	Neurologic
Myocardial infarct	Thoracic outlet syndrome
Dissecting aortic aneurysm	Neuritis
Epigastric/Upper GI	Shingles (herpes zoster)
Esophagitis	Dorsal nerve root irritation
Upper GI index	
Breast	
Breast tumor	
Abscess	
Mastitis	
Lactation problems	
Mastodynia	
Trigger point	
Other	
Rheumatic diseases	
Anxiety	

From Goodman CC, Snyder TE: *Differential diagnosis in physical therapy*, p 532, Philadelphia, 1995, WB Saunders.
GI, Gastrointestinal

If the answer to any of these questions is yes, the examiner must consider the possibility of cardiomyopathy, conduction abnormalities, arrhythmias, valvular problems, coronary artery defects, and lung or related problems.[64] If cardiovascular problems are suspected, the examiner may organize further tests (e.g., ECG, treadmill stress tests, laboratory tests)[65] to detect cardiac abnormalities.

Examples of Cardiovascular Conditions or Signs and Symptoms Requiring Further Examination

- Chest pain
- Dizziness with activity or vertigo
- Irregular heartbeat (rate, rhythm)
- Hypertension (labile or organic)
- Heart murmur
- Family history of heart problems
- Hypertrophic cardiomegaly
- Conduction abnormalities
- Arrhythmias
- Myocarditis
- Valvular problems
- Aortic coarctation
- Marfan syndrome
- Enlarged (athlete's) heart
- Atherosclerotic disease (positive ankle-arm index)
- Mitral insufficiency
- Anemia
- Enlarged spleen
- Unexplained fatigue
- Hypertension

13. Have you had a severe viral infection (myocarditis, mononucleosis) within the last month?
14. Has a physician denied or restricted your participation in any activity for any heart problems?
15. Do your ankles and/or legs swell?[63]

When looking for cardiovascular problems, the examiner should be alert for the following unusual or abnormal findings:

1. Heart rate faster than 120 beats/min or inappropriate tachycardia for a specific activity

Table 17-6

Characteristics of Cardiac Chest Pain

Angina	Myocardial Infarct (MI)	Mitral Valve Prolapse	Pericarditis
1–5 min	30 min to hours	Hours	Hours to days
Moderate intensity	Severe (can be painless)	Rarely severe	Varies; mild to severe
Tightness, chest discomfort	Crushing pain; intolerable (can be painless)	May be asymptomatic; unlike angina in quality or quantity	Asymptomatic; varies; can mimic MI
Subsides with rest or nitroglycerin	Unrelieved by rest or nitroglycerin	Unrelieved by rest or nitroglycerin	Relieved by kneeling on all fours, leaning forward, or sitting upright
Pain related to tone of arteries (spasm)	Pain related to heart ischemia	Mechanism of pain unknown	Pain related to inflammatory process

From Goodman CC, Snyder TE: *Differential diagnosis in physical therapy*, p 94, Philadelphia, 1995, WB Saunders.

2. Arrhythmias or irregular beats[66]
3. Midsystolic clicks, indicating a leaky valve or mitral valve prolapse
4. Murmurs that are grade 3 or louder

The loudness of **systolic murmurs** is graded from 1 to 6, with grade 1 being a very faint murmur requiring concentration to be heard. A grade 2 murmur is a faint murmur but one that is heard immediately after the stethoscope is placed on the chest. Grade 3 is an intermediate murmur louder than grade 2. Most human dynamically significant murmurs are at least grade 3. Grade 4 is a loud murmur, frequently associated with palpable sensation, known as a thrill. A grade 5 murmur is a very loud murmur still requiring at least the edge of the stethoscope to remain in contact with the chest. The grade 6 murmur is a murmur audible with the stethoscope just breaking contact with the chest.[67] **Diastolic murmurs** are graded from 1 to 4, 1 representing the faintest and 4 the loudest murmur. A benign functional murmur or systemic mitral valve prolapse does not preclude exercise or sports but must be evaluated on an individual basis.

The examiner must be aware of congenital heart abnormalities, such as aortic coarctation (stenosis of the artery), which may be revealed by a difference in the femoral and brachial pulses. In such a case, strenuous activity is contraindicated. As another example, 90% of patients with Marfan syndrome (an autosomal dominant condition) have cardiac abnormalities. The examiner must be aware of atrial septal defects (an abnormal communication between the chambers of the heart), dextrocardia (the heart is moved within the thoracic cavity), and paroxysmal auricular tachycardia (an abnormal increase in heartbeat for short periods). Patients with these conditions should be cleared by a specialist before any strenuous activity because of the possibility of fainting in a stressful situation. The examiner must also be aware of heart enlargement (athlete's heart). This condition does not necessarily preclude activity but should be investigated further if found. If any of these abnormalities have been surgically corrected, they should be evaluated by a specialist on an individual basis to determine whether the patient can take part in the proposed activity.

Hypertrophic cardiomyopathy is the most common cause of sudden death in athletes, followed by aortic rupture associated with Marfan syndrome, congenital coronary artery anomalies, and atherosclerotic coronary artery disease.[29,68] If any of these conditions is present, strenuous activity is precluded.

Other cardiovascular problems include thromboembolic disease, pulse irregularities, valvular problems such as mitral insufficiency or mitral valve prolapse, and abnormally high blood pressure (hypertension). Systolic pressure of 140 mm Hg on repeated measurements is considered abnormal (see Chapter 1, Table 1-8).[58] Also, patients with labile hypertension (an unstable condition of free and rapid change in tension) or organic hypertension caused by structural problems should be investigated further. These patients should have a complete comprehensive coronary risk factor work-up. Mild hypertension does not preclude strenuous activity, but this slight abnormality should be noted and evaluated on an individual basis.[29] When taking blood pressure, a proper cuff size must be used to ensure an accurate reading. If the initial reading is high, the reading should be repeated two or three times after the patient has been lying supine for 20 to 30 minutes. Only if the blood pressure is elevated after the third reading should the patient be considered hypertensive.

Another condition the examiner should be aware of is anemia. If anemia is suspected, the level of hemoglobin (the oxygen-carrying pigment in human blood) is tested. Anemia is more likely to be seen in women during menstruation, and sickle cell anemia is more common in black individuals. In some cases, anemia is caused by an increase in blood volume, which decreases the concentration of red blood cells. In this case, the individual has normal red blood cells but appears to be anemic.

Detecting Cardiac Risks in Examinations: Key Physical Findings of Cardiac Evaluation by Physician

Heart rate faster than 120 beats/min
- If repeated tests on second occasion are high, suggest monitoring and recording of pulse at home by a trained parent or nurse friend.
- Pulse recovery tests after jumping or hopping exercises are useless routines except for multiple extrasystoles or arrhythmias.

Multiple extrasystoles or arrhythmias. Check after jumping or hopping 20 times to ascertain if arrhythmias appear or disappear.

Resting blood pressure higher than 130/80 mm Hg for students aged 6 to 11 years, 140/90 mm Hg for students aged 12 to 18 years.
- For validity, be certain that the pressure cuff covers at least two thirds of the upper arm, from elbow to shoulder (adult cuff = 30 × 13 cm; pediatric cuff = 22 × 10 cm; obese cuff = 39 × 15 cm).
- If high, repeat test three times and take average.

All systolic murmurs grade 3 to 6 or louder at any location; all diastolic murmurs of any intensity at any location; or any continuous murmur. Heart should be auscultated at four chest locations:
- Pulmonic area (second intercostal space at left sternal border)
- Aortic area (second intercostal space at right sternal border)
- Tricuspid area (fourth intercostal space at left sternal border)
- Mitral area (fourth intercostal space at left midclavicular line)

Routinely palpate femoral and brachial pulses. Note if absent or if large discrepancy exists between them.

Modified from Schell NB: Cardiac evaluation of school sports participants: guidelines approved by the Medical Society of New York, *NY State J Med* 78:942–943, 1978.

Detecting Cardiac Risks in Examinations: Key Historical Facts Obtained from Students, Parents, and School Health Records

- Cyanotic heart disease early in life
- Murmur early in life based on anatomical diagnosis of left-to-right shunt or pulmonic or aortic stenosis
- Rheumatic heart disease
- Fainting spells (syncope)
- Chest or abdominal pains (not otherwise diagnosed)
- Dyspnea on exertion
- Cardiac surgery
- Enlarged heart
- Cardiac rhythm disturbances
- Familial heart disease* or rhythm disturbances
- Functional or innocent murmur of 4 or more years' duration

Modified from Schell NB: Cardiac evaluation of school sports participants: guidelines approved by the Medical Society of New York, *NY State J Med* 78:942-943, 1978.
*Hypertension, early stroke (before 50 years), or early coronary (before 50 years) in close relatives.

Risk factors for coronary heart disease

Hyperlipidemia
Cigarette smoking
Hypertension
Hyperglycemia or diabetes mellitus
Hyperuricemia or gout
Obesity

Health problems

Cardiopulmonary disease
Neurological disease
Endocrinopathy
Musculoskeletal disorder
Psychiatric disorder
Renal or hepatic disease
Anemia
Current drug use
Other acute or chronic disease

* Exercise stress testing is recommended if patient has cardiopulmonary disease

** Diagnostic laboratory testing is indicated if CDH risk factors include hyperlipidemia, hyperglycemia, or hyperuricemia

Figure 17-1

Preexercise evaluation flow sheet. *CDH*, Coronary heart disease; *CPE*, comprehensive physical examination; *DLT*, diagnostic laboratory testing; *ECG*, resting electrocardiogram; *EST*, exercise stress test; *LPE*, limited physical examination; *MLT*, minimal laboratory testing. (Redrawn from Taylor RB: Pre-exercise evaluation: Which procedures are really needed? *Consultant*, pp. 94–101, April 1983.)

If cardiovascular or cardiopulmonary disease is suspected, an exercise stress test is often recommended.[34,69] Figure 17-1 outlines a flowchart for considerations before doing such a test. Twenty to thirty-five percent of those with heart disease will have a normal stress test, so it is important to remember that any stress test is only valid to the load at which the heart has been stressed when doing the test. Forty-five percent of runners older than 40 years of age have irregular results on ECGs. Further, different types of activity (e.g., static or dynamic) lead to different stresses on the heart.

Contraindications to Exercise Testing

- Physical inability to walk on the treadmill
- Unstable angina or new resting ECG changes
- Acute pericarditis, myocarditis, endocarditis
- Uncompensated CHF, S3 gallop, rales
- Severe aortic stenosis
- Hypertrophic cardiomyopathy
- Known LMCA or equivalent stenoses
- Uncooperative patient
- Other serious medical problem or problems

From Cavell RM: The exercise treadmill test for diagnosis and prognosis of coronary artery disease, *J La State Med Soc* 147:198, 1995.
CHF, congestive heart failure; *ECG*, electrocardiogram; *LMCA*, left main coronary artery

Common Causes of False-Positive Exercise Tests

- Congenital and valvular heart disease
- Digoxin
- Electrolyte abnormalities
- Nonfasting state
- Pre-excitation syndromes, WPW
- Bundle branch block
- Mitral valve prolapse
- Left ventricular hypertrophy
- Hyperventilation

From Cavell RM: The exercise treadmill test for diagnosis and prognosis of coronary artery disease, *J La State Med Soc* 147:198, 1995.
WPW, Wolff-Parkinson-White syndrome.

Indications for Termination of the Exercise Test

- Patient's request
- Achievement of maximum effort
- Appearance of serious arrhythmia, multiform PVCs, triplets, rapid SVT
- Fall in systolic BP in the face of increasing work load
- Progressive anginal pain
- CNS symptoms, dizziness, ataxia
- Signs of poor perfusion, pallor, cyanosis, cool extremities
- More than 0.3 mV of horizontal or down-sloping ST depression
- Technical loss of monitoring ability

From Cavell RM: The exercise treadmill test for diagnosis and prognosis of coronary artery disease, *J La State Med Soc* 147:198, 1995.
BP, Blood pressure; *CNS*, central nervous system; *PVC*, premature ventricular contraction; *SVT*, supraventricular tachycardia.

Examples of Pulmonary Conditions or Signs and Symptoms Requiring Further Examination

- Abnormal coughing
- Abnormal shortness of breath
- Abnormal breath sounds (e.g., wheezing, rhonchi, rales)
- Asthma (uncontrolled or exertional)
- Exercise-induced bronchospasm
- Pulmonary insufficiency
- Severe allergies
- Nasal deviation or occlusion
- Chronic sinusitis

The ankle-arm index (AAI) may also be used to screen for atherosclerotic (cardiovascular) disease.[70,71] This is the ratio of the ankle to arm systolic pressure when measured using a Doppler ultrasound device.[70] The lower the AAI, the greater the risk of disease.[71]

Pulmonary Examination

The pulmonary examination is often done in conjunction with the cardiovascular examination in a quiet area. Questions related to the pulmonary system may include the following:[13,27,32]

1. Have you ever had trouble breathing?
2. Have you ever had a pulmonary disease?
3. Do you use any breathing aids?
4. Have you ever had a chest x-ray? When?
5. Have you ever experienced long periods of intermittent coughing?
6. Do you cough anything up? Have you had a recent productive cough (e.g., sputum, blood, what color?)?
7. Have you ever experienced coughing at work or during or after activity, exercise, or sports?
8. Have you ever experienced shortness of breath or wheezing at work or during or after activity, exercise, or sports?
9. Is your breathlessness related to anything (e.g., exercise, pollen, emotion)?
10. Do you have asthma? If so, how do you treat it?
11. Have you ever broken your nose?
12. Do you suffer from chronic sinus irritation or a runny nose?

The examiner auscultates for clear breath sounds and watches for symmetrical diaphragm excursion.[29] Any required controlling medications should be noted and

Table 17-7

Arterial Blood Gas Values

pH	7.35–7.45
PCO_2 (partial pressure of carbon dioxide)	35–45 mm Hg
HCO_3 (bicarbonate ion)	22–26 mEq/L
PO_2 (partial pressure of oxygen)	80–100 mm Hg
O_2 saturation (oxygen saturation)	95%–100%
Critical Values	
pH	<7.25 or >7.45
PCO_2	<20 or >60 mm Hg
HCO_3	<15 or >40 mEq/L
PO_2	<40 mm Hg
O_2 saturation	<75%

From Goodman CC, Snyder TE: *Differential diagnosis in physical therapy*, p 151, Philadelphia, 1995, WB Saunders. Adapted from Pagana D, Pagana T: *Mosby's diagnostic and laboratory test reference*, p 104, St Louis, 1992, Mosby–Year Book.

recorded. The ears, nose, and mouth may also be checked during this examination. If abnormalities are found, appropriate lung function tests or arterial blood gases may be ordered (Table 17-7).[72] If there is concern about an active disease process, a chest x-ray may be in order.

Respiratory problems such as tuberculosis, uncontrolled asthma, exertional asthma, exercise-induced bronchospasm, pulmonary insufficiency resulting from a collapsed lung, or bronchial asthma should be checked and discussed with the patient.[34,73,74]

Gastrointestinal Examination

The gastrointestinal examination involves evaluation of the digestive system, eating habits, and nutrition.

Some of the questions that may be asked include the following:[13,27,78]

1. Do you have a problem with bowel movements (e.g., diarrhea, constipation)?
2. Do you have any problems chewing or swallowing food?
3. Have you been vomiting lately?
4. Do you have any pain related to eating?
5. Do your stools appear normal?
6. Do you feel you eat regularly and have a well-balanced diet?
7. Are there certain food groups you will not eat?
8. Have you ever been on a diet?
9. Do you view yourself as too thin, too fat, or just right?
10. Have you ever tried to control your weight? If so, how?
11. Have you ever had excessive heartburn or indigestion?
12. Have you had any heartburn or dyspepsia after using anti-inflammatory medications?

A positive answer to any of these questions requires further investigation.

Examples of Gastrointestinal Conditions or Signs and Symptoms Requiring Further Examination

- Organomegaly (e.g., enlarged liver, spleen)
- Anorexia
- Bulimia
- Female athlete triad (anorexia/bulimia, amenorrhea, osteoporosis)
- Ulcers
- Blood in stools

The examiner should palpate the abdomen for masses or organomegaly.[1] The examiner has to ensure that there is no inflammation of the liver (hepatitis, enlarged liver) or enlarged spleen, especially if the patient is involved in contact sports.

In some cases, it is advisable to check the patient's nutritional status, especially if there appears to be a tendency toward eating disorders such as anorexia or bulimia.[79] This is best done by having the patient record his or her food intake for at least 3 days and having the record analyzed by a nutritionist, who can then calculate dietary intake in relation to the activity level of the patient. It also provides an opportunity to determine what supplements the patient is using, in case they contain banned substances.

Urogenital Examination

Depending on whether the patient is male or female, the examination is modified to meet the individual needs. For example, females may be asked about their menstrual history (e.g., when did menses begin? when was the last period? are there any abnormalities?) or about gynecological problems. Males may be given a genital examination looking for abnormalities, hernias, or absence of a testicle.[29] Common history questions asked in the urogenital examination (males and females) include the following:

1. Have you ever had any problems with your kidneys or bladder?
2. Has there been a change in the number of times you urinate daily?
3. When you urinate, do you have trouble starting, continuing, or stopping?
4. Have you ever been treated for venereal disease?
5. Is your urine clear?
6. Have you ever been diagnosed as having sugar, albumin, or blood in your urine?
7. Have you felt any bulges in your groin, testicle, or abdomen?
8. Have you felt a painless hard mass in your testicle (testicular cancer screen)?
9. Have you had any urethral discharge or dysuria?

The examiner should check for hernias, kidney problems, albuminuria (excessive protein in the urine), and venereal disease if a problem of the urogenital system is suspected.[75] Generally, patients with one kidney should be warned of the danger of contact sports, especially if the kidney is abnormally positioned or is diseased.[76] In males, the examiner should be aware of an undescended or atrophied testicle or testicular torsion. A urinalysis should be performed if diabetes or kidney disease is suspected. These conditions do not preclude activity, exercise, or sports, but they may be amenable to treatment, and the patient must be made aware of potential dangers caused by these conditions.

Examples of Urogenital Conditions or Signs and Symptoms Requiring Further Examination

- Hernia (femoral, inguinal, abdominal, sports)
- Absent or undescended testicle
- Lump in testicle
- One kidney or diseased kidney
- Albuminuria
- Hemoglobinuria
- Nephroptosis
- Hematuria
- Exercise amenorrhea
- Diabetes
- Sexually transmitted diseases

Dehydration, athletic pseudonephritis, hemoglobinuria, nephroptosis, and hematuria are all possible problems of the urogenital system. For females in sports, it is important to determine whether they have a regular period and menstrual pattern because of concern about exercise amenorrhea and its relation to bone density and osteoporosis.[34,77]

Dermatological Examination

The primary care assessment may involve examination for any developing skin conditions and those that may be amenable to treatment. Generally, the questions that relate to the dermatological examination would be the following:[13]

1. Have you had any problems with acne?
2. Have you had any problems with rashes or itching, especially in areas covered by clothes, equipment, or footwear?
3. Do you have a history of fungal infections?

The answers to such questions give the examiner some idea of skin conditions, most of which are easily dealt with by treatment.

Examples of Dermatological Conditions or Signs and Symptoms Requiring Further Examination

- Severe acne
- Dermatitis (e.g., contact, clothes)
- Herpes (e.g., simplex, gladiatorum)
- Fungal infection (tinea capitis or corporis)
- Boils
- Warts
- Impetigo
- Molluscum contagiosum
- Psoriasis

The examiner must ensure that the patient with dermatological problems has them under control, because many of these conditions are contagious, including bacterial, fungal, or viral infections, such as herpes simplex, herpes gladiatorum, boils, impetigo, or warts; and contact dermatitis.

Examination For Heat (Hyperthermic) Disorders

Examination for heat disorders should be included if the patient's work, activity, exercise, or sport has involved working or activity where there is high temperature, high humidity, or a combination of the two (e.g., moderate temperature and high humidity) or where a heat injury is suspected.[80–85] These are often the conditions that lead to heat disorders. Questions in the history related to heat disorders may include the following:

1. Have you ever experienced a heat disorder?
2. Have you ever had muscle cramps?
3. Have you ever participated in an activity, exercise, or sport in a high-temperature, high-humidity environment?
4. Have you ever passed out or become dizzy in the heat?
5. Have you been on medication, or do you drink a lot of caffeinated beverages or use stimulants?
6. Have you recently lost a considerable amount of weight in a short time?

Examples of Heat Disorders or Heat-Related Signs and Symptoms Requiring Further Examination

- Heat exhaustion
- Heat stroke
- Excessive muscle cramps in heat
- Excessive dehydration

Intake of antihistamines or excessive caffeine, as well as lack of fluid and/or metabolites, can increase the risk of heat disorders. If a patient has a history of heat-related disorders, the condition should be thoroughly investigated because it could lead to life-threatening situations.

Examination for Cold (Hypothermic) Disorders

Examination for hypothermia should be included if the patient's work, activity, exercise, or sport involves working or activity where there are low temperatures (below freezing), a significant wind chill factor, high humidity (or patient wearing wet clothes), or a combination of the three.[83,85–91] Any of these may lead to environmental factors such as acute (immersion), chronic (exposure), or urban hypothermia. Questions in the history related to hypothermic (cold) disorders may include the following:

1. Have you ever frozen your ears, toes, or fingers?
2. How long have you been in the cold (NOTE: this could be in a cold building, not just outside)?
3. Were you working or participating in an activity, exercise, or sport in low-temperature, windy conditions and/or a humid environment?
4. Have you been in poor health in the last 6 months?
5. Have you been eating well?
6. Have you consumed any drugs or alcohol in the last 24 hours?
7. Do you smoke?

Factors That Increase Susceptibility to Cold

- General: infancy, advanced age, malnutrition, exhaustion
- Drug use: alcohol, sedatives, meperidine, clonidine, neuroleptic agents
- Endocrine system: hypoglycemia, hypothyroidism, adrenal insufficiency, diabetes
- Cardiovascular system: peripheral vascular disease, nicotine use
- Neurological system: peripheral neuropathy, spinal cord damage, autonomic neuropathy, hypothalamic disease
- Trauma: falls (head or spinal injury), fracture causing immobility
- Infection: sepsis (diaphoresis, hypothalamic dysfunction)

From Biem J, et al: Out of the cold: management of hypothermia and frostbite, *Can Med J* 168:306, 2003.

Table 17-8

Blood Cholesterol Levels

Age (yr)	Values (mg/dl)
<25	125–200
25–40	140–225
40–50	160–245
50–65	170–265
>65	<265

From Goodman CC, Snyder TE: *Differential diagnosis in physical therapy*, p 134, Philadelphia, 1995, WB Saunders.

Questions 4 to 7 are asked because of their effect on the circulation and neurological systems. Often the patient experiencing hypothermia is shivering, is apathetic and lethargic, and may demonstrate an inability to perform simple meaningful tasks.

Laboratory Tests

Laboratory tests are often included in a primary care assessment. If the examiner suspects problems for which laboratory tests can be diagnostic, then they should be ordered. For example, if heart disease is suspected or an older population is being examined, serum cholesterol, triglyceride, or high-density lipoprotein tests may be ordered (Tables 17-8 to 17-11).

The incidence of iron deficiency anemia in postmenarche female athletes is as high as 15%. Plasma ferritin may be used to measure iron status. In males, anemia may occur during a growth spurt, with inadequate diet, or with a peptic ulcer. Hemoglobin is often checked if sickle cell anemia (common in blacks) is suspected. The prepubertal level of hemoglobin is about 11.5 g/dl of blood, and the postpubertal value is 14.5 g/dl of blood for males and 12.0 g/dl or higher for females.

Table 17-9

Triglyceride Levels

Age (yr)	Value (mg/dl)
Female Adult	
20–29	10–100
30–39	10–110
40–49	10–122
50–59	10–134
>59	10–147
Female Child	
1–19	10–121
Male Adult	
20–29	10–157
30–39	10–182
40–49	10–193
50–59	10–197
>59	10–199
Male Child	
1–19	10–103

From Chernecky C et al: *Laboratory tests and diagnostic procedures*, p 932, Philadelphia, 1993, WB Saunders.

Common Laboratory Tests

- Hematocrit
- Urinalysis
- Blood chemistry (glucose, creatine, electrolytes)
- Fasting lipid profile
- Electrocardiogram

Diagnostic Imaging

Diagnostic imaging may also be part of a primary care assessment but should not be used indiscriminately.[92]

Table 17-10

Serum Electrolyte Levels

Test	Normal Values
Serum potassium	3.5–5.3 mEq/L
Serum sodium	136–145 mEq/L
Serum calcium	8.2–10.2 mg/dl
	(4.5–5.5 mEq/L)
Serum magnesium	1.8–3 mg/dl
	(1.5–2.5 mEq/L)

Adapted from Chernecky C et al: *Laboratory tests and diagnostic procedures*, Philadelphia, 1993, WB Saunders.

Table 17-11

Urine Analysis (Urinalysis)

	Test	**Normal Result**
General measurements	Color	Yellow-amber
	Turbidity	Clear
	pH	4.6–8.0
	Specific gravity	1.01–1.025
Other components	Glucose	Negative
	Ketones	Negative
	Blood	Negative
	Protein	Negative
	Bilirubin	Negative
Sediment	RBCs	Negative
	WBCs	Negative
	Casts	Occasional
	Mucous threads	Occasional
	Crystals	Occasional

From Goodman CC, Snyder TE: *Differential diagnosis in physical therapy*, p 258, Philadelphia, 1995, WB Saunders. Normal values are taken from Kee J: *Laboratory and diagnostic tests with nursing implications*, ed 3, Norwalk, Conn, 1991, Appelton & Lange. *RBCs*, Red blood cells; *WBCs*, white blood cells.

For the most part, diagnostic imaging should be used following set guidelines and to confirm a clinical diagnosis. The type of imaging will depend on the information sought. More detailed information on diagnostic imaging may be found in Chapter 1 and other more detailed references.[93–95]

Physical Fitness Profile (Functional Assessment)

In some cases, it may be important for the examiner to establish a physical fitness profile for the patient to determine if he or she can meet the stresses of work or sports or to determine his or her functional level.[96] Basically, profiling is the gathering of information about the physical attributes of the participant.[97] Such profiling helps to determine whether the person possesses the attributes, skills, and abilities necessary for a job or participation in various activities and to meet the demands of the job or activity, and it should be geared to the specific job, activity, exercise, or sport (Table 17-12).[97–103] It should be designed to stress the body so that any weakness or pathology that exists will be apparent. In this way, it may be used as a **screening device** to prevent injury.[97,104] The profile also provides a **baseline** in the event of injury or to demonstrate the need for, or effect of, conditioning necessary to do the job or take part in the activity. A physical fitness profile can involve many parameters or aspects, including strength, endurance, flexibility, cardiovascular fitness, and maturation. To be effective, the program or test must exhibit several characteristics.[105]

Characteristics of Physical Fitness Profile

- The variables being tested must be relevant to the job, activity, exercise, or sport
- The test must be reliable and valid
- Test protocols must be as specific to the job, activity, exercise, or sport as possible
- The test must be standardized and controlled
- The rights of the patient and confidentiality must be respected
- Testing may be repeated at regular intervals if the purpose is to show effectiveness of a training program
- Results must be conveyed to the patient in a meaningful way that the patient can understand

Strength

Strength is one of the attributes that is commonly examined in a physical fitness profile. The way in which the examiner determines strength depends on the job, activity, exercise, or sport; the equipment available; and the demands of the activity. It has been reported that strength declines 1% per year after the age of 30 years.[106] The strength measures may involve isometric, isotonic, or isokinetic testing; functional activities; lifting of free weights; or, in some cases, simply a hand grip test.[107,108] In some cases, it may involve muscle fiber typing. If a general indication of strength is desired, a hand grip is relatively easy, and standard tests can be used (see Chapter 7). For the elderly population, plantar flexor, hip abductor, and hip extensor strengths are important to test.[109] Functional strength tests are often used because they are easy and provide comparable results.[1] However, the examiner should make these tests as job or activity specific as possible.

Examples of Functional Strength Tests

- Bench press, leg press
- Sit-ups
- Push-ups
- Pull-ups
- Grip strength

More sophisticated methods may be used, especially if the patient has a history of injury to specific muscles or joints (see the sections on functional testing in Chapters 3 to 13). Isokinetic testing (i.e., Cybex, KinCom, Biodex) is more likely to be used to test specific joints, looking for potential discrepancies between left and right sides, agonist versus antagonist, and differences in strength and endurance. However, it is important to realize that many of these tests are not usually done in functional job- or activity-specific positions or ways.

Power

Power is the ability to move a weight over a distance. This weight may be an object or the human body.

Table 17-12
Used to Determine Athletic Fitness for Specific Sports*

	Speed	Strength	Muscle Endurance	Power	Quickness and Agility	Reaction Time	Flexibility	Cardio-respiratory Endurance	Balance	Anaerobic Endurance	Body Composition	Kinesthetic Perception
Football	X	X	—	X	X	X	X	—	X	X	X	X
Basketball	X	—	X	X	X	—	X	X	X	X	X	X
Baseball	X	—	—	X	—	X	X	—	—	X	—	—
Track and field												
Sprinters	X	X	—	X	—	X	X	—	—	X	X	—
Throwers	—	X	—	X	X	—	X	—	X	X	X	X
Jumpers	X	X	—	X	—	—	X	—	X	X	X	X
Distance	—	—	X	—	—	X	X	X	—	—	X	—
Volleyball	X	—	X	X	X	X	X	X	X	X	X	X
Soccer	X	X	X	—	X	—	X	X	X	—	X	X
Rodeo	—	X	—	X	X	X	X	—	X	X	—	X
Tennis	—	—	X	X	X	X	X	—	—	X	X	X
Golf	—	—	X	—	—	—	X	X	X	—	X	X
Skiing	—	X	X	X	X	—	X	X	X	—	X	X
Wrestling	—	X	X	X	X	—	X	X	X	—	X	X
Gymnastics	X	X	X	X	X	—	X	—	X	—	X	X

Test examples:

Speed: 20-, 40-, 100-yard dashes

Strength: 1 repetition max

Muscle endurance: 225-pound or 285-pound bench test, sit-up, pull-up, dip, push-up

Power: vertical jump, standing broad jump, two-hand medicine ball put

Agility: 20-yard shuttle run, Semo agility test, T-test

Reaction time: Dekan Auto Performance Analyzer

Flexibility: sit and reach test, shoulder rotation test

Cardiorespiratory endurance: 1.5-mile run, 12-min run

Balance: Nelson balance test

Anaerobic endurance: Margaria-Kalamen leg power test, 40-yard repeated sprint test

Body composition: skinfold measurements

Kinesthetic perception: distance perception jump

From Bridgman R: A coach's guide to testing for athletic attributes, *Natl Strength Conditioning Assoc J* 13:35, 1991.
*Xs denotes areas of physical fitness that are most needed in each sport.

Depending on the job, activity, exercise, or sport, power may be included as part of the physical fitness profile. As with all profile parameters, power measurements should be related to the job, activity, exercise, or sport in which the patient will be participating.

Examples of Power Activities

- Throwing a medicine ball (equivalent to weight the patient would throw on the job)
- Lifting a weight and placing it at a higher level
- Stair climbing or running
- Walking up and down stairs
- Bending and lifting
- Jump for height
- Two-legged hop
- Single-leg hop for distance

Flexibility and Range of Motion

Flexibility is a very important consideration when profiling a patient for a specific job or activity.[110,111] In some cases, less flexibility is better than too much, but in some activities, excessive flexibility (laxity) is necessary to succeed. Therefore flexibility testing must be specific to the job or activity in which the patient wishes to take part, or it may be position specific. For example, in running activities, lower limb flexibility (especially hip flexors, hamstrings, rectus femoris, iliotibial band, and gastrocnemius) is of greatest importance, whereas in swimming, upper limb flexibility (especially shoulder abduction and medial and lateral rotation) is more important, as it is with jobs involving a large amount of overhead work. In some activities, such as ballet, gymnastics, and synchronized swimming, overall flexibility is essential. In baseball, pitchers often require greater shoulder, hip, and trunk flexibility than other players.[18] Flexibility may be measured with the use of devices such as a goniometer, Flexometer, or tape measure.[111]

Determinants of Range of Motion[112]

- Shape of the bone and cartilage
- Muscle power and tone
- Muscle bulk
- Ligaments and joint capsule laxity
- Extensibility of the skin and subcutaneous tissue
- Race (Indians are more mobile than blacks, who are more mobile than Caucasians)
- Gender (women are more mobile than men)
- Age (range of motion decreases with age)
- Genetic makeup
- The dominant limb tends to be less mobile than the nondominant limb
- Day to day stresses on joints

When considering range of motion (ROM), the examiner must realize that hypermobility or laxity in one joint or in one direction of joint movement does not necessarily mean hypermobility in all joints or in all directions. Similarly, normal ROM charts are often not valid when dealing with persons who, by virtue of their job or activities (e.g., ballet, gymnastics, synchronized swimming), are hypermobile. Values that are considered normal for these types of activities would be considered hypermobile or abnormal for the general population. It is also important to realize that hypermobility (laxity) and hypomobility are not necessarily pathological states. In pathological states, hypermobility may lead to instability and is usually the result of the individual being unable to control movement in the available ROM (through strength, endurance, passive stabilizers, and neurological input) (see Chapter 1). The ROM available may be the result of genetic makeup or the stresses placed on individual joints. Tight-jointed people tend to be more susceptible to muscle strains, nerve pinch syndromes, and overstress paratenonitis. Hypermobile, or loose-jointed, people are more susceptible to ligament sprains, chronic back pain, disc prolapse, spondylolisthesis, pes planus, joint effusion, and paratenonitis caused by lack of control of the joint. In the hypermobile individual, if strength and endurance are not at the appropriate level to support the joints, the joints are often unstable or are subjected to potentially injuring loads.

Various criteria can be used to determine a patient's generalized joint laxity. However, the points previously mentioned must be kept in mind when looking at these generalized values. Carter and Wilkinson[113] have developed a five-point system. The patient who meets all criteria is said to exhibit general joint hypermobility.

Carter and Wilkinson's Criteria for Generalized Joint Laxity (Hypermobility)[113]

- Passive apposition of the thumb to the flexor aspect of the forearm
- Passive hyperextension of the fingers so they lie parallel with the extensor aspect of the forearm
- Ability to hyperextend elbows at least 10°
- Ability to hyperextend knees at least 10°
- Excessive passive dorsiflexion of the ankle and eversion of the foot

---

Nicholas[114] established criteria for determining whether a patient is tight jointed (hypomobile). It should be realized, however, that under these criteria, the majority of the North American population today would be classified as hypomobile!

Nicholas's Criteria for Hypomobility[114]

- Patient is unable to touch the floor with the palms, bending at the knees with the waist straight
- Patient is unable to sit comfortably in the lotus position
- Patient demonstrates less than 20° hyperextension at the knees when lying prone with the legs hanging over the end of the table
- Patient is unable to position the feet at 180° while standing with the knees flexed at 15° to 30°
- Patient has no upper limb laxity on shoulder flexion, elbow hyperextension, or forearm hypersupination

---

It is important to understand the principles of hypermobility and hypomobility. A person who is hypermobile must avoid further stretching and support the joint through strengthening (concentric and eccentric exercise) and endurance programs. The patient must be taught proper positioning, and if there are hypermobile joints, there are probably hypomobile joints nearby that need to be mobilized. It is essential to make sure that these patients have improved strength, endurance, muscular speed of reaction, and balanced activities to help support the hypermobile joints.

The person who is hypomobile may be treated by mobilization or manipulation of the affected joint in the direction of tightness. Tight supporting structures also must be stretched, and active exercises must be given to maintain the restored ROM. It is important with these patients to retrain their kinesthetic sense so that they can maintain and control the acquired ROM.

Speed

Speed is often considered an important component of a physical fitness profile, depending on the job, activity, exercise, or sport. It is a function of distance covered per unit of time.[1]

Examples of Functional Speed Tests

- Timed moving things from one station to another
- Time to assemble "something"
- Timed 40-yard (40-m) run or walk
- Timed 100-yard (100-m) run or walk
- Timed 440-yard (400-m) run or walk

Cardiovascular Fitness and Endurance

Because almost every activity involves stresses on the heart and vascular system, it is important to know the level of the stresses produced and whether the cardiovascular system can respond to these stresses. Aerobic fitness has been reported to decline 9% per decade for sedentary adults after the age of 25 years.[115] Therefore the cardiovascular system must be evaluated to determine how it responds to these or equivalent loads.[116,117]

Many methods can be used to determine cardiovascular (aerobic) fitness, but the method chosen must be related to the specific job, activity, or population.[118,119] As an example, ice hockey players who are tested on a bicycle may show very good cardiovascular fitness; however, when they get on the ice and skate, their cardiovascular fitness may not be as evident because they are being tested in a different type of activity.

Examples of Common Endurance Tests

- Harvard step test
- 12-minute walk-run
- 1.5-mile (2.4-km) run
- Submaximal ergometer test
- Treadmill test

The Harvard step test is one of the most common general cardiovascular fitness tests done for a physical fitness profile. It is relatively simple, is easy to set up, and takes a minimal amount of time to do. To set up the test, an 18-inch platform is used. The patient is instructed to step with both feet onto the platform at a rate of about 30 times per minute (a metronome is used for cadence). The patient is made to step for 3.5 minutes at a pace of 2 seconds per step and then sprint as fast as possible for 30 seconds (total time: 4 minutes). The patient then immediately sits down in a chair and relaxes for 3 minutes while the pulse is determined. The pulse is taken at 30, 60, 120, and 180 seconds after the exercise. The index formula for the pulse is as follows:

$$\text{Index} = \frac{\text{Duration of exercise (in sec)} \times 100}{2 \times \text{the sum of any three pulse counts}}$$

The higher the index, the better the person's fitness. If the index is less than 65, the patient is not ready for high-level activity. Cooper[120,121] developed an indirect method for measuring fitness using a 12-minute walk-run test. From the distance covered in 12 minutes, he developed tables for men and women that showed the patient's fitness category. He later went on to use a similar method for activities such as swimming and cycling, thus making the testing more activity specific. For older individuals, the Kasch Pulse-Recovery Test[20,122] can be used (Table 17-13).

Other, more detailed aerobic and anaerobic tests may be performed, including a respiratory quotient test (direct method), the Astrand nomogram (indirect method), or the Sjostrad PWC_{170} test (indirect method).[123]

Table 17-13

How to Administer the Kasch Pulse-Recovery Test

1. Measure pulse at rest
2. Ask the patient to step up and down (with both feet) a 12-inch step 24 times per minute for 3 minutes
3. Measure pulse 1 minute after the test
4. Determine patient's fitness level on the following scale:

	Postexercise Beats/Min	
Fitness Level	Age 56–65 Yr	Age 66+ Yr
Men		
Excellent	72–82	72–86
Good	89–97	89–95
Above average	98–101	97–102
Average	105–111	104–113
Below average	113–118	114–119
Poor	122–128	122–128
Very poor	131–150	133–152
Women		
Excellent	74–92	73–86
Good	97–103	93–100
Above average	106–111	104–114
Average	113–117	117–121
Below average	119–127	123–127
Poor	129–136	129–134
Very poor	142–151	135–151

From Kligman EW, et al: Recommending exercise to healthy older adults—the preparticipation evaluation and exercise prescription, *Phys Sportsmed* 27(11):49, 1999. Reproduced with permission of McGraw-Hill.

Although not commonly done except in high-level sports, maximum tests are necessary to get the most complete diagnostic data on a patient's response to exercise. This is important because half of the heart abnormalities are missed if the test stops at 85% of predicted maximum heart rate, which the simplest tests tend to do.[124] Even if a maximum test is performed, 10% to 15% of the normal population may show an abnormal response.[124] It must be remembered that cardiovascular tests clear the subject only up to the heart rate at which he or she has been tested. In most cases, maximum testing is not done, but if a person is showing abnormalities, such a test may be performed as a second diagnostic procedure. These tests must, however, be performed under very controlled conditions, where there are proper facilities to handle cardiac emergencies.

Although anaerobic fitness is not directly related to the cardiovascular system, it is tested through its effects on the cardiovascular system. If the patient's job, activity, exercise, or sport is primarily anaerobic, consideration must be given to including this measurement as part of the profile.[125] Anaerobic tests can be divided into short-term tests (10 seconds or less), intermediate-term tests (20 to 50 seconds), and long-term anaerobic tests (60 to 120 seconds). Probably the most common anaerobic test used today is the 30-second Wingate test.[126]

Agility, Balance, and Reaction Time

For activities requiring agility, balance, and reaction time, the physical fitness profile should include these items. Balance testing is especially important in the elderly population.[109] O'Brien[109] advocated the Sharpened Romberg test, functional reach test, timed get-up-and-go test (see Chapter 11), and Tinetti assessment tool for balance and gait. The functional reach test involves the patient reaching forward as far as possible without falling forward or taking a step while the examiner measures a horizontal for distance. The Tinetti assessment tool has two parts. One part measures static and dynamic sitting and standing balance (Table 17-14) whereas the second part assesses gait (Table 17-15).[127] Ideally, testing should be related to the specific activity. Agility is defined as the ability to change directions rapidly when moving at a high rate of speed.[1] Agility and balance tests are often measured by time or accuracy (e.g., correct two out of three).[1,128]

Maturation and Growth

Maturation assessment is a method of determining how far a patient has progressed toward physical maturity. It also helps to identify periods of rapid growth.[126,129,130] This is especially important where there is a possibility that there will be stress applied to the growth plate, which is commonly the "weak link" in traumatic injury. That is, during a rapid growth spurt period, the growth

---

Agility and Balance Tests

- Carioca
- Run-and-cut drills
- Back-pedal and throw at stationary or moving target
- Kick at stationary or moving target (different distances)
- One-arm spin
- Shuttle drills
- Pivoting drills
- Blocking drills
- Figure-of-eight running
- Front-to-back and side-to-side hops
- Sidestep tests
- Beam-walking tests

Sharpened Romberg Test[106,109]

1. With eyes open, stand with feet together for 10 seconds
2. Repeat step 1 with eyes closed
3. With eyes open, place one foot halfway in front of the other for 10 seconds
4. Repeat step 3 with eyes closed
5. With eyes open, place one foot directly in front of the other for 10 seconds
6. Repeat step 5 with eyes closed

Table 17-14

Performance-Oriented Assessment of Balance*

Maneuver	Response		
	Normal	**Adaptive**	**Abnormal**
Sitting balance	Steady, stable	Holds onto chair to keep upright	Leans, slides down in chair
Arising from chair	Able to arise in a single movement without using arms	Uses arms (on chair or walking aid) to pull or push up; and/or moves forward in chair before attempting to arise	Multiple attempts required or unable without human assistance
Immediate standing balance (first 3-5 sec)	Steady without holding onto walking aid or other object for support	Steady, but uses walking aid or other object for support	Any sign of unsteadiness†
Standing balance	Steady, able to stand with feet together without holding object for support	Steady, but cannot put feet together	Any sign of unsteadiness regardless of stance or holds onto object
Balance with eyes closed (with feet as close together as possible)	Steady without holding onto any object with feet together	Steady with feet apart	Any sign of unsteadiness or needs to hold onto an object
Turning balance (360°)	No grabbing or staggering; no need to hold onto any objects; steps are continuous (turn is a flowing movement)	Steps are discontinuous (patient puts one foot completely on floor before raising other foot)	Any sign of unsteadiness or holds onto an object
Nudge on sternum (patient standing with feet as close together as possible, examiner pushes with light even pressure over sternum 3 times; reflects ability to withstand displacement)	Steady, able to withstand pressure	Needs to move feet, but able to maintain balance	Begins to fall, or examiner has to help maintain balance
Neck turning (patient asked to turn head side to side and look up while standing with feet as close together as possible)	Able to turn head at least halfway side to side and be able to bend head back to look at ceiling; no staggering, grabbing, or symptoms of lightheadedness, unsteadiness, or pain	Decreased ability to turn side to side to extend neck, but no staggering, grabbing, or symptoms of lightheadedness, unsteadiness, or pain	Any sign of unsteadiness or symptoms when turning head or extending neck
One-leg standing balance	Able to stand on one leg for 5 sec without holding object for support		Unable
Back extension (ask patient to lean back as far as possible, without holding onto object if possible)	Good extension without holding object or staggering	Tries to extend, but decreased range of motion (compared with other patients of same age) or needs to hold object to attempt extension	Will not attempt or no extension seen or staggers
Reaching up (have patient attempt to remove an object from a shelf high enough to require stretching or standing on toes)	Able to take down object without needing to hold onto other object for support and without becoming unsteady	Able to get object but needs to steady self by holding onto something for support	Unable or unsteady
Bending down (patient is asked to pick up small objects, such as pen, from the floor)	Able to bend down and pick up the object and is able to get up easily in single attempt without needing to pull self up with arms	Able to get object and get upright in single attempt but needs to pull self up with arms or hold onto something for support	Unable to bend down or unable to get upright after bending down or takes multiple attempts to get upright

Table 17-14—cont'd

Maneuver	Response		
	Normal	**Adaptive**	**Abnormal**
Sitting down	Able to sit down in one smoother movement	Needs to use arms to guide self into chair or not a smooth movement	Falls into chair, misjudges distances (lands off center)

From Tinetti ME: Performance oriented assessment of mobility problems in elderly patients, *J Am Geriatr Soc* 34(2):119–126, 1986.
*The patient begins this assessment seated in a hard, straight-backed, armless chair.
†Unsteadiness defined as grabbing at objects for support, staggering, moving feet, or more than minimal trunk sway.

Table 17-15

Performance-Oriented Assessment of Gait*

Components†	Observation	
	Normal	**Abnormal**
Initiation of gait (patient asked to begin walking down hallway)	Begins walking immediately without observable hesitation; initiation of gait is single, smooth motion	Hesitates; multiple attempts; initiation of gait not a smooth motion
Step height (begin observing after first few steps: observe one foot, then the other; observe from side)	Swing foot completely clears floor but by no more than 1-2 inches	Swing foot is not completely raised off floor (may hear scraping) or is raised too high (>1-2 inches)‡
Step length (observe distance between two steps of stance foot and heel of swing foot; observe from side; do not judge first few or last few steps; observe one side at a time)	At least the length of individual's foot between the stance toe and swing heel (step length usually longer but foot length provides basis for observation)	Step length less than described under normal‡
Step symmetry (observe the middle part of the path, not the first or last steps; observe from side; observe distance between heel of each swing foot and toe of each stance foot)	Step length same or nearly same on both sides for most step cycles	Step length varies between sides or patient advances with same foot with every step
Step continuity	Begins raising heel of one foot (toe off) as heel of other foot touches the floor (heel strike); no breaks or stops in stride; step lengths equal over most cycles	Places entire foot (heel and toe) on floor before beginning to raise other foot; or stops completely between steps; or step length varies over cycles‡
Path deviation (observe from behind; observe one foot over several strides; observe in relation to line on floor [e.g., tiles] if possible; difficult to assess if patient uses a walker)	Foot follows close to straight line as patient advances	Foot deviates from side to side or toward one direction§
Trunk stability (observe from behind; side to side motion of trunk may be a normal gait pattern, need to differentiate this from instability)	Trunk does not sway; knees or back is not flexed; arms are not abducted in effort to maintain stability	Any of preceding features present§
Walk stance (observe from behind)	Feet should almost touch as one passes other	Feet apart with stepping¶
Turning while walking	No staggering; turning continuous with walking; and steps are continuous while turning	Staggers; stops before initiating turn; or steps are discontinuous

From Tinetti ME: Performance oriented assessment of mobility problems in elderly patients, *J Am Geriatr Soc* 34(2):119–126, 1986.
*The patient stands with examiner at end of obstacle-free hallway. Patient uses usual walking aid. Examiner then asks patient to walk down hallway at his or her usual pace. Examiner observes one component of gait at a time (analogous to heart examination). For some components, the examiner walks behind the patient; for other components, the examiner walks next to patient. May require several trips to complete.
†Also, ask patient to walk at a "more rapid than usual" pace, and observe whether any walking aid is used correctly.
‡Abnormal gait finding may reflect a primary neurological or musculoskeletal problem directly related to the finding or reflect a compensatory maneuver for other, more remote problem.
§Abnormality may be corrected by walking aid, such as cane; observe with and without walking aid if possible.
¶Abnormal finding is usually a compensatory maneuver rather than a primary problem.

plate is weaker and more susceptible to injury than the ligaments and/or capsule. Maturation profiling should not be used to push children into specific activities unless chosen by the child, and it should not be used to exclude a child unless documented evidence demonstrates unacceptable risk for the child.[131] In adolescents, growth patterns can have an effect on participation in activities, exercise, and sports and may affect injury patterns. For example, a growth spurt for a gymnast may adversely affect balance and flexibility. Pubertal growth accounts for 20% to 25% of final adult height, and pubertal weight gain accounts for 50% of ideal adult weight.[78]

Skeletal development is usually measured by wrist x-rays, using the *Radiographic Atlas of Skeletal Development of the Wrist and Hand*, by W.W. Greulich and S.U. Pyle,[132] for interpretation.

The most common method of measuring maturation in males and females is the Tanner scale.[28,126,133] The five stages of the Tanner scale are based on pictorial standards of genitalia and pubic hair for males and breast development and pubic hair for females (Figures 17-2 to 17-4 and Table 17-16). Some people have recommended that collision sports not be allowed for boys until they reach level 5 of development. For females,

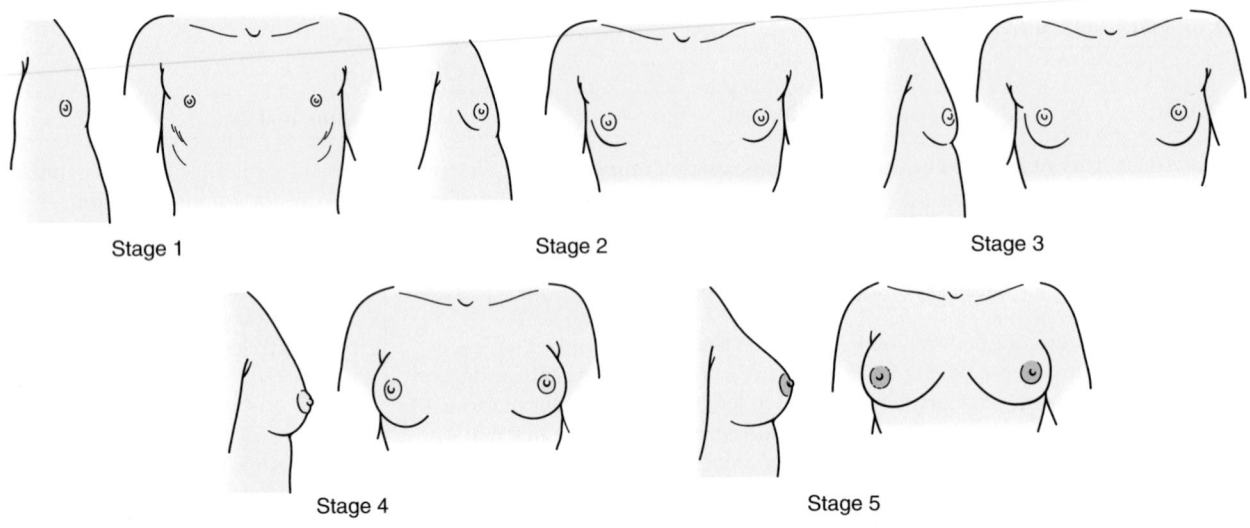

Stage 1   Stage 2   Stage 3

Stage 4   Stage 5

Figure 17-2

Breast development in girls. The development of the mammae can be divided into five stages. In *stage 1*, only the nipple is raised above the level of the breast (as in the child). In *stage 2*, the budding stage, there is bud-shaped elevation of the areola. On palpation, a fairly hard button can be felt that is disk or cherry shaped. The areola is increased in diameter, and the surrounding area is slightly elevated. In *stage 3*, there is further elevation of the mammae; the areolar diameter is further increased, and the shape of mammae is visibly feminine. In *stage 4*, fat deposits increase, and the areola forms a secondary elevation above that of the breast. This secondary mound occurs in approximately half of all girls and in some cases persists in adulthood. In *stage 5*, the adult stage, the areola usually subsides to the level of the breast and is strongly pigmented. (Redrawn from Halpern B, Blackburn T, Incremona B et al: Preparticipation sports physicals. In Zachazewski JE, Magee DJ, Quillen WS, editors: *Athletic injuries and rehabilitation*, p. 855, Philadelphia, 1996, WB Saunders.)

Stage 1   Stage 2   Stage 3   Stage 4   Stage 5

Figure 17-3

Pubic hair development in females. In the development of pubic hair, five stages can be distinguished. In *stage 1*, there is no growth of pubic hair. In *stage 2*, initial, scarcely pigmented hair is present, especially along the labia. In *stage 3*, sparse dark, visibly pigmented, curly pubic hair is present on the labia. In *stage 4*, hair that is adult in type but not in extent is present. In *stage 5*, there is lateral spreading (type and spread of hair are adult). (Redrawn from Halpern B, Blackburn T, Incremona B et al: Preparticipation sports physicals. In Zachazewski JE, Magee DJ, Quillen WS, editors: *Athletic injuries and rehabilitation*, p. 855, Philadelphia, 1996, WB Saunders.)

| Stage 1 | Stage 2 | Stage 3 | Stage 4 | Stage 5 |

Figure 17-4

Genital and pubic hair development in males. The development of external genitalia and pubic hair can be divided into five stages. In *stage 1*, the testes, scrotum, and penis are the same size and shape as in the young child, and there is no growth of pubic hair (hair in pubic area is no different from that on the rest of the abdomen). In *stage 2*, there is enlargement of the scrotum and testes. The skin of the scrotum becomes redder, thinner, and wrinkled. The penis has not grown (or just slightly so). Pubic hair is slightly pigmented. In *stage 3*, there is enlargement of the penis, especially in length, further enlargement of testes, and descent of scrotum. Dark, definitely pigmented, curly pubic hair is present around the base of penis. In *stage 4*, there is continued enlargement of the penis and sculpturing of the glans, with increased pigmentation of the scrotum. This stage is sometimes best described as not quite adult. Pubic hair is definitely adult in type but not in extent (no further than the inguinal fold). In *stage 5*, the adult stage, the scrotum is ample, and the penis reaches almost to the bottom of the scrotum. Pubic hair spreads to the medial surface of the thighs but not upward. In 80% of men, hair spreads along the linea alba. (Redrawn from Halpern B, Blackburn T, Incremona B et al: Preparticipation sports physicals. In Zachazewski JE, Magee DJ, Quillen WS, editors: *Athletic injuries and rehabilitation*, p. 855, Philadelphia, 1996, WB Saunders.)

Table 17-16

Maturity Staging Guidelines

Boys' Stage	Pubic Hair	Penis	Testis	Girls' Stage	Pubic Hair	Breasts
1	None	Preadolescent (infantile)	—	1	Preadolescent (none)	Preadolescent (no germinal button)
2	Slight, long, slight pigmentation	Slight enlargement	Enlarged scrotum, pink slight rugae	2	Sparse, lightly pigmented, straight medial border of labia	Breast and papilla elevated as small mound; areolar diameter increased
3	Darker, starts to curl, small amount	Longer	Larger	3	Darker, beginning to curl, increased	Breast and areola enlarged; no contour separation
4	Coarse, curly, adult type, but less quantity	Increase in glans size and breadth of penis	Larger, darker scrotum	4	Coarse, curly, abundant, but less than adult	Areola and papilla form secondary mound
5	Adult, spread to inner thighs	Adult	Adult	5	Adult female triangle and spread to medial surface	Mature, nipple projects, areola part of general breast contour

From Tanner JM: *Growth and adolescence*, Oxford, England, 1962, Blackwell Scientific.

onset of menstruation is another suitable index of maturity and maturation.

Body Composition and Anthropometry

Body composition profiling is designed to provide a relatively detailed analysis of an individual's muscle, fat, and bone mass.[130,134] Anthropometry may be used to

determine the individual's body type (mesomorphic, endomorphic, ectomorphic) to see whether he or she is properly suited for the desired activity, exercise, sport, or position played in a sport.

Anthropometry also involves body fat measurements, such as skinfold measurements or underwater weighing.[135] Of the two, skinfold measurement is more common because it is easier and faster. Seven skinfold sites are most commonly used (Figure 17-5), although some people believe that measurement at three sites is sufficient (i.e., a different three for males and females).[135] Most males should fall below 12% to 15% body fat. Endurance athletes (e.g., distance runners, gymnasts, wrestlers) are often below 7%. Football, baseball, and soccer players average 10% to 12%.[136] No one should be below 5% body fat. Generally, if the percentage of body fat is greater than the upper normal limit of 14% for males and 17% for females,

the patient should be put on a weight loss program or weight training to increase lean body mass; but again, this depends on the activity in which the patient wishes to participate.

Other methods of body composition measurement include girth measurements, bone diameter measurements, ultrasound measurement, and arm radiograph measurements.[134]

For any primary care evaluation, the physician is the final arbitrator. Any decision as to whether someone

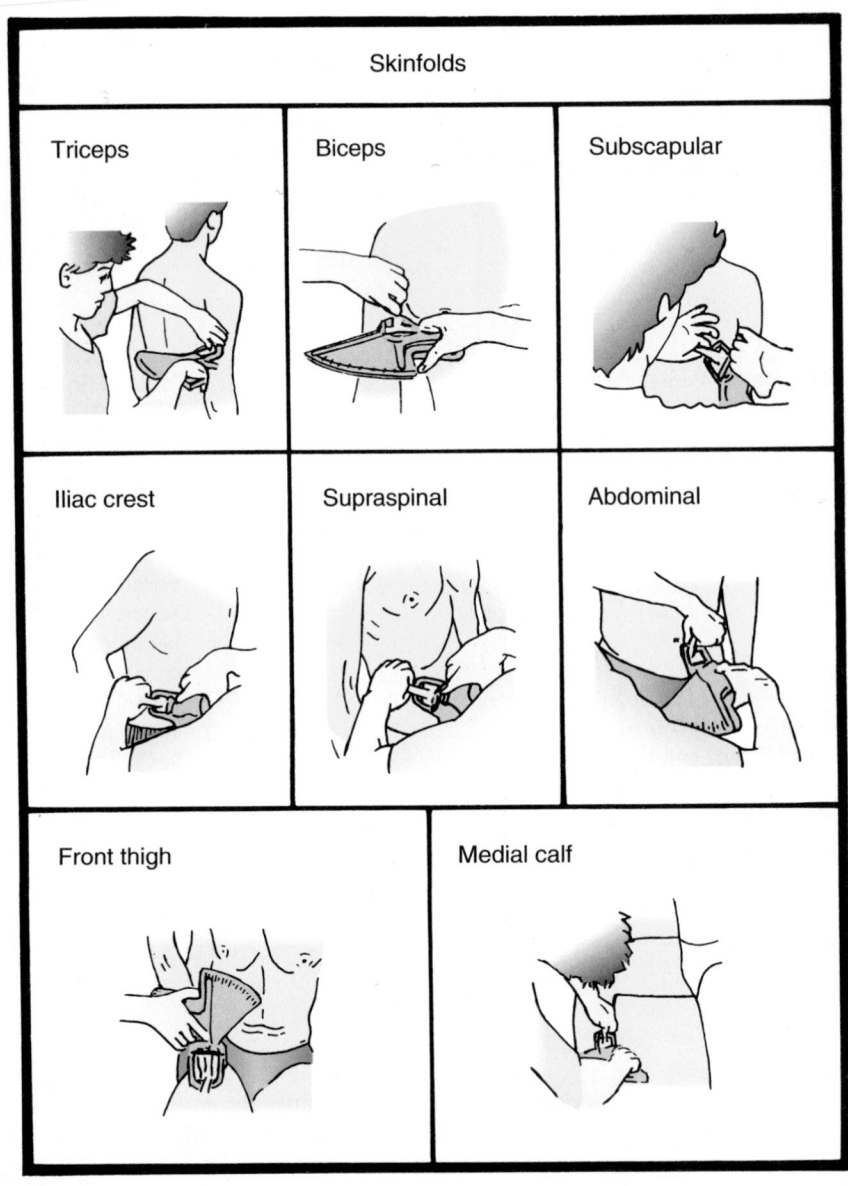

Figure 17-5
Skinfold sites for measuring body fat. (Reprinted, by permission, from Ross WD, Marfell-Jones MJ: Kinanthropometry. In MacDougal JD, Wenger HA, Green HJ, editors: *Physiological testing of the high performance athlete*, ed 2, p. 238, Champaign, Ill, 1991, Human Kinetics.)

should be allowed to work or participate in an activity or as to the patient's functional level must be based on accurate diagnosis of the condition, knowledge of the disease process for the condition, knowledge of the job or sport, knowledge of the physical needs of the patient and the activity, and direct evaluation of the individual.[96] The examiner must also keep in mind the rights of handicapped people and the limits of informed consent. Although standards are often given for participation, in the end, the examiner must make his or her final decision on an individual basis, being primarily concerned with the health and safety of the patient.

Any individual with a solitary paired organ, such as an eye, kidney, or testicle, should not take part in contact sports, especially if the organ is abnormal. Children should be channeled into noncontact sports. High-caliber or older athletes know the rules and should make their own decision. Table 17-17 lists conditions that are contraindications to specific sports, and the level of these activities can be extrapolated to the physical stresses of everyday jobs.[3,28]

Table 17-17

Conditions Commonly Disqualifying an Individual from Participation in Sports

Conditions	Type of Sport			
	Collision*	Contact†	Noncontact‡	Others§
Eyes				
Absence of one eye	??	??	—	—
Congenital glaucoma	X	X	—	—
Retinal detachment	X	X	—	—
Severe myopia	?	?	—	—
Musculoskeletal				
Acute inflammatory conditions	X	X	X	X
Spinal instability	X	X	?	?
Congenital or growth abnormalities that are incompatible with demands of sport	X	X	X	—
Chronic or unhealed conditions (unless cleared by physician)	X	X	X	X
Neurological				
Uncontrolled convulsive disorder	X	X	X	?
Controlled convulsive disorder	?	?	?	?
Repeated concussions	X	X	—	—
Serious head trauma	X	X	—	—
Previous head surgery	X	X	—	—
Transient quadriplegia (unless cleared by physician)	X	X	—	—
Cardiovascular				
Acute infection	X	X	X	X
Cardiomegaly	X	X	X	X
Enlarged spleen	X	X	—	—
Hemorrhage (bleeding) disorders	X	X	X	—
Heart abnormalities (unless cleared by cardiologist)	X	X	X	X
Organic hypertension	X	X	X	X
Previous heart surgery (unless cleared by cardiologist)	X	X	X	X
Pulmonary				
Acute infection	X	X	X	X
Pulmonary insufficiency	X	X	X	X
Uncontrolled asthma (unless cleared by pulmonary physician)	X	X	X	X
Urogenital				
Absence of one kidney	??	??	—	—

Continued

Table 17-17—cont'd

Conditions	Type of Sport			
	Collision*	Contact†	Noncontact‡	Others§
Acute infection	X	X	X	X
Enlarged liver	X	X	—	—
Hernia (inguinal or femoral, unless cleared by physician)	X	X	X	—
Renal disease	X	X	X	X
Absent or undescended testicle (unless cleared by physician)	??	??	—	—
Gastrointestinal				
Jaundice	X	X	X	X
Dermatological				
Acute infection (e.g., boils, herpes simplex, impetigo)	X	X	?	?
General or Systemic Disease				
Acute systemic infection or illness	?	?	?	?
Uncontrolled diabetes	X	X	X	X
Physical immaturity (relative to level of competition)	X	X	—	—

Adapted from the Committee on Medical Aspects of Sports: *Medical evaluation of the athlete: a guide*, American Medical Association, copyright 1966.

?, Depends on individual case and clearance by physician; ??, athlete may compete if athlete knows risks and informed consent form is completed (protective equipment may be necessary); X, participation prohibited; —, participation permitted.

*Examples include boxing, football, hockey (ice and field), and rugby.

†Examples include baseball, basketball, lacrosse, martial arts, rodeo, soccer, volleyball, and wrestling.

‡Examples include dance, rowing, skiing, squash, swimming, tennis, and track/cross-country.

§Examples include archery, bowling, golf, shooting, and track and field events.

References

To enhance this text and add value for the reader, all references have been incorporated into a CD-ROM that is provided with this text. The reader can view the reference source and access it online whenever possible. There are a total of 137 cited references and other general references for this chapter.

APPENDIX 17-1

PRIMARY CARE ASSESSMENT PATIENT QUESTIONNAIRE

DATE: _____/_____/_____

LAST NAME: _____

FIRST NAME: _____

PERMANENT ADDRESS: _____

TELEPHONE NUMBER: _____

DATE OF BIRTH (Day/Month/Year): _____

MARRIED (Yes/No/Spouse's Name): _____

NUMBER OF CHILDREN: _____

MEDICAL INSURANCE COMPANY AND NUMBER: _____

OCCUPATION: _____

IN CASE OF EMERGENCY

PLEASE NOTIFY: _____

NAME OR NAMES: _____

RELATIONSHIP: _____

ADDRESS: _____

_____

TELEPHONE NUMBER: _____

FAMILY DOCTOR'S NAME: _____

FAMILY DOCTOR'S ADDRESS: _____

DATE OF LAST MEDICAL EXAM: _____

ALLERGIES: _____

_____

_____

MEDICATIONS PRESENTLY BEING TAKEN: _____

_____

_____

Continued

APPENDIX 17-1—cont'd

WHY ARE YOU HERE TODAY?

_____

_____

_____

_____

_____

_____

_____

_____

_____

_____

_____

IF YOU WERE INJURED, HOW DID YOU INJURE YOURSELF?

_____

_____

_____

_____

_____

_____

_____

_____

_____

_____

FAMILY HISTORY

PLEASE IDENTIFY ANY HEALTH PROBLEMS THAT HAVE OCCURRED IN YOUR IMMEDIATE FAMILY.

Yes	No		Yes	No	
☐	☐	HAS ANYONE IN YOUR FAMILY (UNDER AGE 50) DIED SUDDENLY?	☐	☐	ALLERGIES / ASTHMA
☐	☐	UNEXPLAINED SEIZURES	☐	☐	ANEMIA
☐	☐	HIGH BLOOD PRESSURE	☐	☐	DIABETES
☐	☐	HEART TROUBLE	☐	☐	EPILEPSY
☐	☐	SUDDEN DEATH	☐	☐	KIDNEY/BLADDER DISORDER
☐	☐	CANCER OR TUMOR	☐	☐	STOMACH DISORDER
☐	☐	MIGRAINE HEADACHES	☐	☐	GENETIC DISORDER
☐	☐	EMOTIONAL PROBLEMS	☐	☐	GOITER
☐	☐	ARTHRITIS	☐	☐	NEUROLOGICAL DISORDERS
☐	☐	OBESITY	☐	☐	TUBERCULOSIS
☐	☐	BLOOD DISORDERS OR EARLY BLEEDING	☐	☐	ABNORMAL NUMBNESS OR ANESTHESIA

SPECIFY: _____

_____

_____

_____

YOUR PRESENT HISTORY (HISTORY OF PRESENT ILLNESS)

ANSWER ALL QUESTIONS CAREFULLY!! FOR "YES" ANSWERS, ELABORATE IN THE FOLLOWING MEDICAL CHART. DO YOU AT THE PRESENT TIME EXPERIENCE:

Yes	No	
☐	☐	DIFFICULTIES WITH YOUR EYES OR VISION?
☐	☐	DIFFICULTIES WITH YOUR NOSE OR THROAT (E.G., TONSILLITIS, SINUSITIS)?
☐	☐	ANY PROBLEM WITH YOUR TEETH OR GUMS?
☐	☐	PROBLEMS WITH HEARING?
☐	☐	HEADACHES, DIZZINESS, WEAKNESS, FAINTING, ANY PROBLEMS WITH COORDINATION OR BALANCE?
☐	☐	NUMBNESS IN ANY PART OF THE BODY?
☐	☐	ANY TENDENCY TO SHAKE OR TREMBLE?
☐	☐	COUGH, SHORTNESS OF BREATH, CHEST PAIN, OR PALPITATIONS?
☐	☐	POOR APPETITE, VOMITING, ABDOMINAL PAIN, ABNORMAL BOWEL HABITS?
☐	☐	ANY SYMPTOMS REFERABLE TO THE MUSCLES, BONES, OR JOINTS (I.E., STIFFNESS, SWELLING, PAIN)?
☐	☐	ANY PROBLEMS WITH THE SKIN, SUCH AS SORES, RASHES, ITCHY OR BURNING SENSATION?
☐	☐	OTHER SYMPTOMS? (SPECIFY ON THE FOLLOWING MEDICAL CHART).

HAVE YOU EVER OR HAVE YOU NOW:

Yes	No	
☐	☐	WORN GLASSES OR CONTACT LENSES?
☐	☐	SUSTAINED AN EYE INJURY?
☐	☐	WORN HEARING AIDS?
☐	☐	SMOKED OR CHEWED TOBACCO?
☐	☐	HAD TO STAY IN THE HOSPITAL?

Continued

APPENDIX 17-1—cont'd

Yes	No	
☐	☐	HAD TO VISIT A HOSPITAL EMERGENCY DEPARTMENT?
☐	☐	HAD AN OPERATION?
☐	☐	BEEN ADVISED TO HAVE ANY OPERATION NOT YET PERFORMED?
☐	☐	HAD PILES OR RECTAL DISEASE?
☐	☐	HAD CHILDHOOD DISEASES (E.G., MUMPS, MEASLES, CHICKENPOX)?
☐	☐	HAD SCARLET FEVER?
☐	☐	HAD HIGH OR LOW BLOOD PRESSURE?
☐	☐	HAD FREQUENT OR PAINFUL URINATION?
☐	☐	HAD A KIDNEY STONE, BLOODY URINE?
☐	☐	HAD VENEREAL DISEASE?
☐	☐	HAD SKIN TROUBLE?
☐	☐	HAVE YOU EVER HAD AN INJURY TO ANY OF YOUR JOINTS? SPECIFY ON THE FOLLOWING MEDICAL CHART.
☐	☐	IF ANSWER TO ABOVE IS "YES," DID THE INJURY INCAPACITATE YOU FOR 1 WEEK OR LONGER?
☐	☐	HAVE YOU EVER BEEN TOLD THAT YOU INJURED A MUSCLE OR LIGAMENT?
☐	☐	DO YOU HAVE A PIN, SCREW, OR PLATE SOMEWHERE IN YOUR BODY AS A RESULT OF BONE OR JOINT SURGERY?
☐	☐	HAVE YOU EVER HAD A BONE GRAFT OR A SPINAL FUSION?
☐	☐	HAVE YOU HAD A FRACTURE DURING THE PAST 2 YEARS?

PAST HISTORY

HAVE YOU EVER HAD, OR BEEN TOLD YOU HAD, OR CONSULTED A PHYSICIAN FOR:

Yes	No	
☐	☐	DIABETES, GOITER, OR ANY OTHER DISEASE OF THE GLANDS (E.G., MONONUCLEOSIS)?
☐	☐	EPILEPSY (SEIZURES)?
☐	☐	NERVOUS DISORDER OR ANY DISEASES OF THE BRAIN OR NERVOUS SYSTEM?
☐	☐	HEART TROUBLE OR RHEUMATIC FEVER?
☐	☐	VARICOSE VEINS, PHLEBITIS, HEMORRHOIDS?
☐	☐	ANY DISEASE OF THE BLOOD, EASY BRUISING, OR BLEEDING TENDENCY?
☐	☐	TUBERCULOSIS, ASTHMA, CHRONIC COUGH, COUGHED-UP BLOOD, PNEUMONIA, OR ANY LUNG DISEASE OR RESPIRATORY DISORDER?
☐	☐	ULCERS, APPENDICITIS, OR ANY DISEASE OF THE STOMACH, INTESTINES, LIVER, OR GALLBLADDER?
☐	☐	SUGAR, ALBUMIN, OR BLOOD IN THE URINE OR ANY DISEASE OF THE KIDNEYS OR GENITOURINARY ORGANS?
☐	☐	ARTHRITIS, RHEUMATISM, OR ANY INJURY OR DISEASE OF THE BONES, PERIPHERAL JOINTS, BACK, OR SPINE?
☐	☐	HERNIA OR ANY DISEASE OF THE MUSCLES OR SKIN?
☐	☐	CANCER, TUMOR, OR GROWTH OF ANY KIND?
☐	☐	A HEAD INJURY CAUSING SEVERE DIZZINESS, LOSS OF MEMORY, VOMITING, UNCONSCIOUSNESS, OR REQUIRING MEDICAL ATTENTION OR HOSPITALIZATION?
☐	☐	CAR, TRAIN, SEA, AIR SICKNESS?
☐	☐	DEPRESSION OR EXCESSIVE WORRY?
☐	☐	LOSS OF MEMORY OR AMNESIA?
☐	☐	GOUT?

Yes	No	
☐	☐	HAVE YOU EVER USED OR ARE YOU PRESENTLY USING ANY HABIT-FORMING DRUGS?
☐	☐	HAVE YOU EVER BLED EXCESSIVELY AFTER TOOTH EXTRACTION?
☐	☐	EVER HAD TROUBLE WITH DEHYDRATION (EXCESS LOSS OF SALT AND WATER)?
☐	☐	BEEN MORE THIRSTY THAN USUAL LATELY?
☐	☐	EVER HAD HEAT STROKE OR ANOTHER HEAT DISORDER (FAILURE OF BODY'S HEAT-REGULATING SYSTEM RESULTING IN THE BODY TEMPERATURE ABOVE 40.5°C (105°F)?
☐	☐	WEIGHT CHANGED IN THE LAST YEAR? GAIN _____ KG; LOSS _____ KG
☐	☐	ANY EXPLANATION FOR THIS WEIGHT CHANGE? (SPECIFY ON THE FOLLOWING MEDICAL CHART.
☐	☐	HAD ANY ADDITIONAL ILLNESS, INJURIES (OTHER THAN CHILDHOOD DISEASE)?
☐	☐	ARE YOU PRESENTLY UNDER A PHYSICIAN'S CARE FOR ANY DIFFICULTY NOT ALREADY DISCUSSED?

MENSTRUAL AND GYNECOLOGICAL HISTORY (IF APPLICABLE)

AT WHAT AGE DID YOU FIRST MENSTRUATE? _____

AT WHAT AGE DID YOUR PERIODS BECOME REGULAR? _____

HOW OFTEN ARE YOUR PERIODS NOW? _____

Yes	No	
☐	☐	EVER HAD A PELVIC EXAMINATION (RECOMMENDED ANNUALLY FOR SEXUALLY ACTIVE INDIVIDUALS 18–35 YR)?
☐	☐	DO YOU HAVE PAINS/CRAMPS DURING YOUR PERIODS?
☐	☐	ANY MENSTRUAL ABNORMALITIES (E.G., ABNORMAL BLEEDING)?
☐	☐	ANY VAGINAL ITCHING OR DISCHARGE?
☐	☐	ARE YOU TAKING THE BIRTH CONTROL PILL?
☐	☐	ANY LUMPS OR PAIN IN YOUR BREASTS?
☐	☐	PREGNANCY? (PAST OR PRESENT) NO. OF CHILDREN _____
☐	☐	OTHER GYNECOLOGICAL PROBLEMS?

INDICATE DATE OF YOUR LAST PAP TEST   _____   _____
                                             MONTH   YEAR

WHAT IS THE INTENSITY OF YOUR PAIN?

Visual Analogue Scale (VAS): Intensity of Pain

|--|

No pain   As bad pain
                                                     as it could
                                                     possibly get

Pain: constant, periodic, episodic, occasional

Continued

APPENDIX 17-1—cont'd

PATIENT-SPECIFIC FUNCTIONAL SCALE [137]

> Baseline Assessment
>
> Please identify important activities that you are unable to do or are having difficulty with as a result of your problem today.

Activity 1 (specify): _____

Patient-Specific Activity Scoring Scheme (circle one number):

0	1	2	3	4	5	6	7	8	9	10

Unable to
perform activity

Able to perform
activity at same
level as before
injury or problem

Activity 2 (specify): _____

Patient-Specific Activity Scoring Scheme (circle one number):

0	1	2	3	4	5	6	7	8	9	10

Unable to
perform activity

Able to perform
activity at same
level as before
injury or problem

Activity 3 (specify): _____

Patient-Specific Activity Scoring Scheme (circle one number):

0	1	2	3	4	5	6	7	8	9	10

Unable to
perform activity

Able to perform
activity at same
level as before
injury or problem

MEDICAL CHART DETAILS IN CONNECTION WITH QUESTIONS ANSWERED "YES"

DATE	NAME AND ADDRESS OF PHYSICIANS, HOSPITAL, ETC.	NATURE OF ILLNESS/INJURY

CERTIFICATION

I certify that I have answered this questionnaire and all questions of the attending health professional completely and correctly to the best of my knowledge. I certify that I have not had any prior illnesses or injuries other than those I have listed on this questionnaire.

Date _____

_____
Patient's signature

_____
Print name

CONSENT FOR TRANSMITTAL OF INFORMATION

I, _____, give my permission for the transmittal of the results of this medical examination to the appropriate health care professional. The confidentiality of these medical records is to be preserved.

Date _____

Signed _____

Place _____

Witness _____

RECORD OF CONSENT FOR MINORS

I, _____, give my permission for emergency medical/surgical care to be given by the appropriate health care professional to

_____ who is my son/daughter.

It is understood that wherever possible I shall be contacted, informed of the problem, diagnosis, treatment required, and the hoped-for results.

Date _____

Signed _____

Place _____

Witness _____

PRIMARY HEALTH CARE EXAMINATION

DATE _____/_____/_____

TEMP_____°F_____°C   HEIGHT_____METERS_____CM   WEIGHT_____KILOGRAMS

MENTAL STATUS _____

☐ SKIN   ☐ PERSONALITY   ☐ MOOD   ☐ GAIT

PRESENT HISTORY

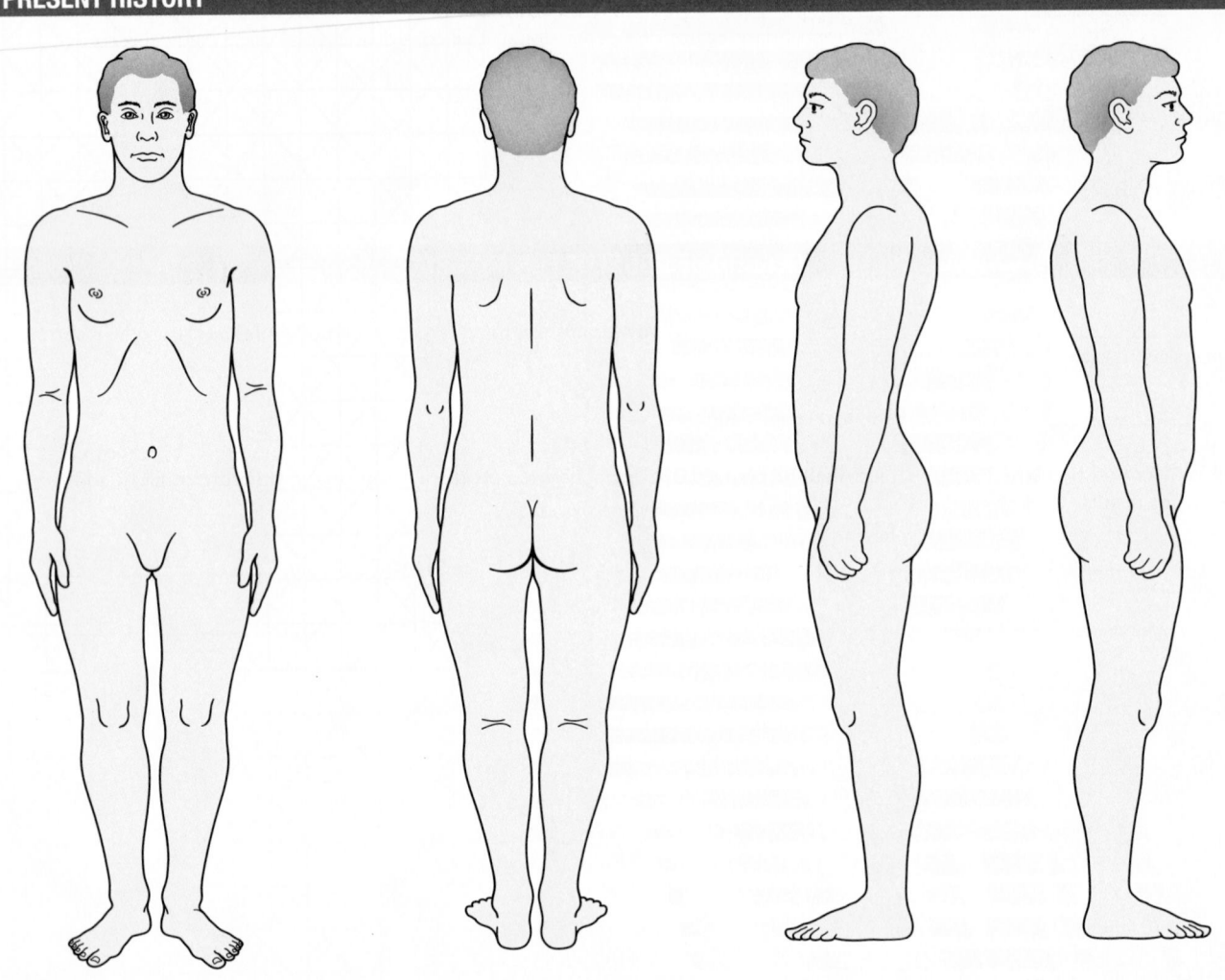

PLEASE ENTER IN BOXED AREAS   "N" IF NORMAL, "A" IF ABNORMAL.

Central Nervous System

☐ REFLEXES   ☐ PROPRIOCEPTION   ☐ BALANCE

☐ MYOTOMES   ☐ SENSORY   ☐ NERVE ROOT   ☐ PERIPHERAL NERVE

IF ABNORMAL FINDINGS ARE PRESENT, PLEASE SPECIFY

Ear, Eye, Nose, and Throat

☐ EYE—VISUAL ACUITY ☐ L ☐ R

☐ NYSTAGMUS

☐ HEARING

☐ TONSILS

☐ FALSE TEETH _____

IF ABNORMAL FINDINGS ARE PRESENT, PLEASE SPECIFY.

IF ABNORMAL FINDINGS ARE PRESENT, PLEASE SPECIFY.

Respiratory

☐ LUNGS ☐ CHEST—SYMMETRY AND WALL ☐ CHEST AUSCULTATION

☐ CHEST EXPANSION _____

IF ABNORMAL FINDINGS ARE PRESENT, PLEASE SPECIFY.

Cardiovascular

BLOOD PRESSURE: _____/_____ HEART RATE: _____ _____ SITE: _____

SUPINE UPRIGHT

PERIPHERAL PULSES ☐_____

CHARACTER RHYTHM

PRECORDIUM	☐ ABNORMAL SOUNDS ☐	☐ ATYPICAL BEAT ☐	☐ THRILLS ☐
	ABSENT PRESENT	NORMAL DISPLACED	ABSENT PRESENT

VARICOSITES ☐ _____

IF ABNORMAL FINDINGS ARE PRESENT, PLEASE SPECIFY.

Abdominal

☐ ABDOMINAL WALL ☐	☐ TENDERNESS ☐	☐ ORGANOMEGALY ☐	☐ MASSES ☐
NORMAL ABNORMAL	ABSENT PRESENT	ABSENT PRESENT	ABSENT PRESENT

Genitourinary

☐ HERNIA ☐ ☐ GENITALIA

ABSENT   PRESENT

☐ BLOOD IN URINE

☐ RECTAL

☐ SACRAL ☐ COCCYX

Musculoskeletal System

☐ CERVICAL ☐ THORACIC ☐ LUMBAR

☐ CHEST/RIBS

IF ABNORMAL FINDINGS ARE PRESENT, PLEASE SPECIFY.

Continued

APPENDIX 17-2—cont'd

Joints

PLEASE EXAMINE FOR PATHOLOGY, RANGE OF MOTION, SWELLING, STABILITY, TENDERNESS OF EACH JOINT. PLEASE ENTER IN BOX "N" IF NORMAL, "AB" IF ABNORMAL.

	LEFT		RIGHT		
	N	AB	N	AB	
SHOULDER					
STERNOCLAVICULAR					
CLAVICLE					
ACROMIOCLAVICULAR					
SCAPULA					
GLENOHUMERAL					
INSTABILITY TESTING					
ROM					
ROTATOR CUFF					
SCAPULAR CONTROL					
MUSCLES					
BURSA					
END FEELS					
UPPER ARM					
ELBOW					
ROM					
MEDIAL EPICONDYLE					
LATERAL EPICONDYLE					
OLECRENON BURSA					
RADIAL HEAD					
END FEELS					
FOREARM					
WRIST					
CARPAL JOINTS					
END FEELS					
HAND AND FINGERS					
END FEELS					
PELVIS					
SACROILIAC					
PUBIS					
ABDOMINAL MUSCLES					
GROIN					
HIP JOINT					
MUSCLE BALANCE					
PATTERNS					
END FEELS					
OTHER					

THIGH					
QUADRICEPS					
HAMSTRINGS					
FEMUR					
KNEE					
ROM					
EFFUSION					
ANTERIOR STABILITY					
POSTERIOR STABILITY					
MEDIAL STABILITY					
LATERAL STABILITY					
MENISCUS					
JOINT LINE					
TENDERNESS					
CREPITUS					
END FEELS					
–PATELLA					
–LATERAL APPREHENSION					
–TENDERNESS					
–Q-ANGLE					
–PATELLA CREPITUS					
–POPLITEAL FOSSA					
LOWER LEG					
TIBIA OR FIBULA					
ANT. COMPARTMENT					
POST. COMPARTMENT					
TENDO ACHILLES					
ANKLE					
ROM					
MEDIAL OR LATERAL MALLEOLUS					
ANT. DRAWER					
BURSA					
END FEELS					
FOOT					
INVERSION					
EVERSION					
MEDIAL LONGITUDINAL ARCH					
LATERAL LONIGTUDINAL ARCH					
PES PLANUS					
PES CAVUS					

Continued

APPENDIX 17-2—cont'd

METATARSAL ARCH				
END FEELS				
TOES				
LOWER LEG ALIGNMENT				

LABORATORY STUDIES

Urinalysis

SG _____ _____RECORD TIME OF EXAM

ALBUMIN _____

GLUCOSE _____

MICROSCOPIC _____

Pelvic

CYTOLOGY _____

Hematology

SERUM FERRITIN _____

HEMOGLOBIN _____

Blood Chemistry

SMA 12 (OPTIONAL) _____

VACCINATIONS

POLIO VACCINE _____ DATE_____

TETANUS TOXOID _____ DATE _____

OTHERS _____

DIAGNOSTIC IMAGING

RECOMMEND:

☐ RADIOGRAPHS   VIEWS: _____

☐ CT SCAN   _____

☐ MRI   _____

☐ BONE SCAN   _____

☐ OTHER _____ _____
          (SPECIFY)

TENTATIVE DIAGNOSIS

ACTION TAKEN

☐ TREATMENT AS INDICATED   ☐ NO FOLLOW-UP   REFERRAL: ☐ GENERAL PRACTITIONER

☐ SPECIALIST (SPECIFY: _____)

NOTES: _____   ☐ NURSE

_____   ☐ DENTIST

_____   ☐ NUTRITION

_____   ☐ PSYCHOLOGY

_____   ☐ PHYSICAL THERAPY

_____   ☐ OCCUPATIONAL THERAPY

_____   ☐ SPEECH PATHOLOGIST

☐ OTHER _____
SPECIFY:

_____
SIGNATURE

PRINT NAME: _____

Ant., Anterior; *CT*, computed tomography; *MRI*, magnetic resonance imaging; *Post.*, posterior; *ROM*, range of motion; *SG*, specific gravity.

CHAPTER 18

EMERGENCY SPORTS ASSESSMENT

This chapter will enable the health care professional to immediately assess a patient before applying first aid or transportation to the hospital. This assessment should be divided into two parts. The first part concerns the primary evaluation or survey, which usually takes place at the location in which the patient is found to ensure that life-threatening situations are handled immediately. The second part of the assessment is performed when the examiner has more time and the patient is not under immediate threat of death or permanent disability.

Pre-Event Preparation

Before any sporting event, the examiner should establish and practice **emergency protocols**.[1,2] This preparation includes designating personnel for specific tasks and establishing emergency vehicle routes and entrances. The examiner and the assistants should know the location of additional medical assistance, emergency equipment (e.g., spinal board, neck supports, sandbags, stretchers, blankets, emergency first-aid kit), and a telephone. The equipment must be compatible with the needs, size, and age of the athletes, and with the equipment of other health care professionals. Near the telephone, the examiner should post emergency telephone numbers (e.g., ambulance, physician, dentist), identify the name and address of the sports facility, specify the entrance to be used, and note any obvious landmarks, because the person making the emergency call may forget information or give inappropriate information when under stress (Figure 18-1). Included in the preparation is a communication plan for on-field or at-site injuries. This plan may involve preestablished hand signals (e.g., crossed arms may mean "send a physician out," whereas a hand on top of one's

head may signify "send ambulance or emergency medical services [EMS] personnel") or walkie-talkies to communicate with other professionals working on the sideline.[3]

Emergency Protocol

- Designated personnel
- Emergency vehicle access routes
- Location of emergency equipment
- Location of telephone
- Communication plan

The examiner should take the time to give the facility a **safety check** by looking for potential hazards. Visiting teams should also be informed of emergency protocols. In addition, emergency situations and protocols must be practiced repeatedly to ensure that proper care will be given in an emergency.

Primary Assessment

After an injury occurs, the examiner must first take control of the situation and ensure that no additional harm comes to the patient. The primary survey, which takes 30 seconds to 2 minutes, with the maximum on-scene time being 10 minutes, is carried out with little or no movement of the patient.[4] It is used to determine whether injuries are life threatening, the severity of injury, and how the patient can be moved. With severe injuries, the longer the assessment takes, the higher the mortality rate is likely to be. If, at any time, the examiner finds that a major injury has occurred (Table 18-1), he or she may

---

Emergency Telephone Numbers

Ambulance _____   Fire/Inhalator _____

Acute Care Hospital (who will receive your athletes)

_____

Emergency Protocol

When you call the ambulance, state:

1. Your name

2. "There has been a suspected _____
   (*insert injury*)

   at _____ (*location*).

   Please send an ambulance to _____
   (*designated meeting spot*)

   I will meet the ambulance there."

3. Ask the estimated time of arrival (ETA).

4. Give them your phone number.

5. DO NOT HANG UP UNTIL THE OTHER PARTY DOES!

Note: If this information cannot be kept by the telephone it should be kept in your first-aid kit with a quarter ($0.25) in case you need to phone the ambulance from a pay phone.

Ambulance Route

Draw a map of the ambulance route to your facility and the designated meeting location.

Figure 18-1 �
Telephone emergency protocol (to be put near emergency telephones or taped to mobile phone). (Modified from Sports Physiotherapy Division Newsletter, Canadian Physiotherapy Association, p. 3, July/August 1991.)

Emergency Evaluation

Airway evaluation (A):	5 to 7 seconds
Ventilation check (B):	5 to 8 seconds
Circulation/heart rate (C):	20 to 30 seconds
Blood loss:	20 to 30 seconds
Neurological injury:	10 to 20 seconds
TOTAL TIME:	60 to 95 seconds

Table 18-1

Priorities in the Management of Injuries: Beware of Injury to the Cervical Spine!

Highest Priority
1. Respiratory and cardiovascular impairment: facial, neck, and chest injuries
2. Hemorrhage: external, severe

High Priority
3. Retroperitoneal injuries: shock, hemorrhage
4. Intraperitoneal injuries: shock, hemorrhage
5. Craniocerebral spinal cord injuries: open or closed, observation
6. Severe burns: extensive soft-tissue wounds

Low Priority
7. Lower genitourinary tract: hemorrhage, extravasation
8. Peripheral vascular, nerve, locomotor injuries: open or closed
9. Facial and neck injuries: except priorities 1 and 2
10. Cold exposure

Special
11. Fractures, dislocations: splinting
12. Tetanus prophylaxis

From Steichen FM: The emergency management of the severely injured, *J Trauma* 12:787, 1972.

---

terminate the assessment process and ensure the patient receives higher levels of care by calling for the ambulance or EMS. The examiner is designated as the **charge person,** or person in control. The examiner takes control by not allowing the patient to be moved until some type of assessment is made, the spine is supported as much as possible, and, if required, assistance is obtained.

For the primary emergency assessment, the examiner should call at least one person to provide immediate assistance, relay messages, and obtain additional help, if necessary. This person is designated the **call person,** and he or she should know the location of the closest telephone (a cell phone would be ideal) and what telephone numbers to call in specific emergencies. This information can be posted on or by the telephone (see Figure 18-1). When telephoning, the call person should state the caller's name, the number of the telephone being used, the exact emergency (type of injury), the degree of urgency, and the exact location of the facility; ask for an estimated time of arrival; and explain which is the best entrance to the facility for responding emergency personnel. Other individuals (as many as six or seven) may be called as necessary to act as transporters or help move the patient.

While performing the initial assessment, the examiner must keep in mind that six situations can immediately threaten the life of a patient: airway obstruction, respiratory failure, cardiac arrest, severe heat injury, head (craniocerebral) injury, and cervical spine injury.[5] It is for these situations, along with severe bleeding,

Figure 18-2
Stabilization of the patient's head and neck before initial assessment.

that the examiner must be most prepared, because they are the most common emergency life-threatening situations. Only practice can ensure proper care in an emergency.

Life-Threatening Emergency Situations

- Airway obstruction
- Respiratory failure
- Cardiac arrest
- Severe heat injury
- Head (craniocerebral) injury
- Cervical spine injury
- Severe bleeding

Initially, the examiner **stabilizes and immobilizes** the patient's head and cervical spine in case the patient has suffered a cervical spine injury (Figure 18-2).[6] If the patient has suffered trauma above the clavicles, he or she should be considered to have suffered a spinal injury to the cervical spine until proven otherwise.[7] Simultaneously, the examiner **talks to the patient.** If the patient replies in a normal voice and gives logical answers to questions, the examiner can assume that the airway is patent and the brain is receiving adequate perfusion. The examiner asks the patient what happened to determine how the injury occurred (mechanism of injury). The patient is asked to describe the symptoms (e.g., pain, numbness) and how severe he or she thinks the injury is. The examiner then explains what he or she is going to do and reassures the patient.[8] If the patient is unable to speak or is unconscious, the examiner must ask witnesses what happened. If the patient is unconscious ("collapsed athlete"), the examiner must work with the assumption that a neck (cervical spine) injury has occurred until proven otherwise.[9]

While the examiner is talking to the patient, he or she should be observing whether the patient moves, is still, or is having a seizure. If the patient moves, it means he

or she is at least partially conscious, has no apparent neurological dysfunction, and has some cardiopulmonary function. If the patient is still, it means he or she is unconscious, has some neurological dysfunction, or has some other major system failure. A seizure indicates neurological, systemic, or psychological dysfunction. The examiner should also observe the position of the patient (e.g., normal, deformity) and look for altered joint alignment (e.g., fracture, dislocation), swelling, or discoloration.[3] In case there is a spinal cord injury, the patient should be left in the original position until the nature and severity of the injury have been determined, except in cases of respiratory or cardiac distress. A rapid assessment of the **brain and spinal** cord can be accomplished by asking the patient to do simple movements such as sticking out the tongue[10] (see the discussion on the assessment for spinal cord injury, presented later).

Emergency on-Field Procedures

- Stabilize head and spine (do not move patient)
- Talk to patient and determine level of consciousness
- Move patient only if in respiratory or cardiac distress
- Check or establish airway
- Check heartbeat
- Check for bleeding, shock, cerebrospinal fluid
- Check pupils
- Check for spinal cord injury (neural watch)
- Position the patient
- Check for head injury
- Assess for heat injury
- Assess movement

Level of Consciousness

The examiner must quickly determine whether the patient is conscious. At no time during the initial assessment should ammonia inhalants be used to arouse the patient. Inhalants should be used only after the examiner is absolutely sure there is no spinal injury, because the fumes may cause a reflex head jerk, complicating the possible neck injury.[8] At this early stage, the examiner simply determines whether the patient is alert (fully conscious), confused (drowsy), in delirium, in obtundation (dulled sensations, especially pain and touch), in a stupor, or in a coma. A patient is classified as **alert** if he or she is able to carry on an appropriate conversation with no delays and is aware of time, place, and identity. See Chapter 2 for an explanation of the levels of consciousness.

The examiner determines the level of consciousness or arousal by talking to the patient, not by moving the patient. This stage is sometimes referred to as the "shake and shout" stage, in which the examiner tries to arouse the unconscious individual by gentle shaking (without allowing movement of the head and neck) and by shouting into each ear. If the patient does not respond to this verbal stimulus, the examiner can, at least initially, assume that the patient is unconscious or not fully conscious and proceed under that assumption. Further neurological assessment is left until the examiner is sure that the patient has a patent airway, is breathing normally, and has a heartbeat. If the patient is conscious, the examiner should reassure the patient that help has arrived. The patient should be informed of what the examiner is doing and proposes to do in terms of examining and moving the patient. Regardless of the patient's state of consciousness, he or she should not move or be moved until the examination has been completed.

Establishing the Airway

While waiting for assistance, the examiner can immediately begin to check for abnormal or arrested breathing, abnormal or arrested pulse, internal and external bleeding, and shock. This initial assessment is called the **ABCs (airway, breathing, and circulation)** of cardiopulmonary resuscitation (CPR). New guidelines also include the use of automated defibrillators if required.[11] The first priority is to maintain an adequate airway, normal ventilation, and hemodynamic stability (see Table 18-1).[12,13] Also, obvious bleeding should be controlled by compression.

While the cervical spine is protected and immobilized, the examiner quickly assesses the airway for patency by looking, listening, and feeling for spontaneous respirations.[4,7] Respirations can be determined by watching for movement of the chest, feeling the breath on the examiner's cheek, or hearing the air move in and out (Figure 18-3). The normal resting ranges of respirations are 10 to 25 breaths per minute for adults and 20 to 25 breaths

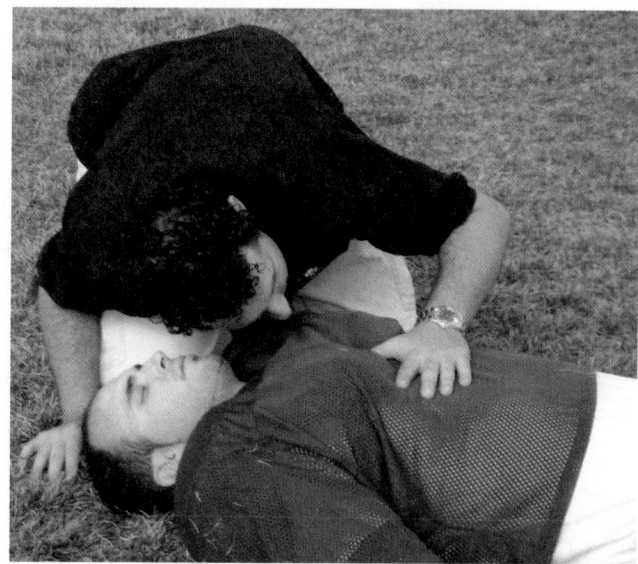

Figure 18-3

Examiner positioning to determine respiration of the patient. The examiner can feel the breath on the cheek, hear the breath, and watch the chest move.

per minute for children. An athlete or someone who has been exerting before injury may show a higher rate. If a patient is not breathing and has no heartbeat, clinical death will occur between 0 and 4 minutes (Figure 18-4). If breathing and heartbeat are not restored within 4 to 6 minutes, brain damage is probable. If there is no breathing and no heartbeat for 6 to 10 minutes, biological death occurs, and brain damage is likely.[14]

If the patient is breathing without difficulty, the rate and rhythm of the respirations and their characteristics should be noted. Cheyne-Stokes and ataxic respirations are often associated with head injuries.[15] Table 18-2 indicates some of the abnormal breathing patterns that may occur in a patient in an emergency situation.

If the conscious patient exhibits abnormal or arrested breathing (asphyxia), the examiner should look for possible causes.[16] Causes include compression of the trachea; tongue falling back, blocking the airway; foreign bodies (e.g., mouthguard, gum, chewing tobacco); swelling of the tissues (e.g., anaphylactic shock after a bee sting); fluid

Causes of Asphyxia

- Compression of trachea
- Tongue blocking airway
- Foreign bodies
- Tissue swelling
- Fluid in air passages
- Harmful gases or fumes
- Suffocation

0 to 4 minutes

4 to 6 minutes

A
Brain damage unlikely

B
Brain damage possible

6 to 10 minutes

C
Brain damage likely

Figure 18-4

If the brain is deprived of oxygen for 4 to 6 minutes, brain damage is possible. After 6 minutes, brain damage is extremely likely.

in the air passages; presence of harmful gases or fumes; pulmonary and chest wall trauma; and suffocation.[16,17]

Falling back of the tongue is the most common cause of airway obstruction after a sport injury, especially in the unconscious patient. Normally, the tone of the tongue muscles ensures airway patency. However, the unconscious person, especially one in the supine position, loses muscle tone and the tongue falls back, potentially leading to an obstruction. If the tongue is the cause of obstruction, the examiner can simply pull the chin forward in a **chin lift** or **jaw thrust maneuver** to restore the airway, being careful to keep movement of the cervical spine to a minimum. The chin lift maneuver is less likely to compromise the cervical spine.[18,19] Either maneuver pulls the retropharyngeal musculature forward, thus opening the airway.[16]

If the examiner can see an object obstructing the airway, an oral screw and tongue forceps can be used to remove the object. The mouth should be held open with the oral screw or something similar, and the examiner can use a finger to sweep the mouth clear of debris (e.g., broken teeth, dentures, mouthguard, chewing gum, tobacco). If the jaw is not held open and blocked from closing, the examiner should put fingers in the patient's mouth only with caution. If the cause of the blockage is something other than the tongue (e.g., foreign body), the patient, if conscious, should be asked to cough. If this does not expel the object, the Heimlich maneuver should be performed until the patient expels the object. If the patient loses consciousness, he or she should be

Table 18-2
Abnormal Breathing Patterns

Term	Description	Location of Possible Neurological Lesions
Hyperpnea	Abnormal increase in the depth and rate of the respiratory movements	
Apnea	Periods of nonbreathing	Pons
Ataxic breathing (Biot's respiration)	Irregular breathing pattern, with deep and shallow breaths occurring randomly	Medulla
Hyperventilation	Prolonged, rapid hyperpnea, resulting in decreased carbon dioxide blood levels	Midbrain, pons
Cheyne-Stokes respirations	Periods of hyperpnea regularly alternating with periods of apnea, characterized by regular acceleration and deceleration in depth	Cerebrum, cerebellum, midbrain, pons
Cluster breathing	Breaths follow each other in disorderly sequence, with irregular pauses between them	Pons, medulla

Adapted from Hickey JV: *The clinical practice of neurological and neurosurgical nursing,* p. 138, Philadelphia, 1986, JB Lippincott.

placed supine and ventilation attempted. If it is unsuccessful, 6 to 10 subdiaphragmatic abdominal thrusts are applied. This sequence of ventilation and subdiaphragmatic abdominal thrusts is repeated until a physician or EMS personnel arrive to perform a laryngoscopy.[20] Other causes of asphyxia may be treated by epinephrine (anaphylaxis) or intubation.[20] If the examiner is concerned about maintaining a patent airway, an oropharyngeal airway may be used. As a last resort, a wide-bore needle (18-gauge or larger) may be inserted into the trachea to ensure an airway.[16]

If the patient is not breathing, artificial ventilation (mouth-to-mouth resuscitation) must be initiated immediately, by using the breathing portion of the CPR techniques or by using a similar artificial breathing method.

If the patient is conscious but obviously in respiratory or cardiac distress, the examiner must deal with the presenting situation immediately (Table 18-3). If the patient does not have a patent airway, an airway must be established, as has been described. If the patient is moving in an attempt to get air into the lungs, the examiner may assume that a severe cervical injury is less likely to have occurred. However, movement of the head in relation to the cervical spine should be kept to a minimum. Keeping in mind the possibility of a cervical injury, the examiner should position the patient so that airway clearance and resuscitation can easily be accomplished. This change in position must be performed carefully to ensure that movement of the cervical spine is kept to a minimum. If the patient is reasonably comfortable in the side-lying

or prone position and there is no problem with cardiac function or breathing, it is not necessary to move the patient to the supine position.

After the airway has been established, whether by the use of an airway device, by proper head or jaw positioning, by the use of tongue forceps, or by a tracheotomy, the examiner must ensure that the airway is maintained and that the patient continues breathing. If respiration is not spontaneous, assisted ventilation (e.g., mouth-to-mouth, bagging) should be instituted. Ventilation can be compromised by a flail chest or pneumothorax (tension or open).[7,17] Endotracheal intubation is necessary if nasopharangeal bleeding, laryngeal trauma, secretions, or aspirations prevent maintenance of an adequate airway or end-ventilation.[12,16,21] Transtracheal ventilation is the treatment of choice for patients with breathing problems caused by brain, cervical spine, or maxillofacial injuries. An endotracheal tube may cause straining and venous hypertension, leading to increased brain edema, and extension of the head and neck to open upper airways may aggravate cervical spine injuries. Also, hemorrhage in maxillofacial injuries prevents the effective use of a breathing mask and does not allow adequate visualization.[13]

Establishing Circulation

While the examiner is determining whether breathing is normal, the patient's circulation should be checked for 10 or 15 seconds using the carotid (preferred), brachial, radial, or femoral pulse (Figure 18-5). For a sedentary adult, the normal heart rate is 60 to 90 beats per minute. For children, the rate is 80 to 100 beats per minute. In the highly trained athlete of either sex, the rate may be as low as 40 beats per minute. With activity, the heart rate will be above these levels, and the examiner should take this fact into account when taking the pulse. Depending on the type and level of the individual's activity, the heart rate for a fit person should decrease to slightly above normal values **within 5 minutes.** The examiner should note whether the pulse is absent, rapid and rebounding, or weak and diminishing.

The pulse is most often checked at the carotid artery because this artery is large and easy to locate. Therefore, the examiner has less chance of missing the pulse and does not have to move from the area of the patient's head to perform palpation. If a pulse cannot be detected, it should be assumed that the patient does not have a heartbeat, and CPR should be initiated using either manual methods or an automated external defibrillator. The use of the defibrillator increases the chance of survival in cardiac arrest.[22] Although cardiac arrest is rare in athletes, sudden death or commotio cordis resulting from low-impact blunt trauma is always a possibility in sports.[23] When the pulse is assessed, the examiner should estimate its rate, strength, and rhythm to obtain an indication of the cardiac output. Circulatory sufficiency may also be determined by squeezing the nail

Table 18-3

Airway Obstruction

Conscious Athlete	Unconscious Athlete
1. If patient is breathing or coughing, leave alone but continue to watch 2. If no air is going in and out of lungs, administer: four abdominal thrusts (Heimlich maneuver); some people also administer four back blows 3. Repeat until patient can breathe independently or patient becomes unconscious	1. Head tilt if no cervical spine injury is suspected 2. No response—try to ventilate 3. No success—reposition head and try to ventilate again 4. If unsuccessful, follow with four abdominal thrusts (Heimlich maneuver); some people also administer four back blows 5. Quick sweep of the mouth 6. If unsuccessful, repeat steps 1 through 5 until there is no longer obstruction or qualified help arrives; a tracheotomy may follow if obstruction continues

Adapted from American Academy of Orthopaedic Surgeons: *Athletic training and sports medicine,* p. 454, Park Ridge, Ill, 1984, AAOS.

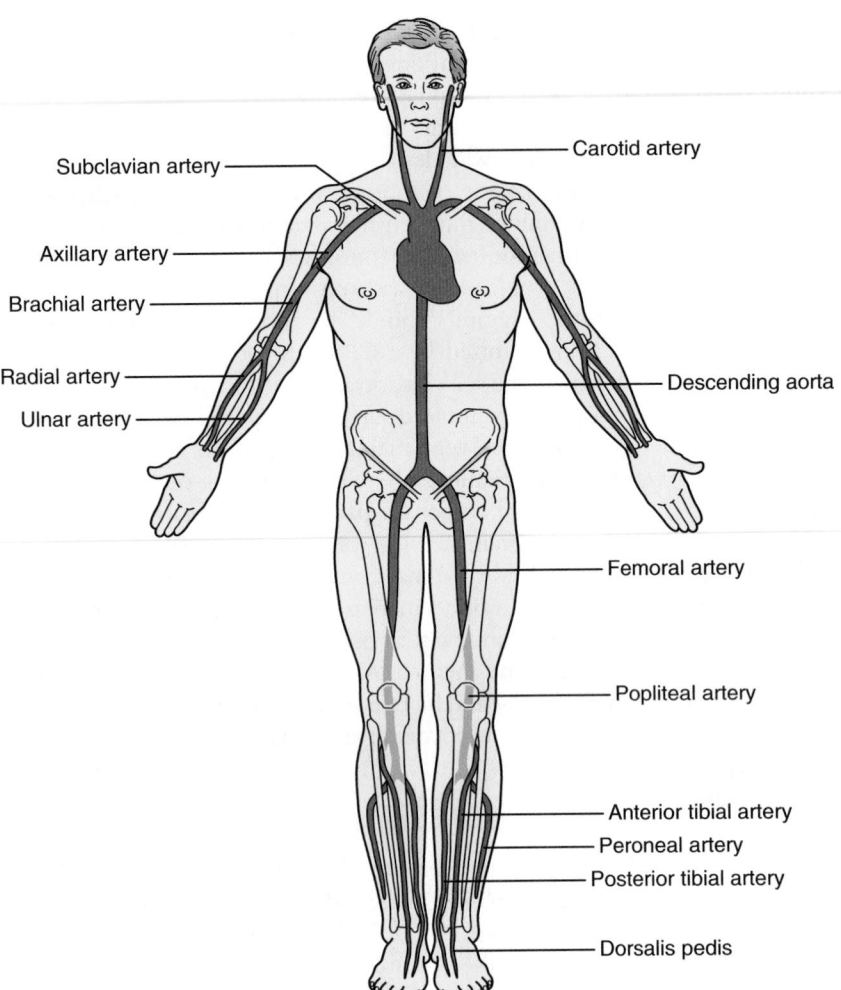

Subclavian artery

Carotid artery

Axillary artery

Brachial artery

Radial artery

Ulnar artery

Descending aorta

Femoral artery

Popliteal artery

Anterior tibial artery

Peroneal artery

Posterior tibial artery

Dorsalis pedis

Figure 18-5

Major arteries in the body. Pressure applied to any of the arteries (pressure points) can decrease bleeding if applied proximal to the bleeding.

bed or hypothenar eminence. **Capillary refill** is delayed if the pink color does not return to the nail bed or hypothenar eminence within 2 seconds after release of the pressure.[24] Squeezing the hypothenar eminence is a better indicator if the patient is hypothermic.

The pulse may also be used to determine the patient's blood pressure. If a carotid pulse can be palpated, systolic blood pressure is 60 mm Hg or higher. If the femoral pulse is palpable, systolic blood pressure is 70 mm Hg or higher. If the radial pulse can be palpated, the systolic blood pressure is 80 mm Hg or higher.[10,15,24] Like heart rate, blood pressure should drop to almost normal levels within 5 minutes following termination of exercise.

A **weak or rapid pulse** usually indicates shock, heat exhaustion, hypoglycemia, fainting, or hyperventilation. A **slowing pulse** is sometimes seen when there is a large increase in intracranial pressure, which usually indicates a severe lower brain stem compression.[25] A pulse that is **rebounding and rapid** is often the result of hypertension, fright, heat stroke, or hyperglycemia.

If the pulse rate is beginning to weaken, the patient may be going into **shock** (Figure 18-6). Shock is characterized by signs and symptoms that occur when the cardiac output is insufficient to fill the arterial tree and the blood is under insufficient pressure to provide organs and tissues with adequate blood flow. It should be noted, however, that patients who maintain pink skin, especially in the face and extremities, are seldom hypovolemic after injury. If the skin of the face or extremities turns ash-gray or white, this usually indicates blood loss of at least 30%.[7] Common types of shock and their causes are shown in Table 18-4. A patient going into shock becomes restless and anxious. The pulse slowly becomes weak and rapid, and the skin becomes cold and wet, often clammy. Sweating may be profuse, and the face is initially pale and later cyanotic (blue) around the mouth. Respirations may be shallow, labored, rapid, or possibly irregular and gasping, especially if a chest injury has occurred. The eyes usually become dull and lusterless, and the pupils become increasingly dilated. The patient may complain

Rapid Assessment Criteria for Circulation

1. Skin color
2. Carotid pulse palpable (systolic blood pressure, ≥ 60 mm Hg)
   Femoral pulse palpable (systolic blood pressure, ≥ 70 mm Hg)
   Radial pulse palpable (systolic blood pressure, ≥ 80 mm Hg)

Modified from Driscoll P, Skinner D: Initial assessment and management: I. Primary survey, *Br Med J* 300:1266, 1990.

Table 18-4

Types of Shock and Their Causes

Type	Cause
Hemorrhagic (hypovolemic)	Blood loss
Respiratory	Inadequate blood supply
Neurogenic	Loss of vascular control by the nervous system
Psychogenic	Common fainting
Cardiogenic	Insufficient pumping of blood by the heart
Septic	Severe infection and blood vessel damage
Anaphylactic	Allergic reaction
Metabolic	Loss of body fluid

of thirst and feel nauseated or vomit. If shock develops quickly, the patient may lose consciousness. To prevent or delay the onset of shock, the examiner may cover the patient, elevate the patient's legs, or attempt to eliminate the cause of the problem.

Signs and Symptoms of Shock

- Increased and weak heart rate
- Cold, clammy, pale skin
- Increased and shallow respiratory rate
- Profuse sweating
- Increased thirst
- Restlessness and anxiousness
- Altered level of consciousness
- Dilated pupils
- Nausea or vomiting

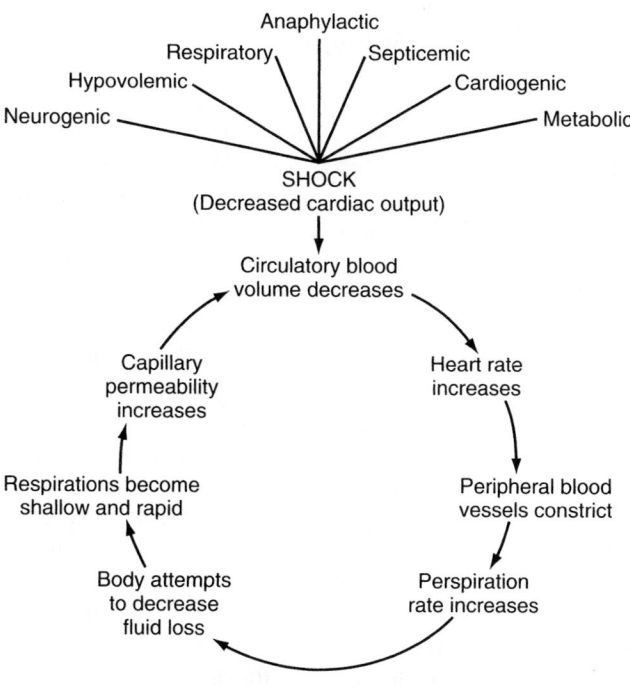

Figure 18-6

The shock cycle.

Circulatory collapse in trauma patients is caused primarily by blood loss from vascular damage or fracture, or **hypovolemic shock,** but the examiner must remember that shock in trauma may also be caused by tension pneumothorax, central nervous system injury, or pericardial tamponade (heart compression resulting from blood in the pericardium)—all emergency conditions that require physician intervention.[26] By the time hypovolemic shock becomes evident, blood loss may be as high as 20% to 25%. The normal range of blood pressure is 100 to 120 mm Hg for systolic pressure and 60 to 80 mm Hg for diastolic pressure. With shock, the blood pressure gradually decreases. If the blood pressure can be measured, it is best to assume that shock is developing in any injured adult whose systolic blood pressure is 100 mm Hg or less.

If the examiner is caring for a dark-skinned person, it may be difficult to determine from observation whether the patient is going into shock. A healthy person with dark skin usually has a red undertone and shows a healthy pink color in the nail beds, lips, and mucous membranes of the mouth and tongue. A dark-skinned patient in shock, however, has a gray cast to the skin around the nose and mouth, especially if experiencing respiratory shock. The mucous membranes of the mouth and tongue, the lips, and the nail beds have a blue tinge. If the shock is caused by hypovolemia, the mucous membranes of the mouth and tongue will not be blue; rather they will have a pale, graying, waxy pallor.[27]

If no pulse is present, then the cardiac portion of CPR techniques should be initiated. Sports equipment such as shoulder pads or rib pads should be removed, at least anteriorly, to give the examiner clear access to the anterior chest wall. CPR provides only approximately 25% of normal cardiac output, so it is imperative that it is performed properly by knowledgeable persons.[28] CPR is maintained until the patient recovers or EMS personnel arrive. If a cervical spine injury is suspected, CPR must be done with care, because compression to the heart can cause repeated flexion-extension of the cervical spine.[13]

Assessment for Bleeding, Fluid Loss, and Shock

The examiner should look for any signs of external bleeding or hemorrhage (Table 18-5). The types of wounds in which external bleeding or hemorrhage may be seen are incisions, which are clean cuts, or lacerations that have jagged edges. A contusion may produce internal bleeding, whereas a puncture or abrasion may also show bleeding or oozing on the surface. Major traumatic injuries such as fractures (e.g., pelvis, femur) can cause a great deal of internal bleeding. Of the five types of wounds, the puncture wound is probably the most difficult to treat because it has the highest probability of infection. The examiner should watch for bleeding from the lungs, the stomach, the upper bowel, the lower bowel, the kidneys, or the bladder. If the liver, spleen, or kidney is injured, serious internal bleeding may result; the blood will not be visible because it is contained within the abdominal cavity. In this case, the patient may experience abdominal rigidity, pain, and difficulty breathing (pressure on diaphragm).

When inspecting a bleeding structure, the examiner should note the type of vessel affected. For example, an artery spurts blood, whereas a vein provides an even flow. Capillaries tend to ooze bright blood (Figure 18-7).[14] Because arterial bleeding is of greatest concern, the examiner must be aware of the pressure points in the body (see Figure 18-5) so that he or she will know where to apply proper treatment. The examiner chooses the pressure point closest to the area of bleeding and applies pressure to the artery to slow or stop the bleeding. Tourniquets should be used only with extreme caution and in selected instances (e.g., accidental amputation of

ARTERIES:
Spurting blood
Pulsating flow
Bright red color

CAPILLARIES:
Slow even flow

VEINS:
Steady flow
Dark red color

Figure 18-7
Bleeding characteristics.

a limb, very severe bleeding from a major artery, or the need to apply CPR with no assistance available) and then only with enough pressure to stop bleeding. If a tourniquet is used, the time of tourniquet application should be noted carefully to prevent unnecessary tissue damage. Hemodynamic stability is best maintained by applying direct pressure to an open wound, keeping the patient in a recumbent position, and minimizing the number of times the patient is moved.[12]

If signs and symptoms of shock are present but visible bleeding is minimal, the examiner should suspect hidden bleeding within the abdomen, chest, or extremities.[15,29] If bleeding is suspected in the abdomen, the examiner should palpate the abdominal wall for shape and distention. To check for bleeding in the chest or extremities, the examiner should look for deformities (e.g., fractures). The fingers may be used to percuss the chest area, noting any loss of hollow sounds, to help locate the presence of fluid or blood. Hyporesonance may indicate a solid organ or the presence of fluid or blood; hyperresonance usually indicates air- or gas-filled spaces.[15]

After the airway and the pulmonary and circulatory systems (ABCs) have been assessed and controlled, the examiner can proceed to the remainder of the primary assessment. The examiner should check the ears and nose for the presence of cerebrospinal fluid. If blood or cerebrospinal fluid leaks from the ear, this may indicate a skull fracture. The examiner should incline the head toward the affected side to facilitate drainage, unless a cervical injury is suspected. The examiner can place a gauze pad over the patient's ear or nose where the bleeding is occurring to collect the fluid on the gauze (Figure 18-8). The examiner should look for an orange halo forming on the pad (see Figure 2-39). The halo is cerebrospinal fluid, the presence of which is a good indication of a skull fracture.[30]

Table 18-5
Bleeding Characteristics and Their Source

Source	Bleeding Characteristics
Artery	Bright red, spurting or pulsating flow
Vein	Dark red, steady flow
Capillary	Slow, even flow
Lungs	Bright red, frothy
Stomach	Coffee grounds–like vomitus
Upper bowel	Tarry black stools
Kidneys	Smoky, red urine
Bladder	Red urine, difficulty urinating
Abdomen	Blood not visible; abdominal rigidity, pain, difficulty breathing

Figure 18-8
Checking the ear for blood or cerebrospinal fluid.

Pupil Check

The examiner checks the pupils for shape and for response to light by using a penlight or by covering the eye with one hand and then taking it away. The pupil normally reacts to the intensity of light or focal distance. The pupils dilate in a dark environment or with a long focal distance, and they constrict in a light environment or with a short focal distance. Normally, the pupils are equally or almost equally dilated (diameter range, 2 to 6 mm; mean of 3.5 mm), but injury to the central nervous system (e.g., head injury) may cause the pupils to dilate unevenly. Some people normally have unequal pupil sizes, and the health care professional must be aware of this possibility. In a fully conscious, alert person who has sustained a blow near the eye, a dilated, fixed pupil is most likely the result of trauma to the short ciliary nerves of that eye rather than the result of third cranial nerve compression caused by brain herniation.[12] Drugs may also affect the pupillary size. For example, opiate drugs cause pinpoint pupils, whereas amphetamines may cause dilated pupils.[15]

To test pupil reaction, the examiner holds one hand over one eye and then moves the hand away quickly, or shines the light from a penlight into the eye, and observes the pupil's reaction when the light is shone on the eye (normal reaction: constriction) or when the light source is removed (normal reaction: dilation). The examiner tests the other eye in a similar fashion and compares the results. The **pupillary reaction** is classified as brisk (normal), sluggish, nonreactive, or fixed. An ovoid or slightly oval pupil or a fixed and dilated pupil indicates increasing

intracranial pressure.[15] If both pupils are midsize, midposition, and nonreactive, midbrain damage is usually indicated. The fixation and dilation of both pupils is a terminal sign of anoxia and ischemia to the brain.[15,31]

Assessment for Spinal Cord Injury

An upper spinal cord injury should be suspected, at least initially, if the patient has neck pain; the patient's head position is asymmetric or abnormal; the patient is having respiratory difficulty, especially if the chest is not moving (absence of abdominal or diaphragmatic breathing); the patient is demonstrating priapism (erection of the penis); or the patient is unconscious after a fall or other contact activity. Other indications of neurological injuries in the conscious patient include numbness, tingling, or burning, especially below the clavicles; muscle weakness; twitching; or paralysis of the arms or legs, especially bilaterally (flaccid paralysis).[15]

The examiner may ask the patient to stick out the tongue, wiggle the toes, move the feet or arms, or squeeze the examiner's fingers.[10] This quick test provides a rapid assessment of the brain and spinal cord by showing whether the patient can follow instructions and can do the activity.

Situations in Which Cervical Spine Injury Must Be Suspected Until Proven Otherwise

- Neck pain or stiffness
- Cervical muscle spasm
- Asymmetric or abnormal head position
- Respiratory difficulty (chest not moving)
- Priapism
- Unconsciousness
- Numbness, tingling, or burning
- Muscle weakness or paralysis
- Loss of bowel or bladder control

If the patient is unconscious (Table 18-6), the examiner should reassess the level of unconsciousness and treat the patient as though a spinal injury has occurred. In the unconscious patient, the examiner should watch for spontaneous limb movement, especially after the application of a painful stimulus, because movement indicates that the patient is less likely to have suffered a severe cervical injury.[15] In addition, the examiner should look for posturing that indicates a severe head injury. **Decerebrate rigidity** is evidenced by all four extremities being in extension. With **decorticate rigidity,** the lower limbs are in extension and the upper limbs are in flexion (see Figure 2-31).

Table 18-6

Some Common Causes of Unconsciousness in Patients

Category	Problem	Cause	Pathophysiology	Management
General	Loss of consciousness	Injury or disease	Shock, head injury, other injuries, diabetes, arteriosclerosis	Need for CPR, triage
Disease	Diabetic coma	Hyperglycemia and acidosis	Inadequate use of sugar, acidosis	Complex treatment for acidosis
	Insulin shock	Hypoglycemia	Excess insulin	Sugar
	Myocardial infarct	Damaged myocardium	Insufficient cardiac output	Oxygen, CPR, transport
	Stroke	Damaged brain	Loss of arterial supply to brain or hemorrhage within brain	Support, gentle transport
Injury	Hemorrhagic shock	Bleeding	Hypovolemia	Control external bleeding, recognize internal bleeding, CPR, transport
	Respiratory shock	Insufficient oxygen	Paralysis, chest damage, airway obstruction	Clear airway, supplemental oxygen, CPR, transport
	Anaphylactic shock	Acute contact with agent to which patient is sensitive	Allergic reaction	Intramuscular epinephrine, support, CPR, transport
	Cerebral contusion, concussion, or hematoma	Blunt head injury	Bleeding into or around brain, concussive effect	Airway, supplemental oxygen, CPR, careful monitoring, transport
Emotions	Psychogenic shock	Emotional reaction	Sudden drop in cerebral blood flow	Place supine, make comfortable, observe for injuries
Environment	Heatstroke	Excessive heat, inability to sweat	Brain damage from heat	Immediate cooling, support, CPR, transport
	Electric shock	Contact with electric current	Cardiac abnormalities, fibrillation	CPR, transport; do not treat until current controlled
	Systemic hypothermia	Prolonged exposure to cold	Diminished cerebral function, cardiac arrhythmias	CPR, rapid transport, warming at hospital
	Drowning	Oxygen, carbon dioxide, breath holding, water	Cerebral damage	CPR, transport
	Air embolism	Intravascular air	Obstruction to arterial blood flow by nitrogen bubbles	CPR, recompression
	Decompression sickness ("bends")	Intravascular nitrogen	Obstruction to arterial blood flow by nitrogen bubbles	CPR, recompression
Injected or ingested agents	Alcohol	Excess intake	Cerebral depression	Support, CPR, transport
	Drugs	Excess intake	Cerebral depression	Support, CPR, transport (bring drug)
	Plant poisons	Contact, ingestion	Direct cerebral or other toxic effect	Support, recognition, CPR, identify plant, local wound care, transport
	Animal poisons	Contact, ingestion, injection	Direct cerebral or other toxic effect	Recognition, support, CPR, identify agent, local wound care, transport
Neurological	Epilepsy	Brain injury, scar, genetic predisposition, disease	Excitable focus of motor activity in brain	Support, protect patient, transport in status epilepticus

From the American Academy of Orthopaedic Surgeons: *Athletic training and sports medicine*, ed 2, pp. 618–619, Park Ridge, Ill, 1991, AAOS.

Assessment for Head Injury (Neural Watch)

The patient's level of consciousness is then reassessed. The examiner should now institute a neural watch (Figure 18-9) or a similar observation scheme to note any changes in the patient over time. The neural watch should initially be performed **every 5 to 15 minutes,** because it also facilitates monitoring of the patient's vital signs.[15] After the patient has stabilized, neural watch recordings may be made **every 15 to 30 minutes.**[25] If possible, reassessment by the same examiner allows the detection of subtle changes.

Neural Watch Chart

Unit		Time 1 ( )	Time 2 ( )	Time 3 ( )
I. Vital signs	Blood pressure Pulse Respirations Temperature			
II. Conscious and	Oriented Disoriented Restless Combative			
	Unconscious			
III. Speech	Clear Rambling Garbled None			
IV. Will awaken to	Name Shaking Light pain Strong pain			
V. Nonverbal reaction to pain	Appropriate Inappropriate "Decerebrate" None			
VI. Pupils	Size on right Size on left Reacts on right Reacts on left			
VII. Ability to move	Right arm Left arm Right leg Left leg			
VIII. Sensation	Right side (normal/abnormal) Left side (normal/abnormal) Dermatome affected (specify) Peripheral nerve affected (specify)			

Figure 18-9

Neural watch chart. (Modified from American Academy of Orthopaedic Surgeons: *Athletic training and sports medicine,* p. 399, Park Ridge, Ill, 1984, AAOS.)

The examination should include an evaluation of the patient's facial expression; a determination of the patient's orientation to time, place, and person; and the presence of both posttraumatic amnesia and retrograde amnesia. Signs and symptoms that demand emergency action in a patient who has sustained a blow to the head are increased headache, nausea and vomiting, inequality of pupils, disorientation, progressive or sudden impairment of consciousness, gradual increase in blood pressure, and diminution of pulse rate.

Emergency Signs and Symptoms of Head Injury

- Increased headache
- Nausea and vomiting
- Inequality of pupils
- Disorientation
- Altered level of consciousness
- Increased blood pressure
- Decreased pulse rate
- Decreased reaction to pain
- Decreased or altered values on neural watch chart or Glasgow Coma Scale

Reaction to pain and the level of consciousness can be determined by the use of physical and verbal stimuli. If there is no cervical injury, the verbal stimuli may include calling the patient's name and shaking and shouting at the patient. Physical stimuli (see Figure 2-30) include squeezing the Achilles tendon, squeezing the trapezius muscle, squeezing the soft tissue between the patient's thumb and index finger, squeezing an object (pen or pencil) between the patient's fingers, squeezing a fingertip, or applying a knuckle to the sternum (this must be done with caution because it may cause bruising). In comatose patients, a motor response to a painful stimulus to an extremity may indicate intact pain appreciation from that site, especially if it is accompanied by a more remote response such as a grimace or a change in respiration or pulse.[12]

The level of consciousness can best be determined with the use of the **Glasgow Coma Scale** (GCS) (see Table 2-18).[32-34] The sooner the patient is tested with the scale, the better, because the initial assessment can be used as a baseline for improvement or deterioration in the patient. The GCS is often used in conjunction with the neural watch. For a description of the test, see Chapter 2.

Deterioration of consciousness may result from many conditions, such as increased intracranial pressure caused by an expanding intracranial lesion, hypoxia (which can aggravate cerebral edema and increase the intracranial pressure), epilepsy, meningitis, or fat embolism. The examiner should always look for signs of expanding intracranial lesions (see Chapter 2), especially if the patient is conscious. These lesions are emergency conditions that must be attended to immediately because of their potentially high mortality rate (up to 50%).

If the patient experiences loss of consciousness or appears to have disturbed senses, is seeing stars or colors, is dizzy, or has auditory hallucinations or a severe headache, the patient should not be left alone or allowed to return to activity (Table 18-7). In addition, nausea, vomiting, lethargy, increasing blood pressure, disturbed sensation of smell, or a diminished pulse should lead the examiner to the same conclusion. Amnesia, hyperirritability, an open wound, unequal pupils, or leaking of cerebrospinal fluid or blood from the ears or nose also indicates an emergency condition. Numbness on one side of the body or a large contusion in the head area should likewise lead the examiner to handle the patient with care. If the frontal area of the brain is affected, the patient may experience lapses of memory, personality changes, or impairment of judgment. If the temporal lobe has been affected, the patient may experience feelings of unreality, déjà vu, or hallucinations involving odors, sounds, or visual disturbances such as macropsia (seeing objects as larger than they really are) or micropsia. The literature indicates that head injury depends not only on the magnitude and direction of impact and the structural features and physical reactions of the skull but also on the state of the head/brain at the moment of impact.[5,35,36]

If the patient has received a head injury and has been checked by a physician and it has been determined that it is not necessary to send the patient to the hospital, the clinician should ensure that the patient and whoever lives with the patient understands what to look for in terms of signs and symptoms that may indicate increasing severity of head injury. Figure 2-32 demonstrates typical home health care guidelines.

Assessment for Heat Injury

If the examiner suspects a heat-type injury with no cervical injury, only heat exhaustion and heat stroke need be considered as life-threatening.[9,37] **Heat fatigue** or exhaustion occurs when a person is exposed to high environmental temperature or humidity and perspires excessively without salt or fluid replacement. **Heat stroke** can occur when a nonacclimatized person is suddenly exposed to high environmental temperature or humidity. The thermal regulatory mechanism fails, perspiration stops, and the body temperature increases. Above 42°C oral body temperature, brain damage occurs, and death follows if emergency measures are not instituted. The diagnostic keys in this situation are the **high body temperature** and the **absence of sweating.** Initial signs of heat injury include muscle cramps, excessive fatigue or weakness, loss of coordination, decreased reaction time, headache, decreased comprehension, dizziness, and nausea and vomiting.

▼ Signs of Heat Injury

- Muscle cramps
- Excessive fatigue or weakness
- Loss of coordination
- Headache
- Decreased comprehension
- Dizziness
- Nausea and vomiting
- Decreased reaction time

Table 18-7

Indications for Immediate Removal from Activity

Area of Injury	Indications for Immediate Removal from Activity
Eye	Blunt trauma, visual difficulty, pain, laceration, obvious deformity
Head	Loss of consciousness, disturbed sensorium, stars or colors being seen, dizziness, auditory hallucinations, nausea, vomiting, lethargy, severe headache, rising blood pressure, disturbed smell, diminishing pulse, amnesia, hyperirritability, large contusion, open wounds, unequal pupils, leakage of cerebrospinal fluid or blood from ears or nose, numbness of one side of body
Spine	Obvious deformity, restricted motion, weakness of extremity, pain on movement, localized tenderness, numbness of extremity (pinched nerve), paresthesias
Extremities	Obvious deformity, crepitus, loss of range of motion, loss of sensation, effusion, pain on use, unstable joint, open wounds, significant tenderness, significant swelling
Abdomen	Dizziness or syncope, nausea, persisting pallor, vomiting, history of infectious mononucleosis, abnormal thirst, muscle guarding, localized tenderness, shoulder pain, distension, rapid pulse, clamminess and sweating

Reprinted by permission from the *New York State Journal of Medicine,* copyright by the Medical Society of the State of New York. Adapted from Greensher J, Mofenson HC, Merlis NJ: First aid for school athletic emergencies, *NY State J Med* 79:1058, 1979.

Table 18-8

Skin Changes and Their Cause

Skin Change	Cause
Hot and dry	Heat stroke, high fever, hyperglycemia
Cold and clammy	Fainting, hypoglycemia, hyperventilation, shock
Cool and moist	Heat exhaustion
Cool and dry	Cold
White pallor	Decreased circulation
Cyanosis (blue pallor)	Respiratory distress
Red pallor	Fever, heat stroke, inflammation, exercise

The body temperature varies according to the site at which the measurement is taken. The oral body temperature is 37°C (98.6°F). Taken in the armpit or axilla, the temperature is 36.4°C to 36.7°C (97.5°F to 98.1°F), and in the rectum, it is 37.3°C to 37.6°C (99.1°F to 99.7°F).

The examiner may palpate the skin to get some idea of the external temperature of the body and possible pathology (Table 18-8). Hot and dry skin is often caused by heat stroke, high fever, or hyperglycemia. Cold and clammy skin is caused by hypoglycemia, shock, fainting, or hyperventilation. Cool and moist skin is often caused by heat exhaustion, whereas cool and dry skin is caused by exposure to cold.

Skin color can also play a significant role. Pallor, or whitish skin, indicates circulatory disturbance or decreased circulation and is most often associated with trauma and shock. Cyanosis, or a blue tint to the skin, indicates respiratory distress, as does a gray tint. Redness indicates an increase in blood flow as a result of fever, heat stroke, or exercise.

Assessment for Movement

While doing the initial assessment, the examiner should also be considering how the patient will be moved and immobilized (e.g., self-ambulation, stretcher, spinal board) depending on the severity of the injury, and whether the patient can move him or herself or can move only with assistance.[38]

If the patient has not already done so, the examiner asks the patient to move the limbs to reassess for a cervical spine injury and look for major trauma (e.g., fracture, dislocation, third-degree strain, third-degree sprain). At the same time, the examiner may palpate the areas of potential injury, noting any pain, abnormal bone or joint alignment, swelling, hypersensitive or hyposensitive areas, or palpable defect (third-degree strain).[3] If movement is relatively normal, the examiner quickly checks

the myotomes of the upper or lower body for any possible motor involvement or motor impairment. Changes in limb power may be caused by a contractile tissue injury, a neurological injury, or an expanding intracranial lesion, which will be displayed as progressive weakness in the contralateral arm or leg.[25] Decreased limb power can also be caused by reflex inhibition as a result of previously unrecognized limb injury. In these cases, contractions are weak and painful. These types of injuries are placed in the low-priority group (see Table 18-1) because they represent a threat to the limb rather than to the life of the patient.[13]

Positioning the Patient

Normally, a patient is left in the position in which he or she is found until the primary assessment is completed. However, if the patient is having difficulty breathing or there is no pulse, the patient must be positioned to do CPR. If the conscious patient is prone and in respiratory difficulty, the examiner, with assistance, should **log-roll** the patient (Figure 18-10) onto a spinal board so that an attempt can be made to restore the airway. During any movement of the patient, the examiner should apply traction of about 4.5 kg (10 lb) to the cervical spine to maintain stability. The patient should be reassured that others are going to carefully move the patient while he or she remains still. Before any movement is attempted, the patient and those who are going to assist the examiner should know what the examiner plans to do and what their jobs are. This requires **frequent practicing of emergency procedures.** The sequence of movement and positioning of the extremities and body of the patient should be thought out beforehand so that everyone is aware of what is going to happen and in what order. The proper procedure for moving the patient should be practiced often to ensure competency.

To roll the patient, at least three assistants are needed. There should be two-way communication between the examiner and the patient at all times to continually evaluate the patient's comfort level and neurological signs. The assistants should place the spinal board beside the patient and then kneel beside the spinal board and patient (see Figure 18-10, A). They should reach over the patient and hold the patient's shoulder, hip, and knees (see Figure 18-10, B). On command from the examiner, the assistants roll the patient toward them while the examiner stabilizes the head (see Figure 18-10, C) until the patient is lying supine on the spinal board (see Figure 18-10, D). Only rolling—not lifting—should occur. With the patient in the supine position, proper CPR techniques may be applied, or the patient may be transported. The patient may also be covered with a blanket to provide warmth.

If a spinal injury is suspected and the conscious patient is in the prone position but has no difficulty breathing,

Figure 18-10

Moving a patient to the supine position after injury. Note that the head and neck are stabilized throughout the movement. **A,** Patient prone, examiner stabilizes head and gives instruction to helpers. **B through D,** Patient is log-rolled onto spinal board.

the patient is log-rolled halfway toward the assistants while another assistant slides the spinal board as close as possible to the patient's side. The patient is then rolled directly onto the spinal board in the prone position. Similarly, if a spinal injury is suspected and the patient is in the supine position and breathing normally, the patient is rolled toward the assistants while another assistant slides the spinal board under the patient as far as possible. The patient is then rolled back onto the spinal board in the supine position. If a spinal injury is suspected and the patient is in side lying, the patient is log-rolled directly onto the spinal board and into the supine position. In each of these cases, the examiner controls the head, applies traction, and instructs the assistants. The patient's head is then stabilized and immobilized with sandbags, a head immobilizer, or triangular bandages, and the patient is strapped to the spinal board with restraining belts. If a collar is used to stabilize the spine, it must do so during movement as well as when the patient is stationary; it must not hinder access to the carotid pulse, airway, or performance of CPR; it must be easy to assemble and apply; it must be adaptable to patients of all ages and sizes; and it must allow radiological examination without removal.[39,40] Any major injury such as a head injury, a spinal injury, or a fracture requires appropriate handling,

slow and deliberate management, and proper transportation to provide a satisfactory outcome. These techniques must be practiced repeatedly.

If possible and if time permits, especially if the assistants are not used to working together, a simulated roll and transport using an uninjured person should be attempted before moving the patient to ensure that all involved know what they are doing in terms of patient positioning, movement sequence, and specific handling (e.g., head, hands, feet), so that any transfer or movement of the patient is effective and organized.

During the emergency assessment, if the patient is nauseated, is vomiting, or has fluid draining from the mouth, and provided breathing and circulation are normal, the patient should be placed in the **recovery position** (Figure 18-11) as long as there is no suspicion of a spinal injury. This side lying position enables the patient to be continually monitored (ABCs) and allows the examiner to easily observe any change in condition while waiting for emergency personnel. The patient's head should be positioned to keep the airway open and to allow drainage from the throat and mouth. If the blood flow to the heart and brain has diminished, circulation can be improved by elevating the lower limbs, provided that the position change can be accomplished without

Figure 18-11
Recovery position.

causing further pain or breathing problems or aggravating an injury. If the patient has breathing difficulties or a chest injury or has experienced a heart attack or stroke, it may be desirable to lower blood pressure in the injured parts by elevating the upper part of the body slightly, if the position change can be accomplished without causing further pain or breathing problems.

If the patient is unconscious and the cardiac and circulatory functions are not compromised, the patient should be left in the original position until consciousness is regained. However, if the patient is unconscious and lying supine, the examiner should always watch for the possibility that the patient may "swallow" the tongue and obstruct the airway. Also, an unconscious patient loses the cough reflex, and if vomiting or bleeding occurs, vomitus, mucus, or blood may enter and obstruct the airway. Therefore, the examiner may elect to put the patient in the recovery position.

If the patient is unconscious and in respiratory or cardiac distress, the examiner must quickly assess the patient and attempt to restore respiratory and cardiac function. This patient is then treated the same as the conscious patient.

If the patient's spine is twisted or flexed and the patient is reasonably comfortable, the patient should be stabilized in that position until a spinal injury is ruled out. If there has been a loss of breathing or cardiac function, the examiner must carefully correct the deformity, place the patient in the supine lying position, and perform the appropriate measures to deal with the problem.

If a cervical spine injury has occurred to a child of 7 years of age or younger, the examiner should realize that in these children, the head is normally larger in proportion to the rest of the body. If the child is positioned on a spinal board without modification, the neck will be forced into some flexion. To alleviate this problem, the spinal board should have a cutout for the head, or a pad for the chest or rest of the body should be added to elevate it in relation to the head.[41]

If the patient is in the water and unconscious, he or she must be reached as quickly as possible. The rescuer should not jump into the water, because this action creates waves that may rock the victim's head and could cause severe consequences if a neck injury has occurred.

The examiner should approach the patient head-on and place an extended arm down the middle of the patient's back with the patient's head in the examiner's axilla. The examiner then grasps the patient's biceps with the forearm around the patient's forehead, slowly lifts the arm, and turns the patient face up. The examiner's forearm locks the patient's head in the examiner's axilla during the turn. Once the patient is supine, both of the examiner's arms support the patient's head and spine in the water. An assistant then slides the spinal board under the patient in the water and blocks the patient's head with towels. The patient is next strapped to the spinal board with restraining straps and is lifted out of the water.[42] If a spinal board is not available and a cervical injury is suspected, the patient should be supported in the water until emergency personnel arrive.

In some sports (e.g., ice hockey, lacrosse, motor car or motorcycle racing, football), the athletes wear helmets. Whether the helmet should be removed to institute emergency procedures is a controversial issue and often depends on the type of training (EMS versus sports therapy) and experience of the health care professional.[2,38,43-46] Generally, if the patient is unconscious, the helmet should not be removed unless the examiner is absolutely certain that there has not been a neck injury. In the patient who wears both helmet and shoulder pads, both should be left on the patient because they help to maintain the cervical sagittal alignment close to normal. Ideally, the helmet and shoulder pads should be removed in a controlled setting such as the emergency department.[2,47,48] Helmets should be removed only if the facemask or visor interferes with adequate ventilation[47,49]; if the facemask interferes with the clinician's ability to restore an adequate airway[47,49]; if the helmet is so loose that it does not provide adequate immobilization of the head when secured to the spinal board[47,49]; if life-threatening hemorrhage under the helmet cannot be controlled[47,49]; if, in children, the helmet is too large and causes flexion of the neck when used as part of the immobilization[41,47,49]; or if it is necessary to defibrillate the patient. In the last case, the shoulder pads must be removed, so the helmet should be removed to maintain spinal position.[3] If the patient is in respiratory distress, facemasks can usually be easily removed with the use of an X-Acto knife or similar device to release the restraining straps while holding the mask in place.

If, for whatever reason, the decision is made to remove the headgear, the neck and head must be held as rigid as possible. Therefore, at least two people are needed: one to stabilize the head and neck and one to remove the facemask. One person, usually the assistant, first applies in-line traction is to the helmet to ensure initial stability. A second person, usually the examiner, then stands at the side of the patient and employs in-line traction by applying a traction force through the patient's chin and occiput. The assistant stops applying traction and, if the helmet is a football helmet, first removes the cheek pads by sliding a flat object (e.g., scissors handle) between the cheek pad and helmet, twisting the object to cause the pads to unsnap. After the pads are removed, the assistant applies bilateral expansion to the helmet so that the ears are cleared as the helmet is removed.[3] After the helmet has been removed, the assistant reapplies in-line traction from the head, and the examiner then releases the traction and continues the primary examination.[36] If desired, the examiner may apply a cervical collar such as the Stifneck collar, but this should be done with caution because cervical collars do not completely eliminate movement in the cervical spine.[50]

If the helmet is removed and the patient is wearing shoulder pads, the person holding the head must ensure that the head does not fall back into extension, and a modification must be made to the spinal board. The shoulder pads should be removed only if it is impossible to do this or if defibrillation is necessary.

If the patient is conscious and there appears to be no cervical injury or other severe injury, the patient may be moved to another area for a more appropriate and complete secondary assessment. If the injury is in the upper limb and the injured part is immobilized, the patient may first be moved from a supine to a sitting or kneeling position, then from sitting or kneeling to supported standing, to unsupported standing, and finally the person may walk off the field. During these changes in position, the examiner or assistants are positioned to provide support and assistance if the patient feels dizzy or unsteady. If the injury is in the lower limb, the athlete may be helped off the field by teammates, stretcher, or cart. Spinal injuries require greater care and the use of a spinal board and cervical collar with support. Again, assistance may be required, and everyone, including the patient and assistants, should be aware of the movement sequence before it is attempted.

Movement Sequence to Remove Conscious, Mobile Athlete from Field of Play

Supine lying

↓

Sitting (supported)

↓

Kneeling (supported, 4 point → 2 point)

↓

Standing (supported)

↓

Standing (unsupported)

↓

Walk off field (assistance ready)

Injury Severity

During the primary assessment, the examiner must use some method of determining the severity of injury. There are several scales that may be used to test the severity of injury or to triage the patient, including the Galveston Orientation and Amnesia Test,[51] which tests for posttraumatic amnesia; the Abbreviated Injury Scale;[52] the Injury Severity Score;[52–54] the Trauma Score;[55] the Triage Index;[56,57] the Circulation, Respiration, Abdomen, Motor, and Speech (CRAMS) Scale;[58,59] and the Trauma Index.[60] Of these, the Trauma Score illustrates the ease of scoring (Figure 18-12) and the survival probabilities (Table 18-9) that can be expected in trauma patients. This tool provides a dynamic score that monitors changes in the patient's condition and is useful in making triage decisions. The CRAMS scale illustrates a similar scoring pattern (Table 18-10).

Secondary Assessment

The examiner can proceed to the secondary assessment if the patient is conscious, is able to respond by talking coherently, shows minimal or no distress in terms of breathing, and displays normal circulation. However, the examiner must keep in mind that the patient may still have suffered a catastrophic injury (e.g., cervical spine injury) that, although not life-threatening at the present time, could lead to significant problems. For the most part, the secondary survey is predicated on the patient's being clinically stable.[7]

If the patient is conscious, the examiner must constantly reassure the patient to reduce potential anxieties. By the time the secondary assessment begins, the examiner should have eliminated any possible life-threatening situations and can then complete the injury assessment. In the case of a sudden injury, the examiner should remember that the patient has had no time to prepare psychologically or practically for the injury. Therefore, the injury can represent a sudden and frightening change in the patient's physical state. Other concerns experienced by the patient may be related to the patient's job, financial situation, family, or prognosis, and these concerns, suddenly magnified, may affect the patient's behavior, especially in later secondary or "sideline" assessments.

The secondary assessment is a head-to-toe rapid physical examination[31] and can be performed after the examiner has ascertained that there is no threat to the patient's life. The patient must be conscious for the examiner to perform the secondary assessment properly. The secondary survey involves a complete body survey to detect other injuries that may cause serious complications or lead to a patient's not being allowed to return to activity. The patient should be instructed not to move unless requested by the examiner, who should also explain to the patient what is being done while the examination is being performed. It is important to maintain communication

Trauma Score

Trauma Score	Value	Points	Score
A. Respiratory rate	10–24	4	
Number of respirations in 15 sec, multiply by four	25–35	3	
	>35	2	
	<10	1	
	0	0	A. _____
B. Respiratory effort	Normal	1	
Shallow—markedly decreased chest movement or air exchange	Shallow or retractive	0	
Retractive—use of accessory muscles or intercostal retraction			B. _____
C. Systolic blood pressure	>90	4	C. _____
Systolic cuff pressure—either arm; auscultate or palpate	70–90	3	
	50–69	2	
	<50	1	
No carotid pulse	0	0	
D. Capillary refill			
Normal—forehead, lip mucosa or nail bed color refill in 2 sec	Normal	2	
Delay—more than 2 sec of capillary refill	Delayed	1	
None—no capillary refill	None	0	D. _____

E. Glasgow Coma Scale (GCS)

Total GCS Points	Score
14–15	5
11–13	4
8–10	3
5–7	2
3–4	1 E. _____

1. Eye opening
   Spontaneous _____ 4
   To voice _____ 3
   To pain _____ 2
   None _____ 1

2. Verbal response
   Oriented _____ 5
   Confused _____ 4
   Inappropriate words _____ 3
   Incomprehensible words _____ 2
   None _____ 1

3. Motor response
   Obeys command _____ 6
   Purposeful movement (pain) _____ 5
   Withdraw (pain) _____ 4
   Flexion (pain) _____ 3
   Extension (pain) _____ 2
   None _____ 1

Trauma Score
(Total points A + B + C + D + E): _____

Total GCS points (1 + 2 + 3) _____

Figure 18-12
Trauma score. (From Champion HR et al: Trauma score, *Crit Care Med* 9:673, 1981.)

with the patient throughout the examination. During this time, the examiner is testing for possible spinal injuries, fractures, dislocations, or soft-tissue injuries. Care must be taken that injuries are not missed.[62]

While performing the secondary assessment, the examiner is considering whether the patient should be allowed to return to activity. The examiner must decide whether further evaluation is required onsite or whether the patient should be taken to some other venue (e.g., training room, hospital). In addition, the examiner should keep in mind that home monitoring may be necessary and therefore should determine whether a responsible person is at home to watch for changing signs and symptoms in the patient (see Figure 2-32).

Musculoskeletal Injuries Commonly Missed during Emergency Assessment[62]

- Closed tendon injuries of the hand
- Carpal bone injuries
- Occult elbow fractures
- Femoral neck fractures
- Posterior shoulder dislocations
- Epiphyseal plate injuries
- Pubic ramus fractures
- Patellar tendon rupture
- Lisfranc (tarsometatarsal) fractures
- Compartment syndromes

Table 18-9

Trauma Score and Probability of Survival Based on the Score

Trauma Score	Probability
16	0.99
15	0.98
14	0.95
13	0.91
12	0.83
11	0.71
10	0.55
9	0.37
8	0.22
7	0.12
6	0.07
5	0.04
4	0.02
3	0.01
2	0
1	0

From Champion HR et al: Trauma score, *Crit Care Med* 9:674, 1981.

Table 18-10

CRAMS Scale

Circulation
2: Normal capillary refill and BP over 100 mm Hg systolic
1: Delayed capillary refill or BP 85–99 systolic
0: No capillary refill or BP less than 85 systolic   _____

Respiration
2: Normal
1: Abnormal (labored, shallow, or rate over 35)
0: Absent   _____

Abdomen
2: Abdomen and thorax not tender
1: Abdomen or thorax tender
0: Abdomen rigid, thorax flail, or deep penetrating injury to either abdomen or thorax   _____

Motor
2: Normal (obeys commands)
1: Responds only to pain—no posturing
0: Posturing or no response   _____

Speech
2: Normal (oriented)
1: Confused or inappropriate
0: No sounds or unintelligible sounds   _____

(Score of 6 or less indicate referral to trauma center should be initiated)
TOTAL   _____

From Hawkins ML, Treat RC, Mansberger AR: Trauma victims: field triage guidelines, *South Med J* 80:564, 1987. Reprinted by permission from the *Southern Medical Journal*.
CRAMS = Circulation, respiration, abdomen, motor, and speech.

Emergency Care Levels of Decision

1. Is the injury life-threatening?
2. What care (first aid) must be given on-site or "on the field"?
3. Can and should the patient be moved?
4. If the patient is to be moved, what is the best way to do it?
5. What steps are to be taken before the patient is moved? Spinal board? Splinting? Instruction?
6. If the patient is to be moved, where to? Sidelines? Locker room? Training room? Hospital?
7. How is the patient to be transported? Ambulance? Parent's vehicle?
8. If the injury is not severe enough to require transportation to the hospital, what protocols are to be followed for return to activity?
9. If the patient is not allowed to return to activity, what protocols are to be followed?

Adapted from Haines A: Principles of emergency care, *Athletic J* 26:66–67, 1984.

When progressing to the secondary assessment, the examiner must continue to do the neural watch or the Glasgow Coma Scale (GCS) and watch for signs of an expanding intracranial lesion or other complications. Advanced cerebral edema may further reduce the perfusion of an already damaged hemisphere of the brain, and compression of the descending motor tracts may decrease limb power. Also, the patient's level of consciousness can reveal a deficit previously overshadowed by other evidence of severe brain injury.

During the secondary assessment, there is time to carry out a more thorough assessment for head injury or perform other tests in addition to the neural watch and GCS. The patient's abilities to assimilate information and act with split-second timing are more likely to be impaired after a concussion than are strength and endurance. If a head injury is suspected, it is important to determine the patient's reasoning and processing ability (see Chapter 2).

The examiner also checks coordination or motor neurological function.[63] When testing for proper neurological function, the examiner should palpate the neck and back for any pain or tenderness.[64] There are a number of tests for eye-hand coordination (see Chapter 2). Balance and motor coordination can be tested by determining whether the patient can maintain balance through unsupported standing, the Romberg test, standing with eyes closed, being pushed from side to side, balancing on one leg, or normal walking. Motor neurological function is tested by checking the patient's grip strength or the various myotomes.

Eye coordination and peripheral vision can be checked by asking the patient to follow the examiner's fingers up and down, side to side, diagonally, and in circles, noting any wandering eye movements. To test visual disturbance, the patient is asked to read or observe something from a short distance (e.g., eye chart, how many fingers the examiner is holding up). To test for vision at distance, the patient can be asked to read the score clock, as an example.

After brain function has been tested, the remainder of the secondary assessment is similar to the "clearing," or scanning, assessments performed for the cervical or lumbar spine. The examiner clears the different areas of the body so that a detailed assessment of the specifically injured joints or structures can be performed. At this stage, the assessment follows the same basic protocol as in the detailed assessment of specific joints—that is, a more detailed history of the injury is taken, the patient is observed for obvious or potential problems, and the entire body is quickly scanned for injury. This is followed by a detailed examination of the specifically injured structures, including active, passive, and resisted isometric movements, special tests, testing of reflexes and cutaneous sensory distribution, joint play movement tests (if applicable), and, finally, palpation and other diagnostic tests such as imaging and laboratory tests (see Chapters 3 to 13).

Because the examiner is one of the first persons to talk to the patient, the examiner will probably obtain the most accurate history. Simple nonleading questions should be asked, and information should be clarified in an attempt to find out what happened and what injury or injuries the patient believes have occurred. Appropriate questions related to specific joints or areas of the body can be found elsewhere in this text. The patient often can provide the examiner with the diagnosis if the examiner listens carefully. After the patient has been thoroughly questioned, others who witnessed the accident or injury may also be questioned to complete the history. Informed conversation with other persons sometimes helps the examiner to detect abnormal behavior that may not be noticed initially. If the patient has a previous medical file, it may also prove beneficial to review the contents for information regarding preexisting conditions, previous trauma, and medications.

While obtaining the patient's history, the examiner continues to observe the patient and notes levels of consciousness, developing symptoms, pain patterns, and altered functional abilities. In addition, the examiner should carefully watch for developing signs and symptoms of an expanding intracranial lesion by noting changes in facial expression, the pupils, and the level of consciousness and by performing the neural watch and GCS several times. The basic observation is the same as that performed during joint assessment and includes observation of bony and soft-tissue contours, scars, deformities, the ability to move, and body alignment.

The next part of the secondary assessment is the scanning examination, in which the examiner quickly scans the entire body through observation, by asking the patient to make particular movements (depending on where the suspected injury has occurred), and by testing myotomes, dermatomes, and reflexes. During this phase, the examiner should explain what is being done and why, not only to reassure the patient but also to ensure cooperation and relaxation. This part of the examination may be done without removing the patient's clothes, although it is better to do so because clothing may obstruct the view of the injured area. However, if the examination is being performed in the presence of other people, clothing removal should be left to a later time, or the patient should be moved to a more appropriate location. If the clothes need to be removed, the patient should be warned, especially if in a public place, and every effort should be made to maintain the patient's dignity.

After the specific area or areas of injury have been narrowed down through the scanning examination, the examiner can perform a detailed assessment of the appropriate parts of the body, as specified in other chapters. Failure to perform a proper examination may lead to a missed assessment and more problems than originally anticipated.

The patient must be immediately sent to a hospital or trauma center if at any time during the primary or secondary evaluation the following signs are exhibited: pupillary or extraocular movement abnormality, facial or extremity weakness, amnesia, confusion or lethargy, sensory or cranial nerve abnormality, positive Babinski sign, deep tendon reflex asymmetry, or posttraumatic seizures.[31,65] Proper care for the patient must always be uppermost in the mind of the examiner.

Signs Indicating Need for Immediate Transport to Hospital

- Abnormal pupil or extraocular movement
- Increasing facial or extremity weakness or flaccid paralysis
- Amnesia, confusion, or lethargy
- Sensory or cranial nerve abnormality
- Decreasing value in Glasgow Coma Scale
- Positive Babinski sign
- Deep tendon reflex asymmetry
- Posttraumatic seizures

After the assessment has been completed and the patient has been stabilized, has returned to competition, or has been referred for further medical care by ambulance, the examiner should be sure to document what happened and the subsequent care that was given, noting any potential difficulties. These notes, if taken at the sideline, should be transferred to the patient's medical record as soon as possible.

Précis of the Emergency Sports Assessment

The sequence to be followed for assessment of acute injury is shown in Figure 18-13.

Figure 18-13

Assessment sequence following acute injury.

Case Studies

When reviewing or practicing these case studies, the examiner should outline the necessary protocol for dealing with the situations described. The examiner can develop different scenarios depending on the degree of severity of the injury. These scenarios, including assessment and movement of the patient, should be practiced often so that the examiner is fully aware of what to do and how to handle emergency situations.

1. A diver misjudges his take-off from the 10-m board, hits his head on the concrete platform, and falls unconscious into the pool, displaying decorticate rigidity as he falls. Describe your emergency protocol for this patient.

2. During squash game, a player is struck near the eye by her opponent's squash racquet. Describe your emergency protocol for this patient.

3. A 22-year-old professional basketball player is under his own net and suddenly collapses and lapses into unconsciousness during a game. Describe your emergency protocol for this patient.

4. During a race on a hot, humid day, a 10,000-m runner collapses on the track during the event and lies motionless. Describe your emergency protocol for this patient.

5. During a baseball game, a batter is hit on the chest by a pitched ball and collapses at home plate. Describe your emergency protocol for this patient.

6. A defensive back tackles a runner and makes the tackle but does not move when the other players get up, even though he is conscious. He is having difficulty breathing. Describe your emergency protocol for this patient.

7. A rugby player hits his head during a collapsing scrum. He is knocked unconscious, is not breathing, and has no pulse. Describe your emergency protocol for this patient.

8. A hockey player receives a deep cut to the neck when another player's skate accidentally cuts him. He is bleeding profusely. Describe your emergency protocol for this patient.

9. A gymnast on the balance beam misses her dismount and lands on her head, neck, and shoulders and is knocked unconscious. Describe your emergency protocol for this patient.

10. A wrestler is thrown to the mat near the end of the first round. He lands hard on the side of his face with his neck twisted. He is lying prone and unconscious. Describe your emergency protocol for this patient.

11. While playing soccer, an athlete is stung by a bee and develops anaphylactic shock. Describe your emergency protocol for this patient.

12. A hockey player is "checked" into the boards from behind. He falls to the ice and has difficulty breathing; he had been chewing gum. Describe your emergency protocol for this patient.

References

To enhance this text and add value for the reader, all references have been incorporated into a CD-ROM that is provided with this text. The reader can view the reference source and access it online whenever possible. There are a total of 64 cited references and other general references for this chapter.

Index

Reinforce

your understanding of

concepts

taught in the book!

This CD provides even more resources for further learning with references from the text that contain links to MEDLINE abstracts.

Try it today!

SL256